SOURCEBOOK FOR ANCIENT MESOPOTAMIAN MEDICINE

SBL PRESS

Writings from the Ancient World

Theodore J. Lewis, General Editor

Associate Editors

Daniel Fleming
Theo van den Hout
Martti Nissinen
William Schniedewind
Mark S. Smith
Emily Teeter
Terry Wilfong

Number 36
Sourcebook for Ancient Mesopotamian Medicine
Volume Editor: Marten Stol

SOURCEBOOK FOR ANCIENT MESOPOTAMIAN MEDICINE

by JoAnn Scurlock

SBL Press

Atlanta, Georgia

SOURCEBOOK FOR ANCIENT MESOPOTAMIAN MEDICINE

Library of Congress Cataloging-in-Publication Data

Scurlock, Jo Ann, 1953-
Sourcebook for ancient Mesopotamian medicine / by JoAnn Scurlock.
pages cm. — (Writings from the ancient world ; number 36)
ISBN 978-1-58983-969-4 (paper binding : alk. paper) — ISBN 978-1-58983-971-7 (electronic format) — ISBN 978-1-58983-970-0 (hardcover binding : alk. paper)
1. Medicine, Assyro-Babylonian—Sources. I. Title.
R135.3.S287 2014
610.935—dc23

2014013642

Printed on acid-free, recycled paper conforming to ANSI/NISO Z39.48-1992 (R1997) and ISO 9706:1994 standards for paper permanence.

CONTENTS

Part 2: Therapeutics

SERIES EDITOR'S FOREWORD

Writings from the Ancient World is designed to provide up-to-date, readable English translations of writings recovered from the ancient Near East.

The series is intended to serve the interests of general readers, students, and educators who wish to explore the ancient Near Eastern roots of Western civilization or to compare these earliest written expressions of human thought and activity with writings from other parts of the world. It should also be useful to scholars in the humanities or social sciences who need clear, reliable translations of ancient Near Eastern materials for comparative purposes. Specialists in particular areas of the ancient Near East who need access to texts in the scripts and languages of other areas will also find these translations helpful. Given the wide range of materials translated in the series, different volumes will appeal to different interests. However, these translations make available to all readers of English the world's earliest traditions as well as valuable sources of information on daily life, history, religion, and the like in the preclassical world.

The translators of the various volumes in this series are specialists in the particular languages and have based their work on the original sources and the most recent research. In their translations they attempt to convey as much as possible of the original texts in fluent, current English. In the introductions, notes, glossaries, maps, and chronological tables, they aim to provide the essential information for an appreciation of these ancient documents.

The ancient Near East reached from Egypt to Iran and, for the purposes of our volumes, ranged in time from the invention of writing (by 3000 BCE) to the conquests of Alexander the Great (ca. 330 BCE). The cultures represented within these limits include especially Egyptian, Sumerian, Babylonian, Assyrian, Hittite, Ugaritic, Aramean, Phoenician, and Israelite. It is hoped that Writings from the Ancient World will eventually produce translations from most of the many different genres attested in these cultures: letters (official and private), myths, diplomatic documents, hymns, law collections, monumental inscriptions, tales, and administrative records, to mention but a few.

Significant funding was made available by the Society of Biblical Literature for the preparation of this volume. In addition, those involved in preparing this volume have received financial and clerical assistance from their respective institutions. Were it not for these expressions of confidence in our work, the arduous tasks of preparation, translation, editing, and publication could not have been accomplished or even undertaken. It is the hope of all who have worked with the Writings from the Ancient World series that our translations will open up new horizons and deepen the humanity of all who read these volumes.

Theodore J. Lewis
The Johns Hopkins University

PREFACE

I would like to thank the late, much missed, Raymond Westbrook for asking me to do a volume of medical texts for the WAW series. I would further like to thank Ted Lewis for his support as this volume has proceeded. Marten Stol is to commended for taking on the Herculean task of reading through this volume as the volume editor. His input is much appreciated and has resulted in many valuable corrections and suggestions. Any mistakes that remain are, of course, my own. My husband, Richard H. Beal, helped with planning museum visits, collations, and photography. He also has spent many months of evenings and weekends as we jointly reference checked the transliteration. I wish to thank the Trustees of the British Museum for permission to transliterate and translate unpublished tablets in their collection. Cuneiform tablet curator Jon Taylor has always been a joy to work with during our visits to the museum. His predecessor Christopher Walker and his wife Marie-Christine Ludwig, besides being always helpful in the museum, made us feel at home with a number of delicious dinners and wonderful conversation. Finally, I wish to thank the National Endowment for the Humanities (a US government agency) for aiding research on Assyrian and Babylonian medicine through the grant "Ancient Mesopotamian Medical Therapies" (2000–2003) paying my way to photograph and collate tablets in European and American museums and to make preliminary transliterations of all the known medical texts from ancient Mesopotamia, a selection of which are included here.

A Note on Conventions

For those unfamiliar with conventions in the field of Assyriology, a few notes here should be useful. The scribes wrote the words of the texts both syllabically in Akkadian (Assyro-Babylonian) and using word signs derived from the Sumerian language. In transliterating the text, we write the syllabically written Akkadian in lowercase italics, while the Sumerian derived word signs are written in capital letters. Sumerian word signs would have been read as the underlying

Akkadian word. So, for example, the Sumerian word DINGIR would have been read as the Akkadian word *ilu*, just as the Arabic numeral 1 is read as English "one." Akkadian signs attached to a Sumerian word sign aid in the reading of the underlying Akkadian word, so DINGIR-*li* provides the last consonant of *ilu* and the genitive case ending -*i*. Hyphens divide individual signs making up an Akkadian word, and periods divide individual signs making up a Sumerian word sign. Some word signs, called "determinatives," tell the class that a particular thing belongs to, such as GIŠ "wooden object" or ŠEM "an aromatic." These word signs, which were unpronounced, are written in modern scholarship as superscripts. Since there are often homophonous signs, scholars today differentiate these with accents and subscript numbers: sig = sig$_1$, síg = sig$_2$, sìg = sig$_3$, then sig$_4$, sig$_5$, etc. The most recent and thorough signlist is Rykle Borger, *Mesopotamisches Zeichenlexikon*, 2nd ed., AOAT 305 (Münster: Ugarit-Verlag, 2010).

In transliterating and translating tablets, the following conventions are followed:

[ ]	indicates damage to the clay tablet. Any signs or words within [ ] are missing on the tablet and are restored by the modern editor.
[( )]	indicates that while the signs are missing in a hole on the main tablet, another tablet allows the modern editor to know what is missing in the damaged section.
‹ ›	indicates that the modern editor thinks that the ancient scribe has omitted something, which the modern editor has supplied within ‹ ›
‹( )›	indicates that a tablet duplicating the passage in question contains information that is not in the text at hand and that the modern editor has supplied.
⸢ ⸣	surrounds signs or words that are damaged, but still readable.
( )	indicates information supplied by the modern editor to make something clearer for the reader.
!	indicates that a sign is miswritten by the ancient scribe or miscopied by the modern copiest.
:	used in the tranliteration to indicate a Glossenkeil, a wedge or two used by the ancient scribe to indicate glosses or variants.
x	illegible sign
o	space within a lacuna for a sign
§	new paragraph
//	parallel or duplicate
#	number missing
col.	column
coll.	collated

Medical texts are identified by their publication or, if unpublished, by their museum number.

ABBREVIATIONS

$4R^2$	H. C. Rawlinson, *The Cuneiform Inscriptions of Western Asia* vol. 4, 2nd ed. London: Lithographed by R. E. Bowler, 1891
A	museum number of cuneiform texts in The Oriental Institute of the University of Chicago
ABRT	James A. Craig, *Assyrian and Babylonian Religious Texts.* Leipzig: Hinrichs, 1895–97
AfO	*Archiv für Orientforschung*
AfOB	Archiv für Orientforschung Beiheft
AfOB 3	F. R. Kraus, *Texte zur babylonischen Physiognomatik.* Berlin, 1939
AfOB 11	Erica Reiner, *Šurpu: A Collection of Sumerian and Akkadian Incantations.* Graz: Weidner, 1958
AHw	Wolfram von Soden, *Akkadisches Handwörterbuch* 3 vols. Wiesbaden: Harrassowitz, 1965–81
AJSL	*American Journal of Semitic Languages and Literature*
AMD	Ancient Magic and Divination
AMD 8/1	Tzvi Abusch and Daniel Schwemer, *Corpus of Mesopotamian Anti-Witchcraft Rituals.* Leiden: Brill, 2011
AMT	Reginald Campbell Thompson, *Assyrian Medical Texts from the Originals in the British Museum.* London: H. Milford, Oxford University Press, 1923
AO	museum number of a cuneiform text in the Louvre
AOAT	Alter Orient und Altes Testament
AOS	American Oriental Series
ArOr	*Archiv Orientální*
AS	Assyriological Studies
ASJ	*Acta Sumerologica* (Japan)
AUAM	museum number of the Andrews University Archaeological Museum
AuOr	*Aula Orientalis*
AUWE	Ausgrabungen in Uruk-Warka—Endberichte

BA	Beiträge zur Assyriologie und semitischen Sprachwissenschaft
BAM	Franz Köcher, *Die babylonisch-assyrische Medizin in Texten und Untersuchungen*. Berlin: de Gruyter, 1963–80
BAM VII	Mark Geller, *Renal and Rectal Disease Texts*. Vol. 7 of *Die babylonisch-assyrische Medizin in Texten und Untersuchungen*. Berlin: de Gruyter, 2005
BE	The Babylonian Expedition of the University of Pennsylvania—Series A: Cuneiform Texts
BiOr	*Bibliotheca Orientalis*
BM	museum number of cuneiform tablets in the British Museum
BPOA	Biblioteca del Proximo Oriente Antiguo
BRM	Babylonian Records in the Library of J. Pierpont Morgan
CAD	*The Assyrian Dictionary of the Oriental Institute of the University of Chicago*. Chicago: The Oriental Institute of the University of Chicago, 1956–2010
CBS	cuneiform tablet in the collection of the University Museum, University of Pennsylvania
CM	Cuneiform Monographs
CM 37	Annie Attia and Giles Buisson, editors. *Advances in Mesopotamian Medicine from Hammurabi to Hippocrates: Proceedings of the International Conference "Oeil Malade et Mauvais Oeil," Collège de France, Paris, 23rd June 2006*. Leiden: Brill, 2009
CT	Cuneiform Texts in the British Museum
CTN	Cuneiform Texts from Nimrud
CTN 4	D. J. Wiseman and J. Black. *Literary Texts from the Temple of Nabû*.The British School of Archaeology in Iraq, 1996
DPS	the Diagnosic and Prognostic Series of tablets, edited in this volume 1.1.3 to 1.1.40
FAS	Freiburger Altorientalische Studien
GCCI	Goucher College Cuneiform Inscriptions
Hg	the ancient lexical series HAR.gud = *imrû*
IM	museum number of cuneiform texts in the Iraq Museum
JCS	*Journal of Cuneiform Studies*
JEOL	*Journal Ex Oriente Lux*
JMC	*Le Journal des Médecines Cunéiformes*
JNES	*Journal of Near Eastern Studies*
JRAS	*Journal of the Royal Asiatic Society*
K	museum number of a cuneiform tablet in the Kuyunjik collection of the British Museum

KADP	Franz Köcher, *Keilschrifttexte zur Assyrisch-Babylonischen Drogen- und Pflanzenkunde*. Berlin: Akademie Verlag, 1955
KAL	Keilschrifttexte aus Assur literarischen Inhalts
KAL 2	Daniel Schwemer, *Rituale und Beschwörungen gegen Schadenzauber*. Keilschrifttexte aus Assur literarischen Inhalts 2, WVDOG 117
KAL 4	Stefan M. Maul and Rita Strauß, *Ritualbeschreibungen und Gebete*, vol. 1. WVDOG 133. Wiesbaden: Harrassowitz, 2011
KAR	E. Ebeling, *Keilschrifttexte aus Assur religiösen Inhalts*. WVDOG 28 and 34. Leipzig: Hinrichs, 1915–23
KMI	Erich Ebeling, *Keilschrifttexte medizinischen Inhalts*, Berliner Beiträge zur Keilschriftforschung, Beiheft 1–2. Berlin: Erich Ebeling, 1921–22
KUB	Keilschrifturkunden aus Boghazköi
LKA	Erich Ebeling and Franz Köcher, *Literarische Keilschrifttexte aus Assur*. Berlin: Akademie-Verlag, 1953
LKU	Adam Falkenstein, *Literarische Keilschrifttexte aus Uruk*. Berlin: Vorderasiatische Abteilung der Staatlichen Museen, 1931
MLC	cuneiform tablet in the J. Pierpont Morgan Library Collection, now a siglum of the Yale Babylonian Collection, New Haven
MVEOL	Mededelingen en verhandelingen van het Vooraziatisch-Egyptisch Genootschap "Ex Orient Lux"
MZL	Rykle Borger, *Mesopotamisches Zeichenlexikon*, 2nd ed. AOAT 305. Münster: Ugarit-Verlag, 2010
NABU	*Notes assyriologiques brèves et utilitaires*
ND	cuneiform tablet excavated at Nimrud (ancient Kalhu)
Ni.	cuneiform tablet from Nippur in the Istanbul Museum
OECT	Oxford Editions of Cuneiform Tablets
Or	*Orientalia*
OrAnt	*Oriens Antiquus*
PBS	Publications of the Babylonian Section, University Museum, University of Pennsylvania
RA	*Revue d'assyriologie*
RlA	*Reallexikon der Assyriologie und Vorderasiatischen Archäologie*
Rm	cuneiform tablet in the Russam collection of the British Museum
RS	cuneiform tablet from Ras Shamra/Ugarit
RSO	*Revista degli studi orientali*

SBH	George Reisner, *Sumerisch-babylonische Hymnen nach Thontafeln griechischer Zeit*. Berlin: Spemann, 1896.
Sm	cuneiform text in the Smith collection of the British Museum
SpTU	Spätbabylonische Texte aus Uruk
SpTU 1	Hermann Hunger, *Spätbabylonische Texte aus Uruk 1*. Ausgrabungen der Deutschen Forschungsgemeinschaft in Uruk-Warka 9. Berlin: Gebr. Mann, 1976.
SpTU 2	Egbert von Weiher, *Spätbabylonische Texte aus Uruk* 2. Ausgrabungen der deutschen Forschungsgemeinschaft in Uruk-Warka 10. Berlin: Gebr. Mann, 1983
SpTU 3	Egbert von Weiher, *Spätbabylonische Texte aus Uruk* 3. Ausgrabungen der deutschen Forscungsgemeinschaft in Uruk-Warka 12. Berlin: Gebr. Mann, 1988
SpTU 4	Egbert von Weiher, *Uruk: Spätbabylonische Texte aus dem Planquadrat U 18*. SpTU 4. AUWE 12. Mainz: von Zabern, 1993
SpTU 5	Egbert von Weiher, *Uruk: Spätbabylonische Texte aus dem Planquadrant U 18*. SpTU 5. AUWE 13. Mainz: von Zabern, 1998
StBoT	Studien zu den Boğazköy Texten
StBoT 36	Gernot Wilhelm, *Medizinsche Omina aus Hattuša in akkdischer Sprache*. Wiesbaden: Harrassowitz, 1994
STT	O. R. Gurney and J. J. Finkelstein, *The Sultantepe Tablets*. Occasional Publications of the British Institute of Archaeology at Ankara 3 and 7. London: British Institute of Archaeology at Ankara, 1957, 1964
Šurpu	Erica Reiner, *Šurpu: A Collection of Sumerian and Akkadian Incantations*. AfOB 11. Graz: Weidner, 1958
TAPS	*Transactions of the American Philosophical Society*
TBP	Fritz Rudolf Kraus, *Texte zur babylonischen Physiognomatik*. AfOB 3. Berlin: Ernst Weidner, 1939
TCL	Textes Cunéiformes du Louvre
TCS	Texts from Cuneiform Sources
Labat, *TDP*	René Labat, *Traité akkadien de diagnostics et pronostics médicaux*. Paris: Academie Internationale d'histoire des sciences, 1951.
TUAT	Texte aus der Umwelt des Alten Testaments Neue Folge
UET	Ur Excavation Texts
Uruanna	ancient pharmacological plant-list
VAT	museum number of tablets in the Vorderasiatische Abteilung of the Berlin Museum

VS	Vorderasiatische Schriftdenkmäler
W	museum number of tablets from Uruk/Warka
WMF	Würzburger medizinhistorische Forschungen
WO	*Die Welt des Orients*
WVDOG	Wissenschaftliche Veröffentlichung der Deutsche Orient Gesellschaft
WZKM	*Wiener Zeitschrift für die Kunde des Morgenlandes*
YOS	Yale Oriental Series, Babylonian Texts
ZA	*Zeitschrift für Assyriologie*

Introduction

Ancient Mesopotamia, the "cradle of civilization," preserves a surprisingly large and comprehensive set of medical texts. Unfortunately, physicians, medical specialists, historians of medicine, or just interested laymen with an interest in exploring ancient Mesopotamian medicine soon discover that most of this fascinating material is essentially inaccessible to the uninitiated. Even those who can read cuneiform well find medical texts difficult, and those attempting to learn to read them for the first time are risking a white-knuckle experience. The technical vocabulary used to describe signs and symptoms, procedures, and plants is unfamiliar to nonspecialists, and enlightenment is in many cases less likely to be found in the dictionary than in one of a growing number of scattered articles to be found in a bewildering variety of specialist medical journals. What is needed is an introductory study guide that will allow interested persons at whatever level of proficiency in cuneiform to get a basic working knowledge of ancient Mesopotamian medical texts either as an end in itself or as a foundation for further research.

This book aims to fill this need. It includes transliterations and translations of individual tablets representing the full range of developed Mesopotamian medicine both in time (from Middle Babylonian and Middle Assyrian to Seleucid periods), in space (texts from Assur, Nineveh, Sultantepe, Nippur, Sippar, Babylon, and Uruk), and by type (diagnostic, therapeutic, and pharmacological) to serve as an introduction to the study of these very difficult but ultimately extremely rewarding texts. These transliterations and translations are intended not just for the specialized reader but also for interested public (as, for example, medical doctors and specialists in the history of medicine). Therefore, philological commentary has been kept to a minimum. For the convenience of those who might wish to use this book as an introductory textbook to learn how to read ancient Mesopotamian medical texts, two source lists have been provided. Source List 1 contains a complete listing of all known duplicates of the Diagnostic and Prognostic Series. Source List 2 provides a basic bibliography of editions and translations of each of the texts treated in the volume, as well as a listing of the most significant duplicates, both published and unpublished.

A handful of Old Babylonian (1792–1595 BCE) incantations and the largely unpublished therapeutic texts from the Ur III (2112–2004 BCE) and Isin-Larsa (2017–1763 BCE) periods do not yet allow for any real attempt to understand the development of this medical tradition over the full course of ancient Mesopotamian history. When, as the Mesopotamians did, you do not record things simply to record them but "in order not to be forgotten," what gets recorded is what cannot easily be remembered. As time goes on and knowledge accumulates, more and more will consequently need to be written down. This factor provides an obvious explanation for why, despite the fact that we have therapeutic texts already in the Ur III period, there are so many recitations and so few treatments from the Old Babylonian period. At this point, there were probably already many treatments, but since ancient Mesopotamian plant mixtures rarely contain more than ten ingredients (and earlier treatments often simply one or two), there were probably not so many that a practicing doctor could not remember them all. He also will have known which recitation to use with which treatment. The exact text of these recitations (and in particular the lengthy sections in Sumerian) are the only feature of his practice where a written copy might have come in handy. By the Neo-Assyrian period, by contrast, when there could be hundreds of treatments for any given condition, writing everything down in a convenient handbook form will have become a desideratum.

Forerunners from the Ur III to the Old Babylonian periods are of interest mainly in terms of the developments that preceded systemization, and will not be dealt with here.[1] Similarly omitted are medical omens (the first two tablets of the Diagnostic and Prognostic Series plus scattered sections within this corpus), the physiognomic omens, the malformed birth omens and astrological medicine (which develops in the late periods).[2] These are subjects which were peripheral to the medical duties of the scholar-physician and/or would deserve a study in their own right.

The Practitioners (*Asû* and *Āšipu*)

As I have argued elsewhere,[3] the *asû* was a close equivalent of the European pharmacist. The pharmacological texts outlined in chapter 2 will have been his primary responsibility, along with generally unrecorded information on exactly where medicinal plants grew, when to pick them, and how to store them. Like his modern counterpart, the "pharmacist" will have been a medical expert of first

1. Interested persons are referred to translations of selections of the most important of these texts in TUAT 5 (Heeßel 2011a and 2011c).

2. For sample texts of this type, see Heeßel 2011b, texts 5.1–2.

3. Scurlock 1999, 69–79. No better suggestion for differentiation exists to date.

resort, particularly for simple problems like headaches and upset stomachs, and there is no doubt that these pharmacists were perfectly capable of devising their own treatments using the plants at their disposal.

The *āšipu*'s job was to diagnose and treat diseases, as these were understood by ancient Mesopotamians. For only a little over half of the syndromes recognized by ancient physicians could a plausible connection be made with already known spirits as potential causal agents. The remaing syndromes were either attributed to a malfunctioning body part, for instance "sick gall bladder" or given a name based on some characteristic, for instance "stinking" (*buʾšānu*)[4] for syndromes involving foul smell and grayish lesions in the mouth. For more details on the diagnostic system, see Scurlock and Andersen 2005, ch. 19. The diagnostic and prognostic handbook translated in chapter 1 was certainly intended exclusively for the use of the *āšipu*, as were the commentaries in chapter 4. In short, he was the equivalent of our physician, or would be if there were a less stringent division of labor between modern physicians and pharmacists.

In ancient Mesopotamia, medicine was a team effort, and the therapeutic texts appearing in part 1, chapter 3 and parts 2 and 3, although provably intended for the use of the *āšipu* also, again provably, contained a fair amount of material that was originally intended for the use of the *asû*, and collected (sometimes with attribution) from that source. Identifying pharmacists' treatments in the mass of texts stemming from physicians' archives is a bit troublesome, but not impossible.

Texts almost certainly to be assigned to the *āšipu* are medical texts with the recitation, label and "its ritual" format typical of "magical" texts. This leaves two major categories of text which give clear indications as to the purpose for which they were intended, those that a) list symptoms after which the treatment is described, and those that b) begin with a list of plants, followed by a label (either immediately after the plants or at the end after preparation instructions) that indicates that the treatment is to be used for such-and-such a problem.

As I have argued elsewhere,[5] only the *āšipu* would have had any use for type a), leaving type b) as the prime candidate for origination with the *asû*, particularly those with labels formulated "it is good for such-and-such a problem," a phraseology that is typical of pharmacological texts. In the translations that follow, note has invariably been made of such potential pharmacists' treatments.

As for what these bits of pharmacists' lore are doing in the archives of *āšipu*s, the obvious suggestion is they were intended to be used as what we call a prescription, a type of text which the physician (*āšipu*) had to be able to generate

4. See chapter 5, text 6.
5. Scurlock 2005, 302–15.

(and hence would have been found in great numbers in his archive) but which was actually intended for the use of the pharmacist (*asû*).

PART 1

FOUNDATIONS

GENERAL REMARKS

Before the ancient physician could treat his patient he had to know what was wrong with him. The problem presented by the divine language of medical signs and symptoms was to determine which combinations of animal products, minerals, and plants and which recitations were effective for which medical problems. To answer this question, the ancestor of the *āšipu* began by carefully observing his patients and deriving a vocabulary to describe their signs and symptoms so that any treatments that might subsequently be devised could be applied consistently, past successes reproduced, and repetition of past failures avoided.

As in our own medical tradition, it was sometimes sufficient to institute symptomatic treatment, but in other cases it was found helpful to attempt to identify the causal agent behind the observed symptoms. The polytheistic religions of the ancient world provided a ready made and very flexible explanatory system that allowed for both "natural" (that is, internal) causes and "supernatural" (that is, external) causes for disease. So, the patient might be diagnosed as having "sick liver" or as being the victim of an attack by a god, ghost, demon, or sorceror. For more details on the diagnostic system of ancient Mesopotamia, see Scurlock and Andersen (2005, ch. 19).

Over the course of time, careful observation and a pooling of knowledge allowed ancient physicians to recognize which set of signs and symptoms belonged to a single syndrome, then to watch the progress of easily recognizable syndromes, and finally to be able to recognize favorable and grave signs so as to be able to prognosticate as well as diagnose. In the course of this process of accumulation of knowledge, it first became necessary to record, and subsequently not merely to record, but also to organize the recorded information in some logical fashion.

Scholarly tradition held that a scholar-physician by the name of Esagil-kīn-apli, patronized by the Babylonian king Adad-apla-iddina (1068–1047 BCE), made a complete reorganization of then-current medical knowledge into a diagnostic and prognostic handbook consisting of a series of forty tablets, the number apparently being chosen because it was associated with a god of healing, Ea, lord of the sweet waters so important in purificatory rites. In this handbook, the patient's symptoms were listed, and the physician directed to the correct ancient diagnosis. Since indexes are a modern invention, any entry of relevance to more than one context had to be repeated. So, for example, references to infants appeared scattered throughout the corpus, but were also collected into a dedicated tablet. This practice produced a certain amount of dittography, which occasionally allows for the restoration of broken passages, as noted in the footnotes to individual tablets.

What remains of the diagnostic and prognostic handbook (excluding purely divinatory material contained in the first two tablets) is given in this chapter in its entirety. The text is a combined edition, based, with a few corrections, on the scored edition of Heeßel 2000 for tablets 15–23, 26–31 and 33 and, for the remaining tablets, on an unpublished scored edition by Scurlock starting from the list of duplicates generously provided by Heeßel 2000 (for a full list, see app. 1). A German translation of selected parts of tablets 1, 4, 9, 13, 16, 26, 33, 36, and 40 appear as Heeßel 2011a, nos. 1.4.1–9.[1] Earlier bibliography for individual entries is given in Scurlock and Andersen 2005, but special mention should be made of the pioneering work of Labat 1951 for the whole series, of Stol 1993, 56–909 for tablets 26–30, of Stol 2000, 194–202 for tablets 36–37 and of Cadelli 1997, 11–33 and Volk 1999, 1–30 for tablet 40.

Besides this diagnostic handbook, there are also isolated diagnostic texts, in addition to fragments of what was apparently an earlier attempt at a systematic organization of diagnostic material. So, inter alia, an early pre-Esagil-kīn-apli version of the Diagnostic and Prognostic Handbook was found in the Hittite capital Hattusa,[2] Middle Assyrian fragments have turned up at Assur,[3] and an almost complete text of tablet 24(?) of an outlying version was discovered at Sultantepe.[4] For more details on these matters, the reader is referred to Heeßel 2011a, 8–31, Fincke 2011a, 472–76 and Rutz 2011, 294–308.

The Diagnostic and Prognostic Handbook was divided into six subseries. The first subseries (DPS 1–2) contained all of the ominous occurrences that might take place as the *āšipu* was on his way to the patient's house. This is fascinating material, but belongs to the study of divination, along with scattered references in the Diagnostic and Prognostic Series to the ominous significance of the patient's dreams or noises made by him/her in the course of her/his illness.

The second subseries was organized around an anatomical principle. Since neither the surviving forerunners nor the outlying diagnostic texts are organized in this fashion, this schema would appear to be the contribution of Esagil-kīn-apli. The sequence begins at the top of the head with DPS 3 and proceeds

1. To be precise, DPS 1 lines 1–25, DPS 4 lines 1–27, DPS 9 lines 1–30, DPS 13 ii 9–31, DPS 16 lines 41′–74′, DPS 26 lines 12′–26′, DPS 33 lines 19–32, 97–108, DPS 36 lines 1–12 and DPS 40, lines 1–20.

2. This is edited in Wilhelm 1994.

3. See Heeßel 2010, 168–87.

4. This is edited in Stol 1993, 91–98.

systematically down the body to the blood vessels of the feet in DPS 14. Signs and symptoms were also grouped by broad categories, usually in the order: fever, pain, and varying color or consistency with references to trauma listed at the end of each anatomical section.

This subseries appears to indicate the presence in ancient Mesopotamia of what we would now call primary care physicians or GPs. In addition, some of the individual tablets in the series and elsewhere in the Diagnostic and Prognostic Series may represent potential subspecialties. The large number of therapeutic texts containing treatments exclusively for the eyes would seem to suggest that there were ophthalmologists in ancient Mesopotamia. Similarly, women's diseases are to be found in discrete texts and have their own dedicated subseries, suggesting the presence of gynecologists.

The first section of the third subseries was organized in accordance with time factors. Many of the entries duplicate those of the second subseries as noted, but are differently arranged. DPS 15–16 contained entries mentioning the number of days the patient had been sick, whereas DPS 17 was concerned with phases of illness and times of day. This organization facilitated the addition of later material as when, in DPS 16, a section organized by the number of five-day weeks a patient had been sick ("one to two five-day weeks, one to four five-day weeks") was apparently inserted, set off by paragraph lines, into the appropriate slot (between "more than five days" and "more than six days").

DPS 18 began a section which was designed to introduce the student to febrile diseases, and to make him aware of signs and symptoms, other than elevated temperature, which he might expect to encounter. DPS 22 and 23 were organized in accordance with the god or goddess or demon whom the *āšipu* held responsible for the disease. These tablets most closely resemble the outlying and precursor texts, which similarly organize their material in accordance with the causal agent held responsible for the observed symptoms. The system by which the ancient physician assigned diseases to causal agents is exhaustively discussed in Scurlock and Andersen, 2005, ch. 19.

The fourth subseries (DPS 26–30) collected together entries relating to neurology, an apparent subspecialty of the *ašipu*'s craft. Since neurology is still largely a clinical science, this is probably the area of ancient medicine in which it is easiest to make correlations with modern practice, and the correlation is a striking testimonial to the skill of pre-modern physicians to observe without the advantages of modern technology, but unblinded by theory.

DPS 31 of the fifth subseries dealing with infectious diseases judges the number of days a patient has been sick with some form of enteric fever by the symptoms which have to that date appeared (e.g., chills on the third day and nosebleeds on the seventh). DPS 33 dealt with skin lesions but also covered flesh wounds and soft tissue infections including tetanus.

The sixth and final subseries was devoted to Obstetrics, Gynecology, and Infant Diseases. Thus, DPS 36 attempts to predict whether the unborn child is a boy, girl, a single child or twins and whether it is alive or dead in the womb and needing to be removed to save the life of the mother. The unfortunately fragmentary DPS 37 and missing DPS 38 can be somewhat filled in by the therapeutic texts of which a number deal exclusively with female problems such as irregular menstruation (treated with plant estrogens) and puerperal fever. Last but not least is the baby tablet, DPS 40.

Most helpful to the ancient student of medicine were two overarching principles of organization for individual entries in the diagnostic/prognostic handbook. There are places where a series of entries with only one or two signs or symptoms and the same diagnosis are listed one after the other. These "sequenced references" were probably intended to provide the physician with an understanding of the variations in signs and symptoms that may be seen in a particular disease. They also allowed him/her to prescribe specific treatments for the specific symptoms presented by a patient at a particular stage of her/his illness. So, for example, there are sections in DPS 11 discussing the progression of arthritis from pain to swelling and sluggishness to immobilization of the joints, for all of which separate symptomatic treatments were available.

Another important use of this ancient textbook was for comparisons between different diseases with overlapping signs or symptoms. By placing these references side by side ("contrasted references"), the physician was able to easily make comparisons and to understand significant differences with important implications for treatment. So, for example, there are sections of DPS 13 that attempt to explain the difference between gastro-intestinal ulcers and obstruction on the one hand and between bleeding ulcers and liver problems on the other. This was to know whether it was appropriate to try one of the available treatments for peptic ulcers or one of those for "sick liver."

Texts with differing signs and symptoms and degrees of severity were also juxtaposed to illustrate how these differences affected prognosis. For example, DPS 16 explains which signs and symptoms in biphasic fever are grave and which are not. For a helpful chart outlining the contents of this diagnostic and prognostic handbook in detail, see Scurlock and Andersen 2005, 577–677.

An interesting aspect of ancient Mesopotamian medicine that is often ignored, or even denied, is the close relationship between diagnosis and treatment. Therapeutic texts of the developed tradition list the symptoms and/or disease to be treated using the same technical terminology to describe symptoms, the same grouping of symptoms into syndromes and the same ancient diagnoses as are to be found in the diagnostic texts. All that is, for obvious reasons, missing from the therapeutic texts are the prognostics and treatments for fatal syndromes for which no treatment was available.

In the tablets that formed part of the therapeutic series known to us as UGU (see below, part 1, ch. 3), a particularly close relationship is evident between diagnosis and therapy. This is striking in the case of DPS 4 and BAM 482 and its duplicates, long known to represent tablet 2 of the first subseries of UGU. In therapeutic BAM 482, symptomatic treatments for headache alternate with over thirty specific treatments for the very types of headache described in diagnostic and prognostic DPS 4, and BAM 482 ends with a citation of untreatable fatal headaches drawn directly from DPS 4. Similarly, CTN 4.72 i 3′–14′ and vi 1′–8′ provide treatments for entries preserved in DPS 27:1–17 and DPS 30:1, respectively. DPS 33, the skin tablet (for which see below), is positively bursting with therapeutic text correlations.

Another practice, typified by texts such as CT 53.1–2 and BAM 578 (also known to be part of the UGU series), is the direct citation of entries from the diagnostic and prognostic series by way of introduction to a series of treatments for the condition that is described in the diagnostic and prognostic entry. Thus, CT 53.1-2:1 introduces its section on *sagallu* with a direct citation from DPS 33:98. Similarly, BAM 578 iii 7 and iv 26, cited from DPS 33:92–93, introduce sections of treatments for the two types of jaundice recognized by ancient physicians. The section then finishes (BAM 578 iv 43–46) with an enumeration of the symptoms marking fatal cases of jaundice clearly drawn from diagnostic material that is no longer elsewhere preserved for us, and may have originated in one of the outlying tablets not incorporated into Esagil-kīn-apli's Diagnostic and Prognostic series. *AMT* 77/1 i 1–10 (perhaps, to judge from this format also originally part of UGU) summarizes the opening section of DPS 27 (1–13 omitting 2–4) to introduce the subject of treatments for stroke, and so on.

Even more interesting is Middle Assyrian BAM 66, which seems to have had a close relationship with a pre-Esagil-kīn-apli precursor of DPS 31 from which at least two entries made it into the canonical series. In this text, a lengthy citation of diagnostic and prognostic material of the "sequenced reference" type (BAM 66 obv. 1–rev. 3′) serves as an introduction to treatments for *ṣētu* (rev. 4′–25′) that have duplicates in purely therapeutic texts (*AMT* 14/7:1–2; BAM 174:21′–24′//*AMT* 45/1:2′–5′//*AMT* 14/7:3–6; *AMT* 45/1:6′–15′//*AMT* 14/7:7–11). Unfortunately fragmentary, BAM 146 seems to have had a similar format, beginning with DPS 31-type material, proceeding to therapeutic text material and ending with a citation of the incipit of the next tablet in the series, DPS 32:1. Extract text K 3628+4009+Sm. 1315 not only cites four lines from DPS 40 (obv. 6–9) by way of introduction to proffered treatments for "hand" of Ishtar (obv. 11–16), but even gives us the ancient equivalent of a footnote reference to the source from which these entries had been copied (obv. 10). And, this overview does not include isolated therapeutic texts with treatments for conditions described in the Diagnostic and Prognostic Series, for which partial references are given in the footnotes.

What all of these therapeutic texts make explicit is what should never have required proof, and that is the close relationship between ancient Mesopotamian diagnostic and therapeutic material. Texts phrased as "if your patient has such and such symptoms, it is such and such a disease" were, *a priori*, meant to be consulted first, as necessary, to diagnose illness. This having been accomplished, texts phrased as "if your patient has such and such a disease, you are to institute such and such treatment" were, *a priori*, meant to be consulted, as necessary, to provide treatment. The fact that we have texts in which the two stages (diagnosis and treament) are both given, and in that sequence, should leave no lingering doubts on this subject!

1

THE DIAGNOSTIC AND PROGNOSTIC SERIES

A. HEAD TO TOE: DPS 3–14

DPS TABLET 3

1. [*ana* G]IG *ina* TE-*ka* EN É[N *ana* NÍ-*ka*] ŠUB-*ú ana* G[IG NU TE-*ḫi*]
2. DIŠ *ana* IGI GIG A.MEŠ ŠUB-*ma* NU ⌈MUD⌉ [*u* ZU-*šú l*]*a ú-ád-da* Š[U? …] ⌈NU⌉ D[IN]
3. DIŠ *ana* UGU-*šú* A.MEŠ ŠUB-*ma* GABA-*su u* SAG ŠÀ-*šú i-nar-*⌈*ru*⌉-[*bu* DIN]
4. DIŠ *ana* KA-*šú* A.MEŠ ŠUB-*ma* A.MEŠ *ina* [K]A-*šú ú-kal* [DIN]
5. DIŠ UGU-*šú* KÚM-*em u* ⌈SAG⌉.KI^{II}-*šú ne-eḫ-a* U_4.1.KÁM GIG-[*ma* …]
6. DIŠ UGU-*šú* KÚM-*em u* SAG.KI^{II}-*šú* KÚM *la-aḫ-ḫa-ḫa-šá* U_4.1.KÁM GIG-[*ma* …]
7. DIŠ [U]GU-*šú* KÚM-*em u* SAG.KI^{II}-*šú* KÚM-*ma* U_4.2.KÁM GIG-*ma* […]
8. DIŠ [UG]U-*šú* KÚM-*em u* SAG.KI^{II}-*šú* KÚM *u* IR *ú-kal-la* U_4.3.⌈KÁM⌉ GIG-*ma* […]
9. DIŠ [UG]U-[*šú*] KÚM-*em* SAG.KI^{II}-*šú u bir-ti* Á^{II}-*šú* KÚM *u* IR *ú-kal-la* U_4.5.⌈KÁM GIG⌉-[*ma* …]
10. [DIŠ UGU-*šú*] ⌈KÚM.KÚM⌉-*im* ŠU ^{d}*Nusku*[1]
11. [DIŠ UGU-*šú* GA]BA-*su u ša-šal-la-šu* KÚM.KÚM ⌈$UŠ_{11}$.ZU⌉ DIB-*su*
12. [DIŠ UG]U-*šú* [GAZ.ME SA]G.DU-*su* TAB-*su* ŠÀ-*šú i-ta-na-ši* GIN_7 *šá ana* UGU MUNUS ŠUB-*tu* ÍL ŠÀ TUKU-*ši* ŠU KI.SIKIL.LÍL.LÁ.EN.NA
13. [DIŠ UGU-*šú*] *ka*[*l* U_4 G]AZ.ME ŠÀ-*šú*! *i-ta-na-áš-ši-ma* KI.NÁ *it-ta-na-as-ḫar*!-*šu* GIN_7 *šá ana* UGU MUNUS ŠUB-*tu* ÍL ŠÀ TUKU-*ši*
14. ŠU K[I.[SIKI]L.LÍL.LÁ.EN.NA
15. [DIŠ UGU-*š*]*ú* ⌈GAZ.ME⌉ *ḫi-ḫi-en* KA/KIR_4-*šú i-raš-ši-šú* SÍG GAL_4.LA-*šú* TAB-*su* ŠU-*šú* BAR.ME-*šu*
16. [U]GU-⌈*šú* NU⌉ [ŠUB-*ma*] *sú-ḫur*? *ina* GI_6 DIB.DIB-*su u* LUḪ(!).MEŠ ŠU *Úr-bi-li-ti*
17. DIŠ UGU UGU GÙ.GÙ-*si* ŠU ^{d}60 AŠ DINGIR *šá* ŠÀ

18. DIŠ *ina* U[G]U-*šú* SÌG-*iṣ* ŠU ^{d}*Papsukkal* KI.MIN ŠU ^{d}[…]
19. DIŠ *ina* U[G]U-*šú* SÌG-*ma* GEŠTU^{II}-*šú* NU ŠE.GA-*a* ŠU ^{d}15 *ana* AŠ-*tim*
20. DIŠ *ina* UGU-*šú* SÌG-*ma kìn-ṣa-a-šú* ⸢Á⸣.MEŠ-*šú u* ŠÀ-*šú* DIB.DIB-*su* DIB-*iṭ* […]
21. DIŠ *ina* U[G]U-*šú* SÌG-*ma* ŠÀ.MEŠ-*šú* MÚ.MÚ-*ḫu* DIB-*iṭ* […]
22. DIŠ TA MURUB$_4$ UGU-*šú* TAG-*su-ma šu-ru-*ʾ-*šú* SAG.KI-*šú* IGI-*šú* ÚNU-*šú* GÚ-*su* GABA-*su* ⸢*tu*⸣-[*l*]*u*?-[*šú* …]
23. *kìn-ṣa-a*!-*šú ki-ṣal-la-šú* 1-*niš* GU$_7$.ME-*šú u ina* IGI MAŠ.MAŠ NU DU$_8$ GIDIM$_7$ DIB-*su-ma* ⸢ÚS⸣.[ÚS-*šu*]
24. DIŠ *ši-bit* SAG.DU-*šú paṭ-rat* [GAM]
25. DIŠ *ši-bit* SAG.DU-*šú tur-ru-rat* : *paṭ-rat* [GA]M
26. DIŠ *ši-bit* SAG.DU-*šú šal-mat* [DI]N?
27. DIŠ *ú-ru-uḫ* SAG.DU-*šú bé-e-er* […]
28. DIŠ *ú-ru-uḫ* ‹SAG.DU›[2]-*šú bé-e-er* ŠU ^{d}[…]
29. DIŠ *ú-ru-uḫ* ‹SAG.DU›-*šú bé-e-er ṣi-bit* […]
30. DIŠ *ú-ru-uḫ* SAG.DU-*šú bé-e-er* […]
31a. DIŠ *ú-ru-uḫ* SAG.DU-*šú šá-lim* DIN
31b. DIŠ MUNUS *ú-ru-u*[*ḫ*] SAG.DU-*šá* ⸢x⸣[…]
32a. DIŠ *kal-li* SAG.DU-*šú sa-ḫir* : *is-saḫ-ḫar* GAM
32b. DIŠ *bi-rit* SAG.DU-*šú sa-mi ina* [EDIN TAG-it]
33. DIŠ SAG.DU-*su* 1-*niš* TUK$_4$-*aš ḫi-ḫi-en* KIR$_4$-*šú i-raš-ši-šum-ma* TAB-*su tu*-⸢*gun*⸣-*šú* TAB-*su* K[I.NÁ NU ÍL …]
34. DIŠ SAG.DU-*su i-ṣa-ád u kìn-ṣa-a-šú ka-ṣa-a* ŠU ^{d}[…]
35. DIŠ SAG.DU-*su i-ṭa-mu* GÌR-*šú šá* 15 *ú-kan-na-an-ma* NU LAL *ú-šap-šaq-ma* […]
36. DIŠ SAG.DU-*su i-ṭa-mu* GÌR-*šú šá* 150 *ú-kan-na-an-ma* NU LAL ŠU ^{d}[…]
37. DIŠ SAG.DU-*su i-zaq-qat$_4$-su* SAG.DU-*su i-šag-gúm* GEŠTU^{II}-*šú* GÙ.DÉ.ME U.ME-*šú* ⸢*ú-zaq-qá*⸣-*t*[*a-šú* DIB GIDI]M$_7$[3]
38. DIŠ SAG.DU-*su ana šuk-lul-ti-šú* SA *uk-tal-lim* TI
39. DIŠ SAG.DU-*su ana šuk-lul-ti-šú* SA NU TUKU ÚŠ
40. DIŠ SAG.DU-*su ti-ik-ka-šú u šá-šal-la-šú* 1-*niš* GU$_7$.MEŠ-*šú* SA.DUGUD[4]
41. DIŠ SAG.DU-*su* DIB.DIB-*su* GÚ-*su* TAG.TAG-*su* GABA-*su* GU$_7$.MEŠ-*šú* ŠÀ-*šú* GAZ.MEŠ-*šú pi-qam la pi-qam i*[*t-ta-na-ad-là*]*ḫ*[5]
42. GU$_7$ *u* NAG NU GUR-*ma* GU$_7$ *u* NAG ^{d}15 MU É / SILA *er-bet-tim* ÚS.ME-*šú šá-niš ana* MUNUS MU *a-rin u sa-ma-li* (*ana*) MUNUS.LUGAL *u ana* KI.SIKIL.BÀN.DA MU *ki-gul-lim u áš-tam-mi*[6]
43. DIŠ SAG.DU-*su* DIB.DIB-*su u* KÚM ŠUB.ŠUB-*su* ŠU ^{d}15

44. DIŠ SAG.DU-*su* DIB.DIB-*su u* KÚM NU TUKU ŠU ^{d}15

45. DIŠ SAG.DU-*su* DIB.DIB-*su u* KÚM TÉŠ.BI UNU-*su* (coll.) GIG-*su* TAK$_4$-*šum$_4$-ma* NÍG.NIGIN TUKU-⸢*ma i-ra-ʾu*⸣-*ba* ⸢*šum-ma* KI⸣ LAL-*šú* LAL-*šú*

46. UŠ$_4$-*šú* KÚR-*šum-ma ina* NU ZU-*ú ú-rap-pad* GIN$_7$ DIB-*it* GIDIM$_7$ ^{d}DIM$_{11}$.ME ⸢DIB⸣-[*su uš*]-*te-zib*(coll.)

47. DIŠ SAG.DU-*su* TÉŠ.BI DIB.DIB-*su* ŠU SAG.ḪUL.Ḫ[A.ZA DIN? : ŠU ^{d}]⸢15(?)⸣ (coll.)

48. DIŠ SAG.DU-*su i-tar-ru-ur* GÚ-*su u* GÚ.MUR$_7$-*šú ka-pí-ip* KA-*šú* ⸢*at*⸣-*ma te-ba-a* NU ZU

49. *ina* KA-*šú* ÚḪ.ME-*šú* DU.MEŠ ŠU^{II}-*šú kìn-ṣa-a-šú u* GÌR^{II}-*šú* 1-*niš i-tar-ru-ra ina* DU-*šú ana* IGI-*šú n*[*a-du-ú* … -*m*]*a* ⸢NU⸣.DIN(coll.)

50. DIŠ SAG.DU-*su* ŠU^{II}-*šú u* GÌR^{II}-*šú i-tar-ru-ra* KA-*šú ana a-ma-ti da-a-an i-na* ⸢KA⸣-[*šú it-te-ne-et-bu-ú* DI]B-*tum* DIB-*su*[7]

51. DIŠ SAG.DU-*su* ŠU^{II}-*šú u* GÌR^{II}-*šú* 1-*niš i-tar-ru-ra ina* KA-*šú át-mu-šú it-te-né-ep-r*[*ik-ku* NA BI *lu-ʾ-tu$_4$ ana ma-al-tak-ti š*]*u-kul*[8]

52. DIŠ SAG.DU-*su* ŠU^{II}-*šú u* GÌR^{II}-*šú i-ra-ʾ-u-ba* KA-*šú ana at-me-e il-la-a* U$_4$[…][9]

53. DIŠ SAG.DU-*su* ŠU^{II}-*šú u* GÌR^{II}-*šú* 1-*niš i-ra-ʾ-u-ba* ŠÀ-*šú ana* BURU$_8$ *i-te-ne-il-la-a-ma* ⸢*mim+ma*⸣ [*šá* GU$_7$ ŠÀ-*šú* GUR ŠU ^{d}]20?

54. DIŠ SAG.DU-*su* ŠU^{II}-*šú u* GÌR^{II}-*šú i-rat-tu-ta* KA-*šú ana* DU$_{10}$ *da-an it-te-né-ep-rik*(coll.) ⸢NA?⸣ [BI *lu-ʾ-a-ti šu-k*]*ul*[10]

55. DIŠ SAG.DU-*su* KÚM *ḫa-ḫaš*[11] U$_4$.1.KÁM TAK$_4$-*šum-ma* U$_4$.2.KÁM DUGUD-*su i-re-ḫi-*[*šum-ma*]

56. Á.ÚR.MEŠ-*šú* 1-*niš* GU$_7$.ME-*šú u* A *ana* NAG APIN ŠU […]

57. DIŠ SAG.DU-*su* KÚM *ḫa-ḫaš* U$_4$.1.KÁM TAK$_4$-*šum-ma* U$_4$.2.KÁM DUGUD-*su i-re-eḫ-ḫi-šum-ma* DIB-*i*⸢*t*⸣ GIDIM$_7$ G⸣[ÌR^{II}-*šú* ŠED$_7$?]

58. *ina* BAR-*šú* ŠU^{II}-*šú u* GÌR^{II}-*šú* KÚM-*ma u* IR ŠED$_7$ ŠUB.ŠUB-*su* GIN$_7$ DIB-*it* GIDIM$_7$ ^{d}DÌM.ME.LAGAB U$_4$-*me-šú* GÍ[D]-*m*[*a* GAM]

59. DIŠ SAG.DU-*su* KÚM *ḫa-ḫaš* SA.ME SAG.KI^{II}-*šú* ZI.MEŠ KÚM-*im u* ŠED$_7$ ŠU DINGIR-*š*[*u*]

60. DIŠ SAG.DU-*su* KÚM-*em* SAG KIR$_4$-*šú* ŠU^{II}-*šú u* GÌR^{II}-*šú* ŠED$_7$ DIḪ KUR DIB-*su* KI.MIN *kiš-pi* DIB.MEŠ-[*šú* …]

61. DIŠ SAG.DU-*su* KÚM-*em* SA SAG.KI^{II}-*šú* ŠU^{II}-*šú u* GÌR^{II}-*šú* 1-*niš* ZI.MEŠ GÌR^{II}-*šú* EN *kìn-ṣi-šú* ŠED$_7$-⸢*a*⸣

62. SAG KIR$_4$-*šú* GI$_6$ ŠE U.MEŠ-*šú* SIG$_7$ ŠUB-*ú* ŠÀ IGI^{II}-*šú* SIG$_7$ *u* BABBAR ŠUB PA IGI^{II}-*šú* 2.TA.ÀM DIB.DIB (*ḫi-pí*) x[…]

63. *na-pi-is-su ina* KIR$_4$-*šú* DIB-*ma ina* KA-*šú* GARZA *uš-ti-ṣi mu-tim ana* ZI-*šú ú-šel-la-a* x x[…]

64. DIŠ SAG.DU-*su* KÚM-*em* SA SAG.KI^{II}-*šú* ŠU^{II}-*šú u* GÌR^{II}-*šú* 1-*niš* ZI.MEŠ SA$_5$ *u i-mim* ŠU [DINGIR DIN]
65. DIŠ SAG.DU-*su u* ŠÀ-*šú* KÚM-*em* SA SAG.KI^{II}-*šú* ŠU^{II}-*šú u* GÌR^{II}-⸢*šú* [1-*n*]*iš* [ZI.MEŠ ...] Š[U ...]
66. DIŠ SAG.DU-*su u* ŠÀ-*šú* KÚM-*em* SA SAG.KI^{II}-*šú* ŠU^{II}-⸢*šú u*⸣ [GÌR^{II}-*šú* 1-*niš* ZI.MEŠ]
67. SAG ŠÀ-*šú na-ši* ḪÁŠ-*su da-an* ŠE[D$_7$ ...]
68. DIŠ SAG.DU-*su* KÚM-*em* (*ḫi-pi*) *ḫa-ḫa*[*š*...]
69. DIŠ SAG.DU-*su* KÚM-*em* NUNDUN.MEŠ-*šú* : *ḫi-ip* KA-*šú* BABBAR.MEŠ Š[U?...]
70. DIŠ SAG.DU-*su* KÚM ÚḪ IGI.MEŠ-*šú* SA$_5$.⸢MEŠ⸣ [...]
71. DIŠ SAG.DU-*su* KÚM ÚḪ IGI.MEŠ-*šú* SA$_5$ *u* [...]
72. DIŠ SAG.DU-*su* AD$_6$-*šú u* SAG KIR$_4$-*šú* SÌG.SÌG-*su* NUND[UN.MEŠ-*šú i-ta-na-zu*][12]
73. *u* ZI.IR.MEŠ *ina ni-šu-ti-šú* GIDIM$_7$ *šá ina ṣu-um-m*[*a-mi* ÚŠ DIB-*su*]
74. DIŠ SAG.DU-*su* AD$_6$-*šú* SAG KIR$_4$-*šú* SÌG.SÌG-*su* NUNDUN.MEŠ-[*šú i-ta-na-zu*][13]
75. *ina ni-šu-ti-šú man-ma šá ina ṣu-ma-mi-ti* ÚŠ DIB-*s*[*u*]
76. DIŠ SAG.DU-*su* AD$_6$-*šú* KÚM ÚḪ *u i-ta-na-šu-‹uš›* ŠU ^{d}MAŠ.TAB.BA DIN *šúm-ma* ⸢*ina* DÚR⸣-[*šú* ZÉ SUR ...]
77. DIŠ SAG.DU-*su* KÚM NAR[14] *ina* KÚM-*šú* LUḪ.ME ŠU ^{d}MAŠ.TAB.BA DIN *šum$_4$-ma ina* DÚR-*šú* ZÉ SUR *u* ZÉ *i-ta-n*[*a-ḫu* ...]
78. DIŠ SAG.DU-*su* KÚM ÚḪ *ina* UD.SA$_9$.ÀM TAK$_4$-*šum-ma* A *ana* TU$_5$! UL$_4$.GAL APIN.ME DIB ^{d}[...]
79. DIŠ *ina* SAG.DU-*šú* KÚM ÚḪ U$_4$.1.KÁM TAK$_4$-*šum-ma* U$_4$.2.KÁM DUGUD-*su i-re-eḫ-ḫi-šum-ma* DIB-*i*[*t* GIDIM$_7$] KI.TA! GÌR^{II}-*šú* ŠED$_7$
80. *ina* BAR-*šú* ŠU^{II}-*šú u* GÌR^{II}-*šú* ⸢KÚM-*ma*⸣ GIN$_7$ DIB-*it* GIDIM$_7$ ^{d}DIM$_{10}$.ME.LAGAB *i-sa-dir-*[*ma* DIN]
81. DIŠ *ina* SAG.DU-*šú* SÌG-*iṣ* ŠU ^{d}[x]
82. DIŠ *ina* SAG.DU-*šú šá* 15 SÌG-*iṣ* ŠU ^{d}IM
83. DIŠ *ina* SAG.DU-*šú šá* 150 SÌG-*iṣ* ŠU ^{d}UTU AL.GAM
84. DIŠ *ina* SAG.DU-*šú* SÌG-*iṣ-ma* IGI^{II}-*šú ur-ru-pa* ŠU ^{d}N[IN].GÍR.SU
85. DIŠ *ina* SAG.DU-*šú* SÌG-*iṣ-ma* Á.ÚR.MEŠ-*šú* 1-*niš* GU$_7$.ME-*šú* ŠU ^{d}15 *ana* BÚR *ú-qàt-ti*(coll.) *ni-ši*
86. DIŠ *ina* SAG.DU-*šú* SÌG-*iṣ-ma u i-ṭa-mu pu-qud-de-e* ^{d}15 *ana* ^{d}MAŠ.TAB.BA
87. DIŠ *ina* SAG.DU-*šú* SÌG-*iṣ-ma u* MÚD MUD ŠUB.ŠUB-*a* ŠU ^{d}MAŠ.TAB.BA GAM
88. DIŠ *ina* SAG.DU-*šú* SÌG-*iṣ-ma u* MÚD *i-ḫa-ḫu* ŠU ^{d}MAŠ.TAB.BA GAM

89. DIŠ *ina* SAG.DU-*šú* SÌG-*iṣ-ma ḫa-si-si-šú ṣa-bit* TA KÚM *lam* GUR-*ma* DIB-*bat ú*ʾ-*i* DUG$_4$.GA ŠU DINGIR *šag-g*[*a*]*š-ši na-kud* GAM
90. DIŠ *ina* SAG.DU-*šú* SÌG-*iṣ-ma* SA SAG.KI-*šú* ŠU[^{II}]-*šú u* [GÌ]R^{II}-*šú* 1-*niš* ZI.MEŠ ⸢SA$_5$⸣ *u i-mim* ŠU DINGIR TI
91. DIŠ *ina* SAG.DU-*šú* SÌG-*iṣ-ma* MIR.ŠEŠ ŠUB.ŠUB-*su* IGI.MEŠ-*šú* SA$_5$ *u* SIG$_7$ GIN$_7$ DIB-*su* ŠUB-*šú*
92. UŠ$_4$-*šú* KÚR-*šum-ma i-ṭa-mu* DIB-*it* ^{d}DIM$_{11}$.ME.LAGAB U$_4$-*me-šú* GÍD.DA.MEŠ-*ma* GAM
93. DIŠ *ina* SAG.DU-*šú u* MURUB$_4$-*šú* SÌG-*iṣ* ŠU ^{d}15 *ana* ^{NA_4}NUNUZ.MEŠ
94. DIŠ TA SAG.DU-*šú* EN *šuk-lul-ti-šú* SA.MEŠ-*šú i-nu-uš-šu* NU DIN
95. DIŠ ⸢TA⸣ SAG.DU-*šú* EN MURUB$_4$-*šú* KÚM TA MURUB$_4$-*šú* EN GÌR^{II}-*šú* ŠED$_7$ SAG.KI-*su* ⸢SÌG⸣.SÌG-*su*[15]
96. Á^{II}-*šú ú-na-aš-šak ina* ^{GIŠ}MÁ *iš-riq* DINGIR *ka-a-ri* DIB-*su* BÚR-*ma* DIN
97. [DIŠ T]A SAG.DU-*šú* EN MURUB$_4$-*šú* SIG$_7$ TA MURUB$_4$-*šú* EN GÌR^{II}-⸢*šu*⸣ [SA$_5$?] ŠU^{II}-*šú* KÚM-*ma* PAP.ḪAL-*ma*[16] GAM
98. [DIŠ TA SAG].⸢DU⸣-*šú* EN MURUB$_4$-*šú* GIG TA MURUB$_4$-*šú* EN GÌR^{II}-*šú* DIN ITU GIG GIG-*su* GÍD-*ma* DIN
99. [DIŠ TA SAG].⸢DU⸣-*šú* EN MURUB$_4$-*šú* TI TA MURUB$_4$-*šú* EN GÌR^{II}-*šú* GIG *e-reb* GIG GIG-*su* GÍD-*ma* DIN
100. [DIŠ TA SAG.D]U-*šú* EN GÌR^{II}-*šú* U$_4$.BU.BU.UL SA$_5$ DIRI *u* SU-*šú* BABBAR KI MUNUS *ina* KI.NÁ KUR ŠU 30
101. [DIŠ TA SAG.D]U-*šú* EN GÌR^{II}-*šú* U$_4$.BU.BU.UL SA$_5$ DIRI *u* SU-*šú* GI$_6$ KI.MIN KI.MIN
102. [DIŠ T]A SAG.DU-*šú* EN GÌR^{II}-*š*[*ú*] U$_4$.BU.BU.UL DIRI *u* SU-*šú* SIG$_7$ KI.MIN ŠU ^{d}15
103. [DIŠ T]A SAG.DU-*šú* EN [GÌR^{II}-*šú* U]$_4$.BU.BU.UL BABBAR DIRI *u* SU-*šú* GI$_6$ KI.MIN ŠU ^{d}UTU
104. [DIŠ TA] ⸢SAG⸣.DU-[*šú*] ⸢EN G⸣[ÌR^{II}-*šú* U]$_4$.BU.BU.UL GI$_6$ DIRI *u* SU-*šú* SA$_5$ KI.MIN ŠU ^{d}[UTU]
105. [DIŠ TA SA]G.⸢DU⸣-[*š*]*ú* [E]N? *meš*-⸢*li*⸣-*šú* SA.MEŠ-*šú* TI-*ma* NU DU.MEŠ *šá-pu-la-šú ka-sa-a*
106. GEŠTU^{II}-*šú mim-ma la i-šem-ma-a* NA.BI ḪUL DIB-*su*
107. [DIŠ SA.MEŠ SAG.DU]-*šú* ⸢2⸣ RI.MEŠ GAR.MEŠ-*ma* PA IGI^{II}-*šú* DIB.DIB-*tu* ŠU.LUḪ BAD DIB.DIB-*tu*
108. TA É *ana* É KÚR-*šum-ma* DIN
109. [DIŠ *bi-rit*]⸢SAG.DU⸣-*šú is-sa-na-la-*ʾ *ina* EDIN TAG-*it na-*ʾ*-id*
110. [DIŠ *bi-rit*] SAG.DU-*šú zuq-qú-pat ina* EDIN TAG *na-*ʾ-[*id*]
111. [DIŠ *bi-rit*] SAG.DU-*šú sa-pat ina* EDIN TAG

112. DIŠ *b*[*i-rit*] SAG.DU-*šú i-sal-li-iḫ ina* EDIN TAG
113. DIŠ SÍG.[MEŠ] *šá* SAG.DU-*šú i-saḫ-ḫar ina* EDIN TAG-*it na-ʾ-id*
114. DIŠ SÍG S[AG].⸢DU⸣-*šú ḫa-šat* DIN : DIŠ SÍG SAG.DU-*šú sa-pat* GAM
115. DIŠ SÍG SAG.DU-*šú is-se-ni-ip-pi ina* EDIN TAG-*it na-ʾ-id* (coll.)
116. DIŠ SÍG SAG.DU-*šú is-sa-na-la-ʾ ina* EDIN TAG KI.MIN
117. DIŠ SÍG SAG.DU-*šú zuq-qú-pat ina* EDIN TAG-*it* [KI.MIN]
118. DIŠ SÍG SAG.[DU-*š*]*ú u* SU-*šú* 1-*niš zuq-qú-pat ina* EDIN TAG-*it* ÚŠ
119. DIŠ SÍG S[AG.DU]-*šú i-na* SÍG-*šú zuq-qú-pat ina* EDIN TAG-*it* [ ]
120. DIŠ SÍG S[AG.DU]-*šú i-na* x x a ZI-*at* GAM
121. DIŠ SÍG SAG.DU-*šú* GI[N_7] ⸢*ta-bár-ri-i ṣar*⸣-*pat* […]
122. DIŠ SÍG S[AG.DU-*šú*] SA_5 GAM : DIŠ SÍG SAG.DU-*šú* SA_5 *u saḫ*-[*rat* GAM]
123. DIŠ SÍG [S]AG.⸢DU-*šú*⸣ *ú-maš-šad u* TÚG [o o o] *dib-bu*

Translation

1. When you approach the ⸢patient⸣, [do not approach] ⸢the patient⸣[17] until you have cast a ⸢spell⸣ [over yourself].
2. If you pour water on the patient’s face and he does not shudder [and] he ⸢does not⸣ recognize [one known to him], ⸢“hand”⸣ of […]; he will not ⸢get well⸣.
3. If you pour water over him and his chest and his epigastrium become ⸢soft⸣, [he will get well].
4. If you pour water into his mouth and he can hold the water in his ⸢mouth⸣, [he will get well].[18]
5. If the top of his head is hot and his temples are calm, [if] he has been sick for one day, […].[19]
6. If the top of his head is hot and his temples are lukewarm, [if] he has been sick for one day, […].[20]
7. If the ⸢top of his head⸣ is hot and his temples are also hot, if he has been sick for two/three days, […].[21]
8. If the ⸢top of his head⸣ is hot and his temples are hot and hold sweat, if he has been sick for three days, […].[22]
9. If the ⸢top of his head⸣, his temples, and the region between his arms[23] are hot and hold sweat, [if] he has been sick for five days, […].
10. [If the top of his head] continually gets hot, “hand” of Nusku.[24]
11. [If the top of his head], his ⸢breast⸣ and his upper back are continually feverish, *kišpu* afflicts him.

12. [If] the ⌜top of his head⌝ [continually feels as if split in two], his ⌜head⌝ burns, his stomach is continually nauseous,[25] (and) like one who lays himself down on top of a woman, he has an erection, "hand" of *ardat lilî*.[26]

13–14. [If the top of his head] ⌜continually feels as if split in two all⌝ [day/night long], his stomach is continually nauseous[27] and the bedding is continually turned around him, (and) like one who lays himself down on top of a woman, he has an erection, "hand" of ⌜*ardat lilî*⌝.[28]

15–16. [If the top] of ⌜his⌝ head continually feels as if split in two, the soft parts of his nose/mouth are reddish, the hair of his pubic region burns him, his hand continually hangs down limply, he does not [lay himself down] ⌜on top of⌝ (a woman)[29] but turns away, it continually afflicts him in the night and he continually jerks, "hand" of Ishtar of Arbela.[30]

17. If a person keeps crying out: "the top of my head, the top of my head," "hand" of Anu because he is the god inside.[31]

18. If he was injured[32] on the ⌜top of his head⌝, "hand" of Papsukkal. Alternatively, it is "hand" of [...].[33]

19. If he was injured on the top of his head and, as a consequence, his ears do not hear, "hand" of Ishtar for a gift (which she wants).[34]

20. If he was injured on the top of his head and consequently his legs, his arms and his stomach continually afflict him, affliction by [...].[35]

21. If he was injured on the top of his head and, as a consequence, his insides are continually bloated, affliction by [...].[36]

22–23. If from the middle of his skull it hurts him intensely and his eyelid,[37] his forehead, his eye, his cheek, his neck, his breast his ⌜nipples⌝? [...], his legs (and) his ankles all together hurt him continually and (the pain) does not let up despite (lit.: in the face of) the *āšipu*('s efforts), a ghost afflicts him and [continually] pursues [him].[38]

24. If the seam of his head (feels like it) is open,[39] [he will die].[40]

25. If the seam of his head (feels like it) is made to tremble (var. is open), [he will die].

26. If the seam of his head (feels like it) is intact, ⌜he will get well⌝.

27. If his head hair is fine (lit. select) [...].

28. If his head hair is fine (lit. select), "hand" of [...].[41]

29. If his head hair is fine (lit. select), affliction by [...].

30. If his head hair is fine (lit. select) [...].

31a–b. If his head hair is normal, he will get well. If a woman's head hair [...].

32a. If the (hair on the) crown of his head frizzes, he will die.[42]

32b. If the (hair on the) central area of his head is red,[43] [he was touched] in [the steppe].[44]

33. If his head shakes all together, the soft parts of his nose/mouth are reddish and burn him, his turban(?) burns him, [he cannot stand] the ⸢bed⸣[45] [...].

34. If his head (seems to) spin and his legs are cold, "hand" of [...].

35. If his head twists and he bends his "right" ⸢foot⸣ and then cannot straighten it out, if he experiences difficulty, [...].[46]

36. If his head twists and he bends his "left" foot and then cannot straighten it out, "hand" of [...].

37. If his head stings him, his head (seems) to roar, his ears roar, (and) his finger(s) sting [him, affliction by] a ⸢ghost⸣.[47]

38. If (from) his head on to the rest of him shows (the presence of) blood vessel(s), he will live.

39. If (from) his head on to the rest of him there is no blood vessel (present), he will die.

40. If his head, his neck and his back all continually hurt him at once, *šaššaṭu*.[48]

41–42. If his head continually afflicts him, his neck continually hurts him intensely, his breast continually hurts him, he continually has a crushing sensation in his chest, [he is continually] and incessantly [troubled], he eats and drinks (but) does not eat and drink again, Ishtar continually pursues him because of a house with four (entrances?)[49] (var. crossroads). For a woman, it is because of well and cup; for the queen or an adolescent girl, it is because of place of mourning[50] and tavern.[51]

43. If his head continually afflicts him and fever continually falls upon him, "hand" of Ishtar.[52]

44. If his head continually afflicts him and he does not have a fever, "hand" of Ishtar.[53]

45–46. If his head continually afflicts him and fever (has) its seat[54] equally all over (and) when his illness leaves him, he has dizziness and trembles (and) if, when his confusional state comes over him, his mentation is altered so that he wanders about without knowing (where he is) as in affliction by a ghost, Lamashtu afflicts [him]. [He] will come through.[55]

47. If his head continually afflicts him all over, "hand" of ⸢*mukīl*⸣ *reš lemutti*, [he will get well, var. "hand" of] Ishtar.[56]

48–49. If his head trembles, his ⸢neck⸣ and his spine are bent, he cannot raise his mouth to the words, his saliva continually flows from his mouth, his hands, his legs and his feet all tremble together, (and) when he walks, he ⸢falls⸣ forward, ⸢if⸣ [...] he will not get well.[57]

50. If his head, his hands and his feet tremble, his mouth is (too) strong for the words (and) [they tumble over one another] in [his] ⸢mouth,⸣ the ⸢affliction⸣ afflicts him.[58]

51. If his head, his hands and his feet all tremble at once (and) his words hinder each other[59] in his mouth, [that person] ⸢has been fed⸣ [a dirty substance to test it].[60]

52. If his head, his hands and his feet tremble, he raises his mouth to the words, [(and) he has been sick for …] days, […].[61]

53. If his head, his hands and his feet all tremble together, his stomach continually rises up to vomit and everything [which he eats, his stomach returns, "hand"] of ⸢Shamash?⸣.[62]

54. If his head, his hands and his feet tremble, his mouth is (too) strong for the words (and) they hinder one other, [that] person ⸢has been fed⸣ [dirty substances].[63]

55–56. If his head (has) a very hot temperature (and) over the course of a day it leaves him and then (later) it overpowers him (and) flows over [him] for two days [so that] his limbs all hurt him at once and he asks for water to drink, "hand" of […].[64]

57–58. If his head (has) a very hot temperature (and) over the course of a day it leaves him and then (later) it overpowers him (and) flows over him for two days (as in) affliction by a ghost and [his] ⸢feet⸣ [are cold], (and) when (the fever) releases him, his hands and feet are hot and a cold sweat continually falls on him as in affliction by a ghost, *aḫḫāzu*.[65] ⸢If⸣ it is ⸢prolonged⸣, [he will die].

59. If his head (has) a very hot temperature, the blood vessels of his temples (seem to) pulsate (and) he gets hot and cold, "hand" of ⸢his⸣ god.[66]

60. If his head is hot (and) the bulb of his nose, his hands, and his feet are cold, *liʾbu* (*ṣibit*) *šadî* afflicts him. Alternatively, *kišpu* continually afflicts [him …].[67]

61–63. If his head is hot (and) the blood vessel(s) of his temples, his hands and his feet all (seem to) pulsate together, his feet are cold as far as the legs, the bulb of his nose is dark, the undersides of his fingers[68] are unevenly colored with yellow, there are dots of yellow and white in his eyes, both upper and lower eyelids are seized […] his breath is seized in his nose so that he makes his breath go out through his mouth, it will make death mount to his throat […].[69]

64. If his head is feverish (and) the blood vessel(s) of his temples, his hands and his feet all seem to pulsate together (and) he is flushed and feverish, "hand" of [god; he will get well].[70]

65. If his head and abdomen are feverish (and) the blood vessel(s) of his temples, his hands and his feet all [seem to pulsate] together [...] ⸢"hand"⸣ of [...].

66–67. If his head and abdomen are hot (and) the blood vessel(s) of his temples, his hands and [his feet all seem to pulsate together], his epigastrium is puffed up, his hypogastric region[71] is hard, he has ⸢chills⸣ [...].[72]

68. If his head is hot (and) [...] has a very hot temperature [...].

69. If his head is hot (and) his lips[73] are white, ⸢"hand"?⸣ of [...].

rev.

70. If his head burns with fever,[74] his face is flushed, [...].

71. If his head burns with fever, his face is flushed and [...].

72–73. If his head, his body and the bulb of his nose continually give him a jabbing pain, [his] ⸢lips⸣ [make babbling noises(?)], and (his stomach) is continually upset, among his people, the ghost of (one who) [died] of ⸢thirst⸣ [afflicts him].[75]

74–75. If his head, his body (and) the bulb of his nose continually give him a jabbing pain, (and) [his] lips [make babbling noises(?)], among his people someone who died of thirst afflicts ⸢him.⸣[76]

76. If his head and body burn with fever and (his stomach) is continually upset, "hand" of the twin gods; he will get well. If [bile drips] from [his] anus [...].[77]

77. If his head burns with fever (and) during the course of his fever, he continually jerks, "hand" of the twin gods; he will get well. If bile drips from his anus and he continually ⸢vomits⸣ bile/blood [...].[78]

78. If his head burns with fever, it leaves/releases him at midday and then he continually asks for a lot of water to bathe in, affliction by [...].

79–80. If in his head he burns with fever (and) over the course of a day it leaves him and then (later) it overpowers him (and) flows over him for two days (as in) affliction by [a ghost] and the plantar surfaces[79] of his feet (feel) cold, (and) when (the fever) releases him, his hands and his feet are hot as in affliction by a ghost, *aḫḫāzu*, [if] (the course of the fever) is regular, [he will get well.][80]

81. If he was injured on his head, "hand" of [...].

82. If he was injured on his head to the "right," "hand" of Adad.[81]

83. If he was injured on his head to the "left," "hand" of Shamash; he will die.[82]

84. If he was injured on his head and, as a consequence, his eyes are heavily clouded, "hand" of ⸢Ningirsu⸣.[83]

85. If he was injured on his head and, as a consequence, his limbs all hurt him together, "hand" of Ishtar. (If) it completely goes away, (there will be a) recovery.[84]

86. If he was injured on his head and he twists, a good entrusted by Ishtar to the twin gods.[85]

87. If he was injured on his head and he continually produces dark blood, "hand" of the twin gods; he will die.[86]

88. If he was injured on his head and vomits blood, "hand" of the twin gods; he will die.[87]

89. If he was injured on his head and, as a consequence, his hearing is affected (and) after the fever, before it returns and afflicts him, he says: "Wah," "hand" of a murderous god; it is serious; he will die.[88]

90. If he was injured on his head and, as a consequence, the blood vessel(s) of his temple, his ⸢hands⸣ and his ⸢feet⸣ all (seem to) pulsate together (and) he is flushed and feverish, "hand of god"; he will get well.[89]

91–92. If he was injured on the head and, consequently, chills keep falling on him, his face flushes and turns pale (and) when his affliction falls upon him, his mentation is altered and he twists, affliction by *aḫḫāzu*.[90] His days may be long but he will die (of it).[91]

93. If he was injured on his head and his hip, "hand" of Ishtar for the sake of egg-shaped beads (which she wants).

94. If from his head to the rest of him (lit. "in his entirety") his muscles shake, he will not get well.[92]

95–96. If he is hot from his head to his hip region (and) cold from his hip region to his feet, his temple continually gives him a jabbing pain (text H: continually afflicts him) (and) he chews on his arms, he stole something from a boat[93] and the god of the quay afflicts him; if he relents, (the patient) will get well.[94]

97. [If] he is pale (greenish) ⸢from⸣ his head to his hip region (and) [flushed?] from his hip region to his feet [and] his hands are hot, if he has a difficult time (text H: covers himself), he will die.

98. [If] he is ill [from] his ⸢head⸣ to his hip region (but) well from his hip region to his feet, he has been sick for a month; his illness may be prolonged (but) he will get well.

99. [If] he is well [from] his ⸢head⸣ to his hip region (but) ill from his hip region to his feet, entrance of the illness; his illness may be prolonged (but) he will get well.

100. [If from] his ⸢head⸣ to his feet, he is full of red *bubuʾtu* and his skin/body is white, he was "gotten" in bed with a woman; "hand" of Sîn.[95]

101. [If from] his ⌜head⌝ to his feet, he is full of red *bubuʾtu* and his skin/body is dark, ditto, ditto (he was "gotten" in bed with a woman); ("hand" of Sîn).[96]
102. [If] ⌜from⌝ his head to his feet, he is full of *bubuʾtu* and his skin/body is yellow, ditto (he was "gotten" in bed with a woman), "hand" of Ishtar.[97]
103. [If] ⌜from⌝ his head to [his feet], he is full of white *bubuʾtu* and his skin/body is dark, ditto (he was "gotten" in bed with a woman), "hand" of Shamash.[98]
104. [If from his] head to [his] ⌜feet⌝, he is full of dark[99] *bubuʾtu* and his skin/body is red, ditto (he was "gotten" in bed with a woman), "hand" of [Shamash].[100]
105–106. [If from] ⌜his head⌝ to his mid point(?) his blood vessels are healthy and do not "go" (but) his inguinal regions are "bound" (and) his ears cannot not hear anything, a *gallû*-demon[101] afflicts that person.
107–108. [If the blood vessels of] his [head] run parallel[102] (and) are present and his eyelids are "seized," you wash (him).[103] If (they) continue to be seized, if you move him from one room to another, he will get well.
109. [If the (hair on the) central area of] his head continually becomes abnormal, he was "touched" in the steppe;[104] it is worrisome.
110. [If the (hair on the) central area of] his head (seems to) stand on end, he was "touched" in the steppe; it is ⌜worrisome⌝.
111. [If the (hair on the) central area of] his head is brittle,[105] he was "touched" in the steppe.[106]
112. If the (hair on the) ⌜central area of⌝ his head trembles, he was "touched" in the steppe.[107]
113. If the hair of his head frizzes, he was "touched" in the steppe; it is worrisome.
114. If the hair of his ⌜head⌝ is chopped looking, he will live. If the hair of his head is brittle, he will die.[108]
115. If the hair of his head continually becomes brittle, he was "touched" in the steppe; it is worrisome.
116. If the hair of his head continually becomes abnormal, he was "touched" in the steppe; ditto (it is worrisome).[109]
117. If the hair of his head seems to stand on end, he was "touched" in the steppe; [ditto (it is worrisome)].[110]
118. If the hair of ⌜his head⌝ and his body all (seems to) stand on end together, he was "touched" in the steppe; he will die.[111]
119. If the hair of his ⌜head⌝ (seems to) stand on end on top of his hair, he was "touched" in the steppe; [he will die].

120. If the hair of his ⸢head⸣ [...] is (easily) pulled out, he will die.[112]
121. If the hair of his head is colored as red ⸢as⸣ red-dyed wool [...].
122. If the hair of [his] ⸢head⸣ is red, he will die. If the hair of his head is red and ⸢frizzes⸣, [he will die].[113]
123. If he rubs the hair of his ⸢head⸣ and [... his] garment [...].

Notes

1. The sign on the tablet is a classic example of a little-known phenomenon, and that is the playful invention of new signs by Neo-Assyrian scribes. In this case, the divine name usually rendered as ^{d}PA.KU is instead rendered as a KU with a tiny PA written onto the front of the bottom half of the sign and the two horizontal wedges of the DINGIR sharing a vertical with the spine of the KU.

2. The scribe left a space for the SAG.DU immediately below the SAG.DU of the previous line in this and the following lines in the two preserved exemplars (A & C). Similarly, in line 102, text C rev. 33 omits U_4.BU.BU.UL SA_5 DIRI but leaves a blank space for it directly under the U_4.BU.BU.UL SA_5 DIRI of its preceding line. In this case, we can be certain that this is what was intended, since text A rev. 9′–10′ has U_4.BU.BU.UL SA_5 DIRI in both lines.

3. Reconstructed from the parallel BAM 9:51–52//*AMT* 14/5:1//BAM 481:13′–15′//BAM 493 i 2′–3′.

4. The parallel passage in DPS 33:94 has *šá-aš-[šá-ṭu]*.

5. The restoration is suggested by the commentary *STT* 403 rev. 35.

6. The commentary *STT* 403 rev. 40 has: [KI.SIKIL.B]ÀN.DA = *ba-tul-tu*.

7. Restored from the similar DPS 7: 6′–7′.

8. The restoration is based on the commentary *STT* 403 rev. 43–45.

9. A single *Winkelhacken* is visible at the end of text C 43.

10. The restoration is based on the commentary *STT* 403 rev. 46.

11. The text uses a very unusual *-ḫaš* sign, listed in Fossey 1926 as no. 900.

12. The restoration is suggested by the commentary *STT* 403 rev. 51 which explains this as meaning *ik-[ki]-lu* ŠUB.ŠUB-*di*: "he continually lets out a ⸢mournful cry⸣."

13. The restoration is suggested by the commentary *STT* 403 rev. 51 which explains this as meaning *ik-[ki]-lu* ŠUB.ŠUB-*di*: "he continually lets out a ⸢mournful cry⸣."

14. This is apparently the equivalent of KÚM ÚḪ in other, similar, passages.

15. text H has DIB.DIB-*su* instead.

16. text H has DUL-*ma* instead.

17. See Heeßel 2000, 20 n. 15.

18. See Scurlock and Andersen 2005, 13.289.

19. See Scurlock and Andersen 2005, 3.12.

20. See Scurlock and Andersen 2005, 3.12.

21. See Scurlock and Andersen 2005, 3.12.

22. See Scurlock and Andersen 2005, 3.12.

23. The commentary, *STT* 403 obv.18 explains this as *bi-rit* MAŠ.SÌLA.MEŠ-*šú*: "the region between his shoulders."

24. The entry appears again in DPS 40:117.

25. The commentary, *STT* 403 obv. 19 explains this as ŠÀ-*šú ana* $BURU_8$ *e-te-ni-la-a*: "his stomach continually rises up to vomit."

26. See Scurlock and Andersen 2005, 12.73.

27. The commentary, *STT* 403 obv. 19 explains this as ŠÀ-*šú ana* $BURU_8$ *e-te-ni-la-a*: "his stomach continually rises up to vomit."

28. See Scurlock and Andersen 2005, 12.74.

29. The referent appears to be masculine but the previous entry has the patient having an erection like one who lays himself down on top of a woman.

30. After a suggestion by Stol 1993, 72; cf. Heeßel 2000, 296. See Scurlock and Andersen 2005, 7.17.

31. The expression is a curious one, but is, in my view, a specific reference to an extremely interesting conceptualization of the human head as a microcosmos. For details, see Scurlock and Andersen 2005, 19.369.

32. Most of the injuries described will have been from war wounds. The current translation allows, however, for reference to accidental injuries and blunt instrument trauma.

33. See Scurlock and Andersen 2005, 19.204.

34. See Scurlock and Andersen 2005, 9.93, 13.101, 13.131, 19.156. The entry appears also in one of the precursors to the diagnostic series, Wilhelm 1994, 35 rev. 1//p. 57 rev. 8′.

35. See Scurlock and Andersen 2005, 19.206 but as corrected here.

36. See Scurlock and Andersen 2005, 19.206.

37. The commentary *STT* 403 obv. 21 explains this as *a-gap-pi* IGI^{II}-*šú*.

38. See Scurlock and Andersen 2005, 19.394. The treatment was originally preserved in *AMT* 94/5:1–5 (Scurlock 2006, no. 346).

39. The commentary *STT* 403 obv. 22 has [*ši-bit*] SAG.DU-*šú paṭ-rat* ÚŠ : SAG.DU-*šú* TAG.MEŠ: "[(If) the seam] of his head (feels like it) is open, he will die. (That means) his head continually hurts him intensely."

40. See Scurlock and Andersen 2005, 13.166.

41. This entry also appears in VAT 11122 obv. 1 (Heeßel 2010, 181–84).

42. See Scurlock and Andersen 2005, 7.6.

43. The reading is confirmed by commentaries *STT* 403 obv. 27 and SpTU 1.40 obv. 7.

44. See Scurlock and Andersen 2005, 7.8.

45. The restoration is suggested by the commentary *STT* 403 obv. 29, which has *su-uḫ-ši*: "bed." See Scurlock and Andersen 2005, 7.18.

46. See Scurlock and Andersen 2005, 13.63, 13.77.

47. The treatment for this condition is to be found in therapeutic texts BAM 9:51–54//*AMT* 14/5:1–2//BAM 481:13′–16′//BAM 493 i 2′–4′ (Scurlock 2006, no. 116).

48. See Scurlock and Andersen 2005, 3.198. This entry appears also in DPS 33:94.

49. Literally "house of four." Van der Toorn 1985, 199 n. 311 emends this to É *sa*(!)-*bit-tum*, which would be another tavern.

50. "Place of destruction" does not seem particularly appropriate to the context; perhaps the similar sounding *kiḫullum*: "place of mourning" was meant.

51. See Scurlock and Andersen 2005, 19.5.

52. See Scurlock and Andersen 2005, 19.254.

53. See Scurlock and Andersen 2005, 13.5, 19.12.

54. UNU = *šubtu*; see *CAD* Š/3, 172b s.v. *šubtu* A lex. section.

55. See Scurlock and Andersen 2005, 3.25, 19.227.

56. See Scurlock and Andersen 2005, 13.151.

57. See Scurlock and Andersen 2005, 13.262 as corrected in Scurlock 2010, 57–60.

58. See Scurlock and Andersen 2005, 13.263.

59. For these expressions, see *CAD* A/2, 498b s.v. *atmû* mng. 2.

60. For the reading and interpretation, see Heeßel 2000, 263. For the medical condition being described, see Scurlock and Andersen 2005, 13.85, 13.263. This is similar to another

entry which appears in DPS 22:5.

61. See Scurlock and Andersen 2005, 13.86.

62. See Scurlock and Andersen 2005, 13.86.

63. See Scurlock and Andersen 2005, 13.87. This is similar to another entry which appears in DPS 22:5.

64. See Scurlock and Andersen 2005, 3.28.

65. Labat 1951, 24:49 has Labaṣu (dDÌM.ME.A). Goetze's copy, however, has dDÌM.ME.LAGAB or *Aḫḫāzu*, and this reading has been confirmed by collations (N. Heeßel and J. Scurlock).

66. See Scurlock and Andersen 2005, 3.7.

67. See Scurlock and Andersen 2005, 3.1, 3.15, 19.216.

68. ŠE = *kittabru*. The commentary *STT* 403 rev. 47 explains the "ŠE U.MEŠ" as meaning TA MU *ap-pat* ŠU.SI.MEŠ-*šú* EN SAG *ṣu-ur-ri-šú*: "from the line represented by the tips of his fingers to the beginning of his core" or, in other words, the underside of the finger. For more on this subject, see Rutz 2011, 304–5.

69. See Scurlock and Andersen 2005, 13.219. This entry also appears in CBS 12580:9–13 (Rutz 2011, 300–305).

70. See Scurlock and Andersen 2005, 8.41, 19.133, 19.361.

71. The commentary *STT* 403 rev. 48 explains this as KI.TA LI.DUR-*sa re-di*: "following the lower part of his navel,"

72. See Scurlock and Andersen 2005, 3.202, 6.40.

73. The gloss explains the lips as being the break in the mouth.

74. Pace *CAD* N/1, 268b, these passages are not to be interpreted as the head being swollen. With Heeßel 2000, 162–63, followed by Borger 2010, 314, the ÚḪ is not a phonetic complement but a Sumerogram for *ṣarāḫu* as is indicated by the fact that a Middle Assyrian precursor to the diagnostic series (*KAR* 211 [Heeßel 2010, 171–77]) renders the expression as KÚM *ṣa-ri-iḫ*: "burns with fever."

75. See Scurlock and Andersen 2005, 3.110.

76. See Scurlock and Andersen 2005, 3.110.

77. See Scurlock and Andersen 2005, 19.136, 19.240.

78. The text has the patient vomiting bile, but the commentary *STT* 403 rev. 52 has "he continually vomits blood." For the entry, see Scurlock and Andersen 2005, 19.241.

79. For the interpretation of KI.TA as "plantar surface," see Adamson 1981, 128.

80. See Scurlock and Andersen 2005, 3.30. This entry appears in the Middle Assyrian precursor *KAR* 211 i 4′–6′ (Heeßel 2010, 171–77).

81. See Scurlock and Andersen 2005, 19.142.

82. See Scurlock and Andersen 2005, 19.190.

83. See Scurlock and Andersen 2005, 9.2, 13.89, 19.167. The entry is similar to DPS 19/20:15′.

84. See Scurlock and Andersen 2005, 19.157. The entry also appears in Wilhelm 1994, 35 obv. 16′–17′//p. 57 rev. 6′–7′.

85. See Scurlock and Andersen 2005, 13.122, 19.158, 19.185. This entry also appears in Wilhelm 1994, 34 obv. 5′.

86. See Scurlock and Andersen 2005, 13.134, 19.180. This entry also appears in Wilhelm 1994, 34 obv. 9′.

87. See Scurlock and Andersen 2005, 6.31, 13.135, 19.180.

88. See Scurlock and Andersen 2005, 9.94, 13.132, 19.213.

89. See Scurlock and Andersen 2005, 8.43, 13.128, 19.132.

90. Labat 1951 has Lamashtu.

91. See Scurlock and Andersen 2005, 13.127, 19.187. This entry appears in the Middle Assyrian precursor *KAR* 211 i 7′–9′ (Heeßel 2010, 171–77).

92. See Scurlock and Andersen 2005, 3.200.

93. See the commentary SpTU 1.29 rev. 3′–4′.

94. See Scurlock and Andersen 2005, 16.27.

95. See Scurlock and Andersen 2005, 3.323, 4.18, 10.85.

96. See Scurlock and Andersen 2005, 10.85. The entry appears also in DPS 18:22. Either this or the preceding entry was listed in *KAR* 211 i 19′–20′ (Heeßel 2010, 171–77) and VAT 10748: 4′ (Heeßel 2010, 178–81).

97. See Scurlock and Andersen 2005, 10.86. The entry appears also in DPS 18:23.

98. See Scurlock and Andersen 2005, 10.87, 19.106. This entry also appears in DPS 18:21 and Wilhelm 1994, 40 obv. 9′–10′.

99. GI$_6$ can be either *ṣalmu*: "black" or *tarku*: "dark."

100. See Scurlock and Andersen 2005, 10.87, 19.106.

101. For the reading, see Heeßel 2000, 187 with n. 17.

102. See the commentary SpTU 1.29 rev. 7′.

103. ŠU.LUḪ = *mesû*, which simply means "to wash" without any necessary ritual connotations.

104. The commentaries SpTU 1.29 rev. 8′ and SpTU 1.36 obv. 26 interpret "touched in the steppe" as "struck on the top of the head."

105. The commentary *STT* 403 obv. 28 explains SI *se-pu-u* SI *e-ni-šú* SÍG SAG.DU-*šú en-šat*: "SI/*sepû*; SI means to be weak (as in the phrase) the hair of his head is weak." That the weakness in question refers to brittle hair is suggested by [NA$_4$] GAR-*šú* GIN$_7$ LAG MUN *sà-pi*: "the nature of the [stone] is that it is as brittle as a lump of salt" (BAM 378 iii 10)

106. See Scurlock and Andersen 2005, 7.2.

107. See Scurlock and Andersen 2005, 7.5.

108. See Scurlock and Andersen 2005, 7.3.

109. See Scurlock and Andersen 2005, 7.1.

110. See Scurlock and Andersen 2005, 7.4.

111. This entry also appears in Labat 1956, 125 rev. 5.

112. See Scurlock and Andersen 2005, 7.7.

113. See Scurlock and Andersen 2005, 7.9.

DPS TABLET 4

DPS 3:124 (catchline) = DPS 4:1

1. DIŠ SAG.KI *ḫe-si-ma* KÚM-*im* : ŠED$_7$ ⸢ŠU⸣ ^{d}*Kù-bi*
2. DIŠ SAG.KI *ḫe-si-ma* ŠÀ.MEŠ-*šú* AL.DU ŠU ^{d}*Kù-bi*
3. DIŠ SAG.KI *ḫe-si-ma* ŠÀ.MEŠ-*šú it-te-nen-bi-ṭu* ŠU ^{d}*Kù-bi*
4. DIŠ SAG.KI *ḫe-si-ma* GEŠTU^{II}-*šú* NU ŠE.GA-*a* ŠU DINGIR-*šú* UGU-*šú um-mu-da* GAM
5. DIŠ SAG.KI-*šú šal-mat* DIN : DIŠ SAG.KI-*šú* ŠUB-*ut* GAM
6. DIŠ SAG.KI-*šú* ŠUB-*ut-ma* IGI^{II}-*šú a-ši-a*/ÍR-*a* GAM

7. DIŠ SAG.KI-*šú* DIB-*su-ma* GÙ.GÙ-*si* MÚD *ina* KIR_4-*šú* DU-*ku* ŠU $GIDIM_7$
8. DIŠ SAG.KI-*šú* DIB-*su-ma* KI.MIN SA SAG.KI-*šú ma-gal* ZI.MEŠ UGU SAG.DU-*šú* DU_8 ŠU $GIDIM_7$ GAM
9. DIŠ SAG.KI-*šú* DIB-*su-ma* KI.MIN SA SAG.KI-*šú ma-gal* ZI.MEŠ *u e-li* SAG.DU-*šú ḫa-biš* GAM
10. DIŠ SAG.KI-*šú* DIB-*su-ma* ŠÀ ŠÀ GÙ.GÙ-*si* ŠU $GIDIM_7$ *šá-né-e* ^{d}15 GAM : ŠU GU_4 GÍD-*ma* GAM
11. DIŠ SAG.KI-*šú* DIB-*su-ma* KI.MIN *ma-gal* i_{16}-*à-ru u* KI.NÁ NU ÍL ŠU $GIDIM_7$ GAM
12. DIŠ SAG.KI-*šú* DIB-*su-ma* TA ^{d}UTU.ŠÚ.A EN EN.NUN UD.ZAL.LI *ur-rak* : *ú-šam-šá* GAM
13. DIŠ SAG.KI-*šú* DIB-*su-ma* TA ^{d}UTU.È EN ^{d}UTU.ŠÚ.A GU_7-*šú* : NU *ina-aḫ ina-aḫ* ŠU $GIDIM_7$
14. DIŠ SAG.KI-*šú* DIB-*su-ma ina* KIR_4-*šú* MÚD DU-*ku* ŠU $GIDIM_7$
15. DIŠ SAG.KI-*šú* DIB-*su-ma* SA GÚ-*šú* GU_7.MEŠ-*šú* ŠU $GIDIM_7$
16. DIŠ SAG.KI-*šú* DIB-*su-ma* SA IGI^{II}-*šú* GU_7.MEŠ ŠU $GIDIM_7$
17. DIŠ SAG.KI-*šú* DIB-*su-ma* KÚM $ŠED_7$ *u* IGI^{II}-*šú nu-up-pu-ḫa* ŠU $GIDIM_7$
18. DIŠ SAG.KI-*šú* DIB-*su-ma* IGI^{ME}-*šú* NIGIN-*du* ZI-*bi u* ŠUB-*ut* ŠU $GIDIM_7$
19. DIŠ SAG.KI-*šú* DIB-*su-ma* SU-*šú šim-ma-tú ú-kal u* IR NU TUKU ŠU $GIDIM_7$
20. DIŠ SAG.KI-*šú* SAG ŠÀ-*šú* NA_4.KIŠIB GÚ-*šú* DIB.DIB-*su* KÚM *la ḫa-aḫ-ḫaš u* IR NU TUKU
21. *ina ma-rak* U_4-*mi* SÍG *šá-pu-li-šú i-šaḫ-ḫu-uḫ* ŠU KI.SIKIL.LÍL.LÁ.EN. NA *la-ʾ-bi*
22. DIŠ SAG.KI-*šú šá* 15 $ŠED_7$-*át šá* 150 KÚM-*e-et* ŠU $GIDIM_7$
23. DIŠ SAG.KI-*šú šá* 15 *i-rad-ma šá* 150 KÚM-*e-et* KI.ÚS SAG.TUKU KI.ÚS-*us* DIN
24. DIŠ SAG.KI-*šú šá* 150 GU_7-*šú u* DIR.MEŠ-*pú* U_4.5.KÁM ŠU ^{d}30 […]
25. DIŠ SAG.KI-*šú šá* 15 GU_7-*šú* ŠU ^{d}UTU DIN
26. DIŠ SAG.KI-*šú šá* 150 GU_7-*šú* ŠU ^{d}15 DIN
27. DIŠ SAG.KI-*šú šá* 15 GU_7-*šú u* IGI-*šú šá* 15 GISSU DÙ ⌜EZEN⌝ *ana* DINGIR URU-*šú iq-bi* BÚR-*ma* DIN
28. DIŠ SAG.KI-*šú šá* 150 GU_7-*šú u* IGI-*šú šá* 150 GISSU DÙ ŠU ^{d}*Šul-pa-è-a* BÚR-*ma* DIN
29. DIŠ SAG.KI-*šú šá* 15 *u* 150 GU_7.MEŠ-*šú* IGI^{II}-*šú šá* 15 *u* 150 GISSU DÙ-*a*

30. LÚ.BI DINGIR-*šú u* DINGIR URU-*šú iz-zur ik-ri-ba ana* DINGIR-*šú iq-bi* BÚR-*ma* DIN
31. DIŠ SAG.KI 15-*šú* GU$_7$-*šú-ma* IGI 15-*šú nap-ḫat u* ÍR DÉ-*qí* ŠU GIDIM$_7$ *šá-‹né-e* ^{d}15›
32. DIŠ SAG.KI 150-*šú* GU$_7$-*šú-ma* IGI 150-*šú nap-ḫat u* ÍR DÉ-*qí* ŠU GIDIM$_7$ *šá-né-e* ^{d}15
33. DIŠ SAG.KI^{II}-*šú šá* 15 *u* 150 GU$_7$.MEŠ-*šú-ma* KÚM-*šú mit-ḫar* ŠU DINGIR-*šú* DIN
34. DIŠ SAG.KI^{II}-*šú šá* 15 *u* 150 GU$_7$.MEŠ-*šú-ma* KÚM-*šú* NU *mit-ḫar* ŠU DINGIR URU-*šú* GIG-*su* GÍD.DA-*ma* : […]-*ma* DIN
35. DIŠ SAG.KI-*šú* GU$_7$-*šú ú-maḫ-ḫa-ṣa-šú* SA.MEŠ IGI^{II}-*šú ú-z*[*aq-qa-tu*]-*šú*
36. SA GÚ-*šú* GU$_7$.MEŠ-*šú* ŠU GU$_4$
37. DIŠ *ina* SAG.KI-*šú* SÌG-*iṣ* ŠU ^{d}*Kù-bi*
38. DIŠ *ina* SAG.KI-*šú šá* 15 SÌG-*iṣ* ŠU ^{d}EN.x NIN.x DIN
39a. DIŠ *ina* SAG.KI-*šú šá* 150 SÌG-*iṣ* ŠU DINGIR-*šú*
39b. DIŠ *ina* SAG.KI-*šú šá* 15 SÌG-*iṣ* ŠU GIDIM ŠU DINGIR DIN
40. DIŠ *ina* SAG.KI-*šú šá* 150 SÌG-*iṣ u* IGI^{I}[^{I}-*šú* ÍR ŠU ^{d}EN.ZU][1]
41. DIŠ *ina* SAG.KI-*šú šá* 150 SÌG-*iṣ u* IGI^{II}-*šú* DIRI.MEŠ-*ḫa* [ŠU ^{d}EN.ZU][2]
42. DIŠ *ina* SAG.KI-*šú šá* 15 SÌG-*iṣ u i-ṭa-mu* […]
43. DIŠ *ina* SAG.KI-*šú šá* 150 SÌG-*iṣ u i-ṭa-mu* […]
44. DIŠ *ina* SAG.KI-*šú* SAG ŠÀ-*šú u* TI-*šú* SÌG-*iṣ* [ŠU ^{d}*Ereš-ki-gal* GAM][3]
45. DIŠ *ina* SAG.KI-*šú* SÌG-*iṣ-ma* ŠÀ.MEŠ-*šú it-te-*[*nen-bi-ṭu* …]
46. DIŠ *ina* SAG.KI-*šú* SÌG-*iṣ-ma* SA SAG.KI-*šú* ŠU^{II}-*šú u* GÌ[R^{II}-*šú* ZI.MEŠ …]-⸢*is-su* ⸣ TI
47. DIŠ *ina* SAG.KI-*šú* SÌG-*iṣ-ma* SA SAG.KI-*šú* ŠU^{II}-*šú u* GÌ[R^{II}-*šú* ZI.MEŠ … *i-bal*]-*lu-uṭ*
48. DIŠ *ina* SAG.KI-*šú* MURUB$_4$-*š*[*ú* SÌG-*iṣ*]-*ma* […]x TI
49. DIŠ *ina* SAG.KI-*šú* […]-*šú* GU.MEŠ TU[R.MEŠ …] TI-*uṭ*
50. DIŠ *ina* SAG.KI-*šú* KIR$_4$-*šú* ŠÀ-*šú* GU.MEŠ TU[R.MEŠ …] ⸢^{d}⸣UTU
51. DIŠ *ina* SAG.KI-*šú u pu-ti-šú* ŠU^{II}-*šú* […]x DU GAM
52. DIŠ SAG.KI^{II}-*šú* KÚM.MEŠ-*ma* GEŠTU^{II}-*šú* ŠED$_7$.M[EŠ …]GAM
53. DIŠ SAG.KI^{II}-*šú* ŠED$_7$.MEŠ-*ma* GEŠTU^{II}-*šú* KÚM.MEŠ […]GAM
54. DIŠ SAG.KI^{II}-*šú* KÚM *la ḫa-aḫ-ḫa-šú* GEŠTU^{II}[-*šú* …]
55. GIG-*su šu-*[…] ŠU! ⸢^{d}AMAR.UTU⸣
56. DIŠ SAG.KI^{II}-*šú* GEŠTU^{II}-*šú* KÚM *la ḫa-aḫ-ḫaš* […] DU$_8$ DIB-*it* SAG.DU TUKU.TUKU-*ši*
57. *lu* ŠU ^{d}30 *l*[*u* ŠU ^{d}]20

58. DIŠ SAG.KI^{II}-*šú* GEŠTU^{II}-*šú* KÚM *la ḫa-aḫ-ḫaš lu* ŠU DINGIR-*šú lu* ŠU DINGIR URU-*šú* TAG-*ma* ÚŠ
59. DIŠ SAG.KI^{II}-*šú* GEŠTU^{II}-*šú mit-ḫa-riš em-ma* ŠU ^{d}30 DIŠ *ša-at* ^{d}UTU
60. DIŠ SAG.KI^{II}-*šú* GEŠTU^{II}-*šú* GU_7.MEŠ-*šú u* AD_6-*šú* KÚM *šá-né-e* ^{d}30
61. DIŠ SAG.KI^{II}-*šú* ‹$MURUB_4$.MEŠ-*šú*› GU_7.MEŠ-*šú u* AD_6-*šú* KÚM *ana* U_4.3.KÁM ŠU DINGIR ÚŠ
62. DIŠ SAG.KI^{II}-*šú* GU_7.MEŠ-*šú u* $ŠED_7$.MEŠ ŠU ^{d}A.ZU
63. DIŠ SAG.KI^{II}-*šú* $MURUB_4$.MEŠ-*šú*[4] GU_7.MEŠ-*šú u* $ŠED_7$.MEŠ U_4.5.KÁM ŠU ^{d}A.ZU
64. DIŠ SAG.KI^{II}-*šú* KÚM-*ma* GEŠTU^{II}-*šú* $ŠED_7$.MEŠ[5] *lu* ŠU DINGIR-*šú lu* ŠU ^{d}*Kù-bi*
65. DIŠ SAG.KI^{II}-*šú* 1-*niš* DU.MEŠ *u* IR-*su it-ta-nag-ra-ár ú-gaš* ŠU ^{d}15 : ŠU ^{d}20
66. DIŠ SAG.KI^{II}-*šú ki-lat-tan* 1-*niš i-rad-da-šú* : DU.MEŠ
67. *u* IR-*su it-ta-nag-ra-ár* U_4.5.KÁM ŠU ^{d}15 *u* ‹^{d}›20
68. DIŠ SAG.KI^{II}-*šú ma-aq-ta* IGI^{II}-*šú ú-tar-ra-aṣ* TU.RA BI NU DIN
69. DIŠ *ina* SAG.KI 15-*šú* SA.MEŠ GIB.MEŠ DIN
70. DIŠ *ina* SAG.KI 150-*šú* SA.MEŠ GIB.MEŠ GIG-*su* GÍD.DA-*ma* DIN
71. DIŠ *ina* SAG.KI^{II}-*šú* SA.MEŠ GIB.MEŠ GIG-*su* GÍD.DA
72. DIŠ *ina* SAG.KI-*šú* SA.MEŠ SA_5.MEŠ GIB.MEŠ DIN
73. DIŠ SA SAG.KI-*šú* [...] *zi-iz* DIŠ KÚM-*im* DI-*ma* DIN
74. DIŠ SA SAG.KI-*šú zi-iz u* GI_6 GIG-*su* DUGUD GABA.RI SÌG-*iṣ*
75. DIŠ SA SAG.KI-*šú* 15 DIB-*su-ma* IGI 15-*šú* MÚD *ú-kal* ŠU $GIDIM_7$
76. DIŠ SA SAG.KI-*šú* 150 DIB-*su-ma* IGI 150-*šú* MÚD *ú-kal* ŠU $GIDIM_7$
77. DIŠ SA SAG.KI-*šú* DIB-*su-ma* IGI^{II}-*šú* MÚD *ú-kal-la* ŠU $GIDIM_7$
78. DIŠ SA SAG.KI 15-*šú* DIB-*su-ma* IGI 15-*šú* ÍR *ú-kal* ŠU $GIDIM_7$
79. DIŠ SA SAG.KI 150-*šú* DIB-*su-ma* IGI 150-*šú* ÍR *ú-kal* ŠU ⸢ $GIDIM_7$⸣
80. DIŠ SA SAG.KI-*šú* DIB-*su-ma* IGI^{II}-*šú* ÍR *ú-kal-la* ŠU [$GIDIM_7$]
81. DIŠ SA SAG.KI-*šú* DIB-*su-ma u* MÚD *i-ḫa-ru* ŠU $GIDIM_7$
82. DIŠ SA SAG.KI-*šú* D[IB].DIB-*su-ma u* MÚD *i-à-ru* NINDA! *u* KAŠ NU IGI-*ár* ŠU $GIDIM_7$
83. DIŠ SA SAG.KI-*šú šá* 15 *ka-bar ma-mál-li-šú* IGI *šá* 15 ŠU $GIDIM_7$
84. DIŠ SA SAG.KI-*šú šá* 150 *ka-bar ma-mál-li-šú* IGI *šá* 150 ŠU $GIDIM_7$
85. DIŠ SA SAG.KI-*šú šá* 15 *tar-ku ta-ḫi-iz* GIG ÚŠ
86. DIŠ SA SAG.KI-*šú šá* 150 *tar-ku na-šar* GIG
87. DIŠ SA SAG.KI-*šú tar-ku* GAM
88. D[IŠ SA] S[AG.KI^{II}-*šú* SA_5.MEŠ ...] *šá* 15 GI_6 *ni-di-it* ‹KIR_4›[6]
89. [DIŠ SA SAG.KI^{II}-*šú* SA_5.MEŠ ...]⸢*šá*⸣ 150 GI_6 GIG-*su* GÍD.DA-*ma* DIN

90. [DIŠ SA SAG.KI^{II}-*šú* SA$_5$.MEŠ …]-*šú* GI$_6$.MEŠ [GAB]A.RI SÌG-*iṣ* GIG-*su* DUGUD-*ma* DIN
91. [DIŠ SA SAG.K]I^{II}-*šú šá* [15 DU.D]U-*ma šá* 150 GAR-*nu* GAB[A.RI] SÌG-*iṣ* GIG-*su* DUGUD-*ma* GAM
92. [DIŠ SA SAG.KI^{II}]-*šú šá* ⸢150 DU-*ku-ma*⸣ *šá* 15 GAR-*nu* GABA.RI SÌG-*iṣ* DIN
93. [DIŠ SA SAG.KI^{II}]-*šú šá* 15 [DU].⸢DU⸣-*ma šá* 150 *n*[*e-e-ḫu* … *m*]*a-aq-tu* GAM
94. [DIŠ SA SAG.KI]-*šú šá* 150 *gal-tiš* GU$_4$.UD.MEŠ *u* ŠE U.MEŠ […] GAM
95. [DIŠ SA SAG.KI^{II}-*š*]*ú ip-te-ru-nim* […] GAM
96. [DIŠ SA SAG.KI^{II}]-*šú* ŠUB-*tu*[$_4$ …] GAM
97. [DIŠ SA SAG.KI^{II}]-*šú* ⸢MÚD⸣ *il-qú-m*[*a* …] GAM
98. [DIŠ SA SAG.KI]^{II}-*šú* ⸢*tar-ku*⸣ *šu-nu-*[…] GAM
99. [DIŠ SA SAG.KI]^{II}-*šú* ⸢GAR-*nu-ma* SA.MEŠ […] : DIN
100. [DIŠ SA] SAG.KI^{II}-*šú* […] *u* IGI^{II}-*šú* [… *na*]-*kid*
101. [DIŠ SA SAG].KI^{II}-*šú u* UZU.BI 1-*n*[*iš* …] GAM
102. [DIŠ SA SAG].KI^{II}-*šú šá* 15 *u* 150 GAR-*n*[*u* …] GAM
103. [DIŠ SA SAG].KI^{II}-*šú šá* 15 *u* 150 ⸢ZI.MEŠ⸣ […] GAM
104. [DIŠ SA SAG].KI^{II}-*šú šá* 15 *u* 150 ZI.MEŠ GI$_6$.MEŠ […*na*]-⸢ʾ-*id*⸣
105. [DIŠ SA SAG].KI^{II}-⸢*šú*⸣[*šá* 15] *u* 150 ZI.MEŠ *u* SAG ŠÀ-*šú* […]
106. [DIŠ SA SA]G.KI^{II}-*šú* ⸢*šá*⸣ 15 *u* 150 *ina* DU-*ki im-taḫ-ru*
107. SÌG-*iṣ* [MA]ŠKIM SÌG-*iṣ* ^{LÚ}MAŠ.MAŠ DÙ-*uš* DIN⸣ [: GAM]
108. [DIŠ SA] ⸢SAG⸣.KI^{II}-*šú šá* 15 *u* 150 DU.MEŠ-*ma* SAG.KI-*šú ú-sa-dar-šu* GAM
109. [DIŠ S]A ⸢SAG⸣.KI^{II}-*šú šá* 15 *u* 150 DU.ME-*ma u* IGI^{II}-*šú ú-rat-ta* GAM
110. [DIŠ SA] ⸢SAG⸣.KI^{II}-*šú šá* 15 *u* 150 DU.ME-*ma u* ŠÀ-*šú* DIB-*su* GAM
111. [DIŠ SA] ⸢SAG⸣.KI^{II}-*šú šá* 15 *u* 150 DU.ME-*ma* DUL.DUL *u* BAL.BAL GAM
112. [DIŠ SA S]AG.KI^{II}-*šú šá* 15 *u* 150 1-*niš* DU.MEŠ SAG ŠÀ-*šú* DIB. DIB-*su* SÌG-*iṣ* MAŠKIM SÌG-*iṣ* ⸢MAŠ⸣.MAŠ-*su* DÙ-*ma* DIN
113. [DIŠ SA S]AG.KI^{II}-*šú šá* 15 *u* 150 1-*niš* DU.ME-*ma u šu-ú* BAL.BAL SÌG-*iṣ* MAŠKIM GAM
114. [DIŠ SA S]AG.KI^{II}-*šú* ŠU^{II}-*šú u* GÌR^{II}-*šú it-ta-*[*na*]-⸢*lak*⸣-*ku*[7] GAM
115. DIŠ SA SAG.KI^{II}-*šú* ŠU^{II}-*šú u* GÌR^{II}-*šú* ‹*šá* 150› DU-*ku-ma šá* 15 GAR-*nu* ŠU DINGIR URU-*šú* : ŠU ^{d}UTU
116. DIŠ SA SAG.KI^{II}-*šú* ŠU^{II}-*šú u* GÌR^{II}-*šú šá* 15 *u* 150 *it-ta-na-aš-gag-gu u* BAL.MEŠ
117. ⸢*e-sa*⸣ *ú-šaq-qa-ma* AD$_6$-*šú* IGI.BAR.MEŠ ŠU ^{d}UTU MU DAM LÚ

118. DIŠ SA SAG.KI^{II}-*šú* ŠU^{II}-*šú* GÌR^{II}-*šú* GÚ-*šú u* SAG ŠÀ-*šú* DU.MEŠ U$_4$.7.KÁM SAL.KALAG.GA ⸢IGI-*ma*⸣ ‹NU› DIN
119. DIŠ SA SAG.KI^{II}-*šú* ŠU^{II}-*šú* GÌR^{II}-*šú* GÚ-*šú pa-pan* ŠÀ-*šú* DU.MEŠ *u* SU-*šú* ŠED$_7$ *za-mar* IGI DU$_8$ DUL-*ma ni-š*[*i*]
120. DIŠ SA SAG.KI^{II}-*šú* ŠU^{II}-*šú* RI.MEŠ GAR.MEŠ-*ma* PA IGI^{II}-*šú*
121. DIB.DIB-*tu* ŠU.LUḪ *ina* KI DIB-*tu* TA É *ana* É KÚR-*šú-ma* DIN
122. DIŠ SA SAG.KI^{II}-*šú tal-lu la ip-rik-u* TAB-*su ra-mu-ú* ÉN ŠUB-*šum-ma* DIN
123. DIŠ ZI SAG.KI TUKU-*ši-ma u* SU-*šú* GU$_7$-*šú* ŠU GÍDIM
124. DIŠ ZI SAG.KI TUKU-*ši-ma* ŠU^{II}-*šú u* GÌR^{II}-*šú i-šam-ma-ma-šú* ŠU GÍDIM
125. DIŠ ZI SAG.KI *šim-ma-tú u ri-mu-tú* TUKU.TUKU-*ši* ŠU GÍDIM
126. DIŠ *ú-ru-uḫ* SAG.KI-*šú šá* 15 *bé-e-er* SA.MEŠ-*šú šá* 150 ZI.MEŠ
127. DIB-*it* ŠÀ TUKU *u* SAG ŠÀ-*šú i-ru-ur* SÌG-*iṣ* ⸢MAŠKIM⸣ GAM
128. DIŠ SAG.KI-*su* KÚM *ú-kal* DIN
129. DIŠ SAG.KI-*su* IR *ú-kal* DIN
130. DIŠ SAG.KI-*su ka-ṣa-at* DIN
131. DIŠ SAG.KI-*su* BABBAR EME-*šú* BABBAR GIG-*su* GÍD-*ma* DIN
132. DIŠ SAG.KI-*su* BABBAR *u i-riš-tú* ŠÀ TUKU-*ši ina* U$_4$-*me-šú-ma bi-bil* ŠÀ APIN-*iš*
133. DIŠ SAG.KI-*su u pa-nu-šú* BABBAR *ina* U$_4$-*me-šú-ma* A.GEŠTIN.NA APIN-*iš*
134. DIŠ SAG.KI-*su* SIG$_7$-*at ina* U$_4$-*me-šú-ma* ^{GIŠ}NU.ÚR.MA APIN-*iš*
135. DIŠ SAG.KI-*su* SA$_5$ *u* SIG$_7$ *ina* U$_4$-*me-šú-ma* KU$_6$ APIN-*iš*
136. DIŠ SAG.KI-*su* SA$_5$ *ina* U$_4$-*me-šú-ma* ZAG.ḪI.LI APIN-*iš*
137. DIŠ SAG.KI-*su* GI$_6$ *u* SA$_5$ *ina* U$_4$-*me-šú-ma* UZU *u* ZAG.ḪI.LI APIN-*iš*
138. DIŠ SAG.KI-*su* GI$_6$ *ina* U$_4$-*me-šú-ma* ^{GIŠ}GEŠTIN *u* ZAG.ḪI.LI APIN-*iš*
139. DIŠ SAG.KI-*su bar-mat ina* U$_4$-*me-šú-ma* ^{GIŠ}GEŠTIN APIN-*iš*
140. DIŠ SAG.KI-*su šal-mat ina* U$_4$-*me-šú-ma* ^{GIŠ}GEŠTIN APIN-*iš*
141. DIŠ SAG.KI-*su* GIN$_7$ *si-ka-a-t*[*i* …]⸢x-*ma*?⸣ ZÚ.LUM.MA APIN-*iš*
142. DIŠ SAG.KI-*su* GIN$_7$ *si-ka-a-t*[*i* …] IGI^{II}-*šú ip-rik* GAM

Translation

1. If he has a vise-like headache[8] and he gets hot (var. cold), "hand" of Kubu.[9]
2. If he has a vise-like headache and his bowels are loose,[10] "hand" of Kubu.[11]

3. If he has a vise-like headache and his insides are continually cramped, "hand" of Kubu.[12]
4. If he has a vise-like headache, and his ears do not hear, the "hand" of his god has been imposed on him; he will die.[13]
5. If his temple is normal, he will get well; if his temp(oral blood vessels) have collapsed,[14] he will die.[15]
6. If his temp(oral blood vessels) have collapsed and his eyes are blurred/ shed tears,[16] he will die.[17]
7. If his temple afflicts him so that he continually cries out (and) blood runs out of his nose, "hand" of ghost.[18]
8. If his temple afflicts him so that ditto (he continually cries out), his temporal blood vessels (feel like they) are pulsating greatly (and) the upper part of his head (feels like it) is open, "hand" of ghost; he will die.[19]
9. If his temple afflicts him so that ditto (he continually cries out), his temporal blood vessels (feel like they) are pulsating greatly (and) the upper part of his head (feels like it) is broken in pieces, he will die.[20]
10. If his temple afflicts him and he keeps crying out: "my insides, my insides," "hand" of ghost, deputy of Ishtar; he will die. Variant: "hand" of ghost; if it is prolonged, he will die.[21]
11. If his temple afflicts him and ditto (he keeps crying out: "my insides, my insides"), he vomits a lot and cannot (stand to) wear the bedding,[22] "hand" of ghost; he will die.[23]
12. If his temple afflicts him and (the affliction) lasts from sunset till the third night watch (var. it keeps him up all night), he will die.[24]
13. If his temple afflicts him and from sunrise to sunset it hurts him (var. it does not let up) it will let up; "hand" of ghost.[25]
14. If his temple afflicts him and blood flows from his nose, "hand" of ghost.
15. If his temple afflicts him and his neck muscles continually hurt him, "hand" of ghost.[26]
16. If his temple afflicts him and his eye muscles continually hurt, "hand" of ghost.[27]
17. If his temple afflicts him and he gets hot (and then) cold and his eyes are swollen, "hand" of ghost.[28]
18. If his temple afflicts him and his face (seems) continually to spin (and) he gets up but then falls down, "hand" of ghost.[29]
19. If his temple afflicts him and numbness grips his body but he does not sweat, "hand" of ghost.[30]

20–21. If his temples, his epigastrium, (and) the vertebrae of his neck continually afflict him, his temperature is lukewarm and he does not sweat (but) over a long period of time[31] the hair of his inguinal regions[32] falls out, "hand" of infectious[33] *ardat lilî*.[34]

22. If his "right" temple (seems) cold and his "left" one (seems) hot, "hand" of ghost.[35]

23. If his "right" temple (seems to) shake[36] and the "left" one seems hot, he has trod in the footsteps of a *rābiṣu*,[37] he will get well.[38]

24. If his "left" temple hurts him and ‹his eyes› drift downstream for five days, "hand" of Sîn [...].[39]

25. If his "right" temple hurts him, "hand" of Shamash; he will get well.[40]

26. If his "left" temple hurts him, "hand" of Ishtar; he will get well.[41]

27. If his "right" temple hurts him and his "right" eye makes an opaque spot, he promised a festival to the god of his city. If it goes away, he will get well.

28. If his "left" temple hurts him and his "left" eye makes an opaque spot, "hand" of Šulpaea. If it goes away, he will get well.

29–30. If his "right" and "left" temple hurt him and his "right" and "left" eye make an opaque spot, that person cursed his god and the god of his city; he made a vow to his god. If it goes away, he will get well.[42]

31. If his "right" temple hurts him and his "right" eye is swollen and sheds tears, "hand" of ghost, deputy of Ishtar.[43]

32. If his "left" temple hurts him and his "left" eye is swollen and sheds tears, "hand" of ghost, deputy of Ishtar.[44]

33. If his "right" and "left" temples hurt him and his temperature is even, "hand" of his god; he will get well.[45]

34. If his "right" and "left" temples hurt him and his temperature is not even, the "hand" of the god of his city; his illness may be prolonged (var. ...) but he will get well.[46]

35–36. If his temple hurts him and gives him jabbing pains, his eye muscles ⸢sting⸣ him (and) his neck muscles continually hurt him, "hand" of ghost.[47]

37. If he was injured[48] on his temple, "hand" of Kubu.[49]

38. If he was injured on his "right" temple, "hand" of Enlil(?) (and) Ninlil(?), he will get well.

39a. If he was injured on his "left" temple, "hand" of his god.[50]

39b. If he was injured on his "right" temple, "hand" of ghost, (or) "hand" of god; he will get well.[51]

40. If he was injured on his "left" temple and [his] eyes [shed tears, "hand" of Sîn].[52]

41. If he was injured on his "left" temple and [his] eyes are suffused,[53] ["hand" of Sîn].[54]

42. If he was injured on his "right" temple and he twists [...].[55]

43. If he was injured on his "left" temple and he twists [...].[56]

44. If he was injured on his temple, his epigastrium and his rib, ["hand" of Ereškigal; he will die].

45. If he was injured on his temple and, consequently, his insides are continually [cramped ...].

46. If he was injured on his temple and, consequently, the blood vessel(s) of his temple, his hands and his ⸢feet⸣ [(feel like they) are pulsating (and) ... afflicts?] him, he will get well.

47. If he was injured on his temple and, consequently, the blood vessel(s) of his temple, his hands and his ⸢feet⸣ [(feel like they) are pulsating (and) ...], ⸢he will get well⸣.

48. If he was [injured?] on his temple and his hip region and [...], he will get well.

49. If ⸢small⸣ webs [...] on his temple (and) his [...], he will get well.[57]

50. If ⸢small⸣ webs [...] on his temple, his nose (and) his abdomen, ["hand" of] Shamash.[58]

51. If [small webs ...] on his temple and his front side, his hands [...], he will die.[59]

52. If his temples are hot and his ears are cold [...], he will die.

53. If his temples are cold and his ears are hot [...], he will die.

54–55. If his temples are lukewarm (and) his ears [are hot/cold ...], [(if)] his illness is [...], "hand" of Marduk.

56–57. If his temples (and) his ears are lukewarm [...] is uncongested[60] (and) he continually has "affliction of the head," either "hand" of Sîn ⸢or⸣ ["hand" of] Shamash.[61]

58. If his temples (and) his ears are lukewarm, either "hand" of his god or "hand" of the god of his city. If it "touches" (him), he will die.

59. If his temples (and) his ears are equally hot, "hand" of Sîn or[62] that of Shamash.

60. If his temples (and) his ears continually hurt him and his body is hot, a deputy of Sîn.[63]

61. If his temples ‹(and) the middle parts (of his ears)› continually hurt him and his body is hot, (and he has been sick) for three days,[64] "hand" of god; he will die.

62. If his temples continually hurt him and he continually has chills, "hand" of Azu.

63. If his temples (and) the middle parts (of his ears) (var. text E: his ears) continually hurt him and he continually has chills, (and he has been sick for) five days, "hand" of Azu.

64. If his temples are hot and his ears continue to be cold (var. A&F: his temples are cold like his ears), either "hand" of his god or "hand" of Kubu.

65. If his temples "go" at the same time and his sweat rolls down (and) he vomits,[65] "hand" of Ishtar (var. "hand" of Shamash).[66]

66–67. If both temples shake (var. "go") at the same time and his sweat rolls down (and he has been sick for) five days, "hand" of Ishtar or Shamash.[67]

68. If his temp(oral blood vessels) have collapsed[68] (and) he stretches out his eyes (towards the darkness), that sick person will not recover.[69]

69. If in his "right" temple, the blood vessels cross, he will get well.

70. If in his "left" temple, the blood vessels cross, his illness may be prolonged (but) he will get well.

71. If in (both) his temples, the blood vessels cross, his illness will be prolonged.[70]

72. If in his temple, the blood vessels are red and cross, he will get well.

73. If a blood vessel of his temple [...] was cut through,[71] if he (merely) gets feverish, he is safe and so will get well.[72]

74. If a blood vessel of his temple was cut through and is dark, his illness will be difficult; he was injured on the front side.[73]

75. If a blood vessel of his "right" temple afflicts him and his "right" eye contains blood, "hand" of ghost.[74]

76. If a blood vessel of his "left" temple afflicts him and his "left" eye contains blood, "hand" of ghost.[75]

77. If a blood vessel of his temple afflicts him and (both) his eyes contain blood, "hand" of ghost.[76]

78. If a blood vessel of his "right" temple afflicts him and his "right" eye contains tears, "hand" of ghost.[77]

79. If a blood vessel of his "left" temple afflicts him and his "left" eye contains tears, "hand" of ghost.[78]

80. If a blood vessel of his temple afflicts him and (both) his eyes contain tears, "hand" of [ghost].[79]

81. If a blood vessel of his temple afflicts him and he also vomits blood, "hand" of ghost.

82. If a blood vessel of his temple continually afflicts him and he also vomits blood (and his stomach) will not accept bread or beer, "hand" of ghost.

83. If the muscles of his "right" temple are thickened (over) the "right" eye, "hand" of ghost.[80]

84. If the muscles of his "left" temple are thickened (over)[81] the "left" eye, "hand" of ghost.[82]
85. If the muscle(s)/blood vessel(s) of his "right" temple are dark, holding fast[83] of the illness; he will die.
86. If the muscle(s)/blood vessel(s) of his "left" temple are dark, diminution (caused by) the illness.
87. If the muscle(s)/blood vessel(s) of (both) his temple(s) are dark, he will die.
88. ⸢If⸣ the [muscles/blood vessels of his] ⸢temples⸣ [are red and his] "right" [temple] is dark, (it means) dejection (var. H: it is worrisome).
89. [If the muscles/blood vessels of temples are red and his] "left" [temple] is dark, his illness may be prolonged (but) he will get well.
90. [If the muscles/blood vessels of his temples are red and] his [temples] are dark, he was injured ⸢on the front side⸣, his illness may be difficult, but he will get well.
91. [If the blood vessel(s) of] his ⸢temples⸣, the ones on the ["right" continually] ⸢"go"⸣ and the ones on the "left" are present, he was injured ⸢on the front side⸣; if he has a difficult time of it, he will die.[84]
92. [If the blood vessel(s) of] his [temples], the ones on the "left" "go" and the ones on the "right" are present, he was injured on the front side; he will get well.[85]
93. [If the blood vessel(s) of] his [temples], the ones on the "right" [continually] "go" and the ones on the "left" are ⸢slow⸣ [and (the blood vessels of) his temples] ⸢have collapsed⸣, he will die.
94. [If the blood vessel(s) of] his [temples], the ones on the "left" pulse very rapidly (lit. "jump" and the undersides of his fingers[86] [...], he will die.
95. [If the blood vessel(s)] of ⸢his⸣ [temples] vomit forth [...], he will die.[87]
96. [If the blood vessel(s)] of his [temples] have collapsed [...], he will die.[88]
97. [If the blood vessel(s) of] his [temples] take away the blood [...], he will die.[89]
98. [If the blood vessel(s) of] his [temples] are dark (and) [...], he will die.
99. [If the blood vessel(s) of] his [temples] are present and the blood vessels of [...], (var. he will get well).
100. [If the blood vessel(s)] of his temples [...] and his eyes [...], ⸢it is worrisome⸣.
101. [If the blood vessel(s)] of his ⸢temples⸣ and his flesh all [...] together, he will die.
102. [If the blood vessel(s) of] his ⸢temples⸣, the ones on the "right" and the ones on the "left" are present [but ...], he will die.

103. [If the blood vessel(s) of] his ⸢temples⸣, the ones on the "right" and the ones on the "left" (feel like they are) pulsating [...], he will die.

104. [If the blood vessel(s) of] his ⸢temples⸣, the ones on the "right" and the ones on the "left" continually (feel like they are) pulsating (and) are continually dark [...], ⸢it is worrisome⸣.

105. [If the blood vessel(s) of] his ⸢temples⸣, [the ones on the "right"] and the ones on the "left" (feel like they are) pulsating and his epigastrium [...].

106–107. [If the blood vessel(s) of] his ⸢temples⸣, the ones on the "right" and the ones on the "left" "go" to an equal extent, he was struck with the blow of a ⸢*rābiṣu*⸣. You may do his medical treatment; he will get well [var. he will die].[90]

108. [If the blood vessel(s)] of his temples, the ones on the "right" and the ones on the "left" "go" and his temple does this to him several times in a row, he will die.[91]

109. [If] the ⸢blood vessel(s)⸣ of his temples, the ones on the "right" and the ones on the "left" "go" and he fixes his eyes, he will die.[92]

110. [If the blood vessel(s)] of his temples, the ones on the "right" and the ones on the "left" "go" and his abdomen afflicts him, he will die.[93]

111. [If the blood vessel(s)] of his temples, the ones on the "right" and the ones on the "left" "go" and he veils himself (i.e., withdraws from social intercourse) and has changes of mood, he will die.[94]

112. [If the blood vessel(s)] of his ⸢temples⸣, the ones on the "right" and the ones on the "left" "go" at the same time (and) his epigastrium continually afflicts him, he was struck with the blow of a *rābiṣu*. If you do his medical treatment (right away), he will get well.[95]

113. [If the blood vessel(s)] of his ⸢temples⸣, the ones on the "right" and the ones on the "left" "go" at the same time and he has continual changes of mood, blow of a *rābiṣu*; he will die.[96]

114. [If the blood vessel(s)] of his ⸢temples⸣, his hands and his feet continually "go," he will die.[97]

115. If the blood vessels of his temples, his hands and his feet, ‹the ones on the "left"› "go" but the ones on the "right" are present, "hand" of the god of his city (var. "hand" of Shamash).[98]

116–117. If the blood vessels of his temples, his hands, or his feet, the ones on the "right" or "left" ‹"go" but the ones on the "left" or "right" are present and the muscles of the feet› on the "right" or "left" side continually become stiff and continually shift under (him),[99] (his feet) have a vise-like pain(?)[100] (but) he can lift (them) and he continually gazes at his body, "hand" of Shamash on account of a man's wife.[101]

118. If the blood vessel(s) of his temples, his hands, his feet, his neck and his epigastrium "go," if he has a very hard time of it for seven days, he will ‹not› get well.[102]
119. If the blood vessels of his temples, his hands, his feet, his neck and his umbilical area "go" and his body is cold, if he occasionally opens and closes his eyes, there will be a recovery.[103]
120–121. If the blood vessel(s) of his temples (and) his hands run parallel (and) are present but his eyelids are "seized," you wash (him). He is at an acute stage of the illness;[104] if you move him from one room to another, he will get well.[105]
122. If the blood vessel(s) of his temples run parallel (and) do not cross (and) his burning (fever?) has slackened, if you cast a spell over him, he will get well.
123. If he experiences pulsating of the temples and his body hurts him, "hand" of ghost.[106]
124. If he experiences pulsating of the temples and his hands and feet go numb, "hand" of ghost.[107]
125. If he continually experiences pulsating of the temples (and) numbness or limpness,[108] "hand" of ghost.[109]
126–127. If the hair of his "right" temple is fine (lit. select), the blood vessels of his "left" (temple feel like they) are pulsating, he has affliction of the abdomen and his epigastrium rumbles,[110] blow of a *rābiṣu*; he will die.[111]
128. If his forehead holds fever, he will get well.
129. If his forehead holds sweat, he will get well.
130. If his forehead is cold, he will get well.[112]
131. If his forehead is white (and) his tongue is white, his illness may be prolonged but he will get well.[113]
132. If his forehead is white and he has some craving, on that same day, he will ask for what he wants.
133. If his forehead and his face are white, on that same day, he will ask for vinegar.
134. If his forehead is yellow, on that same day, he will ask for pomegranate.
135. If his forehead is red and yellow, on that same day, he will ask for fish.
136. If his forehead is red, on that same day, he will ask for *saḫlû*-cress.
137. If his forehead is dark and red, on that same day, he will ask for meat and *saḫlû*-cress.
138. If his forehead is dark, on that same day, he will ask for grapes and *saḫlû*-cress.[114]
139. If his forehead is multicolored, on that same day, he will ask for grapes.

140. If his forehead is healthy, on that same day, he will ask for grapes
141. If his forehead is [...] like brewer's yeast [...] he will ask for dates.
142. If his forehead is [...] like brewer's yeast (and) his eyes cross, he will die.[115]

Notes

1. The restoration is based on *KAR* 211 i 21′ (Heeßel 2010, 171–77).
2. The restoration is based on *KAR* 211 i 22′ (Heeßel 2010, 171–77).
3. The restoration is confirmed by the commentary SpTU 1.30 obv. 2.
4. Text E has GEŠTU^{II}-*šú*.
5. Texts A and F have SAG.KI^{II}-*šú ki-ma* GEŠTU^{II}-*šú* ŠED$_7$.MEŠ.
6. Text H has *na-kid*.
7. With *CAD* A/2, 481a, this is from *alāku* and not *etēqu*, as the immediately preceding and following entries show.
8. Literally: "his temple (feels) squeezed."
9. See Scurlock and Andersen 2005, 19.339.
10. The commentary, SpTU 1.30 obv. 2 explains that AL.DU means *il-la-ku*: "they run." Normal bowel movements are not described in this fashion.
11. See Scurlock and Andersen 2005, 13.13, 19.339.
12. See Scurlock and Andersen 2005, 19.339.
13. See Scurlock and Andersen 2005, 13.14, 19.212, 19.292, 20.64.
14. Literally: "fallen down."
15. See Scurlock and Andersen 2005, 14.24.
16. The commentary CT 51.136 obv. 12 shows that even ancient scribes were unsure as to the correct reading.
17. See Scurlock and Andersen 2005, 14.25.
18. See Scurlock and Andersen 2005, 15.23.
19. See Scurlock and Andersen 2005, 13.167. This entry is cited in therapeutic text BAM 482 iv 49′//*AMT* 19/1 iv! 32′–33′.
20. See Scurlock and Andersen 2005, 13.168, 20.63.
21. This entry is cited in therapeutic text BAM 482 iv 47′//*AMT* 19/1 iv! 30′.
22. Normal bedding was a reed mat which you wrapped round yourself on cold nights. The point is that he is having a hard night's sleep.
23. See Scurlock and Andersen 2005, 6.28, 19.302, 20.70. This entry is cited in therapeutic text BAM 482 iv 48′//*AMT* 19/1 iv! 31′.
24. See Scurlock and Andersen 2005, 13.165. This entry is cited in therapeutic text BAM 482 iv 46′//*AMT* 19/1 iv! 29′.
25. A treatment for this condition appears in BAM 482 iii 7–9 (Scurlock 2006, no. 68).
26. A treatment for this condition appears in BAM 482 iv 44′–45′//*AMT* 19/1 iv! 27′–28′. (Scurlock 2006, no. 84).
27. See Scurlock and Andersen 2005, 19.247.
28. See Scurlock and Andersen 2005, 19.247. A treatment for this condition appears in BAM 482 iii 5–6 (Scurlock 2006, no. 83).
29. See Scurlock and Andersen 2005, 19.43. Treatments for this condition appear in BAM 482 iv 40′–41′//*AMT* 19/1 iv! 23′//Jastrow 1913, rev. 28′ (Scurlock 2006, no. 90) and BAM 482 iv 42′–43′//*AMT* 19/1 iv! 24′–26′ (Scurlock 2006, no. 89) and with very slightly varying

symptoms in *AMT* 97/4: 6′–8′ (Scurlock 2006, no. 88).

30. See Scurlock and Andersen 2005, 19.86.

31. The reading is indicated by the commentary SpTU 1.30 obv. 6: [*ina ma-rak*] U_4-*mi* = *ina*(?) [*a-r*]*a-ku* U_4-*mu*.

32. For the translation of *šāpulu* as "inguinal region," see Heeßel 2000, 168 ad 57′. Adamson 1984, 7–8 proposes an alternative translation of "scrotal sac." However, in this passage, the hair of the *šāpulu* is described as falling out. Since the scrotal sac has minimal or no hair, "inguinal region" appears to be the preferable translation.

33. KI.TAG.GA = *la'bu* (5R 116 i 37). The commentary to this line (SpTU 1.30 obv. 7d) defines *la'bu* as "what the *lilû* left behind."

34. See Scurlock and Andersen 2005, 4.26.

35. See Scurlock and Andersen 2005, 13.158.

36. See the commentary SpTU 1.30 obv. 9.

37. This interpretation of SAG.TUKU follows the commentary, SpTU 1.30 obv. 9–11. The spirit in question is a "demon-bailiff." Just as human courts sent out human *rābiṣu*'s to bring miscreants to justice, so too the gods. Pace *CAD* R, this is not an attorney, a class of persons who did not exist at any period in Mesopotamian history and who do not, in any case, perform the functions attested for the *rābiṣu*.

38. See Scurlock and Andersen 2005, 19.82. This entry appears also in Ni. 470:8 (Kraus 1987, 196–202).

39. This entry also appears in *STT* 89:209.

40. See Scurlock and Andersen 2005, 19.253.

41. See Scurlock and Andersen 2005, 19.253. The commentary, SpTU 1.30 obv. 11–12 cites this and the previous line with the following explanation: If his "right" temple hurts him, "hand" of Shamash; he will get well. [If his] ⌈"left"⌉ [temple] hurts him, "hand" of Ishtar; he will get well. This is because the right eye is Ishtar and the left eye is Shamash. This proves beyond the shadow of a doubt that the "right" and "left" designations in medical symptomology refer to the doctor's point of view. Modern medicine phrases its symptoms from the patient's point of view.

42. See Scurlock and Andersen 2005, 9.91, 19.350.

43. Treatments for this condition appear in BAM 482 ii 62′–64′a (Scurlock 2006, no. 79) and BAM 482 ii 64′b–65′ (Scurlock 2006, no. 81).

44. Treatments for this condition appear in BAM 482 iii 1–2, 3–4 (Scurlock 2006, nos. 82, 80).

45. See Scurlock and Andersen 2005, 3.3, 13.164, 16.6, 19.35, 19.211.

46. See Scurlock and Andersen 2005, 13.164.

47. See Scurlock and Andersen 2005, 9.52. A treatment for this condition appears in *AMT* 19/1 iv! 9′–13′//BAM 482 iv 30′–32′ (Scurlock 2006, no. 118).

48. Most of the injuries described will have been from war wounds. The current translation allows, however, for reference to accidental injuries and blunt instrument trauma.

49. See Scurlock and Andersen 2005, 19.188.

50. See Scurlock and Andersen 2005, 19.210.

51. See Scurlock and Andersen 2005, 19.169, 19.210.

52. See Scurlock and Andersen 2005, 19.200. This entry appears also in Middle Assyrian precursors *KAR* 211 i 21′ (Heeßel 2010, 171–77) and VAT 10748:5′ (pp. 178–81) except that the entry has the "right" temple being injured.

53. Literally: "soaked." This entry appears also in Middle Assyrian precursors *KAR* 211 i 22′ (Heeßel 2010, 171–77) and VAT 10748:6′ (pp. 178–81).

54. See Scurlock and Andersen 2005, 19.200.
55. See Scurlock and Andersen 2005, 13.123.
56. See Scurlock and Andersen 2005, 13.123.
57. See Scurlock and Andersen 2005, 6.153.
58. See Scurlock and Andersen 2005, 6.153.
59. See Scurlock and Andersen 2005, 6.153.
60. Literally: "open." The translation assumes that the lungs are being referred to.
61. See Scurlock and Andersen 2005, 19.270.
62. The reading is confirmed by lines 56-57.
63. See Scurlock and Andersen 2005, 3.2
64. The positioning of the "hand" would seem to indicate that this was intended as a diagnosis (what is the cause) and not a prognosis ("he will die within three days").
65. See Scurlock and Andersen 2005, p. 122.
66. See Scurlock and Andersen 2005, 19.252.
67. See Scurlock and Andersen 2005, 19.257.
68. Literally: "have fallen."
69. See Scurlock and Andersen 2005, 9.16.
70. This entry also appears in Labat 1956, 125 rev. 10.
71. Literally, "divided."
72. See Scurlock and Andersen 2005, 14.4.
73. See Scurlock and Andersen 2005, 14.4.
74. A treatment for this condition appears in BAM 3 iii 28–30//BAM 482 ii 26–27//*AMT* 20/1 ii! 3′–4′//K 19766:1′ (Scurlock 2006, no. 73). Similarly, *AMT* 20/1 ii! 9′–10′//K 19766:6′–7′, which has pulsating blood vessels in the temples.
75. A treatment for this condition appears in BAM 3 iii 31–33//BAM 482 ii 28–29//*AMT* 20/1 ii! 5′–6′//K 19766:2′–3′ (Scurlock 2006, no. 74). Similarly, *AMT* 20/1 ii! 11′–12′, which has pulsating blood vessels in the temples.
76. Treatments for this condition appear in BAM 3 iii 15–17 (Scurlock 2006, no, 72) and BAM 3 iii 34–36//*AMT* 20/1 ii! 7′–8′//K 19766:4′–5′ (Scurlock 2006, no. 75).
77. A treatment for this condition appears in BAM 482 ii 20–21//BAM 9:14–15 (Scurlock 2006, no. 76). Similarly, BAM 3 iii 20–23//BAM 35 iv 1′–3′//*AMT* 20/1 ii! 13′–14′ (Scurlock 2006, no. 93) and BAM 6:1–6 (Scurlock 2006, no. 94), which have pulsating blood vessels in the temples.
78. A treatment for this condition appears in BAM 482 ii 22–23//BAM 9:16–17 (Scurlock 2006, no. 77). Similarly, BAM 3 iii 24//BAM 35 iv 4′//*AMT* 20/1 ii! 15′ (Scurlock 2006, no. 95) and BAM 6:7–11 (Scurlock 2006, no. 96), which have pulsating blood vessels in the temples.
79. A treatment for this condition appears in BAM 482 ii 24–25//BAM 9:18–20//*AMT* 20/1 ii! 1′–2′ (Scurlock 2006, no. 78). Similarly, BAM 3 iii 25–27//BAM 35 iv 5′–7′//*AMT* 20/1 ii! 16′–17′ (Scurlock 2006, no. 97), which have pulsating blood vessels in the temples.
80. See Scurlock and Andersen 2005, 9.55.
81. Literally, "is thick to an equal extent with."
82. See Scurlock and Andersen 2005, 9.55.
83. *tāḫīzu* from *aḫāzu*, here in a more literal sense than the otherwise attested "learning" (actually "retention"). See *CAD* T, 50.
84. See Scurlock and Andersen 2005, 8.58.
85. See Scurlock and Andersen 2005, 8.59.
86. ŠE = *kittabru*. *STT* 403 rev. 47 explains the "ŠE U.MEŠ" as meaning TA MU *ap-pat* ŠU.SI.MEŠ-*šú* EN SAG *ṣu-ur-ri-šú*: "from the line (represented by) the tips of his fingers to

the beginning of his core" or, in other words, the underside (belly) of the finger. For more on this subject, see Rutz 2011, 304–5.

87. See Scurlock and Andersen 2005, 14.30. This entry appears also in Labat 1956, 125 rev. 10.

88. This entry appears also in Labat 1956, 125 rev. 11.

89. See Scurlock and Andersen 2005, 14.31 as corrected here. This entry appears also in Labat, *Syria* 33.125 rev. 12.

90. See Scurlock and Andersen 2005, 19.116, 20.25. This entry appears also in Labat1956, 125 rev. 13 and Ni. 470:5–6 (Kraus 1987, 196–202).

91. See Scurlock and Andersen 2005, 20.25. This entry appears also in Labat 1956, 125 rev. 14 and Ni. 470:7 (Kraus 1987, 196–202).

92. See Scurlock and Andersen 2005, 20.23. This entry appears also in SpTU 3.86 obv. 1–2.

93. See Scurlock and Andersen 2005, 20.24.

94. See Scurlock and Andersen 2005, 20.24.

95. See Scurlock and Andersen 2005, 19.117.

96. See Scurlock and Andersen 2005, 19.118.

97. See Scurlock and Andersen 2005, 8.55.

98. See Scurlock and Andersen 2005, 19.124.

99. The Akkadian leaves out everything which will have been obvious to an ancient reader including the fact that the same word indicates blood vessels and muscles, making it possible to considerably shorten the sentence.

100. The translation assumes that *esû* is a variant of *ḫesû* as suggested in *CAD* E, 338a.

101. See Scurlock and Andersen 2005, 16.55, 19.125. The commentary to tablet 4, SpTU 1.30 obv. 14–15 explains the supplementary diagnosis "on account of a man's wife" in this "hand" of Shamash reference where the temples (SAG.KI) are involved by pointing out that SAG ("head") is equivalent to "man" and KI ("earth") to "woman."

102. See Scurlock and Andersen 2005, 8.56.

103. See Scurlock and Andersen 2005, 8.57, 20.12, 20.21.

104. For the interpretation, see Heeßel 2000, 187.

105. See Scurlock and Andersen 2005, 2.7.

106. A treatment for this condition appears in BAM 11:30–31 (Scurlock 2006, no. 99).

107. See Scurlock and Andersen 2005, 15.22. Treatments for this condition appear in BAM 482 i 60′–61′ (Scurlock 2006, no. 102) and BAM 482 i 62′–63′ (no. 103).

108. The pulsating temples with numbness are treated separately from the pulsating temples with limpness.

109. Treatments for this condition appear in BAM 11:34–35//BAM 482 i 54′–55′//*AMT* 20/1 i! 42′–43′ (Scurlock 2006, no. 100), BAM 482 i 56′–58′//*AMT* 20/1 i! 44′–46′ (Scurlock 2006, no. 104) and BAM 489 i 59′//*AMT* 20/1 i! 47′ (Scurlock 2006, no. 101) for the numbness and in BAM 11:32–33//BAM 482 i 49′–50′//*AMT* 20/1 i! 36′–37′ (Scurlock 2006, no. 105), BAM 482 i 51′//*AMT* 20/1 i! 38′–39′ (Scurlock 2006, no. 106) and BAM 482 i 52′-53′//*AMT* 20/1 i! 40′–41′ (Scurlock 2006, no. 107) for the limpness.

110. Ni. 470:3–4 (Kraus 1987, 196–202) has "protrudes."

111. See Scurlock and Andersen 2005, 7.27, 19.115. This entry also appears in Ni. 470:3–4 (Kraus 1987, 196–202).

112. See Scurlock and Andersen 2005, 20.19.

113. See Scurlock and Andersen 2005, 18.38.

114. For the creative use of this passage to argue for a correspondence between the new Hellenistic sciences and those of ancient Mesopotamia, see Scurlock and al-Rawi 2006, 375–78.

115. See Scurlock and Andersen 2005, 13.92.

DPS TABLET 5

DPS 4: 143 (catchline) = DPS 5:1

1. DIŠ GIG IGI 15-*šú* GU$_7$-*šú* ŠU DINGIR AD-*šú* GIG-*ma* DIN
(gap of unknown length)
1′. [DIŠ] IGI^{I} [^{I}…]
2′. [o o] LÚ-x[…]
3′. [DIŠ IG]I 15-*šú pa-*[*ʾa-ṣa-at-ma* …]
4′. [DIŠ IG]I 150-*šú pa-*[*ʾa-ṣa-at-ma* …]
5′. [DIŠ I]GI^{II} -*šú pa-ʾa-*[*ṣa-ma* …]
6′. [DIŠ] IGI 15-*šú pa-ʾa-ṣa-a*[*t-ma* IM.GÚ DIRI …]
7′. DIŠ IGI 150-*šú pa-ʾa-ṣa-at-m*[*a* IM.GÚ DIRI …]
8′. DIŠ IGI^{II} -*šú pa-ʾa-ṣa-ma* IM.G[Ú DIRI …]
9′. DIŠ IGI 15-*šú* IM.GÁ.LI ŠUB-*át* […]
10′. DIŠ IGI 150-*šú* IM.GÁ.LI ŠUB-*át* […]
11′. DIŠ IGI^{II} -*šú* IM.GÁ.LI ŠUB.MEŠ […]
12′. DIŠ IGI 15-*šú tar-kàt* [GÍD-*ma* …]
13′. DIŠ IGI 150-*šú tar-kàt* GÍD-*ma* […]
14′. DIŠ IGI^{II} -*šú tar-ka* GÍD-*ma* […]
15′. DIŠ IGI 15-*šú tar-kàt-ma* NU BAD *qu-t*[*u-*…]
16′. [DIŠ IGI 150-*šú tar*]-*kàt-ma* NU BAD […]
17′. [DIŠ IGI^{II} -*šú tar-ka-ma* N]U BAD […]
18′–36′. (fragmentary)
37′. [DIŠ IGI-*šú šá* 15 *i*]-*la-wi u i-su-šú nu-*⸢*šá-át* DIN⸣
38′. [DIŠ NA IGI-*šú šá* 150 *u i-su-šú* K]I.MIN GIG-*su* DUGUD-*ma* DIN
39′. [DIŠ IGI-*šú šá* GÙB *kap-ṣa-at u i-s*]*a-šú nu-uš-šá* ŠU 30[1]
40′. [DIŠ … IGI ZA]G-*šú kap-ṣa-at pu-us-su*
41′. [… NU]NDUN-*su šá* 15 *na-šal-lu-lu*
42′. […]*šá* 15 IM *ina ṣi-im-ri-šú*
43′. […*na-*]*ša-a* NU ZU-*e*
44′. […]ÚḪ-*su ina* ŠUB-*e*
45′. […]*ana* EGIR SÌG-*iṣ*
46′. […]x-*su šu-ru-ʾ-šú*
47′. […*šá*] 150 *i-šag-gúm*
48′. […]x-*šú šá* 15
49′. […] x x
50′. ⸢DIŠ⸣ [IGI-*š*]*ú* x […]
51′. DIŠ IGI^{II} -*šú* I[M.GÚ DIRI …]

52′. DIŠ IGI^{II}-*šú* IM.G[Ú …]
53′. DIŠ IGI^{II}-*šú* IM.GÚ D[IRI …]
54′. GIG BI DIN
55′. DIŠ IGI^{II}-*šú* MÚD DIRI.MEŠ […]
56′. DIŠ IGI^{II}-*šú* MÚD DIRI.MEŠ […]
57′. DIŠ IGI^{II}-*šú* MÚD DIRI […]
58′. DIŠ IGI^{II}-*šú* MÚD DIRI.ME[Š …]
59′. IM.RI.A […]
60′. DIŠ IGI^{II}-*š*[*ú*…]
61′. DIŠ […]
62′. DIŠ IGI^{I} [^{I}…]
63′. DIŠ IGI^{II}-*š*[*ú*…]
64′. DIŠ IGI^{II}-*šú a-ši-a* GI$_6$ […]
65′. DIŠ IGI^{II}-*šú a-ši-a bir-d*[*u* …]
66′. DIŠ IGI^{II}-*šú* ÍR TUKU.TUK[U …]
67′. DIŠ IGI^{II} [-*šú*] ÍR ŠUB.ŠUB x […]
68′. DIŠ IGI^{II}-*šú* […]
69′. GIG-*s*[*u*…]
70′. DIŠ IGI^{II}-*šú bal-*[*ṣa-a-ma* …]
71′. DIŠ IGI^{II}-*šú bal-*[*ṣa-a-ma* …]
72′. DIŠ IGI^{II}-*šú na-pa*[*l-ka-a*…][2]
73′. DIŠ IGI^{II}-*šú na-pa*[*l-ka-a*…]
74′. DIŠ IGI^{II}-*šú* ŠUB-*ta*$_5$ *ina pi-*[*qam la pi-qam*…]
75′. DIŠ IGI^{II}-*šú* ŠUB-*ma* […]
76′. DIŠ IGI^{II}-*šú* ŠUB-*ma* […]
77′. DIŠ IGI^{II}-*šú* ŠUB-*ma* […]
78′. DIŠ IGI^{II}-*šú* ŠUB-*ma* […]
79′. DIŠ IGI^{II}-*šú* ŠUB-*ma* […]
80′. [*ina*] ⸢IGI⸣ […]
81′. ⸢DIŠ IGI⸣[…]
82′. DIŠ IGI^{II} […]
83′. ta[…]
84′. ZU.AB […]
85′. ⸢DIŠ⸣ [IGI^{II}]-⸢*šú*⸣ *it-te*[*-né-ep-rik-ka-a-ma* …]
86′. DIŠ IGI^{II} -[*šú i*]*t-te-né-*[*ep-rik-ka-a-ma* …]
87′. DIŠ IGI^{II}-*šú i*[*t-te-né-ep-rik-ka-a-ma* …]
88′. DIŠ IGI^{II}-*šú iṣ-ṣa-nun-d*[*a* …]
89′. *u* UB.NIGIN.NA.BI D[U.MEŠ …]
90′. DIŠ IGI^{II}-*šú iṣ-ṣa-nun-da u* […]

91′. DIŠ IGI^{II}-*šú iz-za-naq*!-*qá*!-*p*[*a*! …].
92′. DIŠ IGI^{II}-*šú ú*-⸢*am*⸣-*ma-aṣ* […].
93′. *ina* KA-*šú* DU-[*k*]*u* […]
94′. DIŠ IGI^{II}-*šú be-e-r*[*a* …]
95′. DIŠ IGI^{II}-*šú* DUGUD-*ma* […]
96′. DIŠ IGI^{II}-*šú* UGU […]
97′. DIŠ IGI^{II}-*šú tar*[-*ka*…]
98′. DIŠ IGI^{II}-*šú t*[*ar-ka*…]
99′. […]
100′. […] x SIG$_7$ *qa* x[…]
101′. […] SIG$_7$ *ba-am* x […]
102′. [DIŠ BABBAR IGI^{II}]-*šú* BAL-*ut* […]
103′. [DIŠ BABBAR IG]I^{II}-*šú* BAL-*ut-ma* AN.TA *u* K[I.TA …]
104′. DIŠ BABBAR IGI^{II}-*šú* BAL-*ut-ma* GÌR^{II}-*šú* ŠED[$_7$…]
105′. DIŠ BABBAR IGI^{II}-*šú* BAL-*ut-ma* GÌR^{II}-*šú* ZI x […]
106′. DIŠ GI$_6$ IGI^{II}-*šú* BAL-*ut* […]
107′. DIŠ GI$_6$ IGI^{II}-*šú* BAL-*ut-ma* IGI^{II}-*šú ana* ⸢ŠÀ⸣ […]
108′. DIŠ SA IGI^{II}-*šú* GIN$_7$ ŠU.GUR *kup-pu*-[*pu* …]
109′. *na-kid* […]
110′. DIŠ SA IGI^{II}-*šú* GIN$_7$ *ši-te-e* […]
111′. ŠU DINGIR-*šú lu* ŠU DINGIR UR[U-*šú*]
112′. DIŠ SA IGI^{II}-*šú* DU.ME-*ma šá* SAG.KI.ME-*š*[*ú* …]

113′. DIŠ SA *kak-kul-ti* IGI 15-*šú* GI$_6$.MEŠ […]
114′. DIŠ SA *kak-kul-ti* IGI 150-*šú* GI$_6$.MEŠ […]
115′. DIŠ SA *kak-kul-ti* IGI^{II}-*šú* GI$_6$.MEŠ […]
116′. DIŠ SA *kak-kul-ti* IGI 15-*šú tar-ku* […]
117′. DIŠ SA *kak-kul-ti* IGI 150-*šú tar-ku* […]
118′. DIŠ SA *kak-kul-ti* IGI 15-*šú* x[…]
119′. DIŠ SA *kak-kul-ti* IGI 150-*šú* […]
120′. DIŠ SA *kak-kul-ti* IGI^{II}-*š*[*ú* …]
121′. DIŠ KI.A IGI^{II}-*šú* MÚ.ME[Š …]
122′. MÚ.MEŠ-*ḫu* x[…]
123′. DIŠ PA IGI^{II}-*šú* MIN SU […]
124′. ⸢DIŠ⸣ PA IGI^{II}-*šú šá* 1[5…]
125′. ŠU ^{d}[…]
126′. [o o o I]G[I…]

TRANSLATION

(DPS 4: 143) If the patient's "right" eye hurts him, if he is sick with "hand" of his father's god, he will get well. (catchline)

1′. [If] his eyes […].
2′. [If] … […].
3′. [If] his "right" ⌈eye⌉ was ⌈smashed⌉ [and …].
4′. [If] his "left" ⌈eye⌉ was ⌈smashed⌉ [and …].
5′. [If] (both) his ⌈eyes⌉ were ⌈smashed⌉ [and …].
6′. [If] his "right" eye was ⌈smashed⌉ [and, as a consequence, is full of sediment …].
7′. If his "left" eye was smashed ⌈and⌉, [as a consequence, is full of sediment …].
8′. If (both) his eyes were smashed and, as a consequence, [are full] of ⌈sediment⌉ […].[3]
9′. If his "right" eye is unevenly colored with *kalû*-clay yellow[4] […].
10′. If his "left" eye is unevenly colored with *kalû*-clay yellow […].
11′. If (both) his eyes are unevenly colored with *kalû*-clay yellow […].[5]
12′. If his "right" eye is dark (i.e., has a black patch),[6] [(if) it is prolonged, …].
13′. If his "left" eye is dark, (if) it is prolonged, […].
14′. If (both) his eyes are dark, (if) it is prolonged, […].
15′. If his "right" eye is dark and he cannot open (it) […].[7]
16′. [If his "left" eye] is ⌈dark⌉ and he cannot open (it) […].
17′. [If his eyes are dark and he] ⌈cannot⌉ open (them) […].
18′–36′. *(no symptoms preserved)*
37′. [If his "right" eye] ⌈goes round⌉ and his jaw shakes, he will get well.[8]
38′. [If his "left" eye] ⌈ditto⌉ (goes round and [his jaw] shakes), his illness may be difficult but he will get well.
39′. [If his "left" eye droops and] his ⌈jaws⌉ shake, "hand" of Sîn.[9]
40′–41′. [If his "left" eye …], his ⌈"right"⌉ [eye] droops, his forehead […] (and) his "right" ⌈lip⌈ is slippery […].[10]
42′–50′. *(too broken to translate)*
51′. If his eyes [are full] of ⌈sediment⌉ […].
52′. If his eyes [are full] of ⌈sediment⌉ […].
53′–54′. If his eyes are ⌈full⌉ of sediment […] that patient will get well.
55′. If his eyes are full of blood […].[11]
56′. If his eyes are full of blood […].
57′. If his eyes are full of blood […].
58′–59′. If his eyes are full of blood […] slime […].

60′. If his eyes [...].
61′. If [his eyes ...].
62′. If [his] eyes [...].
63′. If his eyes [...].
64′. If his eyes are "confused" (and) the pupil [...].
65′. If his eyes are "confused" (and) ⸢*birdu*⸣ [...].[12]
66′. If his eyes continually have tears [...].
67′. If [his] eyes continually shed tears [...].
68′–69′. If his eyes [...] ⸢his⸣ illness [...].
70′. If his eyes are ⸢dilated⸣ [...].
71′. If his eyes are ⸢dilated⸣ [...].
72′. If his eyes are ⸢opened wide⸣ [...].
73′. If his eyes are ⸢opened wide⸣ [...].
74′. If (he lets) his eyes fall (and) he [...] ⸢incessantly⸣ [...].
75′. If (he lets) his eyes fall and [...].
76′. If (he lets) his eyes fall and [...].
77′. If (he lets) his eyes fall and [...].
78′. If (he lets) his eyes fall and [...].
79′–80′. If (he lets) his eyes fall and [... in] the eye [...].
81′. If [his] eye [...].
82′–84′. If [his] eyes [...] ... [...].
85′. If his [eyes] are continually [crossed ...].
86′. If [his] eyes are continually [crossed ...].
87′. If his eyes are [continually crossed ...].
88′–89′. If his eyes (seem to) spin [...] and his limbs continually ⸢move⸣ [...].
90′. If his eyes (seem to) spin and [...].
91′. If (the pupils of) his eyes are continually ⸢constricted⸣ [...].[13]
92′–93′. If he stares fixedly(?)[14] and [...] flows from his mouth [...].
94′. If his eyes leave a space between (the lids)[15] [...].[16]
95′. If his eyes (feel) heavy and [...].
96′. If his eyes ... [...].
97′. If his eyes are ⸢dark⸣ [...].
98′. If his eyes are ⸢dark⸣ [...].
99′. [...]
100′. [...] yellow/green [...].
101′. [...] yellow/green [...].
102′. [If] he rolls the [whites] of his [eyes] [...].
103′. [If] he rolls the [whites] of his ⸢eyes⸣ and above and ⸢below⸣ [...].
104′. If he rolls the whites of his eyes and his feet are ⸢cold⸣ [...].

105′. If he rolls the whites of his eyes and he raises his feet […].
106′. If he rolls his pupils […].
107′. If he rolls his pupils so that his eyes [look] inward […].[17]
108′–109′. If the blood vessel(s) of his eyes are ⸢curved⸣ like a ring,[18] […] it is worrisome […].[19]
110′–111′. If the blood vessels of his eye are […] like a web, "hand" of his god or "hand" of the god of [his] ⸢city⸣.[20]
112′. If the blood vessel(s) of his eyes "go" and those of ⸢his⸣ temples […].

113′. If the muscle(s) of his "right" iris are black […].[21]
114′. If the muscle(s) of his "left" iris are black […].[22]
115′. If the muscle(s) of (both) his irises are black […].
116′. If the muscle(s) of his "right" iris are dark […].[23]
117′. If the muscle(s) of his "left" iris are dark […].[24]
118′. If the muscle(s) of his "right" iris are […].
119′. If the muscle(s) of his "left" iris are […].
120′ If the muscle(s) of (both) ⸢his⸣ irises are […].
121′–122′. If the rims of his eyes are swollen (and) […] are swollen/bloated […].
123′. If the rims of his eyes ditto (are swollen) (and) [his] body […].
124′–125′. If the rim of his ⸢"right"⸣ eye […], "hand" of […].
126′. […]

Notes

1. Restored from *STT* 89:208.
2. Restorations are based on the commentary SpTU 1.31 obv. 12.
3. See Scurlock and Andersen 2005, 9.85, 14.5.
4. Stol 1998, 347–48 suggests that *kalû*-clay is yellow ochre.
5. See Scurlock and Andersen 2005, 9.41.
6. The commentary SpTU 1.31 obv. 4 indicates that the reference is to a black patch.
7. See Scurlock and Andersen 2005, 9.25, 10.37.
8. See the commentary SpTU 1.31 obv. 10.
9. This entry also appears in *STT* 89:208.
10. See Scurlock and Andersen 2005, 13.235.
11. One of these entries also appears in Wilhelm 1994, 23 rev. 5′a.
12. See Scurlock and Andersen 2005, 3.279, 10.76.
13. See Scurlock and Andersen 2005, 3.216.
14. Literally, "he strips his eyes naked."
15. The commentary SpTU 1.31 rev. 30–31 confirms that this expression means that the eyes are (partially) open.
16. See Scurlock and Andersen 2005, 9.51.
17. See Scurlock and Andersen 2005, 13.93.

18. See *CAD* K, 175b; Labat 1956, 125.
19. The entry appears also in Labat 1956, 125 rev. 7.
20. See Scurlock and Andersen 2005, 9.73.
21. See Scurlock and Andersen 2005, 9.71.
22. See Scurlock and Andersen 2005, 9.71.
23. See Scurlock and Andersen 2005, 9.72.
24. See Scurlock and Andersen 2005, 9.72.

DPS TABLET 6

1. [DIŠ GIG KIR$_4$-*šú* SA$_5$ DI]N : DIŠ KIR$_4$-*šú* GI$_6$ ⸢GAM⸣[1]
2. [DIŠ KIR$_4$-*šú* ... G]AM? : DIŠ KIR$_4$-*šú* *du-ʾ-um* GAM
3. [DIŠ KIR$_4$-*šú* KÚM DI]N : DIŠ KIR$_4$-*šú* ŠED$_7$ GAM
4. [DIŠ KIR$_4$-*šú* ... G]AM? : DIŠ KIR$_4$-*šú* BAD.BAD-*ir* GAM
5. [DIŠ KIR$_4$-*šú* ...] : DIŠ KIR$_4$-*šú* *ur-ru-ub* GAM
6. [DIŠ KIR$_4$-*šú* *šá* 1]5 *it-te-né-ek-dar* GAM
7. [DIŠ KIR$_4$-*šú* *šá* 1]50 *it-te-né-ek-dar* GAM
8. [DIŠ KIR$_4$-*šú* UD.A(?) SA$_5$(?).M]EŠ DIRI DIN[2]
9. [DIŠ KIR$_4$-*šú* UD.A(?) BABBAR(?).M]EŠ DIRI DIN
10. [DIŠ KIR$_4$-*šú* UD.A(?) GI$_6$(?).M]EŠ DIRI GAM
11. [DIŠ KIR$_4$-*šú* ...] *ú-ád-da na-kud* NU TE-*šú*
12. [DIŠ KIR$_4$-*šú* ... .ME]Š-*šú* *bu-ʾ-ra* GAM
13. [DIŠ KIR$_4$-*šú* ...] *ú-ṣa-an-dar* GA[M]
14. [DIŠ KIR$_4$-*šú* ... N]A BI *ana* UD.25.KÁM GAM : A ŠÙD ^{d}20 (coll.) UGU-*šú* GÁL-*ú*
15. [...] *u ú-rap-pad* GAM
16. DIŠ *in*[*a* KIR$_4$-*šú* U$_4$ *u* GI$_6$ MÚD *la i*]*k-kal-lu-ú* ŠU ^{d}*Uraš* MU DAM LÚ GÍD-*ma* GAM
17. DIŠ *in*[*a* KIR$_4$-*šú* MÚD DU-*ku* oooo] *pa-ru-ud* SIG$_7$ *im-ta-lu-ú* GAM
18. DIŠ *ina* ⸢KIR$_4$-*šú* MÚD DU⸣-*k*[*u* ZI-*šú* *pa*]-*áš-qa-a*[*t*] GEŠTU^{II}-*šú* BABBAR-*at u* GÌR^{II}-*šú* *nu-up-pu-ḫa* GAM
19. DIŠ *ina* KIR$_4$-*šú* IGI^{II}-*šú* *u* GEŠTU[^{II}-*šú* MÚD] 1-*niš* DU-*ku* ŠU ^{d}ME.ME SÌG-*su* KI-*šú* *uš-ta-ad* GAM
20. DIŠ *ina* KIR$_4$-*šú* A DU-*ku-ma* KÚM-*mu u* SAG KIR$_4$-*šú* *na-ši* GAM
21. DIŠ *ina* KIR$_4$-*šú* A SA$_5$.MEŠ DU-*ku* GAM
22. DIŠ SAG KIR$_4$-*šú* *na-ru-ub* KÚM-*im u* ŠED$_7$ ŠU DINGIR-*šú* DIN
23. DIŠ SAG KIR$_4$-*šú* KÚM-*im u* ŠED$_7$ ^{GIŠ}GIDRU *šá* DINGIR-*šú*
24. DIŠ SAG KIR$_4$-*šú* *ku-uṣ ba-lil ina* U$_4$-*mi-šú-ma* EGIR MAŠ.MAŠ LÍL-*ma* DIN
25. DIŠ SAG KIR$_4$-*šú* : ŠÀ-*šú* SIG$_7$ GAM : DIŠ SAG KIR$_4$-*šú* *ma-qit* GAM

26. DIŠ *ina* SAG KIR$_4$-*šú* ḪÁD.A SA$_5$.MEŠ *it-tab-šu-ú* LÚG NU TUKU
27. DIŠ *ina* SAG KIR$_4$-*šú* ḪÁD.A BABBAR.MEŠ *it-tab-šu-ú* DIN
28. DIŠ *ina* SAG KIR$_4$-*šú* ḪÁD.A SA$_5$ *u* BABBAR *it-tab-šu-ú* LÚG NU TUKU
29. DIŠ *ina* SAG KIR$_4$-*šú* ḪÁD.A GI$_6$.MEŠ *it-tab-šu-ú ana* U$_4$.3.KÁM GAM
30. DIŠ *ina* SAG KIR$_4$-*šú* ḪÁD.A GI$_6$.MEŠ *it-tab-šu-ú u* IGI^{II}-*šú* MÚD DIRI.MEŠ GAM
31. DIŠ *ina* SAG KIR$_4$-*šú* SÌG-*iṣ* ŠU DINGIR-*šú* : DIŠ *ina* SUḪUŠ KIR$_4$-*šú* SÌG-*iṣ ana* U$_4$.15 ŠU ^{d}*Papsukkal*
32. DIŠ IM KIR$_4$-*šú ina* KA-*šú* È-*a ana* U$_4$.3.KAM GAM
33. DIŠ IM KIR$_4$-*šú šam-ru* GIG-*su* ‹*nu*›-*uk-ku-up* GAM
34. DIŠ IM KIR$_4$-*šú* ZI.MEŠ GIG-*su i-na-šu um-mu* GAM
35. DIŠ IM KIR$_4$-*šú us-sur-ma* KÚM-*em ù* KÚM NA DIB-*ta*$_5$ GAM
36. DIŠ IM ⸢KIR$_4$⸣-*šú ep-qá-ma* GÍD ⸢IM⸣ [K]IR$_4$-*šú* KÚM-⸢*em*⸣ [...] *ina* IGI GI$_6$ T[AG? GAM]

37′–59′. (fragmentary)

60′. DIŠ *na-ḫir-šú šá* GÙB *ú-zaq-qat-s*[*u* ...]
61′. DIŠ *na-ḫi-ra-šú sa-an-qa* [...]
62′. DIŠ *na-ḫi-ra-šú šat-qa* [...]
63′. DIŠ *na-ḫi-ra-šú áš-ṭa* : D[IB ...]
64′. DIŠ *na-ḫi-ra-šú it-ta-n*[*a-* ...]
65′. DIŠ *na-ḫi-ra-šú* DIB.DIB-*ta*$_5$ [...]
66′. DIŠ *na-ḫi-ra-*⸢*šú*⸣ [... : ...]
67′. DIŠ *na-*[*ḫi-ra-šú* ...]

68″–69″ *(lost)*

70″–81″ all begin with DIŠ NUNDUN but are too fragmentary to translate.

82″. DIŠ NUNDUN-[*šú* ... *li*]*q* KA-*šu* KÚM ŠU ⸢^{d}⸣[DN GIG]-*su* NU B[ÚR]
83″. DIŠ NUNDUN-[*šú* ... *l*]*iq* KA-*šú šá-bu-ul* [U$_4$].⸢3⸣7.KÁM ŠU [...]
84″. DIŠ NUNDUN-[*šú* ...] DIN : DIŠ NUNDUN.MEŠ-*šú u liq* KA-*šú* K[ÚM...]
85″. DIŠ NUNDUN-[*šú* ...] GAM : DIŠ NUNDUN.MEŠ-*šú* IM SIG$_7$.SIG$_7$ Š[UB ...]

86″–88″ all begin with DIŠ NUNDUN but are too fragmentary to translate.

89″. DIŠ NUNDUN-[*šú* ...]-*aṣ* : *ú-ḫa-an-na-*[*aṣ* ...]

90″–96″ all begin with DIŠ NUNDUN but are too fragmentary to translate.

97″. DIŠ ZÚ-*šú* GU$_7$-*š*[*ú*] *u* ÚḪ-*su* ŠUB-*di* [...]
98″. DIŠ ZÚ.MEŠ-*šú nam-*[*r*]*a* DIN : DIŠ ZÚ.MEŠ-*šú* [...]
99″. DIŠ ZÚ.MEŠ-*šú i-ri-*[*r*]*a* GIG-*su* GÍD : DIŠ ZÚ.MEŠ-*šú* [...]
100″. DIŠ ZÚ.MEŠ-*šú tar-k*[*a*] GIG-*su* GÍD : DIŠ ZÚ.MEŠ-*šú* [...]

101″. DIŠ ZÚ.MEŠ-*šú* *pu-uḫ-*[*ḫu*]*-ra* GAM : DIŠ ZÚ.MEŠ-*šú* [...] ⸢É⸣ BI BIR-*aḫ*

102″. DIŠ ZÚ.MEŠ-*šú* ZÚ.GUZ GIG-*su* GÍD : DIŠ ZÚ.MEŠ-*šú* Z[Ú.GUZ N]Í-*šú* (coll.) *ma-ši* K⸢I.MIN⸣

103″. DIŠ ZÚ.MEŠ-*šú* ZÚ.GUZ *šu-ú-ra-šú* DU$_8$.MEŠ IGI.MEŠ-*šú* *šu-*[*ú-r*]*a-šú* *tar-ra* GAM

104″. DIŠ ZÚ.MEŠ-*šú* ZÚ.GUZ ŠU^{II}-*šú* *u* GÌR^{II}-*šú* GI$_6$ D[IB] ⸢GIDIM⸣$_7$ GAM

105″. DIŠ ZÚ.MEŠ-*šú* ZÚ.GUZ ŠU^{II}-*šú* *u* GÌR^{II}-*šú* *ú-n*[*a-aš* ŠU] ^{d}30 GAM

106″. DIŠ ZÚ.[ME]Š-*šú* ZÚ.GUZ SAG.DU-*su* ŠUB.ŠU[B-*di*] ŠU ^{d}15

107″. DIŠ ZÚ.⸢MEŠ⸣-*šú* ZÚ.GUZ ŠU-*su* ŠUB.Š[UB-*d*]*i* ŠU ^{d}15

108″. DIŠ ZÚ.[MEŠ]-*šú* ZÚ.GUZ *u* G[ÌR]-*su* ŠUB.ŠUB-*di* GA[M KI.MIN] ŠU ^{d}15 MU TAG-*te*

109″. DIŠ ⸢ZÚ⸣.[MEŠ-*šú*] *ig-ta-na-*[*aṣ*]*-ṣa-aṣ* IGI.[MEŠ-*šú*] ŠED$_7$.MEŠ GIG. [BI DIB.D]IB-*su* ŠU ^{d}15 BI GAR-*šú*

Translation

1. [If the patient's nose is red,] he will get well. If his nose is dark, he will die.[3]
2. [If the patient's nose is ...], ⸢he will die?⸣. If his nose is dark (red), he will die.
3. [If his nose is hot], ⸢he will get well⸣. If his nose is cold, he will die.[4]
4. [If his nose was ...], ⸢he will die?⸣. If his nose is completely blocked off, he will die.[5]
5. [If his nose was ...]. If his nose was knocked in all over, he will die.[6]
6. [If his] ⸢"right"⸣ [nostril] is continually closed in (lit. "bounded"), he will die.
7. [If his] ⸢"left"⸣ [nostril] is continually closed in (lit. "bounded"), he will die.
8. [If a person's nose] is full of [red *ramīṭu*-lesions], he will get well. [7]
9. [If a person's nose] is full of [white *ramīṭu*-lesions], he will get well.
10. [If a person's nose] is full of [black *ramīṭu*-lesions], he will die.

11–15. *(fragmentary)*

16. If [day and night blood does not] ⸢stop⸣ (flowing) ⸢from⸣ [his nose], "hand" of Uraš on account of a man's wife. If it is prolonged, he will die.[8]
17. If [blood flows] ⸢from⸣ [his nose], he shudders [incessantly?] (and) he has become full of yellow (spots), he will die.
18. If blood flows from his nose, [his breathing?] ⸢is labored⸣, his ears are white and his feet are swollen, he will die.

19. If [blood] flows from his nose, his eyes and [his] ears all at the same time, "hand" of Gula has struck him and concerns itself(?) with him; he will die.[9]
20. If fluid flows from his nose and it is hot and the bulb of his nose is puffed up, he will die.
21. If red fluid flows from his nose, he will die.
22. If the bulb of his nose is soft (and) he gets hot and cold, "hand" of his god; he will get well.[10]
23. If the bulb of his nose gets hot and then cold, scepter of his god.
24. If the bulb of his nose is cold mixed (with warm) (i.e., "lukecold"), on the same day, after treatment, he may get worse, (but) he will get well (in the end).[11]
25. If the bulb of his nose (var. his abdomen) is yellow, he will die. If the bulb of his nose (looks) bruised,[12] he will die.[13]
26. If red *ramīṭu*-lesions have appeared on the bulb of a person's nose, it is of no consequence.
27. If white *ramīṭu*-lesions have appeared on the bulb of a person's nose, he will get well.
28. If red or white *ramīṭu*-lesions have appeared on the bulb of a person's nose, it is of no consequence.[14]
29. If black *ramīṭu*-lesions have appeared on the bulb of a person's nose, (if he has been sick) for three days,[15] he will die.[16]
30. If black *ramīṭu*-lesions have appeared on the bulb of a man's nose and his eyes are continually full of blood, he will die.[17]
31. If he was injured on the bulb of his nose, "hand" of his god.[18] If he was injured on the base of his nose, (and he has been sick) for fifteen days, "hand" of Papsukkal.[19]
32. If the breath of his nose comes out of his mouth, (and he has been sick) for three days, he will die.[20]
33. If the breath of his nose is violent, his illness is goring (him); he will die.
34. If the breath of his nose continually rises up (and) his illness carries fever, he will die.
35. If the breath of his nose is stifled and hot and fever afflicts the person, he will die.
36. If the breath of his nose is massive and long, the breath of his ⸢nose⸣ is hot [...] (and) it ⸢"touches"⸣ (him) at the beginning of the night, [he will die].

37–59′. *(fragmentary)*

60′. If his "left" nostril stings, [...].[21]

61′. If his nostrils are fastened together, [...].

62′. If his nostrils are cleft, […].
63′. If his nostrils are stiff (var. "⌈stopped⌉ up"), […].
64′. If his nostrils are continually […].
65′. If his nostrils are continually stopped up […].[22]
66′. If his nostrils […].
67′. If his nostrils […].
68′–69′. *(broken away)*
70″–81″. (*all begin with* "If [his] lips," *but are too fragmentary to translate)*
82″. If his lip(s) […] (and) his ⌈palate⌉ is hot, "hand" of […], his [illness] will not ⌈relent⌉.
83″. If his lip(s) […] (and) his ⌈palate⌉ is dry, (and he has been sick for) thirty seven days, "hand" of […].
84″. If his lip(s) […], he will get well. If his lips and palate are ⌈hot⌉ […]
85″. If his lip(s) […], he will die. If his lips are ⌈unevenly colored⌉ with dark red colored spots […].[23]
86″–88″ *all begin with* "If [his] lips," *but are too fragmentary to translate.*
89″. [If] he [… his] lip[s] (var. he ⌈rubs⌉ (them against each other) […].[24]
90″–96″ *all begin with* "If [his] lips," *but are too fragmentary to translate.*
97″. If his tooth hurts ⌈him⌉ and he lets his spittle fall […].[25]
98″. If his teeth ⌈shine⌉, he will get well; if his teeth […].[26]
99″. If his teeth ⌈tremble⌉, his illness will be prolonged; if his teeth […].
100″. If his teeth are dark, his illness will be prolonged; if his teeth […].[27]
101″. If his teeth are ⌈"gathered together"⌉, he will die; if his teeth [are "scattered"], that household will be scattered.
102″. If he gnashes his teeth, his illness will be prolonged. If he ⌈gnashes his teeth⌉ (and) loses ⌈consciousness⌉, ditto (his illness will be prolonged).
103″. If he gnashes his teeth, his eyelids are continually open (and) his face (and) his ⌈eyelids⌉ tremble, he will die.
104″. If he gnashes his teeth (and) his hands and feet are dark, ⌈affliction⌉ by a ghost; he will die.[28]
105″. If he gnashes his teeth (and) his hands and feet ⌈shake⌉, ["hand"] of Sîn; he will die.[29]
106″. If he gnashes his teeth (and) ⌈continually⌉ lets his head drop, "hand" of Ishtar.[30]
107″. If he gnashes his teeth (and) ⌈continually⌉ lets his hand drop, "hand" of Ishtar.[31]
108″. If he gnashes his teeth and continually lets his ⌈foot⌉ drop, ⌈he will die⌉; [alternatively], "hand" of Ishtar on account of touching the cheek.[32]

109″. If he continually ⸢gnashes⸣ [his] teeth, his face is continually cold (and) [that] illness [continually] afflicts him, that "hand" of Ishtar has been laid on him.[33]

NOTES

1. The restoration is based on citation by the commentary SpTU 1.31:39.
2. Restorations of this and the following lines follows Labat 1951 and is based on lines 26–30.
3. See Scurlock and Andersen 2005, 20.36.
4. See Scurlock and Andersen 2005, 20.18.
5. See Scurlock and Andersen 2005, 20.32.
6. See Scurlock and Andersen 2005, 14.7.
7. Restorations of this and the following lines follows Labat 1951 and is based on lines 26–30.
8. The entry appears also in Wilhelm 1994, 34 obv. 6′.
9. See Scurlock and Andersen 2005, 3.239.
10. See Scurlock and Andersen 2005, 19.215.
11. See Scurlock and Andersen 2005, 3.37.
12. See Scurlock and Andersen 2005, p. 216.
13. See Scurlock and Andersen 2005, 20.44.
14. See Scurlock and Andersen 2005, 10.165.
15. Alternatively: "he will die within three days."
16. See Scurlock and Andersen 2005, 10.169.
17. See Scurlock and Andersen 2005, 10.170.
18. See Scurlock and Andersen 2005, 19.214.
19. See Scurlock and Andersen 2005, 19.205.
20. Alternatively: "he will die within three days."
21. This entry appears in VAT 11122 obv. 2 (Heeßel 2010, 181–84).
22. See Scurlock and Andersen 2005, 9.120.
23. See Scurlock and Andersen 2005, 10.51.
24. This entry appears also in Wilhelm 1994, 67 obv. 9.
25. See Scurlock and Andersen 2005, 18.3.
26. See Scurlock and Andersen 2005, 18.21.
27. See Scurlock and Andersen 2005, 18.20.
28. See Scurlock and Andersen 2005, 19.130, 20.69.
29. See Scurlock and Andersen 2005, 18.27. This entry also appears in Wilhelm 1994, 40 obv. 7′.
30. See Scurlock and Andersen 2005, 19.283.
31. See Scurlock and Andersen 2005, 19.284.
32. See Scurlock and Andersen 2005, 19.285.
33. See Scurlock and Andersen 2005, 19.286.

DPS TABLET 7

DPS 6:110″ (catchline) = DPS 7:1

A obv.

1. DIŠ GIG [EME]-*šú* SA$_5$-*át* DIN[1]
2. DIŠ EME[…]
3. DIŠ EME-*š*[*ú*…]
4. DIŠ EME-*šú* x[…]
5. DIŠ EME-*šú šur*-(?)[…]
6. DIŠ EME-*šú pi*-[…]
7. DIŠ EME-*šú ir-te-d*[*i*…]
8. DIŠ EME-*šú ú-na-at-ta*[…]
9. DIŠ EME-*šú ú-na-at-ta* KI.MIN x[…]
10. DIŠ EME-*šú* ḪÁD.A GI$_6$.MEŠ [D]IRI x[…]
11. DIŠ EME-*šú u* KA-*šú* IM DIRI […]
12. DIŠ E[M]E-*šú i-ta-nab-bal* […]
13. DIŠ EME-*šú u liq* KA-*šú* […]
14. DIŠ EME-*šú ina* ŠU^{II}-*šú ú-mar*-[*raṭ* …]
15. DIŠ EME-*šú ú-qar-ra-aš* ⸢NÍG.GIG⸣ (coll.) [IGI-*ma* DIN]
16. DIŠ EME-*šú ú-na-aš-šak* […]
17. DIŠ EME-*šú ina* ZÚ.MEŠ-*šú na-šik* UGU ⸢SÌG⸣-[*iṣ* …]
18. DIŠ EME-*šú ik-ka-ṣir* […]
19. DIŠ EME-*šú ik-ka-ṣir-ma* KA *la ip-te* (coll.) […]
20. NIN.DINGIR DINGIR-*šú iš-šiq* AZAG [DINGIR-*šú* GU$_7$]
21. DIŠ EME-*šú i-tál-lal* GIG-*su* TAK$_4$-*šum-ma* […]
22. DIŠ EME-*šú i-tál-lal u* UŠ$_4$-*šú* NU DIB […]
23. DIŠ EME-*šú* GI$_6$-*at ina* KA-*šú* S[ÌG-*iṣ* …]
24. DIŠ EME-*šú la ú-tar-ra ina* U[GU? …]
25. DIŠ EME-*šú* GU$_7$-*šú u* ÚḪ-⸢*su*⸣ [ŠUB …]
26. DIŠ *ina* (coll.) EME-*šú* SÌG-*iṣ* ŠU ^{d}IM […]

---

27. DIŠ KA-*šú* SA$_5$ DIN : DIŠ KA-[*šú* …]
28. DIŠ KA-*šú* GI$_6$ GAM : DIŠ KA-*šú* […]
29. DIŠ KA-*šú* KÚM DIN : DIŠ KA-*šú* [ŠED$_7$ GAM]
30. [DIŠ KA-*šú i-ṭ*]*a*?-*ab* DIN : DIŠ KA-*šú* […]
31. [DIŠ KA-*šú* o-]-*i-iḫ* GAM : DIŠ KA-*šú* […]
32. [DIŠ KA-*šú* o o o] KÚM ri x[…]

B obv.

1′ […]

2′ DIŠ KA-*šú* DIB.DIB-*ma mim-ma la i-lim* ŠU DINGIR ⸢URU-*šú*⸣ […]

3′ DIŠ [K]A-*šú* DIB.DIB-*ma an-na ma*!-*gal la ip-pal-lum ana* DINGIR x[…]

4′ DIŠ KA-*šú* U_4.BU.BU.UL DIRI *u il-la-tu-šú* [DU-*ka* …]

5′ DIŠ [K]A-*šú* GU_7-*šú u* ÚḪ-*su* ŠUB-*di* x […]

6′ DIŠ *i*[*na* K]A-*šú at-mu-ú it-te-né-et-bu-ú*[2] SAG.DU-*su* ŠU^{II}[-*šú u* GÌR^{II}-*šu* 1-*niš i-tar-ru-ra*]

7′ [N]A.BI *ana maš-tak-ti ru-*ʾ*-a-t*[*i šu-kul*][3]

8′ DIŠ *ina* KA-*šú i-ḫaš-šal u* MÚD.GI_6 ŠUB.ŠUB-*a* […]

9′ DIŠ *ina* KA-*šú* Ì.GIŠ ŠÀ-*šú i*-[*ú-a* …]

10′ DIŠ *ina* KA-*šú* ZÉ GI_6 *i*-⸢*ú*⸣-[*a* …]

11′ DIŠ *ina* KA-*šú* ZÉ SA_5 *i-ú*-[*a* …]

12′ DIŠ *ina* KA-*šú* ZÉ SIG_7 *i-ú*-[*a* …]

13′ DIŠ *ina* KA-*šú* ZÉ BABBAR *i-ú-a ana* U_4.⸢3⸣.[KÁM …](coll.)

14′ DIŠ *liq* KA-*šú* KÚM-*em u* SAG ŠÀ-*šú za-qir* […]

15′ DIŠ *liq* KA-*šú šá-bu-ul la-ga-a* ŠUB.ŠUB ^{GIŠ}GIDRU ⸢*šá* ^{d}x⸣[…]

16′ DIŠ *liq* KA-*šú i-ta-nab-bal* ŠÀ.MEŠ-*šú* MÚ.ME[Š …]

17′ DIŠ MIN ŠÀ.MEŠ-[*šú*] ⸢MÚ.M⸣Ú-*ḫu u it-te-nen-bi-ṭu u* ⸢*it-te-nen*⸣-[*mi-ru* …]

B rev.

1. DIŠ [MIN ŠÀ.MEŠ-*šú* M]Ú.MEŠ-*ḫu u ma-gal it-ta-na-a-a-al* […]
2. DIŠ *liq* [KA-*šú* o o]-*ta-na-an* ÚŠ *ir-ru-ub-šum-ma ana* UD.3.[KÁM …]
3. DIŠ GIG [INIM-*šú*] KÚR.KÚR-*ir ana* U_4.3.[KÁM …]
4. INIM-*šú* […] *u ra-pa-du su-ud-dur-šú*[4] *ana* U_4.3.K[ÁM …]
5. DIŠ GIG ⸢INIM⸣-[*šú*] ⸢KÚR⸣.KÚ[R-*ir u*] SIG_7.MEŠ *i-ár-ru u* UZU.ME-*šú* SIG_7.MEŠ *ana* U_4.3.K[ÁM …]
6. DIŠ INIM-*šú* KÚR.KÚR-*ir* [*u*] KÚM DIB.DIB-*su u ú-rap-pad ana* U_4.3.K[ÁM …]
7. DIŠ INIM-*šú* KÚR.KÚR-*i*[*r*] *u* ⸢*ḫa-a-šú*⸣ *i-ḫa*-⸢*a*⸣-*šú ana* U_4.3.K[ÁM …]
8. DIŠ INIM-*šú* KÚR.KÚR-[*ir*] *u a-šu-uš-tum* ŠUB.ŠUB-*su ana* U_4.DUG_4.GA-⸢*šú ana*⸣ U_4.3.K[ÁM …]
9. DIŠ INIM-*šú* KÚR.KÚR-[*i*]*r u* ÍR.MEŠ [*ana*] U_4.DUG_4.GA-*šú ana* U_4.3.[KÁM …]
10. DIŠ INIM-*šú* KÚR.[KÚR-*i*]*r* MÚD *ina* KA-*šú* ŠUB.ŠUB-*a u* ŠÀ.MEŠ-*šú* ÍL-*ú ana* U_4.10.[KÁM …]
11. DIŠ INIM-*šú* KÚR.[KÚR-*i*]*r* IM *ina* DÚR-*šú* È.MEŠ-*a u ú-ga-aš-ši ana* U_4.10.[KÁM …]

12. DIŠ INIM-*šú* KÚR[.KÚR-*i*]*r u* KÚM ŠUB.ŠUB-*su* ŠU ^{d}MAŠ *ana* U$_4$.10.[KÁM ...]
13. DIŠ INIM-*šú* KÚR[.KÚR-*i*]*r u* KAŠ APIN.MEŠ-*iš ana* U$_4$.10.[KÁM ...]
14. DIŠ INIM-*šú* K[ÚR.KÚR-*i*]*r u* ^{GIŠ}GEŠTIN APIN.MEŠ-*iš ana* U$_4$.DUG$_4$.GA-[*šú ana* U$_4$.10.KÁM ...]
15. DIŠ INIM-*šú* [KÚR.KÚR-*i*]*r u* ⸢*i-ram*⸣-*mu-um* (coll.) *ana* [U$_4$.10.KÁM ...]
16. DIŠ INIM-*šú* [KÚR.KÚR-*ir u*] x x *u*ʾ-*i* ŠÀ *u*ʾ-*i* ŠÀ-*bi* GÙ.GÙ-*si* x [...]
17. ⸢DIŠ INIM⸣-[*šú* KÚR.KÚR-*ir u* ...] *lu* ŠU ^{d}MAŠ x [...]

A rev.

1′. [DIŠ IN]⸢IM-*šú*⸣ [KÚR.KÚR-*ir* ...]
2′. [DIŠ] INIM-*šú* KÚR.KÚR-*ir u* GUR x[...]
3′. DIŠ INIM-*šú* KÚR.KÚR-*ir u kab-tá-š*[*ú* (coll.) ...]
4′. DIŠ INIM-*šú* KÚR.KÚR-*ir u ú-nam-b*[*a-aḫ* ...]
5′. DIŠ INIM-*šú* [KÚR.KÚR-*ir*] x x[...]
6′. DIŠ IN]IM-*šú* KÚR.KÚR-*ir* ...]
7′. ⸢DIŠ INIM-*šú*⸣ [KÚR.KÚR]-⸢*ir*⸣[...]
8′. DIŠ INIM-*šú* KÚR.KÚR-*ir* x [...]
9′. DIŠ INIM-*šú* KÚR.KÚR-*ir* x [...]
10′. DIŠ INIM-*šú* KÚR.KÚR-*ir u* x[...]
11′. DIŠ GIG *ri-gim-šu* [...]

12′. DIŠ *ri-gim* GIG *taš-me-ma* G[IN$_7$ ...]
13′. DIŠ *ri-gim* GIG *taš-me*-⸢*ma*⸣ [...]
14′. DIŠ *ri-gim* GIG *taš*-⸢*me*⸣-[*ma*...]
15′. DIŠ *ri-gim* GIG *t*[*aš-me-ma* ...]
16′. DIŠ *ri-gim* GIG[...]
17′. DIŠ *ri-gim* GIG[...]

Translation

A obv.

1. If the patient's [tongue] is ⸢red⸣, he will get well.[5]
2. If [his] tongue [....]
3. If ⸢his⸣ tongue [...].
4. If his tongue [...].
5. If his tongue [...].

6. If his tongue […].
7. If he sticks out(?) his tongue […].[6]
8. If he licks(?) with his tongue […].
9. If he licks(?) with his tongue; alternatively, […].
10. If his tongue is ⸢full⸣ of black *ramīṭu*-lesions […].[7]
11. If his tongue and his mouth are full of "clay" […].
12. If his ⸢tongue⸣ keeps drying out […].[8]
13. If his tongue and palate [keep drying out? …].[9]
14. If he ⸢rubs⸣ his tongue with his hands […].
15. If he kneads his tongue, [(even if) he has] a hard time of it, [he will get well(?)].
16. If he habitually bites his tongue […].[10]
17. If his tongue was bitten with his teeth, the top of the head was struck […].[11]
18. If his tongue is tied in knots[12] […].
19–20. If his tongue is tied in knots and he cannot open (his) mouth […], he has kissed the *ēntu*-priestess of his god,[13] [he has done] something offensive [to his god].[14]
21. If his tongue hangs out, his illness is leaving him and […].[15]
22. If his tongue hangs out and he is not in full possession of his faculties[16] […].[17]
23. If his tongue is black, he was ⸢injured⸣ on his mouth […].[18]
24. If he cannot return his tongue to [his mouth …].[19]
25. If his tongue hurts him and [he lets] his spittle [fall …].[20]
26. If he was injured on his tongue, "hand" of Adad […].[21]

---

27. If his mouth is red, he will get well.[22] If [his] mouth is […].
28. If his mouth is black, he will die. If his mouth is […].[23]
29. If his mouth is hot, he will get well; if his mouth is [cold, he will die].[24]
30–32. *(fragmentary)*

B obv.

2′. If his mouth is continually "seized" so that he cannot eat anything, "hand" of the god of his city […].[25]
3′. If his ⸢mouth⸣ is continually "seized" so that he cannot frequently answer: *annu* (yes), [he has …] to a god.[26]
4′. If a person's mouth is full of *bubuʾtu* and his saliva [flows …].[27]
5′. If his ⸢mouth⸣ hurts him and he lets his spittle fall […].[28]

6′–7′. If the words tumble over one another ⸢in his mouth⸣ (and) his head, [his] hands [and his feet all tremble at once], that ⸢person⸣ [has been fed] sorcerous spittle to test it.[29]

8′. If it crushes (him) in his mouth and he continually produces black blood [...].[30]

9′. If he ⸢vomits⸣ his stomach fat from his mouth [...].

10′. If he ⸢vomits⸣ black bile from his mouth [...].

11′. If he ⸢vomits⸣ red bile from his mouth [...].

12′. If he ⸢vomits⸣ yellow bile from his mouth [...].

13′. If he vomits white bile from his mouth, (and he has been sick) for three(?) days [...].[31]

14′. If his palate is hot and his epigastrium protrudes [...].

15′. If his palate is dried up (and) dotted with "slag," scepter of [...].[32]

16′. If his palate continually dries out (and) his insides are continually bloated [...].[33]

17′. If ditto (his palate continually dries out), [his] insides are continually bloated and cramped and ⸢colicky⸣ [...].

B rev.

1. If [ditto (his palate continually dries out), his insides] are continually ⸢bloated⸣ and he continually has to lie down a lot [...].

2. If his ⸢palate⸣ [...], he will die. If it enters him (and he has been sick) for three days, [...].

3. If the patient's [words] are unintelligible, (and he has been sick) for three days [...].[34]

4. ‹If› his words [are unintelligible?] and he experiences (mental) "wandering about"[35] for days in a row (and he has been sick) for three days [...].[36]

5. If the patient's words are ⸢unintelligible⸣ [and] he vomits green stuff and his flesh is yellow (and he has been sick) for three days [...].[37]

6. If his words are unintelligible [and] fever continually afflicts him and he wanders about (and he has been sick) for three days [...].[38]

7. If his words are unintelligible, he is nauseous (and he has been sick) for three days [...].

8. If his words are unintelligible and depression keeps falling on him, (and it is) at his appointed time,[39] (and he has been sick) for three days, [he will die].[40]

9. If a person's words are unintelligible and he continually weeps, (and it is) at his appointed time, (and he has been sick) for three days [he will die].[41]

10. If his words are ⸢unintelligible⸣, he continually produces blood from his mouth, his insides are puffed up, (and he has been sick) for ten days [...].[42]
11. If his words are ⸢unintelligible⸣, he constantly emits "wind" from his anus, he belches, (and he has been sick) for ten days [...].[43]
12. If his words are ⸢unintelligible⸣ and fever continually falls upon him, "hand" of Ninurta. (If he has been sick) for ten days [...].[44]
13. If his words are ⸢unintelligible⸣ and he continually asks for beer, (and he has been sick) for ten days [...].[45]
14. If his words are ⸢unintelligible⸣ and he continually asks for wine, (and it is) at [his] appointed time, [and he has been sick for ten days ...].[46]
15. If his words are ⸢unintelligible⸣, he drones, (and he has been sick) for [ten days ...].[47]
16. If his words are [unintelligible and ...] he continually cries out: "Woe, my heart," "Woe, my heart" [...].[48]
17. If his words [are unintelligible ...] or "hand" of Ninurta [...].[49]

A rev.

1′. [If his] ⸢words⸣ [are unintelligible ...].
2′. If his words are unintelligible and [he has] a return [of the illness ...].
3′. If his words are unintelligible and it is difficult for him to [...].
4′. If his words are unintelligible and he ⸢chokes⸣ [...].
5′–10′ *(all begin* "If his words are unintelligible" *but are otherwise broken)*
11′. If the patient's noise [...].

12′–17′ *(all begin* "If you have heard the patient's noise and it is like [...]"*)*[50]

Notes

1. Restored from the commentary SpTU 1.32 rev. 14.
2. See *CAD* A/2, 498b.
3. Restored from the similar DPS 3:50–51.
4. The commentary SpTU 1.32 rev. 8–9 explains: *ra-pa-du su-ud-dur-*[*šú*] = [*šá-n*]*e-e ṭè-e-me sa-dir-šú*.
5. See Scurlock and Andersen 2005, 18.39.
6. This entry appears also in Wilhelm 1994, 62 J 2:13′–14′.
7. See Scurlock and Andersen 2005, 10.168.
8. See Scurlock and Andersen 2005, 3.104.
9. See Scurlock and Andersen 2005, 3.104.
10. See Scurlock and Andersen 2005, 16.64.
11. See Scurlock and Andersen 2005, 14.10.
12. *Kaṣāru* means literally "to knot," as in making a Turkish carpet.
13. The reference is to the patient's mother.

14. See Scurlock and Andersen 2005, 16.39.
15. See Scurlock and Andersen 2005, 18.35.
16. For a differing interpretation, see Stol 2009, 3–4.
17. See Scurlock and Andersen 2005, 18.34.
18. See Scurlock and Andersen 2005, 14.8, 18.32, 18.42.
19. See Scurlock and Andersen 2005, 18.32.
20. See Scurlock and Andersen 2005, 18.32.
21. See Scurlock and Andersen 2005, 19.143.
22. See Scurlock and Andersen 2005, 18.46.
23. See Scurlock and Andersen 2005, 18.46.
24. See Scurlock and Andersen 2005, 20.17.
25. See Scurlock and Andersen 2005, 13.298
26. See Scurlock and Andersen 2005, 18.48.
27. See Scurlock and Andersen 2005, 3.65, 4.17, 10.81, 18.47. This entry appears also in DPS 33:87.
28. See Scurlock and Andersen 2005, 18.44.
29. For the reading and interpretation, see Heeßel 2000, 263.
30. See Scurlock and Andersen 2005, 14.9.
31. See Scurlock and Andersen 2005, 6.32.
32. See Scurlock and Andersen 2005, 3.105.
33. See Scurlock and Andersen 2005, 3.105.
34. The prognosis is probably grim. This and, indeed, all similar passages in this tablet could also be translated as "he will die within x number of days."
35. The commentary SpTU 1.32 rev. 8–9 explains that the reference is to alteration of mentation.
36. See Scurlock and Andersen 2005, 14.34, 16.48.
37. See Scurlock and Andersen 2005, 6.140.
38. See Scurlock and Andersen 2005, 3.124.
39. Or "within his appointed time."
40. See Scurlock and Andersen 2005, 14.36, 16.85.
41. See Scurlock and Andersen 2005, 16.85.
42. See Scurlock and Andersen 2005, 6.141, 19.366.
43. See Scurlock and Andersen 2005, 19.366.
44. See Scurlock and Andersen 2005, 19.366.
45. See Scurlock and Andersen 2005, 15.14, 19.367.
46. See Scurlock and Andersen 2005, 15.14, 16.82, 19.367.
47. See Scurlock and Andersen 2005, 16.41, 19.367.
48. See Scurlock and Andersen 2005, 19.367.
49. See Scurlock and Andersen 2005, 19.367.
50. Some idea of the nature of this section can be gleaned from commentaries SpTU 1.32 rev. 11–13 and SpTU 1.33 rev. 6′ which reveal that the *āšipu* did not, in contrast to the alleged methods of the Greek Sacred Disease specialists, make a diagnosis on the basis of sounds made by the patient. What he did do was attempt to prognosticate on that basis.

DPS TABLET 8

1. [DI]Š GIG GEŠTU 15-*šú tar-kàt* GIG-*su* DUGUD-*ma* TI-*uṭ*

2. [DI]Š GEŠTU 150-*šú tar-kàt na-kud*
3. DIŠ GEŠTU^{II}-*šú tar-ka* GAM
4. DIŠ GEŠTU 15-*šú* [*t*]*ur-ru-pat* GIG-*su* GÍD-*ma* DIN
5. DIŠ GEŠTU 150-*šú tur-ru-pat na-kud*

6a. DIŠ GEŠTU^{II}-*šú tur-ru-pa* GAM

6b. : DIŠ GEŠTU 15-*šú* DU$_8$-*át* DIN

7a. DIŠ GEŠTU 150-*šú* DU$_8$-*át* GIG-*su* GÍD

7b. : DIŠ GEŠTU^{II}-*šú* DU$_8$.DU$_8$-*ra* GAM

8. DIŠ GEŠTU 15-*šú* GÙ.GÙ-*si* DIN : DIŠ GEŠTU 150-*šú* GÙ.GÙ-*si* GIG-*su* GÍD
9. DIŠ GEŠTU^{II}-*šú* GÙ.GÙ.MEŠ GIG-*su* DUGUD

10a. DIŠ NA GEŠTU 15-*šú* GÙ.GÙ-*si me-sír* IGI

10b. : [DIŠ GE]ŠTU 150-*šú* GÙ.GÙ-*si* Á.TUK IGI

11a. DIŠ NA GEŠTU^{II}-*šú* GÙ.GÙ.MEŠ *ina-an-ziq*

11b. [:] DIŠ GEŠTU 15-*šú sa-ki-ik* GIG.BI DIN

12. DIŠ GEŠTU 150-*šú sa-ki-ik* GIG-*su* DUGUD : DIŠ GEŠTU^{II}-*šú sak-ka* É.BI BIR-*aḫ*
13. DIŠ GEŠTU^{II}-*šú i-šag-gu-mu u* UGU-*šú i-šam-ma-am-ma-šu* ŠU ^{d}15
14. DIŠ GEŠTU^{II}-*šú kab-ta-šú* UŠ$_4$-*šu* KÚR.KÚR-*šú u* KA.KA-*šú it-te-né-ep-rik-ku* GAM
15. DIŠ GEŠTU^{II}-*šú* u SIG$_4$ GÌR^{II}-*šú* 1-*niš* (coll.) ŠED$_7$.MEŠ GIDIM *šu-ru-bat* EDIN DIB-*su*
16. DIŠ GEŠTU^{II}-*šú* GIN$_7$ GEŠTU MÁŠ.TUR *sa-al-ḫa* ŠU GIDIM *ana* U$_4$.3.KÁM *ni-kit-tú* : LÍL TUKU

17a. DIŠ GEŠTU^{II}-*šú it-ta-na-az-qa-pa* ŠU GIDIM$_2$

17b. : [DI]Š GEŠTU^{II}-*šú i-az-za-za* ŠU GIDIM$_2$

18–21. DIŠ GEŠTU^{II}-*šú kir-ra-šu u ki-ṣir* 1.KÙŠ.M[EŠ-*š*]*ú* TA GIG-*su* TAK$_4$-⸢*šu*⸣ 1-*niš*! GU$_7$.MEŠ-*šú ki*-⸢*ma* DU$_8$?-*ra*⸣ GIG-[*su* GUR-*m*]*a ana* É.MEŠ GUR-*šú-ma* GIG SAL.KALAG.GA IGI-*ma* DIN [o o o o] DIŠ ŠU^{II}-*šú u* GÌR^{II}-*šú ana* x-x[…] GIG.BI *šum$_4$-ma* É.MEŠ […]

22. DIŠ *is-sa-a-šú ḫe-sa-a-m*[*a* GEŠTU^{II}-*šú* …]
23. DIŠ GEŠTU-*šú* x […]
24. [DIŠ *i*]*na* GEŠTU-*šú* [15 SÌG-*iṣ* …]
25. [DIŠ *in*]*a* GEŠTU-*šú* [150 SÌG-*iṣ* …]

(remainder of obv. and all of reverse except a line of colophon is broken away)

TRANSLATION

1. ⌜If⌝ the patient's "right" ear is dark, his illness may be difficult (but) he will get well.[1]
2. ⌜If⌝ his "left" ear is dark, it is worrisome.
3. If (both) his ears are dark, he will die.
4. If the patient's "right" ear ⌜looks sprinkled⌝, his illness may be prolonged (but) he will get well.[2]
5. If his "left" ear looks sprinkled, it is worrisome.[3]

6a. If (both) his ears look sprinkled, he will die.[4]
6b. If his "right" ear was (cut/broken) open, he will get well.[5]
7a. If his "left" ear was (cut/broken) open, his illness will be prolonged.
7b. If (both) his ears were (cut/broken) open, he will die.

8. If his "right" ear continually rings, he will get well.[6] If his "left" ear continually rings, his illness will be prolonged.
9. If (both) his ears continually ring, his illness will be difficult.[7]

10a. If a person's "right" ear continually rings, he will experience hard times.[8]
10b. [If] his "left" ⌜ear⌝ continually rings, he will experience profit.[9]
11a. If (both) his ears continually ring, he will have worries.
11b. If his "right" ear is obstructed, that patient will get well.

12. If his "left" ear is obstructed, his illness will be difficult. If (both) his ears are obstructed, his house will be scattered.
13. If his ears roar and his skull goes numb, "hand" of Ishtar.[10]
14. If his ears (feel) heavy, his mentation is continually altered and his words hinder each other (in his mouth),[11] he will die.[12]
15. If his ears and the soles of his feet are cold at the same time, a ghost, one brought into the steppe,[13] afflicts him.
16. If his ears wiggle like the ears of a young goat, "hand" of ghost. (If it is the third day he has been sick), there will be cause for worry (var. crisis).

17a. If his ears continually stand up, "hand" of ghost.[14]
17b. ⌜If⌝ his ears make strange noises, "hand"] of ghost.[15]

18–21. If after his illness has left him his ears, his throat and his elbows all hurt him at the same time (and) after it has let up, [his] illness [returns] ⌜and⌝ comes back inside him[16] so that he gets sick (again), he may have a difficult time of it, but he will get well. [...] If his hands and feet [...]. If his illness [comes back] inside him [a third time ...].[17]

22. If his jaws are pressured and, ⌜consequently⌝, [his ears ...].
23. If his ears [...].
24. [If he was injured] ⌜on⌝ his ["right"] ear [...].

25. [If he was injured] ⌜on⌝ his ["left"] ear [...].
(the remainder of obverse and all of reverse except a line of colophon are broken away)

NOTES

1. This line is cited in the commentary to DPS 7, SpTU 1.33 rev. 7′.
2. See Scurlock and Andersen 2005, 10.52.
3. See Scurlock and Andersen 2005, 10.52.
4. See Scurlock and Andersen 2005, 10.52.
5. See Scurlock and Andersen 2005, 9.95, 14.6.
6. See Scurlock and Andersen 2005, 20.2.
7. See Scurlock and Andersen 2005, 9.116.
8. See Scurlock and Andersen 2005, 20.3. Treatments for this condition appear in BAM 155 ii 5′–11′//RSO 32.109–22 iii 10′–15′, BAM 155 ii 12′–13′ and BAM 506:8′–9′.
9. Treatments for this condition appear in BAM 506:10′–11′ and RSO 32.109–22 iii 16′–19′. Note the contrast between line 10 and the remaining entries which attempt a distinction between right and left sides. In most of the entries, right is good and left is bad, whereas in line 10, left is good and right is bad. The reason for this is, quite simply, that prognoses were taken from the doctor's point of view, whereas omens were taken from the affected person's perspective. Thus a sign on the doctor's left but the patient's right was good if omens were being taken, as in line 10, but bad if a prognosis was called for, and vice versa.
10. See Scurlock and Andersen 2005, 19.287. This entry also appears in VAT 11122 obv. 6 (Heeßel 2010, 181–84).
11. Heeßel 2000, 261: 53 suggests interpreting this as his words continually failing.
12. See Scurlock and Andersen 2005, 13.220.
13. *CAD* Š/3 recognizes both a *šuribtu*, which seems to mean something like "terror" and *šūrubtu* which is from *erēbu*: "to enter." Unaccountably, this reference is cited under *šuribtu* and not *šūrubtu*.
14. See Scurlock and Andersen 2005, 9.112.
15. See Scurlock and Andersen 2005, 9.113, 19.379.
16. The translation in *CAD* U/W, 132b takes this phrase out of context and translates it as if it were a separate sentence completely unrelated to what precedes and follows it.
17. See Scurlock and Andersen 2005, 3.54, 11.38.

DPS TABLET 9

1. [DIŠ GIG IGI.M]EŠ-*šú* IR *ú-kal u* DUL.DUL-*tam*
2. ŠU ^{d}MAŠ.TAB.BA [MAŠ].⌜MAŠ-*su*⌝ DÙ-*uš u* ŠU.GUR.GUR-*šu-ma* DIN
3. [DIŠ ... I]GI.MEŠ-*šú* SA_5 GAM
4. DIŠ [IGI.MEŠ-*šú* S]A_5.MEŠ *u i-šap-pu-ú* GAM
5. DIŠ ⌜IGI.MEŠ-*šú*⌝ SA_5.MEŠ *u* SIG_7.MEŠ ZI-*ma* MAN-*ma* GIG
6. DIŠ IGI.MEŠ-*šú* SA_5.MEŠ *u* GI_6.MEŠ SUMUN-*ma* EGIR-*šú* MAN-*ma* GAM

7. DIŠ IGI.MEŠ-*šú* BABBAR.MEŠ DIN
8. DIŠ IGI.MEŠ-*šú* BABBAR *u* SIG$_7$ ŠUB.ŠUB-*ú* KA-*šú* NUNDUN.ME-*šú* *ši-ši-tu*
9. IGI-*šú šá* 150 *i-ṣap-par* GAM
10. DIŠ IGI.MEŠ-*šú* BABBAR GI$_6$ SA$_5$ *u* SIG$_7$ ŠUB : *ú-kal-lu* GIG-*su* GÍD-*ma* DIN
11. DIŠ IGI.MEŠ-*šú* SIG$_7$.MEŠ ^{d}DIM$_{11}$.ME DIB-*su*
12. DIŠ IGI.MEŠ-*šú* SIG$_7$.MEŠ *u* IGI^{II}-*šú šap-la* GAM
13. DIŠ IGI.MEŠ-*šú* SIG$_7$.MEŠ ŠÀ IGI^{II}-*šú* SIG$_7$.ME SUḪUŠ EME-*šú* GI$_6$ *aḫ-ḫa-zu*
14. DIŠ IGI.MEŠ-*šú* SIG$_7$.MEŠ *u* GI$_6$.MEŠ GAM
15. DIŠ IGI.MEŠ-*šú* GI$_6$.MEŠ GIG-*su* GÍD-*ma* GAM
16. DIŠ IGI.MEŠ-*šú* GI$_6$.MEŠ EME-*šú* SA$_5$ GIG-*su* GÍD-*ma* GAM
17. DIŠ IGI.MEŠ-*šú* GI$_6$.MEŠ *u* BABBAR.MEŠ GAM
18. DIŠ IGI.MEŠ-*šú* GI$_6$.MEŠ ŠÀ.MEŠ-*šú nap-ḫu* GAM
19. DIŠ IGI.MEŠ-*šú* GI$_6$.MEŠ NINDA APIN-*ma* GU$_7$ GAM
20. DIŠ IGI.MEŠ-*šú* GI$_6$.MEŠ-*ma* MÚD *i-par-ri* GABA.RI SÌG-*iṣ* GAM
21. DIŠ IGI.MEŠ-*šú* GI$_6$.MEŠ-*ma* GIN$_7$ *šá-lam-ti ib-šu-ú*
22. IGI.MEŠ-*šú i-te-eb-ṭú* NUNDUN.MEŠ-*šú ma-diš ik-tab-ra*
23. IGI.MEŠ-*šú iš-ta-na-an-nu-ú mu-du-šú ul* GIG-*ma*
24. *i-qab-bi* ÚŠ *ug-ga-ti* GAM EGIR-*su na-ʾ-da-at* É-*su* BIR-*aḫ*
25. DIŠ IGI.MEŠ-*šú* DAR$_4$ GÍR-*iš* GAM
26. DIŠ IGI.MEŠ-*šú* DAR$_4$ ZÚ.LUM.MA APIN-*ma* GU$_7$ GAM
27. DIŠ IGI.MEŠ-*šú še-bu-ú* : *te-bu-ú* DIN : GAM
28. DIŠ IGI.MEŠ-*šú ṣar-pu u i-ša-ap-pu-ú* ŠU ^{d}IM GAM
29. DIŠ IGI.MEŠ-*šú* IM.GÁ.LI ŠUB-*ú* NUNDUN.MEŠ-*šú ši-ši-tu* DIRI.MEŠ IGI^{II}-*šú* SIG$_7$ ŠUB.ŠUB-*a u* IGI-*šú šá* 15 *i-ṣa-par* GAM
30. DIŠ IGI.MEŠ-*šú* KÚR.KÚR-*ru* GAM
31. DIŠ IGI.MEŠ-*šú* KÚR.KÚR-*ru* EME-*šú* SIG$_7$: SU-*šú* SIG$_7$ TÙN.GIG *ana* U$_4$.3.KÁM GAM
32. DIŠ IGI.MEŠ-*šú ṣe-em-ru* : *ma-⸢lu⸣-ú* DIN-*uṭ*
33. DIŠ IGI.MEŠ-*šú* IR *ú-kal-lu* DIN-*uṭ*
34. DIŠ IGI.MEŠ-*šú* KÚM *ú-kal-lu* DIN-*uṭ*
35. DIŠ IGI.MEŠ-*šú* KÚM.MEŠ IGI^{II}-*šú um-mu-ra ina ú-kul-ti* : *ina qú-ul-ti* SÌG-*iṣ* GAM
36. DIŠ IGI.MEŠ-*šú* ŠED$_7$.MEŠ GAM
37. DIŠ IGI.MEŠ-*šú ma-aq-tu* GAM
38. DIŠ IGI.MEŠ-*šú ma-aq-tu-ma su-qat-su ṣab-ta-at u* UŠ$_4$-*šú* NU DIB GAM

39. DIŠ IGI.MEŠ-*šú šal-mu* DIN
40. DIŠ IGI.MEŠ-*šú šal-mu* EME-*šú* SA$_5$ GIG-*su* GÍD-*ma* DIN-*uṭ*
41. DIŠ IGI.MEŠ-*šú ad-ru* DIN
42. DIŠ IGI.MEŠ-*šú* GIN$_7$ Ì.GIŠ È-*ú* DIN
43. DIŠ IGI.M[EŠ-*šú*] ḪÁD.A SA$_5$.MEŠ DIRI.MEŠ GIG-*su* GÍD-*ma* DIN
44. DIŠ IGI.MEŠ-*šú* ḪÁD.A BABBAR.MEŠ DIRI.MEŠ DIN
45. DIŠ IGI.MEŠ-*šú* ḪÁD.A SIG$_7$.MEŠ DIRI.MEŠ ŠU ^{d}BAD DIN
46. DIŠ IGI.MEŠ-*šú* ḪÁD.A GI$_6$.MEŠ DIRI.MEŠ GAM
47. DIŠ IGI.MEŠ-*šú* U$_4$.BU.BU.UL SA$_5$ DIRI.MEŠ ŠU ^{d}30 DIN
48. DIŠ IGI.MEŠ-*šú* U$_4$.BU.BU.UL BABBAR DIRI.MEŠ ŠU ^{d}UTU DIN
49. DIŠ IGI.MEŠ-*šú* BU.BU.UL GI$_6$ DIRI.MEŠ ŠU ^{d}15 GAM
50. DIŠ IGI.MEŠ-*šú bir-di* DIRI.MEŠ ŠU DINGIR-*šú* DIN KI.MIN UD.DA TAB.BA ŠU DINGIR AD-*šú*
51. DIŠ IGI.MEŠ-*šú ziq-ti* DIRI.MEŠ ŠU ^{d}AMAR.UTU DIN KI.MIN ŠU ^{d}IM
52a. DIŠ IGI.MEŠ-*šú ri-šu-tú* DIRI.MEŠ DIN
52b : DIŠ IGI.MEŠ-*šú i-ši-tú* DIRI.MEŠ DIN
53. DIŠ IGI.MEŠ-*šú* NIGIN.ME *ina* SAG GI$_6$ TAG-*it*
54. DIŠ IGI.MEŠ-*šú* NIGIN.ME *u ú-šam-šá* ŠU DINGIR URU-*šú ana* ÚŠ GAR-*šú*
55. DIŠ IGI.MEŠ-*šú* NIGIN.MEŠ-*du u* IGI^{II}-*šú ur-ru-pa* ŠU DINGIR AD-*šú*
56. DIŠ IGI.MEŠ-*šú* NIGIN.ME *u su-qat-su* DU$_8$-*át ina* GIG-*šu* ÚŠ
57. DIŠ IGI.MEŠ-*šú* NIGIN.ME SAG.DU-*su* ŠU^{II}-*šú u* GÌR^{II}-*šú i-tar-ru-ra*
58. ŠU ^{d}LUGAL.GÌR.RA *u* ^{d}MEŠ.LAM.TA.È.A
59. DIŠ IGI.MEŠ-*šú* NIGIN.MEŠ ŠU^{II}-*šú u* GÌR^{II}-*šú i-ra-ʾ-ú-ba* U$_4$.59.KÁM ŠU ^{d}UD.AL.TAR
60. DIŠ IGI.MEŠ-*šú* NIGIN.MEŠ GEŠTU^{II}-*šú* GÙ.DÉ.MEŠ UB.NÍGIN.NA-*šú* DUB.DUB-*ka* ŠU GIDIM$_7$
61. DIŠ IGI.MEŠ-*šú* NIGIN.MEŠ GEŠTU^{II}-*šú i-šag-gu-ma* SAG.KI^{II}-*šú ú-maḫ-ḫa-ṣa-šú u i-rad-da-šú* ŠU GIDIM$_7$
62. DIŠ IGI.MEŠ-*šú* NIGIN.MEŠ ZI.ME-*šú* LÚGUD.MEŠ ZI-*šú* GIN$_7$ *šá* A *ṣa-mu-ú i-te-ner-ru-ub* ŠU GIDIM$_7$ *mur-tap-pi-di ina* EDIN DIB-*su*
63. DIŠ IGI.MEŠ-*šú* NIGIN.MEŠ *ina* KI.NÁ-*šú* ZI-*ma* ŠUB-*ut* ŠU GIDIM$_7$
64. DIŠ IGI.MEŠ-*šú* NIGIN.ME UB.NÍGIN.NA-*šú i-tar-ru-ra u i-ṭa-ma-a*
65. ŠU ^{d}LUGAL.GÌR.RA *u* ^{d}MEŠ.LAM.TA.È.A : ^{d}LUGAL.BÀN.DA
66a. DIŠ IGI.MEŠ-*šú* ⸢*nap*⸣-*ḫu u* IGI^{II}-*šú* MÚ.MEŠ GAM
66b. : DIŠ IGI.ME-*šú nap-ḫu u* ŠÀ.ME-*šú* MÚ.MEŠ GAM
67. DIŠ IGI.MEŠ-*šú u* ⸢ŠÀ⸣.MEŠ-*šú* MÚ.ME-*ḫu* TÙN.GIG *ana* U$_4$.3.KÁM GAM

68. DIŠ IGI.MEŠ-*šú* ŠÀ.MEŠ-*šú* ⸢ŠU^{II}⸣-*šú u* GÌR^{II}-*šú* MÚ.ME *nap-paḫ-tú* GIG ŠU 20
69. DIŠ IGI.MEŠ-*šú u* IGI^{II}-*šú* MÚ.MEŠ KI.A IGI^{II}-*šú* SA_5 IM KIR_4-*šú* KÚM.ME (coll.) : *ṣa-bit*
70. ⸢KÀŠ⸣.MEŠ-*šú ta-ba-ka* NU ZU-*e* GABA.RI SÌG-*iṣ* ŠU ᵈMAŠ
71. DIŠ IGI.MEŠ-*šú* ZIB-*ru ta-lam-ma-šú pur-ru-ur* ŠU-*su šá* 150 *na-ša-a* NU ZU-*e* GÌR^{II}-*šú i-maš-šar* GAM
72. DIŠ IGI.MEŠ-*šú ṣap-ru* ⸢*ta*⸣-*lam-ma-šú pur-ru-ur* ŠU-*su šá* NÍG.GIG-*ti-šú* ŠUB-*ma* NU ÍL-*ši*
73. GÌR-*šú i-maš-šar* ŠU *mi-šit-tú* U_4.ME-*šú* GÍD.ME NU SI.SÁ
74. DIŠ IGI.MEŠ-*šú* GIN_7 *ḫi-in-qí* UDU.NITÁ GÁL-*ú ú-šam-šá u* MÚD *i-ḫa-ḫu* GAM
75. DIŠ IGI.MEŠ-*šú ú-maš-šad* GIDIM *šá ina* A ÚŠ DIB-*su*
76. DIŠ IGI.MEŠ-*šú* SÌG.SÌG-*aṣ u* GÙ.DÉ.DÉ.ME-*si* GIDIM *qá-li-i* DIB-*su*
77. DIŠ *ina* SAG IGI.MEŠ-*šú* ḪÁD.A SA_5.MEŠ È.MEŠ GAM/DIN
78. DIŠ *ina* SAG IGI.MEŠ-*šú* ḪÁD.A.MEŠ GI_6.MEŠ È.ME GAM
79. DIŠ A.SAG-*šú* ŠÚ-*ip ina* EDIN TAG-*it* GAM

Translation

1–2. [If a patient]'s [face] holds sweat and he veils himself (i.e., withdraws from social intercourse), "hand" of the twin gods. If you do his ⸢treatment⸣ and you continually wipe him off, he will get well.[1]
3. [If …] (and) his ⸢face⸣ is red, he will die.
4. If [his face] is continually ⸢red⸣, and swells up like a cloud, he will die
5. If his face flushes and turns pale, (the illness) may be removed but he will be ill again.
6. If his face flushes and turns black, if he lingers and afterwards he takes a change (for the worse), he will die.
7. If his face is white, he will get well.
8–9. If his face is unevenly colored with white and yellow, his mouth (and) his lips (have) a glaze and his "left" eye flutters, he will die.[2]
10. If his face is unevenly colored with (var. contains) white, black, red and yellow, his illness may be prolonged, (but) he will get well.[3]
11. If his face is yellow, Lamashtu afflicts him.[4]
12. If his face is yellowish and his eyes are sunken, he will die.[5]
13. If his face is yellow and the inner part of his eyes is yellow (and) the base of the tongue is black, *aḫḫāzu*.[6]
14. If his face is yellow and black, he will die.

15. If his face is dark/black, if his illness is prolonged, he will die.
16. If his face is dark/black (and) his tongue is red, if his illness is prolonged, he will die.
17. If his face turns black and turns white, he will die.[7]
18. If his face turns black (and) his insides are bloated, he will die.
19. If his face turns black (and) he asks for bread and eats it, he will die.
20. If his face turns black and he vomits blood, he was injured on the front side; he will die.[8]
21–24. If his face turns black and becomes like (that of) a corpse, his face is continually frowning, his lips are very much thickened, his face keeps changing (and) one who knows him says: "Is he not sick?,"[9] death from (divine) anger; he will die. His inheritance will be in danger; his house will be scattered.[10]
25. If his face is dark red, he will speedily die.
26. If his face is dark red, he asks for dates and eats them, he will die.
27. If his face swells up like a cloud (var. rises), he will get well (var. he will die).
28. If his face looks died red and swells up like a cloud, "hand" of Adad; he will die (var. B: live).[11]
29. If his face is unevenly colored with *kalû*-clay yellow, his lips are full of glaze, his eyes are continually colored with yellow (and) his "right" eye flutters, he will die.[12]
30. If his face continually alters, he will die.
31. If his face continually alters, his tongue is yellow (var. his body is yellow), "sick liver." (If he has been sick) for three days, he will die.[13]
32. If his face is distended (var. full), he will get well.
33. If his face holds sweat, he will get well.
34. If his face holds fever, he will get well.
35. If his face is continually warm (and) his eyes are prominent[14] (and) he was stricken in the dead of night, he will die.[15]
36. If his face is continually cold, he will die.[16]
37. If his face has fallen in, he will die.
38. If his face has fallen in and his chin is "seized" and he is not in full possession of his faculties, he will die.
39. If his face is healthy, he will get well.
40. If his face is healthy (and) his tongue is red, his illness may be prolonged but he will get well.[17]
41. If a person's face is mournful, he will get well.[18]
42. If his face exudes something like oil,[19] he will get well.[20]

43. If [his] face is full of red *ramīṭu*-lesions, his illness may be prolonged but he will get well.[21]
44. If his face is full of white *ramīṭu*-lesions, he will get well.[22]
45. If his face is full of yellow *ramīṭu*-lesions, "hand" of Bel; he will get well.[23]
46. If his face is full of black *ramīṭu*-lesions, he will die.[24]
47. If his face is full of red *bubuʾtu*, "hand" of Sîn; he will get well.[25]
48. If his face is full of white *bubuʾtu*, "hand" of Shamash; he will get well.[26]
49. If his face is full of black *bubuʾtu*, "hand" of Ishtar; he will die.[27]
50. If his face is full of *birdu*, "hand" of his god; he will get well. Alternatively, burning of *ṣētu*, "hand" of the god of his father.[28]
51. If his face is full of *ziqtu*, "hand" of Marduk; he will get well. Alternatively, "hand" of Adad.[29]
52a. If his face is full of redness, he will get well.[30]
52b. If his face is full of *išītu*, he will get well.[31]
53. If his face (seems) continually to be spinning, he was "touched" at the beginning of the night.
54. If his face (seems) continually to be spinning and it keeps him up all night, the "hand" of the god of his city has been placed on him for death.
55. If his face (seems) continually to be spinning and his eyes are heavily clouded, "hand" of the god of his father.
56. If his face (seems) continually to be spinning and his chin was (cut) open, he will die during his illness.[32]
57–58. If his face (seems) continually to be spinning (and) his head, his hands and his feet tremble, "hand" of LUGAL.GÌR.RA and MEŠ.LAM.TA.È.A.[33]
59. If his face (seems) continually to be spinning (and) his hands and his feet tremble (and he has been sick for) fifty-nine days, "hand" of Dapinu.[34]
60. If his face (seems) continually to spin, his ears roar, (and) his limbs get tense,[35] "hand" of ghost.[36]
61. If his face (seems) continually to spin, his ears roar (and) his temples give him jabbing pains and seem to shake, "hand" of ghost.[37]
62. If his face seems continually to be spinning (and) his breaths have become short (and) his breath constantly enters his throat as if he were thirsting for water,[38] the hand of a ghost roving in the steppe afflicts him.[39]
63. If his face seems continually to be spinning (and) he gets up from his bed and then falls down (again), "hand" of ghost.[40]

64–65. If his face (seems) continually to be spinning (and) his limbs tremble and twist, "hand" of LUGAL.GÌR.RA and MEŠ.LAM.TA.È.A (var. LUGAL.BÀN.DA).[41]

66a. If his face is swollen and his eyes are swollen, he will die.

66b. If his face is swollen and his insides are bloated, he will die.[42]

67. If his face and his insides are continually swollen/bloated, "sick liver"; (if he has been sick) for three days, he will die.[43]

68. If his face, his insides, his hands and his feet are continually swollen/bloated, he is ill with swelling/bloating, "hand" of Shamash.[44]

69–70. If his face and his eyes are swollen, the rims of his eyes are red, the breath of nose is continually hot (var. "seized") (and) he is not able to pour out his urine, he was injured on the front side; "hand" of Ninurta.[45]

71. If his face twitches, his torso is powerless, he is unable to lift his "left" hand (and) he drags his feet, he will die.[46]

72–73. If his face twitches, his torso is powerless, he lets the affected hand drop and is unable to lift (it) (and) he drags his foot, "hand" of a stroke. ‹Even if› he lives for a long time, he will not straighten up.[47]

74. If his face looks like that of a strangled sheep, it keeps him up all night and he vomits blood, he will die.[48]

75. If he massages his face, the ghost (of one) who died in water afflicts him.[49]

76. If he continually strikes his face and screams, the ghost of someone burned to death afflicts him.[50]

77. If red *ramīṭu*-lesions erupt at the upper part of his face, he will die (var. B: he will live).[51]

78. If black *ramīṭu*-lesions erupt at the upper part of his face, he will die.[52]

79. If (his face) falls flat against his skull, he was "touched" in the steppe; he will die.[53]

Notes

1. See Scurlock and Andersen 2005, 19.239.
2. See Scurlock and Andersen 2005, 6.149, 18.30.
3. See Scurlock and Andersen 2005, 10.49.
4. See Scurlock and Andersen 2005, 3.26, 19.223.
5. See Scurlock and Andersen 2005, 3.106, 20.80.
6. See Scurlock and Andersen 2005, 6.117. The entry appears also in DPS 33:93.
7. See Scurlock and Andersen 2005, 19.321.
8. See Scurlock and Andersen 2005, 8.92. The entry appears also in DPS 15:5′.
9. With Heeßel, 2011a, 21. *CAD* M/2, 165a's translation makes no sense whatsoever.
10. See Scurlock and Andersen 2005, 8.91, 10.38.
11. See Scurlock and Andersen 2005, 20.42.

12. See Scurlock and Andersen 2005, 6.148, 18.29.

13. Alternatively: "he will die within three days." See Scurlock and Andersen 2005, 6.138, 18.41, 20.45.

14. For a discussion of this verb, see Civil 1974, 338.

15. See Scurlock and Andersen 2005, 7.25.

16. See Scurlock and Andersen 2005, 20.20.

17. See Scurlock and Andersen 2005, 18.40.

18. See Scurlock and Andersen 2005, 16.30.

19. It would be nice if this could be the patient's face shining (i.e., happy), reading *ne-per-du-ú*. This does not, however, account for the "like" and the text has not "*du*" but "È." Suggestion courtesy M. Stol.

20. See Scurlock and Andersen 2005, 10.9.

21. See Scurlock and Andersen 2005, 10.161.

22. See Scurlock and Andersen 2005, 10.162.

23. See Scurlock and Andersen 2005, 10.163, 19.102.

24. See Scurlock and Andersen 2005, 10.164.

25. See Scurlock and Andersen 2005, 3.232, 4.16, 10.82.

26. See Scurlock and Andersen 2005, 10.83.

27. See Scurlock and Andersen 2005, 10.84.

28. See Scurlock and Andersen 2005, 10.72.

29. See Scurlock and Andersen 2005, 10.109.

30. See Scurlock and Andersen 2005, 10.13.

31. See Scurlock and Andersen 2005, 10.174.

32. See Scurlock and Andersen 2005, 13.133.

33. See Scurlock and Andersen 2005, 3.45, 13.82.

34. See Scurlock and Andersen 2005, 13.82, 13.102, 19.88.

35. Literally: "all heaped up (in a bunch)."

36. See Scurlock and Andersen 2005, 19.278.

37. See Scurlock and Andersen 2005, 19.278.

38. *AHw* 238 takes this as thirsty people's souls being proverbially clouded.

39. See Scurlock and Andersen 2005, 8.78.

40. See Scurlock and Andersen 2005, 13.104.

41. See Scurlock and Andersen 2005, 3.46, 13.76.

42. See Scurlock and Andersen 2005, 8.24

43. See Scurlock and Andersen 2005, 6.150.

44. See Scurlock and Andersen 2005, 19.104.

45. See Scurlock and Andersen 2005, 5.38, 19.138.

46. See Scurlock and Andersen 2005, 13.50.

47. See Scurlock and Andersen 2005, 13.80, 13.242.

48. See Scurlock and Andersen 2005, 8.90.

49. The entry appears also in DPS 26:42′a.

50. See Scurlock and Andersen 2005, 16.63, 19.27.

51. See Scurlock and Andersen 2005, 10.166.

52. See Scurlock and Andersen 2005, 10.167.

53. See Scurlock and Andersen 2005, 7.10.

DPS TABLET 10

DPS 9:80 (catchline) = DPS 10:1

1. DIŠ GIG GÚ-*su ana* 15 NIGIN.ME ŠU^{II}-*šú u* GÌR^{II}-*šú am-šá* IGI^{II}-*šú* DUL-*ma*
2. ⸢BAL-*ma*⸣ *ina* KA-*šú* ÚḪ DU-*ak i-ḫar-ru-ur* AN.TA.ŠUB.BA
3. *šum-ma e-nu-ma* DIB-*šú* ŠÀ-*šú e-er* ZI-*aḫ šum-ma e-nu-ma* DIB-*šú* NÍ-*šú* NU ZU-*e* NU ZI
4. DIŠ GÚ-*su ana* 150 NIGIN.ME ŠU^{II}-*šú u* GÌR^{II}-*šú tar-ṣa* IGI^{II}-*šú ana* IGI AN-*e na-pal-ka-a*
5. *ina* KA-*šú* ÚḪ DU-*ak i-ḫar-ru-ur* NÍ-*šú* NU ZU *ina taq-ti-it* [LÁ-*š*]*ú*
6. *iḫ-ta-niṭ-ṭa-áš-šú* AN.TA.ŠUB.BA ŠU ^{d}30 (coll.)
7. DIŠ GÚ-*su* GU$_7$-*su* ŠU DINGIR-*šú* : ⸢ŠU⸣ ^{d}UTU *ana* ŠÙD *qí-bit* KA-*šú* DIN
8. DIŠ GÚ-⸢*su*⸣ GU$_7$-*su-ma* ⸢A⸣.[MEŠ API]N.MEŠ-*iš* ŠU ^{d}15 *ina* GÚ-*šú* SÌG-*iṣ* GAM
9. DIŠ GÚ-*su u* MUR[U]B$_4$.MEŠ-*šú* 1-*niš* GU$_7$.MEŠ-*šú* ŠU ^{d}IM
10. DIŠ GÚ-*su* MU[R]UB$_4$.MEŠ-*šú* ŠU^{II}-*šú u* GÌR^{II}-*šú aš-ṭa* SA.DUGUD
11. DIŠ ⸢GÚ⸣-*su i-zur-ma* IGI-*šú gal-ta-át pi-qam* NU *pi-qam* LUḪ-*ut* SA.DUGUD
12. ⸢DIŠ GÚ⸣-*su i-tar-rak* SAG.DU-*su* ŠUB.ŠUB-*ut* ŠU^{II}-*šú u* GÌR^{II}-*šú it-ta-na-aš-gag-gu*
13. *u ana qaq-qa-ru ú-ḫa-an-na-aṣ* KI.SIKIL.LÍL.LÁ DIB-*su*

14a. DIŠ GÚ-*su* 15 *u* 150 *ut-ta-nar* GAM
14b. : DIŠ GÚ-*su* 15 *u* 150 ŠUB.ŠUB-*di* GAM
15a. DIŠ GÚ-*su* 15 *u* 150 ŠUB.ŠUB-*ut* GAM
15b. : DIŠ GÚ-*su* TA 15 *ana* 150 *suḫ$_4$-ḫur-ma* ŠUB-*ut* [G]AM

16. DIŠ *ina* GÚ-*šú* SÌG-*iṣ* ŠU ^{d}IM
17. DIŠ *ina* GÚ-*šú* SÌG-*iṣ u* GABA-*su* GU$_7$-*šú* ŠU ^{d}15 *ana* NA$_4$.NUNUZ.MEŠ
18. DIŠ *ina* GÚ-*šú* SÌG-*iṣ-ma u du-us-su KAR-et* ŠU ^{d}15 GAM
19. DIŠ *ina* GÚ-*šú* SÌG-*ma* ŠÀ.MEŠ-*šú it-te-nen-bi-ṭu u* GÌR^{II}-*šú na-šá-a* DIB GIDIM$_7$
20. DIŠ *ina* GÚ-*šú* SÌG-*iṣ-ma* GÌR^{II}-*šú i-ra-ʾ-ú-ba* ŠÀ.MEŠ-*šú it-te-nen-bi-ṭu* DIB GIDIM$_7$
21. DIŠ *ina* GÚ-*šú* SÌG-*iṣ-ma e-lat* IGI^{II}-*šú* GU$_7$.ME-*šú* MÚD *ina* KA-*šú* ŠUB.ŠUB-*a* ŠU^{II}-*šú u* GÌR^{II}-*šú eṣ-la* NA BI ḪUL DIB-*su*

22a. DIŠ ^{NA_4}KIŠIB GÚ-*šú* DU$_8$ GAM

22b. : DIŠ ^{NA_4}KIŠIB GÚ-*šú* DU$_8$ *na-ḫi-ra-šú* DIB.DIB GAM
23. DIŠ ^{NA_4}KIŠIB GÚ-*šú* DU$_8$ SA.MEŠ-*šú* GAR-*nu u na-ḫi-ra-šú* DIB.DIB GAM
24. DIŠ ^{NA_4}KIŠIB GÚ-*šú* DU$_8$ SA.MEŠ-*šú* GAR-*nu u* PA.AN.BI *ina* KIR$_4$-*šú* DIB.DIB GIG BI NU DIN
25. DIŠ ^{NA_4}KIŠIB GÚ-*šú* DU$_8$ SA.MEŠ-*šú* GAR-*nu* KA-*šú ṣa-pir*[1] *mu-dá-a-šu la-a* [...]
26. DIŠ *pur-qí-dam* ŠUB-*ma* BIR-*iḫ* GÚ-*su* 15 *u* 150 ŠUB.ŠUB-*di* GAM
27. DIŠ TA SA.GÚ-*šú* EN SÌL.MUD-*šú* SA.MEŠ-*šú šag-gu šu-ʾ-ra-šú kaṣ-ra* ME.ZÉ-*šú hé-sa$_5$* SA.DUGUD

---

28. DIŠ GÚ.MUR-*su ḫa-niq* NÍG.GIG DINGIR-*šú* GU$_7$: *uš-te-zeb*
29. DIŠ GÚ.MUR-*su i-ḫar-ru-ur* GAM

---

30. DIŠ ZI-*šú* GU$_4$.UD.ME *u* ŠÀ.MEŠ-*šú it-te-nen-bi-ṭu* GAM
31a. DIŠ ZI-*šú* GU$_4$.UD.ME *u* SA.MEŠ-*šú šap-ku* GAM
31b. : DIŠ ZI-*šú i-tar-rak-ma qit-ru-bat* [G]AM
32a. DIŠ ZI-*šú ú-šel-li* NU DIN
32b. : DIŠ ZI-*šú* GIN$_7$ *šá* TA A E$_{11}$-*a* LÚGUD.MEŠ ŠU DINGIR.[MAḪ?]
33. : ŠU ^{d}*Nin-giz-zi-da* : ŠU GIDIM$_4$ *šá ina* A [ÚŠ DIB-*su*]
34a. DIŠ *ina* ZI-*šú* GÚ.MUR-*su i-ḫar-ru-ur* GAM
34b. : DIŠ *ni-ip-qú-šú qit-ru-bu u* UŠ$_4$-*šú* NU DIB [GAM]

---

35. DIŠ ZI.ḪA.ZA SAG.ÚS DIB.DIB-*su* KÚR DINGIR.MEŠ-*ma* [...]
36. DIŠ ZI.ḪA.ZA SAG.ÚS DIB.DIB-*su u ug-gag* [...]
37. DIŠ ZI.ḪA.ZA SAG.ÚS DIB.DIB-*su u* MUD-*ud* ŠU ^{d}15 [GAM]
38. DIŠ ZI.ḪA.ZA SAG.ÚS DIB.DIB-*su u* ÍR ÚŠ-*ma* E[G]IR-*šú* AD-*šú* [GAM]
39. DIŠ ZI.ḪA.ZA SAG.ÚS DIB.DIB-*su u i-ṭa-mu* ÚŠ-*ma* EGIR-*šú* AMA-*šú* [GAM]
40. DIŠ ZI.ḪA.ZA SAG.ÚS DIB.DIB-*su u* GÙ.⸢DÉ⸣.ME ÚŠ-*ma* EGIR-*šú* ŠEŠ-*šú* [GAM]

---

41. DIŠ *gir-ri* 15-*šú* SA$_5$ DIN : DIŠ *gir-ri* 150-*šú* SA$_5$ DUGUD-*ma* DIN
42. DIŠ ⸢*gir*⸣-*ra-šú* SA$_5$.ME DIN : DIŠ *gir-ri* 15-*šú* SIG$_7$ GIG-*su* GÍD : DIŠ *gir-ri* 150-*šú* SIG$_7$ GAM
43. DIŠ *gir-ra-šú* SIG$_7$.MEŠ GÍD-*ma* GAM : DIŠ *gir-ri* 15-*šú* GI$_6$ GIG-*su* MAN-*ni*
44. DIŠ *gir-ri* 150-*šú* GI$_6$ GIG-*su* GÍD : DIŠ *gir-ra-šú* GI$_6$.MEŠ GAM

45. DIŠ *gir-ri* 15-*šú tar-kát* GIG-*su ú-ša-an-na-aḫ* : [DIŠ *g*]*ir-ri* 150-*šú tar-kát* GAM
46. DIŠ *gir-ra-šú tar-ka* GAM : DIŠ *gir-ri* 15-*šú nap-ḫat* DIN [:] DIŠ *gir-ri* 150-*šú nap-ḫat* GAM
47. DIŠ *gir-ra-šú nap-ḫa ú-ša-an-na-aḫ-ma* GAM : DIŠ *gir-ri* 1[5-*šú* M]Ú.⸢ME GIG-*su* KI⸣.[MIN]
48. DIŠ *gir-ri* 150-*šú* MÚ.ME GIG-*su* ⸢DUGUD⸣ : DIŠ *g*[*i*]*r-ra-šú* MÚ.ME GAM
49. DIŠ *gir-ri* 15-*šú šu-uḫ-ḫu-ṭa-át ú-šá-an-na-aḫ-ma* DIN
50. DIŠ *gir-ri* 150-*šú šu-uḫ-ḫu-ṭa-át* ⸢GAM⸣ : DIŠ *gir-ra-šú šu-uḫ-ḫu-ṭa* GAM
51. DIŠ *gir-ra-šú šu-uḫ-ḫu-ṭa u* UZU.ME-*šú šal-mu* DIN : *na-*⸢*kid*⸣
52. ⸢DIŠ *gir*⸣*-ra-a-šú šu-uḫ-ḫu-ṭa u* UZU.ME-*šú* ŠUB-*tu u ṣi-rip-tu* ŠUB.ŠUB-*a* [KI.MI]N
53. DIŠ *gir-ra-a-šú ma-aq-ta* GÌR^{II}-*šú na-šá-a ú-šam-šá* ŠU DINGIR URU-*šú ana* ÚŠ GAR-[*šú*]
54a. DIŠ *gir-ra-a-šú* ŠUB.MEŠ-*ma* GU$_7$.ME-*šú* ŠU GIDIM$_7$
54b. ⸢DIŠ *ina gir*⸣*-ri-šú* SÌG-*iṣ* ŠU ^{d}MAŠ.T[AB.BA GAM]
55. [DIŠ Á-*šú šá* 15 GI$_6$-*át* EME-*šú kaṣ-rat ina* EGIR-*šú* SÌG-*iṣ* GAM][2]
56. [DIŠ Á-*šú šá* 150 GI$_6$-*át* EME-*šú kaṣ-rat* GABA.RI-*šú* SÌG-*iṣ* GAM]
57. [DIŠ Á-*šú šá* 15 GI$_6$-*át u i-ṭa-mu* …]

B rev.

1. ⸢DIŠ Á-*šú šá* 150⸣ [GI$_6$-*át i-ṭa-mu* SÌG-*iṣ* ^{d}30 G]AM[3]
2. DIŠ Á^{II}-*šú tur-ra* NU ⸢ZU-*e u* [DÚR]-*su* ŠE$_{10}$-*šú u*⸣ MÚD SUR GAM
3. DIŠ Á^{II}-*šú tur-ra* NU ZU-*e u* MÚD *i-te-ez-zi* EGIR-*tú* SÌG-*iṣ* GAM
4. DIŠ Á^{II}-*šú tur-ra* NU ZU-*e u* MÚD BURU$_8$ ŠU ^{d}15 GÍD-*ma* GAM
5. DIŠ Á^{II}-*šú* IGI.BAR.MEŠ ŠED$_7$ ŠUB.ŠUB-*su* ŠU ^{d}15 MU TAG-*te u* NA$_4$.NUNUZ.MEŠ
6. DIŠ Á^{II}-*šú ú-na-aš-šak ina šag-gaš-ti* LÚ *ú-šaḫ-niq-ma ár-da-na-an* ÚŠ DIB-*su*
7. DIŠ A^{II}-*šú ik-ta-na-ṣa-a* ŠU ^{d}MAŠ.TAB.BA
8. DIŠ Á^{II}-*šú bir-ka-šú i-ta-na-na-ḫa ina pi-qam* ŠÀ-*šú* MUD-*ud*
9. *ina* KI.N[Á-*š*]*ú il-la-tu-šú* DU-*ak pi-qam la pi-qam in-né-ṣil* KÚM ŠÀ-*šú* TUKU.MEŠ
10. NA BI ÚḪ DIB-*su* KI.MIN GIDIM$_7$ DIB-*su*
11. DIŠ *ina* Á-*šú* SÌG-*iṣ* ŠU ^{d}MAŠ.TAB.BA
12. DIŠ *ina* Á-*šú u ki-ṣir* 1 KÙŠ.MEŠ-*šú* SÌG-*iṣ* ŠU ^{d}15
13. DIŠ MUD Á-*šú šá* 15 *ú-za-qat-su* ŠU ^{d}1[5]
14. DIŠ TA MUD Á-*šú* EN MURUB$_4$-*šú* KÚM TA MURUB$_4$-*šú* EN GÌR^{II}-*šú* ŠED$_7$ PAP.ḪAL.ME-*ma* SUR-*ma* DIN

15. DIŠ KÙŠ.MEŠ-*šú ana* SU-*šú* NU TE-*ḫi* ŠU 20 MU KÙ.BABBAR ZAG. GAR.RA
16. DIŠ KÙŠ.MEŠ-*šú kin-ṣi-šú u* GÌR^{II}-*šú* GU$_7$.MEŠ-*šú* ŠU ^{d}UTU
17. DIŠ KÙŠ.MEŠ-*šú* MURUB$_4$.ME-*šú u* GÌR^{II}-*šú* 1-*niš* GU$_7$.MEŠ-*šú* ŠU ^{d}15 MU TAG-*te*
18. DIŠ *ki-ṣir* KÙŠ.MEŠ-*šú ana* SAG-*šú* GAR.GAR-*an* ÚḪ.ME-*šú i-s*[*al-l*]*u* GIG *na-kam-ti* ŠU.ZAG.GAR.RA DIN

Translation

1–3. If the patient continually turns his head to the "right," his hands and his feet are immobilized, he closes and rolls his eyes and spittle flows from his mouth (and) he makes rumbling noises, AN.TA.ŠUB.BA. If when it afflicts him, his heart is awake, it can be removed. If when it afflicts him, he does not know who he is, it cannot be removed.[4]

4–6. If he continually turns his head to the "left," his hands and his feet are stretched out, his eyes are opened wide towards the sky, spittle flows from his mouth, he makes rumbling noises, he does not know who he is at the beginning when ⸢his⸣ [confusional state] comes over him, AN.TA.ŠUB. BA, "hand" of Sîn.[5]

7. If his neck hurts him, "hand" of his god (var. "hand" of Shamash on account of a vow promised by him); he will get well.[6]

8. If his neck hurts him (and) he continually ⸢asks⸣ for water, "hand" of Ishtar. He was injured on his neck; he will die.[7]

9. If his neck and his hips continually hurt him at once, "hand" of Adad.

10. If his neck, his hips, his hands and his feet are stiff, *šaššaṭu*.[8]

11. If he twists his neck and his eye jerks (and) he jerks (var. A: shudders) incessantly, *šaššaṭu*.[9]

12–13. If his neck throbs, his head continually drops, his hands and feet are continually stiff and he rubs (them) on the ground, *ardat lilî* afflicts him.[10]

14a. If he continually turns his head to "right" or "left," he will die.[11]

14b. If he continually lets his neck drop to the "right" or "left," he will die.[12]

15a. If his neck drops to the "right" or "left," he will die.[13]

15b. If his neck, whenever it is turned from "right" to "left," drops, ⸢he will die⸣.[14]

16. If he was injured on his neck, "hand" of Adad.[15]

17. If he was injured on his neck and his breast hurts him, "hand" of Ishtar for the sake of egg-shaped beads (which she wants).[16]

18. If he was injured on his neck and his virility is taken away "hand" of Ishtar; he will die.[17]
19. If he was injured on his neck and consequently his insides are continually cramped and his feet are raised up, affliction by a ghost.[18]
20. If he was injured on his neck and consequently his feet tremble (and) his insides are continually cramped, affliction by a ghost.[19]
21. If he was injured on his neck and consequently the upper part of his eyes continually hurts him, he continually produces blood from his mouth (and) his hands and his feet are sluggish, a *gallû* afflicts that person.[20]
22a. If a vertebra of his neck was (cut) open, he will die.[21]
22b. If a vertebra of his neck was (cut) open (and) his nostrils are continually "seized," he will die.[22]
23. If a vertebra of his neck was (cut) open, (and) his blood vessels are present, but his nostrils are continually "seized," he will die.
24. If a vertebra of his neck was (cut) open (and) his blood vessels are present but his breath is continually "seized" in his nose, that patient will not get well.[23]
25. If a vertebra of his neck was (cut) open (and) his blood vessels are present (but) his nose/mouth twitches (and) he does not [recognize] one known to him, [he will die].[24]
26. If he falls backwards and (lies) stretched out (and) he continually lets his neck drop to the "right" and "left," he will die.
27. If a person's muscles are stiff from his neck to his heel, his eyebrows are knitted (and) his jaws (feel like they) are pressured, *šaššaṭu*.[25]

---

28. If his larynx is constricted, he ate something offensive to his god (var. he will get through).[26]
29. If his larynx makes a croaking noise, he will die.[27]

---

30. If his breath becomes rapid and his insides are continually cramped, he will die.[28]
31a. If his breath becomes rapid (lit. "jumps"), and his muscles are tense,[29] he will die.[30]
31b. If his breath throbs and comes closely spaced, ⸢he will die.⸣[31]
32a. If he makes his breath go up, he will not get well.[32]
32b–33. If his breath is continually short like one who has just come up from the water, "hand" of ⸢Dingirmaḫ⸣, "hand" of Ningizzida or the "hand" of the ghost of one who [died] in the water [afflicts him].[33]
34a. If his larynx makes a croaking noise when he breathes, he will die.[34]

34b. If his chokings come close together and he is not in full possession of his faculties, [he will die].[35]

---

35. If persistent "grabbing of the throat"[36] continually afflicts him, the enmity of the gods [...]
36. If persistent "grabbing of the throat" continually afflicts him and he scratches [...]
37. If persistent "grabbing of the throat" continually afflicts him and he shudders, "hand" of Ishtar; [he will die].[37]
38. If persistent "grabbing of the throat" continually afflicts him and he wails, he will die and ⸢afterwards⸣ his father [will die].[38]
39. If persistent "grabbing of the throat" continually afflicts him and he twists, he will die and afterwards his mother [will die].[39]
40. If persistent "grabbing of the throat" continually afflicts him and he roars, he will die and afterwards his brother [will die].[40]

---

41. If the "right" side of his throat is red, he will get well. If the "left" side of his throat is red, even if it becomes difficult for him, he will get well.
42. If (both) sides of his throat are red, he will get well. If the "right" side of his throat is yellow, his illness will be prolonged. If the "left" side of his throat is yellow, he will die
43. If (both) sides of his throat are yellow, if it is prolonged, he will die. If the "right" side of his throat is black his illness will alter (for the worse).
44. If the "left" side of his throat is black his illness will be prolonged. If both sides of his throat are black, he will die.
45. If the "right" side of his throat is dark, his illness will exhaust (him). [If] the "left" ⸢side of his throat⸣ is dark, he will die.
46. If (both) sides of his throat are dark, he will die. If the "right" side of his throat is swollen, he will get well. If the "left" side of his throat is swollen, he will die.
47. If (both) sides of his throat are swollen, it will exhaust him so that he dies. If the ⸢"right"⸣ side of [his] throat is continually ⸢swollen⸣, his illness (will exhaust him so that he dies).
48. If the "left" side of his throat is continually swollen, his illness will be difficult. If ⸢(both) sides of his throat⸣ are continually swollen, he will die.[41]
49. If the "right" side of his throat (looks) skinned, it may exhaust him but he will get well.[42]
50. If the "left" side of his throat (looks) skinned, he will die. If both sides of his throat (look) skinned, he will die.

51. If (both) sides of his throat (look) skinned but his flesh is healthy, he will get well (var. it is worrisome).[43]
52. If (both) sides of his throat (look) skinned and his flesh (looks) bruised[44] and is spotted with red dye-red spots, ⌜(it is worrisome)⌝.[45]
53. If (both) sides of his throat (look) bruised, his feet are raised up (and) it keeps him awake all night, the "hand" of the god of his city (var. A: "hand" of his god) has been placed [on him] for death.[46]
54a. If (both) sides of his throat (look) bruised and continually hurt him, "hand" of ghost.[47]
54b. If he was injured on his throat, "hand" of the ⌜twin gods⌝; [he will die].[48]
55. [If his "right" arm is dark (and) he is tongue-tied, he was injured from behind; he will die.] [49]
56. [If his "left" arm is dark (and) he is tongue-tied, he was injured on the front side; he will die.]
57. [If his "right" arm is dark and he twists ...]

B rev.

1. If his "left" arm [is dark (and) he twists, blow of Sîn]; ⌜he will die⌝.[50]
2. If he is ⌜unable⌝ to turn his arms and his [anus] drips his excrement and blood, he will die.[51]
3. If he is unable to turn his arms and he excretes blood, he was injured on the back side; he will die.[52]
4. If he is unable to turn his arms and he vomits blood, "hand" of Ishtar. If it is prolonged, he will die.[53]
5. If he continually gazes at his arms (and) cold continually falls upon him, "hand" of Ishtar on account of touching the cheek and egg-shaped beads.
6. If he chews on his arms, he had a person strangled to death in a brawl and the "double" of the dead person afflicts him.[54]
7. If his arms are continually cold, "hand" of the twin gods.[55]
8–10. If his arms and knees continually become tired, his heart flutters suddenly, his spittle flows (when he is) in ⌜his bed⌝, he is incessantly sluggish (and) he continually has intestinal fever, sorcerous spittle afflicts that person. Alternatively, a ghost afflicts him.[56]
11. If he was injured on his arm, "hand" of the twin gods.[57]
12. If he was injured on his arm and his elbows, "hand" of Ishtar.
13. If his "right" arm socket stings him, "hand" of ⌜Ištar⌝.[58]
14. If he is hot from his arm socket to his hip (and) cold from his hip to his feet, he may have a difficult time of it, but if he comes through, he will get well.

---

15. If he does not bring his forearms close to his body, "hand" of Shamash on account of silver for a tithe.[59]
16. If his forearms, his shins and his feet continually hurt him, "hand" of Shamash.[60]
17. If his forearms, his hip region and his feet all continually hurt him at the same time, "hand" of Ishtar on account of touching the cheek.[61]
18. If he continually places his elbows on his head (and) he ⌜sprays⌝ his spit, he (has) a sickness of excess(?),[62] "hand" of a tithe; he will get well.[63]

Notes

1. The remainder of this line was broken away "*he-pí*" on the tablet from which the ancient scribe copied our tablet. It can be restored from a precursor to the Diagnostic and Prognostic Series, which was found at the Hittite capital Ḫattuša (Wilhelm 1994, 62: obv. 4).
2. Restored from a parallel passage DPS 15:9.
3. Restored from a parallel passage DPS 15:10.
4. See Scurlock and Andersen 2005, 8.5, 13.118, 13.193.
5. See Scurlock and Andersen 2005, 13.116, 13.194, 19.266.
6. See Scurlock and Andersen 2005, 11.42.
7. See Scurlock and Andersen 2005, 13.138, 19.150. This entry also appears in DPS 15:6′.
8. See Scurlock and Andersen 2005, 3.199. This entry also appears in DPS 33:95.
9. See Scurlock and Andersen 2005, 3.197, 13.68, 13.107. This entry also appears in DPS 33:96.
10. See Scurlock and Andersen 2005, 4.30, 16.65.
11. See Scurlock and Andersen 2005, 13.251, 13.283.
12. See Scurlock and Andersen 2005, 13.246, 13.283.
13. This entry appears also in Wilhelm 1994, 62 J 1:5.
14. See Scurlock and Andersen 2005, 13.246, 13.284.
15. See Scurlock and Andersen 2005, 19.148. This entry also appears in Wilhelm 1994, 35 obv. 15′//Wilhelm 1994, 57 obv. 5′
16. See Scurlock and Andersen 2005, 19.274.
17. See Scurlock and Andersen 2005, 5.68, 13.139, 19.149, 19.274.
18. See Scurlock and Andersen 2005, 13.140.
19. See Scurlock and Andersen 2005, 13.83, 19.171.
20. See Scurlock and Andersen 2005, 13.46, 13.141, 19.171.
21. See Scurlock and Andersen 2005, 13.143. This is similar to DPS 21:16 and Wilhelm 1994, 60 obv. 7.
22. See Scurlock and Andersen 2005, 13.143.
23. See Scurlock and Andersen 2005, 13.144, 20.33. This entry also appears in SpTU 3.86 obv. 3–4.
24. The entry appears also in Wilhelm 1994, 62 obv. 4.
25. See Scurlock and Andersen 2005, 3.196. This entry appears also in DPS 33:97 and Arnaud 1987, 694 obv. 6′.
26. See Scurlock and Andersen 2005, 8.88, 16.26. This entry appears also in DPS 15:7′.
27. See Scurlock and Andersen 2005, 3.58, 20.31.
28. See Scurlock and Andersen 2005, 8.18, 13.278.

29. See Scurlock and Andersen 2005, p. 212.
30. See Scurlock and Andersen 2005, 8.19, 13.278, 20.34.
31. See Scurlock and Andersen 2005, 8.19, 13.278, 20.34.
32. See Scurlock and Andersen 2005, 8.20.
33. See Scurlock and Andersen 2005, 8.77.
34. See Scurlock and Andersen 2005, 3.57.
35. See Scurlock and Andersen 2005, 3.57. This entry also appears in DPS 15:8′.
36. Pace *CAD* D, 80a, this is not "shortness of breath" for which there is a different expression.
37. See Scurlock and Andersen 2005, 19.288.
38. See Scurlock and Andersen 2005, 20.30.
39. See Scurlock and Andersen 2005, 2.11, 3.59.
40. See Scurlock and Andersen 2005, 2.11, 3.60.
41. See Scurlock and Andersen 2005, 3.56.
42. See Scurlock and Andersen 2005, 3.50.
43. See Scurlock and Andersen 2005, 3.51.
44. See Scurlock and Andersen 2005, p. 216.
45. See Scurlock and Andersen 2005, 3.52, 10.59.
46. See Scurlock and Andersen 2005, 19.293.
47. See Scurlock and Andersen 2005, 19.248.
48. See Scurlock and Andersen 2005, 14.11, 19.182.
49. This entry appears in DPS 15:9′.
50. See Scurlock and Andersen 2005, 19.201. This entry appears in DPS 15:10′.
51. This entry appears in DPS 15:11′.
52. See Scurlock and Andersen 2005, 13.136. This or the following entry appears in DPS 15:12′.
53. See Scurlock and Andersen 2005, 19.160.
54. See Scurlock and Andersen 2005, 16.79, 19.28. A similar entry appears in DPS 11 obv. 40.
55. See Scurlock and Andersen 2005, 19.134, 19.237.
56. See Scurlock and Andersen 2005, 8.10.
57. See Scurlock and Andersen 2005, 19.135.
58. This entry appears in VAT 11122 obv. 4 (Heeßel 2010, 181–84).
59. See Scurlock and Andersen 2005, 19.3. This entry may be cited in VAT 10748: 12′ (Heeßel 2010, 178–81).
60. See Scurlock and Andersen 2005, 11.43.
61. See Scurlock and Andersen 2005, 11.52.
62. Literally: "store house, reserves."
63. See Scurlock and Andersen 2005, 19.4.

DPS TABLET 11

DPS 10 B rev. 19 (catchline) = DPS 11:1

1. DIŠ GIG *rit-ta-šú šá* 15 GU_7-*šú* ŠU ^{d}UTU *ana ik-rib qí-bit* KA-*šú* DIN
2. DIŠ *rit-ta-šú šá* 150 GU_7-*šú* [...]

3. DIŠ *rit-ta-a-šú* GU$_7$.MEŠ-*šú* [...]
4. DIŠ IGI KIŠIB.MEŠ-*šú ana* UD.5.KAM *im-ta*-x-[...]

---

5. DIŠ ŠU-*su šá* 15 GU$_7$-*šú* ŠU ^{d}UTU
6. DIŠ ŠU-*su šá* 150 GU$_7$-*šú* [...]
7. DIŠ ŠU-*su šá* 15 *ana* KA-*šú tur-ra* NU ZU-*e šá* 150 *ana tur-ra aš*-⸢*ṭa*⸣-[*át* ...]
8. DIŠ ŠU-*su šá* 150 *ana* KA-*šú tur-ra* NU ZU-e *šá* 15 *ana tur-ra aš-ṭa-át* KI.[MIN]
9. DIŠ ŠU-*su ina* LI.DUR-*šú* GAR-*at-ma* ŠU^{II}-*šú u* GÌR^{II}-*šú* ŠED$_7$ *ina* NU ZU DUG$_4$.DUG$_4$-*ub* ZI-*bi* [*u* TÚŠ-*ab ina* LI.DUR-*šú* SÌG-*iṣ* ŠU ^{d}*Dil-bat* GAM]
10. DIŠ ŠU^{II}-*šú* SA$_5$.MEŠ *u* UZU.MEŠ-*šú ṣar-pu* [...]
B9 DIŠ ŠU^{II}-*šú* SA$_5$.MEŠ *u* UZU.MEŠ-*šú* S[IG$_7$ ...]
11. DIŠ ŠU^{II}-*šú* SIG$_7$.MEŠ *u* UZU.MEŠ-*šú* SIG$_7$.MEŠ [...]
12. DIŠ ŠU^{II}-*šú* SIG$_7$.MEŠ *u* U.MEŠ-*šú pu-ṣa* ŠUB [...]
B11. DIŠ ŠU^{II}-*šú* SIG$_7$.MEŠ *u* IGI^{II}-*šú pu-ṣa* ŠU[B ...]
13. DIŠ ŠU^{II}-*šú* GI$_6$.MEŠ SÌG-*iṣ* SAG.[TUKU ...]
14. DIŠ ŠU^{II}-*šú* GI$_6$.MEŠ-*ma* AD$_6$-*šú ma-ši* SÌG-*i*[*ṣ* SAG.TUKU ...]
15. DIŠ ŠU^{II}-*šú* GI$_6$.MEŠ-*ma* AD$_6$-*šú* KÚM-*im* [...]
16. DIŠ ŠU^{II}-*šú* GI$_6$.MEŠ-*ma u* UZU.MEŠ-*šú* SIG$_7$.MEŠ [...]
17. DIŠ ŠU^{II}-*šú i-ra-ʾ-ú-ba* ŠU DINGIR TI.[LA]
18. DIŠ ŠU^{II}-*šú it-te-nen-ṣi-la-šú u it-ta-nak-na-an-na* ŠU ^{d}*D*[*il-bat* ...]
19. DIŠ ŠU^{II}-*šú ana* SU-*šú* NU TE-*a* ŠU ^{d}UTU MU KÙ.BABBAR [ZAG.GAR.RA]
20. DIŠ ŠU^{II}-*šú am-šá-ma ta-ra-ṣa* NU ZU-*e u* UŠ$_4$-*šú* NU DIB Š[U 20 GAM][1]
21. DIŠ ŠU^{II}-*šú ina* IGI.MEŠ-*šú* NU DU$_8$.MEŠ MAŠKIM ÍD [...]
22. DIŠ ŠU^{II}-*šú ina* UGU-*šú* NU DU$_8$.MEŠ MAŠKIM SÌG ŠU [...]
23. DIŠ ŠU^{II}-*šú ina* SAG.DU-*šú* NU DU$_8$.MEŠ-*ni* ŠU ^{d}DÌM.ME *ú*-[...]
24. DIŠ ŠU^{II}-*šú ina* SAG.DU-*šú* GAR-*na-ma la ur-ra-da-ni* ŠU ^{d}LUGAL.GÌR.RA *u* ^{d}MES.L[AM.TA.È.A ...]
25. DIŠ ŠU^{II}-*šú ina* SAG.DU-*šú* GAR-*na-ma la ur-ra-da-ni* ŠÀ.MEŠ-*šú na-šú-u* KÚM *ṣa-ri-i*[*ḫ ina* SAG ŠÀ-*šú* SÌG-*iṣ* GAM][2]
26. DIŠ ŠU^{II}-*šú ina* KA-*šú* GAR-*na-ma ta-tab-bal-ma ana* KA-*šú ú-tar* [GAM]
27. [DIŠ Š]U^{II}-*šú ina* KA-*šú ú-man-zaq* KÚM ÚḪ ŠÀ.ME-*šú* ÍL-*ú u ú-ra*[*p-pad* ...]

28. [DIŠ] ŠU^{II}-*šú ana* KA-*šú ú-ṭeb-be* TÚG-*su it-ta-na-suk u* UŠ$_4$-*šú* NU [DIB *lu-ʾ-a-tú šu-kul* GAM][3]
29. [DIŠ] ŠU^{II}-*šú* AD$_6$-*šú* TAG.MEŠ GÍD-[*ma* GAM]
30. [DIŠ ŠU^{II}-*šú*] AD$_6$-*šú ma-gal* TAG.MEŠ GIN$_7$ TAG.MEŠ NU ZU [GAM]
31. [DIŠ ŠU^{II}-*š*]*ú* SAG.DU-*su ma-gal* TAG.MEŠ [...]
32. [DIŠ Š]U^{II}-*šú ka-ma-ma* GÌR^{II}-*šú šad-da* : *šad-na* DINGIR [...]
33. [DIŠ ŠU^{II}-*š*]*ú it-ta-na-aš-gag-ga* [...]
34. [DIŠ ŠU^{II}-*šú i*]*t-ta-na-aš-gag-ga ù* GÌR^{II}-*šú nu-up-pu-ḫ*[*a* ...]
35. [DIŠ ŠU^{II}-*šú*] ⸢*ú*⸣-*ta-ṣa-la* : *ú-ta-ka-ṣa ut-tap-pa-ḫ*[*a* ...]
36. [DIŠ ŠU^{II}-*šú ú-ḫa-a*]*m-ma-aṣ* EME-*šú* ⸢*ú*⸣-*na-aṭ-ṭa* ÚḪ-[*su* ...]
37. [DIŠ ŠU^{II}-*šú* IGI.BA]R.MEŠ *u uš-ta-*[*na*]*b-lak-kát* [...]
38. [DIŠ ŠU^{II}-*šú* IG]I.BAR.MEŠ BAL.BAL Z[I]-*bi u* DU$_{10}$.GAM *ina* SAG [GI$_6$ TAG-*it* ...]
39. [DIŠ ŠU^{II}-*šú u* G]ÌR^{II}-*šú* GI$_6$.MEŠ *uš-ta-nab-lak-kát* ZI-*bi u* D[U$_{10}$.GAM ...]
40. [DIŠ ŠU^{II}-*šú*] ⸢*ú*⸣-*na-aš-šak ina šag-gaš-*[*ti* LÚ *ú-šaḫ-niq-ma ár-da-na-an* ÚŠ DIB-*su*][4]
41. [DIŠ ŠU^{II}-*šú*] ⸢*ú-na*⸣-[*aš*]-⸢*šak*⸣ [...]
42. [DIŠ ŠU^{II}-*š*]*ú* KÚM-*ma* [GÌR]^{II}-*šú us-su-la* [...]
43. [DIŠ ŠU^{II}-*š*]*ú* KÚM-*ma* GÌR^{II}-*šú* ŠED$_7$.ME [...]
44. [DIŠ ŠU^{II}-*š*]*ú* ŠED$_7$.ME GÌR^{II}-*šú* KÚM-*ma* [...]
45. [DIŠ ŠU^{II}]-*šú u* GÌR^{II}-*šú* ŠED$_7$ GIG-*su* KÚR-*šum-ma* UGU-[*šú i-sap-pi-du-ma* DIN][5]
46. [DIŠ ŠU^{II}]-*šú u zu-ḫar* GÌR^{II}-*šú* ŠED$_7$.ME [...]
47. [DIŠ ŠU^{II}]-*šú* ŠED$_7$.ME-*a* [...]
48. [DIŠ ŠU^{II}]-*šú i-nap-pa-ṣa u* GÌR^{II}-*šú* KÚM-*ma* [...]
49. [DIŠ ŠU^{II}-*šú u* G]ÌR^{II}-*šú i-nap-pa-ṣa u* GÌR^{II}-*šú am-*[*šá* ...]
50. [DIŠ ŠU^{II}-*šú u* GÌR^{II}-*šú*] ⸢*i*⸣-*nap-pa-ṣa u zu-ḫar* GÌR^{II}-*šú* [...]
51. [DIŠ ŠU^{II}-*šú u* GÌR^{II}-*šú i*]-⸢*nap*⸣-*pa-ṣa u* SU-*šú* ŠED[$_7$ ...]
52. [DIŠ ŠU^{II}-*šú* ...]x.MEŠ-*šú* [...]
53. [DIŠ ŠU^{II}-*šú u* GÌR^{II}-*šú* M]Ú.MEŠ-*ḫa* [...]
54. [DIŠ ŠU^{II}-*šú u* GÌR^{II}-*šú* MÚ.M]EŠ-*ḫa u* KÚM *la ḫa-*[*aḫ-ḫaš* ...]
55. [DIŠ ŠU^{II}-*šú u* GÌR^{II}-*šú it-te-n*]*en-ṣi-la*[-*šú* ...]
56. (broken)

rev.

1 (broken)

2. [DIŠ ŠU^{II}-*šú u* GÌR^{II}-*šú*] ⸢*ú*⸣-*za-ár* ÚḪ *ina* KA-*š*[*ú* ...]
3. [DIŠ ...-*š*]*ú ik-tap-pa* : DIŠ *i*[*m-* ...]
4. [DIŠ ...] *i-kas-sa-sa* NIN-x[...]

5. [...G]ÌR-*šú a-ku-tam* DU-*ak* [...]
6. [DIŠ SA.MEŠ ŠU^{II}-*šú*] SA$_5$.MEŠ [...]
7. [DIŠ SA.MEŠ ŠU^{II}-*šú*] SIG$_7$.MEŠ [...]
8. [DIŠ SA.MEŠ ŠU^{II}]-*šú* MÚD *il-te-qu-ú* [...]
9. [DIŠ SA.MEŠ Š]U^{II}-*šú* DIB.MEŠ [...]
10. [DIŠ SA.MEŠ Š]U^{II}-*šú* AN.TA DU.MEŠ-*ma* KI.TA [...]
11. [DIŠ SA.MEŠ Š]U^{II}-*šú* KI.TA DU.MEŠ-*ma* AN.TA [...]
12. [DIŠ SA.MEŠ Š]U^{II}-*šú* AN.TA *u* KI.TA DU.[MEŠ ...]
13. [DIŠ SA.MEŠ Š]U^{II}-*šú tab-ku šá* GÌR^{II}-*šú* ZI.MEŠ IGI^{II}-*š*[*ú* ...]
14. [DIŠ SA.MEŠ Š]U^{II}-*šú šá* 15 *tab-ku-ma* : DU-*ku-ma ù* [...]
15. [DIŠ SA.MEŠ ŠU^{I}]^{I}-*šú šá* 15 DU-*ku-ma* SAG ŠÀ-*šú* G[U$_7$-*šú* ...]
16. [DIŠ SA.MEŠ ŠU^{I}]^{I}-*šú* DU.MEŠ-*ma šá* GÌR^{II}-*šú ne*[*-e-ḫu* ...]
17. [DIŠ SA.MEŠ ŠU^{I}]^{I}-*šú* DU.MEŠ-*ma šá* GÌR^{II}-*šú* GAR-*n*[*u* ...]
18. [DIŠ SA.MEŠ ŠU]^{II}-*šú* DU.MEŠ-*ma šá* SAG.KI-*šú* GAR-*nu* : *šá* U[GU-*šú* ...]
19. [DIŠ SA.MEŠ ŠU^{II}]-*šú u* GÌR^{II}-*šú šá* 15 DU.MEŠ-*ma šá* 150 G[AR-*nu* ...]
20. [DIŠ SA.MEŠ ŠU^{II}]-*šú u* GÌR^{II}-*šú* AN.TA DU.MEŠ-*ma* KI.TA *n*[*e-e-ḫu* ...]
21. [DIŠ SA.MEŠ ŠU^{II}]-*šú u* GÌR^{II}-*šú* AN.TA *u* KI.TA DU.ME SÌG-*iṣ* MAŠKIM MAŠ.M[AŠ-*su* DÙ-*ma* DIN] (coll.)
22. [DIŠ SA.MEŠ ŠU^{II}-*š*]*ú u* GÌR^{II}-*šú* 1-*niš* DU.MEŠ [...]
23. [DIŠ SA.MEŠ ŠU^{II}-*š*]*ú u* GÌR^{II}-*šú* 1-*niš* DU.MEŠ KÚM ÚḪ *u* SA[G ...]
24. [DIŠ SA.MEŠ ŠU^{II}]-*šú u* GÌR^{II}-*šú* 1-*niš* DU.MEŠ KÚM ÚḪ *u* SAG [...]
25. [DIŠ SA.MEŠ ŠU^{II}-*š*]*ú u* GÌR^{II}-*šú* 1-*niš* DU.MEŠ KÚM ÚḪ *u* SAG-*š*[*ú*...]
26. [DIŠ SA.MEŠ ŠU^{II}-*š*]*ú u* GÌR^{II}-*šú* 1-*niš* DU.MEŠ KÚM ÚḪ *ina* SU-*šú* [...]
27. [DIŠ SA.MEŠ Š]U^{II}-*šú u* GÌR^{II}-*šú* 1-*niš* DU.MEŠ KÚM ÚḪ *ina* SU-*šú* [...]
28. [DIŠ SA.MEŠ Š]U^{II}-*šú u* GÌR^{II}-*šú* 1-*niš* DU.MEŠ-*ma* KI.TA GÌR^{II}-*šú* x[...]
29. [DIŠ SA.ME]Š ŠU^{II}-*šú u* GÌR^{II}-*šú* ZI.MEŠ-*ma* IGI^{II}-*šú* DUGUD-*šú* SAG.DU [...]
30. [DIŠ MURU]B$_4$ ŠU^{II}-*šú* SIG$_7$ ŠUB-*di u* U.MEŠ-*šú* ÚḪ!.MEŠ [...]
31. [DIŠ MURU]B ŠU^{II}-*šú* SIG$_7$ ŠUB-*di u* ŠU^{II}-*šú* DU$_8$.DU$_8$-*r*[*a* ...]
32. [DIŠ U].MEŠ ŠU^{II}-*šú pa-áš-ṭa* [...]
33. [DIŠ U.MEŠ] ŠU^{II}-*šú* GI$_6$.MEŠ [...]
34. DIŠ U.MEŠ [Š]U^{II}-*šú* GI$_6$.MEŠ [...]
35. DIŠ U.MEŠ ŠU^{II}-*šú it-te-nen-ṣi-la-šú* [...]

36. DIŠ U.MEŠ ŠU^{II}-*šú ina* KA-*šú ú-man-zaq* KÚM ÚḪ ŠÀ-*šú* [*na-pi-iḫ u ú-rap-pad ina* GÚ-*šú* SÌG-*iṣ* ŠU ^{d}*Ba-ú* GAM][6]
37. DIŠ U.MEŠ ŠU^{II}-*šú šá* 15 MÚD DIRI.MEŠ-*ma* GU$_7$.MEŠ-*šú* […]
38. DIŠ U.MEŠ ŠU^{II}-*šú šá* 150 MÚD DIRI.MEŠ-*ma* GU$_7$.MEŠ-*šú* […]
39. DIŠ U.MEŠ ŠU^{II}-*šú šá* 15 *u* 150 MÚD DIRI.MEŠ-*ma* GU$_7$.MEŠ-*šú* […]
40. DIŠ U.MEŠ ŠU^{II}-*šú u* GÌR^{II}-*šú šá* 15 *u* 150 MÚD DIRI.MEŠ-*ma* GU$_7$.MEŠ-*šú* […]
41. DIŠ U.MEŠ ŠU^{II}-*šú šá* 15 ZÉ DIRI-*ma* GU$_7$.MEŠ-*šú* […]
42. DIŠ U.MEŠ ŠU^{II}-*šú šá* 150 ZÉ DIRI-*ma* GU$_7$.MEŠ-*šú* […]
43. DIŠ U.MEŠ ŠU^{II}-*šú u* GÌR^{II}-*šú* GU$_7$.MEŠ-*šú* […]
44. DIŠ U.MEŠ ŠU^{II}-*šú u* GÌR^{II}-*šú* MÚ.MEŠ-*ḫa* […]
45. DIŠ U.MEŠ ŠU^{II}-*šú u* GÌR^{II}-*šú it-te-nen-ṣi-la-šú* […]
46. DIŠ U.MEŠ ŠU^{II}-*šú u* GÌR^{II}-*šú šàg-ga u* GIŠ.KUN.MEŠ-[*šú* …]
47. DIŠ U.MEŠ ŠU^{II}-*šú u* GÌR^{II}-*šú* SIG$_7$ ŠUB-*a u* GIŠ.KUN.MEŠ-[*šú* ..]
48. DIŠ U.MEŠ-*šú* SIG$_7$ ŠUB-*a* ŠU ^{d}*Iš-ḫa-ra* NU DIN : [DIŠ U.M]EŠ-⸢*šú*⸣ SI[G$_7$ …] / [DIŠ U.MEŠ-*š*]*ú* S[IG$_7$ …]
49. DIŠ U.MEŠ-*šú* GI$_6$.MEŠ GABA.MEŠ U.MEŠ-*šú* DU$_8$.ME[Š …]
50. DIŠ U.MEŠ-*šú ina* KA-*šú* GAR-*na-ma ta-tab-bal-ma a*[*na* KA-*šú ú-tar* ÚŠ-*ma* EGIR-*šú ina* É-*šú* ÚŠ GAM][7]
51. DIŠ U.MEŠ-*šú ú-za-ár* IGI^{II}-*šú it-ta-na-az-*[*qa-pa* …]
52. DIŠ U.MEŠ-*šú i-lam-ma-am u* NUNDUN NÍ-*šú* GU$_7$ […]
53. DIŠ *ap-pat* U.MEŠ-*šú* SA$_5$.MEŠ GAM : […]
54. DIŠ ŠE U.MEŠ-*šú im-taq-tu u* GI$_6$ GAM : DIŠ ŠE U.[MEŠ-*šú* …]
55. DIŠ *kar-ši* U.MEŠ-*šú* SIG$_7$.MEŠ GAM ⸢:⸣ […]
56. DIŠ *kar-ši* U.MEŠ-*šú* GI$_6$ *tur-ru-pa* GAM […]
57. DIŠ *kar-ši* U.MEŠ-*šú* SA$_5$.MEŠ […]
58. DIŠ *kar-ši* U.MEŠ-*šú sa-am-ta im-t*[*aḫ-ṣa* …]
59. DIŠ *kar-ši* U.MEŠ-*šú sa-am-ta i*[*m-taḫ-ṣa* …]
60. DIŠ UMBIN GIG *te-eḫ-*[…

TRANSLATION

obv.

1. If the patient's "right" hand hurts him, "hand" of Shamash because of a vow which he promised; he will get well.[8]
2. If his "left" hand hurts him […].
3. If (both) his hands hurt him […].
4. If the top part of his hands […] for five days […].

---

5. If his "right" hand hurts him, "hand" of Shamash.

6. If his "left" hand hurts him [...].
7. If he is unable to turn his "right" hand to his mouth (and) his "left" turns ⌜stiffly⌝ [...].[9]
8. If he is unable to turn his "left" hand to his mouth (and) his "right" turns stiffly, ⌜ditto⌝.[10]
9. If his hand is placed on his navel and his hands and his feet are cold, he continually talks without knowing (what he is saying and) he gets up [and sits down (again), he was injured on his navel. "Hand" of Ishtar; he will die].[11]
10. If his hands are red and his flesh is bright red [...].
B9. If his hands are red and his flesh is ⌜yellow⌝ [...].[12]
11. If his hands are yellow and his flesh is yellow [...].[13]
12. If his hands are yellow and his fingers are unevenly colored with white spots [...].[14]
B11. If his hands are yellow and his eyes are ⌜unevenly colored⌝ with white spots [...].[15]
13. If his hands are dark/black, blow of a ⌜*rābiṣu*⌝ [...].
14. If his hands are dark/black and he loses consciousness, blow of [a *rābiṣu* ...].[16]
15. If his hands are dark/black and his body is feverish [...].[17]
16. If his hands are dark/black and his flesh is yellow [...].
17. If his hands tremble, "hand" of god; he will get well.
18. If his hands are continually sluggish and are continually contorted, "hand" of ⌜Ištar⌝ [...].[18]
19. If he does not bring his hands close to his body, "hand" of Shamash on account of silver [for a tithe].[19]
20. If his hands are immobilized so that he is unable to stretch (them) out and he is not in full possession of his faculties, ⌜"hand"⌝ of [Shamash; he will die].[20]
21. If his hands never leave his face, the *rābiṣu* of the river [afflicts him].
22. If his hands never leave his skull, a *rābiṣu* has struck (him); "hand" of [...].[21]
23. If his hands never leave his head, "hand" of Lamashtu [...].
24. If his hands are placed on his head and he does not bring them down, "hand" of LUGAL.GÌR.RA and ⌜MES.LAM.TA.È.A⌝ [...].[22]
25. If his hands are continually placed on his head and he does not bring them down, his insides are puffed up, (and) he burns with fever,[23] [he was injured on his epigastrium; he will die].[24]

26. If his hands are placed in his mouth and (if) you take (them) out, he returns (them) to his mouth, [he will die].[25]
27. [If] he sucks his ⸢hands⸣ in his mouth, he burns with fever,[26] his insides are puffed up and he ⸢wanders about⸣ […].
28. [If] he sticks his hands into his mouth, he continually throws off his garment and he is not in full [possession] of his faculties, [he has been made to eat dirty substances; he will die].[27]
29. [If] his hands continually rub his body, [if] it is prolonged, [he will die].[28]
30. [If his hands] continually rub his body a lot (and) he does not realize that they are continually rubbing (it), [he will die].[29]
31. [If his hands] continually rub his head a lot […]
32. [If] his ⸢hands⸣ are "bound" and his feet are pulled taut (var. …) […].[30]
33. [If his hands] continually become stiff […].[31]
34. [If his hands] continually become stiff and his feet are swollen […].
35. If his hands become sluggish (var. become stiff) (and) become swollen, […].[32]
36. [If he ⸢rubs⸣ [his hands (against each other)], he licks(?) with his tongue, his spittle […].
37. [If he] continually ⸢gazes⸣ at [his hands] and he has ⸢changes of mood⸣ […].
38. [If] he continually ⸢gazes⸣ at [his hands], he has changes of mood, he ⸢gets up⸣ and (has to) squat down, (and) [he is particularly affected] at the beginning of [the night …].[33]
39. [If his hands and] his ⸢feet⸣ are dark/black, he has changes of mood (and) gets up and ⸢(has to) squat down⸣ […].[34]
40. [If] he chews on [his hands, he had a person strangled] to ⸢death⸣ in a brawl [and the "double" of the dead person afflicts him].[35]
41. [If] he ⸢chews on⸣ [his hands …].
42. [If his hands] are hot (and) his ⸢feet⸣ are sluggish […].
43. [If his hands] are hot (and) his feet are cold […].
44. [If his hands] are cold (and) his feet are hot […].[36]
45. [If] his [hands] (and) his feet are cold, even if his illness changes on him so that [they beat their breasts] over [him, he will get well].[37]
46. [If] his [hands] and the soles of his feet are cold […].
47. [If] his [hands] are cold […].
48. [If] his [hands] thrash around and his feet are hot […]
49. [If his hands and] his ⸢feet⸣ thrash around and his feet are ⸢immobilized⸣ […].
50. [If his hands and his feet] thrash around and the soles of his feet are […].

51. [If his hands and his feet] ⌜thrash around⌝ and his body is ⌜cold⌝ […].
52. *(fragmentary)*
53. [If his hands (and his feet)] are ⌜swollen⌝ […].
54. [If his hands (and his feet)] are ⌜swollen⌝ and (he has) a ⌜lukewarm temperature⌝ […].
55. [If his hands (and his feet)] are ⌜continually sluggish⌝ […].
56. *(fragmentary)*

rev.

1. *(fragmentary)*
2. [If] he twists [his hands (and his feet)] (and) spittle [flows] from ⌜his⌝ mouth […].

3–5. *(fragmentary)*

6. [If the muscles of his hands] are red […].
7. [If the muscles of his hands] are yellow […].
8. [If the blood vessels] of his [hands] take up blood […].[38]
9. [If the blood vessels] of his ⌜hands⌝ continually afflict him […].
10. [If the blood vessels] of his ⌜hands⌝, the ones above continually "go" but the ones below […].
11. [If the blood vessels] of his ⌜hands⌝, the ones below continually "go" but the ones above […].
12. [If the blood vessels] of his ⌜hands⌝, the ones above and the ones below [continually] "go" […].[39]
13. [If the blood vessels] of his ⌜hands⌝ are tense[40] (and) those of his feet (feel like they are) pulsating, ⌜his⌝ eyes […].[41]
14. [If the blood vessels] of his ⌜hands⌝, the ones on the "right" are tense (var: "go" but) […].[42]
15. [If the blood vessels] of his ⌜hands⌝, the ones on the "right" "go" and his epigastrium ⌜hurts⌝ [him …].
16. [If the blood vessels] of his ⌜hands⌝ "go" and those of his feet are ⌜slow⌝ […].
17. [If the blood vessels] of his ⌜hands⌝ "go" and those of his feet are present […].
18. [If the blood vessels of] his ⌜hands⌝ "go" but those of his forehead (var. his ⌜skull⌝ are present […].
19. [If the blood vessels] of his [hands] and his feet, the ones on the "right" "go" but the ones on the "left" are ⌜present.⌝
20. [If the blood vessels] of his [hands] and his feet, the ones above continually "go" and the ones below are ⌜slow.⌝

21. [If the blood vessels] of his [hands] and his feet, the ones above and the ones below "go," blow of a *rābiṣu*. [If you do his] ⌜treatment⌝, [he will get well].
22. [If the blood vessels] of ⌜his⌝ [hands] and his feet "go" at the same time [...].
23. [If the blood vessels] of ⌜his⌝ [hands] and his feet "go" at the same time, he burns with fever and [his] ⌜head⌝ [...].
24. [If the blood vessels] of his [hands] and his feet "go" at the same time, he burns with fever (and) [his] head [...].
25. [If the blood vessels] of ⌜his⌝ [hands] and his feet "go" at the same time, he burns with fever and ⌜his⌝ head [...].[43]
26. [If the blood vessels] of ⌜his⌝ [hands] and his feet "go" at the same time, he burns with fever (and) in his body [...].
27. [If the blood vessels] of his ⌜hands⌝ and his feet "go" at the same time, he burns with fever (and) in his body [...].[44]
28. [If the blood vessels] of his ⌜hands⌝ and his feet "go" at the same time and the bottoms of his feet [...].[45]
29. [If the blood vessels] of his hands and his feet (feel like they are) pulsating and his eyes (feel) heavy (and) [his] head [...].[46]
30. [If] the ⌜middle part⌝ of his hands is unevenly colored with yellow and his fingers feel burning hot [...].
31. [If the ⌜middle part⌝ of his hands is unevenly colored with yellow and his hands were (cut) open [...].
32. [If the finger]s of his hands are rubbed off [...].[47]
33. [If the fingers] of his hands are dark (and) [...].
34. If the fingers of his ⌜hands⌝ are dark [...].
35. If the fingers of his hands are continually sluggish [...].[48]
36. If he sucks his fingers in his mouth, he burns with fever[49] his abdomen [is bloated and he wanders about, he was injured on his neck. "Hand" of Bau; he will die].[50]
37. If the fingers of his hands, the ones on the "right" are full of blood and continually hurt him [...].[51]
38. If the fingers of his hands, the ones on the "left" are full of blood and continually hurt him [...].[52]
39. If the fingers of his hands, the ones on the "right" and "left" are full of blood and continually hurt him [...].[53]
40. If the digits of his hands and his feet, the ones on the "right" and "left" are full of blood and continually hurt him [....].[54]

41. If the fingers of his hands, the ones on the "right" are full of venom[55] and continually hurt him […].[56]
42. If the fingers of his hands, the ones on the "left" are full of venom and continually hurt him […].
43. If the digits of his hands and his feet continually hurt him […].[57]
44. If the digits of his hands and his feet are continually swollen […].[58]
45. If the digits of his hands and his feet are continually sluggish […].[59]
46. If the digits of his hands and his feet are stiff(?) and [his] pelvis […].
47. If the digits of his hands and his feet are unevenly colored with yellow and [his] pelvis […].
48. If his fingers are unevenly colored with yellow, "hand" of Ishhara; he will not get well.[60] [If] his [fingers are unevenly colored] with ⌈yellow⌉ […] [If] ⌈his⌉ [fingers are unevenly colored] with ⌈yellow⌉ […].
49. If his fingers are dark (and) the "breasts" of his fingers were (cut) open […].
50. If his fingers are placed in his mouth and (if) you take (them) out, [he returns (them)] ⌈to⌉ [his mouth, he will die and afterwards there will be a(nother) death in his household].[61]
51. If he twists his fingers and (the pupils of) his eyes are continually ⌈constricted⌉ […].
52. If he chews his fingers and eats his own lips […].[62]
53. If the tips of his fingers are red, he will die. [If the tips of his fingers …]
54. If the undersides of his fingers[63] (look) bruised[64] and are dark/black, he will die. If the undersides of [his] ⌈fingers⌉ […].
55. If the "bellies" of his fingers are yellow, he will die. [If the "bellies" of his fingers …].
56. If the "bellies" of his fingers are dotted with black, he will die. [If the "bellies" of his fingers …].[65]
57. If the "bellies" of his fingers are red […].
58. If the "bellies" of his fingers are ⌈streaked⌉ with redness […].
59. If the "bellies" of his fingers are ⌈streaked⌉ with redness […].
60. If the patient's nails […].

Notes

1. Restored from parallel passage DPS 15:18′.
2. Restored from parallel passage DPS 15:15′.
3. Restored from parallel passage DPS 15:16′.
4. Restored from the similar entry in DPS 10:6.
5. Restored from parallel passage DPS 16:93′.
6. Restored from parallel passage DPS 15:26′.

7. Restored from parallel passage DPS 15:27′.

8. See Scurlock and Andersen 2005, 11.44.

9. See Scurlock and Andersen 2005, 11.26.

10. See Scurlock and Andersen 2005, 11.26.

11. See Scurlock and Andersen 2005, 3.39, 14.26, 19.64, 19.129, 19.151. This entry appears also in DPS 15:13′–14′.

12. See Scurlock and Andersen 2005, 6.146.

13. See Scurlock and Andersen 2005, 6.147.

14. See Scurlock and Andersen 2005, 10.54.

15. See Scurlock and Andersen 2005, 10.55.

16. This entry appears also in Ni. 470:2 (Kraus 1987, 196–202).

17. See Scurlock and Andersen 2005, 14.40.

18. See Scurlock and Andersen 2005, 13.268. This entry also appears in Wilhelm 1994, 35 obv. 13′//Wilhelm 1994, 57 rev. 2′.

19. This entry may also appear in VAT 10748:12′ (Heeßel 2010, 178–81).

20. See Scurlock and Andersen 2005, 19.271. This entry also appears in DPS 15:18′.

21. This entry also appears in Wilhelm 1994, 62 J 1:6.

22. See Scurlock and Andersen 2005, 19.41.

23. See above, DPS 3:70.

24. See Scurlock and Andersen 2005, 3.210. This entry appears in DPS 15.15′.

25. See Scurlock and Andersen 2005, 16.61.

26. See above, DPS 3:70.

27. See Scurlock and Andersen 2005, 16.59, 16.62 as here corrected. This entry also appears in DPS 15:16′.

28. This entry also appears in DPS 15:17′.

29. See Scurlock and Andersen 2005, 16.60, 20.11.

30. See Scurlock and Andersen 2005, 13.60.

31. See Scurlock and Andersen 2005, 11.15.

32. See Scurlock and Andersen 2005, 11.16.

33. See Scurlock and Andersen 2005, 8.29, 16.54.

34. See Scurlock and Andersen 2005, 8.29, 10.39.

35. A similar entry appears in DPS 10:6.

36. This entry appears also in Wilhelm 1994, 21 obv. 1.

37. This entry appears also in DPS 16:93′.

38. See Scurlock and Andersen 2005, 8.33.

39. This entry appears also in CBS 12580:1 (Rutz 2011, 301–5).

40. See Scurlock and Andersen 2005, p. 212.

41. See Scurlock and Andersen 2005, 8.49. This entry appears also in CBS 12580:3 (Rutz 2011, 301–5).

42. See Scurlock and Andersen 2005, 8.49.

43. See Scurlock and Andersen 2005, 8.51.

44. See Scurlock and Andersen 2005, 8.52.

45. This entry appears also in CBS 12580:2 (Rutz 2011, 301–5).

46. This entry appears also in CBS 12580:4 (Rutz 2011, 301–5).

47. See Scurlock and Andersen 2005, 3.215.

48. See Scurlock and Andersen 2005, 11.19.

49. See the discussion under DPS 3:70.

50. See Scurlock and Andersen 2005, 14.37, 19.166. The entry appears also in DPS 15:26′.

51. See Scurlock and Andersen 2005, 8.60.
52. See Scurlock and Andersen 2005, 8.61.
53. See Scurlock and Andersen 2005, 8.62.
54. See Scurlock and Andersen 2005, 8.63.
55. Kämmerer 1999–2000, 168 interprets this as gall; ZÉ can refer to either.
56. See Scurlock and Andersen 2005, 15.39.
57. See Scurlock and Andersen 2005, 11.27.
58. See Scurlock and Andersen 2005, 11.28.
59. See Scurlock and Andersen 2005, 11.29.
60. See Scurlock and Andersen 2005, 19.289.
61. This entry appears also in DPS 15:27′.
62. See Scurlock and Andersen 2005, 7.31.
63. ŠE = *kittabru*. The commentary *STT* 403 rev. 47 explains the "ŠE U.MEŠ" as meaning TA MU *ap-pat* ŠU.SI.MEŠ-*šú* EN SAG *ṣu-ur-ri-šú*: "from the line represented by the tips of his fingers to the beginning of his core" or, in other words, the underside of the finger. For more on this subject, see Rutz 2011, 304–5.
64. See Scurlock and Andersen 2005, 216.
65. See Scurlock and Andersen 2005, 10.53.

DPS TABLET 12

DPS 11 rev. 61 (catchline) = DPS 12:1

1. DIŠ GIG GABA-*su* GU$_7$-*šú* ŠU DINGIR-*šú ana si-riq* GA[BA.RI]
2. DIŠ GABA-*su* DU$_8$.MEŠ-*át* SAG.KI-*šú* ŠUB-*ut* MÚD *ina* KA-*šú pi-qam la p*[*i-qam*] ⸢DU⸣-*k*[*a*]
3. ŠÀ-*šú pi-qam la pi-qam* MUD-*ud* ŠU ^{d}AMAR.UTU *a-dir-ma* BA.ÚŠ
4. DIŠ *ina* GABA-*šú* SÌG-*iṣ-ma* MÚD *ú-tab-ba-ka u ú-rap-pad* ŠU ^{d}U.GUR GABA.RI SÌG-*iṣ* GAM
5. DIŠ *ina* GABA-*šú* A *i-sal-lu ù* KA-*šú* KIR$_4$.ŠU.GÁL ŠU ^{d}UTU MU KÙ.BABBAR ZAG.GAR.RA
6. DIŠ SA GABA-*šú* SIG$_7$ *il-te-qu-ú* NU DIN
7. DIŠ SA SAG ZI-*šú šá* 15 *u* 150 DU-*ku-ma šá pu-ti-šú* GAR-*nu* ÚŠ
8. DIŠ SÍG GABA-*šú i-ṭa-mu* A GIŠ.BAL ÍD NAG
9. DIŠ UBUR 15-*šú* SA$_5$ AL.TI
10. : DIŠ UBUR 150-*šú* SA$_5$ BA.ÚŠ
11. DIŠ UBUR.MEŠ-*šú* SA$_5$ LÚG NU TUKU
12. : DIŠ UBUR 15-*šú* SIG$_7$ GIG-*su* MAN-*ni*
13. DIŠ UBUR 150-*šú* SIG$_7$ GIG-*su* DUGUD
14. : DIŠ UBUR.MEŠ-*šú* SIG$_7$.MEŠ *na-ḫi-id*
15. DIŠ UBUR 15-*šú* GI$_6$ *na-ḫi-id*
16. : DIŠ UBUR 150-*šú* GI$_6$ GÍD-*ma* BA.ÚŠ

17. DIŠ UBUR.MEŠ-*šú* GI$_6$.MEŠ *ár-ḫiš* GAM
18. : DIŠ UBUR 15-*šú ta-rik* GIG-*su* MAN-*ni*
19. DIŠ UBUR 150-*šú ta-rik ú-zab-bal-ma* GAM
20. : DIŠ UBUR.MEŠ-*šú tar-ka* GAM
21. DIŠ UBUR 15-*šú du-ʾ-um* GIG-*su ú-zab-bal*
22. ⸢: DIŠ UBUR⸣ 150-*šú du-ʾ-um* GIG-*su* MAN-*ni*
23. DIŠ UBUR.MEŠ-*šú du-ʾ-ú-mu na-ḫi-i*[*d*]
24. [DIŠ UBU]R 15-*šú na-pi-iḫ* GIG-*su* MAN-*ni*
25. DIŠ UBUR 150-*šú na-pi-iḫ* GIG [...]
26. [DIŠ UBUR].MEŠ-*šú nap-ḫa* GIG [...]
27. DIŠ UBU[R] 15-*šú muq-qut* [...]
28. [DIŠ UBUR] ⸢1⸣50-*šú muq-qut* GIG [...]
29. [DIŠ UBUR].MEŠ-*šú muq-qu-ta*$_5$ [...]
30. [DIŠ UBUR 1]5-*šú* DU$_8$-*ir* GIG [...]
31. [DIŠ UBUR 1]50-*šú* DU$_8$-*ir* [...]
32. [DIŠ UBUR.MEŠ-*š*]*ú* DU$_8$.MEŠ [...]
33. [DIŠ UBUR? 15-*šú*] *in-ni-ṣil* GI[G...]
34. [DIŠ UBUR? 150-*šú*] *in-ni-ṣil* GI[G ...]
35. [DIŠ UBUR?.MEŠ-*šú in-ni-ṣil-l*]*a* GIG[...]

35a′. [DIŠ o o o 15-*šú ṣa-pir*...]

36′. [DIŠ o o o 150-*šú*] *ṣa-pir* GIG-*s*[*u* ...]

37′. [DIŠ o o o MEŠ-*š*]*ú ṣap-ru* [...]

38′. [DIŠ o o o 15]-*šú pa-šír* [...]

39′. [DIŠ o o] 150-*šú pa-šír* GÍD-*ma* [...]

40′. [DIŠ o]x.ME-*šú pa-áš-ru* LÚG NU T[UKU]

41′. [DIŠ TI 1]5-*šú* SA$_5$ GIG-*su* GÍD

42′. [DIŠ T]I 150-*šú* SA$_5$ GIG-*su* DUGUD

43′. [DIŠ] TI.MEŠ-*šú* SA$_5$.MEŠ DIN

44′. [DIŠ] TI 15-*šú* SIG$_7$ SILIM!-*ma* DIN

45′. [DIŠ] TI 150-*šú* SIG$_7$ *na-ḫi-*⸢*id*⸣

46′. [DIŠ] TI.MEŠ-*šú* SIG$_7$.MEŠ [...]

47′. [DIŠ T]I 15-*šú* GI$_6$ [KA-*šú* ḪÁD.DA.MEŠ *u it-ta-nag-ra-ár* ŠU ^{d}*Da-mu* *ina* ÉLLAG-*šú* SÌG-*iṣ* GAM][1]

48′. [DIŠ TI] 150-*šú* GI$_6$ [MÚD BURU$_8$ *u* ZI.IR.MEŠ *ina* U$_4$ BI SÌG-*iṣ* GAM][2]

49″–55″. (only prognoses preserved)

56″. [DIŠ ÉLLAG 150-*šú* GI$_6$ GÍD-*m*]*a* GAM

57″. ⸢DIŠ⸣ [ÉLLAG.MEŠ-*šú* GI$_6$.MEŠ ...]

58″. ⸢DIŠ⸣ [ÉLLAG 15-*š*]*ú tar-kàt* GIG-[*s*]*u* DUGUD

59″. ⸢DIŠ⸣ [ÉLLAG 150-*šú tar-kàt* ...]

60″. DIŠ [ÉLLAG.ME]Š-*šú tar-ka* B[A.Ú]Š
61″. DIŠ ÉLLAG [15-*šú du-ʾ-ú-mat* G]I[G-*su* …]
62″. DIŠ ÉLLAG 150-*šú du-ʾ-ú-mat* G[IG-*su* M]AN-*ni*
63″. DIŠ ÉLLAG.MEŠ-*šú du-ʾ-*⸢*ú*⸣-[*m*]*a* ⸢*na*⸣-[*ḫi-id*]
64″. DIŠ ÉLLAG 15-*šú nap-ḫat* GIG-*su* [MA]N-*ni*
65″. DIŠ ÉLLAG 150-*šú nap-ḫat* GIG-*su* […]
66″. DIŠ ÉLLAG.MEŠ-*šú nap-ḫa na-ḫi-id*
67″. DIŠ ÉLLAG 15-*šú muq-qú-ta-át* G[IG …]
68″. DIŠ ÉLLAG 150-*šú muq-qú-ta-át* GIG-*su* GÍD
69″. DIŠ ÉLLAG.MEŠ-*šú muq-qú-tà* LÚG NU [TUKU]
70″. DIŠ ÉLLAG 15-*šú ḫé-sa*$_5$*-át* GIG-*su* DUGUD
71″. DIŠ ÉLLAG 150-*šú ḫé-sa*$_5$*-át na-ḫi-i*[*d*]
72″. DIŠ ÉLLAG.MEŠ-*šú ḫé-sa*$_5$ GAM
73″. DIŠ ÉLLAG 15-*šú* GU$_7$-*šú na-kid* : TAG ŠU ^{d}MAŠ.[TAB.BA]
74″. DIŠ ÉLLAG 150-*šú* GU$_7$-*šú* DIN : ^{d}MAŠ.TAB.BA
75″. DIŠ ÉLLAG.MEŠ-*šú* GU$_7$.ME-*šú na-ḫi-id*
76″. DIŠ ÉLLAG 15-*šú* GU$_7$-*šú-ma ina* UGU-*šú* NÁ-*al* ŠU ^{d}MAŠ.TAB.BA DIN
77″. DIŠ ÉLLAG 150-*šú* GU$_7$-*šú-ma ina* UGU-*šú* NÁ-*al* GÍD-*ma* DIN
78″. DIŠ ÉLLAG.MEŠ-*šú* GU$_7$.ME-*šú-ma ina* UGU-*ši-na* NÁ-*al* DIN LÚG NU TUKU
79″. DIŠ ÉLLAG 15-*šú* GU$_7$-*šú-ma ina* UGU-*šú* NU NÁ-*al ina* U$_4$.7.KÁM GAM
80″. DIŠ ÉLLAG 150-*šú* GU$_7$-*šú-ma ina* UGU-*šú* NU NÁ-*al* DIN : GAM
81″. DIŠ ÉLLAG.MEŠ-*šú* GU$_7$.ME-*šú-ma ina* UGU-*ši-na* N[U] NÁ-*al ana* U$_4$.15.KÁM GAM
82″. DIŠ *ina* ÉLLAG-*šú* SÌG-*iṣ* ŠU ^{d}IM : ŠU ^{d}*Kù-bi*
83″. DIŠ *ina* ÉLLAG-*šú šá* 15 SÌG-*iṣ ana* U$_4$.14.KÁM ŠU ^{d}UTU
84″. DIŠ *ina* ÉLLAG-*šú šá* 15 SÌG-*ma* UŠ$_4$-*šú* NU DIB *ina* NU ZU *ú-ra*[*p*]-*pad* ŠU ^{d}MAŠ.TAB.BA GAM
85″. DIŠ *ina* ÉLLAG-*šú šá* 150 SÌG-*iṣ* UŠ$_4$-*šú* NU DIB MÚD BURU$_8$ ŠU ^{d}7.BI GAM
86″. DIŠ *ina šá-šal-li-šú šá* 15 SÌG-*iṣ u ú-rap-pad* ŠU DINGIR URU-*šú ina* EN.NUN.ZALÁG.G[A [SÌG]-⸢*iṣ*⸣ G[AM]
87″. DIŠ *ina šá-šal-li-šú šá* 150 SÌG-*iṣ ú-rap-pad* ŠU DINGIR-*šú ina* EN.NUN MURUB$_4$-*t*[*i* SÌG]-*iṣ* GAM
88″. DIŠ GÚ.MURGU-*šú* SA$_5$ […]
89″. DIŠ GÚ.MURGU-*šú* SIG$_7$ GIG-*su* GÍD.DA
90″. DIŠ GÚ.MURGU-*šú* GI$_6$ GAM

91″. DIŠ GÚ.MURGU-*šú ta-rík na-kid*
92″. DIŠ GÚ.MURGU-*šú du-ʾ-um* GIG-*su* GÍD
93″. DIŠ GÚ.MURGU-*šú šu-uḫ-ḫu-uṭ* GAM
94″. DIŠ GÚ.MURGU-*šú ša-lim* DIN
95″. DIŠ GÚ.MURGU-*šú qa-nin na-ḫi-id*
96″. DIŠ GÚ.MURGU-*šú* GAM-*ma* LAL NU ZU-*e* GÍD-*ma* GAM
97″. DIŠ GÚ.MURGU-*šú* GAM-*ma* LAL NU ZU-*e* UŠ$_4$-*šú* NU DIB GÍD-*ma* GAM
98″. DIŠ *ina* GÚ.MURGU-*šú* SÌG-*ma* BAD-*ma* KI.GUB-*šu* NU È-*a* ŠU GIDIM$_7$ *šag-ga-ši* [GAM]
99″. DIŠ MURUB$_4$.ME-*šú* GU$_7$.ME-*šú* ŠU ^{d}UTU BÚR-*ma* [DIN]
100″. DIŠ MURUB$_4$.ME-*šú* GU$_7$.ME-*šú-ma* KÚM-*šú mit-ḫar* ŠU DINGIR URU-*šú* […]
101″. DIŠ MURUB$_4$.ME-*šú* GU$_7$.ME-*šú-ma* KÚM-*šú* NU *mit-ḫar* […]
102″. DIŠ MURUB$_4$.ME-*šú* GU$_7$.ME-*šú-ma u* GÌR^{II}-š[*ú* …]
103″. DIŠ MURUB$_4$.ME-*šú* ŠUB Í[L NU ZU-*e* …]
104″. DIŠ MURUB$_4$.ME-*šú* Í[L.MEŠ-*šú* GIN$_7$ *i-te-ni-ep-pu-šu* NU ZU GAM]
105″. DIŠ MURUB$_4$.ME-*šú* […]
106″. DIŠ *ina* MUR[UB$_4$.ME-*šú* …]-*šú u ki-ṣir* 1 KÙŠ.MEŠ-*šú* SÌG-*iṣ* [… :] ŠU ^{d}15
107″. DIŠ [*ina* MURUB$_4$.ME-*šú* Á?]^{II}-*šú u ki-ṣir* 1 KÙŠ.MEŠ-*šú* SÌG-*iṣ* ŠU ^{d}15
108″. [DIŠ *ina* MURUB$_4$.ME-*šú u k*]*i-ṣir* 1 KÙŠ.MEŠ-*šú* SÌG-*iṣ* […] *ter-de-e-ti* (coll.)
109″. [DIŠ MURUB$_4$.MEŠ-*šú*] GIG-*ma* ZI-*bi u* DU$_{10}$.GAM *šit-ta-šú* NU *ú-kal*
110″. [*u* KA-*šú*] *ana* KA *da-an* GAM
111″. [DIŠ MU]RUB$_4$ ⸢*u* ŠÀ⸣-*šú* GIG-*ma* ZI-*bi u* DU$_{10}$.GAM NINDA NU GU$_7$
112″. KAŠ NU NAG IGI^{II}-*šú pár-da* GAM
113″. [DIŠ T]A MURUB$_4$.ME-*šú* EN SAG.DU-*šú* GIG *ana* GÌR^{II}-*šú* TI TAG GIG-*su* GÍD-*ma* DIN
114″. [DIŠ T]A MURUB$_4$.ME-*šú* EN SAG.DU-*šú* TI *ana* GÌR^{II}-*šú* GIG TAG GIG-*su* GÍD-*ma* DIN
115″. [DIŠ Ú]R.KUN-*šú* SA$_5$-*át* DIN
116″. [DIŠ] ÚR.KUN-*šú* SIG$_7$-*át* GIG-*su* MAN-*ni*
117″. [DIŠ Ú]R.KUN-*šú* GI$_6$-*át* GAM
118″. [DIŠ Ú]R.KUN-*šú tar-kát na-ḫi-id*
119″. [DIŠ ÚR].KUN-*šú du-ʾ-ú-mat* GIG-*su* MAN-*ni*
120″. [DIŠ ÚR].⸢KUN⸣-*šú nap-ḫat* GIG-*su* DUGUD
121″. [DIŠ ÚR].⸢KUN⸣-*šú muq-qú-ta-át* LÚG NU TUKU
122″. DIŠ ÚR.KUN-*šú šu-uḫ-ḫu-ta-át na-kid*

123″. DIŠ ÚR.KUN-*šú pu-uṭ-ṭu-rat* GAM
124″. DIŠ ⸢ÚR⸣.KUN-*šú* GU_7-*šú* ŠU ᵈ*Gu-la* DIŠ *ni-ri* ÍL-*ma* NIGIN-*šú*
125″. [DIŠ *ina* ÚR].KUN-*šú* SÌG-*iṣ* ŠU ᵈ*Šu-lak ana* NIN-*šú* TE-*ḫi* ŠU ᵈ30 GÍD-*ma* GAM
126″. [DIŠ TA Ú]R.KUN-*šú* EN $GÌR^{II}$-*šú* SA.MEŠ-*šú* GU_7.MEŠ-*šú* SA.GIG
127″. [DIŠ S]U.GAM-*šú šá* 15 GU_7-*šú u ú-rap-pad* GABA.RI SÌG-*iṣ* GAM
128″. [DIŠ S]U.GAM-*šú šá* 150 GU_7-*šú* KÚM NU TUKU *ár-da-na-an* ÚŠ DIB-*su* GAM
129″. [DIŠ SU].GAM-*šú šá* 15 GU_7-*šú u* IGI^{II}-*šú ur-ru-pa* ŠU ᵈDÌM.ME
130″. [DIŠ SU].GAM-*šú šá* 150 GU_7-*šú u* IGI^{II}-*šú ur-ru-pa* ŠU ᵈ*Šul-pa-è-a*
131″. [DIŠ *ina kur-ri-šú šá* 15] SÌG-*iṣ-ma* NÍ-*šú ma-ši* ŠU ᵈUD.AL.TAR GAM
132″. [DIŠ *ina kur-ri-šú šá* 15]0 SÌG-*iṣ* GÌR-*šú* NU ZI-*aḫ ina* ᵈUTU È SÌG-*iṣ* ŠU ᵈ15 GAM
133″. [DIŠ …-*l*]*a-šú-šú šá-bu-la* ŠU ᵈMAŠ.TAB.BA
134″. [DIŠ]-*šú* ta ku GAM

TRANSLATION

1. If the patient's breast hurts him, "hand" of his god for scattered ⸢*miḫru*⸣-offerings[3] (which he wants).[4]
2–3. If his chest is not congested,[5] his temporal (blood vessels) have collapsed, blood incessantly flows from his mouth/nose, (and) his heart incessantly flutters, "hand" of Marduk; there is a danger that he will die.[6]
4. If he was injured on his breast and he continually pours out blood and wanders about, "hand" of Nergal. He was injured on the front side; he will die.[7]
5. If he sprinkles water on his breast[8] and makes gestures of supplication, "hand" of Shamash on account of silver for a tithe.[9]
6. If the muscle(s) of his breast take on a yellow color, he will not get well.
7. If the blood vessel(s) of the upper part of his throat, the ones on the "right" and the ones on the "left" "go" but those of his forehead are present, he will die.
8. If the hair of his breast twines, he drank water from a hoisting device of the river.
9–10. If his "right" nipple is red, he will live. If his "left" nipple is red, he will die.
11. If (both) his nipples are red, it is of no consequence.
12. If his "right" nipple is yellow, his illness will change (for the worse).

13–14. If his “left” nipple is yellow, his illness will be difficult. If (both) his nipples are yellow, it is worrisome.
15–16. If his “right” nipple is black, it is worrisome. If his “left” nipple is black, if it is prolonged, he will die.
17. If (both) his nipples are black, he will quickly die.
18. If his “right” nipple is dark, his illness will change (for the worse).
19–20. If his “left” nipple is dark, he will die a lingering death. If (both) his nipples are dark, he will die.
21–22. If his “right” nipple is dark red, his illness will last a long time. If his “left” nipple is dark red, his illness will change (for the worse).
23. If (both) his nipples are dark red, it is ⌜worrisome⌝.
24. [If] his “right” ⌜nipple⌝ is swollen, his illness will change (for the worse).
25. If his “left” nipple is swollen, [his] illness […]
26. If (both) his nipples are swollen, [his] illness […]
27. If his “right” ⌜nipple⌝ was bruised all over[10] […]
28. [If] his “left” [nipple] was bruised all over, [his] illness […]
29. [If] (both) his [nipples] were bruised all over […]
30. [If] his ⌜“right”⌝ [nipple] was (cut) open, [his] illness […]
31. [If] his ⌜“left”⌝ [nipple] was (cut) open, […]
32. [If] (both) ⌜his⌝ [nipples] were (cut) open, […]
33. [If his “right” nipple(?)] is sluggish, [his] ⌜illness⌝ […]
34. [If his “left” nipple(?)] is sluggish, [his] ⌜illness⌝ […]
35. [If (both) his nipples(?)] are ⌜sluggish⌝, [his] illness […]
35a′. [If his “right” … twitches …]
36′. [If his “left” …] twitches ⌜his⌝ illness […]
37′. [If (both)] ⌜his⌝ […-s] twitch […]
38′. [If] his [“right” …] is relaxed […]
39′. [If] his “left” […] is relaxed, it may be prolonged but [he will get well.]
40′. [If] (both) his […-s] are relaxed, it is of no ⌜consequence.⌝
41′. [If] his ⌜“right”⌝ [rib] is red, his illness will be prolonged.
42′. [If] his “left” ⌜rib⌝ is red, his illness will be difficult.
43′. [If] (both) his ribs are red, he will get well.
44′. [If] his “right” rib is yellow, (if) it heals, he will get well.[11]
45′. [If] his “left” rib is yellow, it is worrisome.
46′. [If] (both) his ribs are yellow […]
47′. [If] his “right” ⌜rib⌝ is black, [his mouth is continually dry and he rolls over and over, “hand” of Damu. He was injured on his kidney; he will die][12]
48′. [If] his “left” [rib] is black, [he vomits blood and (his stomach) is continually upset (and) he was injured that same day, he will die].[13]

49″–55″. *(only the prognosis is preserved)*

56″. [If his “left” kidney (= the lower back over the kidney) is black], ⸢(if)⸣ [it is prolonged], he will die.

57″. If [(both) his kidneys are black …]

58″. If [his] “right” kidney is dark, ⸢his⸣ illness will be difficult.

59″. If [his “left” kidney is dark …].

60″. If (both) his [kidneys] are dark, ⸢he will die⸣.

61″. If [his “right”] kidney [is dark red], [his] ⸢illness⸣ […]

62″. If his “left” kidney is dark red, [his] ⸢illness⸣ will ⸢change⸣ (for the worse).

63″. If (both) his kidneys are ⸢dark red, it is worrisome⸣.

64″. If his “right” kidney is swollen, his illness ⸢will change⸣ (for the worse)

65″. If his “left” kidney is swollen, his illness […].

66″. If (both) his kidneys are swollen, it is worrisome.

67″. If his “right” kidney was bruised all over, [his] ⸢illness⸣ […]

68″. If his “left” kidney was bruised all over, his illness will be prolonged.

69″. If (both) his kidneys were bruised all over, [it is] of no consequence.

70″. If his “right” kidney (feels) pressured, his illness will be difficult.

71″. If his “left” kidney (feels) pressured, it is ⸢worrisome⸣.

72″. If (both) his kidneys (feel) pressured, he will die.[14]

73″. If his “right” kidney hurts him, it is worrisome (var: “touch” of the “hand” of ⸢the twin gods⸣).

74″. If his “left” kidney hurts him, he will get well (var: twin gods).[15]

75″. If (both) his kidneys hurt him, it is worrisome.[16]

76″. If his “right” kidney hurts him so that he can lie on it, “hand” of the twin gods; he will get well.[17]

77″. If his “left” kidney hurts him so that he can lie on it, it may be prolonged, but he will get well.

78″. If (both) his kidneys hurt him so that he can lie on them, he will get well; it is of no consequence.[18]

79″. If his “right” kidney hurts him so that he cannot lie on it, on the seventh day, he will die.[19]

80″. If his “left” kidney hurts him so that he cannot lie on it, he will get well (var. he will die).

81″. If (both) his kidneys hurt him so that he ⸢cannot⸣ lie on them (and he has been sick) for fifteen days, he will die.[20]

82″. If he was injured on his kidney, “hand” of Adad (var. “hand” of Kubu).[21]

83″. If he was injured on his “right” kidney (and he has been sick) for fourteen days (var. G_2: fifteen days; var. E: five days), “hand” of Shamash.[22]

84″. If he was injured on his "right" kidney, he is not in full possession of his faculties (and) he wanders about without knowing (where he is), "hand" of the twin gods; he will die.[23]

85″. If he was injured on his "left" kidney, he is not in full possession of his faculties (and) he vomits blood, "hand" of the Sibitti; he will die.[24]

86″. If he was injured on his "right" upper back and he wanders about, "hand" of the god of his city. (If) he was ⌜injured⌝ in the dawn watch, ⌜he will die⌝.[25]

87″. If he was injured on his "left" upper back (and) he wanders about, "hand" of his god. (If) he was ⌜injured⌝ in the middle watch, he will die.[26]

88″. If his spine is red [...]

89″. If his spine is yellow, his illness will be prolonged.

90″. If his spine is black, he will die.

91″. If his spine is dark, it is worrisome.

92″. If his spine is dark red, his illness will be prolonged.

93″. If his spine was skinned, he will die.

94″. If his spine is normal, he will live.

95″. If his spine is curved, it is worrisome.[27]

96″. If his spine is curved so that he cannot straighten it out, if it is prolonged, he will die.[28]

97″. If his spine is curved so that he cannot straighten it out (and) he is not in full possession of his faculties, if it is prolonged, he will die.[29]

98″. If he was injured on his spine and he is blocked off so that his excrement cannot come out, "hand" of a murderous ghost; [he will die].[30]

99″. If his hips continually hurt him, "hand" of Shamash; if it goes away, [he will get well].[31]

100″. If his hips continually hurt him (and) his temperature is even, "hand" of the god of his city [...].

101″. If his hips continually hurt him (and) his temperature is not even [...]

102″. If his hips continually hurt him and ⌜his⌝ feet [...].

103″. If he continually lets his pelvic region drop (and) [cannot] ⌜lift (it)⌝ [...].

104″. If his pelvic region is [continually] ⌜lifted up⌝ (and) [he does not realize that he is continually doing (this), he will die].[32]

105″. If his hips [...]

106″. If he was injured on [his] ⌜hips⌝, his [...] and his elbows, [...] (var. "hand" of Ishtar)

107″. If he was injured [on his hips], his ⌜arms⌝ and his elbows, "hand" of Ishtar.[33]

108″. [If] he was injured [on his hips and] his elbows [...] sequellae.

109″–110″. [If his hips] are so sick that he gets up and (has to) kneel down (again), he cannot retain his shit[34] [and his mouth] is too strong for the words, he will die.[35]

111″–112″. [If] his ⌜pelvic region⌝ and abdomen are so sick that he gets up and (has to) kneel down (again), he will not eat bread, he will not drink beer (and) his eyes shudder,[36] he will die.[37]

113″. [If] he is ill ⌜from⌝ his hips to his head (but) well to his feet, he was "touched"; his illness may be prolonged but he will get well.

114″. [If] he is well ⌜from⌝ his hips to his head (but) ill to his feet, he was "touched"; his illness may be prolonged but he will get well.

115″. [If] his ⌜coccyx⌝[38] is red, he will get well.[39]

116″. [If] his coccyx is yellow, his illness will change (for the worse).[40]

117″. [If] his ⌜coccyx⌝ is black, he will die.[41]

118″. [If] his ⌜coccyx⌝ is dark, it is worrisome.[42]

119″. [If] his ⌜coccyx⌝ is dark red, his illness will change (for the worse).[43]

120″. [If] his ⌜coccyx⌝ is swollen, his illness will be difficult.[44]

121″. [If] his ⌜coccyx⌝ was bruised all over, it is of no consequence.[45]

122″. If his coccyx was skinned, it is worrisome.[46]

123″. If his coccyx was (cut) open, he will die.[47]

124″. If his coccyx hurts him, "hand" of Gula. If a yoke-shaped lesion rises and curves round, ("hand" of Gula).[48]

125″. [If] he was injured [on] his ⌜coccyx⌝, "hand" of Shulak; he approached his sister (sexually); "hand" of Sîn. If it is prolonged, he will die.[49]

126″. [If from] his ⌜coccyx⌝ to his feet his muscles continually hurt him, *maškādu*.[50]

127″. [If] his "right" ⌜armpit⌝ hurts him and he wanders about, he was injured on the front side; he will die.[51]

128″. [If] his "left" ⌜armpit⌝ hurts him (but) he does not have a fever, the "double" of a dead man afflicts him; he will die.[52]

129″. [If] his "right" ⌜armpit⌝ hurts him and his eyes are clouded, "hand" of Lamashtu.

130″. [If] his "left" ⌜armpit⌝ hurts him and his eyes are clouded, "hand" of Šulpaea.

131″. [If] he was injured [on his "right" femural crease] and, as a consequence, he is unconscious, "hand" of Dapinu; he will die.[53]

132″. [If] he was injured [on his] ⌜"left"⌝ [femural crease] (and) he cannot uproot his foot (from the ground) (and) he was injured at sunrise, "hand" of Ishtar; he will die.[54]

133″. [If …] his […] are dried up, "hand" of the twin gods.

134″. *(fragmentary)*

Notes

1. Restored from parallel passage DPS 15:42′.
2. Restored from parallel passage DPS 15:43′.
3. Suggestion courtesy M. Stol.
4. See Scurlock and Andersen 2005, 19.209.
5. Literally: “is clear.”
6. See Scurlock and Andersen 2005, 3.237, 8.6, 19.235, 20.28.
7. See Scurlock and Andersen 2005, 14.32, 19.174. This entry appears also in DPS 15:32′.
8. See *CAD* S s.v. *saʾālu*.
9. See Scurlock and Andersen 2005, 19.2. This entry appears also in VAT 10748:11′ (Heeßel 2010, 178–81).
10. See Scurlock and Andersen 2005, p. 216.
11. See Scurlock and Andersen 2005, 20.43.
12. This entry appears also in DPS 15:42′.
13. This entry appears also in DPS 15:43′.
14. See Scurlock and Andersen 2005, 13.15.
15. See Scurlock and Andersen 2005, 5.57.
16. See Scurlock and Andersen 2005, 20.60.
17. See Scurlock and Andersen 2005, 19.368.
18. See Scurlock and Andersen 2005, 20.61.
19. See Scurlock and Andersen 2005, 5.56.
20. Alternatively, “he will die within fifteen days.” See Scurlock and Andersen 2005, 20.62.
21. See Scurlock and Andersen 2005, 19.141, 19.189.
22. See Scurlock and Andersen 2005, 19.191.
23. See Scurlock and Andersen 2005, 14.33, 19.179, 20.8. This entry appears also in DPS 15:39′.
24. See Scurlock and Andersen 2005, 14.27, 19.178. This entry appears also in DPS 15:40′.
25. See Scurlock and Andersen 2005, 19.207. This entry appears also in DPS 15:44′.
26. See Scurlock and Andersen 2005, 19.207. This entry appears also in DPS 15:45′.
27. See Scurlock and Andersen 2005, 11.23.
28. See Scurlock and Andersen 2005, 11.24, 20.84. This entry appears also in DPS 15:47′.
29. See Scurlock and Andersen 2005, 11.25.
30. See Scurlock and Andersen 2005, 5.40, 6.155, 13.142, 19.172. This entry appears also in DPS 15:46′.
31. See Scurlock and Andersen 2005, 11.47.
32. See Scurlock and Andersen 2005, 13.88. This entry appears also in DPS 15:48′.
33. This entry may have appeared in VAT 11122 obv. 11 (Heeßel 2010, 181–84).
34. Reading courtesy M. Stol.
35. See Scurlock and Andersen 2005, 13.216 as here corrected.
36. Scurlock and Andersen 2005, 294–96. The reference is to nystagmus.
37. See Scurlock and Andersen 2005, 13.105, 13.216
38. Literally: “tail region.”
39. See Scurlock and Andersen 2005, 10.45.
40. See Scurlock and Andersen 2005, 10.45.
41. See Scurlock and Andersen 2005, 10.45.

42. See Scurlock and Andersen 2005, 10.45.
43. See Scurlock and Andersen 2005, 10.45.
44. See Scurlock and Andersen 2005, 10.45.
45. See Scurlock and Andersen 2005, 10.45.
46. See Scurlock and Andersen 2005, 10.45.
47. See Scurlock and Andersen 2005, 10.45.
48. See Scurlock and Andersen 2005, 10.102, 19.238.
49. This entry also appears in DPS 15:41′.
50. See Scurlock and Andersen 2005, 11.60. This entry appears also in DPS 33:100.
51. This entry also appears in DPS 15:30′.
52. See Scurlock and Andersen 2005, 19.391.
53. See Scurlock and Andersen 2005, 14.16, 19.197. This entry appears also in DPS 15:49′.
54. See Scurlock and Andersen 2005, 14.18, 19.153. This entry appears also in DPS 15:50′.

DPS TABLET 13

DPS 12:135″ (catchline) = DPS 13:1

1. [DIŠ G]IG SA[G] ŠÀ-*šú* SA$_5$ DIN
2. [DIŠ S]AG ⸢ŠÀ-*šú*⸣ GI[$_6$-*ma* EME-*šú ḫe-em-ret ana* GIZKIM GIG GAM]
3. [DIŠ S]AG ŠÀ-*šú* x[...]
4. DIŠ SAG ŠÀ-*šú* SIG$_7$.SIG$_7$ [...] TAG *si-li-ʾ-ti-šú* GÚ-*su* [...]
5. IM KIR$_4$-*šú šá* [...]⸢15⸣ *u* 150 ŠED$_7$ ŠU KI-*ti* : ŠU GUNNI GAM
6. DIŠ SAG ŠÀ-*šú* GU$_7$!.[MEŠ-*šú*] SAG.KI 150-*šú* TAG.TAG-*su in-da-na-ag-ga-ag*
7. [KA.DIB DIB-*su* SU-*šú* KÚM-*e*]*m u ši-ḫat* UZU TUKU NA BI GIG *na-ki* GIG
8. [DIŠ SAG ŠÀ-*šú*] *i-ḫa-am-maṭ-su u* KÚM NINDA GU$_7$-*ma* UGU-*šú* NU DU-*ak*
9. [A NAG-*m*]*a* UGU-*šú* NU ŠE.GA *u* SU-*šú* SIG$_7$ NA BI GIG *na-ki* GIG
10. [DIŠ SAG Š]À-*šú* DIB.DIB-*su* DIB GIDIM$_7$
11. [DIŠ SA]G ŠÀ-*šú* DIB.DIB-*su u* EME-*šú ḫe-em-ret ana* KI GIG GAM
12. [DIŠ S]AG ŠÀ-*šú* DIB.DIB-*su u* ŠÀ.MEŠ-*šú* MÚ.MEŠ-*ḫu* GIG-*su* GÍD.DA
13. *ana* UD.31.KAM ŠU ZAG 10 GAL.MEŠ
14. DIŠ SAG ŠÀ-*šú* DIB.DIB-*su* ŠÀ.MEŠ-*šú* KÙŠ.ME-*šú kin-ṣa-a-šú u* GÌR^{II}-*šú* GU$_7$.MEŠ-*šú* ŠU DINGIR-*šú ni-ši*
15. DIŠ SAG ŠÀ-*šú e-bi-iṭ ša-šal-la-šú* GU$_7$.MEŠ-*šú* ŠU GIDIM$_7$
16. DIŠ SAG ŠÀ-*šú a-šá-áṭ* NU DIN DIŠ SAG ŠÀ-*šú na-pi-iḫ na-kid*
17. DIŠ SAG ŠÀ-*šú* MÚ.MEŠ DIB GIDIM$_7$
18. DIŠ SAG ŠÀ-*šú za-qir u* ŠÀ.MEŠ-*šú* MÚ.MEŠ-*ḫu* GIG-*su* GÍD

19. DIŠ SAG ŠÀ-*šú za-qir* KÚM NU TUKU $UŠ_4$-*šú* KÚR.KÚR ŠÚ.ŠÚ A.GA.NU.TIL-*le-e*
20. SI-*šum-ma ina* U_4-*um* BI.IZ AN-*e* GAM
21. DIŠ SAG ŠÀ-*šú* ÍL-*ma* IGI.MEŠ-*šú* MÚ.MEŠ-*ḫu ina* IGI^{II}-*šú* ÍR DU GÍD-*ma* GAM
22. DIŠ SAG ŠÀ-*šú* ÍL-*ma* ḪÁŠ-*su da-an* U_4.27.KÁM GIG ŠU ZAG.ME GAL.MEŠ
23. DIŠ SAG ŠÀ-*šú* ÍL-*ma* ḪÁŠ-*su da-an* KÚM *u* $ŠED_7$ *ana* NIN.DINGIR DINGIR-*šú* TE-*ḫi*
24. *ana* U_4.31.KÁM BÚR-*ma* DIN
25. DIŠ SAG ŠÀ-*šú* ÍL-*ma* ḪÁŠ-*su* DIG-*ub* ŠU ZAG 10 GAL.MEŠ
26. DIŠ SAG ŠÀ-*šú* DU_8-*ma* ḪÁŠ-*su da-an* U_4.27.KÁM ŠU ZAG 10 GAL. MEŠ
27. DIŠ SAG ŠÀ-*šú* DU_8-*ma i-ár-ra-ár* ŠU ZAG 10 GAL.MEŠ
28. DIŠ SAG ŠÀ-*šú* DIG-*ub i-mim u* $ŠED_7$ ^{GIŠ}GIDRU *šá* DINGIR-*šú ana* GAL *u* TUR 1-*ma*
29. DIŠ SAG ŠÀ-*šú* KÚM *u* ŠÀ.MEŠ-*šú* MÚ.MEŠ-*ḫu* DIB $GIDIM_7$
30. DIŠ SAG ŠÀ-*šú* KÚM-*ma* SA $SAG.KI^{II}$-*šú* $ŠU^{II}$-*šú u* $GÌR^{II}$-*šú* ZI.ME IGI^{II}-*šú* DUGUD-*šú*
31. DIŠ SAG ŠÀ-*šú* ÍL ḪÁŠ-*su da-an* $ŠED_7$ *u* KÚM-*im* ŠU *ìl-ti* NU DIN
32. DIŠ SAG ŠÀ-*šú* KÚM *ú-kal* $UŠ_4$-*šú* KÚR.KÚR-*šú* A GIŠ.BAL ÍD NAG *ana* ⸢MÁ.ÚR.RA TAG-*ma*⸣ GAM
33. DIŠ SAG ŠÀ-*šú* GIG ZI-*bi u* TUŠ-*ab* $GIDIM_7$ ŠEŠ *u* NIN DIB-*su*
34. DIŠ SAG ŠÀ-*šú* DIŠ *em-ši-šú* DU-*ak u* AD_6-*šú* $ŠED_7$ GAM
35. DIŠ *ina* SAG ŠÀ-*šú* SÌG-*iṣ* ŠU ^{d}IM : *pu-qud-de-e* ^{d}UTU *ana* ^{d}MAŠ.TAB. BA
36. DIŠ *ina* SAG ŠÀ-*šú* SÌG-*iṣ* $ŠU^{II}$-*šú u* $GÌR^{II}$-*šú am-šá* ŠU ^{d}DUMU. MUNUS ^{d}*A-nim*
37. DIŠ *ina* SAG ŠÀ-*šú u su-ḫa-ti-šú* SÌG-*iṣ* DAM LÚ *it-ta-na-a-a-ak*
38. DIŠ *ina* SAG ŠÀ-*šú* SAG.KI-*šú u* TI-*šú* SÌG-*iṣ* ŠU ^{d}*Ereš-ki-gal* GAM
39. DIŠ *ina* SAG ŠÀ-*šú* ^{GIŠ}NÍG.GIDRU GAR-*su-ma u* MÚD MUD ŠUB. ŠUB-*a* GAM
40. DIŠ *ina* SAG ŠÀ-*šú* ^{GIŠ}NÍG.GIDRU GAR-*su-ma* MÚD MUD *i-ʾa-ḫa u* SAG.KI-*šú ḫe-sa-át* GAM
41. DIŠ *ina* SAG ŠÀ-*šú di-ik-šú u* ^{GIŠ}NÍG.GIDRU GAR-*nu-šum-ma* MÚD *i-te-zi* GAM
42. DIŠ *ina* SAG ŠÀ-*šú di-ik-šú u* ^{GIŠ}NÍG.GIDRU GAR-*nu-šum-ma* MÚD *i-ḫa-ḫu ana* U_4.2.KÁM *ana* U_4.3.KÁM GAM

43. DIŠ *ina* SAG ŠÀ-*šú di-i*[*k-š*]*ú* [*u* ^{GIŠ}NÍG.GIDRU GAR-*nu*]-*šum-ma e-sil* GAM

44. DIŠ *ina* SAG ŠÀ-*šú d*[*i-ik-šú* GAR-*su-ma* NU D]U$_{8}$-*ir ana* U$_{4}$.31.KÁM ŠU ^{d}IM GAM

45. DIŠ *ina* SAG ŠÀ-*šú* [... *ur*]-*qá* ŠUB-*a* ŠU ^{d}AMAR.UTU : ŠU ^{d}15 GAM

46. DIŠ *ina* SAG Š[À-*šú* ...] ŠU ^{d}TIR.AN.NA DIN : GAM

47. DIŠ ŠÀ-*šú* [15 *na-pi-iḫ* GIG-*s*]*u* MAN-*ni*

48. DIŠ ŠÀ-*šú* 150 *na-pi-iḫ* GIG-[*s*]*u* DUGUD

49. DIŠ ŠÀ.[MEŠ-*šú nap-ḫ*]*a* ŠU ^{d}KÙ.BI NIG.GIG IGI-*ma* DIN

50. DIŠ ŠÀ-*š*[*ú* ... Š]U ^{d}*Iš-tar*

51. DIŠ ŠÀ-*š*[*ú* ...] ŠU ^{d}*Da-mu*

52. DIŠ ŠÀ-*šú* GU$_{7}$-*šú* ŠU ^{d}20

53. DIŠ ŠÀ-*šú* [DIB-*su*] ŠU ^{d}*Ba-ú* DIŠ ŠU-*šú* NU ÍL-*e*

54. [DIŠ] ŠÀ-*šú* DIB-[-*su-ma ú-a* D]UG$_{4}$.GA ŠU ^{d}ME.ME DIŠ *ni-ri ina* GÚ-*šú* GAR-*ma* NIGIN

55. [DIŠ ŠÀ]-*š*[*ú*] KÚM *r*[*uq-q*]*í* GEŠTU^{II}-*šú* ŠED$_{7}$.MEŠ

56. *ḫaṭ-ṭu* ŠED$_{7}$.MEŠ *ina* KA-*šú* DU.MEŠ GÍD-*ma* GAM

57. [DIŠ ŠÀ-*šú*] KÚM [TUKU].MEŠ *ruq-qí* GEŠTU^{II}-*šú* KÚM.MEŠ

58. *ḫaṭ-ṭu* KÚM.MEŠ *ina* KA-*šú* DU.MEŠ *ni-ši*

59. DIŠ ŠÀ-*šú* KÚM ⸢*u*⸣ SAG ŠÀ-*šú za-qir* DIN

60. DIŠ ŠÀ-*šú* KÚM ÚḪ U.MEŠ GÌR^{II}-*šú* ŠED$_{7}$ *ina* U$_{4}$.3.KÁM : U$_{4}$.4.KÁM

61. *i-la-az-za-az-ma* DIN : GAM

62. DIŠ ŠÀ-*šú* KÚM IR GIN$_{7}$ *lu-ba-ṭi* ŠUB.ŠUB-*su u* ZI.IR.MEŠ GAM

63. DIŠ ŠÀ-*šú* KÚM IR GIN$_{7}$ *lu-ba-ṭi* ŠUB.ŠUB-*su u* ZI.IR.MEŠ ŠU 20

64. MAŠ.MAŠ-*su* DÙ-*uš u* ŠU.⸢ÚR⸣-*šú-ma* DIN

65. DIŠ ŠÀ-*šú* KÚM-*ma* IR GIN$_{7}$ *lu-ba-ṭi* ŠUB.ŠUB-*su u* ZI.IR.MEŠ-*aš* ⸢ŠÀ-*šú*⸣

66. KÚM ÚḪ U.MEŠ GÌR^{II}-*šú* ŠED$_{7}$.MEŠ U$_{4}$.3.KÁM ZAL-*ma* DIN

67. DIŠ ŠÀ-*šú* KÚM-*ma* IR GIN$_{7}$ *lu-ba-ṭi* ŠUB.ŠUB-*su u* ŠED$_{7}$ U$_{4}$.31.KÁM ŠU ^{d}20

68. DIŠ ŠÀ-*šú* KÚM IR ŠUB.ŠUB-*su lu* ŠU ^{d}UTU *lu* ^{d}*Šu*-⸢*lak*⸣ GABA.RI ⸢SÌG⸣-*iṣ*

69. DIŠ ŠÀ-*šú* KÚM-*im u* ŠED$_{7}$ A UL$_{4}$-*gal* APIN-*ma* NAG ŠU ^{d}DÌM.ME

70. DIŠ ŠÀ-*šú* KÚM-*im u* ŠED$_{7}$ A *ana* TU$_{5}$ UL$_{4}$-*gal* APIN.MEŠ ŠU ^{d}DÌM.ME DIN

71. DIŠ ŠÀ-*šú* DIG-*ub* A UL$_{4}$-*gal* APIN-*eš* KÚM-*šú mit-ḫar* TA *taš-ri-ti* EN SAG GI$_{6}$

72. DIŠ GIG-*su id-da-lip* SÌG-*iṣ* MAŠKIM : GIDIM SÌG-*iṣ* GAM

73. DIŠ ŠÀ-*šú* MUD.MUD-*ud* SAG ŠÀ-*šú* GU$_{4}$.UD.MEŠ IGI^{II}-*šú*

74. *ana e-ṭú-ti* NIR.NIR-*aṣ* ŠU GIDIM$_7$
75. DIŠ *ina* ŠÀ-*šú* SÌG-*iṣ* U$_4$.9.KÁM ŠU ^{d}MAŠ.TAB.BA DIŠ TAB-*i* ŠU ^{d}IM
76. DIŠ *šal-šú* ŠU ^{d}*É-a* DIŠ 4 ŠU DINGIR.MAḪ DIŠ 5 ŠU ^{d}*Papsukkal*
77. DIŠ *ina* ŠÀ-*šú* SÌG-*iṣ e-mir u e-sil* GAM : DIŠ *ina* ŠÀ-*šú* SÌG-*ma u* ZI.IR.MEŠ ŠU ^{d}MAŠ.TAB.BA GAM
78. DIŠ *ina* ŠÀ-*šú* SÌG-*ma u* MÚD MUD ŠUB.ŠUB-*a* DIB-*it* ^{d}MAŠ.TAB.BA GAM
79. DIŠ *ina* ŠÀ-*šú u ri-bit* 150-*šú* SÌG-*iṣ-ma u* MÚD *i-ḫa-ḫu ana* U$_4$.31.KÁM ŠU ^{d}⸢U.GUR⸣ GAM
80. DIŠ *ina* ŠÀ-*šú* Á 15-*šú di-ik-šu* GAR-*nu-ma u* BURU$_8$.MEŠ ŠU ^{d}15 DIN
81. DIŠ *ina* ŠÀ-*šú* Á 150-*šú di-ik-šu* GAR-*nu-ma u* NU BURU$_8$ ŠU ^{d}15 GAM
82. DIŠ *ina* ŠÀ-*šú* Á 15-*šú* ^{GIŠ}GIDRU GAR-*su-ma u* BURU$_8$ ŠU ^{d}15 GAM
83. DIŠ *ina* ŠÀ-*šú* Á 150-*šú* ^{GIŠ}GIDRU GAR-*su-ma u* BURU$_8$ ŠU ^{d}15 GAM
84. DIŠ *ina* ŠÀ-*šú* Á 15-*šú* ^{GIŠ}GIDRU GAR-*su-ma u* MÚD BURU$_8$ ŠU ^{d}15 GAM
85. DIŠ *ina* ŠÀ-*šú* Á 150-*šú* ^{GIŠ}GIDRU GAR-*su-ma u* MÚD *i-ḫa-ḫu* ŠU ^{d}15[1] GAM
86. DIŠ *ina* ŠÀ-*šú* Á 150-*šú* ^{GIŠ}GIDRU GAR-*su-ma u* MÚD SUR ŠU ^{d}IM GAM
87. DIŠ *ina* ŠÀ-*šú* Á 150-*šú* ^{GIŠ}GIDRU GAR-*su-ma* IGI^{II}-*šú* GU.MEŠ SIG$_7$.MEŠ DIRI.MEŠ
88. ŠU ^{d}15 GAM
89. DIŠ *ina* ŠÀ-*šú* Á 150-*šú* MIN-*ma* NUNDUN.MEŠ-*šú ši-qá* ŠUB-*a* ŠU ^{d}30 *lu* ŠU ^{d}15 GAM
90. DIŠ *ina* ŠÀ-*šú* Á 15-*šú u* 150-*šú di-ik-šú u* ^{GIŠ}GIDRU GAR-*nu-šum-ma* MÚD MUD ŠUB.ŠUB GAM
91. DIŠ *ina* ŠÀ-*šú* KI.MIN-*ma* EME-*šú ú-na-aṭ-ṭa* ÁŠ-*át* AD-*šú* KUR-*su* PÚŠ.ME-*ma* GAM : DIN
92. DIŠ *ina* ŠÀ-*šú ši-qu ina* ŠÀ IGI^{II}-*šú* GU.MEŠ SIG$_7$.MEŠ *ip-ri-ku* GAM
93. DIŠ ŠÀ.MEŠ-*šú* SA$_5$.MEŠ DIN
94. DIŠ ŠÀ.MEŠ-*šú* SIG$_7$.MEŠ *na-kid*
95. DIŠ ŠÀ.MEŠ-*šú* GI$_6$.MEŠ GAM
96. DIŠ ŠÀ.MEŠ-*šú* GI$_6$.MEŠ-*ma* SA.MEŠ ŠÀ-*šú šu-ud-du-du*
97. *ina* KA-*šú* IM *i-giš-šú ana* U$_4$.3.KÁM GAM
98. DIŠ ŠÀ.MEŠ-*šú tar-ku na-ʾ-id*
99. DIŠ ŠÀ.MEŠ-*šú du-ʾ-um-mu* GIG-*su* GÍD
100. DIŠ ŠÀ.MEŠ-*šú raq-qu* LÚG NU TUKU
101. DIŠ ŠÀ.MEŠ-*šú i-tab-lu* GAM
102. DIŠ ŠÀ.MEŠ-*šú suk-ku-ru* ŠU ^{d}*Da-mu*

103. DIŠ ŠÀ.MEŠ-*šú nap-ḫu* GIG-*su* GÍD : *na-ʾ-id*
104. DIŠ ŠÀ.MEŠ-*šú nap-ḫu-ma* SA.MEŠ ŠÀ-*šú šu-ud-du-du* ŠU ^{d}15 NU ⸢DIN⸣
105. DIŠ ŠÀ.MEŠ-*šú nap-ḫu-ma* SA.MEŠ ŠÀ-*šú šu-ud-du-du* SIG$_7$ ŠUB-*ú* KÚM *mit-ḫar*
106. *ana mál-*[*da-riš*] GUR-*šum-ma* GAM
107. DIŠ ŠÀ.MEŠ-*šú nap-ḫu-ma* SA ŠÀ-*šú* SIG$_7$ ŠUB-*ú*
108. *ana* U$_4$.31.KÁM ŠU ^{d}*I*[*š-ḫa-ra* …] za x
109. DIŠ ŠÀ.MEŠ-*šú nap-ḫu-ma* SA ŠÀ-*š*[*ú*] SIG$_7$ SA$_5$ ŠUB-*ú* ⸢GAM⸣
110. DIŠ ŠÀ.MEŠ-*šú nap-ḫu-*⸢*ma* S⸣[A ŠÀ-*šú*] SIG$_7$ *u pa-*IGI^{II} ⸢ŠÁ-*šú* SA$_5$⸣
111. GIDIM$_4$ EŠ xxx *niš-šu-tim*??
112. DIŠ ŠÀ.MEŠ-*šú* ⸢*nap-ḫu-m*⸣*a* IM DIRI.GA x x
113. DIŠ ŠÀ.MEŠ-*šú nap-ḫu-ma* MIN *lu* ŠU DINGIR-*šú lu* ^{d}15-*šú*
114. : ŠU ^{d}EŠ$_4$.DAR
115. DIŠ ŠÀ.MEŠ-*šú nap-ḫu-ma* KÚM NU *mit-ḫar* ⸢GÍD-*ma*⸣ […]
116. DIŠ ŠÀ.MEŠ-*šú nap-ḫu-ma nag-la-bu-šu* […]
117. DIŠ ŠÀ.MEŠ-*šú* MÚ.MÚ-*ḫu* ŠU ^{d}*Kù-bi* : […]
118. [DI]Š ŠÀ.MEŠ-*šú* MIN *u* ÍR.MEŠ ŠU ^{d}*Kù-bi* : ŠU […]
119. [DI]Š ŠÀ.MEŠ-*šú* MIN *u* IGI^{II}-*šú* DUGUD-*šú* ŠU ^{d}*Kù-bi* : ŠU ^{d}[…]
120. [DIŠ ŠÀ.MEŠ-*šú* MÚ].⸢MÚ⸣ IGI^{II}-*šú kab-*⸢*ta* ŠU⸣ ^{d}[*K*]*ù-bi* DIN
121. [DIŠ ŠÀ.MEŠ-*šú i*]*t-te-nen-bi-ṭu mim-ma* NU GU$_7$ […]
122. [DIŠ ŠÀ.MEŠ-*š*]*ú* MIN Á^{II}-*šú tab-ka* […]
123. [DIŠ ŠÀ.ME]Š-*šú* MIN IGI^{II}-*šú* DUGUD-*šú* […]
124. [DIŠ Š]À.MEŠ-*šú nàr-bu-ma* A UL$_4$-*gal* APIN.MEŠ-*ma* NAG K[ÚM …]
125. [DIŠ] ŠÀ.MEŠ-*šú* MIN-*ma* A UL$_4$-*gal* APIN.MEŠ KÚM *mit-ḫar* TA SAG GI$_6$ EN […]
126. DIŠ ŠÀ.MEŠ-*šú* MIN-*ma* A *ana* NAG UL$_4$-*gal* APIN.MEŠ KÚM *mit-ḫar* TA ŠÀ *taš-rit* GI$_6$ EN EN!.[NUN?! …]
127. DIŠ ŠÀ.MEŠ-*šú* ŠU^{II}-*šú u* GÌR^{II}-*šú it-te-nen-bi-ṭu* U$_4$.32.KÁM *lu* NITA *l*[*u* MUNUS …]
128. DIŠ ŠÀ.MEŠ-*šú* ŠU^{II}-*šú u* GÌR^{II}-*šú* UL$_4$-*gal* TAG.TAG-*at ši-gu-ú* GÙ.[GÙ …]
129. DIŠ ŠÀ.MEŠ-*šú* ŠU^{II}-*šú* GÌR^{II}-*šú* MIN *u rik-su-šú ir-mu-ú* PÚŠ.ME-*m*[*a* …]
130. DIŠ ŠÀ.MEŠ-*šú* GIN$_7$ ŠU.SI.MEŠ-*šú it-te-nen-ṣi-la ana* U$_4$.31.KÁM […]
131. DIŠ ŠÀ.MEŠ-*šú iṣ-ṣa-na-pu-ú* KÀŠ.MEŠ-*šú ta-ba-ka* NU ZU-*e* ŠU ⸢^{d}⸣[EŠ$_4$.D]AR
132. DIŠ ŠÀ ŠÀ GÙ.GÙ-*si* LÚG NU [TU]KU

133. DIŠ ŠÀ ŠÀ MIN NÍG.GIG DINGIR-*šú* GIG GU$_7$ *ana* NÍTA *u* MUNUS ŠU-*su ú-bil* ŠU […] GAM
134. DIŠ ŠÀ ŠÀ GÙ.GÙ-*si u* SÍG-*su ú-baq-qa-an ina ban-ti-šú* SÌG-*iṣ* GAM
135. DIŠ ŠÀ ŠÀ GÙ.GÙ-*si u gi-lid-su* GU$_7$-*šú* ŠU ^{d}15
136. DIŠ ŠÀ ŠÀ GÙ.GÙ-*si* MURUB$_4$.ME-*šú* ÍL.ME IGI.LÁ-*šú* LÁ-*šú* U$_4$ LÁ-*šú* LÁ-*šú par-di-iš* DUG$_4$.DUG$_4$-*ub* ŠU KI.SIKIL.LÍL.LÁ
137. DIŠ ŠÀ ŠÀ GÙ.GÙ *it-bi-ma il-su-um* GIDIM *ár-da-na-an* ÚŠ DIB-*su*
138. [DIŠ] ŠÀ ŠÀ *rab-biš* : *rap-diš* GÙ.GÙ-*si* ŠU GIDIM$_7$ *šag-ga-ši* [GAM]
139. [DIŠ] ŠÀ ŠÀ TA U$_4$.SA$_9$ GÙ.GÙ-*si ma-mit* ^{d}30 : 20 DIB-*su*
140. [DIŠ ŠÀ Š]À *lu* U$_4$.2.KÁM *lu* U$_4$.3.KÁM GÙ.GÙ-*si* NÍG.GIG DINGIR-*šú* GIG GU$_7$
141. ⸢DIŠ⸣ ŠÀ ŠÀ GÙ.GÙ-*si ana* U$_4$.5.KÁM GAM
142. DIŠ *ina* MURUB$_4$-*ti* ŠÀ ŠÀ GÙ.GÙ IGI^{II}-*šú* ⸢*e*⸣?-*ša di-ig-la* DUGUD
143. GÌR 150-*šú* DIB.DIB-*šú ug-gàt* MAŠKIM DIB.[D]IB-*su ár-ḫiš* ⸢GAM⸣
144. DIŠ *ana* BAR-*ti* È-*ma* ŠÀ ŠÀ GÙ.GÙ ŠU ⸢^{d}MAŠ.TAB.BA⸣ *ana* U$_4$.⸢7⸣.K[Á]M GAM
145. DIŠ TA ^{d}UTU.ŠÚ *ter$_4$-di-it-ma* ŠÀ ŠÀ GÙ.GÙ ŠU GIDIM$_7$
146. DIŠ *kal* U$_4$-*mi ḫa-niq-ma ina* GI$_6$ ŠÀ ŠÀ GÙ.GÙ-*si* ŠU GIDIM$_7$
147. DIŠ TÙN ŠÀ-*šú ta-kád* GAM
148. DIŠ TÙN ŠÀ-*šú* GU$_7$-*šú niš-mu-šú* DUGUD *ina* LÍL-*šú* GÚ-*su* ŠUB. ŠUB-*su* […]
149. […] ⸢*šá*⸣ 150 ŠED$_7$ ŠU NAM.ERÍM GAM
150. [DIŠ … SA]G ŠÀ-*šú za-qir* [GAM]
151. [DIŠ …]x BÀD ŠÀ-*šú ana* ḪAR-*šú is-niq* GAM
152. [DIŠ …] ÍL ŠÀ-*šú ṣa-bit* ŠU ^{d}15 *ana* KI G[IG! GAM]
153. [DIŠ …]KA ÍL ŠÀ-*šú* A *tab-ku* ŠU [^{d}…]TI
154. [DIŠ … *ḫ*]*u-uṣ-ṣa* GAZ ŠÀ TUKU.MEŠ ŠU ^{d}15 : ŠU [^{d}…]x
155. [DIŠ SA *šá*] *pa-pan* ŠÀ-*šú* DU-*ak* ŠU [^{d} …]
156. [DIŠ LÚ.TUR S]A ŠÀ-*šú* SA$_5$ *u* SIG$_7$ ŠUB-*ú* ŠU [^{d}*Kù-bi*]
157. [DIŠ SA.MEŠ ŠÀ].MEŠ-*šú šá* 15 *u* 150 *ana pi-rik* ŠÀ-*šú šu-ud-*[*du-du*]
158. NAM.ERÍM DI[B-*su*]

---

159. [DIŠ]x-*šú* GU$_7$.MEŠ-*šú u uš-ta-kal* […]
160. [ ] x x x x x […]
161. ⸢DIŠ⸣ MIN-*šu* x ku ku x

---

162. DIŠ *i-me-es-su u* SAG ŠÀ […]
163. DIŠ *ina em-ši-šú* SÌG-*iṣ* ŠU ^{d}MAŠ.[TAB.BA …]
164. DIŠ *ina em-ši-šú* SÌG-*iṣ-ma u du-u*[*s-su KAR-et* …]

165. DIŠ *ina em-ši-šú* SÌG-*iṣ-ma u* GÌR^{II}-*šú* [...]

---

166. DIŠ *e-mir u e-sil* [...]
167. DIŠ *e-mir u e-sil* ŠÀ.MEŠ-*šú e[b-ṭu* ...]
168. DIŠ *e-mir u e-sil* ŠÀ.MEŠ-*šú eb-[ṭu* ...]
169. DIŠ *e-mir u du-us-su* K[AR-*et* ...]
170. DIŠ *e-mir u tu-[l]im-šú* GU$_7$.MEŠ-*šú* ŠU [...]
171. DIŠ *ma-gal it-te-nen-sil re-du-ut ir-[ri* TUKU ...]

---

172. DIŠ *ir-ru-šú i-ḫar-ru-ru u* Á^{II}-[*šú* ...]
173. DIŠ *ir-ru-šú i-ḫar-ru-ru u* ŠÀ-*šú* [...]
174. DIŠ *ir-ru-šú i-ḫar-ru-ru* [...]
175. DIŠ *ir-ru-šú i-ḫar-ru-ru* Š[À-*šú*...]
176. DIŠ *ir-ru-šú it-ta-na-ʾ-ra-[ru* ...]
177. DIŠ *ir-ru-šú paṭ-ru na-kid* [...]
178. DIŠ *ir-ru-šú* SI.SÁ *u* Á^{II} [...]
179. DIŠ *ir-ru-šú* SI.SÁ [*u*] ŠÀ.MEŠ-*šú* [...]
180. [DIŠ *ir*]-⸢*ru*⸣-*šú* ⸢DÙ⸣-x[...]
181. [...]x[...]

TRANSLATION

1. [If] the ⸢patient's epigastrium⸣ is red, he will get well.
2. [If] his ⸢epigastrium⸣ is ⸢dark⸣ [and his tongue is shriveled, he is at an acute stage of the illness;[2] he will die].[3]
3–5. If his epigastrium is [unevenly colored] with yellow (spots), [when] his illness "touches" him, his neck [...] (and) the breath of his "right" and "left" nostril is cold, "hand" of the Netherworld (var.: "hand" of the brazier[4]); he will die.
6–7. If his epigastrium [continually] hurts [him], his "left" temple continually hurts him intensely, he is continually rigid, [inability to open the mouth afflicts him, his body] is ⸢feverish⸣ and he has wasting away of the flesh, that person is sick with a venereal disease.[5]
8–9. [If his epigastrium] gives him a burning pain and he is feverish, he eats bread and it does agree with him, [he drinks water] ⸢and⸣ it does not taste good to him and his body is yellow, that person is sick with a venereal disease.[6]
10. [If] his ⸢epigastrium⸣ continually afflicts him, affliction by a ghost.[7]

11. [If] his ⸢epigastrium⸣ continually afflicts him and his tongue is shriveled, he is at an acute stage of the illness;[8] he will die.[9]

12–13. [If] his ⸢epigastrium⸣ continually afflicts him and his insides are bloated, his illness will be prolonged. (If he has been sick) for thirty-one days, "hand" of a tithe owed to the great (gods).[10]

14. If his epigastrium continually afflicts him (and) his insides, his upper arms, his shins, and his feet continually hurt him, "hand" of his god; (there will be) recovery.[11]

15. If his epigastrium is cramped (and) his upper back continually hurts him, "hand" of ghost.[12]

16. If his epigastrium (feels) stiff, he will not get well. If his epigastrium is bloated, it is worrisome.

17. If his epigastrium is continually bloated, affliction by a ghost.[13]

18. If his epigastrium protrudes and his insides are bloated, his illness will be prolonged.

19–20. If his epigastrium protrudes (but) he does not have a fever (and) his mentation is altered, overwhelming of *aganutillû*. If it increases on him, he will die on a day when it is raining/hailing.[14]

21. If his epigastrium is puffed up and his face is swollen (and) tears flow from his eyes, if it is prolonged, he will die.[15]

22. If his epigastrium is puffed up and his hypogastric region is hard, (and he has been sick for) twenty-seven days, "hand" of a tithe owed to the great (gods).[16]

23–24. If his epigastrium is puffed up and his hypogastric region is hard (and) he gets hot and gets cold, he has approached the *ēntu* priestess of his god.[17] If it lets up within 31 days, he will get well.[18]

25. If his epigastrium is puffed up and his hypogastric region is soft, "hand" of a tithe owed to the great (gods).[19]

26. If his epigastrium is uncongested[20] and his hypogastric region is hard (and he has been sick for) twenty-seven days, "hand" of a tithe owed to the great (gods).[21]

27. If his epigastrium is uncongested but rumbles,[22] "hand" of a tithe owed to the great (gods).[23]

28. If his epigastrium is soft (and) he gets hot and gets cold, scepter of his god. It is the same for adults and children.[24]

29. If his epigastrium is hot and his insides are continually bloated, affliction by a ghost.[25]

30. If his epigastrium is hot and the blood vessels of his temples, his hands and his feet continually (feel like they) are pulsating (and) his eyes (feel) heavy (affliction by a ghost).[26]
31. If his epigastrium is puffed up and his hypogastric region is hard (and) he gets cold and gets hot, "hand" of the goddess; he will not get well.[27]
32. If his epigastrium holds fever (and) his mentation is altered, he drank water from a hoisting device of the river. If it affects the diaphragm, he will die.[28]
33. If his epigastrium is sore (and) he gets up and (has to) sit down, the ghost of (his) brother or sister afflicts him.
34. If his epigastrium or his hypogastric region "goes" and his body is cold, he will die.[29]
35. If he was injured on his epigastrium, "hand" of Adad (var. a good entrusted by Shamash to the twin gods).[30]
36. If he was injured on his epigastrium (and) his hands and his feet are immobilized, "hand" of the daughter of Anu.[31]
37. If he was injured on his epigastrium and his armpit, he makes a habit of intercourse with (another) man's wife.
38. If he was injured on his epigastrium, his temple and his rib, "hand" of Ereškigal; he will die.[32]
39. If a burning pain[33] is firmly established in his epigastrium and he continually produces dark blood, he will die.[34]
40. If a burning pain is firmly established in his epigastrium and he vomits dark blood and he has a vise-like headache, he will die.
41. If a needling pain or burning pain is firmly established in his epigastrium and he excretes blood, he will die.[35]
42. If a needling pain or burning pain is firmly established in his epigastrium and he vomits blood, (and he has been sick) for two or three days, he will die.[36]
43. If a ⌜needling pain⌝ [or burning pain is firmly established] in his epigastrium and he is constipated, he will die.[37]
44. If a ⌜needling pain⌝ [is firmly established] in his epigastrium [and will not] ⌜let up⌝, (and he has been sick) for thirty-one days, "hand" of Adad; he will die.[38]
45. If [a needling pain is firmly established] in his epigastrium (and) it is unevenly colored with ⌜yellow spots⌝, "hand" of Marduk (var. "hand" of Ishtar); he will die.[39]
46. If in [his] ⌜epigastrium⌝ [...], "hand" of the rainbow; he will get well (var. he will die).

47. If his abdomen [is bloated on the "right" side] ⸢his⸣ [illness] will alter (for the worse).

48. If his abdomen is bloated on the "left" side, ⸢his⸣ illness will be difficult.

49. If [both sides of his] abdomen ⸢are bloated⸣, "hand" of Kubu; he may have a hard time of it but he will get well.

50. If ⸢his⸣ abdomen [...], ⸢"hand"⸣ of Ishtar.

51. If his abdomen is [...], "hand" of Damu.

52. If his abdomen hurts him, "hand" of Shamash.

53. If his abdomen [afflicts him], "hand" of Bau. If he cannot lift his hand ("hand" of Bau).

54. [If] his abdomen afflicts [him so that] he ⸢says⸣ [Wah!], "hand" of Gula. If a yoke is established on his neck and goes round (it, "hand" of Gula).[40]

55–56. [If] ⸢his⸣ [abdomen] is hot (but) his ear ⸢canals⸣ are cold (and) the scepter of the cold goes to his mouth, if it is prolonged, he will die.[41]

57–58. [If his abdomen] continually [holds] fever (and) his ear canals are hot (and) the scepter of the heat goes to his mouth, (there will be a) recovery.[42]

59. If his abdomen is hot and his epigastrium protrudes, he will get well.

60–61. If his abdomen burns with fever[43] (and) his toes are cold, if he lasts for three or four days, he will get well (var. die).

62. If his abdomen is hot, sweat keeps falling upon him as in *lubāṭu* and (his stomach) is continually upset, he will die.

63–64. If his abdomen is hot, sweat keeps falling upon him as in *lubāṭu* and (his stomach) is continually upset, "hand" of Shamash. You do his treatment and if you continually wipe him off, he will get well.[44]

65–66. If his abdomen is hot, sweat keeps falling upon him as in *lubāṭu* and (his stomach) is continually upset, his abdomen burns with fever[45] (and) his toes are cold, if he lasts for three days, he will get well.[46]

67. If his abdomen is hot, sweat keeps falling upon him as in *lubāṭu* and he is cold (and he has been sick for) thirty-one days, "hand" of Shamash.[47]

68. If his abdomen is hot (and) sweat keeps falling on him, either "hand" of Shamash or "hand" of Shulak; he was injured on the front side.[48]

69. If his abdomen gets hot and gets cold (and) he asks for a lot of water and then drinks it, "hand" of Lamashtu.[49]

70. If his abdomen gets hot and gets cold (and) he continually asks for a lot of water to bathe in, "hand" of Lamashtu; he will get well.[50]

71–72. If his abdomen is soft, he asks for a lot of water (but) his temperature is even, (and) if his illness has kept him awake from the beginning to the middle of the night, he was stricken with the blow of a *rābiṣu*[51]-demon (var. a ghost); he will die.[52]

73–74. If his heart flutters, his epigastrium pulses rapidly (and) he continually stretches out his eyes toward the darkness, "hand" of ghost.[53]

75–76. If he was injured on his abdomen (and he has been sick for) nine days, "hand" of the twin gods.[54] If (it is) the second (day), "hand" of Adad. If the third, "hand" of Ea. If the fourth, "hand" of Dingirmaḫ. If the fifth, "hand" of Papsukkal.

77. If he was injured on his abdomen (and it) is colicky and constipated, he will die. If he was injured on his abdomen and, consequently, (it) is also continually upset, "hand" of the twin gods; he will die.[55]

78. If he was injured on his abdomen and, consequently, he also continually produces dark blood, affliction by the twin gods; he will die.[56]

79. If he was injured on his abdomen or on the "left" side of his abdomen and, consequently, he also vomits blood, (and he has been sick) for thirty-one days, "hand" of Nergal; he will die.[57]

80. If needling pains are firmly established in his abdomen on the "right" side and he continually vomits, "hand" of Ishtar; he will live.[58]

81. If needling pains are firmly established in his abdomen on the "left" side and he does not vomit, "hand" of Ishtar; he will die.

82. If a burning pain is firmly established in his abdomen on the "right" side and he vomits, "hand" of Ishtar; he will die.[59]

83. If a burning pain is firmly established in his abdomen on the "left" side and he vomits, "hand" of Ishtar; he will die.

84. If a burning pain is firmly established in his abdomen on the "right" side and he vomits blood, "hand" of Ishtar; he will die.[60]

85. If a burning pain is firmly established in his abdomen on the "left" side and he vomits blood, "hand" of Adad (var. G. Ishtar); he will die.[61]

86. If a burning pain is firmly established in his abdomen on the "left" side and he drips blood, "hand" of Adad; he will die.[62]

87–88. If a burning pain is firmly established in his abdomen on the "left" side and his eyes are full of yellow threads, "hand" of Ishtar; he will die.[63]

89. If in his abdomen on the "left" side ditto (a burning pain is firmly established) and his lips produce *šīqu*, "hand" of Sîn or "hand" of Ishtar; he will die.[64]

90. If needling pains or burning pains are firmly established in his abdomen on the "right" or "left" side and he continually produces dark blood, he will die.[65]

91. If in his abdomen ditto (a needling pain or burning pain is firmly established) and he kneads his tongue, the curses of his father have "gotten" him. If he has a difficult time of it, he will die (var. even if he has a difficult time of it, he will get well).
92. If there is *šīqu* in his abdomen (and) yellow threads cross in his eyes, he will die.
93. If his chest and abdomen are red, he will get well.
94. If his chest and abdomen are yellow, it is worrisome.
95. If his chest and abdomen are black, he will die.
96–97. If his chest and abdomen are black, the muscles of his abdomen are pulled taut, (and) he belches "wind" from his mouth, (once he has been sick) for three days, he will die.[66]
98. If his chest and abdomen are dark, it is worrisome.
99. If his chest and abdomen are dark red, his illness will be prolonged.
100. If his chest and abdomen are flat, it is of no consequence.[67]
101. If his insides have dried up, he will die.[68]
102. If his insides are stopped up, "hand" of Damu.[69]
103. If a person's insides are bloated, his illness will be prolonged (var. it is worrisome).
104. If his insides are bloated and the muscles of his abdomen are pulled taut, "hand" of Ishtar; he will not get well.[70]
105–6. If his insides are bloated and the muscles of his abdomen are pulled taut (and) unevenly colored with yellow, (and) his temperature is even, if it keeps coming back ⌈again and again⌉, he will die.[71]
107–8. If his insides are bloated and the muscles of his abdomen are unevenly colored with yellow, (and he has been sick) for thirty-one days, "hand" of ⌈Ishhara⌉; [...].[72]
109. If his insides are bloated and the muscles of his abdomen are unevenly colored with yellow, he will die.
110–11. If his insides are bloated, the ⌈muscles⌉ of [his abdomen are yellow (and) his umbilical area is red, a ghost [...].
112. If his insides are bloated and full of "wind" [...].
113–14. [If] his ⌈insides⌉ are bloated and ditto (full of "wind"), either "hand" of his god ⌈or⌉ ["hand" of his goddess] (var. "hand" of Ishtar).
115. ⌈If⌉ his insides are bloated and (full of "wind" and) his temperature is not ⌈even⌉, if it is prolonged [...].
116. ⌈If⌉ his insides are bloated and his shoulders [...].
117. ⌈If⌉ his insides are continually bloated, "hand" of Kubu (var. [...]).[73]

118. ⸢If⸣ his insides (are continually bloated) and he continually wails, "hand" of Kubu (var. "hand" of […]).[74]
119. ⸢If⸣ his insides (are continually bloated) and his eyes (feel) heavy, "hand" of Kubu (var. "hand" of […]).[75]
120. [If his insides] are [continually] bloated and) his eyes (feel) heavy, "hand" of Kubu; he will get well.
121. [If his insides] are continually cramped (and) he cannot eat anything […].
122. [If his insides] ditto (are continually cramped) and his arms are tense[76] […].
123. [If] his ⸢insides⸣ ditto (are continually cramped and) his eyes (feel) heavy […].
124. [If] his ⸢chest and abdomen⸣ are soft and he continually asks for a lot of water and drinks (it) [and he has/does not have] a ⸢fever⸣ […].
125. [If] his chest and abdomen ditto (are soft) and he continually asks for a lot of water (but) his temperature is even, (and) [his illness has kept him awake] from the middle of the night till […].
126. If his chest and abdomen (are soft) and he continually asks for a lot of water to drink (but) his temperature is even, (and) [his illness has kept him awake] from the beginning of the night till […].
127. If his insides, his hands and his feet are continually cramped (and he has been sick for) thirty-two days, either a man ⸢or⸣ [a woman …].
128. If he continually rubs his chest and abdomen, his hands and his feet a lot, (and) he ⸢utters⸣ a *šigû*-prayer, […].
129. If ditto (he continually rubs) his chest and abdomen, his hands (and) his feet and his tendons[77] are limp, ⸢if⸣ he has a difficult time of it, […].
130. If his insides are as sluggish as his fingers (and he has been sick) for thirty one days[78] […].
131. If his insides are continually purged[79] (but) he is not able to pour out his urine, "hand" of ⸢Ištar⸣.[80]
132. If he keeps crying out: "My insides, my insides," ⸢it is⸣ of no consequence.
133. If ditto (he keeps crying out): "My insides, my insides," the patient has done something offensive to his god; he has raised his hand against (another) man or woman; "hand" of […]; he will die.
134. If he keeps crying out: "My insides, my insides!" and he tears his hair, he was injured on his thorax; he will die.[81]
135. If he keeps crying out: "My insides, my insides" and his hip socket hurts him, "hand" of Ishtar.

136. If he keeps crying out: "My insides, my insides!," his hips are raised up, his confusional state(s)[82] come over him (and) when they come over him, he continually talks in a frightful manner, "hand" of *ardat lilî*.[83]
137. If he keeps crying out: "My insides, my insides" and he gets up and runs, a ghost, the "double" of a dead person afflicts him.[84]
138. [If] he keeps crying out softly (var. intermittently?): "My insides, my insides," "hand" of a murderous ghost; [he will die].[85]
139. [If] he has been continually crying out: "My insides, my insides" for half a day, a curse of Sîn (var: Shamash) afflicts him.
140. [If] he keeps crying out: ["My insides, my] ⸢insides⸣" for two or three days, the patient has done something offensive to his god.
141. If he keeps crying out: "My insides, my insides" for five days, he will die.
142–43. If in the middle (watch), he keeps crying out: "My insides, my insides," his eyes are confused (and) his eyesight is difficult (and) his "left" foot continually afflicts him, anger of a *rabiṣu* continually afflicts him; he will speedily die.
144. If he comes to the dusk(-watch) and he keeps crying out: "My insides, my insides," hand of the twin gods. (Once he has been sick) for seven days, he will die.
145. If from sunset on, there is an increase (of the illness) and he keeps crying out: "My insides, my insides," "hand" of ghost.
146. If all day he chokes and in the night, he keeps crying out : "My insides, my insides," "hand" of ghost.
147. If his liver is … , he will die.
148–149. If his liver hurts him (and) his ⸢hearing⸣ is difficult, during the course of his illness, his neck continually "falls," [his "right" temple (feels like it) is hot], (and) his "left" one (feels like it) is cold, "hand" of curse; he will die.[86]
150. [If he keeps crying out: "My insides, my insides"] (and) his ⸢epigastrium⸣ protrudes, [he will die].[87]
151. [If he keeps crying out: "My insides, my insides"] (and) the wall of his abdomen approaches his lung (i.e., his diaphragm breaks), he will die.[88]
152. [If he keeps crying out: "My insides, my insides"] (and) he is impotent, "hand" of Ishtar, he is at an acute stage of the ⸢illness⸣;[89] [he will die].[90]
153. *(unclear and broken)*
154. [If he keeps crying out: "My insides, my insides"] (and) he continually has a crushing sensation[91] in his chest, "hand" of Ishtar (var. "hand" of […]).
155. [If the blood vessel(s) of] his umbilical area "go," "hand" of […].

156. [If] the ⸢muscle(s)⸣ of [an infant's] abdomen are unevenly colored with red and yellow, "hand" of [Kubu].[92]

157–158. [If the muscles] of his [abdomen], those of the "right" and "left" sides are ⸢drawn taut⸣ across his abdomen, a curse ⸢afflicts⸣ [him].[93]

159–161. *(too broken to translate)*

---

162. If his hypogastric region and [his] epigastrium [...].
163. If he was injured on his hypogastric region, "hand" of the ⸢twin gods⸣ [...].
164. If he was injured on his hypogastric region and [his] ⸢virility⸣ [is taken away ...].[94]
165. If he was injured on his hypogastric region and his feet [...].

---

166. If he is colicky[95] and constipated [...].
167. If he is colicky and constipated (and) his insides are ⸢cramped⸣ [...].
168. If he is colicky and constipated (and) his insides are ⸢cramped⸣ [...].
169. If he is colicky and his virility is ⸢taken away⸣ [...].
170. If he is colicky and his spleen continually hurts him, "hand" of [...].
171. If he is continually very sluggish (and) [has] "flowing of the ⸢bowels⸣" [...]

---

172. If his bowels rumble[96] and [his] arms [...].
173. If his bowels rumble and his stomach [...].
174. If his bowels rumble [...].
175. If his bowels rumble (and) [his] ⸢stomach⸣ [...].
176. If his bowels continually vomit [...].
177. If his bowels were (cut) loose, it is worrisome.[97]
178. If his bowels are loose[98] and [his] arms [...].
179. If his bowels are loose [and] his insides [...].

180-181.If his bowels [...].

Notes

1. Text G has ŠU ^{d}IM.
2. For the reading and interpretation, see Heeßel 2000, 164 (after Landsberger).
3. See Scurlock and Andersen 2005, 18.37.
4. The commentary, GCCI 2 406 obv. 2, explains this as "hand" of Nusku.
5. A quite similar entry appears in DPS 22:10–11.
6. See Scurlock and Andersen 2005, 4.35, 13.27. This entry appears also in DPS 22:12–13.
7. See Scurlock and Andersen 2005, 19.386.
8. For the interpretation, see Heeßel 2000, 187.

9. See Scurlock and Andersen 2005, 3.103, 18.36.

10. See Scurlock and Andersen 2005, 3.211.

11. See Scurlock and Andersen 2005, 19.363.

12. See Scurlock and Andersen 2005, 19.297.

13. See Scurlock and Andersen 2005, 6.33, 19.298. This entry also appears in Wilhelm 1994, 41 rev. 8′–9′.

14. See Scurlock and Andersen 2005, 8.22.

15. See Scurlock and Andersen 2005, 6.36, 8.21, 20.83. This entry appears also in DPS 15:34′.

16. See Scurlock and Andersen 2005, 3.212.

17. I.e., incestuously approached his mother.

18. See Scurlock and Andersen 2005, 6.41.

19. See Scurlock and Andersen 2005, 3.213.

20. Literally: "clear."

21. See Scurlock and Andersen 2005, 3.213.

22. See *AHw* 171, 65b.

23. See Scurlock and Andersen 2005, 3.213.

24. See Scurlock and Andersen 2005, 19.362.

25. See Scurlock and Andersen 2005, 19.388.

26. See Scurlock and Andersen 2005, 6.79, 8.42, 19.388.

27. See Scurlock and Andersen 2005, 19.347.

28. See Scurlock and Andersen 2005, 15.31.

29. See Scurlock and Andersen 2005, 20.22.

30. See Scurlock and Andersen 2005, 19.139, 19.183.

31. See Scurlock and Andersen 2005, 19.159.

32. See Scurlock and Andersen 2005, 19.173.

33. For this interpretation of ^{GIŠ}NÍG.GIDRU/*ḫaṭṭu*: "sceptre" as a punning writing for *ḫaṭṭu*/*ḫanṭu* from *ḫamāṭu*, see *CAD* D, 137 s.v. *dikšu* mng. 1a1′.

34. See Scurlock and Andersen 2005, 6.93, 20.51.

35. See Scurlock and Andersen 2005, 6.94, 20.65.

36. Alternatively: "he will die within two or three days." See Scurlock and Andersen 2005, 6.95, 20.52.

37. See Scurlock and Andersen 2005, 6.91.

38. The positioning of the "hand" would seem to indicate that this was intended as a diagnosis (what is the cause) and not a prognosis ("he will die within thirty-one days").

39. See Scurlock and Andersen 2005, 19.113.

40. See Scurlock and Andersen 2005, 10.103, 19.329.

41. See Scurlock and Andersen 2005, 14.45, 20.16.

42. See Scurlock and Andersen 2005, 14.46, 20.16.

43. See above, DPS 3:70.

44. See Scurlock and Andersen 2005, 6.80, 19.256.

45. See above, DPS 3:70.

46. See Scurlock and Andersen 2005, 10.26.

47. See Scurlock and Andersen 2005, 19.193, 19.258.

48. See Scurlock and Andersen 2005, 19.192.

49. See Scurlock and Andersen 2005, 19.230.

50. See Scurlock and Andersen 2005, 19.231.

51. This demon served for the gods the same service supplied by his human counterpart, who was a court bailiff.

52. See Scurlock and Andersen 2005, 6.42.

53. See Scurlock and Andersen 2005, 8.9, 9.15, 13.215.

54. See Scurlock and Andersen 2005, 19.146.

55. See Scurlock and Andersen 2005, 3.204, 19.137. This entry appears also in DPS 15:35′–36′.

56. See Scurlock and Andersen 2005, 19.181., 20.50.

57. The positioning of the "hand" would seem to indicate that this was intended as a diagnosis (what is the cause) and not a prognosis ("he will die within thirty-one days"). See Scurlock and Andersen 2005, 19.175.

58. See Scurlock and Andersen 2005, 20.66.

59. See Scurlock and Andersen 2005, 20.67.

60. See Scurlock and Andersen 2005, 19.373.

61. See Scurlock and Andersen 2005, 19.373.

62. See Scurlock and Andersen 2005, 6.152.

63. See Scurlock and Andersen 2005, 6.126, 9.38, 19.374.

64. See Scurlock and Andersen 2005, 19.376.

65. See Scurlock and Andersen 2005, 6.7.

66. Alternatively, "he will die within three days." See Scurlock and Andersen 2005, 3.208. This entry appears also in DPS 15:37.

67. See Scurlock and Andersen 2005, 7.16.

68. See Scurlock and Andersen 2005, 3.109, 20.81.

69. See Scurlock and Andersen 2005, 17.120.

70. See Scurlock and Andersen 2005, 19.152.

71. See Scurlock and Andersen 2005, 6.144.

72. The positioning of the "hand" would seem to indicate that this was intended as a diagnosis (what is the cause) and not a prognosis ("he will die within thirty-one days").

73. See Scurlock and Andersen 2005, 19.337.

74. See Scurlock and Andersen 2005, 19.337.

75. See Scurlock and Andersen 2005, 19.337.

76. See Scurlock and Andersen 2005, p. 212.

77. See the commentary GCCI 4.406 obv. 7.

78. Alternatively, "he will […] within thirty-one days."

79. The translation "purge" is based on etymological connection with Syr. *ṣebʿ*. Suggestion courtesy W. G. Lambert.

80. See Scurlock and Andersen 2005, 5.28.

81. See Scurlock and Andersen 2005, 14.12. The entry appears also in BAM 15:38′.

82. See the commentary GCCI 4.406 obv. 9.

83. See Scurlock and Andersen 2005, 13.264.

84. See Scurlock and Andersen 2005, 19.30.

85. See Scurlock and Andersen 2005, 19.385.

86. See Scurlock and Andersen 2005, 13.222, 19.314.

87. This entry appears also in Wilhelm 1994, 48 obv. 5.

88. See Scurlock and Andersen 2005, 14.13.

89. For the interpretation, see Heeßel 2000, 187.

90. See Scurlock and Andersen 2005, 19.162.

91. The commentary GCCI 4.406 obv. 10 explains this as "roasting" (pain).

92. This entry appears also in DPS 40:32.

93. See Scurlock and Andersen 2005, 19.307.

94. See Scurlock and Andersen 2005, 5.69, 19.161.

95. See *CAD* E, 148.
96. See *AHw* 171, 65b.
97. See Scurlock and Andersen 2005, 3.203.
98. I.e., he has diarrhea.

DPS TABLET 14

1. [DIŠ GIG *gi-l*]*iš* 15-*šú* SA$_5$ [DIN : GIG-*su ú-zab-bal-ma* DIN][1]
2. [DIŠ *gi-liš* 1]50-*šú* SA$_5$ GIG-*su ú-za-bal*
3. [DIŠ TUGUL.M]EŠ-*šú* SA$_5$ LÚG [N]U TUKU
4. [DIŠ *gi*]-*liš* 15-*šú* SIG$_7$ GI[G]-*su* MAN-*ni*
5. [DIŠ *gi*]-*liš* 150-*šú* SIG$_7$ [GIG]-*su* DUGUD-*it*
6. [DIŠ TUGUL].MEŠ-*š*[*ú* SIG$_7$ *n*]*a-ḫi-id*
7. [DIŠ *gi-liš* 15-*šú* GI$_6$ GIG]-*su* DUGUD
8. [DIŠ *gi-liš* 150-*šú* GI$_6$ *n*]*a-ḫi-id*
9. [DIŠ TUGUL.MEŠ-*šú* GI$_6$] BA.ÚŠ
10. [DIŠ *gi-liš* 15-*šú tar-kat* GI]G-*su* MAN-*ni*
11. [DIŠ *gi-liš* 150-*šú tar-kat* GI]G-*su* DUGUD
12. [DIŠ TUGUL.MEŠ-*šú tar-ka n*]*a-ḫi-id*
13. DIŠ [*gi-liš* 15-*šú du-ʾ-mat* GI]⸢G-*su ú-zab-bal*⸣[2]
14. DIŠ [*gi-liš* 150-*šú du-ʾ-mat* GIG-*su*] MAN-*ni*
15. DIŠ [TUGUL.MEŠ-*šú du-ʾ-ma* GIG-*s*]*u* DUGUD
16. [DIŠ *gi-liš* 15-*šú nap-ḫat* GIG]-*su* MAN-*ni*
17. [DIŠ *gi-liš* 150-*šú nap-ḫat* GIG]-*su* DUGUD
18. DIŠ [TUGUL.MEŠ-*šú nu-up-pu-ḫa* GIG]-*su* MAN-*ni*
19. [DIŠ *gi-liš* 15-*šú muq-qu-ta-á*]*t*[3] TI
20. DIŠ [*gi-liš* 150-*šú muq-qu-ta-at* GIG-*s*]*u* MAN-*ni*
21. DIŠ [TUGUL.MEŠ-*šú muq-qu-ta n*]*a-ḫi-id*
22. DIŠ *gi*[-*liš* 15-*šú* DU$_8$-*rat* GIG]-*su* DUGUD[4]
23. DIŠ *gi-l*[*iš* 150-*šú* DU$_8$-*rat n*]*a-ḫi-i*[*d*(coll.)]
24. DIŠ TUGUL.MEŠ-[*šú* DU$_8$-*ra* GIG-*s*]*u* [DUGUD]
25. DIŠ *gi-liš* 1[5-*šú in-ni-ṣil* GI]G-*s*[*u* DUGUD][5]
26. DIŠ *gi-liš* 150-*šú* [*in-ni-ṣil* …]
27. DIŠ TUGUL.MEŠ-*šú in*-⸢*ni*⸣-*ṣ*[*i-la* …]
28. DIŠ MUNUS TUGUL.MEŠ-*šá it-te-né-ṣ*[*i-la* …][6]
29. DIŠ TUGUL.MEŠ-*šú šal*-[*ma* DIN]
30. DIŠ TA TUGUL-*šú* EN U.MEŠ GÌR^{II}-*šú* SA.MEŠ-*š*[*ú* …]
31. *ki-is-sat* [UD.DA]
32. ⸢DIŠ GU⸣.DU 15-*šú* SA$_5$-*át* [DIN]

33. [DIŠ G]U.DU 150-*šú* SA$_5$-*át* GIG-*su ú*-[*zab-bal*]
34. [DIŠ G]U.DU.MEŠ-*šú* SA$_5$.MEŠ LÚG [NU TUKU]
35. [DIŠ G]U.DU 15-*šú* SIG$_7$-*át* GIG-*su* MAN-*ni*
36. [DIŠ G]U.DU 150-*šú* SIG$_7$-*át* GIG⸢-*su*⸣ DUGUD
37. [DIŠ GU].DU.MEŠ-*šú* SIG$_7$.MEŠ *na-ḫi-id*
38. [DIŠ GU.D]U 15-*šú* GI$_6$-*át* GIG-*su* DUGUD
39. [DIŠ GU.DU] 150-*šú* GI$_6$-*át na-ḫi-id*
40. [DIŠ GU.DU.MEŠ]-*šú* GI$_6$.MEŠ ⸢BA.ÚŠ⸣
41. [DIŠ GU].⸢DU⸣ 15-*šú* ⸢*tar*⸣-*kat ú-zab-bal-ma* DIN
42. [DIŠ GU.DU 150-*šú tar-kat* …]
43. [DIŠ GU].DU.MEŠ-*šú tar-ku* GAM
44. [DIŠ GU.DU 15-*šú du-ʾ-ú-mat* GIG-*su ú-zab-bal*]
45. [DIŠ GU].⸢DU 150⸣-*šú du-ʾ-ú-mat* GIG-*su* MAN-*ni*
46. [DIŠ GU.DU.MEŠ-*šú du-ʾ-ú-ma* GIG-*su* DUGUD]
47. [DIŠ] GU.DU 15-*šú nap-ḫat* GIG-*su* MAN-*ni*
48. [DIŠ GU.DU 150-*šú nap-ḫat* GIG-*su* DUGUD]
49. [DIŠ] GU.DU.MEŠ-*šú nu-up-pu-ḫu* GIG-*su* MAN-*ni*
50. [DIŠ GU.DU 15-*šú muq-qú-ta-át* …]
51. [D]IŠ GU.DU 150-*šú muq-qú-ta-át* GIG-*su* GÍD
52. [DIŠ GU.DU.MEŠ-*šú muq-qú-ta na-ḫi*]-*id*
53. [DIŠ] ⸢GU.DU 15⸣-*šú šu-uḫ-ḫu-ṭa-át* GIG-*su* MAN-*ni*
54. [DIŠ GU.DU 150-*šú šu-uḫ-ḫu-ṭa*]-⸢*át*⸣ [GIG-*s*]*u* DUGUD
55. DIŠ G[U].⸢DU.MEŠ-*šú šu*⸣-*uḫ-ḫu-ṭa na-ḫi-id*
56. DIŠ GU.DU 15-*šú* DU$_8$-*át* GIG-*su* MAN-*ni*
57. DIŠ GU.DU 150-*šú* DU$_8$-*át* GIG-*su na-ḫi-id*
58. DIŠ GU.DU.MEŠ-*šú* DU$_8$.MEŠ BA.ÚŠ
59. DIŠ GU.DU.MEŠ-*šú šal-ma* DIN
60. [DIŠ G]U.[D]U.MEŠ-*šú* GI$_6$.MEŠ-*ma* KI.GUB-*su* NU È-*a u* A NU *ú-še-rid* A GA SÌG-*iṣ* GAM
61. [DIŠ *ina*] ⸢TUGUL⸣-*šú u* GU.DU-*šú* SÌG-*iṣ* ŠU ^{d}15
62. [DIŠ *ina* TU]GUL-*šú u kin-ṣi-šú* SÌG-*iṣ* ŠU ^{d}15
63. [DIŠ *šá-p*]*u-la-šu* BAL.BAL-*ut* GIG-*su* MAN-*ni*
64. [DIŠ *šá*]-*pu-la-šu* BAL.BAL-*ut u* UŠ$_4$ LÍL-*šú* KÚR-*šú* ŠU ^{d}UTU DIN
65. […]-*am* DIŠ GUB-*ma ár*!-*ḫiš*! GAM
66. [DIŠ *ina šá*]-*pu-li-šu šá* 15 SÌG-*iṣ* UŠ$_4$-*šú* NU DIB-*bat-ma ina* NU ZU *ú-rap-pad* GAM
67. DIŠ *ina šá-pu-li-šu šá* 150 SÌG-*iṣ-ma* GIN$_7$ GÙ.GÙ NU ZU BA.ÚŠ
68. ⸢DIŠ SA *šá-pu-li-šu*⸣ *šá* 15 ZI.MEŠ *u* GI$_6$.MEŠ *ana* U$_4$.2.KAM BA.ÚŠ
69. [DIŠ SA] ⸢*šá-pu-li-šu*⸣ *šá* 150 ZI.MEŠ *u* GI$_6$.MEŠ *ár-hiš* BA.ÚŠ

70. ⸢DIŠ DÚR-*šú* GUB-*iz* GAM⸣
71. ⸢DIŠ DÚR-*šú* GUB-*iz u* IM⸣ […] ⸢DUGUD-*ma*⸣ GAM
72. ⸢DIŠ DÚR-*šú* BAD.BAD-*ir*⸣ GAM[7]
73. ⸢DIŠ DÚR-*šú ṣu*⸣-[*dur*? …] GAM
74. ⸢DIŠ *ina* DÚR-*šú* A⸣.M[EŠ] ⸢SA$_{5}$.MEŠ DU-*ku* GIG-*su* GÍD⸣
75. : ⸢DIŠ⸣ [*ina* DÚR]-⸢*šú* [A].MEŠ SIG$_{7}$.MEŠ DU-*ku* NA⸣.B[I …]
76. ⸢DIŠ *ina* DÚR-*šú* ZÉ⸣ [S]A$_{5}$ ⸢DU-*ak* GÍD-*ma* DIN⸣
77. : ⸢DIŠ⸣ [*ina*] ⸢DÚR-*šú*⸣ [Z]É ⸢SIG$_{7}$⸣ DU-*ak k*[*a*]? *lu*? *mir-riš* BA.ÚŠ
78. ⸢DIŠ *ina* DÚR-*šú* ZÉ⸣ G[I$_{6}$ D]U-⸢*ak* GAM⸣
79. DIŠ *ina* DÚR-*šú* ⸢Ì ŠÀ-*šú* DU-*ku* GAM⸣
80. DIŠ *ina* DÚR-*šú d*[*a*]-*ku-ti*[8] ŠÀ-*šú* ŠUB.ŠUB-*a* GAM⸣
81. DIŠ *ina* DÚR-*šú* ⸢UZU ŠUB.ŠUB⸣-[*a* …]
82. DIŠ *ina* DÚR-*šú* MÚD ⸢MUD ŠUB.ŠUB-*a* GAM⸣
83. DIŠ *ina* DÚR-*šú* MÚD ⸢*u* IM ŠUB.ŠUB⸣-[*a*…]
84. DIŠ *ina* DÚR-*šú* MÚD *it*-⸢*te*⸣-*eṣ-ṣí* ŠU […]
85. DIŠ *ina* DÚR-*šú* MÚD MUD *it-te-ez-zi* Š[U …]
86. DIŠ *ina* DÚR-*šú* MÚD *u* ÚŠ.BABBAR *it-te-ez-zi* ŠU ^{d}[…]

---

87. DIŠ DÚR-*šú is-s*[*e-kir* DÚR.GI]G GAM
88. DIŠ ŠE$_{10}$-*šú* SA$_{5}$.MEŠ DIN
89. DIŠ ŠE$_{10}$-*šú* SIG$_{7}$.[MEŠ …]
90. DIŠ ŠE$_{10}$-*šú* [GI$_{6}$].MEŠ GAM
91. DIŠ ŠE$_{10}$-*šú du-ʾ-ú-*[*mu* …]
92. DIŠ ŠE$_{10}$-*š*[*ú* …] GIG-*su* GÍD
93. : DIŠ ŠE$_{10}$-*ú-šú* ŠÀ[…]
94. [DIŠ DÚR?-*šú*] *i*[*t-te-n*]*ek-ki-ik* ḪAR.GIG [GIG]
95. [DIŠ GÌŠ-*šú* SA$_{5}$-*át* GIG-*su*] GÍD-*ma* DIN
96. DIŠ GÌŠ-*šú* SIG$_{7}$-⸢*át*⸣ G[IG-*su* …]
97. [DIŠ GÌŠ-*šú* GI$_{6}$-*a*]*t* GAM
98. DIŠ GÌŠ-*šú tar-kát na-*[*ḫi*]-*i*[*d*]
99. [DIŠ GÌŠ-*šú du-ʾ-ú-mat*] GIG-*su ú-ša-an-na-aḫ*
100. DIŠ GÌŠ-*šú nap-ḫat na-ḫi-id*
101. [DIŠ GÌŠ-*šú muq-qú-t*]*a-át* DIN
102. DIŠ GÌŠ-*šú šu-uḫ-ḫu-ṭ*[*a-at-ma* NU DU$_{8}$]-*ir* GAM

---

103. [DIŠ GÌŠ-*šú šal-mat*] DIN
104. DIŠ GÌŠ-*šú is-se-kir* GAM
105. DIŠ GÌŠ-*šú* bar/maš […] GAM

---

106. [DIŠ GÌŠ-*šú u* SAG ŠÀ-*šú* KÚM ÚḪ *ú-kal* TÙN ŠÀ-*šú* GU$_7$-*šú u* ŠÀ-*šú* *ma-ḫu*
107. Á^{II}-*šú* GÌR^{II}-*šú* ŠÀ-*šú* KÚM NA BI GIG *na-a-ki* GIG
108. ŠU DINGIR-*šú* : ^{d}15-*šú*
109. DIŠ *ina mu-šar-ri-šú* MÚD SUR ŠU ^{d}UTU MU KI MUNUS(!)[9] GI GAM
110. DIŠ *mu-šar-šú u* ŠIR^{II}-*šú nap-ḫu* ŠU ^{d}*Dil-bat ina* KI.NÁ-*šú* KUR-*su*

---

111. DIŠ KÀŠ.MEŠ-*šú* SA$_5$.MEŠ ŠU DINGIR-*šú* DIN
112. DIŠ KÀŠ.MEŠ-*šú* SIG$_7$.MEŠ GIG-*su* GÍD KI.MIN UD.DA TAB-*iṭ* GAM
113. [DIŠ K[ÀŠ.MEŠ-*šú* GI$_6$.MEŠ TAG ÚŠ TAG-*it* GAM
114. DIŠ KÀŠ.MEŠ-*šú tar-ka* GAM
115. [DIŠ KÀ]Š.MEŠ-*šú it-te-né-es-ki-ra* GAM
116. DIŠ KÀŠ.MEŠ-*šu* DU.MEŠ GAM
117. [DIŠ KÀ]Š.MEŠ-*šú u* A.RI.A-*su* DU-*ak* GAM
118. DIŠ [K]ÀŠ.MEŠ-*šu* GI[N$_7$ …] x GAM
119. [DIŠ K]ÀŠ.MEŠ-*šú* GIN$_7$ A.MEŠ GIG-*su* GÍD-*ma* DIN
120. DIŠ KÀŠ.MEŠ-*šú* GIN$_7$ A GAZI[^{SAR}] KI.MIN
121. [DIŠ K]ÀŠ.MEŠ-*šú* GIN$_7$ GEŠTIN GIG-*su* DUGUD-*ma*[10] DIN
122. DIŠ KÀŠ.MEŠ-*šú* GIN$_7$ GA DIN
123. DIŠ KÀŠ.MEŠ-*šú taq-na* [GIG-*su* GÍD-*ma* DIN]
124. DIŠ KÀŠ.MEŠ-*šú* IGI-*ma li-piš-tú* È.MEŠ-*ni ina* EDIN TA[G-*it*]
125. DIŠ KÀŠ.MEŠ-*šú* IGI-*ma* UZU.ME-*šú* È.ME-*ni ina* EDIN T[AG-*it*]

---

126. DIŠ ŠIR^{II}-*šú* SA$_5$.MEŠ DIN
127. DIŠ ŠIR^{II}-*šú* SIG$_7$.MEŠ […]
128. DIŠ ŠIR^{II}-*šú* GI$_6$.MEŠ GAM
129. DIŠ ŠIR^{II}-*šú tar-ka* […]
130. DIŠ ŠIR^{II}-*šú du-ʾ-um-ma* GIG-*su* DUGUD
131. DIŠ ŠIR^{II}-*šú muq-qú-ta$_5$* […]
132. DIŠ ŠIR^{II}-*šú šu-uḫ-ḫu-ṭa* GAM
133. DIŠ ŠIR^{II}-*šú šal-*[*ma* DIN]
134. DIŠ ŠIR^{II}-*šú ze-ra* GAM : *ana* NIN.DINGIR.RA [DINGIR-*šú* TE-*ḫi*]
135. DIŠ ŠIR^{II}-*šú ze-ra* EME-*šú i-te-níq-qí-iq*
136. NUNDUN.MEŠ-*šú ú-na-*[*aš-ša-ak*][11]
137. DIŠ ŠIR^{II}-*šú nap-ḫu na-ḫi-iṭ* : *ana* NIN.DINGIR.RA [DINGIR-*šú* TE-*ḫi*]
138. DIŠ ŠIR^{II}-*šú* MÚ.MEŠ-*ḫa* GÌŠ-*šú sik-ka-ta$_5$* DIRI *ana* N[IN.DINGIR.RA DINGIR-*šú* TE-*ḫi*]
139. DIŠ *ina* ŠIR^{II}-*šú* SÌG-*iṣ ana* NIN.DINGIR.RA DINGIR-*šú* TE-*ḫi* : […]
140. DIŠ *ina* ŠIR^{II}-*šú* SÌG-*iṣ* (*ḫi-pi*) *ana* x[…]-*šú it-te-né-*[…]

141. DIŠ ÉLLAG *zi-kar-ti-šú* GAZ-*át pa-pa-a*[*n* ŠÀ-*šú* …]
142. KÀŠ.MEŠ-*šú* DIB.DI[B …]
143. DIŠ *šap-la-tu-šú nap-ḫ*[*a* …]

---

144. DIŠ ÚR 15-*šú* SA$_5$-*át ú-pa-su* ⸢*e*⸣-[…]
145. DIŠ ÚR 150-*šú* SA$_5$[-*át* …]
146. DIŠ ÚR.MEŠ-*šú* SA$_5$.MEŠ *na-ʾ-iṭ*
147. DIŠ ÚR 15-*šú* [SIG$_7$-*át* …]
148. DIŠ ÚR 150-*šú* SIG$_7$-*át* x […]
149. DIŠ ÚR.MEŠ-*šú* SIG$_7$.MEŠ *na-ḫi-iṭ*
150. DIŠ ÚR 15-*šú* GI$_6$-*át* GIG-*s*[*u* …]
151. [DI]Š ÚR 150-*šú* GI$_6$-*át na-ḫi-iṭ*
152. : DIŠ ÚR.MEŠ-*šú* GI$_6$.MEŠ […]
153. [DI]Š ÚR 15-*šú tar-kat* GIG-*su* MAN-*ni*
154. : DIŠ ÚR 150-*šú tar-kat* GIG-*s*[*u* …]
155. [DI]Š ÚR.MEŠ-*šú tar-ka na-ḫi-iṭ*
156. DIŠ ÚR 15-*šú du-ʾ-ú-mat* GIG-[*su* …]
157. [DI]Š ÚR 150-*šú du-ʾ-mat ú-šá-an-na-*[*aḫ*]
158. DIŠ ÚR.MEŠ-*šú du-ʾ-ú-ma na-ḫi-*[*iṭ*]
159. DIŠ ÚR 15-*šú nap-ḫat ú-za-bal-ma* […]
160. DIŠ ÚR 150-*šú nap-ḫat* GIG-*su* […]
161. DIŠ ÚR.MEŠ-*šú nap-ḫa na-ḫi-iṭ*
162. : DIŠ ÚR 1[5-*šú muq-qú-ta-át* …]
163. DIŠ ÚR 150-*šú muq-qú-ta-át* GI[G-*su* …]
164. DIŠ ÚR.MEŠ-*šú muq-qú-ta$_5$* […]
165. DIŠ ÚR 15-*šú šu-uḫ-ḫu-*⸢*ṭa-át*⸣ […]
166. DIŠ ÚR 150-*šú šu-uḫ-*[*ḫu-ṭa-át* …]
167. [DI]Š ÚR.MEŠ-*š*[*ú šu-uḫ-ḫu-ṭa* …]
168′. [DIŠ ÚR-*šú ú-maḫ-ḫaṣ* ŠU^{II}-*šú ú-na-aš*]-*šak*
169′. [Á^{II}-*šú ana ku-tal-li-šú* GUR ŠU] ⸢^{d}⸣[MAŠ.TAB].BA GAM[12]
170′. [DIŠ SA.MEŠ ^{UZU}ÚR-*šú* TA *giš-ši-šú* EN ZI.IN.G]I-*šú* GU$_7$-*šú*
171′. [ZI-*a u* DU.MEŠ-*ka*] ZU SA.GIG[13]
172′. [DIŠ SA.MEŠ ^{UZU}ÚR-*šú* 1-*niš* GU$_7$.MEŠ-*šú* ZI-*a u* D]U.MEŠ-*ka* NU ZU SA.GAL[14]
173′. [DIŠ *ina* ÚR-*šú šá* 15] SÌG-⸢*iṣ u*⸣ *e-sil* GAM[15]
174′. [DIŠ *ina* ÚR-*šú šá* 150 SÌG-*iṣ* ŠÀ-*šú eb-ṭú*] SAG.KI-*šú ḫe-sa-át* GAM[16]

175′. [DIŠ *ri-bit-su šá* 15 G]U$_7$-*šú* ŠU DINGIR-*šú* DIN
176′. [DIŠ *ri-bit-su šá* 150 GU$_7$-*šú*] ŠU ^{d}15-*šú* DIN

177′. [DIŠ *ri-bit-su šá* 15 *n*]*ap-ḫat-ma* GI$_6$-*át u ina* NU ZU *ú-rap-pad*
178′. [ŠU ^{d}IŠKUR *ina* A]N.BAR$_7$ SÌG-*iṣ* GAM[17]
179′. [DIŠ *ri-bit-su šá*] 150 *nap-ḫat-ma* GI$_6$-*át u ina* NU ZU *ú-rap-pad*
180′. [ŠU ^{d}DIL.BAT *ina*] *šat ur-ri* SÌG-*iṣ* GAM[18]
181′. DIŠ *r*[*i-biti r*]*i-biti* GÙ.GÙ-*si ina* DÚR-*šú* ZÉ *i-te-ez-zi*
182′. *u* ŠIR-*šú ze-ra* ⸢GAM⸣
183′. DIŠ *ina ri-biti-šú* SÌG-*iṣ* ŠU ^{d}IM
184′. DIŠ *ina ri-biti-šú* SÌG-*iṣ-ma ina* KA-*šú* MÚD MUD ŠUB.ŠUB-*a* ŠU ^{d}IM GAM
185′. DIŠ *ina ri-biti-šú* SÌG-*iṣ-ma* DÚR-*šú* BAD.BAD-*ir* ŠU ^{d}*Nin-giz-zi-da*
186′. DIŠ *ina ri-biti-šú* SÌG-*iṣ-ma* MÚŠ-*šú uš-qa-ma-am-ma ina* EDIN TAG-⸢*it*⸣ KI.MIN
187′. DIŠ *ina ri-biti šú* SÌG-*iṣ-ma* MÚŠ-*šú i-na-ḫi-su* (coll.) SUḪUŠ.MEŠ-*šú i-tar-ru-*[*ra* …]
188′. DIŠ *ina ri-biti-šú* SÌG-*iṣ-ma ri-biti ri-biti* GÙ.GÙ-*si*
189′. *ina a-zi-ri-šú* ZÉ *i-ḫa-ḫu* ŠU ⸢^{d}⸣[…]
190′. DIŠ *ina ri-biti-šú u su-ḫa-ti-šú* SÌG-*iṣ* ŠU ^{d}[…]

191′. [DI]Š *bir-ka-a-šú* GU$_7$.MEŠ-*šú* AZAG ^{d}UTU KÙ
192′. DIŠ *bir-ka-a-šú u* MURUB$_4$.MEŠ-*šú ina* GI$_6$ GU$_7$.ME-*šú*
193′. SU-*šú* KÚM NU TUKU DIB-*šú* ⸢AZAG⸣ ‹^{d}›UTU DIB-[*su*]

194′. DIŠ *pu-qa-a-šú it-te-né-ep-ta-a* GAM
195′. DIŠ *pu-qa-a-šú it-ta-na-az-qa-pa* DIN

196′. DIŠ *ki-is-su šá* 15 GU$_7$-*šú* KÚM-*šú mit-ḫar* ŠU ^{d}*Eš$_4$-dar* MU […]
197′. [DIŠ *k*]*i-is-su šá* 150 GU$_7$-*šú* KÚM-*šú* NU *mit-ḫar* GIG-*su* GÍD-*ma* D[IN?]
198′. DIŠ *kin-ṣa-a-šú* GU$_7$.MEŠ-*šú* KÚM-*šú* NU *mit-ḫar* [Š]U DINGIR-*šú* BÚR
199′. ⸢DIŠ *kin-ṣa-a*⸣-*šú* GU$_7$.MEŠ-*šú* ⸢ŠU⸣ DINGIR ⸢URU⸣-*šú* : ŠU DINGIR-*šú*
200′. DIŠ *kin-ṣa-a-šú* GU$_7$.MEŠ-*šú* ŠU ^{d}UTU MU KÙ.BABBAR ZAG.10.MEŠ D[IN]
201′. DIŠ *kin-ṣa-a-šú ki-iṣ-ṣa-ta$_5$-am* DIRI[19] *ina* DUG$_4$.DUG$_4$-*šú* ÚḪ-*su* ŠUB-*d*[*i-ma*]
202′. BÚR ŠUB-⸢*di-ma*⸣ KA BAD NU DU$_8$ DIŠ ÚḪ SUD *pi-šu* N[U BAD…]
203′. DIŠ *kin-ṣa-a-šu ki-is-*[*sa-tum* DI]RI.MEŠ UZU.MEŠ-*šú* KÚM.MEŠ *u mim-ma šá* GU$_7$ *i-ḫa-*[*ru* …]
204′. DIŠ *ina kin-ṣi-šu* SÌG-*iṣ* ŠU ^{d}[…]

205′. DIŠ *ina kin-ṣi-šú šá* 15 [SÌG-*i*]*ṣ u ina* KA-*šú* MÚD BURU$_{8}$ [GÍD-*ma*? GAM]
206′. DIŠ *ina kin-ṣi-šú šá* 150 SÌG-*iṣ u ina* KA-*šú* MÚD MUD [ŠUB-*di* GAM]
207′. DIŠ GÌR-*šu šá* 15 GU$_{7}$-*šu* ŠU ^{d}*Eš$_{4}$-dar*
208′. DIŠ GÌR-*šu šá* 1[50 GU$_{7}$-*šu* …] DIŠ GÌR^{II}-*šu* GU$_{7}$.MEŠ-*šu* [… -*m*]*a* DIN
209′. DIŠ GÌR-*šu šá* 15 *i-maš-š*[*ar* K]A-*šú ṣu-un-dur*
210′. [*mi-šit*]-*ti* MAŠKIM GÍD-*ma* GAM
211′. ⸢DIŠ GÌR⸣-*šu šá* 150 *i-maš-šar* SÌG-*iṣ* ^{d}*Ba-ú* SÌG-*iṣ* GAM
212′. ⸢DIŠ GÌR⸣-*šu*⸣ *šá* 15 *ik-te-ner-ru* ŠU ^{d}15 : DIB GIDIM$_{7}$ GAM
213′. [DIŠ GÌR-*šu*] ⸢*šá* 150⸣ *ik-te-ner-ru* ŠU ^{d}15
214′. DIŠ GÌR^{II}[-*šú i*]*k-te-ner-ra-a* ⸢ŠU DINGIR ḪUL DIB-*su*⸣
215′. [DIŠ GÌR-*šú*] *šá* 15 *ana šá* 150 LAL-*át* ⸢ŠU⸣ […]
216′. DIŠ GÌR^{II}-*šú tur-ra* NU ZU-*ú u* x […]
217′. DIŠ GÌR^{II}-*šú am-šá-ma ana* ⸢LAL⸣ NU ZU-*e u* UŠ$_{4}$-*šú* (coll.) NU DIB [GAM]
218′. DIŠ GÌR^{II}-*šú it-t*[*e*]-⸢*nin*⸣-*gi-ra* ŠU ^{d}UTU
219′. DIŠ NA GÌR^{II}-*šú it-te-nen-ṣi-la u it-ta-nak-na-an-na*
220′. ŠU ^{d}[…] x *ana* kur me ru
221′. DIŠ GÌR^{II}-*šú it-t*[*a-n*]*a-aš-gag-ga ina* KI.ÚS MAŠKIM GUB-*iz* DIN
222′. DIŠ GÌR^{II}-*šú i-*[*šam-ma*]-*ma-šú ru-mi-ka-a-ti ik-bu-us*
223′. DIŠ GÌR^{II}-*šú i-*[*nap-p*]*a-ṣa* ŠU^{II}-*šú ne-e-ḫa na-ḫi-iṭ*
224′. [DIŠ GÌR]^{II}-*šú i-*[*mim-ma* ŠU^{II}-*š*]*ú* ŠED$_{7}$.MEŠ DU$_{8}$-*ár* GIG
225′. […] ⸢DIB⸣-*su* BÚR-*ma* DIN
226′. […]x DIB-*su* BÚR-*šú-ma* DIN
227′. […*ana* NÍTA *u* MUN]US 1-*ma*
228′. […] it? GABA.RI […]x NA.BI […]
229′. […] LÚG NU.TUKU *ki-iṣ-ṣ*[*a-tum*]
230′. [DIŠ GÌR]⸢^{II}-*šu áš-ṭa*⸣-*a* GIG-*su* ⸢MAN-*ni*⸣
231′. DIŠ G[ÌR^{II}-*šu áš-ṭa-a-ma*] GUB [NU ZU ŠU ^{d}15]
232′. [DIŠ GÌR^{II}]-*šu* […]ta[…]
233′. DIŠ *ina* GÌR-*šu* SÌG-*iṣ* ŠU ^{d}MAŠ.TAB.BA
234′. [DIŠ *ina* GÌR-*š*]*u šá* 15 SÌG-*iṣ* ŠU ^{d}UTU *ana* [U$_{4}$.3.KÁM GAM]
235′. DIŠ *ina* GÌR-*šu šá* 150 SÌG-*iṣ* ŠU ^{d}15 GÍD-*ma* GAM
236′. [DIŠ *ina* GÌR-*š*]*u šá* 15 SÌG-*iṣ u* GÙ.[GÙ]-*si pu-qud-de-e* ^{d}UTU
237′. DIŠ *ina* G[ÌR-*š*]*u šá* 150 SÌG-*iṣ u* GÙ.[GÙ]-*si*
238′. *pu-qud-de-e* ^{d}15 *ana* ^{d}MAŠ.TAB.BA
239′. DIŠ *ina* GÌR-*šú* SÌG-*iṣ u* GÙ.GÙ-*si pu-qud-*[*d*]*e-e ana*
240′. DIŠ *ina* GÌR-*šú* MURUB$_{4}$.MEŠ-*šú* Á.MEŠ-*šú u* GÚ-*šú* SÌG-*iṣ*
241′. U$_{4}$.41.KÁM ŠU ^{d}15

242′. DIŠ U.MEŠ GÌR^{II}-*šú* GI$_6$.MEŠ ⸢GÍD⸣-*ma* GAM
243′. DIŠ U.MEŠ GÌR^{II}-*šú uṣ*-⸢*ṣu*?⸣-*la-šú* ŠU ^{d}*Iš-ha-ra*
244′. DIŠ U.MEŠ GÌR^{II}-*šú šu-ut-tu-qa ina* [...]
245′. *ina* AN.BAR$_7$ SÌG-*iṣ* ŠU ^{d}U.GUR GAM
246′. DIŠ U.MEŠ GÌR^{II}-*šú* MÚD DIRI.MEŠ-*ma* ⸢GU$_7$⸣.MEŠ-*šú*
247′. *ana la-ba-ṣu* GUR-*šum-ma* GAM
248′. DIŠ UMBIN U.MEŠ GÌR^{II}-*šú* SIG$_7$.M[EŠ] GAM
249′. DIŠ UMBIN U.MEŠ GÌR.MEŠ-*šú* SA$_5$.MEŠ *i-šar-*[*r*]*ù* DIN
250′. DIŠ *kar-ši* U.MEŠ GÌR^{II}-*šú* GI$_6$.MEŠ *i-ṭa-mu* GAM
251′. DIŠ KIR$_4$ U.MEŠ GÌR^{II}-*šú* ŠED$_7$.MEŠ-*šú* ÚŠ-*šú* GAM
252′. DIŠ GABA.MEŠ *šá* GÌR^{II}-*šú* GI$_6$.MEŠ ŠU ^{d}15 GÍD-*ma* GAM
253′. DIŠ *su-ḫar* GÌR^{II}-*šú* ŠED$_7$ KI.A IGI^{II}-*šú nu-up-pu-ḫa* GÌŠ-*šú aš-ṭa-at*
254′. LI.DUR-*su* DU$_8$-*át* ŠU NAM.ÉRIM.MA *ú-zab-bal-ma* GAM
255′. DIŠ KUŠ *šá* KI.TA-*nu* GÌR^{II}-*šú te-bi* SAG.DU-*su* DIB.DIB-*su*
256′. *u* ŠÀ-*šú tur-ru-ur* GAM
257′. DIŠ *ka-bit-ma* GÌR-*šú šá* 150 : 15 *i-kan-na-an*
258′. *u i-tar-ra-aṣ* BA.ÚŠ
259′. [DIŠ] SA GÌR^{II}-*šú* DU-*ku-ma šá* ŠU^{II}-*šú ne-e-ḫu ár-ḫiš* ÚŠ : AL.TI
260′. ⸢DIŠ SA⸣ GÌR^{II}-*šú* DU-*ku-ma šá* ŠU^{II}-*šú* GAR-*nu*
261′. KI.TA-*nu* GIG KU$_4$-*šú* NÍG.GIG IGI-*ma* DI[N]
262′. DIŠ SA GÌR^{II}-*šú* ZI.MEŠ-*ú* IGI^{II}-*šú ana* ÍL DUGUD
263′. SAG.DU-*su u* SAG ŠÀ-*šú e-em* ŠU ⸢20?⸣ [: AL].TI
264′. DIŠ *ta-bi* (coll.) : SA ZI.IN.GI-*šú* KÚM NU TUK[U ...]
265′. DIŠ *ta-bi* (coll.) : SA ZI.IN.GI-*šú* KÚM TUKU ⸢ḪAR⸣.MEŠ-*š*[*ú* GIG].MEŠ
266′. *u* UGU(!)-*šú i-šag-gúm* TI-*uṭ šum*$_4$-*ma* GIG-*su* ⸢GÍD⸣-*ma* GAM

DPS TABLET 14

1. [If the patient]'s "right" ⸢hip socket⸣ is red, [he will get well (var. his illness may last a long time but he will get well)].
2. [If] his ⸢"left"⸣ [hip socket] is red, his illness will last a long time.
3. [If] (both) his [hip sockets] are red, it is of ⸢no⸣ consequence.
4. [If] his "right" [hip] socket is yellow, his ⸢illness⸣ will change (for the worse).
5. [If] his "left" [hip] socket is yellow, his [illness] will be difficult.
6. [If] (both) his [hip sockets are yellow], it is ⸢worrisome⸣.
7. [If his "right" hip socket is black], his [illness] will be difficult.
8. [If his "left" hip socket is black], it is ⸢worrisome⸣.

9. [If (both) his hip sockets are black], he will die.
10. [If his "right" hip socket is dark], his ⌜illness⌝ will change (for the worse).
11. [If his "left" hip socket is dark], his ⌜illness⌝ will be difficult
12. [If (both) his hip sockets are dark], it is ⌜worrisome⌝.
13. If [his "right" hip socket is dark red], his ⌜illness⌝ will last a long time.
14. If [his "left" hip socket is dark red, his illness] will change (for the worse).
15. If [(both) his hip sockets are dark red], ⌜his⌝ [illness] will be difficult.
16. [If his "right" hip socket is swollen], his [illness] will change (for the worse).
17. [If his "left" hip socket is swollen], his [illness] will be difficult.
18. [If (both) his hip sockets are swollen], his [illness] will change (for the worse).
19. [If his "right" hip socket was bruised[20] all over], he will get well.
20. If [his "left" hip socket was bruised all over], ⌜his⌝ [illness] will change (for the worse).
21. If [(both) his hip sockets were bruised all over], it is ⌜worrisome⌝.
22. If [his "right"] ⌜hip socket⌝ [was (cut) open], his [illness] will be difficult.
23. If [his "left"] ⌜hip socket⌝ [was (cut) open], it is ⌜worrisome⌝.
24. If (both) [his] hip sockets [were (cut) open], ⌜his⌝ [illness will be difficult].
25. If [his] ⌜"right"⌝ hip socket [is sluggish], ⌜his illness⌝ [will be difficult].
26. If his "left" hip socket [is sluggish …].
27. If (both) his hip sockets are ⌜sluggish⌝ […].
28. If a woman's hip sockets are continually ⌜sluggish⌝ […].
29. If his hip sockets are ⌜normal⌝[21] [he will get well].

30–31. If from his hip socket to his toes, ⌜his⌝ muscles [are continually sluggish], "gnawing" [of *ṣētu*].[22]

32. If his "right" buttock is red, [he will get well].
33. [If] his "left" ⌜buttock⌝ is red, his illness may ⌜last a long time⌝.
34. [If] (both) his ⌜buttocks⌝ are red, [it is of no] consequence.
35. [If] his "right" ⌜buttock⌝ is yellow, his illness will change (for the worse).
36. [If] his "left" ⌜buttock⌝ is yellow, his illness will be difficult.
37. [If] (both) his ⌜buttocks⌝ are yellow, it is worrisome.
38. [If] his "right" ⌜buttock⌝ is black, his illness will be difficult.
39. [If] his "left" [buttock] is black, it is worrisome.
40. [If] (both) his [buttocks] are black, he will die.
41. [If] his "right" ⌜buttock⌝ is dark, he may be ill a long time, but he will get well.
42. [If his "left" buttock is dark …].

43. [If] (both) his ⸢buttocks⸣ are dark, he will die.
44. [If his "right" buttock is dark red, his illness will last a long time].
45. [If] his "left" ⸢buttock⸣ is dark red, his illness will change (for the worse).
46. [If (both) his buttocks are dark red, his illness will be difficult].
47. [If] his "right" buttock is swollen, his illness will change (for the worse).
48. [If his "left" buttock is swollen, his illness will be difficult].
49. [If] his buttocks are swollen, his illness will change (for the worse).
50. [If his "right" buttock was bruised all over ...].
51. ⸢If⸣ his "left" buttock was bruised all over, his illness will be prolonged.
52. [If (both) his buttocks were bruised all over], it is ⸢worrisome⸣.
53. [If] his "right" buttock was skinned,[23] his illness will change (for the worse).
54. [If his "left" buttock] was ⸢skinned, his⸣ [illness] will be difficult.
55. If (both) his ⸢buttocks⸣ were skinned, it is worrisome.
56. If his "right" buttock was (cut) open, his illness will change (for the worse).
57. If his "left" buttock was (cut) open, his illness is worrisome.
58. If (both) his buttocks were (cut) open, he will die.
59. If his buttocks are intact,[24] he will get well.
60. [If] his ⸢buttocks⸣ are dark so that his excrement cannot come out[25] and he cannot pass water, he was injured[26] on the back side; he will die.[27]
61. [If] he was injured [on] his hip socket and his buttock, "hand" of Ishtar.[28]
62. [If] he was injured [on] his ⸢hip socket⸣ and his leg, "hand" of Ishtar.[29]
63. [If] his ⸢inguinal regions⸣ shift constantly under him, his illness will change (for the worse).[30]
64. [If] his ⸢inguinal regions⸣ shift constantly under (him) but the nature of his disease alters, "hand" of Shamash; he will get well.[31]
65. [...] (If) it persists,[32] he will speedily? die"
66. [If] he was injured [on] his "right" ⸢inguinal region⸣,[33] he is not in full possession of his faculties and he wanders about without knowing (where he is), he will die.[34]
67. If he was injured on his "left" inguinal region (and) he does not know that he is continually crying out,[35] he will die.[36]
68. If the blood vessel(s) of his "right" inguinal region (feel like they are) pulsating and they are dark/black (once he has been sick) for two (var. C: three) days, he will die.[37]
69. If the blood vessel(s) of his "left" inguinal region (feel like they are) pulsating and they are dark/black, he will speedily die.[38]
70. If his anus stands still, he will die.[39]

71. If his anus stands still and wind […], if he has a difficult time of it, he will die.
72. If his anus is continually blocked off, he will die.[40]
73. If his anus ⸢twitches?⸣ […], he will die.
74. If red liquid flows from his anus, his illness will be prolonged.[41]
75. If yellow liquid flows [from] his [anus], ⸢that person⸣ […].[42]
76. If ⸢red⸣ bile flows from his anus, (his illness) may be prolonged, but he will get well.[43]
77. If yellow ⸢bile⸣ flows [from his anus] … he will die.[44]
78. If ⸢black⸣ bile ⸢flows⸣ from his anus, he will die.[45]
79. If his body fat flows from his anus, he will die.[46]
80. If he continually produces material removed from his insides(?) from his anus, he will die.
81. If he continually produces flesh from his anus, […].[47]
82. If he continually produces dark red blood from his anus, he will die.
83. If he continually produces blood and wind from his anus […].
84. If he excretes blood from his anus, "hand" of […].[48]
85. If he excretes dark blood from his anus, ⸢"hand"⸣ [of …].[49]
86. If he excretes blood and pus from his anus, "hand" of […].[50]

---

87. If his anus is ⸢blocked off, ⸢DÚR.GIG⸣?; he will die.
88. If his excrement is red, he will get well.[51]
89. If his excrement is yellow […].[52]
90. If his excrement is [black], he will die.[53]
91. If his excrement is ⸢dark red⸣ […].[54]
92. If ⸢his⸣ excrement […], his illness will be prolonged.
93. If his excrement […] within […].
94. [If he continually] ⸢scratches⸣ [his anus?, he is sick with] "sick entrails."[55]
95. [If his penis is red, his illness] may be prolonged, (but) he will get well.
96. If his penis is yellow, [his] ⸢illness⸣ […].
97. [If his penis is black], he will die.
98. If his penis is dark, it is ⸢worrisome⸣.
99. [If his penis is dark red], his illness will exhaust (him).
100. If his penis is swollen, it is worrisome.
101. [If his penis] was ⸢bruised all over⸣, he will get well.
102. If his penis was ⸢skinned⸣ [and it does not] ⸢let up⸣, he will die.

---

103. [If his penis is intact], he will get well.
104. If his penis is blocked off, he will die.[56]

105. If his penis is […], he will die.

106–108. [If his penis and his epigastrium] hold ⸢burning⸣ [fever], his liver hurts him and his stomach goes crazy (and) his arms, his feet, (and) his stomach are feverish, that person is sick with disease of intercourse; "hand" of his god (var. his goddess).[57]

109. If blood drips from his penis, "hand" of Shamash on account of sexual intercourse with a woman; he will die.[58]

110. If his penis and his testicles are swollen, "hand" of Ishtar has gotten him in his bed.[59]

---

111. If his urine is reddish, "hand" of his god; he will get well.[60]

112. If his urine is (dark) yellow, his illness will be prolonged. Alternatively, he burns with *ṣētu*; he will die.[61]

113. [If] his ⸢urine⸣ is black, he was touched with the touch of death; he will die.[62]

114. If his urine is dark, he will die.[63]

115. [If] his ⸢urine⸣ is continually blocked off, he will die.[64]

116. If his urine continually flows, he will die.

117. [If] his ⸢urine⸣ or his semen (continually) flows, he will die.[65]

118. If his ⸢urine⸣ is like […], he will die.

119. [If] his ⸢urine⸣ is like water, his illness may be prolonged, but he will get well.[66]

120. If his urine is like *kasû* juice, ditto (his illness may be prolonged, but he will get well).[67]

121. [If] his ⸢urine⸣ is like wine, his illness may be difficult, (var. A: "prolonged") (but he will get well.[68]

122. If his urine is like milk, he will get well.[69]

123. If his urine is normal, [his illness may be prolonged, (but) he will get well].[70]

124. If you examine his urine and *lipištu* comes out of it, he was ⸢"touched"⸣ in the steppe.[71]

125. If you examine his urine and (bits of) his flesh come out of it, he was ⸢"touched"⸣ in the steppe.[72]

---

126. If his testicles are red, he will get well.[73]

127. If his testicles are yellow […].

128. If his testicles are black, he will die.[74]

129. If his testicles are dark […].

130. If his testicles are dark red, his illness will be difficult.[75]
131. If his testicles were bruised all over […].
132. If his testicles were skinned, he will die.
133. If his testicles are ⸢intact⸣, [he will get well].
134. If his testicles are twisted, he will die (var. [he approached] the *ēntu* [of his god]).[76]
135–136. If his testicles are twisted, his tongue continually stammers? (and) he [bites?] his lips […].
137. If his testicles are swollen, it is worrisome (var. [he approached] the *ēntu* [of his god]).
138. If his testicles are continually swollen (and) his penis is full of *sikkatu*, [he approached] the ⸢*ēntu*⸣ [of his god]).[77]
139. If he was injured in his testicles, he approached the *ēntu* of his god (var. […]).[78]
140. If he was injured in his testicles […] his […] is continually [blocked off? …].
141–142. If his testicle was crushed, [his] ⸢umbilical area⸣ […] he ⸢continually⸣ retains his urine […].[79]
143. If the lower parts (of his body) are swollen […].[80]

---

144. If his "right" thigh is red, his snot? […].
145. If his "left" thigh is red […]
146. If (both) his thighs are red, it is worrisome.
147. If his "right" thigh [is yellow …].
148. If his "left" thigh is yellow […].
149. If (both) his thighs are yellow, it is worrisome.
150. If his "right" thigh is black, ⸢his⸣ illness […].
151. ⸢If⸣ his "left" thigh is black, it is worrisome.
152. If (both) his thighs are black […].
153. ⸢If⸣ his "right" thigh is dark, his illness will change (for the worse).
154. If his "left" thigh is dark, ⸢his⸣ illness […].
155. ⸢If⸣ (both) his thighs are dark, it is worrisome.[81]
156. If his "right" thigh is dark red, [his] illness […].
157. ⸢If⸣ his "left" thigh is dark red, it will ⸢exhaust⸣ (him).
158. If (both) his thighs are dark red, it is ⸢worrisome.⸣
159. If his "right" thigh is swollen, he will/may linger and/but […].
160. If his "left" thigh is swollen, his illness […].
161. If (both) his thighs are swollen, it is worrisome.
162. If [his] ⸢"right"⸣ thigh [was bruised all over …].

163. If his "left" thigh was bruised all over, [his] illness [...].
164. If (both) his thighs were bruised all over [...].
165. If his "right" thigh was skinned [...].
166. If his "left" thigh was ⸢skinned⸣ [...].
167. ⸢If⸣ (both) ⸢his⸣ thighs [were skinned ...].
168′–169′. [If he strikes his crotch], ⸢chews⸣ [on his hands (and) they have to put his arms behind him, "hand"] of the ⸢twin gods⸣; he will die.[82]
170′–171′. [If the muscles of his thigh from his hip sockets to] his ⸢ankles⸣ hurt him (but) he can [stand and walk], *maškādu*.[83]
172′. [If the muscles of his thigh all hurt him at once (and)] he cannot [stand up or] ⸢walk about⸣, *sagallu*.[84]
173′. [If] he was injured [on his "right" thigh] and he is constipated, he will die.[85]
174′. [If he was injured on his "left" thigh, his stomach is cramped] (and) he has a vise-like headache, he will die.[86]

175′. [If the "right" side of his abdomen] ⸢hurts⸣ him, "hand" of his god; he will get well.
176′. [If the "left" side of his abdomen hurts him], "hand" of his goddess; he will get well.
177′–178′. [If the "right" side of his abdomen] is ⸢swollen⸣ and dark and he wanders about without knowing (where he is), ["hand" of Adad]. (If) he was injured [at] ⸢noon⸣, he will die.[87]
179′–180′. [If] the "left" [side of his abdomen] is swollen and dark/black and he wanders about without knowing (where he is), ["hand" of Ishtar]. (If) he was injured [in] the morning, he will die.[88]
181′–182′. If he continually cries out: "⸢the side of my abdomen, the side of my abdomen!⸣," he excretes bile from his anus and his testicle(s) are twisted, he will die.
183′. If he was injured on the side of his abdomen, "hand" of Adad.[89]
184′. If he was injured on the side of his abdomen and, consequently, he continually produces black blood from his mouth, "hand" of Adad; he will die.[90]
185′. If he was injured on the side of his abdomen and, consequently, his anus is continually stopped up, "hand" of Ningizzida.[91]
186′. If he was injured on the side of his abdomen and, consequently, his countenance becomes subdued and he is "touched in the steppe"; ditto ("hand" of Ningizzida).[92]
187′. If he was injured on the side of his abdomen and, consequently, his countenance becomes withdrawn (and) his foundations ⸢tremble⸣ [...].

188′–189′. If he was injured on the side of his abdomen and he continually cries "the side of my abdomen, the side of my abdomen" (and) he vomits bile from his …, "hand" of […].

190′. If he was injured on the side of his abdomen and his armpit, "hand" of […].

191′. ⌈If⌉ his knees continually hurt him, he has done something offensive to Shamash.[93]

192′–193′. If his knees and his hips continually hurt him in the night (and) his body has no fever, an offense against Shamash afflicts [him].[94]

194′. If his anal opening is continually opened, he will die.[95]

195′. If his anal opening is continually constricted, he will live..[96]

196′. If his "right" leg hurts him (and) his temperature is even, "hand" of Ishtar on account of […].[97]

197′. If his "left" ⌈leg⌉ hurts him (and) his temperature is not even, (even if) his illness is prolonged, ⌈he will get well⌉.

198′. If (both) his legs continually hurt him (and) his temperature is not even, ⌈"hand"⌉ of his god; it will let up.

199′. If his legs continually hurt him, "hand" of the god of his city (var. "hand" of his god).

200′. If his legs continually hurt him, "hand" of Shamash on account of silver for a tithe; ⌈he will get well⌉.[98]

201′–202′. If his legs are full of "gnawing," [if] when he speaks, he lets his spittle fall, it will let up but (if) he lets (it) fall (and his) mouth is open, it will not relent. If he sprinkles (his) spittle (and) his mouth ⌈is not⌉ [open …].

203′. If his legs are continually ⌈full⌉ of ⌈"gnawing"⌉, his flesh is continually hot, and he ⌈vomits⌉ whatever he eats […].

204′. If he was injured on his leg, "hand" of […]

205′. If he was ⌈injured⌉ on his "right" leg and he vomits blood from his mouth, [(if) it is prolonged?, he will die].[99]

206′. If he was ⌈injured⌉ on his "left" leg and he [produces] dark blood from his mouth, [he will die].[100]

207′. If his "right" foot hurts him, "hand" of Ishtar.[101]

208′. If his ⌈"left"⌉ foot [hurts him …]. If (both) his feet continually hurt him, ⌈if⌉ […] he will get well.[102]

209′–210′. If he ⌈drags⌉ his "right" foot (and) his ⌈mouth⌉ twitches, ⌈stroke⌉ of a *rābiṣu*; if it is prolonged, he will die.[103]

211′. If he drags his “left” foot, he was struck by a blow of Bau; he will die.[104]

212′. If his “right” foot gets shrunken, “hand of Ishtar” (var. affliction by a ghost); he will die.[105]

213′. [If] his “left” [foot] gets shrunken, “hand” of Ishtar.[106]

214′. If (both) [his] feet get shrunken, “hand” of an evil god afflicts him.[107]

215′. [If his] “right” [foot] is stretched out towards his “left,” “hand” of [...].[108]

216′. If he is unable to turn his feet and [...].

217′. If his feet are immobilized so that he is unable to stretch (them) out and he is not in full possession of his faculties, [he will die].[109]

218′. If his feet are continually twisted, “hand” of Shamash.[110]

219′–220′. If a person’s feet are continually sluggish and continually contorted, “hand” of [...] ... .[111]

221′. If his feet ⸢continually⸣ become stiff, he stood in the footsteps of a *rābiṣu*; he will get well.[112]

222′. If his feet ⸢go numb⸣, he stepped in (dirty) bath water.

223′. If his feet ⸢thrash around⸣ and his hands are quiet, it is worrisome.

224′–225′. [If] his [feet] get ⸢hot⸣ (and) ⸢his⸣ [hands] are cold, letting up of the illness; if the [...] which afflicts him goes away, he will get well.

226′. [...]; (if) the [...] which afflicts him goes away, he will get well.

227′. [...] it is the same [for a man or] a ⸢woman⸣.

228′. *(fragmentary)*

229′. [...] it is of no consequence; it is called ⸢“gnawing”⸣.[113]

230′. [If] his [feet] are stiff,[114] his illness will change (for the worse).

231′. If his ⸢feet⸣ [are so stiff that he cannot] stand, [“hand” of Ishtar]

232′. *(fragmentary)*

233′. If he was injured on his foot, “hand” of the twin gods.

234′. [If] he was injured [on] ⸢his⸣ “right” [foot], “hand” of Shamash. (If he has been sick) for [three days, he will die].[115]

235′. If he was injured on his “left” foot, “hand” of Ishtar. If (his illness) is prolonged, he will die.[116]

236′. [If] he was injured [on] ⸢his⸣ “right” [foot] and he [continually] cries out, a good entrusted by Shamash to the twin gods.[117]

237′–238′. If he was injured on ⸢his⸣ “left” ⸢foot⸣ and he [continually] cries out, a good entrusted by Ishtar to the twin gods.[118]

239′. If he was injured on his foot and he continually cries out, a good entrusted (by Shamash) to the twin gods.[119]

240′–241′. If he was injured on his foot, his hips, his arms (and) his neck (and he has been sick for) forty-one days, “hand” of Ishtar.[120]

242′. If his toes are dark/black, if it is prolonged, he will die.

243′. If his toes are ⌜sluggish⌝, "hand" of Ishhara.

244′–245′. If his toes were split in [...] places (and) he was injured at noon, "hand" of Nergal; he will die.

246′–247′. If his toes are continually full of blood and continually hurt him, if it turns to Labaṣu on him, he will die.[121]

248′. If his toenails are continually yellow, he will die.[122]

249′. If his toenails are continually red, he will get rich (var. he will get well).[123]

250′. If the "bellies" of his toes are dark/black (and) he twists, he will die.[124]

251′. If the tips of his toes are cold, he will die his death.

252′. If the "breasts" of his feet are dark/black, "hand" of Ishtar; if it is prolonged, he will die.[125]

253′–254′. If the soles of his feet are cold, the rims of his eyes are swollen, his penis is stiff (but) his navel is not stiff, "hand" of curse; he will die a lingering death.[126]

255′–256′. If the skin on the bottom of his feet continually (feels like it) is pulsating, his head continually afflicts him and his abdomen trembles, he will die.[127]

257′–258′. If it is difficult (for him) to bend and straighten out his "left" (var: "right") foot, he will die.

259′. [If] the blood vessels of his feet "go" and those of his hands are slow, he will speedily die (var: he will get well).[128]

260′–261′. If the blood vessels of his feet "go" and those of his hands are present, his illness has entered him from below; he may have a difficult time of it but ⌜he will get well⌝.[129]

262′–263′. If the blood vessels of his feet (feel like they are) pulsating, it is difficult for him to raise his eyes, (and) his head and his epigastrium are feverish, "hand" of Shamash (var. he will get well).[130]

264′. If it (that is) a blood vessel (in his feet) (feels like it) is pulsating, his ankles are not feverish [...].

265′–266′. If it (that is) a blood vessel (in his feet) (feels like it) is pulsating, his ankles are feverish, ⌜his⌝ lungs are continually [sick] and his head(!)[131] roars, he will get well. If his illness is prolonged, he will die.[132]

NOTES

1. Restored from commentary SpTU 1.36 obv. 1.
2. The restoration is confirmed by the commentary SpTU 1.36 obv. 2-3.
3. The restoration is confirmed by the commentary SpTU 1.36 obv. 4.
4. The restoration is confirmed by the commentary SpTU 1.36 obv. 4.
5. Restoration is based on the commentary SpTU 1.36 obv. 5.
6. Restoration is based on the commentary SpTU 1.36 obv. 5.

7. Geller's copy has a DIN; the text has a GAM (coll.)

8. Geller, BAM 7 no. 49′s reading and interpretation of this as referring to the patient continually producing a figurine(!) is patent nonsense.

9. After a suggestion of Buisson 2006, 187.

10. Text A has GÍD-*ma*.

11. For the reading, see *CAD* E, 249a.

12. Restored from DPS 15:56′.

13. Restored from DPS 33:99.

14. Restored from DPS 33:98.

15. Restored from DPS 15:54′.

16. Restored from DPS 15:56′.

17. Restored from DPS 15:52′.

18. Restored from DPS 15:53′.

19. The original is very badly effaced. Geller (BAM 7 no. 49) saw *i-šá-a*.

20. See Scurlock and Andersen 2005, 216.

21. The commentary SpTU 1.36 obv. 5-6 explains: *šá* TUGUL.MEŠ-*šú* GIG *u líp-tu ina* ŠÀ *la i-šu-ú*: "whose hips are sore but there is no intense pain there."

22. See Scurlock and Andersen 2005, 3.129 as here corrected. The entry appears also in DPS 33:102, Arnaud 1987, 694 obv. 5′ and Wilhelm 1994, 48 D 2:13′.

23. The commentary SpTU 1.36 obv. 9 explains: *šá maš-ku ina* UGU *iš-šaḫ-ṭu*: "whose skin has been stripped from it."

24. The commentary SpTU 1.36 obv. 9-10 explains: *šá pi-ṭir-*[*šú*] *la ib-šu-ú*: "that does not have a hole in it."

25. See the commentary SpTU 1.36 obv. 10.

26. The commentary, SpTU 1.36 obv. 11, indicates that the "striking" in question was done with a weapon.

27. See Scurlock and Andersen 2005, 5.41. The entry also appears in DPS 15:51′.

28. See Scurlock and Andersen 2005, 19.163.

29. See Scurlock and Andersen 2005, 19.163.

30. See Scurlock and Andersen 2005, 19.272.

31. See Scurlock and Andersen 2005, 19.272.

32. Literally: "stands."

33. See Heeßel 2000, 168 ad 57′.

34. See Scurlock and Andersen 2005, 14.14. The entry appears also in DPS 15:57′.

35. Geller, BAM 7 no. 49′s translation does not account for the end of the line.

36. See Scurlock and Andersen 2005, 14.15. The entry also appears in DPS 15:58′.

37. Alternatively, "he will die within two/three days." See Scurlock and Andersen 2005, 3.230.

38. See Scurlock and Andersen 2005, 3.231.

39. See Scurlock and Andersen 2005, 6.154.

40. See Scurlock and Andersen 2005, 6.89.

41. See Scurlock and Andersen 2005, 6.14.

42. See Scurlock and Andersen 2005, 6.21.

43. See Scurlock and Andersen 2005, 6.15.

44. See Scurlock and Andersen 2005, 6.22.

45. See Scurlock and Andersen 2005, 6.18.

46. See Scurlock and Andersen 2005, 6.23.

47. See Scurlock and Andersen 2005, 6.19.

48. See Scurlock and Andersen 2005, 6.16.

49. See Scurlock and Andersen 2005, 6.16.
50. See Scurlock and Andersen 2005, 6.16.
51. See Scurlock and Andersen 2005, 6.13.
52. See Scurlock and Andersen 2005, 6.20.
53. See Scurlock and Andersen 2005, 6.13.
54. See Scurlock and Andersen 2005, 6.13.
55. This is usually "sick lungs" but the series is rather too far down the body for this to be the correct reading.
56. See Scurlock and Andersen 2005, 5.35.
57. See Scurlock and Andersen 2005, 2.18, 4.34, 19.348. This entry appears also in DPS 22:14-15.
58. See Scurlock and Andersen 2005, 4.4, 5.18, 19.108. Similar entries appear in VAT 10748:14′–15′ (Heeßel 2010, 178–81).

KAR 211 i 17′–18′ [If] a ⌜falling⌝ spell falls on him so that he ⌜trembles⌝ (and) shakes and his eyes [...] or are "soaked," ⌜"hand"⌝ of Sîn.

59. See Scurlock and Andersen 2005, 4.1, 5.76.
60. See Scurlock and Andersen 2005, 5.2, 20.54.
61. See Scurlock and Andersen 2005, 3.168, 5.4.
62. See Scurlock and Andersen 2005, 5.5, 7.32.
63. See Scurlock and Andersen 2005, 5.7.
64. See Scurlock and Andersen 2005, 5.36, 20.82.
65. See Scurlock and Andersen 2005, 4.8.
66. See Scurlock and Andersen 2005, 5.6.
67. See Scurlock and Andersen 2005, 5.9.
68. See Scurlock and Andersen 2005, 5.3.
69. See Scurlock and Andersen 2005, 5.11.
70. See Scurlock and Andersen 2005, 5.1.
71. See Scurlock and Andersen 2005, 7.30.
72. See Scurlock and Andersen 2005, 5.27, 7.29.
73. See Scurlock and Andersen 2005, 5.84, 20.41.
74. See Scurlock and Andersen 2005, 5.84, 20.37.
75. See Scurlock and Andersen 2005, 20.39.
76. See Scurlock and Andersen 2005, 5.83. The entry also appears in DPS 21:19.
77. See Scurlock and Andersen 2005, 4.28, 10.149.
78. See Scurlock and Andersen 2005, 5.87.
79. See Scurlock and Andersen 2005, 5.86.
80. See Scurlock and Andersen 2005, 8.26.
81. See Scurlock and Andersen 2005, 20.38.
82. See Scurlock and Andersen 2005, 16.78, 19.238. The entry appears also in DPS 15:56′.
83. See Scurlock and Andersen 2005, 11.59. This entry appears also in DPS 33:99.
84. See Scurlock and Andersen 2005, 11.58. This entry also appears in DPS 33:98. It is cited in *AMT* 42/6:1 and CT 23.1–2:1 as a sort of introduction to treatments for *sagallu*. It also appears in the UGU Catalogue (9c16′+9d12′), for which see ch. 3, text 1.
85. See Scurlock and Andersen 2005, 14.19. This entry appears also in DPS 15:54′.
86. See Scurlock and Andersen 2005, 14.20. This entry also appears in DPS 15:55′.
87. See Scurlock and Andersen 2005, 14.38, 19.144. This entry appears also in DPS 15:52′.
88. See Scurlock and Andersen 2005, 3.206, 19.155. This entry also appears in DPS 15:53′.
89. The entry appears also in Labat 1974, no. XI ii 2.
90. See Scurlock and Andersen 2005, 3.205, 19.140.

91. See Scurlock and Andersen 2005, 3.209, 6.156, 19.203.
92. See Scurlock and Andersen 2005, 3.309
93. See Scurlock and Andersen 2005, 11.17.
94. See Scurlock and Andersen 2005, 11.45.
95. See Scurlock and Andersen 2005, 6.162.
96. See Scurlock and Andersen 2005, 6.161.
97. See Scurlock and Andersen 2005, 11.53.
98. See Scurlock and Andersen 2005, 11.46.
99. See Scurlock and Andersen 2005, 14.17. This entry appears also in DPS 15:59′.
100. See Scurlock and Andersen 2005, 14.17. The entry also appears in DPS 15:60′.
101. See Scurlock and Andersen 2005, 11.50.
102. See Scurlock and Andersen 2005, 11.50.
103. See Scurlock and Andersen 2005, 13.55, 13.79, 13.243, 20.86. This entry appears also in DPS 15:63′.
104. See Scurlock and Andersen 2005, 19.165. The entry also appears in DPS 15:64′a.
105. See Scurlock and Andersen 2005, 11.51.
106. See Scurlock and Andersen 2005, 11.51.
107. See Scurlock and Andersen 2005, 11.20.
108. See Scurlock and Andersen 2005, 13.64.
109. This entry appears also in DPS 15:64′b.
110. See Scurlock and Andersen 2005, 11.21, 11.48.
111. See Scurlock and Andersen 2005, 13.269.
112. See Scurlock and Andersen 2005, 11.40, 19.83.
113. The entry also appears in DPS 33:101.
114. Geller reads *ú-ḫúl-a* which he takes from *eʾēlu* and interprets as "coagulate." His feet coagulate?!
115. See Scurlock and Andersen 2005, 19.186, 19.194. The entry appears also in DPS 15:61′.
116. See Scurlock and Andersen 2005, 19.154, 19.186, 20.85. The entry also appears in DPS 15:62′.
117. See Scurlock and Andersen 2005, 19.186.
118. See Scurlock and Andersen 2005, 19.186.
119. This entry appears also in Wilhelm 1994, 34 obv. 4′.
120. See Scurlock and Andersen 2005, 19.164.
121. See Scurlock and Andersen 2005, 3.35.
122. See Scurlock and Andersen 2005, 10.204.
123. See Scurlock and Andersen 2005, 10.205.
124. See Scurlock and Andersen 2005, 14.42. This entry appears also in DPS 15:66′.
125. See Scurlock and Andersen 2005, 14.44, 19.128, 20.87. This entry also appears in DPS 15:65′.
126. See Scurlock and Andersen 2005, 5.59, 19.316.
127. See Scurlock and Andersen 2005, 20.29.
128. See Scurlock and Andersen 2005, 8.53, 20.27.
129. See Scurlock and Andersen 2005, 8.54.
130. See Scurlock and Andersen 2005, 19.255.
131. Suggestion courtesy M. Stol.
132. See Scurlock and Andersen 2005, 8.83 as here corrected.

B. TIME: DPS 15–17

DPS 15

DPS 14:267′ (catchline) = DPS 15:1

1. [DIŠ] U$_4$.1.KÁM GIG-*ma ina* SAG.DU-*šú* SÌG-*iṣ* za/ḫa?[…].

(gap of unknown length)

1′–3′. (fragmentary)

4′. DIŠ KI.MIN-*ma* [*i-ṭa-mu u* MÚD *i-ḫa-ḫu*] SÌG-*iṣ* NAM.TAR SÌG-*iṣ* GAM

5′. DIŠ KI.MIN-⸢*ma*⸣ IGI.MEŠ-*šú* G[I$_6$.MEŠ-*ma* MÚD *i-ḫa-ḫu*] GABA.RI SÌG-*iṣ* GAM[1]

6′. DIŠ KI.MIN-⸢*ma*⸣ ⸢GÚ-*su*⸣ [G]U$_7$-*šú*-[*ma* A APIN.MEŠ ŠU] ^{d}15 *ina* GÚ-*šú* SÌG-*iṣ* GAM[2]

7′. DIŠ KI.MIN-⸢*ma*⸣ G[Ú.ḪAR-*s*]*u* ⸢*ḫa-niq* NÍG.GIG DINGIR-*šú*⸣ GU$_7$ ŠU DINGIR-*šú* GA[M].

8′. DIŠ KI.MIN-⸢*ma ni-ip-qu-šú qit*⸣-*ru-bu u* UŠ$_4$-*šú* NU DIB [GAM]

9′. DIŠ KI.MIN-*ma* ⸢Á-*šú šá* 15 GI$_6$⸣-*át* EME-*šú kaṣ-rat ina* EGIR-*šú* SÌG-*iṣ* GAM

10′. DIŠ KI.MIN-*ma* ⸢Á⸣-*šú šá* 150 GI$_6$-*át i-ṭa-mu* [SÌG-*i*]*ṣ* ^{d}30 *u uš-te-zeb* [: GAM]

11′. DIŠ KI.MIN-*ma* Á^{II}-*šú tur-ra* NU ZU-*e* [*u ina* DÚR]-*šú* MÚD SUR [GAM]

12′. DIŠ KI.MIN-*ma* Á^{II}-*šú tur-ra* NU ZU-*e* […]

13′–14′. DIŠ KI.MIN-*ma* ŠU-*su ina* LI.DUR-*šú* GAR-*at-ma* ŠU^{II}-*šú u* GÌR^{II}-*šú ka-ṣa-a ina* NU ⸢ZU-*e*⸣ [DUG$_4$.DUG$_4$-*ub*] ZI-*bi u* TÚŠ-*ab ina* LI.DUR-*šú* SÌG-*iṣ* ŠU ^{d}*Dil-bat* [GAM]

15′. DIŠ KI.MIN-*ma* ŠU^{II}-*šú ina* SAG.DU-*šú* GAR.MEŠ-*ma la ur-ra-da-ni* ŠÀ.MEŠ-*šú* ÍL.MEŠ KÚM ÚḪ *ina* SAG ⸢ŠÀ-*šú*⸣ [SÌG-*iṣ* GAM]

16′. DIŠ KI.MIN-*ma* ŠU^{II}-*šú ana* KA-*šú ú-ḫab-bat* TÚG-*su it-ta-na-suk lu-ʾ-a-tú šu-k*[*ul* GAM]

17′. DIŠ KI.MIN-*ma* ŠU^{II}-*šú* AD$_6$-*šú ú-lap-pa-ta$_5$ ina* GIG.BI GÍD-[*ma* GAM]

18′. DIŠ KI.MIN-*ma* ŠU^{II}-*šú am-šá-ma* LAL NU ZU-*e u* UŠ$_4$-*šú* NU DIB ŠU 20 [GAM]

19′. DIŠ KI.MIN-*ma* ŠU^{II}-*šú u* GÌR^{II}-*šú am-šá-ma* LAL NU ZU-*e u* UŠ$_{4}$-*šú* NU DIB *ana* GIZKIM GIG [GAM]

20′. DIŠ KI.MIN-*ma* ŠU^{II}-*šú u* GÌR^{II}-*šú* ⸢*am*⸣-*šá* ⸢DUG$_{4}$⸣ [*ne*]-⸢*e-ḫe*⸣-*e* DUG$_{4}$.GA DINGIR URU-*šú* SÌG-*su* [GAM]

21′. DIŠ KI.MIN-*ma* ŠU^{II}-*šú u* GÌR^{II}-*šú* [...] DUG$_{4}$-*šú ú-rap-pad ina* AN.BAR$_{7}$ SÌG-*iṣ* ŠU ^{d}⸢10⸣ [GAM]

22′. DIŠ KI.MIN-*ma* ŠU^{II}-*šú u* G[ÌR]^{II}-*š*[*ú* ... *ḫ*]*a* MÚD BURU$_{8}$ ŠU ^{d}U.GUR ⸢GAM⸣

23′. DIŠ KI.MIN-*ma* ŠU^{II}-*šú u* [GÌR^{II}-*šú* ...] *ú-ḫar-ra-aṣ* ŠU ^{d}*be-en-nu šá-né* ^{d}30 GAM

24′. DIŠ KI.MIN-*ma* ŠU^{II}-*šú u* [GÌR^{II}-*šú* ... N]AG *u* UŠ$_{4}$-*šú* NU DIB GAM : DIŠ KI.MIN-*ma* ŠU^{II}-*šú u* GÌR^{II}-*šú ú-lap-pa-ta*$_{5}$ *ina* GIG.BI GÍD-*ma* GAM

25′. DIŠ KI.MIN-*ma* U.MEŠ-*šú ú*-[...] *ú-te-né-eṭ-ṭe* : ZI.ZI-*bi* ŠUB AN-*e* TAG-⸢*su* ŠU⸣ DINGIR-*šú* GAM

26′. DIŠ KI.MIN-*ma* U.MEŠ ŠU^{II}-*šú ina* [KA-*šú ú-man-zaq* KÚM] ⸢ÚḪ⸣ ŠÀ-*šú na-pi-iḫ u ú-rap-pad ina* GÚ-*šú* SÌG-*iṣ* ⸢ŠU⸣ ^{d}⸢*Ba*⸣-*ú* GAM

27′. DIŠ KI.MIN-*ma* U.MEŠ-*šú ina* KA-*šú* ⸢GAR⸣-*n*[*a*]-*ma* ⸢*ta*⸣-*tab-bal-ma ana* KA-*šú ú-tar* ÚŠ-*ma* ⸢EGIR⸣-*šú ina* ⸢É⸣-*šú* ÚŠ GAM

28′. DIŠ KI.MIN-*ma* GABA.MEŠ *šá* ŠU^{II}-*šú* GI$_{6}$.MEŠ ŠU DINGIR ⸢URU⸣-*šú* GAM

29′. DIŠ KI.MIN-*ma kar-ši* U.MEŠ ŠU^{II}-*šú* GI$_{6}$.MEŠ *u i-ṭa-me* ŠU.GÍDIM.⸢MA⸣ GAM

30′. DIŠ KI.MIN-*ma šá-ḫat-su* : *šá-ḫaš-šú šá* 15 GU$_{7}$-*šú u ú-rap-pad* GABA.RI SÌG-*iṣ* GAM

31′. DIŠ KI.MIN-*ma šá-ḫat-su* : *šá-ḫaš-šú šá* 150 GU$_{7}$-*šú u* KÚM NU TUKU *ár-da-na-an* ÚŠ DIB-⸢*su*⸣

32′. DIŠ KI.MIN-*ma ina* GABA-*šú* SÌG-*ma* MÚD *ú-tab-ba-ka u ú-rap-pad* ŠU ^{d}U.GUR GABA.RI ⸢SÌG⸣-*iṣ* GAM

33′. DIŠ KI.MIN-*ma* SAG ŠÀ-*šú* GI$_{6}$-*ma* EME-*šú ḫe-em-ret ana* GIZKIM GIG GAM

34′. DIŠ KI.MIN-*ma* SAG ŠÀ-*šú* ÍL-*ma* IGI.ME-*šú nu-up-pú-ḫu ina* IGI^{II}-*šú* ÍR DU-*ak* GÍD-*ma* GAM

35′. DIŠ KI.MIN-*ma ina* ŠÀ-*šú* SÌG-*iṣ-ma e-mir u e-sil* GAM

36′. DIŠ KI.MIN-*ma ina* ŠÀ-*šú* SÌG-*iṣ-ma u* ZI.IR.MEŠ ŠU ^{d}MAŠ.TAB.BA GAM

37′. DIŠ KI.MIN-*ma* ŠÀ.MEŠ-*šú* GI$_{6}$.MEŠ-*ma* SA ŠÀ-*šú šu-ud-du-du ina* KA-*šú* IM *ú-ga-áš-šá ana* U$_{4}$.3.KÁM GAM

38′. DIŠ KI.MIN-*ma* ŠÀ ŠÀ GÙ.GÙ-*si u* SÍG-*su ú-ban-qam ina ban-ti-šú* SÌG-*iṣ* GAM

39′. DIŠ KI.MIN-*ma ina* ÉLLAG-*šú šá* 15 SÌG-*iṣ* UŠ$_4$-*šú* NU DIB *ina* NU ZU *ú-rap-pad* ŠU ^{d}MAŠ.TAB.⸢BA⸣ GA[M]

40′. DIŠ KI.MIN-*ma ina* ÉLLAG-*šú šá* 150 SÌG-*iṣ* UŠ$_4$-*šú* NU DIB *u* MÚD BURU$_8$ ŠU ^{d}7.BI GAM

41′. DIŠ KI.MIN-*ma ina* GIŠ.KUN-*šú* SÌG-*iṣ* : *ina* ŠIR-*šú* ŠU ^{d}30 GÍD-*ma* GAM

42′. DIŠ KI.MIN-*ma* TI-*šú šá* 15 GI$_6$ KA-*šú* ḪÁD.DA.MEŠ *u it-ta-nag-ra-ár* ŠU ^{d}*Da-mu ina* ÉLLAG-*šú* SÌG-*iṣ* GAM

43′. DIŠ KI.MIN-*ma* TI-*šú šá* 150 GI$_6$ MÚD BURU$_8$ *u* ZI.IR.MEŠ *ina* U$_4$ BI SÌG-*iṣ* GAM

44′. DIŠ KI.MIN-*ma ina šá-šal-li-šú šá* 15 SÌG-*iṣ u ú-rap-pad* ŠU DINGIR URU-*šú ina šat ur-ra* SÌG-*iṣ* GAM

45′. DIŠ KI.MIN-*ma ina šá-šal-li-šú šá* 150 SÌG-*iṣ u ú-rap-pad* ŠU DINGIR-*šú ina* ‹EN.NUN› MURUB$_4$-*ti* SÌG-*iṣ* GAM

46′. DIŠ KI.MIN-*ma ina* GÚ.SIG$_4$-*šú* SÌG BAD-*ir-ma* KI.GUB-*su* NU ⸢È⸣-*a* ŠU GIDIM$_7$ *šag-ga-ši* GAM

47′. DIŠ KI.MIN-*ma* GÚ.SIG$_4$-*šú* GÚR-*ma* LAL NU ZU-*e* GÍD-*ma* GAM

48′. DIŠ KI.MIN-*ma* MURUB$_4$.MEŠ-*šú* ÍL.MEŠ-*šú* GIN$_7$ *i-te-né-ep-pu-šu* NU ZU GAM

49′. DIŠ KI.MIN-*ma ina kur-ri-šú šá* 15 SÌG-*iṣ-ma* NÍ-*šú ma-ši* ŠU ^{d}ŠUL.PA.È.A GAM

50′. DIŠ KI.MIN-*ma ina kur-ri-šú šá* 150 SÌG-*iṣ-ma* GÌR-*šú* NU ZI-*aḫ ina* ^{d}UTU È ‹SÌG-*iṣ*› ŠU ^{d}15 GAM

51′. DIŠ KI.MIN-*ma* GU.DU.MEŠ-*šú* GI$_6$.MEŠ-*ma* KI.GUB-*su* NU È-*a u* A NU *ú-še-rid* EGIR-*ta*$_5$ SÌG-*iṣ* GAM

52′. DIŠ KI.MIN-*ma ri-bit-su šá* 15 *nap-ḫat-ma* GI$_6$-*át ina* NU ZU *ú-rap-pad* ŠU ^{d}IŠKUR *ina* AN.BAR$_7$ SÌG-*iṣ* GAM

53′. DIŠ KI.MIN-*ma ri-bit-su šá* 150 *nap-ḫat-ma* GI$_6$-*át ina* NU ZU *ú-rap-pad* ŠU ^{d}DIL.BAT *ina šat ur-ri* SÌG-[*i*]*ṣ* GAM

54′. DIŠ KI.MIN-*ma ina* ÚR-*šú šá* 15 SÌG-*iṣ u e-sil* GAM

55′. DIŠ KI.MIN-*ma ina* ÚR-*šú šá* 150 SÌG-*iṣ* ŠÀ.MEŠ-*šú eb-ṭú* SAG.KI-*šú ḫe-sa-át* [GAM]

56′. DIŠ KI.MIN-*ma* ÚR-*šú ú-maḫ-ḫaṣ* ŠU^{II}-*šú ú-na-aš-šak* Á^{II}-*šú ana ku-tal-li-šú* GUR ŠU ^{d}MAŠ.T[AB.BA GAM]

57′. DIŠ KI.MIN-*ma ina* ḪÁŠ.‹GAL›-*šú šá* 15 SÌG-*iṣ* UŠ$_4$-*šú* NU DIB [*ina* NU ZU *ú-rap-pad* GAM]

58′. DIŠ KI.MIN-*ma ina* ḪÁŠ.GAL-*šú šá* 150 SÌG-*iṣ* GIN$_{7}$ GÙ.GÙ N[U ZU GAM]
59′. DIŠ KI.MIN-*ma ina* DU$_{10}$.GAM-*šú šá* 15 SÌG-*iṣ u ina* KA-*šú* MÚD BURU$_{8}$ [GÍD-*ma* GAM]
60′. DIŠ KI.MIN-*ma ina* DU$_{10}$.GAM-*šú šá* 150 SÌG-*iṣ u ina* KA-*šú* MÚD MUD ŠUB-[*di* GAM]
61′. DIŠ KI.MIN-*ma ina* GÌR-*šú šá* 15 SÌG-*iṣ* ŠU ^{d}UTU *ana* U$_{4}$.⸢3⸣.[KÁM GAM]
62′. DIŠ KI.MIN-*ma ina* GÌR-*šú šá* 150 SÌG-*iṣ* ŠU ^{d}15 GÍD-[*ma* GAM]
63′. DIŠ KI.MIN-*ma* GÌR-*šú šá* 15 *i-maš-šar* KA-*šú ṣu-dur mi-šit-ti* [MAŠKIM GÍD-*ma* GAM]
64′a. DIŠ KI.MIN-*ma* GÌR-*šú šá* 150 *i-maš-šar* SÌG-*iṣ* ^{d}*Ba-ú* SÌG-*iṣ* GAM
64′b. DIŠ KI.MIN-‹*ma*› GÌR^{II}-*šú am-šá-ma* LAL NU [ZU-*e u* UŠ$_{4}$-*šú* NU DIB GAM]
65′. DIŠ KI.MIN-*ma* GABA.MEŠ *šá* GÌR^{II}-*šú* GI$_{6}$.MEŠ ŠU ^{d}[15 GÍD-*ma* GAM]
66′. DIŠ KI.MIN-*ma kar-ši* U.MEŠ GÌR^{II}-*šú* GI$_{6}$.MEŠ [*i-ṭa-mu* GAM]
67′. DIŠ KI.MIN-*ma* UZU.MEŠ-*šú i-šam-ma-mu-šú* IGI^{II}-*šú* MÚD D[IRI.MEŠ GAM]
68′. DIŠ KI.MIN-⸢*ma* UZU⸣.MEŠ-*šú ug-gag* GIN$_{7}$ *ug-ga-*⸢*gu*⸣ [NU ZU GAM]
69′–75′. (fragmentary)
76′. DIŠ KI.MIN-*ma i-b*[*ak-ki* …]
77′. DIŠ KI.MIN-*ma iṣ-ṣe-ni-iḫ* […]
78′. DIŠ KI.MIN-*ma de-ki-šu la i*[*p-pal* …]
79′. DIŠ KI.MIN-*ma* ŠUB.ŠUB-*ut* […]
80′. DIŠ KI.MIN-*ma* DUL.DUL […]
81′. DIŠ KI.MIN-*ma il-ta-na-*⸢*as*⸣-[*si* …]
82′. DIŠ KI.MIN-*ma* MUD.MUD-*u*[*d* …]
83′. DIŠ KI.MIN-*ma* LUḪ.LUḪ-[*ut* …]
84′. DIŠ KI.MIN-*ma i-ṭ*[*a-mu* …]
85′. DIŠ KI.MIN-*ma pit-*⸢*ru*⸣-[*ud* …]
86′–87′. (fragmentary)
88′. DIŠ KI.MIN-*ma* […] ⸢GÙ.GÙ-*si*⸣ GAM
89′. DIŠ KI.MIN-*ma i-*[*na* KI.NÁ-*šú* G]Ù.GÙ-*si u di-ki-šu la ip-pal* ŠU DINGIR-*šú* GAM
90′. DIŠ KI.MIN-*ma i-*[*na* KI.NÁ]-*šú* GIN$_{7}$ MUŠEN *ù*ʾ GÙ.GÙ-*si u* LUḪ.LUḪ-*ut ana* U$_{4}$.3.KÁM GAM
91′. DIŠ KI.MIN-*ma i*[*-siḫ-ti* KI.MA]Ḫ-*šú i-si-iḫ* SÌG-*iṣ* ^{d}DIM$_{11}$.ME GAM : SÌG-*iṣ* ^{d}IM DUMU ^{d}*A-nim* GA[M]

92′. DIŠ KI.MIN-*ma* […] ḫal zu *na-kud* GAM : *pú-qud-de-e* ^{d}15 *ana* ^{d}MAŠ.TAB.BA GAM

Translation

DPS 14:267′ (catchline) = DPS 15:1

1. [If] it is the ⸢first⸣ [day] he is sick and he was injured on his head …
(gap of unknown length)
1′–3′. *(fragmentary)*
4′. If ditto (it is the first day he has been sick) and [he twists and vomits blood], he was injured with the wound of (his own) personal death demon; he will die.
5′. If ditto (it is the first day he has been sick) and his face turns ⸢black⸣ [and he vomits blood], he was injured on the front side; he will die.[3]
6′. If ditto (it is the first day he has been sick) and his neck ⸢hurts⸣ him [and he continually asks for water, "hand"] of Ishtar. He was injured on his neck; he will die.[4]
7′. If ditto (it is the first day he has been sick) and ⸢his larynx⸣ is constricted, he ate something offensive to his god; "hand" of his god; he will ⸢die⸣.[5]
8′. If ditto (it is the first day he has been sick) and his chokings come close together and he is not in full possession of his faculties, [he will die].[6]
9′. If ditto (it is the first day he has been sick) and his "right" arm is dark (and) his tongue is tied in knots, he was injured from behind; he will die.[7]
10′. If ditto (it is the first day he has been sick) and his "left" arm is dark (and) he twists, ⸢blow⸣ of Sîn but he will get through [(var. he will die)].[8]
11′. If ditto (it is the first day he has been sick) and he is unable to turn his arms [and] blood drips [from] his [anus, he will die].[9]
12′. If ditto (it is the first day he has been sick) and he is unable to turn his arms […].[10]
13′–14′. If ditto (it is the first day he has been sick) and his hand is placed on his navel and his hands and his feet are cold, [he talks] without knowing (what he is saying and) he gets up and sits down (again), he was injured on his navel; "hand" of Ishtar; [he will die].[11]
15′. If ditto (it is the first day he has been sick) and his hands are continually placed on his head and he does not bring them down, his insides are puffed up, (and) he burns with fever,[12] [he was injured] on his ⸢epigastrium⸣; [he will die].[13]

16′. If ditto (it is the first day he has been sick) and he moves his hands across his mouth[14] (and) continually throws off his garment, he has been made [to eat] dirty substances;[15] [he will die].[16]

17′. If ditto (it is the first day he has been sick) and his hands rub his body, [if] his illness is prolonged, [he will die].[17]

18′. If ditto (it is the first day he has been sick) and his hands are immobilized so that he is unable to stretch (them) out and he is not in full possession of his faculties, "hand" of Shamash; [he will die].[18]

19′. If ditto (it is the first day he has been sick) and his hands or feet are immobilized so that he is unable to stretch (them) out and he is not in full possession of his faculties, he is at an acute stage of the illness; [he will die].

20′. If ditto (it is the first day he has been sick) and (either or both of) his hands or feet are immobilized (and) he speaks ⸢calmly(?)⸣; the god of his city has stricken him; [he will die].[19]

21′. If ditto (it is the first day he has been sick) and his hands and his feet [...], his speech wanders about (and) he was injured at noon, "hand" of Adad; [he will die].[20]

22′. If ditto (it is the first day he has been sick) and his hands and his ⸢feet⸣ ... and he vomits blood, "hand" of Nergal; he will die.

23′. If ditto (it is the first day he has been sick) and his hands and [his feet ... (and) it itches, "hand" of *bennu*, deputy of Sîn; he will die.

24′. If ditto (it is the first day he has been sick) and his hands and [his feet rub (each other)(?) (and)] he ⸢drinks⸣ [a lot of water?] and he is not in full possession of his faculties, he will die. If ditto (it is the first day he has been sick) and his hands and feet rub (each other), if his illness is prolonged, he will die.

25′. If ditto (it is the first day he has been sick) and he [sucks?] his fingers [...], he continually becomes darkened (and) he continually gets up (afterwards), *miqit šamê* has "touched" him; "hand" of his god; he will die.

26′. If ditto (it is the first day he has been sick) and he sucks his fingers in his mouth, he burns with fever, his abdomen is bloated and he wanders about, he was injured on his neck; "hand" of Bau; he will die.[21]

27′. If ditto (it is the first day he has been sick) and his fingers are placed in his mouth and (if) you take (them) out, he returns (them) to his mouth, he will die and afterwards there will be a(nother) death in his household.[22]

28′. If ditto (it is the first day he has been sick) and the "breasts" of his hands are dark/black, "hand" of the god of his city; he will die.[23]

29′. If ditto (it is the first day he has been sick) and the "bellies" of the fingers of his hands are dark/black and he twists, "hand" of ghost; he will die.[24]

30′. If ditto (it is the first day he has been sick) and his "right" armpit hurts him and he wanders about, he was injured on the front side; he will die.[25]

31′. If ditto (it is the first day he has been sick) and his "left" armpit hurts him (but) he does not have a fever, the "double" of a dead man afflicts him.[26]

32′. If ditto (it is the first day he has been sick) and he was wounded on his breast and, as a consequence, he continually pours out blood and wanders about, "hand" of Nergal; he was wounded on the front side; he will die.[27]

33′. If ditto (it is the first day he has been sick) and his epigastrium is dark/black and his tongue is shriveled, he is at an acute stage[28] of the illness, he will die.[29]

34′. If ditto (it is the first day he has been sick) and his epigastrium is puffed up and his face is swollen (and) tears flow from his eyes, if it is prolonged, he will die.[30]

35′. If ditto (it is the first day he has been sick) and he was injured on his abdomen and, as a consequence, he is colicky and constipated, he will die.[31]

36′. If ditto (it is the first day he has been sick) and he was injured on his abdomen and, as a consequence, (his stomach) is continually upset, "hand" of the twin gods; he will die.[32]

37′. If ditto (it is the first day he has been sick) and his chest and abdomen are dark/black and the muscles of his abdomen are pulled taut (and) he belches "wind" from his mouth, (once he has been sick) for three days, he will die.[33]

38′. If ditto (it is the first day he has been sick) and he cries: "My insides, my insides!" and he tears his hair, he was injured on his thorax; he will die.[34]

39′. If ditto (it is the first day he has been sick) and he was injured on his "right" kidney (= lower back), he is not in full possession of his faculties (and) he wanders about without knowing (where he is), "hand" of the twin gods; he will die.[35]

40′. If ditto (it is the first day he has been sick) and he was injured on his "left" kidney, he is not in full possession of his faculties and he vomits blood, "hand" of the Sibitti; he will die.[36]

41′. If ditto (it is the first day he has been sick) and he was injured on his coccyx (var. testicle), "hand" of Sîn. If it is prolonged, he will die.[37]

42′. If ditto (it is the first day he has been sick) and his "right" rib is dark/black, his mouth is continually dry and he rolls over and over, "hand" of Damu. He was injured on his kidney; he will die.[38]

43′. If ditto (it is the first day he has been sick) and his "left" rib is dark, he vomits blood and (his stomach) is continually upset (and) he was injured that same day, he will die.[39]

44′. If ditto (it is the first day he has been sick) and he was injured on his "right" upper back and he wanders about, "hand" of the god of his city. (If) he was injured in the dawn watch, he will die.[40]

45′. If ditto (it is the first day he has been sick) and he was injured on his "left" upper back and he wanders about, "hand" of his god. (If) he was injured in the middle watch, he will die.[41]

46′. If ditto (it is the first day he has been sick) and he was injured on his spine and he is blocked off so that his excrement cannot come out, "hand" of a murderous ghost; he will die.[42]

47′. If ditto (it is the first day he has been sick) and his spine is curved so that he cannot straighten it out, if it is prolonged, he will die.[43]

48′. If ditto (it is the first day he has been sick) and his pelvic region is continually lifted up (and) he does not realize that he is continually doing (this), he will die.[44]

49′. If ditto (it is the first day he has been sick) and he was injured on his "right" femural crease and, as a consequence, he is unconscious, "hand" of Šulpaea; he will die.[45]

50′. If ditto (it is the first day he has been sick) and he was injured on his "left" femural crease and, as a consequence, he cannot uproot his foot (from the ground) (and) he ‹was injured› at sunrise, "hand" of Ishtar; he will die.[46]

51′. If ditto (it is the first day he has been sick) and his buttocks are dark/black so that his excrement cannot come out and he cannot pass water, he was injured on the back side; he will die.[47]

52′. If ditto (it is the first day he has been sick) and the "right" side of his abdomen is swollen and dark/black (and) he wanders about without knowing (where he is), "hand" of Adad. (If) he was injured at noon, he will die.[48]

53′. If ditto (it is the first day he has been sick) and the "left" side of his abdomen is swollen and dark/black (and) he wanders about without knowing (where he is), "hand" of Ishtar. (If) he was injured in the morning, he will die.[49]

54′. If ditto (it is the first day he has been sick) and he was injured on his "right" thigh and he is constipated, he will die.[50]

55′. If ditto (it is the first day he has been sick) and he was injured on his "left" thigh, his stomach is cramped (and) he has a vise-like headache, [he will die].[51]

56′. If ditto (it is the first day he has been sick) and he strikes his crotch, chews on his hands (and) they have to put his arms behind him, "hand" of the ⌜twin⌝ [gods; he will die].[52]

57′. If ditto (it is the first day he has been sick) and he was injured on his "right" inguinal region, he is not in full possession of his faculties [(and) he wanders about without knowing (where he is), he will die].[53]

58′. If ditto (it is the first day he has been sick) and he was injured on his "left" inguinal region (and) he does ⌜not⌝ [know] that he is continually crying out, [he will die].[54]

59′. If ditto (it is the first day he has been sick) and he was injured on his "right" leg and he vomits blood from his mouth, [if it is prolonged(?), he will die].[55]

60′. If ditto (it is the first day he has been sick) and he was injured on his "left" leg and he produces dark blood from his mouth, [he will die].[56]

61′. If ditto (it is the first day he has been sick) and he was injured on his "right" foot, "hand" of Shamash. (Once he has been sick) for three days, [he will die].[57]

62′. If ditto (it is the first day he has been sick) and he was injured on his "left" foot, "hand" of Ishtar. [If] (his illness) is prolonged, [he will die].[58]

63′. If ditto (it is the first day he has been sick) and he drags his "right" foot (and) his mouth twitches, stroke of [a *rābiṣu*; if it is prolonged, he will die].[59]

64′a. If ditto (it is the first day he has been sick) and he drags his "left" foot, he was injured with a wound of Bau; he will die.[60]

64′b. If ditto (it is the first day he has been sick) and his feet are immobilized so that he is ⌜unable⌝ to stretch (them) out [and he is not in full possession of his faculties, he will die].[61]

65′. If ditto (it is the first day he has been sick) and the "breasts" of his feet are dark, "hand" of [Ishtar; if it is prolonged, he will die].[62]

66′. If ditto (it is the first day he has been sick) and the "bellies" of his toes are dark [(and) he twists, he will die].[63]

67′. If ditto (it is the first day he has been sick) and his flesh goes numb (and) his eyes are ⌜full⌝ of blood, [he will die].

68′. If ditto (it is the first day he has been sick) and he scratches his flesh (and) [he does not realize] that he is scratching (it), [he will die].

69′–75′. *(fragmentary)*

76′. If ditto (it is the first day he has been sick) and he ⌜wails⌝ [...].

77′. If ditto (it is the first day he has been sick) and he laughs [...].

78′. If ditto (it is the first day he has been sick) and he does not ⸢answer⸣ the one trying to wake him […].

79′. If ditto (it is the first day he has been sick) and he continually falls down […].

80′. If ditto (it is the first day he has been sick) and he continually veils (himself) […].

81′. If ditto (it is the first day he has been sick) and he continually cries out […]

82′. If ditto (it is the first day he has been sick) and he continually shudders […].

83′. If ditto (it is the first day he has been sick) and he continually jerks […].

84′. If ditto (it is the first day he has been sick) and he ⸢twists⸣ […].

85′. If ditto (it is the first day he has been sick) and he ⸢is confused⸣ […]

86′–87′. *(fragmentary)*

88′. If ditto (it is the first day he has been sick) and he […] (and) continually cries out, he will die.

89′. If ditto (it is the first day he has been sick) and he continually cries out ⸢in⸣ [his sleep] and does not answer the one trying to wake him, "hand" of his god; he will die.[64]

90′. If ditto (it is the first day he has been sick) and like a bird he continually cries out "Oh, woe" ⸢in⸣ his [sleep] and he continually jerks, (once he has been sick) for three days, he will die.[65]

91′. If ditto (it is the first day he has been sick) and he makes the ⸢assignments⸣ [for] his ⸢tomb⸣, wound of Lamashtu; he will die (var. wound of Adad, son of Anu; he will die).[66]

92′. [If …]. it is worrisome; he will die (var. it is a good entrusted by Ishtar to the twin gods).[67]

Notes

1. Restored from DPS 9:20.
2. Restored from DPS 10:8.
3. See Scurlock and Andersen 2005, 8.92. The entry appears also in DPS 9:20.
4. See Scurlock and Andersen 2005, 13.138, 19.150. This entry appears also in DPS 10:8.
5. See Scurlock and Andersen 2005, 8.89. This entry appears also in DPS 10:28.
6. See Scurlock and Andersen 2005, 3.57. This entry appears also in DPS 10:34.
7. This entry also appeared in DPS 10:55.
8. See Scurlock and Andersen 2005, 19.201. This entry also appears in DPS 10B rev. 1.
9. This entry also appears in DPS 10B rev. 2.
10. This entry also appears in DPS 10B rev. 3 or 4.
11. See Scurlock and Andersen 2005, 3.39, 14.26, 19.64, 19.129, 19.151. This entry also

appears in DPS 11 obv. 9.

12. See the discussion under DPS 3:70.

13. See Scurlock and Andersen 2005, 3.210. This entry also appears in DPS 11 obv. 25.

14. For the reading and discussion, see Heeßel 2000, 164.

15. For the reading, see Heeßel 2000, 163 (after a suggestion by M. Stol).

16. See Scurlock and Andersen 2005, 16.59, 16.62. This entry also appears in DPS 11 obv. 28.

17. This entry appears also in DPS 11 obv. 29.

18. See Scurlock and Andersen 2005, 19.271. This entry appears also in DPS 11 obv. 20.

19. See Scurlock and Andersen 2005, 19.126.

20. See Scurlock and Andersen 2005, 14.38, 19.145.

21. See Scurlock and Andersen 2005, 14.37, 19.166. The entry appears also in DPS 11 rev. 36.

22. This entry appears also in DPS 11 rev. 50.

23. See Scurlock and Andersen 2005, 14.43, 19.127.

24. See Scurlock and Andersen 2005, 14.41, 19.131.

25. This entry appears also in DPS 12:127″.

26. See Scurlock and Andersen 2005, 19.391. This entry appears also in DPS 12:128″.

27. See Scurlock and Andersen 2005, 14.32, 19.174. This entry appears also in DPS 12:4.

28. For the reading and interpretation, see Heeßel 2000, 164 (after Landsberger).

29. See Scurlock and Andersen 2005, 18.37. This entry appears also in DPS 13:2.

30. See Scurlock and Andersen 2005, 6.36, 8.21, 20.83. This entry also appears in DPS 13:21.

31. See Scurlock and Andersen 2005, 3.204. This entry also appears in DPS 13:77a.

32. See Scurlock and Andersen 2005, 3.204, 19.137. This entry also appears in DPS 13:77b.

33. See Scurlock and Andersen 2005, 3.208. This entry appears also in DPS 13:96–97.

34. See Scurlock and Andersen 2005, 14.12. This entry also appears in DPS 13:134.

35. See Scurlock and Andersen 2005, 14.33, 19.179, 20.8. This entry appears also in DPS 12:84″.

36. See Scurlock and Andersen 2005, 14.27, 19.178. This entry appears also in DPS 12:85″.

37. See Scurlock and Andersen 2005, 19.198. This entry appears also in DPS 12:125″.

38. See Scurlock and Andersen 2005, 10.36, 14.28. This entry appears also in DPS 12:47′.

39. See Scurlock and Andersen 2005, 14.29. This entry appears also in DPS 12:48′.

40. See Scurlock and Andersen 2005, 19.207. This entry appears also in DPS 12:86″.

41. See Scurlock and Andersen 2005, 19.207. This entry appears also in DPS 12:87″.

42. See Scurlock and Andersen 2005, 5.40, 6.155, 13.142, 19.172. This entry appears also in DPS 12:98."

43. See Scurlock and Andersen 2005, 11.24, 20.84. This entry appears also in DPS 12:96″.

44. See Scurlock and Andersen 2005, 13.88. This entry also appears in DPS 12:104″.

45. See Scurlock and Andersen 2005, 14.16, 19.197. This entry appears also in DPS 12:131″.

46. See Scurlock and Andersen 2005, 14.18, 19.153. This entry appears also in DPS 12:132″.

47. See Scurlock and Andersen 2005, 5.41. This entry appears also in DPS 14:60.

48. See Scurlock and Andersen 2005, 14.38, 19.144. This entry appears also in DPS 14:177′–178′.

49. See Scurlock and Andersen 2005, 3.206, 19.155. The entry appears also in DPS 14:179′–180′.

50. See Scurlock and Andersen 2005, 14.19. The entry appears also in DPS 14:173′.

51. See Scurlock and Andersen 2005, 14.20. The entry also appears in DPS 14:174′–175′.
52. See Scurlock and Andersen 2005, 16.78, 19.238. The entry also appears in DPS 14:168′–169′.
53. See Scurlock and Andersen 2005, 14.14. The entry also appears in DPS 14:66.
54. See Scurlock and Andersen 2005, 14.15. The entry also appears in DPS 14:67.
55. See Scurlock and Andersen 2005, 14.17. The entry appears also in DPS 14:205′.
56. See Scurlock and Andersen 2005, 14.17. The entry also appears in DPS 14:206′.
57. See Scurlock and Andersen 2005, 19.186, 19.194. The entry appears also in DPS 14:234′.
58. See Scurlock and Andersen 2005, 19.154, 19.186, 20.85. The entry also appears in DPS 14:235′.
59. See Scurlock and Andersen 2005, 13.55, 13.79, 13.243, 20.86. The entry appears also in DPS 14:209′–210′.
60. See Scurlock and Andersen 2005, 19.165. This entry also appears in DPS 14:211′.
61. The entry appears also in DPS 14:217′.
62. See Scurlock and Andersen 2005, 14.44, 19.128, 20.87. The entry also appears in DPS 14:252′.
63. See Scurlock and Andersen 2005, 14.42. The entry appears also in DPS 14:250′.
64. See Scurlock and Andersen 2005, 19.294, 20.101.
65. See Scurlock and Andersen 2005, 13.208.
66. See Scurlock and Andersen 2005, 19.147.
67. See Scurlock and Andersen 2005, 19.184.

DPS 16

DPS 15:93′ (catchline) = DPS 16:1

1. DIŠ U$_4$.1.KÁM GIG-*ma* SAG.DU-*su* GU$_7$-*šú* UD.DA TAB.BA ŠU DINGIR AD.A.NI DIN GAM
2. DIŠ U$_4$.1.KÁM GIG-*ma ina* ŠÀ-*šú* ŠU^{II}-*šú* GAR.GAR-*an ši-gu-ú* GÙ-*si* ŠU^{II}-*šú* NIR.NIR-*aṣ* GAM
3. DIŠ KI.MIN-*ma ina* ŠÀ-*šú* ŠU^{II}-*šú* GAR.GAR U.MEŠ-*šú ú-na-ṣab* ŠU DINGIR *rab-bu-ti* GAM
4. DIŠ KI.MIN-*ma ana* É-*šú* ÍR GAM
5. DIŠ KI.MIN-*ma ana* DUMU.MEŠ-*šú* ÍR GAM
6. DIŠ KI.MIN-*ma* ŠE$_{10}$ *ma-ru-ti-šú*[1] *iz-zi* GAM
7. DIŠ KI.MIN-[*m*]*a ina* KÀŠ-*šú* MÚD *iš-tin ana* KI GIG GAM
8. DIŠ KI.MIN-*ma i-leb-bu u i-sa-a*ʾ GAM
9. DIŠ KI.MIN-*ma a-a* GÙ.GÙ-*si-ma* NU NAG ŠU DINGIR.GAL.GAL GAM
10. DIŠ KI.MIN-*ma* MÚD MUD *iz-zi* GAM : *ana* GAL$_5$.LÁ ÚŠ *pa-qid* GAM
11. DIŠ KI.MIN-*ma* GIG-*su* DUGUD-*su-ma* ZU-*šú* NU *ú-ad-da* GAM

12. DIŠ U$_4$.1.KÁM TAG$_4$-*šú-ma* U$_4$.1.KÁM LÁ-*šú* NÍG.GU$_7$ ^{d}DÌM.ME.LAGAB ŠU DINGIR.GAL.MEŠ GAM
13. DIŠ U$_4$.1.KÁM DIB-*su* U$_4$.1.KÁM BAR-*šú* ZI DINGIR DIB-*su*
14–15. DIŠ U$_4$.1.KÁM DIB-*su* U$_4$.1.KÁM BAR-*šú* U$_4$ LÁ-*šú* LÁ-*šú* UB.MEŠ-*šú* GU$_7$.MEŠ-*šú* KÚM-*ma i-ra-ʾu-ub* IR ŠUB-*su-ma ina-aḫ u* A *ana* NAG *ma-gal* APIN.MEŠ ŠU ^{d}DÌM.ME (var. ^{d}AMAR.UTU) DIN
16. DIŠ U$_4$.1.KÁM GIG-*ma* U$_4$.1.KÁM *ba-liṭ* GIDIM AD *u* AMA DIB-*su*
17. DIŠ U$_4$.1.KÁM U$_4$.2.KÁM *i-re-eḫ-ḫi-šum-ma ina* U$_4$.3.KÁM DIB-*su* DIB GIDIM$_7$
18. DIŠ U$_4$.1.KÁM U$_4$.2.KÁM GIG-*ma* ŠÀ-*šú* DIB.DIB-*su* DIB-*su* ŠUB.ŠUB-*šú* GAM
19–20. DIŠ U$_4$.1.KÁM U$_4$.2.KÁM U$_4$.3.KÁM GIG-*ma* KÚM ÚḪ *ina* SU-*šú* DU$_8$-*ma* EGIR DU$_8$ KÚM ÚḪ *ina* SAG.DU-*šú* NU DU$_8$ *ana* U$_4$.3.KÁM *ana* U$_4$.6.KÁM (var. U$_4$.4.KÁM) GAM
21. DIŠ U$_4$.2.KÁM GIG-*ma* SAG.KI-*šú šá* 15 GU$_7$-*šú* IGI-*šú šá* 15 GISSU DÙ ŠU ^{d}UD.AL.TAR BÚR-*ma* DIN
22. DIŠ U$_4$.2.KÁM GIG-*ma* SAG.KI-*šú šá* 150 GU$_7$-*šú* IGI-*šú šá* 150 GISSU DÙ ŠU ^{d}UD.AL.TAR BÚR-*ma* DIN
23–24. DIŠ U$_4$.2.KÁM GIG-*ma* SAG.KI-*šú šá* 15 *u* 150 GU$_7$.MEŠ-*šú* IGI^{II}-*šú šá* 15 *u* 150 GISSU *ib-na-a* NA BI DINGIR-*šú u* DINGIR URU-*šú iz-zur* BÚR-*ma* DIN
25–27. DIŠ U$_4$.2.KÁM ŠUB-*šú-ma ina* U$_4$.3.KÁM DIB-*su* U$_4$-*ma* DIB-*šú im-ta-na-ag-ga-gu* EGIR *im-ta-na-gag-ga ra-ʾ-i-ba* TUKU-*ši* UB.MEŠ-*šú* GU$_7$.MEŠ-*šú* ŠU^{II}-*šú u* GÌR^{II}-*šú* ŠED$_7$-*a* EGIR-*nu* KÚM 1-*niš i-rak-kab-šú* : *i-re-eḫ-ḫi-šú u* IR ŠUB-*su-ma ina-aḫ* DIB KUR-*i* DIB-*su*
28. DIŠ U$_4$.2.KÁM DIB-*su*-⸢*ma*⸣ *ina* U$_4$.3.KÁM *i-re-eḫ-ḫi-šú* DIB-*it* KUR-*i* : GAM
29. DIŠ U$_4$.2.KÁM U$_4$.3.KÁM GIG-*ma uš-tar-di-ma* ŠÀ-*šú* DIB.DIB-⸢*su*⸣ MÚD *ina* KIR$_4$-*šú* ŠUB.Š[UB]-⸢*a* GIG⸣ *ki-is-sa-tú* GIG
30. DIŠ U$_4$.2.KÁM U$_4$.3.KÁM GIG-*ma uš-tar-di-ma ḫu-qu* DIB-*su ina* U$_4$.7.KÁM *ina* [… -*m*]*a* GAM
31–32. DIŠ U$_4$.2.KÁM U$_4$.3.KÁM GIG-*ma* KÚM *ṣar-ḫu ina* SU-*šú* DU$_8$-*ma* EGIR DU$_8$ *ina* [SAG.DU-*šú* NU DU$_8$ G]IG-*s*[*u* …]
33. DIŠ *ina* U$_4$.2.KÁM *ina* U$_4$.3.KÁM KÚM ŠED$_7$ *u* IR-*su* GIN$_7$ *lu-ba-ṭi* [ŠUB.ŠUB-*su* …]
34. DIŠ *ina* ⸢U$_4$⸣.2.KÁM *ina* U$_4$.3.KÁM *šá* DIB ŠUB.ŠUB-*su* KÚM *u* IR TU[KU …]
35. [DIŠ *ina* U$_4$.2.K]ÁM *ina* U$_4$.3.KÁM [… K]ÚM? *u* IR TUKU […]

(break of unknown length)

36′. DIŠ U$_4$.2.KÁM GIG-*ma ina* ⸢U$_4$⸣.[3.KÁM ...]

37′. DIŠ U$_4$.2.KÁM GIG-*ma ina* U$_4$.3.KÁM ⸢*it*⸣-*te-bi* [...]

38′. DIŠ U$_4$.3.KÁM GIG-*ma ina* U$_4$.4.KÁM *it-te-bi* [...]

39′. DIŠ U$_4$.3.KÁM GIG-*ma ina* U$_4$.4.KÁM MÚD *ina* KIR$_4$ -*šú* DU-*ku* [...]

40′. DIŠ U$_4$.3.KÁM GIG-*ma u* ZI-*bi ina t*[*am-ḫ*]*e-e* [DU$_8$] GIG

41′. DIŠ U$_4$.3.KÁM GIG-*ma u* UZU.MEŠ-*šú šal-mu ana* GIG-⸢*šú* GUR⸣-[*m*]*a* GAM

42′. DIŠ U$_4$.3.KÁM ŠÀ.ŠÀ GÙ.GÙ-*si u* ŠÀ.MEŠ-*šú nap-ḫu* GAM

43′. DIŠ U$_4$.4.KÁM GIG-*ma* ŠU^{II}-*šú ina* ŠÀ-*šú* GAR.GAR-*an* IGI.MEŠ-*šú* SIG$_7$ ŠUB-*ú* GAM

44′. DIŠ U$_4$.4.KÁM U$_4$.5.KÁM GIG-*ma* IR ŠUB.ŠUB-*su* DU$_8$-*ár* GIG

45′. DIŠ U$_4$.4.KÁM U$_4$.5.KÁM GIG-*aṣ* ŠU ^{d}DÌM.ME.LAGAB

46′. DIŠ U$_4$.5.KÁM GIG-*ma ina* U$_4$.6.KÁM MÚD *ina* KIR$_4$-*šú* DU-*ku* GIG-*su* DU$_8$-*ár* TAB UD.DA

47′. DIŠ U$_4$.5.KÁM GIG-*ma* UZU.MEŠ-*šu* SIG$_7$ ŠUB-*ú* IGI^{II}-*šú* MÚD DIRI. MEŠ GAM

48′. DIŠ U$_4$.5.KÁM U$_4$.6.KÁM GIG-*ma uš-tar-di-ma ia-ú ia-ú la ú-kal-la* GAM

49′. DIŠ U$_4$.5.KÁM U$_4$.10.KÁM GIG-*ma uš-tar-di-ma ḫu-qu ka-a-a-man-šú* GAM

50′–51′. DIŠ U$_4$.5.KÁM U$_4$.10.KÁM GIG *dan-na* GIG-*ma uš-tar-di-ma* MÚD *ka-a-a-na* U$_4$.5.KÁM *ina* KIR$_4$-*šú* DU-*ku u ik-ka-la* GIG-*su* DU$_8$-*ár* UD.DA *ḫa-miṭ ba-liṭ* LÚG NU TUKU

52′. DIŠ U$_4$.5.KÁM U$_4$.10.KÁM GIG *dan-na* GIG-*ma uš-tar-di-ma* GIG *dan-na ka-a-a-na* U$_4$.5.KÁM DIB.DIB-*su ba-liṭ* LÚG NU TUKU

53′–54′. DIŠ U$_4$.5.KÁM U$_4$.10.KÁM GIG *dan-na* GIG-*ma uš-tar-di-ma* GI$_6$ IGI^{II}-*šú uš-ter-di-a* U$_4$.2.KÁM *ḫu-qu* DIB.DIB-*su ina* U$_4$.3.KÁM GAM

55′. DIŠ U$_4$.5.KÁM U$_4$.10.KÁM GIG-*ma* EGIR-*nu* MÚD *pe-lu-tu ina* KIR$_4$-*šú* DU-*ku* DIN

56′. DIŠ U$_4$.5.KÁM U$_4$.10.KÁM GIG-*ma* KÚM *u* IR NU TUKU ŠU ^{d}30 GAM

57′. DIŠ U$_4$.5.KÁM U$_4$.10.KÁM U$_4$.15.KÁM GIG-*ma ḫu-qu* DIB.DIB-*su u* BAR-*šú* PAP.ḪAL.MEŠ-*ma* GAM

58′. DIŠ KI.MIN-*ma* GI$_6$ IGI^{II}-*šú* E$_{11}$-*a u ḫu-qu* DIB.DIB-*su ana* U$_4$.3.KÁM GAM

59′–60′. DIŠ U$_4$.5.KÁM U$_4$.10.KÁM U$_4$.15.KÁM U$_4$.20.KÁM U.MEŠ ŠU^{II}-*šú u* GÌR^{II}-*šú am-šá aš-ṭa-a-ma*[2] BAD-*a u* GUB-*za* NU ZU-*e* ŠU ^{d}15 *uš-šar-ma* : *iš-šìr-ma* DIN

61′. DIŠ U$_4$.6.KÁM GIG-*ma u* UZU.MEŠ-*šú šal-mu ana* GIG-*šú* GUR-*ma ni-kit-tam* TUKU-*ši* ŠÀ-*šú* DIB.DIB-*su* GAM

62′. DIŠ U$_4$.6.KÁM U$_4$.10.KÁM NÍG.GI TUKU-*ši šum-ma* SAG ŠÀ-*šú* DIB-*su* GAM

63′–64′. DIŠ U$_4$.6.KÁM LÍL-*ma ina* U$_4$.7.KÁM NU PA.AN-*uš* A *ana* IGI.MEŠ-*šú i-sal-la-ú-ma šum$_4$-ma* IGI^{II}-*šú* NU BAD GAM *šum$_4$-ma* IGI^{II}-*šú* BAD *u* DUL-*tam ana* A *šá is-lu-ḫu-šú* ÍR DIN

65′–66′. DIŠ U$_4$.6.KÁM GIG-*ma ina* U$_4$.7.KÁM *ḫur-ba-šú* ŠUB.ŠUB-*su* EGIR *ḫur-ba-šú* IR TA SAG.DU-*šú* EN *kin-ṣi-šú*[3] GÁL GIG-*su* DU$_8$-*ár-ma* DIN

67′–68′. [DIŠ U$_4$.6.KÁM GIG-*ma ina* U$_4$.7.KÁM GIG TI U$_4$-*ma* TI GIG] IR TA SAG.DU-*šú* [EN …] GAM

69′. [DIŠ U$_4$.6.KÁM] GI[G]-*ma ina* U$_4$.7.KÁM DIN-*uṭ* ⸢GIG⸣ TI U$_4$-*ma*[4] TI GIG SAG ŠÀ-*šú* DIB-*su* GAM

70′. DIŠ [U$_4$.6.KÁM] G[IG-*m*]*a ina* U$_4$.7.⸢KÁM DIN⸣ [KI.MIN-*ma ṣ*]*a-lim* ZÉ *ina* DÚR-*šú* SI.SÁ-*am-ma* GAM

71′. DIŠ U$_4$.⸢6⸣.[KÁM] G[IG-*ma ina* U$_4$.7.KÁM DIN KI.MIN-*ma* DUG$_4$]-*su im-ta-aš-šu* ZÉ *ina* DÚR-*šú* KI.MIN-*ma* GAM

72′. DIŠ U$_4$.6.KÁM GIG-⸢*ma ina* U$_4$.7⸣.[KÁM KI.MIN-*ma* IGI]⸢^{II}⸣-*šú* IM.GÚ DIRI.DIRI.MEŠ MÚD *ina* KIR$_4$-*šú* DU-*ku-ma* DIN

73′–74′. DIŠ U$_4$.6.KÁM GIG-*ma ina* U$_4$.7.KÁM DIN-*uṭ ina* U$_4$.8.KÁM GIG-*ma ina* U$_4$.9.KÁM DIN-*uṭ* U$_4$.10.KÁM GIG-*ma ina* U$_4$.11.KÁM DIN-*uṭ* GIG-*su ni-kit-tú* TUKU-*ši* ^{LÚ}MAŠ.MAŠ *ana* DIN-*šú* ME.A NU GAR-*an*

75′. DIŠ *ina* U$_4$.15.KÁM GIG-*su* ŠUB-*su na-šar* GIG

76′. DIŠ *a-di-na* ITU NU GIG-*ma iṣ-lim-ma*[5] *kir-ra-šú šu-uḫ-ḫu-ṭa* GIG-*ma* GAM

77′. DIŠ KI.MIN-*ma iṣ-lim-ma* IGI^{II}-*šú rab-ṣa* GIG-*ma* GAM

78′–79′. DIŠ ITI.1.KÁM ITI.2.KÁM GIG-*ma* GIG-*su* TAK$_4$-*šú-ma ina* ŠÀ-*šú* DIB.DIB-*su ina* KIR$_4$-*šú* MÚD *pe-la-a* ŠUB.ŠUB-*a* GIG *ki-iṣ-ṣa-ti* GIG DIN

80′. DIŠ ITI.1.KÁM ITI.2.KÁM *ina* GI$_6$ ŠUB-*su u* GÙ-*si pi-rit-tu* ŠU ^{d}15 ZI-*bé*

81′–82′. DIŠ U$_4$-*mi-šam ana* GIZKIM-*šú* LAL-*šú u* BAR-*šú* U$_4$ LAL-*šú* KÚM-*ma* SA.MEŠ-*šú* GU$_7$.MEŠ-*šú* IR ŠUB-*su-ma ina-aḫ* LAL-*ti* UD.DA

83′–84′. DIŠ U$_4$-*mi ma-ʾ-du-ti* GIG-*ma* A.MEŠ SA$_5$.MEŠ *ina* DÚR-*šú* DU-*ku* GIG-*su* DU$_8$ UD.DA TAB.BA DIN U$_4$.MEŠ-*šú* GÍD.DA.MEŠ LÚG NU TUKU

85′. DIŠ KI.MIN-*ma* SA.MEŠ-*šú* SIG$_7$ ŠUB-*ú* IGI^{II}-*šú* MÚD DIRI.MEŠ GAM

86′. DIŠ KI.MIN-*ma* UZU.MEŠ-*šú ur-qá it-ta-du-ni* IGI^{II}-*šú* SA$_5$ ŠUB.MEŠ NU DIN

87′. DIŠ U$_4$.MEŠ-*šú* GÍD.DA.MEŠ-*ma ana* É-*šú* ÍR GAM

88′. DIŠ U$_4$.MEŠ-*šú* GÍD.DA.MEŠ-*ma ana* É-*šú u* DUMU.MEŠ-*šú* ÍR GAM

89′. DIŠ U$_4$.MEŠ-*šú* GÍD.DA.MEŠ-*ma i-siḫ-ti* KI.MAḪ-*šú i-siḫ* GAM

90′. DIŠ U$_4$.MEŠ-*šú* GÍD.DA.MEŠ-*ma* ŠE$_{10}$ *ma-ru-ti-šú*[6] *iz-zi* GAM

91′. DIŠ KI.MIN-*ma* IGI^{II}.MEŠ-*šú* GIN$_7$ *si-ka-a-ti ana* GA.RAŠ^{SAR} SIG$_7$.ME GAM

92′. DIŠ KI.MIN SU-*šú* GIN$_7$ KI.MIN SIG$_7$ ŠÀ.MEŠ-*šú nap-ḫu* SA ŠÀ-*šú* SIG$_7$ GIB.MEŠ GAM

93′. DIŠ KI.MIN ŠU^{II}-*šú u* GÌR^{II}-*šú* ŠED$_7$?! GIG-*su* KÚR-*šum-ma* UGU-*šú i-sap-pi-du-ma* DIN

94′. DIŠ KI.MIN ŠU^{II}-*šú u* GÌR^{II}-*šú ik-tap-pá* GIG-*su* KÚR-*šum-ma* UGU-*šú* KI.MIN DIN

95′. DIŠ KI.MIN ŠU^{II}-*šú u* GÌR^{II}-*šú ik-ra-a* GIG-*su* KÚR-*šum-ma* UGU-*šú* KI.MIN DIN

96′. DIŠ KI.MIN MÚD *ina* KIR$_4$ DU-*ku* DIN

97′. DIŠ KI.MIN GU$_7$ *u* NAG NU ZU ŠUK KI.MAḪ-*šú* (*ḫi-pi*)

98′–99′. DIŠ KI.MIN *ḫu-qu* DIB.DIB-*su* ^{GIŠ}NU.ÚR.MA APIN-*iš* GAM : DIŠ KI.MIN ZÚ.LUM.MA APIN-*ma* GU$_7$ DIN

100′–101′. DIŠ KI.MIN-*ma* DÍLIM NINDA APIN-*ma* Ì GU$_7$ GAM : DIŠ KI.MIN-*ma* GA APIN-*ma* Ì GU$_7$ *ana* KI GIG GAM

TRANSLATION

1. If it is the first day he has been sick and his head hurts him, he burns with *ṣētu* (or) "hand" of his father's god; he will get well or die.[7]
2. If it is the first day he has been sick and his hands are continually placed on his abdomen, he utters a *šigu*-prayer and stretches out his hands (in supplication), he will die.

3. If ditto (it is the first day he has been sick) and his hands are continually placed on his abdomen (and) he sucks his fingers, "hand" of the great gods; he will die.
4. If ditto (it is the first day he has been sick) and he wails for his household, he will die.[8]
5. If ditto (it is the first day he has been sick) and he wails for his children, he will die.
6. If ditto (it is the first day he has been sick) and he excretes the excrement of his body fat, he will die.[9]
7. If ditto (it is the first day he has been sick) and he urinates blood in his urine, he is at an acute stage of the illness;[10] he will die.[11]
8. If ditto (it is the first day he has been sick) and he groans and cries out, he will die.
9. If ditto (it is the first day he has been sick) and he cries out "Ah" and will not drink, "hand" of the great gods; he will die.
10. If ditto (it is the first day he has been sick) and he excretes dark blood, he will die (var: he was entrusted to a *gallû* of death; he will die).[12]
11. If ditto (it is the first day he has been sick) and his illness becomes so difficult for him that he does not recognize person(s) known to him, he will die.[13]
12. If over the course of a day it leaves him and then later (febrile convulsions) come over him for one day, "eating" of *aḫḫāzu*; "hand" of the great gods, he will die.[14]
13. If it afflicts him for one day (and) for one day it releases him, an oath by a god afflicts him.

14–15. If it afflicts him for one day (and) for one day it releases him (and) when his confusional states come over him, his limbs continually hurt him, he is feverish and trembles, sweat falls upon him and then he finds relief and continually asks for a great deal of water to drink, "hand" of Lamashtu (var. Marduk); he will get well.[15]

16. If he is sick for one day and then he is well for one day, the ghost of his father or mother afflicts him.
17. If it flows over him for one or two days and afflicts him on the third day, affliction by a ghost.
18. If he has been sick for one or two days and his abdomen continually afflicts him and his affliction continually falls upon him, he will die.

19–20. If he is sick for one, two, (and then) three days and subsequently the burning fever lets up from his body but after it has left, the burning fever does not let up from his head (and he continues this way) for three days (or) for six (var. four) days (altogether), he will die.[16]

21. If he has been sick for two days and his "right" temple hurts him and his "right" eye makes a "shadow," "hand" of Dapinu. If it goes away, he will get well.[17]

22. If he has been sick for two days and his "left" temple hurts him and his "left" eye makes a "shadow," "hand" of Dapinu. If it goes away, he will get well.[18]

23–24. If he has been sick for two days and his "right" and "left" temple continually hurt him and his "right" and "left" eye make a "shadow," he cursed his god and the god of his city. If it goes away, he will get well.[19]

25–27. If it falls upon him for two days and then afflicts him on the third day and when it afflicts him, he continually becomes rigid and after he continually becomes rigid, he has a trembling, his limbs continually hurt him, his hands and his feet are cold (and) afterwards fever rides (var. flows over) him everywhere at once and sweat falls upon him and then he finds relief, *ṣibit šadî* afflicts him.[20]

28. If it afflicts him for two days and flows over him on the third day, *ṣibit šadî* (var. he will die).[21]

29. If he has been sick for two or three days and his abdomen persists in continually afflicting him (and) he ⸢continually⸣ produces blood from his nose, he is sick with an illness of "gnawing."

30. If he has been sick for two or three days and *ḫūqu* persists in afflicting him, on the seventh day in [...], he will die.

31–32. If he has been sick for two or three days and the burning fever lets up from his body but after it has left [it does not let up] from [his head], hi[s] ⸢illness⸣ [...].

33. If on the second or third day, he is hot and then cold and his sweat [keeps falling upon him] as in *lubāṭu* [...].

34. If on the second or third day of the affliction, it continually falls upon him, he is feverish and ha[s] sweat [...].

35. [If on] the ⸢second⸣ or third day [...] and he has ⸢fever⸣? and sweat [...].

(unknown number of lines broken away)

36′. If he has been sick for two days and on the [third] day [...].

37′. If he has been sick for two days and he gets up on the third day [...].

38′. If he has been sick for three days and he gets up on the fourth day [...].

39′. If he has been sick for three days and on the fourth day blood flows from his nose [...].

40′. If he has been sick for three days and then gets up in the ⸢evening⸣, [letting up] of the illness.

41′. If he has been sick for three days and his flesh is normal, ⸢if⸣ he returns into his illness, he will die.

42′. If for three days he continually cries out: "My insides, my insides" and his insides are bloated, he will die.

43′. If he has been sick for four days and his hands are continually placed on his abdomen (and) his face is unevenly colored with yellow, he will die.[22]

44′–45′. If he has been sick for four or five days and subsequently sweat continually falls upon him, letting up of the illness. If he has been sick for four or five days, "hand" of *aḫḫāzu*.[23]

46′. If he has been sick for five days and on the sixth day, blood flows from his nose, his illness will let up; "burning" of *ṣētu*.

47′. If he has been sick for five days and his flesh is unevenly colored yellow (and) his eyes are full of blood, he will die.[24]

48′. If he has been sick for five or six days and he persists in not being able to stop (crying out): "Yow, Yow," he will die.[25]

49′. If he has been sick for five or ten days and *ḫūqu* persists in being continuous for him, he will die.[26]

50′–51′. If he has been sick with a mighty sickness for five or ten days and blood persists in continually flowing for five days from his nose but it stops, his illness will let up; he burns with *ṣētu*; he will get well; it is of no consequence.[27]

52′. If he has been sick with a mighty sickness for five or ten days and the mighty sickness persists in continually afflicting him (for) five (more days), he will get well; it is of no consequence.[28]

53′–54′. If he has been sick with a mighty sickness for five or ten days and the pupils of his eyes persist in (moving) downward (and) *ḫūqu* continually afflicts him for two days, he will die on the third day.[29]

55′. If he has been sick for five or ten days and afterwards red blood flows from his nose, he will get well.

56′. If he has been sick for five or ten days and he does not have a fever or sweat, "hand" of Sîn; he will die.[30]

57′. If he has been sick for five, ten, or fifteen days and *ḫūqu* continually afflicts him and releases him, if he continually has a difficult time of it, he will die.

58′. If ditto (he has been sick for five, ten, or fifteen days) and the pupils of his eyes (move) upward and *ḫūqu* continually afflicts him for three days, he will die.[31]

59′–60′. If he has been sick for five, ten, fifteen (and then) twenty days (and) the digits of his hands and his feet are immobilized (and) so stiff that he cannot open (them) or stand (on them), "hand" of Ishtar. If it leaves him (var. he comes through), he will get well.[32]

61′. If he is sick for six days and his flesh is normal, if he returns into his illness and has a turn for the worse (and) his abdomen continually afflicts him, he will die.[33]

62′. If in six days or ten days he has a return (of the illness and) if his epigastrium afflicts him, he will die.[34]

63′–64′. If he has been sick for six days and he does not get a respite on the seventh, they throw water on his face and if he does not open his eyes, he will die. If he opens and closes his eyes at the water which they throw over him (and) wails, he will get well.[35]

65′–66′. If he has been sick for six days and, on the seventh, chills continually fall upon him (and) after the chills, there is sweat from his head to his shins, his illness will let up and he will get well.[36]

67′–68′. [If he has been sick for six days and, on the seventh, he gets well (and) he recovers from the illness (but) when he has recovered, he gets sick (again and) there is] sweat from his head [to his shins and his abdomen afflicts him], he will die.

69′. [If] he has been ⸢sick⸣ [for six days] and, on the seventh, he gets well (and) he recovers from the illness (but) when he has recovered, he gets sick (again and) his epigastrium afflicts him, he will die.[35]

70′. If he has been ⸢sick⸣ [for six days] ⸢and⸣, on the seventh, he gets well [(and) he recovers from the illness (but) when he has recovered, he gets sick (again and)], he (looks) dark, if he excretes bile from his anus, he will die.

71′. If he has been ⸢sick⸣ for six days [and, on the seventh, he gets well (and) he recovers from the illness (but) when he has recovered, he gets sick (again and)] he forgets what he has [said], if ditto (he excretes bile) from his anus, he will die.

72′. If he has been sick for six days and on the seventh, [he gets well (and) he recovers from the illness (but) when he has recovered, he gets sick (again and)] his [eye]s are continually full of sediment, if blood flows from his nose, he will get well.[38]

73′–74′. If he is sick for six days and on the seventh he gets well, on the eighth day he is sick and on the ninth he gets well, on the tenth day he is sick and on the eleventh he gets well (and) his illness has turn for the worse, the *āšipu* shall not make a prognosis as to his recovery.[39]

75′. If on the fifteenth day, his illness falls upon him, (it means) diminution (caused by) the illness.

76′. If he has not yet been sick for a month and he turns black[40] and his throat (looks) skinned, (if) he worsens, he will die.

77′. If (he has not yet been sick for a month) and he turns black and his eyes "lie down," if he worsens, he will die.

78′–79′. If he has been sick for one or two months and his illness leaves him and then it continually afflicts him in his abdomen (and) he continually produces red blood from his nose, he is sick with an illness of "gnawing"; he will get well.

80′. If it falls upon him in the night for one or two months and he cries out, it is shuddering of "hand" of Ishtar; he can get up (afterwards).[41]

81′–82′. If daily, at the expected time, it comes over him and leaves him (and) when it comes over him, he becomes hot and his muscles continually hurt him (and) sweat comes out on him and then he finds relief, confusional state due to *ṣētu*.[42]

83′–84′. If he has been sick for a long time and red liquid flows from his anus, his illness will let up. He burns with *ṣētu*; he will get well. His days will be long; it is of no consequence.[43]

85′. If ditto (he has been sick for a long time) and his muscles are unevenly colored yellow (and) his eyes are full of blood, he will die.

86′. If ditto (he has been sick for a long time) and his flesh is unevenly colored yellow (and) his eyes are colored with red, he will not get well.[44]

87′. If he is in his seventies[45] and he wails for his household, he will die.

88′. If he is in his seventies and he wails for his household and his children, he will die.[46]

89′. If he is in his seventies and he makes the assignments for his tomb, he will die.[47]

90′. If he is in his seventies and he excretes the excrement of his body fat, he will die.[48]

91′. If ditto (he is in his seventies) and his eyes are as yellow as the "peg" on a leek, he will die.[49]

92′. If ditto (he is in his seventies and) his body is as yellow as ditto (the "peg" on a leek), his insides are bloated (and) yellow crosses the muscles of his abdomen, he will die.[50]

93′. If ditto (he is in his seventies and) his hands and feet are cold, (even if) his illness changes on him so that they beat their breasts over him, he will get well.[51]

94′. If ditto (he is in his seventies and) his hands and feet have become bent, even if his illness changes on him so that they ditto (beat their breasts) over him, he will get well.[52]

95′. If ditto (he is in his seventies) and his hands and feet become shrunken, even if his illness changes on him so that they ditto (beat their breasts) over him, he will get well.[53]

96′. If ditto (he is in his seventies and) blood flows from his nose, he will get well.[54]

97′. If ditto (he is in his seventies and) he is unable to eat or drink, [he has eaten] the provisions for his grave; [he will die].[55]

98′–99′. If ditto (he is in his seventies and) *ḫūqu* continually afflicts him (and) he asks for pomegranates, he will die. If ditto (he is in his seventies and) he asks for dates and eats them, he will get well.

100′–101′. If ditto (he is in his seventies) and he asks for a spoonful of bread and eats fat (with it), he will die. If ditto (he is in his seventies) and he asks for milk and eats the cream, he is at an acute stage of the illness; he will die.[56]

Notes

1. Correcting the reading of Heeßel 2000, 172.
2. Correcting the reading of Heeßel 2000, 177.
3. Correcting the reading of Heeßel 2000, 178.
4. Correcting the reading of Heeßel 2000, 178.
5. Correcting the reading of Heeßel 2000, 179
6. Correcting Heeßel 2000, 180.
7. See Scurlock and Andersen 2005, 3.142, 19.222.
8. See Scurlock and Andersen 2005, 20.103.
9. See Scurlock and Andersen 2005, 6.24, correcting Heeßel 2000, 172.
10. For the reading and interpretation, see Heeßel 2000, 187.
11. See Scurlock and Andersen 2005, 5.19, 5.52, 20.55
12. See Scurlock and Andersen 2005, 6.17.
13. See Scurlock and Andersen 2005, 3.112.

14. See Scurlock and Andersen 2005, 6.131.
15. See Scurlock and Andersen 2005, 3.20, 13.84, 19.225.
16. See Scurlock and Andersen 2005, 3.8.
17. See Scurlock and Andersen 2005, 9.90, 19.87.
18. See Scurlock and Andersen 2005, 9.90, 19.87.
19. See Scurlock and Andersen 2005, 19.349.
20. See Scurlock and Andersen 2005, 3.10, 19.218.
21. See Scurlock and Andersen 2005, 3.21, 19.220.
22. See Scurlock and Andersen 2005, 6.143.
23. See Scurlock and Andersen 2005, 3.31, 6.132. The entry appeared also in *KAR* 211 i 1′–3′. (Heeßel 2010, 171–77).
24. See Scurlock and Andersen 2005, 6.123, 9.36, 20.56.
25. See Scurlock and Andersen 2005, 20.58.
26. See Scurlock and Andersen 2005, 8.84.
27. See Scurlock and Andersen 2005, 3.138.
28. See Scurlock and Andersen 2005, 20.88.
29. See Scurlock and Andersen 2005, 13.119, 13.279, 20.35.
30. See Scurlock and Andersen 2005, 19.262.
31. See Scurlock and Andersen 2005, 13.120, 13.280.
32. See Scurlock and Andersen 2005, 11.6, 11.49, 13.40.
33. See Scurlock and Andersen 2005, 3.27, 3.32.
34. See Scurlock and Andersen 2005, 3.32.
35. See Scurlock and Andersen 2005, 13.286, 20.102.
36. See Scurlock and Andersen 2005, 3.29, 3.33, 3.40.
37. See Scurlock and Andersen 2005, 3.34.
38. See Scurlock and Andersen 2005, 9.86.
39. See Scurlock and Andersen 2005, 3.44.
40. Correcting Heeßel 2000, 79.
41. See Scurlock and Andersen 2005, 19.15.
42. See Scurlock and Andersen 2005, 3.123, 13.173.
43. See Scurlock and Andersen 2005, 3.139, 3.151.
44. See Scurlock and Andersen 2005, 6.124. This entry may appear in SpTU 1.145:5–6 (Cavigneaux 1988).
45. "70 = *ūmū arkūtu*" (*STT* 400:46).
46. See Scurlock and Andersen 2005, 2.40.
47. See Scurlock and Andersen 2005, 20.104.
48. See Scurlock and Andersen 2005, 6.25, 20.93, correcting Heeßel 2000, 180.
49. See Scurlock and Andersen 2005, 2.41, 6136.
50. See Scurlock and Andersen 2005, 6.145, 20.94.
51. See Scurlock and Andersen 2005, 2.42, 20.15. This entry also appears in DPS 11 obv. 45.
52. See Scurlock and Andersen 2005, 11.30, 20.97.
53. See Scurlock and Andersen 2005, 2.43, 11.31.
54. See Scurlock and Andersen 2005, 2.44, 20.47, 20.98.
55. See Scurlock and Andersen 2005, 2.44, 20.95.
56. See Scurlock and Andersen 2005, 20.96.

DPS 17

DPS 16:102′ (catchline) = DPS 17:1

1–3. DIŠ *ina* SAG GIG-*šú* IR *bu-úḫ-bu-ú*[*ḫ*]-*ta*[1] TUKU-*ma* IR *ši-i* TA *kìn-ṣi-šú* EN ZI.IN.GI-*šú* KI.TA GÌR^{II}-*šú* NU KUR-*ád* GIG.BI LÍL-*ti* U$_4$.2.KÁM U$_4$.3.KÁM LÍL-*ma* DIN

4–7. DIŠ *ina taš-rit* GIG-*šú* TA TAG-*šú* ⸢EN *ik*⸣-*lu-ú* 1-*is-su* KÚM 1-*is-su* ŠED$_7$ *a-ḫu ma-la a-ḫi* TUKU.MEŠ-*ši* EGIR KÚM *u* IR *ip-ṭú-ru* UB.NÍGIN.NA-*šú um-ma ub-la-nim-ma um-ma ma-la um-mi maḫ-ri-i ir-ši-ma ip-ta-ṭar* EGIR-*nu* ŠED$_7$ *u* IR *ir-ta-ši di-ḫu e-ri-bu wa-ṣú-u* UD.DA TAB.BA U$_4$.7.KÁM LÍL-*ma* DIN

8–9. DIŠ *ina taš-rit* GIG-*šú* ⸢SAG.KI^{II}⸣-*šú um-ma* ⸢*ub*⸣-*la-nim-ma* EGIR KÚM *u* IR *it-tab-la-ni* LÍL-*ti* UD.DA U$_4$.2.KÁM U$_4$.3.KÁM LÍL-*ma* DIN

10–13. DIŠ *ina taš-rit* GIG-*šú* KÚM ÚḪ NINDA KAŠ GURUN *ma-da* GU$_7$ *ina* ŠÀ-*šú* NU ḪUN DUB-*ka* U-*šú* LAL-*aṣ* IGI^{II}-*šú* BAD.BAD-*te ana* ⸢AKKIL⸣ *i-qal* NÍ-*šú ú-dam-ma-aq* ZI.IR.MEŠ *u* IGI.MEŠ-*šú i-ta-nar-ri-qu* MAŠKIM SÌG-*su* TA TAG-*ma* KI-*šú* [K]EŠDA *ina* NINDA *ik-ka-lu* GU$_7$ *ina* A NAG-*ú* NAG NA BI *ana* U$_4$.5.KÁM : *ana* U$_4$.7.KÁM DIN

---

14. DIŠ *ina* GIG-*šú i-leb-bu* GIG A.ZA.AD GIG DIN
15. DIŠ *ina* GIG-*šú* GÙ.GÙ-*si* GIG UB.NÍGIN.NA GIG DIN
16. DIŠ *ina* GIG-*šú* ZI.ZI-*bé* GIG UB.NÍGIN.NA GIG DIN
17. DIŠ *ina* GIG-*šú* DUG$_4$.DUG$_4$-*ub* GIDIM *ár-da-na-an* ÚŠ DIB-*su* DIN
18. DIŠ *ina* GIG-*šú* GÙ.DÉ-*šú-ma* NU *ip-pal ù* DIB-*it* KÚM NU TUKU DIN
19. DIŠ *ina* GIG-*šú* ʾ*ua* GÙ-*si ina ban-ti-šú ana* GÍR *ṣa-líl-ma* NU BAL-*it* ŠU ^{d}MAŠ.TAB.BA GAM
20. DIŠ *ina* GIG-*šú* ʾ*ua* GÙ-*si ina ban-ti-šú* NÁ-*ma* NU BAL-*it u* TU.ME-*šú* ŠU ^{d}MAŠ.TAB.BA
21. DIŠ *ina* GIG-*šú i-ṣa-ad* A ^{GIŠ}BAL ÍD NAG
22. DIŠ *ina* GIG-*šú i-ṭa-mu* A ^{GIŠ}BAL ÍD NAG
23. DIŠ *ina* GIG-*šú pa-rid* ZI-*bi u* DU$_{10}$.GAM-*is* GAM
24. DIŠ *ina* GIG-*šú* LUḪ.LUḪ-*uṭ* ZI-*bi u* TUŠ-*ab* NINDA GU$_7$ A NAG ŠUK *qu-bu-ri-šú il-qí* GAM

25–26. DIŠ *ina* GIG-*šú* IGI^{II}-*šú* NU ÍL-*ši ina* IGI^{II}-*šú* KIR$_4$-*šú* KA-*šú* GEŠTU^{II}-*šú u* GÌŠ-*šú* MÚD TÉŠ.BI È.ME-*a* ŠU ^{d}7-*bi* : U$_4$.31.KÁM ŠU ^{d}MAŠ.TAB.⸢BA⸣

27. DIŠ *ina* GIG-*šú* 1-*šú* 2-*šú ina* IGI ZÉ *i-ḫa-ḫu* EGIR-*nu* MÚD *i-ḫa-ḫu* GAM

28. DIŠ *ina* GIG-*šú* ḪÁŠ.MEŠ-*šú* GU_7.MEŠ-*šú* EGIR-*nu* MÚD *i-ḫa-ḫu* GAM
29. DIŠ *ina* GIG-*šú* *pa-su-šú ir-mu-ú u* ZI.IR.MEŠ GIG-*su* TAG_4-*šú*
30. DIŠ *ina* GIG-*šú* KA-*šú* DIB-*ma* $ŠU^{II}$-*šú u* $GÌR^{II}$-*šú ik-ta-ra-a ul mi-šit-ti* GIG-*su* DIB-*iq*
31. DIŠ *ina* GIG-*šú lu* ŠU-*su lu* GÌR-*šú a-ku-tam* DU-*ak ul mi-šit-ti* GIG-*su* DIB-*iq-šu-ma* DIN

---

32. DIŠ GIG-*su ina* EN.NUN.$MURUB_4$.BA ZI.ZI-*šú ana* DAM LÚ TE-*ḫi* ŠU ^{d}*Uraš*
33. DIŠ GIG-*šú* DU_8-*ma* $BURU_8$ NU KUD-*us* GAM
34. DIŠ GIG-*su* KU_4 *u* È U_4 LAL-*šú* LAL-*šú* ÍL IGI^{II}-*šú* DUGUD ŠU ^{d}UTU
35–36. DIŠ GIG-*su* KU_4 *u* È U_4 LAL-*šú* LAL-*šú* MIN KA-*šú* DIB.DIB-*ma* U_4.1.KÁM U_4.2.KÁM NU DUG_4.DUG_4 ŠU 20
37. DIŠ GIG-*su* KU_4 *u* È KI.MIN Á.ÚR.MEŠ-*šú* TÉŠ.BI GU_7.MEŠ-*šú* ŠU ^{d}UTU
38–39. DIŠ GIG-*su* KU_4 *u* È KI.MIN ÍL IGI^{II}-*šú* DUGUD ŠÀ.MEŠ-*šú* MÚ.ME-*ḫu* SA.MEŠ-*šú kìn-ṣa-a-šú* ZI.IN.GI.MEŠ-*šú* $MURUB_4$.MEŠ-*šú* 1-*niš* GU_7.MEŠ-*šú* ^{GIŠ}GIDRU ŠU ^{d}UTU GAR-*su*
40. DIŠ GIG-*su* KU_4 *u* È KI.MIN *par-diš* DUG_4.DUG_4-*ub* ŠU KI.SIKIL.LÍL.LÁ

41–42. DIŠ GIG-*ma ina* GIG-*šú* GIN_7 *šá* DIN-*šú* KI DAM-*šú* DUMU-*šú* DUMU.MUNUS-*šú* SIG_5-*iš i-ta-mu* NINDA NU GU_7 *di-ḫu* D[IN]
43. DIŠ GIG-*ma* GIG-*su* ŠUB-*šum-ma ina* KA-*šú* MÚD *pe-la-a i-sal-la-a ina* U_4-*mi-šú-ma* GAM : D[IN]
44–45. DIŠ GIG-*ma* GIG-*su i-re-eḫ-ḫi-šum-ma* MÚD.MEŠ MEŠ *ina* KI.NÁ-*šú* IGI.MEŠ *ana* U_4.3.KÁM GAM : NA BI *ina* GIG-*šú* [NU Z]I-*bi*
46. DIŠ GIG-*ma* GIG-*su* NÍG.GI TUKU-*ši u* SAG ŠÀ-*šú* DIB-*su* GAM
47. DIŠ GIG-*ma* DIN-*ma* GIG-*su* NÍG.GI TUKU-*šu* TU BI NU DIN
48–49. DIŠ GIG-*ma* DIN EGIR DIN ŠÀ-*šú* SI.SÁ-*šú* U_4.3.KÁM U_4.4.KÁM *ka-ma-su u la sa-ka-pu* GAR.GAR-*šú ana* U_4.5.KÁM : *ana* U_4.6.KÁM […]
50. DIŠ GIG-*ma* Ù.SÁ DIB-*su* GIG-*su* GÍD
51. DIŠ GIG-*ma* AD_6-*šú ma-gal* $ŠED_7$ GIG-*su* GÍD-*ma* GAM
52–53. DIŠ GIG-*ma* NINDA *šá* GU_7 *ina* ŠÀ-*šú la i-kal-la-ma bal-ṭa ina* KA-*šú* NU GIN-*an ina* KA-*šú* ŠUB-*a* GAM
54–55. DIŠ GIG $MURUB_4$ GIG-*ma* ZI-*bi u* DU_{10}.GAM GABA-*su* BAD.BAD-*te* KA-*šú ana* DUG_4.DUG_4 *da-an* IGI^{II}-*šú* GUB.GUB-*za* GAM
56. DIŠ GIG $MURUB_4$ *u* ŠÀ GIG-*ma* ZI-*bi u* DU_{10}.GAM *rit-ta-šú paṭ-rat* KA-*šú ana* DUG_4.DUG_4 *da-an* GAM

57–58. DIŠ GIG MURUB$_4$ *u* ŠÀ GIG GU$_7$ *u* NAG BAR-*us*^{2} KA-*šú ana a-wa-ti da-an* IGI.MEŠ-*šú* MÚ.MEŠ-*ḫu* ^{LÚ}TU.RA BI NU D[IN]

---

59. DIŠ TA GIG *šap-ti-šú uš-ta-nat-tak u ṣa-lil* ŠU ^{d}*ra-ʾi-i-bi*
60. DIŠ TA GIG *ip-ru-ma ana ḫu-ḫa-ti-šú* NIM *la* TE-*ḫi* GAM
61. DIŠ TA GIG U$_4$.1.KÁM U$_4$.2.KÁM ZI-*ma* DU.DU-*ak ana* GIG-*šú* GUR-*ma* GAM
62. DIŠ TA GIG *it-til-ma i-ra-am* : *ra-ḫi* DU$_8$-*ár* GIG
63. DIŠ TA *re-še-ti ana še-pe-ti* TA *še-pe-ti ana re-še-ti ina* NU ZU BAL.BAL GAM
64. DIŠ TA A *ina* E$_{11}$-*šú* ŠÀ.MEŠ-*šú nap-ḫu* A ^{GIŠ}BAL ÍD NAG
65–66. DIŠ *ina* ÍD A ^{GIŠ}BAL ÍD NAG *su-ḫar* GÌR^{II}-*šú* ŠED$_7$ *ruq-qí* GEŠTU-*šú* KÚM-*em* KIR$_4$-*šú šá* 15 ŠED$_7$ *šá* 150 KÚM-*em ana* U$_4$.31.KÁM GAM
67. DIŠ *ina* U$_4$-*mi šá* GIG ŠU.GÍD.GÍD KU$_4$ TU.BI
68. DIŠ *ina* U$_4$-*mi šá* GIG KA-*šú* NU BAD KU$_4$ TU.BI
69. DIŠ *ina* U$_4$-*mi šá* GIG KA-*šú* BAD.BAD-*te* KU$_4$ TU.BI
70. DIŠ *ina* U$_4$-*mi šá* GIG *kap-pi-šú u* KA-*šú* BAD.BAD-*te* TU.BI ŠUB-*šú*
71. DIŠ *ina* U$_4$-*mi šá* GIG *kap-pi-šú* ÍL.MEŠ-*ši* TU.BI DU$_8$-*ár*
72. DIŠ *ina* U$_4$-*mi šá* GIG *kap-pi-šú* KA-*šú* : EME-*šú* ÍL.MEŠ-*ši* GIG.BI DU$_8$-*ár*
73. DIŠ *ina* U$_4$-*mi šá* GIG GIG-*su* DUGUD-*su-ma* ZU-*šú* NU *ú-ád-da* GAM

---

74. DIŠ *kal* U$_4$-*mi* GIG-*ma ina* GI$_6$ *ba-liṭ* UD.DA GIG-*su*
75. DIŠ *kal* U$_4$-*mi* TI-*ma ina* GI$_6$ GIG UD.DA GIG-*su* U$_4$.27.KÁM ŠU ^{d}MAŠ
76. DIŠ *kal* U$_4$-*mi* ŠED$_7$-*ma kal* GI$_6$ *e-em* U$_4$.7.KÁM GIG-*ma* D[IN]
77. DIŠ *kal* U$_4$-*mi* ŠED$_7$-*ma ḫur-ba-šú* ŠUB.ŠUB-*su* IGI^{II}-*šú* GU.MEŠ SA$_5$.MEŠ DIRI (coll.) [...]

---

78. DIŠ *ina* GI$_6$ GIG-*ma ina šèr-ti ba-liṭ u ú-šam-šá* ŠU LÍL.LÁ.[EN.NA] (coll.)
79. DIŠ *ina* GI$_6$ GIG-*ma ina ka-ṣa-a-ti ba-liṭ* ŠU ^{d}*Uraš* MU D[AM LÚ]
80. DIŠ *ina* GI$_6$ GIG-*su* DIB.DIB-*su u* LUḪ.LUḪ NAM.ÉRIM DIB-*su* : DIB
81. DIŠ *ina* GI$_6$ GIG-*su* DIB.DIB-*su* MAŠKIM ⸢SÌG-*iṣ*⸣ (coll.) [...]
82. DIŠ *ina ši-mi-tan* GIG-*su* DIB.DIB-*su* M[AŠKI]M ⸢SÌG-*iṣ*⸣ (coll.) [...]
83–85. DIŠ *ina ši-mi-tan lu* LÚ.TI *lu* LÚ.ÚŠ *lu* ⸢*mu-da-šú lu*⸣ (coll.) *la m*[*u-da-šú*] *lu mam-ma lu mim-ma* IGI-*ma* LUḪ-*ut i-tu-ram-ma* GIN$_7$ *šá* Ì.ḪAB tu [...] KA-*šú* DIB-*ma šá i-ta-a-šú ṣal-lu šá-sa-a* NU ZU-*e* ŠU GIDIM$_7$: ŠU [...]
86. DIŠ *ina ši-mi-tan* ÍR.MEŠ ŠU [...]

87. DIŠ *ina ši-mi-tan* ÍR.MEŠ *u* GA NU NAG ŠU ⸢^{d}*Kù*⸣-[*bi*]
88. DIŠ *ina* IGI NÁ-*šú ú-na-ʾ-aš* ŠU ^{d}*Kù*-⸢*bi*⸣
89. DIŠ ÍR.MEŠ *u ú-na-ʾ-aš* ŠU ^{d}*Kù-bi*
90. DIŠ *ina šèr-ti* KÚM-*em ina le-lá-a-ti* ŠED$_7$ *u i-ra-ʾ-ub* ŠU ^{d}30
91–92. DIŠ *ina šèr-ti* KÚM-*em ina le-lá-a-ti* ŠED$_7$ *ina* ⸢GI$_6$⸣ *ma-šil ù ʾ-a*(coll.) DUG$_4$.GA ŠEŠ-*šú ma-a-a-ta-nu* KI-*šú* KEŠDA
93. DIŠ *ina šèr-ti* KÚM-*em ina le-lá-a-ti* ŠED$_7$ ŠU ^{d}30
94. DIŠ *ina šèr-ti* KÚM-*ma* ŠU^{II}-*šú u* GÌR^{II}-*šú i-ra-ʾ-ú-ba* ŠU ^{d}30
95–99. DIŠ *ina šèr-ti* GIG-*ma ina kin-zi-gi* GIG-*su* TA[K$_4$]-*šú-ma za-mar-ra-nu-um-ma* GUR-*šú niš-rat* GIG-*šú ina* U$_4$.2.KÁM EN UD.SA$_9$.ÀM *ina* U$_4$.3.KÁM EN *kin-zi-gi ina* U$_4$.4.KÁM EN *ši-mi-tan ina* U$_4$.5.KÁM EN *a-dan-ni-šú ina* U$_4$.6.KÁM EN BAR EN.NUN *ina* U$_4$.7.KÁM EN EN.NUN.MURUB$_4$.BA *ina* U$_4$.8.KÁM [E]N *šat ur-ri ina* U$_4$.9.K[ÁM] EN *na-mir ina* U$_4$.10.KÁM ZI-*ma* DIN
100–105. DIŠ TA *šèr-ti* EN *le-lá-a-ti di-ḫu ina* SU-*šú ú-šar-r*[*i*]-*ma* LÍL-*ti* ŠÀ *ir-ta-ši ir-ra-šú i-te-šír ina* KA-*šú ig-di-šá-a ina* DÚR-*šú uš-te-ši-ra* TAG-*ti* UD.DA *šá ina mi-ni-a-ti-šú la rak-sat* GIG.BI LÍL-*ti* U$_4$.1.KÁM DIŠ *uq-ta-ta$_5$ ina šèr-ti* GIG-*ma* ŠU^{II}-*šú i-nap-pa-aṣ* GÌR^{II}-*šú* KÚM-*ma* GIG-*su* KI.TA E$_{11}$-*šú* DU-*ak*

Translation

1–3. If at the beginning of his illness,[3] he has sweat (and) *bubuʾtu*-blisters and that sweat does not reach from his shins to his ankles and the soles of his feet, if that illness has reached the critical stage by the second or third day, he will get well.[4]

4–7. If at the beginning of his illness from the time it "touches" him till it stops, he continually has now fever, now chills in equal proportions (and) after the fever and sweat have left, his limbs produce heat so that he has a fever to the same degree as the previous fever and it leaves (and) afterwards he has chills and sweat, *diʾu*-fever coming in and going out (or) he burns with *ṣētu*-fever; if he is has reached the critical stage by the seventh day, he will get well.[5]

8–9. If at the beginning of his illness his temples produce heat so that afterwards it has brought fever and sweat, if he has reached the critical stage of *šētu*-fever by the second or third day, he will get well.[6]

10–13. If at the beginning of his illness he burns with fever, he eats a lot of bread, beer and fruit (but) it does not rest easy in his stomach (and) he pours it out, he can stretch out his finger, he continually opens his eyes, at a mournful cry, he is silent, he treats himself well, (his stomach) is continually upset and his face continually turns yellow, a *rābiṣu* has struck him (and) after it touched him, it was ⸢bound⸣ with him (or) he ate it with the bread he ate (or) drank it with the water he drank; (once he has been sick) for five (var. seven days), he will get well.[7]

---

14. If during his illness he groans (and) he is sick with an illness (with) ice cold, he will get well.[8]
15. If during his illness, he continually cries out, he is ill with an illness of the limbs (only); he will get well.
16. If during his illness, he always gets up (afterwards), he is ill with an illness of the limbs (only); he will get well.
17. If during his illness, he continually talks, a ghost, the "double" of a dead person afflicts him; he will get well.[9]
18. If during his illness, you shout at him and he does not answer but he does not have affliction by fever, he will get well.
19. If during his illness he cries out: "Ua" (and) he sleeps briefly on his thorax and will not turn over, "hand" of the twin gods; he will die.[10]
20. If during his illness he cries out: "Ua" (and) he sleeps on his thorax and will not turn over and it makes him ill, "hand" of the twin gods.
21. If during his illness he (feels like he) is spinning, he drank water from a hoisting device of the river.[11]
22. If during his illness he twists, he drank water from a hoisting device of the river.[12]
23. If during his illness he shudders (and) he gets up and (has to) squat down, he will die.[13]
24. If during his illness he continually jerks, he gets up and (has to) sit down (and) he eats bread (and) drinks water, he has eaten provisions for his grave; he will die.[14]

25–26. If during his illness, he does not raise his eyes (and) blood comes out of his eyes, his nose, his mouth, his ears, and his penis all at the same time, "hand" of the Sibitti.[15] (If he has been sick for) thirty-one days (when this happens), "hand" of the twin gods.[16]

27. If once or twice during (the course of) his illness, he first vomits bile and afterwards vomits blood, he will die.[17]
28. If during (the course of) his illness, his inguinal regions continually hurt him (and) afterwards he vomits blood, he will die.

29. If during (the course of) his illness, his insides are (alternatively) relaxed and upset, his illness is leaving him.[18]
30. If during (the course of) his illness, his mouth is seized and his hands and his feet become shrunken, it is not a stroke; his illness will pass.
31. If during (the course of) his illness, either his hand or his foot becomes weak, it is not a stroke; his illness will pass and he will get well.[19]

---

32. If his illness continually rises on him in the middle watch of the night, he approached a(nother) man's wife; "hand" of Uraš.
33. If his illness lets up but he cannot stop vomiting, he will die.[20]
34. If his illness enters and leaves (and) when his confusional state comes over him, lifting his eyes is difficult, "hand" of Shamash.[21]
35–36. If his illness enters and leaves (and) when his confusional state comes over him, ditto (lifting his eyes is difficult and) is mouth is continually "seized" so that he cannot talk for one or two days, "hand" of Shamash.[22]
37. If his illness enters and leaves ditto (and when his confusional state comes over him), his limbs all hurt him at once, "hand" of Shamash.[23]
38–39. If his illness enters and leaves ditto (and when his confusional state comes over him), lifting his eyes is difficult, his insides are continually bloated (and) his muscles, his shins, his ankles (and) his hips all hurt him at once, the sceptre, "hand" of Shamash, has been laid upon him.
40. If his illness enters and leaves ditto (and when his confusional state comes over him), he continually talks in a frightful manner, "hand" of *ardat lilî*.[24]

41–42. If he is sick and, during his sickness, he speaks in a friendly way with his wife, son (and) daughter just as if he were feeling well (but) he does not eat bread, *di'u*; he will get ⌈well⌉.[25]
43. If he is sick and his illness falls on him so that red blood sprays from his mouth, he will die on that same day (var. he will get ⌈well⌉).
44–45. If he is sick and his illness flows over him so that a great deal of blood is found in his bed, (once he has been sick) for three days, he will die (variant: he will [not] ⌈get up⌉ from his illness).
46. If he is sick and he has a return of his illness and his epigastrium afflicts him, he will die.
47. If he is sick and then well and then he has a return of the illness, that patient will not get well.
48–49. If he is sick and then well (and) after he gets well his bowels are loose for three or four days and squatting but not lying down to rest are continu-

ally established for him, (once he has been sick) for five days (var. six days)[…].[26]

50. If he is sick and a stupor afflicts him, his illness will be prolonged.

51. If he is sick and his body is very cold, if his illness is prolonged, he will die.[27]

52–53. If he is sick and he cannot retain the food which he eats in his stomach and he cannot (even) put anything raw into his mouth (but) he produces it from his mouth, he will die.[28]

54–55. If he is sick with an illness of the hips and he gets up and (has to) squat down, his chest is not congested (but) his mouth is too strong for the words (and) his eyes continually stand (still), he will die.[29]

56. If he is sick with an illness of the hips and abdomen and he gets up and (has to) squat down, his hand will open (but) his mouth is too strong for the words, he will die.[30]

57–58. If he is sick with an illness of the hips and abdomen, he stops eating and drinking, his mouth is too strong for the words (and) his face is continually swollen, that patient will not ⸢get well⸣.

---

59. If after falling ill, he keeps moistening his lips while he sleeps, "hand" of "the trembler."

60. If after falling ill, he vomits and flies will not come near his vomitus, he will die.[31]

61. If after falling ill, he gets up for one or two days and walks about, if he has a return of his illness, he will die.

62. If after falling ill, he lies down and (in his dream) he makes love (var. is spattered with semen), letting up of the illness.

63. If he keeps turning round from the head end to the foot end of the bed (and) from the foot end to the head end without realizing it, he will die.[32]

64. If when he comes up from the water, his insides are bloated, he drank water from a hoisting device of the river.[33]

65–66. If, in the river, he drank water from a hoisting device of the river, the soles of his feet are cold, his ear canal is hot, his "right" nostril is cold (and) the "left" one is hot, (once he has been sick) for thirty-one days, he will die.

67. If on the day he becomes ill[34] he continually pulls himself taut(?), entrance of his illness.

68. If on the day he becomes ill he does not open his mouth, entrance of his illness.

69. If on the day he becomes ill he continually opens his mouth, entrance of his illness.[35]
70. If on the day he becomes ill he continually opens his (eye)lids and mouth, his illness is falling on him.
71. If on the day he becomes ill he continually lifts his (eye)lids, his illness will let up.
72. If on the day he becomes ill he continually lifts his (eye)lids (and) his mouth (var. his tongue), his illness will let up.
73. If on the day he becomes ill, his illness becomes so difficult for him that he does not recognize person(s) known to him, he will die.[36]

---

74. If he is sick all day and well in the night, *ṣētu* has made him ill.
75. If he is well all day and sick in the night, *ṣētu* has made him ill. (If he has been sick for) twenty-seven days, "hand" of Ninurta.
76. If he is cold all day and hot all night, if he has been sick (for) seven days, he will get ⌜well⌝.[37]
77. If he is cold all day and chills continually fall upon him (and) his eyes are full of red threads [...].[38]

---

78. If (she) is sick in the night and well in the morning and it keeps (her) up all night, "hand" of the *lilû*-demon.
79. If he is sick in the night and well in the early morning, "hand" of Uraš on account of [a(nother) man's] ⌜wife⌝.
80. If his illness continually afflicts him in the night and he continually jerks, a curse afflicts him (var. affliction by [...]).
81. If his illness continually afflicts him in the night, he was struck by a *rābiṣu* [...].[39]
82. If his illness continually afflicts him in the evening, he was struck by a ⌜*rābiṣu*⌝; [...].[40]
83–85. If in the evening, he sees either a living person or a dead person or someone known to him or someone not ⌜known to him⌝ or anybody or anything and jerks; he turns around but, like one who has [been hexed with(?)] rancid oil, his mouth is seized so that he is unable to cry out to one who sleeps next to him, "hand" of ghost or "hand" of [...].[41]
86. If in the evening he continually wails, "hand" of [...].
87. If in the evening he continually wails and will not drink milk, "hand" of ⌜Kubu⌝.[42]
88. If before he goes to bed he shakes, "hand" of Kubu.[43]
89. If he continually wails and shakes, "hand" of Kubu.[44]

90. If in the morning he is hot (and) in the evening he is cold and trembles, "hand" of Sîn.[45]

91–92. If in the morning he is hot, in the evening he is cold (and) in middle of the night he says, "Ua," his dying brother is bound with him.[46]

93. If in the morning he is hot (and) in the evening he is cold, "hand" of Sîn.[47]

94. If in the morning he is hot and his hands and his feet tremble, "hand" of Sîn.[48]

95–99. If he is sick in the morning and in the late afternoon his illness leaves him and then suddenly it returns on him (and he has) a reduced form of his illness the second day until noon, the third day until late afternoon, the fourth day until evening, the fifth day until its normal term,[49] the sixth day until the middle of the (first) watch (of the night), the seventh day until the middle watch (of the night), the eighth day until the dawn watch (and) the ninth day until it is light, if he gets up on the tenth day, he will get well.[50]

100–105. If from morning till evening, *diʾu* starts in his body so that he gets an acute attack of the stomach (and when) his bowels move, he belches from his mouth and emits (wind) from his anus, "touch" of *ṣētu* which is not (yet) bound to his limbs; his sickness is an acute attack of one day. If it (seems to) have finished, (but) on the (next) morning, he is so sick that his hands thrash around (and) his feet are hot, his illness is going down and up on him.[51]

Notes

1. Collated in *CAD* B, 300; the collation is confirmed by the quotation of this line by incipit in Kinnier Wilson 1956, 133:17 (Heeßel 2000, 14–17) and by the catchline of SpTU 2.44 rev. 23.

2. Both parallels have BAR rather than the expected TAR for *parāsu*; see Heeßel 2000, 214.

3. For a discussion of Akkadian terms for illness, see Stol 2009b, 30–46. See Scurlock and Andersen 2005, 10.79.

4. For *salāʾu* = LÍL "to enter a critical stage of an illness" see *CAD* S, 96–97. My translation assumes that the noun *salītu* when used with the verb from which it comes takes on the specific coloring of the verb. Correct Scurlock and Andersen 2005, 10.79.

5. See and correct Scurlock and Andersen 2005, 3.163, 20.90.

6. See and correct Scurlock and Andersen 2005, 3.143, 20.89.

7. See Scurlock and Andersen 2005, 6.127, 19.233.

8. See Scurlock and Andersen 2005, 3.41.

9. See Scurlock and Andersen 2005, 16.45, 19.29.

10. See Scurlock and Andersen 2005, 20.68.

11. See Scurlock and Andersen 2005, 15.29.

12. See Scurlock and Andersen 2005, 15.30.
13. See Scurlock and Andersen 2005, 8.30.
14. See Scurlock and Andersen 2005, 8.30.
15. See Scurlock and Andersen 2005, 3.236, 9.26, 19.234.
16. See Scurlock and Andersen 2005, 3.236, 9.26, 19.236.
17. See Scurlock and Andersen 2005, 6.5, 20.53.
18. See Scurlock and Andersen 2005, 6.48.
19. See Scurlock and Andersen 2005, 20.75.
20. See Scurlock and Andersen 2005, 6.62, 20.79.
21. See Scurlock and Andersen 2005, 13.189.
22. See Scurlock and Andersen 2005, 13.190.
23. See Scurlock and Andersen 2005, 13.191.
24. See Scurlock and Andersen 2005, 13.265.
25. See Scurlock and Andersen 2005, 3.22, 3.162, 6.50. This entry also appears in Labat 1956, 121 obv. 15.
26. See Scurlock and Andersen 2005, 3.113.
27. See Scurlock and Andersen 2005, 3.38.
28. See Scurlock and Andersen 2005, 6.61.
29. See Scurlock and Andersen 2005, 13.90, 13.217.
30. See Scurlock and Andersen 2005, 13.218, 20.6.
31. See Scurlock and Andersen 2005, 6.12.
32. See Scurlock and Andersen 2005, 20.9.
33. See Scurlock and Andersen 2005, 15.32.
34. One of this or the following entries was referenced in Labat 1956, 121 obv. 18.
35. This entry appears in Labat 1956, 121 obv. 19.
36. See Scurlock and Andersen 2005, 20.10.
37. See Scurlock and Andersen 2005, 20.91.
38. See Scurlock and Andersen 2005, 9.17.
39. This entry appears in Ni. 470:12 (Kraus 1987, 197).
40. This entry appears in Wilhelm 1994, 21 obv. 4.
41. See Scurlock and Andersen 2005, 16.19, 19.32.
42. See Scurlock and Andersen 2005, 19.340.
43. See Scurlock and Andersen 2005, 19.340.
44. See Scurlock and Andersen 2005, 19.340.
45. See Scurlock and Andersen 2005, 19.261. The entry appears also in *KAR* 211 i 12' (Heeßel 2010, 171–77).
46. See Scurlock and Andersen 2005, 2.12, 19.261.
47. See Scurlock and Andersen 2005, 19.261.
48. See Scurlock and Andersen 2005, 3.23, 19.261.
49. Stol 1983–84, 57–58 suggests that this refers to the patient and means something like "until the normal time (for the patient to go to bed)"; see also Heeßel 2000, 216.
50. See Scurlock and Andersen 2005, 20.92. This entry appears in Labat 1956, 121 obv. 10–12.
51. See Scurlock and Andersen 2005, 3.164.

C. FEVER/NO FEVER: DPS 18–23

DPS 18

DPS 17:106 (catchline) = DPS 18:1

1. DIŠ GIG SU-*šú* KÚM-*im* ŠED$_7$ *u* DIB-*su* KÚR.KÚR-*ir* ŠU ^{d}30
2. [DIŠ SU-*š*]*ú* ⸢KÚM⸣-*im* ⸢ŠED$_7$⸣ *u* IR NU TUKU ŠU [GI]DIM$_7$? DUMU *šip-ri šá* DINGIR-*šú*
3–4. [DIŠ SU-*šú* KÚM-*i*]*m u* ŠED$_7$ KIN-*šú ma-a-ád* LÁ-[*š*]*ú qer-bet* U$_4$ *u* GI$_6$ *la ina-aḫ* GÙ-*šú* GIN$_7$ GÙ ÙZ [ŠU GIDIM] *a-ḫi-i ina ḫar-ba-ti* DIB-*su*
5–6. [DIŠ SU-*šú* KÚ]M ÚḪ TUKU-*ma* ŠU^{II}-*šú u* GÌR^{II}-*šú*-[*ma*] *mar-ṣa it-te-nin-ṣi-la-šú* [...]-*a-šú* GU$_7$.MEŠ-*šú* GÌR^{II}-*šú* x.[M]EŠ ŠU 15 : ŠU ^{d}*Kù-bi*
7. [DIŠ SU-*šú* K]ÚM NU TUKU IR *ma-at-tú* [TU]KU.TUKU-*ši* ŠU ^{d}DIM$_{11}$.ME
8–9. [DIŠ SU-*šú* K]ÚM NU TUKU GU$_7$ NAG *muṭ-ṭu* [*šá i*]-*lam-mu*[1] UGU-*šú* GIG *ik-ki ku-ri iq-ta-nab-bi* [*u i-ta*]-*na-aš-šá-aš* NA BI GIG [*r*]*a-a-me* GIG *u ana* NÍTA *u* MUNUS 1-*ma*
10–11. [DIŠ SU-*šú* KÚM] ⸢NU⸣ TUKU GU$_7$ *u* NAG SA SAG.DU-*šú* x [x *ša*]*l-mu-ma* ŠÀ-*bi* SAG.DU DUG$_4$ *up-ta-sa-am* NA B[I] *ḫi-pí* [...] aš ḫul *u* šur ra [...] GIG *uš-te-di*
12–14. [DIŠ SU-*šú* K]ÚM NU TUKU SA SAG.[DU-*šú* ... -*š*]*ú šal-mu-ma* IGI.MEŠ-*šú i-sim-mu* [...] as sa bat [... KIR$_4$-*šú ú*]-⸢*gan*⸣-*na-aṣ* SAG.KI-*su ú-sa-ʾ-ar* [...] ^{LÚ}A.ZU ^{LÚ}MAŠ.‹MAŠ› ^{LÚ}ḪAL ^{LÚ}ENSI *šu-ud-di*
15–16. [DIŠ ... KÚM]-*em* IGI^{II}-*šú it-te-ni-ip-rik-ka-a* [... ŠU] ^{d}MAŠ MU DAM LÚ
17–18. [DIŠ ...]^{II}-*šú* ŠED$_7$-*ma* IGI^{II}-*šú it-te-né-ep-rik-ka-a* [... GIDIM *mu-ša*]*m-šu-u* DIB-*su*
19. [...]-*uš* ŠU ^{d}15 *ana* TAG TE
20. [DIŠ ... Z]É BABBAR[2] SIG$_7$-*tú ba-lil* ŠU ^{d}15
21. [DIŠ TA SAG.DU-*šú* EN GÌR^{II}-*šú* U$_4$.BU.BU.UL BABBAR DIRI *u* SU-*šú* GI$_6$] ⸢KI⸣ MUNUS *ina* KI.NÁ *ka-šid* ŠU 20 DIN
22. [DIŠ TA SAG.DU-*šú* EN GÌR^{II}-*šú* U$_4$.BU.BU.UL SA$_5$ DIRI *u* SU-*šú*] ⸢GI$_6$⸣ KI MUNUS *ina* KI.NÁ *ka-šid* ŠU 30 DIN
23. [DIŠ TA SAG.DU-*šú* EN GÌR^{II}-*šú* KI.MIN *u* SU-*šú*] SIG$_7$ KI MUNUS *ina* KI.NÁ *ka-šid* ŠU ^{d}15 DIN

24. [DIŠ SU-*šu* S]IG$_7$ IGI^{II}-*šú* SIG$_7$.MEŠ *šiḫ-ḫat* UZU TUKU.MEŠ *a-mur-ri-qa-nu*

25–26. [DIŠ …]-⸢*su*⸣ IGI^{II}-*šú* MÚD DIRI.MEŠ *mim-ma šá* GU$_7$ *ina* ŠÀ-*šú la i-kam-ma* […]x GIG BI *ana* U$_4$.3.KÁM NU IGI

---

27. [DIŠ …] ŠED$_7$-*a* ÚŠ KU$_4$-*ub-šú*

28. [DIŠ … ŠE]D$_7$-*a* GIG-*su* MAN-*ni*

29. [DIŠ … Š]U ^{d}15 MU *mé-reš-ti*

30. [DIŠ …] : ŠU ^{d}15 *ana* NÍTA *u* MUNUS 1-*ma*

31. [DIŠ … ^{GIŠ}GID]RU *šá* ^{d}UTU GAR-*su*

32′–36′. (fragmentary)

37′. [DIŠ …]x-⸢*ub*⸣ ŠU LÍL.LÁ.EN.NA : ŠU DINGIR-*šú* GAM

38′. [DIŠ …]x-⸢*šu* U$_4$.31.KÁM⸣ ŠU ^{d}*Iš-ḫa-ra* DU$_6$.DU$_6$-*ma* : NU DIN : DIN

39′. [DIŠ… SAG.D]U-*su* DIB.DIB-*su* GIG-*su* GIG UD.DA

40′–41′. […] 3 U$_4$-*me* DIŠ NA$_4$ *muš-tin-ni* GAR-*šú* DIŠ NA BI KAŠ NAG [NA$_4$.BI *i-š*]*aḫ-ḫu-uḫ* NA BI KAŠ NU NAG-*ma* A UL$_4$.GAL NAG *ana* NAM-*šú* GAR-*šú*

42′. [DIŠ … S]IG$_7$ DIRI IGI^{II}-*šú* MÚD DIRI.MEŠ NINDA *šá* GU$_7$ *ina* ŠÀ-*šú* NU *ina-aḫ is-ḫur-ma* DUB-*ka* GAM

43′. [DIŠ …]-*tú sa*-⸢*li-iḫ*⸣ ŠU ^{d}NIN.GEŠTIN.AN.NA

44′. [DIŠ …]-*tú s*[*a-li-iḫ liq* K]A-*šú šá-bul* ŠU ^{d}NIN.GEŠTIN.AN.NA

45′. [DIŠ *i-mim u* ŠED$_7$ …]-⸢*ma*⸣ DIN

TRANSLATION

1. If the patient's body gets hot (and then) cold (and) his affliction keeps changing (for the worse), "hand" of Sîn.[3]

2. [If] ⸢his⸣ [body] gets hot (and then) cold but he does not have sweat, "hand" of ⸢ghost⸣? messenger of his god.

3–4. [If his body] gets ⸢hot⸣ and then cold, his attack(s) are numerous, his confusional state(s) are close together, he gets no rest day or night (and) his cry is like the cry of a goat, ["hand" of] a strange [ghost] has seized him in the wasteland.[4]

5–6. [If his body] burns with ⸢fever⸣, his hands and his feet are sore and sluggish, his [legs?] continually hurt him (and) his feet […], "hand" of Ishtar (var. "hand" of Kubu).[5]

7. [If his body] does not have ⸢fever⸣ (but) he continually has a lot of sweat, "hand" of Lamashtu.

8–9. [If his body] does not have ⸢fever⸣, his desire for food and drink is diminished, [whatever he] eats[6] does not taste good to him, he is short tempered, he talks continually, [and (his stomach)] is ⸢continually⸣ upset, he is sick with ⸢love⸣ sickness and it is the same for a man and a woman.

10–11. [If his body] does not have [fever], he can eat and drink, (and) the blood vessels of his head (and) [his abdomen?] are healthy but he says: "My heart, my head" (and) he veils himself, ⸢that⸣ person [...] ... marks the illness.

12–14. [If his body] does not have ⸢fever⸣, the blood vessels of his ⸢head⸣ (and) ⸢his⸣ [...] are healthy but his face flushes, [...], he wrinkles [his nose] (and) wipes his forehead [...] inform the *asû*, the *āšipu*, the diviner (and) the dream interpreter.

15–16. [If] ... he is ⸢feverish⸣ (and) his eyes are continually crossed ... ["hand"] of Ninurta on account of a man's wife.

17–18. [If] his [...] are cold and his eyes are continually crossed [... a ghost who wanders about] at ⸢night⸣ afflicts him.[7]

19. [...], "hand" of Ishtar on account of touching the cheek.

20. [If ...] white ⸢bile⸣ mixed with yellow, "hand" of Ishtar.[8]

21. [If from his head to his feet, he is full of white *bubu᾽tu* and his skin/body is dark], he was "gotten" in bed with a woman, "hand" of Shamash; he will get well.[9]

22. [If from his head to his feet, he is full of red *bubu᾽tu* and his skin/body] is dark, he was "gotten" in bed with a woman, "hand" of Sîn; he will get well.[10]

23. [If from his head to his feet, ditto (he is full of red *bubu᾽tu*) and his skin/body] is yellow, he was "gotten" in bed with a woman, "hand" of Ishtar; he will get well.[11]

24. [If a person's body] is ⸢yellow⸣, his eyes are yellow (and) he has wasting of the flesh, *amurriqānu*.[12]

25–26. [If] his [...], his eyes are full of blood (and) whatever he eats he does not retain in his stomach [...] he will not experience that illness for three days.

---

27. [If ...] are cold, death enters him.

28. [If ... are] ⸢cold⸣, his illness will change (for the worse).

29. [If ...] ⸢"hand"⸣ of Ishtar on account of (an unfulfilled) request.

30. [If ...] (var. "hand" of Ishtar); it is the same for a man and a woman.

31. [If ...] the ⸢scepter⸣ of Shamash has been laid on him.

32–36′. *(fragmentary)*

37′. [If ...], "hand" of *lilû* (var. "hand" of his god); he will die.

38′. [If] ... thirty one days, "hand" of Ishhara. If he is continually overwhelmed, he will not get well (var. he will get well).[13]

39′. [If ... (and)] his ⸢head⸣ continually afflicts him, his illness is an illness of *ṣētu*.

40′–41′. [If ... he has been sick for] three days. If he has a stone in the urethra, if that person drinks beer, [that stone] will ⸢fall⸣ out. If that person does not drink beer but drinks a lot of water, he will certainly die.[14]

42′. [If ...] is full of ⸢yellow⸣ spots, his eyes are full of blood, the bread which he eats does not rest easy in his stomach but it turns about and pours out, he will die.[15]

43′. [If ...] shakes, "hand" of Ningeštinanna.

44′. [If ...] ⸢shakes⸣ (and) his ⸢palate⸣ is dried up, "hand" of Ningeštinanna.

45′. [If he gets hot and then cold ...], (if) [...], he will get well

NOTES

1. Differently, Heeßel 2000, 218.
2. Correcting Heeßel 2000, 219.
3. This entry appears also in *STT* 89:205 and Wilhelm 1994, 40 obv. 6′.
4. A treatment for this condition appears in BAM 323:65-68//BAM 471 ii 26′–29′//BAM 385 i 23′–26′ (see Scurlock 2006, no. 225).
5. See Scurlock and Andersen 2005, 19.250, 19.341.
6. Differently, Heeßel 2000, 220.
7. See Scurlock and Andersen 2005, 19.279.
8. The entry appears also in VAT 11122 obv. 7 (Heeßel 2010 181–84).
9. This entry appears also in DPS 3:103.
10. The entry appears also in DPS 3:101.
11. The entry appears also in DPS 3:102.
12. See Scurlock and Andersen 2005, 6.121. This entry also appears in DPS 33:92 (q.v.).
13. See Scurlock and Andersen 2005, 20.72.
14. Lit. "(going) to his fate is established for him." See Scurlock and Andersen 2005, 5.34.
15. See Scurlock and Andersen 2005, 6.125, 20.57.

DPS 19–20

DPS 18:45′ (catchline) = DPS 19/20:1

1. [DIŠ *i-mim u* ŠED$_7$ ...]-⸢*ma*⸣ DIN

2′–4′. (fragmentary)

5′. [DIŠ ... Š]À.[M]EŠ-*šú eb-ṭú-ma* SIG[$_7$] ⸢ŠUB-*ú*⸣ [Š]U ^{d}[...]

6′. [DIŠ ...] TUKU.MEŠ-*ši* ŠU ^{d}[...]

7′. [DIŠ ...] *ana* NAG APIN.MEŠ ŠU ^{d}[...]

8′. [DIŠ ...] ⸢KÚM⸣.MEŠ ŠU ^{d}DIM[$_{11}$.ME]

9′. [DIŠ KÚM-*im u* ŠED$_{7}$^{1} A *a*]*na* ⸢TU$_{5}$ UL$_{4}$.GAL APIN⸣.MEŠ [Š]U ^{d}DIM$_{11}$.ME : ŠU ^{d}30 x [...]

10′. [DIŠ ...*i*]-*bal-luṭ* ŠU ^{d}DI[M$_{11}$.ME]

11′. [DIŠ ... IR] NU TUKU ŠU ^{d}30 DIN KI.MIN *ana* GAL *u* TU[R] 1-[-*ma*]

12′. [DIŠ ... G]IG-*su* KÚR.KÚR-*ir* U$_{4}$.5.KÁM ŠU ^{d}30 [...]

13′. [DIŠ ...] DIB-*su* KÚR.KÚR-*ir* : UŠ$_{4}$-*šú* KÚR.KÚR-*ir* ŠU ^{d}30 [...]

14′. [DIŠ ...] *u da-bab-šú* KÚR.KÚR-*ir* U$_{4}$.3.KÁM GIG ⸢ŠU⸣ ^{d}[...]

15′. [DIŠ ...] *u* IGI^{II}-*šú ur-ru-pa* U$_{4}$.12.KÁM ŠU ^{d}NIN.GÍR.[SU]

16′. [DIŠ ...] *u* IGI.MEŠ-*šú ur-ru-pú ina* U$_{4}$.1.KÁM 2-*šú* LAL-*šú* ŠU ^{d}[...]

17′. [... *m*]*a* ZI-*bi u* TÚŠ-*ab* U$_{4}$.59.KÁM GIG ŠU ^{d}*Dil-bat* : ITI U$_{4}$.15.KÁM GIG [...]

18′. [DIŠ ... *ri-b*]*it-su šá* 15 GU$_{7}$-*šú* ŠU DINGIR-*šú* [...]

19′. [DIŠ ... *ri*]-*bit-su šá* 150 GU$_{7}$-*šú* ŠU ^{d}15-[*šú* ...]

20′. [DIŠ KÚM-*ma*] AD.BI ÚḪ [KUD^{2}...]

21′. [DIŠ ...] AL.ZU.BI NAM.BA.ZU.ZU[...]

22′. [DIŠ ...] UŠ$_{4}$.BI NAM.BA.ḪA.ZA [...]

23′. [DIŠ ...] AD$_{6}$-*šú ú-lap-pat* [...]

24′. [DIŠ ...] GÌR-*šú šá* 15 *ú*-[*l*]*ap-pat* [...]

25′. [DIŠ ...] *u ú-nap-paq ina* SAG GI$_{6}$ TAG [...]

26′. [DIŠ ...] *su-ḫar* GÌR^{II}-*šú ka-ṣi* ŠU DUMU.MUNUS ^{d}*A*-[*nim*]

27′. [DIŠ ... G]U.DU.MEŠ-*šú u* MURUB$_{4}$.M[E]-*š*[*ú*] *ka-ṣa-a* ŠU DUMU.MUNUS ^{d}[*A-nim*]

28′. [DIŠ ... G]U.DU.MEŠ-*šú ka*-[*ṣa-a* Š]U GIDIM$_{7}$ GIG-*su* [...]

29′. [DIŠ ...] ŠU^{II}-*šú u* GÌR^{II}-*šú ka*-[*ṣa-a* S]ÌG ^{d}30

30′–36′. (fragmentary, blamed on Lamashtu)

37′. [DIŠ ...]^{II}-*šú muq-qú-ta$_{5}$* ŠÀ.MEŠ-*šú* x [...]

38′. [DIŠ ... Š]À.MEŠ-*šú eb-ṭú-ma* SIG$_{7}$ ŠUB-*ú ina* GI$_{6}$ ÍL *ú*-[...]

39′. [DIŠ ... *i*]*r* KI.MIN *ba-de* LUL.AŠ *i-ši* DIB-*iṭ* GÌR^{II}-*šú* [...]

40′. [DIŠ ...] TA GIŠ.KUN-*šú ana* GÌR^{II}-*šú* ŠE[D$_{7}$ ...]

41′. [DIŠ ...] U$_{4}$.1.KÁM DIB-*su* U$_{4}$.1.KÁM ŠUB-*šú* NINDA *u* KAŠ UL[$_{4}$.GAL ...]

42′. [DIŠ ...]x *taš-li-ma-ti* DUG$_{4}$.DUG$_{4}$-*ub* TÚG-*su* [...]

43′. [DIŠ ...] *šá* x-*šú šá* 150-*ma š*[*i* ...]

44′. [DIŠ ...] 1.KÙŠ.MEŠ-*šú* ŠED$_{7}$.MEŠ x x GIG.BI [...]

45′. [DIŠ ...] ŠU DINGIR-*šú* DIN : DIŠ KÚM *mit-ḫar* ZAG GU.DU-*šú u* GEŠTU^{II} ŠED$_7$-*a* ŠU ^{d}DI[M$_9$.ME]

46′. [DIŠ ...]x.ME-*šú* ŠU^{II}-*šú u* GÌR^{II}-*šú* ŠED$_7$-*a* ŠU ^{d}DIM$_9$.ME

47′. [DIŠ ...]-su ud *u* a ár ^{GIŠ}GIDRU DUMU *šip-ri šá* DINGIR-*šú* KI.MIN U$_4$.31.KÁM GI[G ...]

48′. [DIŠ ...]x A NAG-*ma* UGU-*šú* DÙG.GA GIG-*su* ŠUB-*šú lu* ŠU DINGIR-*šú lu* ŠU ^{d}[15-*šú*]

49′. [DIŠ ...] KÚM [*mi*]*t*-⸢*ḫar*⸣ [...] ⸢UGU-*šú*⸣ DÙG.GA *šá-né-e* ^{d}[...]

50′. [DIŠ ... *m*]*a* UGU-*šú* GIG GIG-*su* [...]

51′. [DIŠ ...] A *ir-muk-ma* UGU-*šú* GIG *u* ZI.IR.MEŠ ŠU ^{d}[...]

52′. [DIŠ ... K]ÁM GIG-*aṣ* ^{GIŠ}GIDRU *šá* D[INGIR-*šú* ...]

53′. [DIŠ ...] *ku-uṣ-ṣu-ru* x-*ta-šú u* ŠÀ.MEŠ-*šú* MÚ.MEŠ-*ḫu mu-kil* SAG ŠU DINGIR-*šú* : Š[U ...]

54′–87′. (fragmentary)

88′–99′. (Hemerology = ominous significance of fevers in various months and on various days of the month)

100′. [DIŠ] *ina* SAG.DU-*š*[*ú* D]IB-*su* DIB DINGIR-*ti* : DIŠ *ina* SAG.KI-*šú* DIB-*su* DIB DINGIR-*t*[*i*]

101′–103′. (medical omens)

104′–105′. (fragmentary)

106′. [DIŠ DIB-*su-ma* A AP]IN-*eš ḫi-miṭ* UD.DA : DIŠ DIB-*su-ma* KAŠ APIN-*eš u* BE-*sa-a* x x

107′. [DIŠ DIB-*su-ma* ŠE$_{10}$-*šú i*]*z-zi ana* TI.BI GAR-*šú* : DIŠ DIB-*su-ma* KÀŠ-*šú* SUR *ana* TI.⸢BI⸣ [GAR-*š*]*ú*

108′. [DIŠ DIB-*su-ma* ŠÀ.MEŠ]-*šú i-ši-ru* DIB DINGIR-*ti* : DIŠ DIB-*su-ma ip-ta-ru* DIB DI[NGIR-*š*]*ú* GAM

109′. [DIŠ DIB-*su-ma* SA.MEŠ?] *nu-uḫ-ḫu-ú* DIB DINGIR-*šú* GAM : DIŠ DIB-*su-ma i-ta-ru*-⸢*ur*⸣ [D]IB DINGIR-*šú* GAM

110′. [DIŠ ... DIB-*s*]*u* ŠU ^{d}DIM$_9$.ME : DIŠ *ki-ma* ^{d}UTU *šá-qé-e* DIB-*su* ŠU ^{d}DIM$_9$.ME

111′. [DIŠ...]x DIB-*su* ŠU ^{d}DIM$_9$.ME : DIŠ *ina ši-mi-tan* DIB-*su* ŠU ^{d}DIM$_9$.ME

112′. [DIŠ *ina* EN.NUN.AN.USAN^{3} DIB-*su*] ŠU ^{d}DIM$_{9}$.ME DUMU *šip-ri šá* ^{d}30 : DIŠ *ina* EN.NUN.MURUB$_{4}$.BA DIB-*su* ŠU ^{d}DIM$_{9}$.ME DUMU *šip-ri šá* ^{d}30

113′. [DIŠ *ina* EN.NUN.ZALAG.GA DIB-*s*]*u* ŠU ^{d}DIM$_{9}$.ME DUMU *šip-ri šá* ^{d}30 : DIŠ GIN$_{7}$ DIB-*it* ^{d}DIM$_{9}$.ME U$_{4}$-*me-šam-ma* DIB.DIB-*su* ŠU ^{d}DIM$_{9}$.ME.A

114′. [DIŠ IR *ina*] *um-ma-a-ti* TUKU.TUKU-*ši* NA BI *ḫi-miṭ ka-ṣab šam-ra-a-ti* GI[G] ŠU ^{d}30 *u* ^{d}UTU : ŠU DINGIR AD-*šú*

115′. [DIŠ ... G]IG-*su* ŠUB-*šú* : DIŠ IR-*su i-ta-nab-bal* GIG-*su* GÍD

116′. [DIŠ IR TA S]AG.DU-*šú* EN GÌR^{II}-*šú* NU GÁL *na-kid*

117′. [DIŠ DIB-*su* DIB].DIB-*su ir-te-né-éḫ-ḫi-šu u iš-ta-na-da-as-su* MÁ[ŠK]IM KI-*šú* KEŠDA *ina* SAG-*šú* GUB-*az* GAM

118′–124′. (fragmentary)

Translation

1′. [If he gets hot and then cold …], if […], he will get well

2′–4′. *(fragmentary)*

5′. [If …] his ⌜insides⌝ are cramped and (his abdomen) is unevenly colored with yellow, ⌜“hand”⌝ of […].

6′. [If …] (and) he continually has […], “hand” of […].

7′. [If …] he asks for a lot of water to drink, “hand” of […].

8′. [If …] is continually hot, “hand” of ⌜Lamaštu⌝.

9′. [If he is hot and then cold (and)] he continually asks for a lot of [water] ⌜to⌝ bathe in, ⌜“hand”⌝ of Lamashtu (var. “hand” of Sîn), […].[4]

10′. [If … he] will get well; “hand” of ⌜Lamaštu⌝.

11′. [If he has been sick for only one or two? days (and) he is hot but] he does not have [sweat], “hand” of Sîn; he will get well. Alternatively, it is the same for adults and children.[5]

12′. [If …] his ⌜illness⌝ keeps changing (for the worse and) it is the fifth day (he has been sick), “hand” of Sîn; [he will die].

13′. [If …] his affliction keeps changing (for the worse) (var. his mentation is continually altered, “hand” of Sîn […].

14′. [If …] and his words are unintelligible (and) it is the third day he has been sick, “hand” of […].

15′. [If …] and his eyes are heavily clouded (and) it is the twelfth day (he has been sick), “hand” of ⸢Ningirsu⸣.[6]

16′. [If …] and his eyes are clouded (and his confusional state) comes over him twice in one day, “hand” of […].

17′. [If …] he gets up and (has to) sit down (and) it is the fifty-ninth day he has been sick, “hand” of Ishtar (var. once he has been sick for a month and fifteen days […]).

18′. [If …] (and) the “right” side of his ⸢abdomen⸣ hurts him, “hand” of his god; […].[7]

19′. [If …] (and) the “left” side of his ⸢abdomen⸣ hurts him, “hand” of [his] goddess; […].[8]

20′. [If he is hot and] …[…].

21′. [If …] (and) he does not recognize person(s) known to him […].

22′. [If …] (and) he is not in full possession of his faculties […].

23′. [If …] (and) he rubs his body, […].

24′. [If …] (and) he rubs his “right” foot, […].

25′. [If …] and he chokes, he was “touched” at the beginning of the night […].

26′. [If …] (and) the soles of his feet are cold, “hand” of the daughter of A[nu].

27′. [If …] his buttocks and ⸢his hips⸣ are cold, “hand” of the daughter of [Anu].

28′. [If …] his buttocks [are] ⸢cold⸣, [“hand”] of ghost. [If] his illness […].

29′. [If …] (and) his hands and his feet are ⸢cold, blow⸣ of Sîn […].

30′–36′. *(syndromes caused by Lamashtu, fragmentary)*

37′. [If …], his […] (look) bruised (and) his insides […].

38′. [If …], his insides are cramped and (his chest and abdomen) are unevenly colored with yellow, he gets himself up in the night to […].

39′. [If …] he has a lot of ditto in the evening, the affliction of his feet […].

40′. [If he is hot from his head to his pelvis] (and) ⸢cold⸣ from his pelvis to his feet […].

41′. [If …] it afflicts him for one day (and) for one day it falls on him, he […] a lot of bread and beer […].

42′. [If …] he continually says greetings (and) […] his garment […].

43′. [If] his “left” […].

44′. [If …] his forearms are cold … that illness […].

45′. [If …], "hand" of his god; he will get well. If (his) temperature is even but the "right" side of his buttocks and his ears are cold, "hand" of ⌜Lamaštu⌝.

46′. [If …], his […], his hands and his feet are cold, "hand" of Lamashtu.

47′. [If …] … scepter, messenger of his god. Alternatively, [if] it is the thirty-first day he has been sick […].

48′. [If …] (and) he drinks water and it tastes good to him, his illness is falling on him; either "hand" of his god or "hand" [of his goddess].

49′. [If …] his temperature is ⌜even⌝, […] tastes good to him, deputy of […].

50′. [If …] does not taste good to him, his illness […].

51′. [If …] he bathes in water and it makes him feel worse and (his stomach) is continually upset, "hand" of […].

52′. [If …] it is the [… day] he has been sick, scepter of [his] ⌜god⌝ […].

53′. [If …] (feel like) they are tied together, his […] and his insides are continually bloated, assistant of the "hand" of his god (var. ⌜"hand"⌝ [of …]

54′–87′. *(fragmentary)*

88′–99′. *(Hemerology—ominous significance of fevers in various months and on various days of the month)*

100′. [If] it afflicts him in ⌜his⌝ head, affliction of godship. If it afflicts him in his temple, affliction of ⌜godship⌝.[9]

101′–103′. *(medical omens)*

104′–105′. *(signs of death or recovery, fragmentary)*

106′. [If it afflicts him and] he ⌜asks⌝ [for water], burning of *ṣētu*. If it afflicts him and he asks for beer, […].

107′. [If it afflicts him and he] excretes [his excrement], it is a sign that he will live. If it afflicts him and his urine flows, [it is a sign] that he will live.[10]

108′. [If it afflicts him and] his [bowels] are loose,[11] affliction of godship. If it afflicts him and he continually vomits, affliction by ⌜his god⌝; he will die.

109′. [If it afflicts him and the blood vessels?] are slow, affliction by his god; he will die.[12] If it afflicts him and he trembles, ⌜affliction⌝ by his god; he will die.

110′. [If it afflicts] ⌜him⌝ [at sunrise(?)], "hand" of Lamashtu. If it afflicts him after the sun has gotten high, "hand" of Lamashtu.

111′. [If] it afflicts him [at noon(?)], "hand" of Lamashtu. If it afflicts him in the evening, "hand" of Lamashtu.

112′. [If] it afflicts him [in the early evening watch], "hand" of Lamashtu, messenger of Sîn. If it afflicts him in the middle watch (of the night), "hand" of Lamashtu, messenger of Sîn.

113′. [If it afflicts him in the last watch of the night], "hand" of Lamashtu, messenger of Sîn. If it continually afflicts him daily as in affliction by Lamashtu, "hand" of *labaṣu*.

114′. [If] he continually has [sweat during] bouts of fever, that person is ⸢sick⸣ with burning of the cutting short(?) of bouts of "raging"; "hand" of Sîn or Shamash (var. "hand" of the god of his father).

115′. [If …] his ⸢illness⸣ is falling on him. If his sweat keeps drying out, his illness will be prolonged.

116′. [If] there is no [sweat from] his ⸢head⸣ to his feet, it is worrisome.

117′. [If his affliction? continually] afflicts him, flows over him and pulls him taut, a ⸢*rābiṣu*⸣ is bound with him (and) stands at his head; he will die.[13]

118′–124′. *(fragmentary)*

Notes

1. Restored from the commentary SpTU 1.38:1–2.
2. Restorations are based on SpTU 1.38:5.
3. Restored from SpTU 1.38:30′.
4. The entry appears also in *KAR* 211 i 10′–11′ (Heeßel 2010, 171–77) but with "touch" of Sîn.
5. See Scurlock and Andersen 2005, 19.263. The entry appears in *STT* 89:212.
6. See Scurlock and Andersen 2005, 19.168. The entry is similar to DPS 3:84.
7. The entry appears also in DPS 14:175′.
8. The entry appears also in DPS 14:176′.
9. See Scurlock and Andersen 2005, 16.5
10. See Scurlock and Andersen 2005, 5.37.
11. I.e., he has diarrhea.
12. See Scurlock and Andersen 2005, 20.26.
13. See Scurlock and Andersen 2005, 19.120.

DPS 21

DPS 19/20:125′ (catchline) = DPS 21:1

1. [DIŠ GIG NIGI]N SA.MEŠ-*šú šal-mu-ma* SÍG S[AG.DU-*šú in*]*a* GEŠTU-*šú zaq-pat* GAM
2. DIŠ K[I].MIN-⸢*ma*⸣ [SÍG SAG.DU-*šú* SA$_5$-*át* SAG.KI-*su* x x x UZU *ina muḫ-ḫi ia-a-nu*[1] GAM]
3. DIŠ KI.MIN-*ma ka-ra-an* IGI^{II}-*šú* [*šad-du* …][2]
4. DIŠ KI.MIN-*ma* KA-*šú ṣu-dur* […]
5. DIŠ KI.MIN-*ma* MÚD *ina* KIR$_4$-*šú* DU-*ku* […]

6–7. DIŠ KI.MIN-*ma* MÚD *ina* KIR$_4$-*šú* DU-⸢*ku*⸣-*ma* U$_4$ *u* [GI$_6$ …] ŠU ^{d}MAŠ BUR-*ma* DIN

8. DI[Š] KI.MIN-*ma* MÚD *ina* KIR$_4$-*šú* U[$_4$] *u* GI$_6$ DU-*ku-m*[*a* …]
9. D[IŠ] KI.MIN-*ma* MÚD *ina* KIR$_4$-*šú* U$_4$ *u* GI$_6$ DU-*k*[*u-ma* …]
10. [DIŠ] KI.MIN-*ma* ZÚ.MEŠ-*šú ub-tar-r*[*a-ru* …]
11. [DIŠ KI.MI]N-*ma* KA-*šú* DA[D]AG.MEŠ x[…]
12. [DIŠ KI.MI]N-*ma ina* DÚR-*šú* ZÉ G[I$_6$ *i-te-ez-zi*? …]
13. [DIŠ KI.MIN]-*ma* [IGI].M[EŠ-*šú*] UD.A [GI$_6$.MEŠ[3] DIRI.MEŠ GAM]
14. [DIŠ KI.MI]N-[*m*]*a* IGI.MEŠ-*šú* S[IG$_7$.MEŠ …]
15. [DIŠ KI.MIN]-*ma* IGI.MEŠ-*šú* SA$_5$.MEŠ [IGI^{II}-*šú pur-ru-ku* …][4]
16. [DIŠ KI.MI]N-*ma* NA$_4$.KIŠIB GÚ-*šú* DU[$_8$ GAM]
17. [DIŠ KI.MI]N-*ma* ŠU^{II}-*šú u* GÌR^{II}-*šú ut-tu-*[*qa* …]
18. [DIŠ KI.M]IN-*ma* GÌR^{II}-*šú nu-up-pu-ḫa* GAM : [D]IŠ [KI.MIN-*ma* …]
19. [DIŠ K]I.⸢MIN⸣-*ma* ŠIR.MEŠ-*šú zi-ir* GAM : DIŠ K[I.MIN-*ma* …]
20. [DIŠ K]I.[MI]N-*ma ina* DÚR-*šú* MÚD *i-a-ú ana ḫu-*[*ḫa-ti-šú* NIM NU TE GAM]
21. [DIŠ KI].MIN-*ma* GIG-*su iš-ta-na-*[*ad-da-as-su* …][5]
22. [DIŠ KI.MI]N-*ma mim-ma* GU$_7$ *ina* ŠÀ-*šú* N[U *ina-aḫ is-ḫur-ma* DUB-*ka* GAM]
23. [DIŠ KI.MIN]-⸢*ma* NINDA⸣ Ì GU$_7$ KAŠ […]

TRANSLATION

1. [If the patient]'s blood vessels are healthy but the hair of [his] ⸢head⸣ stands on end ⸢at⸣ his ear, he will die.[6]
2. If ditto (his blood vessels are healthy) but [the hair of his head is red … (and) there is no flesh on his forehead, he will die].[7]
3. If ditto (his blood vessels are healthy) but the grapes of his eyes [are pulled taut[8] …].[9]

4. If ditto (his blood vessels are healthy) but his mouth twitches […].

5. If ditto (his blood vessels are healthy) but blood flows from his nose […].

6–7. If ditto (his blood vessels are healthy) but blood flows from his nose and it [does not stop?] day or [night], "hand" of Ninurta; if it lets up, he will get well.[10]

8. ⸢If⸣ ditto (his blood vessels are healthy) but blood flows from his nose ⸢day⸣ and night ⸢and⸣ […].

9. I[f] ditto (his blood vessels are healthy) but blood flows from his nose day and night […].

10. [If] ditto (his blood vessels are healthy) but his teeth have turned ⸢dusky⸣ […].

11. [If] ⸢ditto⸣ (his blood vessels are healthy) and his mouth is ⸢pure⸣ (i.e., his teeth shine) […].

12. [If] ⸢ditto⸣ (his blood vessels are healthy) but [he excretes?] ⸢black⸣ bile from his anus […].

13. [If ditto (his blood vessels are healthy)] but [his face is full of black] *ramīṭu*-lesions, [he will die].

14. [If] ⸢ditto⸣ (his blood vessels are healthy) ⸢but⸣ his face is ⸢yellow⸣ […].

15. [If [(his blood vessels are healthy)] but his face flushes [(and) his eyes are crossed[11] …].

16. [If ditto (his blood vessels are healthy)] but his vertebra is (cut) ⸢open⸣, [he will die].[12]

17. [If] ⸢ditto⸣ (his blood vessels are healthy) but his hands and his feet are ⸢paralyzed(?)⸣[13] […].

18. [I] ⸢ditto⸣ (his blood vessels are healthy) but his feet are swollen, he will die. ⸢If⸣ [ditto (his blood vessels are healthy) but …].

19. [If ditto (his blood vessels are healthy)] but his testicles are twisted, he will die. If [ditto (his blood vessels are healthy) but …].[14]

20. [If ditto (his blood vessels are healthy)] but he vomits blood from his anus (and) [flies will not approach his] ⸢vomitus⸣, [he will die].[15]

21. [If ditto (his blood vessels are healthy)] but his illness ⸢draws⸣ [him taut …].

22. [If] ⸢ditto⸣ (his blood vessels are healthy) but whatever he eats does ⸢not⸣ [rest easy] in his stomach [but it turns about and pours out, he will die].[16]

23. [If ditto (his blood vessels are healthy)] and he eats bread and fat (and) [drinks] beer […]

NOTES

1. Restored after the commentary, Leichty 1973, 82–86:1–3; cf. *pe-ret* SAG.DU-*šú sa-mat* SpTU 1.40:7.

2. *ka-ra-an* IGI^{II}-*šú šad-du* : *kak-kul-tu$_4$ i-ni-šú ú-ṣa-a* (SpTU 1.40:8–9) *ka-ra-an* IGI^{II}-*šú šad-du* [...] *šá kak-kul-tu*$_4$ IGI^{II}-*šú a-na bi-ta-nu i-ru-*[*bu*] (Leichty 1973, 82–86:3–4).

3. Restored from the commentary Leichty 1973, 82–86:5

4. Restored from Wilhelm 2004, 60:3.

5. Restored from the commentary Leichty 1973, 82–86:7.

6. See Scurlock and Andersen 2005, 10.189.

7. Restored after the commentary, Leichty 1973, 82–86:1–3; cf. "the hair of his head is red" (SpTU 1.40:7).

8. Commentary SpTU 1.40 obv. 9 has: "The grapes of his eyes are pulled taut." (That means that) his eye balls stick out. Commentary Heeßel 2000, 247:3–4 has: "The grapes of his eyes are pulled taut." (That means that) his eye balls turn inwards.

9. See Scurlock and Andersen 2005, 9.74.

10. See Scurlock and Andersen 2005, 20.48.

11. Restored from Wilhelm 1994, 60:3.

12. See Scurlock and Andersen 2005, 13.143. This is similar to DPS 10:22a.

13. The translation assumes a connection with *etēqu* B which is equated lexically with *ramû* (Ludlul Comm. 86, apud *CAD* B, 395b). The commentary, Leichty 1973, 82–86:6 explains the expression as meaning "seized, said of an attack."

14. See Scurlock and Andersen 2005, 5.83. The entry also appears in DPS 14:134.

15. For the fly test, see also DPS 17:60.

16. See Scurlock and Andersen 2005, 20.78.

DPS 22

1. DIŠ GIG *ina še-re-e-ti il-te-né-eb-bu u* A *ma-gal* NAG *li-ʾ-bu* DIB-*su* GIG-*su* ŠU.NAM.LÚ.U$_{18}$.LU

2–3. DIŠ *rì-mu-tu* ŠUB.ŠUB-*su* SAG ŠÀ-*šú* DIB.DIB-*su ma-gal in-né-sil* GIG-*su* ŠU.NAM.LÚ.U$_{18}$.LU NU.MEŠ-*šú šu-nu-lu* MAŠ.MAŠ *ana* DIN-*šú* ME-*a* NU GAR-*an*

4. DIŠ *i-riš-ti* ŠÀ APIN-*ma* NU GU$_7$ *ú-gan-na-aḫ u* KÚM DIB.DIB-*su* GIG-*su* ŠU.NAM.LÚ.U$_{18}$.LU

5. DIŠ *ina* DUG$_4$.DUG$_4$-*šú it-te-né-ep-rik-ku* NA BI *ana maš-tak-ti kiš-pu šu-kul*

6–7. DIŠ *iš-ta-na-ʾ-i* KA ŠUB.ŠUB-*su* KI ŠÀ-*šú* DUG$_4$.DUG$_4$-*ub ṣu-uḫ la pak-ki iṣ-ṣe-ni-iḫ* GIG *ra-mi* GIG *ana* NITA *u* MUNUS 1-*ma*

8–9. DIŠ NÍG.ZI.IR ŠUB.ŠUB-*su* ZI.MEŠ-*šú* LÚGUD.MEŠ(coll.) NINDA GU$_7$ A (var. A&D: KAŠ) NAG-*ma* UGU-*šú* NU DU-*ak* *ʾú-a* ŠÀ-*bi i-qab-bi u uš-tan-na-aḫ* GIG *ra-a-mi* GIG *ana* NITA *u* MUNUS 1-*ma*

10–11. DIŠ NA SA.MEŠ ŠÀ-*šú* GU$_7$.MEŠ-*šú* SAG.KI GÙB-*šú* TAG.TAG-*su im-ta-nag-ga-ag* KA DIB SU-*šú* KÚM-*em u ši-ḫat* UZU.MEŠ TUKU NA BI GIG *na-a-ki* GIG

12–13. DIŠ NA SAG ŠÀ-*šú i-ḫa-am-maṭ-su u* KÚM-*em* NINDA GU$_7$-*ma* UGU-*šú* NU DU-*ak* A NAG-*ma* UGU-*šú* NU DÙG.GA *u* SU-*šú* SIG$_7$ NA BI GIG *na-a-ki* GIG

14–15. DIŠ NA GÌŠ-*šú u* SAG ŠÀ-*šú* KÚM *ṣar-ḫa ú-kal* TÙN ŠÀ-*šú* GU$_7$-*šú u* ŠÀ-*šú ma-ḫu* Á^{II}-*šú* GÌR^{II}-*šú u* ŠÀ-*šú* KÚM-*em* NA BI GIG *na-a-ki* GIG ŠU ^{d}15

---

16. DIŠ *ina* DUG$_4$.DUG$_4$-*šú il-la-tu-šú* DU.MEŠ *aḫ-ḫa-zu* IGI.MEŠ-*šú* DIRI.MEŠ ŠÀ.MEŠ-*šú i-šá-ru-šú* ŠU *ma-mit* GAM

17. DIŠ *taš-*⸢*li-ma*⸣*-ti* DUG$_4$.DUG$_4$-*ub* GIG *ma-mit* GIG

18. DIŠ [*taš-l*]*i-*⸢*ma*⸣*-ti* DUG$_4$.DUG$_4$-*ub* GIG TI-*ma* TI GIG-*ma* GAM

19–20. [DIŠ D]IRI.MEŠ-*pú* ŠÀ.MEŠ-*šú* MÚ.MEŠ-*ḫu* PIŠ$_{10}$ IGI^{II}-*šú* MÚ.MEŠ-*ḫu* MURGU GÌR^{II}-*šú* MÚ.MEŠ *u* MÚD *ina* KIR$_4$-*šú šá* GÙB DU-*ku* ŠU NAM.ÉRIM.MA GAM

21. DIŠ *za-mar* KÚM-*em za-mar* ŠED$_7$ UZU.ME-*šu* SIG$_7$ ŠUB-*ú ga-ṣu u qá-ti-ir* ŠU *ma-mit* GAM

22–23. DIŠ NU *pa-tan* UZU.ME-*šú uš-ta-nak-ta-tu i-riš-ti* SUM^{SAR} : ^{Ú}[Z]AG.ḪI.LI^{SAR} UGU-*šu* GIG *ap-*[*p*]*at* U.MEŠ ŠU^{II}-*šú u* GÌR^{II}-*šú ḫu-ul-la-a* ŠU NAM.ÉRIM.MA

24. DIŠ U$_4$ *u* G[I]$_6$ NAM.ÉRIM DIB-*su* : *lu-ʾa-ti* DIB-*su*

---

25. DIŠ NA KÚM-*im* ŠÀ-*šú i-ta-na-aš ú-gan-na-aḫ u ki-ṣir-ta-šú* GI$_6$ NA BI *ma-mit* GIG

26–27. DIŠ NA KÚM *ma-dam* TUKU-*ma la i-na-aḫ ú-na-ḫaṭ u i-sa-ul u* ŠÀ-*šú ana a-re-e i-ta-na-šá-a* NAM.ÉRIM GIG

---

28. DIŠ GABA-*su u šá-šal-la-šú* GU$_7$.ME-*šú ki-ṣir-ti* ŠÀ GI$_6$ ⸢TUKU⸣.ME ⸢ŠÀ-*šú i-ta-na*⸣*-áš* NA BI NAM.TAG.GA : NAM.ÉRIM DIB-⸢*su*⸣

29–30. DIŠ ŠÀ-*šú* KÚM-*ma* NINDA GU$_7$-*ma* KAŠ NAG-*ma ú-gan-na-aḫ* SAG ŠÀ-*šú u* MAŠ.SÌLA.MEŠ-*šú* GU$_7$.MEŠ-*šú ú-sa-al ú-na-ḫaṭ u* ÚḪ-*su i-šal-lu* : NA BI ⸢NAM.ÉRIM⸣ *u* NAM.TAG.GA DIB-*su*

31–32. DIŠ SAG ŠÀ-*šú i-kàṣ-ṣa-su* ŠÀ-*šú* KÚM *ú-kal* KÚM *la ḫa-ḫaš* ÚḪ GI$_6$ ŠUB.ŠUB-*a u i-ta-nar-ru* NA BI NAM.ÉRIM DIB-*su*

---

33. DIŠ NA SAG ⸢ŠÀ⸣-*bi-šú š*[*á-b*]*ul* SAG ŠÀ-*š*[*ú* G]U$_7$-*šú* KÚM *la ḫa-ḫaš* MÚD *iš-tan* NA BI DU$_8$ GIG DIḪ

34–35. DIŠ UB.MEŠ-*š*[*ú*] ⸢DU$_8$⸣.MEŠ SAG ŠÀ-*šú di-ik-*⸢*šá* TUKU⸣ *pi-qam la pi-qam* (coll.) MÚD *ina* KIR$_4$-*šú* DU-*ku* Á^{II}-*šú* SIG.MEŠ NÍG.ZI.[IR] ŠUB.ŠUB-*su* IGI^{II}-*šú* MÚD *šu-un-nu-ʾ-a* ŠU ^{d}AMAR.UTU *a-dir-ma* GAM

36–37. DIŠ UB.MEŠ-*š*[*ú* DU$_8$].MEŠ SAG.KI^{II}-*šú* ŠUB-*ta*$_5$ *gir-ra-šú šu-uḫ-ḫu-ṭa* ŠÀ^{II}-*šú it-te-nen-bi-ṭu kal* U[$_4$] *u kal* GI$_6$ GIG ŠU ^{d}AMAR.UTU *a-dir-ma* GAM

38. DIŠ UB.ME-*š*[*ú ir*]-*mu-ú u* MÚD *i-te-ez-zi* EGIR-*ta*$_5$ SÌG-*iṣ* GAM

39a. DIŠ UB.ME-*šú* GU$_7$.MEŠ-*šú* ŠU ^{d}15 *ana* TAG-*te* TI-*uṭ* (var. GAM)

39b. DIŠ *i-ṭa-mu u* MÚD *i-ḫa-ḫu* SÌG-*iṣ* NAM.TAR SÌG-*iṣ* GAM

40. DIŠ *i-ṭa-mu* A *u* K[A]Š(coll.) APIN.MEŠ-*iš* : NU APIN-*iš* MAŠKIM *ur-ḫi* SÌG-*su*

41. DIŠ UL$_4$.GAL BAL.BAL DUL.DUL-*tam u* ŠUB.ŠUB-*ut* GAM

42a. DIŠ UL$_4$.GAL BAL.BAL *u* ŠÀ.GAL *ma-gal* APIN-*iš* NU DIN

42b. DIŠ EGIR.MEŠ-*šú ú-ḫa-as-sa-as* TI-*uṭ* (var. ÚŠ.MEŠ) MAN TAG-*ma* GAM

43. DIŠ EGIR.MEŠ-*šú ú-ḫa-as-sa-as* ŠUK-*su* APIN-*ma* GU$_7$ GAM

44. ⸢DIŠ⸣ TÚG-*su ú-na-kas*$_4$ *u* UB.NÍGIN.NA-*šú i-ṭa-ma-a* ŠU ^{d}*Šul-pa-è-a*

45. [DIŠ T]ÚG-*su ú-na-kas*$_4$ *u* UB.NÍGIN.NA-*šú na-šá-a* ŠU ^{d}*Šul-pa-è-a*

46. [DIŠ TÚ]G-*su* ŠUB.ŠUB-*di u i-te-ner-ru-ub* ŠU ^{d}MAŠ.TAB.BA GAM

47a. [DIŠ U]Š$_4$-*šu šá-ni-šu-ma* UŠ$_4$-*šú* NU DIB ŠU GIDIM *mur-tap-pi-du* GAM

47b. DIŠ UŠ$_4$-*šu* MAN.MAN-*šu uz-zi* DINGIR

48. [DIŠ UŠ$_4$]-*šu* MAN.MAN-*šu u* EME-*šú ir-ta-nap-pu-ud* GAM

49–50. [DIŠ UŠ$_4$]-*šu* MAN.MAN-*ni* DU$_{11}$.DU$_{11}$-*šú* KÚR.KÚR *mim-mu-ú i-qab-bu-ú i-ma-áš-šú* IM *ku-tal-li* DIB-*su* 1-*ma* KÚR-*iš* GAM

51–52. DIŠ UŠ$_4$-[*šu* KÚR-*ir* IN]IM.MEŠ-*šú it-te-né-ep-rik-ka-a* GIDIM *mu-šam-šu-ú* DIB-*su* [:] KI.SIKIL.LÍL.LÁ *šum*$_4$-*ma* LÚ.LÍL.LÁ

53–54. DIŠ UŠ$_4$-*šú* KÚR-⸢*ir*⸣ [...] x *maš-u-tú* INIM.MEŠ-*šú it-te-né-ep-rik-ka-a* GIDIM$_7$ *mut-tag-gi-šú* DIB-*su* [...].MEŠ-*ma* DIN KI.MIN ŠU LÚ.LÍL.LÁ

55a. DIŠ UŠ$_4$-*šú* KÚR.KÚR-*šú* ŠU ^{d}UTU AZAG GU$_7$

55b. DIŠ NÍ-*šú i-*[*maš-ši* ...] *ḫi-pi eš-šú* GAM

56. DIŠ AL.ZU.BI NAM.BA.ZU.BI *u* DU$_{11}$-*šú* KÚR.KÚR-*ir* GAM

57. DIŠ *ú-rap-pad ú-ma-aq it-ta-na-an-di* : ŠUB.ŠUB-*ut* GAM

58. DIŠ *i-leb-bu* KÚM U_5-*šú* : DIŠ GÙ.GÙ-*si* ŠU MU DINGIR-*šú* GAM
59. DIŠ *ma-gal* GÙ.GÙ-*si* KÚM.KÚM-*im* ŠU.GIDIM.MA GAR-*e* ᵈ*É-a*
60. DIŠ *ina kal* Á.KAL-*šú* GÙ-*si* U_4.1.K[Á]M U_4.2.KÁM GIG-*ma* GÙ-*šú* *im-ṭi* GAM
61. DIŠ *i-nam-gag* $ŠU^{II}$-*šú u* KI.TA $GÌR^{II}$-*šú* $ŠED_7$-*a* GAM
62. DIŠ *iṣ-ṣe-ni-iḫ* ŠU ᵈSAG.ḪUL.ḪA.ZA GAM : ŠU ᵈ*Iš-tar*
63. DIŠ *ḫa-di u pa-rid* ŠU SAG.ḪUL.ḪA.ZA GAM : ŠU ᵈ*Iš-tar*
64a. DIŠ *ud-daḫ-ḫa-as* GAM : ŠU SAG.ḪUL.ḪA.ZA
64b. DIŠ ZI-*bi u* DU_{10}.GAM-*is* ŠU-*su* LAL-*át* GAM
65. DIŠ ZI-*bi-ma* ŠU *ti-iṣ-bat* ᴸᵁ́TU.RA BI ÚŠ-*ma* EGIR-*šú* GIG GÁL-*ši*
66. DIŠ GÍR-*iš* ZI-*bi* GIG-*su* GÍD-*ma* GAM
67. DIŠ *ú-ta-aṭ-ṭal u im-ta-nag-ga-ag ina di-ʾi* TAG-*it*
68. DIŠ *ú-te-eṭ-ṭe* ZI.IR.MEŠ SÍG UGU-*šú it-ta-na-az-qap ina* GI_6 GAM
69–70. DIŠ SAL.KALAG.GA IGI-*ma ib-luṭ* EGIR *ib-lu-ṭu* $GÌR^{II}$-*šú it-te-né-eb-ṭa-ni* GIG.BI *šum-ma* É.MEŠ EN LÍL-*šú i-qat-tu-ú* EN.TE.NA RI-*šum-ma* NU DIN
71–72. DIŠ NAM.KALAG DIB-*su-ma a-ka-la muṭ-ṭu ḫa-šu-šu i-ḫal-lu-la* U_4-*mu-us-su* KÚM DIB.DIB-*su ina ku-uṣ-ṣi* GAM
73. DIŠ [*u*]*š-ta-na-aḫ u i-na-iš* GAM : DIŠ [N]A BI *it-ta-bi-ik* GAM
74. DIŠ *it-te-ni-in-sír* DIN (var. A GAM) : DIŠ *še-e-ṭú* GAM : DIŠ *i-par-ru-ur* GAM
75. DIŠ BAL.BAL-*at* DIN : DIŠ ŠÚ-*ap* DIN : DIŠ *i-na-ḫu-ur* DIN
76. DIŠ *i-*[*š*]*a-al u i-tap-pa-al* DIN
77. DIŠ *i*-x […] *ṭi-ib u i-geš-šú na-šar* GIG
78. DIŠ DINGIR[.MEŠ URU?]-*šú ul-la-nu iḫ-ṭú-u* È.MEŠ

Translation

1. If the patient continually groans in the mornings and drinks a lot of water (and) *liʾbu* afflicts him, his illness is "hand" of mankind.
2–3. If limpness continually falls upon him, his epigastrium continually afflicts him (and) he is very sluggish, his illness is "hand" of mankind. His figurines have been made to lie (with a corpse); the *āšipu* should not make a prognosis as to his recovery.[1]
4. If he asks for something he has a craving for and then does not eat (it), he *guḫḫu*-coughs and fever continually afflicts him, his illness is "hand" of mankind.

5. If (the words) hinder each other (in his mouth) when he speaks, that person has been fed *kišpu* to test it.[2]

6–7. If he continually flutters about, he is continually insolent, he continually talks with himself (and) he continually laughs for no reason, he is sick with love sickness; it is the same for a man and a woman.[3]

8–9. If depression continually falls upon him, his breath is continually short, he eats bread (and) drinks water (var. beer) but it does not agree with him, he says "Ua my heart" and he is dejected, he is sick with love sickness; it is the same for a man and a woman.[4]

10–11. If the muscles of his abdomen continually hurt him, his "left" temple continually hurts him intensely, he is continually stiff/rigid, inability to eat afflicts him, his body is feverish and he has wasting away of the flesh, that person is sick with a venereal disease (lit. "disease of intercourse").[5]

12–13. If his epigastrium gives him a burning pain and he is feverish, he eats bread and it does agree with him, he drinks water and it does not taste good to him and his body is yellow, that person is sick with a venereal disease.[6]

14–15. If a person's penis and his epigastrium hold burning fever, his liver hurts him and his stomach goes crazy (and) his arms, his feet, and his stomach are feverish, that person is sick with a venereal disease; "hand" of Ishtar.[7]

---

16. If a person's spittle flows when he speaks, *aḫḫāzu* fills his face (and) his bowels are loose, "hand" of curse; he will die.[8]

17. If he continually says greetings,[9] he is sick with an illness of curse.

18. If he continually says ⸢greetings⸣, if the patient gets well (and) if, once well, he gets sick (again), he will die.

19–20. [If (his eyes]] drift downstream, his insides are bloated, the rims of his eyes are swollen, the soles of his feet are swollen and blood flows from his "left" nostril, "hand" of curse; he will die.[10]

21. If he is sometimes hot and sometimes cold, his flesh is unevenly colored with yellow, he (looks white as) whitewash and (dark as) the color of smoke, "hand" of curse; he will die.

22–23. If, without (his) having[11] eaten, his flesh is continually thickened, the smell of garlic (var. *saḫlû*) bothers him (and) the tips of his fingers and his toes (appear to be) made to dissolve,[12] "hand" of curse.[13]

24. If (it afflicts him) day and night, a curse afflicts him (var. dirty substances afflict him).

---

25. If a person becomes feverish, his stomach is continually nauseous, he *guḫḫu*-coughs and his thick sputum is dark, that person is sick with a curse.[14]

26–27. If a person is very feverish and cannot find rest, he breathes deeply[15] and *su'alu*-coughs and his stomach is nauseous to the point of vomiting, he is sick with a curse.[16]

---

28. If his breast and his upper back continually hurt him, he has dark thick sputum (and) his stomach is continually nauseous, wrongdoing or a curse afflicts that person.

29–30. If his stomach feels hot, he eats bread and drinks beer and then *guḫḫu*-coughs, his epigastrium and his shoulders continually hurt him, he *su'ālu*-coughs, he breathes deeply and he sprays his saliva, curse or wrongdoing afflicts that person.[17]

31–32. If his epigastrium gnaws at him, fever grips his stomach, his temperature is lukewarm, he continually produces dark phlegm and he continually vomits, a curse afflicts that person.[18]

---

33. If his epigastrium (looks) ⌜dried⌝ out, ⌜his⌝ epigastrium ⌜hurts⌝ him, his temperature is lukewarm (and) he urinates blood, that man (is experiencing) a letting up of an illness of *li'bu*.[19]

34–35. If his limbs are supple, his epigastrium has a needling pain, blood incessantly flows from his nose, his arms are continually weak, ⌜depression⌝ continually falls upon him (and) his eyes are suffused with blood, "hand" of Marduk; he is in danger of dying.[20]

36–37. If his limbs [are supple], (the blood vessels of) his temples have collapsed, his throat (looks) skinned, his insides are continually cramped (and) he is sick all ⌜day⌝ and all night, "hand" of Marduk; he is in danger of dying.[21]

38. If ⌜his⌝ limbs become ⌜limp⌝ and he excretes blood, he was wounded from behind; he will die.[22]

39a. If his limbs continually hurt him, "hand" of Ishtar on account of touching the cheek; he will get well (var: die).

39b. If he twists and vomits blood, he was struck with the blow of (his own) personal death demon; he will die.

40. If he twists (and) continually asks for water and beer (var. does not ask) the *rābiṣu* of the road has struck him.

41. If he has frequent changes of mood and veils himself (i.e., withdraws from social intercourse) and continually falls down, he will die.

42a. If he has frequent changes of mood and asks for a lot of food, he will not get well.

42b. If he thinks seriously about arranging his affairs, he will get well. If it changes (for the worse and) "touches" him, he will die.

43. If he thinks seriously about arranging his affairs, asks for his travel provisions (to the Netherworld) and eats them, he will die.[23]

44. If he tears his garment and his limbs twist, "hand" of Šulpaea.[24]

45. [If] he tears his ⸢garment⸣ and his limbs are raised up, "hand" of Šulpaea.[25]

46. [If] he keeps taking off and getting into his ⸢garments⸣, "hand" of the twin gods; he will die.[26]

47a. [If] his ⸢mentation⸣ is altered[27] so that he is not in full possession of his faculties, "hand" of a roving ghost; he will die.[28]

47b. If his mentation is continually altered, anger of a god.[29]

48. [If] his [mentation] is continually altered and his tongue continually roves about, he will die.[30]

49–50. [If] his [mentation] is continually altered, his words are unintelligible and he forgets whatever he says, a wind from behind afflicts him; he will die alone like a stranger.[31]

51–52. If [his] mentation [is altered] (and) his ⸢words⸣ hinder each other (in his mouth), a ghost who wanders about at night afflicts him ([var.] *ardat lilî* or *lilû*).[32]

53–54. If his mentation is altered, ... forgetfullness? (and) his words hinder each other in his mouth, a roaming ghost afflicts him. If [...] he will get well. Alternatively, "hand" of *lilû*.[33]

55a. If his mentation continualy alters, "hand" of Shamash; he has transgressed a taboo.[34]

55b. If he loses consciousness [...], ... he will die.

56. If he does not recognize person(s) known to him and his words are unintelligible, he will die.[35]

57. If he wanders about, he does things slowly (and) he is continually thrown down (var. falls down), he will die.[36]

58. If he groans (and) fever rides him, (var. If he continually cries out), "hand" of an oath (sworn by) his god; he will die.[37]

59. If he cries out a lot (and) continually gets feverish, "hand" of ghost, deputy of Ea.[38]

60. If he cries out with all his force, he is sick for one or two days and his crying gets softer, he will die.[39]

61. If he brays (like a donkey and) his hands and the bottoms of his feet are cold, he will die.
62. If he continually laughs, "hand" of *mukīl rēš lemutti*; he will die; var. "hand" of Ishtar.[40]
63. If he rejoices and is terrified, "hand" of *mukīl rēš lemutti*; he will die; var. "hand" of Ishtar.[41]
64a. If he feels harassed, he will die; var. "hand" of *mukīl rēš lemutti*.[42]
64b. If he gets up and (has to) squat down (and) his hand is stretched out, he will die.[43]
65. If he gets up and (his) hand is grasped (by others), if that patient dies, there will be another patient after him.[44]
66. If he gets up (too) quickly, if his illness is prolonged, he will die.[45]
67. If he continually lays himself down[46] and he continually becomes rigid, he was "touched" by *diʾu*.[47]
68. If he continually becomes darkened (i.e., passes out), (his stomach) is continually upset (and) the hair of his scalp continually stands on end, he will die in the night.
69–70. If he experiences a mighty illness and then gets well (and) after he gets well, his feet are continually cramped, if the summer finishes before his illness does, the cold will fall upon him so that he will not get well.[48]
71–72. If a mighty illness afflicts him so that he has a reduced appetite for bread, his lungs sing like a reed flute (and) fever continually afflicts him daily in winter, he will die.[49]
73. [If he] is continually exhausted and shakes, he will die. If that ⸢person⸣ falls over in a heap, he will die.[50]
74. If he is continually bunched up,[51] he will get well (var. he will die). If he is spread out, he will die. If he lies still, he will die.
75. If he tosses and turns, he will get well. If he falls out of bed,[52] he will get well. If he snores, he will get well.
76. If he asks questions and answers (them), he will get well.
77. If [...], he feels better and he belches, diminution of the illness.
78. If they have a long history of sinning against the ⸢gods⸣ [of] his [city(?)], they (the gods) will leave.

Notes

1. See Scurlock and Andersen 2005, 19.122.
2. The described symptoms also appear as part of DPS 3:51 and DPS 3:54.
3. See Scurlock and Andersen 2005, 16.23.

4. See Scurlock and Andersen 2005, 6.83, 16.24.

5. A quite similar entry appears in DPS 13:6–7.

6. See Scurlock and Andersen 2005, 4.35, 13.27. This entry appears also in DPS 13:8–9.

7. See Scurlock and Andersen 2005, 2.18, 4.34, 19.378. This entry appears also in DPS 14:106–108.

8. See Scurlock and Andersen 2005, 19.312.

9. The commentary explains: [*taš-l*]*i-ma-a-ti* $DUG_4.DUG_4$-*ub* … [*taš-li-ma*]-*ti* : *nu-ul-at ina ṣa-a-tú* E: "He continually says ⸢greetings⸣" : "'⸢greetings⸣' means 'untruths.'" (SpTU 1.38:15–17).

10. See Scurlock and Andersen 2005, 19.313, 20.40.

11. The translation assumes a direct connection with the Arabic cognate which means "to become thick or dense" (Lane, *Arabic-English Lexicon*, 2591). *CAD* K, 304b s.v. *katātu* mng. 1b interprets this as the patient's flesh collapsing. Heeßel 2000, 259 translates "vibrate."

12. The translation assumes a D-stem from *ḫâlu*.

13. See Scurlock and Andersen 2005, 3.214.

14. See Scurlock and Andersen 2005, 3.79.

15. The Aramaic cognate means "to sigh."

16. See Scurlock and Andersen 2005, 3.80, 6.54, 8.66.

17. See Scurlock and Andersen 2005, 19.309.

18. See Scurlock and Andersen 2005, 3.4, 3.81.

19. Correcting Heeßel 2000, 254.

20. See Scurlock and Andersen 2005, 3.238, 9.24.

21. See Scurlock and Andersen 2005, 3.238.

22. See Scurlock and Andersen 2005, 13.51.

23. See Scurlock and Andersen 2005, 20.105.

24. See Scurlock and Andersen 2005, 13.258.

25. See Scurlock and Andersen 2005, 13.74, 13.258.

26. See Scurlock and Andersen 2005, 16.57.

27. Stol 2009a, 3–6 argues that the particular way of expressing alteration of mentation in lines 47–50 indicates a serious and irrevocable condition as opposed to the less serious expression used in lines 51–55.

28. See Scurlock and Andersen 2005, 16.35, 19.33, 19.281, 20.5.

29. See Scurlock and Andersen 2005, 16.34.

30. See Scurlock and Andersen 2005, 16.40, 19.281.

31. See Scurlock and Andersen 2005, 13.252, 20.7 correcting Heeßel 2000, 255.

32. See Scurlock and Andersen 2005, 16.36, 19.22, 19.282.

33. See Scurlock and Andersen 2005, 16.37, 19.34.

34. See Scurlock and Andersen 2005, 16.38, 19.1.

35. See Scurlock and Andersen 2005, 16.42.

36. See Scurlock and Andersen 2005, 16.50, 20.74.

37. See Scurlock and Andersen 2005, 19.291.

38. See Scurlock and Andersen 2005, 19.242.

39. See Scurlock and Andersen 2005, 20.59.

40. See Scurlock and Andersen 2005, 16.74, 19.7, 19.63.

41. See Scurlock and Andersen 2005, 16.75, 19.9, 19.63.

42. See Scurlock and Andersen 2005, 19.63.

43. See Scurlock and Andersen 2005, 20.71.

44. See Scurlock and Andersen 2005, 2.16.

45. See Scurlock and Andersen 2005, 20.76.

46. The translation assumes an otherwise unattested form of *itulu*.
47. See Scurlock and Andersen 2005, 3.158.
48. See Scurlock and Andersen 2005, 2.8, 20.77.
49. See Scurlock and Andersen 2005, 8.98.
50. See Scurlock and Andersen 2005, 20.73.
51. Differently Heeßel 2000, 257.
52. Correcting Heeßel 2000, 257.

DPS 23

DPS 22:79 (catchline) = DPS 23:1

1. DIŠ GIG [ZÉ][1] *ip-ru* UD.DA TAB.BA ŠU DINGIR AD-*šú*
2. [DIŠ *it-te-né*]-*ep-ru* ŠU NAM.ÉRIM.MA *šá* […]
3. [DIŠ *ip-ra-am*]-*ma ana* ZAG-*šú* BAL-*it u* ZI-*b*[*i* …]
4. [DIŠ *ip-ru-ma* ZA]G *u* GÙB SÌG-*iṣ* ŠU! *šag-ga-š*[*i* GAM]
5. [DIŠ *ip-ru-ma*] *ana ḫu-ḫa-ti-šú* NIM *la is-niq* Ú[Š]

---

6. [DIŠ …]x DU-*ak* IGI^{II}-*šú bal-ṣa* : *na-bal-ku-ta*$_5$ Š[U …]
7. [DIŠ …]x DU-*ak* IGI.MEŠ-*šú* : UZU.MEŠ-*šú* GI$_6$.MEŠ *u* x[…]
8. [DIŠ … DU.M]EŠ SAG.KI GÙB SÌG-*iṣ* BA.ÚŠ
9. [DIŠ … *ina*] KA/KIR$_4$-*šú* MÚD *pe-la-a* ŠUB.ŠUB BA.ÚŠ
10. [DIŠ … *ina* KA/KIR$_4$-*šú* MÚD MUD ŠU]B.ŠUB-*a* BA.ÚŠ
11. [DIŠ …]x AD$_6$-*šú* KÚM-*em* ŠU DINGIR-*šú ana* U$_4$.32.KÁM B[A.Ú]Š
12. [DIŠ …] *ka-si* DIB-*su*

---

13. (fragmentary)

(gap of 35 entries)

14′. (fragmentary)

15′. DIŠ […]x *u* ⸢A⸣ UL$_4$.GAL APIN⸣-[*iš*…]

16′. DIŠ *i*-⸢x x⸣ *u* A UL$_4$.GAL APIN-*iš-ma* NAG ŠU DINGIR-*šú* x[…]

17′. DIŠ *ir-te*-⸢*eq*⸣ *u* A UL$_4$.GAL APIN-*iš* : *i-la-ab*-[*bi* …]

18′. DIŠ GA UGU-*šú* DÙG-*ab* GIG-*su* GÍD.DA-*ma ni-kit-tú* T[UKU-*ši*]

19′. [DIŠ] GIG ^{GIŠ}ḪAŠḪUR APIN-*iš*

TRANSLATION

1. If the patient vomits [bile] (and) he burns with *ṣētu*, "hand" of his father's god.[2]

2. [If he continually] ⸢vomits⸣, “hand” of the curse of […].
3. [If he vomits] and then rolls to his “right” and gets up […].
4. [If he vomits(?) and] he was wounded on the ⸢“right”⸣ or “left” side, “hand” of a murderous (ghost); [he will die].[3]
5. [If he vomits and] flies will not come near his vomitus, he will die.[4]

---

6. [If] … flows, his eyes are dilated (var. roll), ⸢“hand”⸣ [of …].
7. [If] … flows (and) his face (var. flesh) is dark/black and […].
8. [If … flows] continuously (and) he was wounded (on) his “left” temple; he will die.
9. [If …] (and) he produces red blood [from] his nose/mouth, he will die.
10. [If …] (and) he produces dark blood [from] his nose/mouth, he will die.
11. [If …] (and) his body is hot, “hand” of his god. (If he is sick) for thirty-two days, he will die.
12. [If …] afflicts him.

(gap of 37 entries)

15′. If […] and he asks for a lot of water […].
16′. If […] and he asks for a lot of water and drinks it, “hand” of his god […].
17′. If he is withdrawn and he asks for a lot of water (var. he ⸢groans⸣) […].
18′. If milk tastes good to him (and) if his illness is prolonged, he will ⸢have⸣ a cause for worry.

19′. If the patient asks for an apple […].

NOTES

1. Restored from commentary Cornell University 193:1 (Heeßel 2000, 273).
2. See Scurlock and Andersen 2005, 3.133.
3. See Scurlock and Andersen 2005, 19.170.
4. This entry appears also in PBS 2/2 104:1.

D. NEUROLOGY: DPS 26–30

DPS 26

2′. [DIŠ ŠUB-*ti* ŠUB-*su-ma* …]-*ut* [ŠU] ^{d}[…]

3′. [DIŠ ŠUB-*ti* ŠUB-*su-ma* U$_4$ ŠUB-*šú*] IGI.MEŠ-[*šú*] SA$_5$ SIG$_7$ [ŠU] KI.SIKIL.LÍL.[LÁ.EN.NA]

4′. [DIŠ ŠUB-*ti* ŠUB-*su-ma* U$_4$ ŠUB-*š*]*ú an-nu-ú šu-ú i-qab-bi be-en-nu ṣa-i-du* DIB-*su uš-*[*t*]*e-*⸢*zeb*⸣

5′. [DIŠ ŠUB-*ti* ŠUB-*su-ma*] *ina* U$_4$.1.KÁM 2-*šú* 3-*šú* KÚR(var. LÁ)-*šum-ma ina šér-ti* SA$_5$ *ina* AN.USAN SIG$_7$ AN.TA.ŠUB.BA

6′. [DIŠ ŠUB-*ti* ŠUB-*su-ma ina* U]$_4$.1.KÁM 2-*šú* 3-*šú* DIB-*su u i-ri-iq* GÍD-*ma ina* ŠUB-*ti* TAB.TAB-*šú*

7′. [DIŠ ŠUB-*ti* ŠUB-*su-ma ina*] ⸢U$_4$⸣-*mi šu-a-tum* 7-*šú uš-ter-de-ma* DIB-*su uš-te-zeb šum-ma* 8-*šú-nu*[1] ŠUB-*aš-šú ul uš-te-*[*zib*]

8′. [DIŠ ŠUB-*ti* ŠUB]-*su-ma* MU.1.KÁM ŠUB-*šú-ma ana* GIZKIM-*šú-ma* LÁ-*šú na-kid* AN.TA.ŠUB.BA *ina ma-šal* U$_4$-*mi uš-ta-qar-rab-šú-ma* DUGUD-*su*

9′–10′. [DIŠ ŠUB]-*ti* ŠUB-*su-ma ina* U$_4$ *šú-a-tum* 7-*šú uš-ter-di-ma i-ḫi-is-su e-nu-ma um-taš-ši-ru-šú i-ṭi-ib* ŠU *šag-ga-ši* GAM

11′–13′. [DIŠ G]IN$_7$ ŠUB-*ti* ŠUB.ŠUB-*su* IGI^{II}-*šú* MÚD DIRI.MEŠ : IGI^{II}-*šú* BAD-*te u* DUL-*am* UNU^{II}-*šú* (var. [M]E.ZÉ-*šú*) *nu-uš-šá* ŠU^{II}-*šú u* GÌR^{II}-*šú tar-ṣa ina sa-naq a-ši-pi i*ʾ*-a-bat ša* DIB-*šú ina-ṭal* ŠU GIDIM$_7$ *šag-ga-ši*

14′. D[IŠ] ⸢GIN$_7$⸣ ŠUB-*šú i-ri-iq-ma ma-gal i-ṣi-iḫ u* GÌR^{II}-*šú it-ta-naq-na-an-na* : ŠU^{II}-*šú u* GÌR^{II}-*šú* ŠU LÍL.LÁ.EN.NA

15′. [DIŠ] LÁ-*šú* LÁ-*šum-ma ina* KA-*šú* ÚḪ DU-*ak* AN.TA.ŠUB.BA

16′. DIŠ [L]Á-*šú* LÁ-*šum-ma* ŠU^{II}-*šú u* GÌR^{II}-*šú ana* GÚ-*šú ik-tab-ba* AN.TA.ŠUB.BA

17′. D[IŠ U]$_4$ LÁ-*šú a-šiš-tum* DIB-*su* ÚḪ *ina* KA-*šú* DU-*ak* ŠÙD AD-*šú* DIB-*su* GAM

18′. [DIŠ U$_4$ L]Á-*šú* TA *iṣ-ṣab-tu-šú* ÚḪ *ina* KA-*šú* DU-*ak* ŠU LÍL.LÁ.EN.NA

19′. [D]IŠ U$_4$ LÁ-*šú* UB.NÍGIN.NA-*šú i-šaḫ-ḫu-ḫa* ŠÀ-*šú* DIB.DIB-*su* ŠÀ.MEŠ-*šú* SI.SÁ.MEŠ-*šú* ŠU GIDIM$_7$

20′–21′. DIŠ U[$_4$] LÁ-*šú* UB.NÍGIN.NA-*šú i-šam-ma-ma-šú* IGI.MEŠ-*šú* NIGIN.MEŠ-*du* ŠÀ-*šú i-šaḫ-ḫu-uḫ u mim-ma šá ana* KA-*šú* GAR-*ár ina* U$_4$-*me-šú ma-ti-ma ina* DÚR-*šú* ŠUB-*šú* ŠU GIDIM$_7$ *šá ina šag-gaš-ti* GAM

22′–25′. ⸢DIŠ⸣ U$_4$ LÁ-*šú* UB.NÍGIN.NA-*šú i-šam-ma-ma-šú i-re-eḫ-ḫi-šum-ma* NÍ-*šú i-maš-ši* U$_4$ *ir-te-ḫu-šú* IGI^{II}-*šú* SAR-*ṭa* IGI.MEŠ-*šú* SA$_5$: *suḫ$_4$-ḫu-ru* SA.MEŠ-*šú* ZI.MEŠ *u i-leb-bu ap-pat* U.MEŠ ŠU^{II}-*šú u* GÌR^{II}-*šú ka-ṣa-a* GIG BI MAŠ.MAŠ *ú-šad-bab-šú-ma ša ú-šad-ba-bu-šú i-qab-bi* U$_4$ *un-deš-ši-ru-šú šá id-bu-bu* NU ZU ŠU LÍL.LÁ.EN.NA *la-ʾ-bi*

26′–27′. DIŠ U$_4$ LÁ-*šú ta-lam-ma-šú* DUGUD-*su u ú-zaq-qat-su* EGIR-*nu* LÁ-*šum-ma* NÍ-*šú i-maš-ši* AN.TA.ŠUB.BA *ina ma-šal* U$_4$-*mi* DUGUD-*su*

28′–29′. DIŠ U$_4$ LÁ-*šú* SAG.KI^{II}-*šú* GU$_7$.MEŠ-*šú* ŠÀ-*šú* GAZ.MEŠ-*šú* EGIR-*nu* ŠU^{II}-*šú u* GÌR^{II}-*šú ú-kap-p*[*ár*] BAL.BAL-*ut* ÚḪ NU TUKU : *it-ta-nag-ra-ár* ŠUB-*tu* : *ḫa-mi-tum* ŠU ^{d}15 ZI-*bi*

30′. DIŠ U$_4$ LÁ-*šú* ŠU^{II}-*šú* IGI.BAR-*as* BABBAR IGI^{II}-*šú* BAL-*ut u* MÚD *ina* KIR$_4$-*šú* DU-*ku ana* MUNUS LÍL.LÁ.EN.NA *ana* NITA MUNUS. LÍL.LÁ.EN.NA

31′. DIŠ DIB-*su ina* AN.USAN DIB.DIB-*su* DIB GIDIM$_7$

32′. DIŠ DIB-*su ina* AN.USAN DIB.DIB-*su* SAG.ŠÀ-*šú* MÚ.MEŠ-*aḫ u* GÌR^{II}-*šú* ÍL-*a* DIB GIDIM$_7$

33′. DIŠ DIB-*su ina* AN.USAN DIB.DIB-*su* ŠÀ.MEŠ-*šú* MÚ.MEŠ-*ḫu* EN EN.NUN.MURUB$_4$.BA *id-lip* DIB GIDIM$_7$

34′. DIŠ DIB-*su ina* AN.USAN DIB.DIB-*su* IGI^{II}-*šú ur-ru-pa* GEŠTU^{II}-*šú* GÙ.DÉ.MEŠ DIB GIDIM$_7$

35′. DIŠ DIB-*su ina* AN.USAN DIB.DIB-*su u* GEŠTU^{II}-*šú* GÙ.DÉ.MEŠ DIB GIDIM$_7$

36′. DIŠ DIB-*su ina* AN.USAN DIB.DIB-*su u* GEŠTU^{II}-*šú i-šam-ma-ma-šú* DIB GIDIM$_7$

37′. DIŠ DIB-*su ina* AN.USAN DIB.DIB-*su u* SAG.KI-*šú* GU$_7$-*šú* DIB GID[IM$_7$]

38′. DIŠ KI.MIN U$_4$ DIB-*šú* KÚM TA EN.NUN.AN.USAN EN EN.NUN. MURUB$_4$.BA *id-da-lip-šú* DIB GID[IM$_7$]

39′. DIŠ KI.MIN U$_4$ DIB-*šú an-nu-ú šu-ú i-qab-bi* ŠU KI.SIKIL.LÍL.L[Á. EN.NA]

40′. DIŠ *šá* DIB DIB.DIB-*su* U$_4$ DIB-*šú* IGI.MEŠ-*šú* SA$_5$ *u* SIG$_7$ ŠU KI.SIKIL. LÍL.[LÁ.EN.NA]

41′. DIŠ *šá* DIB DIB.DIB-*su* U$_4$ DIB-*šú* ŠU^{II}-*šú u* GÌR^{II}-*šú* SIG$_7$.MEŠ ŠU LÍL.LÁ.EN.N[A]

42′. DIŠ *šá* DIB DIB.DIB-*su* U$_4$ DIB-*šú* ŠU^{II}-*šú u* IGI.ME-*šú ú-maš-šad* GIDIM$_7$ *šá ina* A ÚŠ DIB-*su ina ma-šal* U$_4$-*mi* DUGUD-*su* : MAŠKIM ÍD SÌG-*s*[*u*]

43′–44′. DIŠ *šá* DIB-*šú šu-te-eq-ru-ub* U$_4$ LÁ-*šú* ŠU^{II}-*šú* GIN$_7$ *šá ku-uṣ-ṣú* DIB-*šú i-ḫe-es-*⸢*si*⸣ GÌR^{II}-*šú* LAL-*aṣ u ma-gal* LUḪ-*ut-ma ina-aḫ* DIB-*su* IGI.BAR-*as* ŠU *ʾe-e-li*

45′–47′. DIŠ *ina* EN.NUN.MURUB$_4$.BA *šá* DIB DIB.DIB-*su* U$_4$ DIB-*šú* ŠU^{II}-*šú u* GÌR^{II}-*šú ka-ṣa-a ma-gal ú-te-te-eṭ-ṭe* KA-*šú* BAD.BAD-*te* IGI.MEŠ-*šú* SA$_5$ *u* SIG$_7$ MURUB$_4$.ME-*šú* ŠUB.ŠUB-*di* ŠU KI.SIKIL.LÍL.LÁ.EN.NA GÍD-*ma* GAM : *ana* MUNUS LÍL.LÁ.EN.NA *ana* NITA MUNUS.LÍL.LÁ.EN.NA

48′–49′. DIŠ *ina ṣa-lu-ti-šú* DIB-*su-ma* DIB-*su* IGI.BAR-*as i-re-eḫ-ḫi-šum-ma* NÍ-*šú i-maš-ši* GIN$_7$ *šá id-ku-šú* MUD-*ud* ZI.ZI-*bi* : U$_4$ *id-de-ku-šú re-ḫi* ŠU LÍL.LÁ.EN.NA *sar-ru ana* MUNUS LÍL.LÁ.EN.NA ZI.ZI-*bi*

50′. DIŠ *ina* U$_4$.GURUM.MA DIB-*su* DIB.DIB-*su* U$_4$ DIB-*šú* KÚM NU *ma-dam-ma u* IR.ME[Š] SAG.KI-*šú* IGI^{II}-*šú i-se-ʾa u* ŠÀ-*šú* GU$_7$-*šú* ŠU GIDIM$_7$

51′–52′. DIŠ *la-am* DIB-*šú ru-qiš* GI[N$_7$ ⸢x x x x⸣-*ki it-tap-la-as* GIN$_7$ *it-tap-la-su da-da-nu-šú* GU$_7$.MEŠ-*šú ba-mat-s*[*u* …] ŠUB-*ti* ŠUB.ŠUB-*su* ŠU GIDIM$_7$ *šag-ga-ši* GAM

53′–55′. DIŠ *la-ma* DIB-*šú* IGI.MEŠ[-*šú* …]-*su ne-ḫu* ŠU^{II}-*šú u* GÌR^{II}-*šú am-šá mi-na-tu-šú i-ṭa-ma-a* [… ŠU LÍL.LÁ.EN.N]A *la-ʾ-bi šum-ma* U$_4$ DIB-*š*[*ú* …]-*ku* […] G[IG.BI …]

56′–57′. (fragmentary)

58′. [… G]U$_4$.UD.MEŠ […]-*šú* ŠU^{II}-*šú u* GÌR^{II}-*šú* […]

59′–60′. (fragmentary)

61′. […] x-*šú* GU$_7$.MEŠ-*šú-ma la i-ṣal-*[*la*]*l* ŠU GI[DIM$_7$]

62′–63′. [DIŠ U$_4$] DIB-*šú* GIN$_7$ *áš-bu-ma* IGI-*šú i-ṣap-par* NUNDUN-*su ip-paṭ-ṭar* ÚḪ *ina* KA-*šú* DU-*ak* ŠU-*su* GÌR-*šú ta-lam-ma-šú šá* 150 GIN$_7$ UDU.NÍTA *ṭa-ab-ḫi i-nap-pa-aṣ* AN.TA.ŠUB.B[A] *šum-ma* U$_4$ DIB-*šú* ŠÀ-*šú e-er* ZI-*aḫ šum-ma* U$_4$ DIB-*šú* ŠÀ-*šú* NU *e-er* NU ZI-*aḫ*

64′–65′. DIŠ U$_4$ DIB-*šú* ŠÀ-*bi* ŠÀ-*bi* GÙ.GÙ-*si* IGI^{II}-*šú* BAD-*te u* DUL-*am* KÚM *li-ʾ-ba i-šu* SAG KIR$_4$-*šú ú-lap-pat ap-pat* ŠU.SI.MEŠ ŠU^{II}-*šú u* GÌR^{II}-*šú* ŠED$_7$-*a* GIG *šú-a-tu tu-šad-bab-šú-ma la ip-pal* ŠU LÍL.LÁ.EN.NA

66′–68′. DIŠ U$_4$ DIB-*šú* ŠÀ-*bi* ŠÀ-*bi* GÙ.GÙ-*si* IGI^{II}-*šú* BAD-*te u* DUL-*am* KÚM *li-ʾ-ba i-šu* SAG KIR$_4$-*šú ú-lap-pat ap-pat* ŠU.SI.MEŠ ŠU^{II}-*šú u* GÌR^{II}-*šú ka-ṣa-a* GIG DIB-*šú ina-ṭal* KI-*šú* DUG$_4$.DUG$_4$-*ub u* NÍ-*šú ut-ta-na-kar* ŠU LÍL.LÁ.EN.NA *la-ʾ-bi*

69′–70′. DIŠ U$_4$ U$_6$.SÁ *i-re-eḫ-ḫu-šu* U.MEŠ ŠU^{II}-*šú u* GÌR^{II}-*šú i-nap-pa-ṣa* AN.TA.ŠUB.BA *ina ni-du-ti* KI.MIN *ina túb-qí* DIB-*su*

71′. DIŠ UB.NÍGIN.NA-*šú i-tar-ru-ra i-ṭa-ma-a u* IGI.MEŠ-*šú* NIGIN. MEŠ-*du* AN.TA.ŠUB.BA *ina ma-šal* U$_4$-*mi* DUGUD-*su*

72′. DIŠ UB.NÍGIN.NA-*šú i-šam-ma-ma-šú ú-zaq-qa-ta-šú u* IGI.ME-*šú* NIGIN.ME-*du* AN.TA.ŠUB.BA *ina ma-šal* U$_4$-*mi* DUGUD-*su*

73′–74′. DIŠ UB.NÍGIN.NA-*šú* GIN$_7$ *šá bal-ṭi ne-ḫa* IGI^{II}-*šú* BAD.MEŠ-*ma* U$_4$ DIB-*su ina-ṭal* KI-*šú* DUG$_4$.DUG$_4$-*ub u* NÍ-*šú ut-ta-na-kar* ŠU LÍL. LÁ.EN.NA DUMU *šip-ri šá* DINGIR-*šú*

75′. DIŠ UB.NÍGIN.NA-*šú* GIN$_7$ *šá bal-ṭi ne-ḫa* KA-*šú* DIB-*ma* NU DUG$_4$. DUG$_4$-*ub* ŠU GIDIM$_7$ *šag-ga-ši* : ŠU GIDIM$_7$ *qa-li-i*

76′. DIŠ UB.NÍGIN.NA-*šú* GIN$_7$ *šá bal-ṭi ne-ḫa-ma i-qá-al u mim-ma la i-lim* ŠU GIDIM$_7$ *šag-ga-ši šá-niš* ⌈ŠU GIDIM$_7$ *qa-li-i*⌉

77′. DIŠ *u$_8$-a a-i* GÙ.GÙ-*si i-leb-bu* ÚḪ *ina* KA-*šú* DU-*ak u* GÚ-*su ana* 150 *zi-ir* AN.TA.ŠUB.B[A]

78′–79′. DIŠ *i-te-ner-ru-ub* TÚG-*su* ŠUB.ŠUB-*di iš-ta-na-su ma-gal* DU[G$_4$. DUG$_4$-*ub*] NINDA *u* KAŠ NU GUR-*ma* GU$_7$ *u la i-ṣal-lal* ŠU ^{d}15 GAR ⌈TI⌉

80′. DIŠ KI.MIN IGI^{II}-*šú ú-zaq-qap* SÌG-*su ina* SAG-*šú* GUB-*az* GAM

81′. DIŠ *i-ta-nar-ra-ar* IGI^{II}-*šú ú-zaq-qap* SÌG-*su ina* SAG-*šú* GUB-*ma* ⌈GAM⌉

82′–83′. DIŠ *pa-rid-ma it-te-né-et-bi ma-gal* DUG$_4$.DUG$_4$-*ub u i*[*g-d*]*a*-⌈*na*⌉-*al-lu-u*[*t*] *ana* MUNUS LÍL.L[Á].EN.NA *ana* NITA MUNUS.LÍL.LÁ.EN. NA ZI.ZI-*bi*

84′. DIŠ *ina* GIG-*šú* M[UD].MUD-*ud* : *ina* KI.NÁ-*šú* LUḪ.LUḪ *u* GIŠ.KUN. ME-*šú* ÍL.MEŠ *ù* KI.SIKIL.LÍL.LÁ.EN.NA *ina* [...] TAG-*ma be-en-nu*

85′. DIŠ MUD.MUD-*ud* ŠU ^{d}*Ur-bi-li-ti*

86′–87′. DIŠ *ik-kil-lu* GÙ.GÙ-*šú u šu-ú i-ta-nap-pal-šú* U_4 GÙ.GÙ-*šú at-ta*$_5$ *man-nu* DUG_4.GA *mu-ut-til*(!)-*lu*^{MUŠEN} TAG-*ma* KI-*šú* KEŠDA *ina* SAG-*šú* GUB-*az* GAM

88′. DIŠ *ik-kil-lu* GÙ.GÙ-*šú u šu-ú i-ta-nap-pal-šú* ZI-*bi u* DU_{10}.GAM-*is* MAŠKIM *ḫur-ba-ti* DIB-*su*

89′–90′. DIŠ *ik-kil-lu* GÙ.GÙ-*šú* U_4 GÙ.GÙ-*šú i-ta-nap-pal-šú it-ta-na-as-pak* ZI-*ma i-káš-šú-uš* ZI-*bi u* DU_{10}.GAM GIG-*su uš-te-zeb* MAŠKIM *mur-tap-pi-du* DIB-*su*

Translation

2′. [If a falling spell falls upon him and …] he [continually jerks(?)], [“hand”] of […].

3′. [If a falling spell falls upon him and when it falls upon him, his] face flushes and turns pale, [“hand”] of *ardat lilî*.[2]

4′. [If a falling spell falls upon him and when it falls upon] ⌜him⌝, he says “This is it,” spinning *bennu* afflicts him; ⌜he will come through⌝.[3]

5′. [If a falling spell falls upon him and] (his mentation) alters (var. [the falling spell] comes over him) two or three times a day and in the morning he flushes (and) in the evening he turns pale, AN.TA.ŠUB.BA.[4]

6′. [If a falling spell falls upon him and] it afflicts him two or three times a ⌜day⌝ and he turns pale, if it is prolonged, it begins with/grows out of the falling spell.[5]

7′. [If a falling spell falls upon him and] it afflicts him seven times on the same day one after the other, he will come through. If eight of them[6] fall on him, he will not ⌜come through⌝.[7]

8′. [If a falling spell falls] upon him and it has been falling upon him for one year and as its sign it comes over him, it is worrisome. If the AN.TA.ŠUB.BA comes closely spaced (and) in the middle of the day, it will be difficult for him.[8]

9′–10′. [If a falling] spell falls on him and, on the same day, (confusional states) come over him seven times one right after the other (and), when (the confusional state) has left him, he feels better, “hand” of a murderous (ghost); he will die.[9]

11′–13′. [If] it continually falls upon him ⌜like⌝ a falling spell (and) his eyes are full of blood var. he opens and closes his eyes, his cheeks (var. ⌜jaws⌝) shake, his hands and his feet are stretched out, he collapses at the approach of the *āšipu* (and) he can see the one who afflicts him, "hand" of a murderous ghost.[10]

14′. ⌈If⌉ when (a falling spell) falls upon him, he turns pale and laughs a lot and his feet (var. his hands and his feet) are continually contorted, "hand" of *lilû*.[11]

15′. [If] his confusional state comes over him and spittle flows from his mouth, AN.TA.ŠUB.BA.[12]

16′. If his ⌈confusional⌉ state comes over him and he bends his hands and his feet towards his neck,[13] AN.TA.ŠUB.BA.[14]

17′. ⌈If when⌉ (a confusional state) comes over him, depression afflicts him (and) spittle flows from his mouth, a vow made by his father afflicts him; he will die.

18′. [If when (a confusional state)] ⌈comes⌉ over him, after it afflicts him, spittle flows from his mouth, "hand" of *lilû*.

19′. ⌈If⌉ when it comes over him, his limbs waste away (and) his abdomen continually afflicts him (and) his bowels are continually loose,[15] "hand" of ghost.[16]

20′–21′. If ⌈when⌉ it comes over him, his limbs go numb, his face seems continually to spin, his abdomen wastes away and whatever he puts to his mouth is always excreted from his anus on the very same day, "hand" of a ghost who died through murder.[17]

22′–25′. If when it comes over him, his limbs go numb, as it flows over him he "forgets himself," when it has flowed over him, his eyes (look) "(wind) blasted,"[18] his face flushes (var. he turns away), his blood vessels (feel like they) are pulsating and he groans, the tips of his fingers and toes are cold (and) the *āšipu* makes that patient say (something) and (the patient) says what (the *āšipu*) has him say (but) when (the confusional state) has left him, (the patient) does not know what he said, "hand" of *lilû* (of) *li*ʾ*bu*.[19]

26′–27′. If when (a confusional state) comes over him, his torso (feels) heavy and stings him (and) afterwards it comes over him and he loses consciousness, AN.TA.ŠUB.BA. (If this happens) in the middle of the day, it will be difficult for him.[20]

28′–29′. If when (a confusional state) comes over him, his temples continually hurt him, he continually has a crushing sensation in his heart (and) afterwards he ⌈rubs⌉ his hands and his feet, he rolls over and over (but) he does not have any spittle, var. he rolls over and over, falling spell, var. paralysis, of "hand" of Ishtar; he can get up (afterwards).[21]

30′. If when (a confusional state) comes over him, he gazes at his hands, he rolls the whites of his eyes and blood runs from his nose, for a woman, *lilû*; for a man, a *lilītu*.[22]

31′. If his affliction always afflicts him in the evening, affliction by a ghost.[23]

32′. If his affliction always afflicts him in the evening (and) his epigastrium is continually bloated and his feet are puffed up, affliction by a ghost.[24]

33′. If his affliction always afflicts him in the evening (and) his insides are continually bloated (and) it keeps (him) awake until the middle watch, affliction by a ghost.[25]

34′. If his affliction always afflicts him in the evening (and) his eyes are clouded (and) his ears roar, affliction by a ghost.[26]

35′. If his affliction always afflicts him in the evening and his ears roar, affliction by a ghost.[27]

36′. If his affliction always afflicts him in the evening and his ears go numb, affliction by a ghost.[28]

37′. If his affliction always afflicts him in the evening and his temples continually hurt him, affliction by a ⸢ghost⸣.[29]

38′. If ditto (his affliction always afflicts him in the evening and) when it afflicts him, fever keeps him awake from the evening watch till the middle watch of the night, affliction by a ⸢ghost⸣.[30]

39′. If ditto (his affliction always afflicts him in the evening and) when it afflicts him, he says "This is it," "hand" of *ardat* ⸢*lilî*⸣.[31]

40′. If that which afflicts continually afflicts him (and) when it afflicts him, his face flushes and turns pale, "hand" of *ardat* ⸢*lilî*⸣.

41′. If that which afflicts continually afflicts him (and) when it afflicts him, his hands and his feet turn pale, "hand" of ⸢*lilû*⸣.

42′. If that which afflicts continually afflicts him (and) when it afflicts him, he rubs his hands and face, the ghost (of one) who died in the water afflicts him. (If this happens) in the middle of the day, it will be difficult for him, var. the *rābiṣu* of the river has struck ⸢him⸣.[32]

43′–44′. If what afflicts him does so in close sequence (and) when it comes over him, he wrings his hands like one whom cold afflicts, he stretches out his feet, he jerks a lot and then is quiet, (and) he gazes at the one who afflicts him, "hand" of the binder.[33]

45′–47′. If that which afflicts continually afflicts him during the middle watch of the night (and) when it afflicts him his hands and his feet are cold, he continually becomes darkened (i.e., loses consciousness), he continually opens his mouth, his face flushes and turns pale (and) he continually lets his hips drop, "hand" of *ardat lilî*. If it is prolonged, he will die, var. for a woman, a *lilû*; for a man, a *lilītu*.[34]

48′–49′. If it afflicts him in his sleep and he gazes at the one who afflicts him, it flows over him and he forgets himself, he shudders like one whom they have awakened (and) he can still get up (var. when they try to wake him, he is groggy), false "hand" of *lilû*. For a woman, a *lilû*; he can get up (afterwards).[35]

50′. If his affliction always afflicts him at midday (and) when it afflicts him, his temperature does not seem very high but sweat presses down on his temples (and) his eyes, and his abdomen hurts him, "hand" of ghost.[36]

51′–52′. If before it afflicts him, he gazes at something very far off ⸢like⸣ [a ...] (and) when he gazes at it, his neck muscles continually hurt him, ⸢his⸣ chest [...] (and) a falling spell continually falls upon him, "hand" of a murderous ghost; he will die.[37]

53′–55′. If, before it afflicts ⸢him⸣, [his] face [...], his [...] is calm, his hands and his feet are immobilized, his limbs twist [... "hand" of *lilû*] (of) *li ʾbu*. If when it afflicts ⸢him⸣ [...], [that] ⸢patient⸣ [will not live].[38]

56′–57′. *(fragmentary)*

58′. [If ...] jump ... his hands and feet [...].

59′–60′. *(fragmentary)*

61′. [If ...] his [ears?] hurt him so that he cannot ⸢sleep⸣, "hand" of ⸢ghost⸣.

62′–63′. [If when] it afflicts him, as he is sitting, his eye flutters, his lips come apart, his spittle flows from his mouth, his hand, his foot (and) his "left" torso thrash around like (those of) a slaughtered sheep, AN.TA.ŠUB.BA. If, when it afflicts him, his heart is awake, it can be removed; if, when it afflicts him, his heart is not awake, it cannot be removed.[39]

64′–65′. If when it afflicts him, he continually cries out: "My insides, my insides!," he opens and shuts his eyes, he has *li ʾbu* fever, he rubs the bulb of his nose, the tips of his fingers and toes are cold (and if) you try to make that patient talk, he does not answer, "hand" of *lilû*.[40]

66′–68′. If when it afflicts him, he continually cries out: "My insides, my insides!," he opens and shuts his eyes, he has *li ʾbu* fever, he rubs the bulb of his nose, the tips of his fingers and toes are cold, he can see the illness which afflicts him, he talks with it and continually changes his self, "hand" of *lilû* (of) *li ʾbu*.[41]

69′–70′. If, when a stupor flows over him, his fingers and toes thrash around, AN.TA.ŠUB.BA. It afflicted him in an abandoned place or in a corner.[42]

71′. If his limbs tremble (and) twist and his face seems continually to spin,[43] AN.TA.ŠUB.BA. (If this happens) in the middle of the day, it will be difficult for him.

72′. If his limbs go numb (and) sting him and his face seems continually to spin, AN.TA.ŠUB.BA. (If this happens) in the middle of the day, it will be difficult for him.[44]

73′–74′. If his limbs are as still as those of a healthy person, (and) he continually opens his eyes and, when he sees the one who afflicts him, he talks with him and continually changes his self, "hand" of *lilû*, messenger of his god.[45]

75′. If his limbs are as still as those of a healthy person (but) his mouth is "seized" so that he cannot talk, "hand" of a murderous ghost, variant: hand of the ghost of someone burned to death.[46]

76′. If his limbs are as still as those of a healthy person (but) he is silent and does not take any food, "hand" of a murderous ghost, variant: "hand" of the ghost of someone burned to death.[47]

77′. If he continually cries out: "Oh woe!," he groans, his spittle flows from his mouth and his neck is twisted to the "left," AN.TA.ŠUB.BA.[48]

78′–79′. If he keeps beginning to put on and throwing off his garments, he continually cries out(!), he ⸢talks⸣ a lot, bread and beer do not come back up on him so that he can eat but he cannot sleep, the "hand" of Ishtar is laid (on him); he will get well.[49]

80′. If ditto (he continually goes through the motions of getting into and out of his clothing and) he makes (the pupils of) his eyes constrict, the one who strikes him stands at his head; he will die.[50]

81′. If he continually trembles (and) makes (the pupils of) his eyes constrict, the one who strikes him stands at his head and consequently he will die.[51]

82′–83′. If he shudders and he can get up (afterwards), he talks a lot and he continually ⸢jerks⸣, for a woman, a *lilû*, for a man, a *lilītu*; he can get up (afterwards).[52]

84′. If during his illness, he continually shudders (var. he jerks in his bed), and he raises his pelvis, (and) if *ardat lilî* "touches" (him) during [the night? …], *bennu*.[53]

85′. If he continually shudders, "hand" of Ishtar of Arbela.

86′–87′. If a mournful cry continually cries out to him and he continually answers it (and) when it cries out to him, he says: "Who are you?," a *muttillu* has touched him and is bound with him (and) stands at his head; he will die.[54]

88′. If a mournful cry continually cries out to him and he continually answers it (and) he gets up and (has to) squat down, the *rābiṣu* of the wastes afflicts him.[55]

89′–90′. If a mournful cry continually cries out to him (and) when it cries out to him, he continually answers it, he behaves like an animal caught in a trap[56] (and) when he gets up, he feels exhausted, he gets up and (has to) squat down, he will come through his illness; a roving *rābiṣu* afflicts him.[57]

Notes

1. Correcting Heeßel 2000, 279.
2. See Scurlock and Andersen 2005, 19.58.
3. See Scurlock and Andersen 2005, 3.269, 13.202. The entry appears also in Arnaud 1987, 694 obv. 7′–8′.
4. See Scurlock and Andersen 2005, 13.188, 19.57. The entry appears also in Arnaud 1987, 694 obv. 9′.
5. See Scurlock and Andersen 2005, 13.187. The entry appears also in Arnaud 1987, 694 obv. 10′.
6. Heeßel 2000, 279 follows Stol 1993, 58 in reading *šum-ma* 8-*šú* NU ŠUB-*aš-šú ul uš-te*-[*zib*]: "If it does not fall on him eight times, he will not come through." This makes no sense at all, which led Stol to suggest omitting the "not" from the translation. However, reading instead 8-*šú-nu*: "eight of them" (von Soden, *GAG* §139j) restores the sense, and makes this emendation unnecessary.
7. See Scurlock and Andersen 2005, 13.207.
8. See Scurlock and Andersen 2005, 13.224, 20.13.
9. See Scurlock and Andersen 2005, 13.209.
10. See Scurlock and Andersen 2005, 13.81, 13.204.
11. See Scurlock and Andersen 2005, 13.206, 19.56.
12. See Scurlock and Andersen 2005, 13.171.
13. The reference is to "fetal positon."
14. See Scurlock and Andersen 2005, 13.172.
15. I.e., he has diarrhea.
16. See Scurlock and Andersen 2005, 3.101, 3.116, 19.296.
17. See Scurlock and Andersen 2005, 3.111, 19.296.
18. Correcting Heeßel 2000, 280.
19. See Scurlock and Andersen 2005, 4.29, 13.290.
20. See Scurlock and Andersen 2005, 13.201.
21. See Scurlock and Andersen 2005, 13.42, 16.66.

22. See Scurlock and Andersen 2005, 19.21.
23. See Scurlock and Andersen 2005, 0.2, 19.273.
24. See Scurlock and Andersen 2005, 0.2, 19.273.
25. See Scurlock and Andersen 2005, 0.2, 19.273.
26. See Scurlock and Andersen 2005, 0.2, 19.273.
27. See Scurlock and Andersen 2005, 0.2, 19.273.
28. See Scurlock and Andersen 2005, 0.2, 19.273.
29. See Scurlock and Andersen 2005, 0.2, 19.273.
30. See Scurlock and Andersen 2005, 0.2, 3.9, 19.273.
31. See Scurlock and Andersen 2005, 13.203, 19.55.
32. See Scurlock and Andersen 2005, 19.46.
33. See Scurlock and Andersen 2005, 13.69, 13.199.
34. See Scurlock and Andersen 2005, 19.59.
35. See Scurlock and Andersen 2005, 12.71, 13.73, 16.51, 19.19.
36. See Scurlock and Andersen 2005, 15.17.
37. See Scurlock and Andersen 2005, 13.205.
38. See Scurlock and Andersen 2005, 4.31.
39. See Scurlock and Andersen 2005, 8.4.
40. See Scurlock and Andersen 2005, 19.25.
41. See Scurlock and Andersen 2005, 16.92, 19.24.
42. See Scurlock and Andersen 2005, 13.186
43. See Scurlock and Andersen 2005, 13.198, 20.14.
44. See Scurlock and Andersen 2005, 13.198.
45. See Scurlock and Andersen 2005, 16.69, 16.90, 19.23.
46. See Scurlock and Andersen 2005, 16.46, 19.31.
47. See Scurlock and Andersen 2005, 16.22, 16.47.
48. See Scurlock and Andersen 2005, 13.192.
49. See Scurlock and Andersen 2005, 16.56, 16.88, 19.6.
50. See Scurlock and Andersen 2005, 13.276.
51. See Scurlock and Andersen 2005, 13.277.
52. See Scurlock and Andersen 2005, 12.72, 16.44, 19.20.
53. See Scurlock and Andersen 2005, 3.273.
54. See Scurlock and Andersen 2005, 16.71.
55. See Scurlock and Andersen 2005, 16.72.
56. The verb is otherwise used to describe the action of animals caught in a trap. (see *AHw*; *CAD* S, 157).
57. See Scurlock and Andersen 2005, 13.211, 16.72, 19.61.

DPS 27

DPS 26:86′ (catchline) = DPS 27:1

1. DIŠ *mi-šit-ti pa-ni ma-šid-ma ta-lam-ma-šú i-šam-ma-am-šú* KIN *mi-šit-ti* GIG

2–3. DIŠ *m*[*i-šit-ti im*]*-šid-su-ma ib-ta-luṭ* SAG.KI-*šú* DIB.DIB-*su u* MUD.MUD-*ud m*[*u-ki*]*l* SAG-*šu* NU *pa-ṭir*

4. DIŠ *mi-šit-ti im-šid-su-ma* SAG.KI-*šú* DIB.DIB-*su mu-kil* SAG-*šú ina-ṭal* GAM : SAG.ḪUL.ḪA.ZA IGI GAM

5–7. DIŠ *mi-šit-ti im-šid-su-ma lu* 15 *lu* 150 SÌG-*iṣ* MUD Á-*šú* NU *pa-ṭir* ŠU.SI.MEŠ-*šú* NIR.NIR-*aṣ* ŠU-*su ú-šaq-qá u* NIR-*aṣ* GÌR-*šú i-qan-na-an u* NIR-*aṣ* [NIN]DA *u* KAŠ NU TAR-*us* DIB GIDIM$_7$ *ana* EDIN ‹U$_4$›.3.KÁM *ni-ši*

8. DIŠ *k*[*a-b*]*it-ma lu* ŠU-*su lu* GÌR-*šú iq-ta-na-an mi-šit-ti im-šid-su* DIN

9. DIŠ Z[A]G-*šú tab-kát mi-šit-ti* MAŠKIM DIN

10. [DIŠ ZA]G AD$_6$-*šú ka-lu-šú-ma tab-kát mi-šit-ti* MAŠKIM EGIR-*ta*$_5$ SÌG-*iṣ*

11. [DIŠ GÙ]B-*šú tab-kát-šú* ŠU ^{d}*Šu-lak*

12–13. DIŠ ⸢GÙB⸣ AD$_6$-*šú ka-lu-šú-ma tab-kát* GABA.RI SÌG-*iṣ* ŠU ^{d}Šu-lak MAŠKIM *mu-sa-a-ti* MAŠ.MAŠ *ana* DIN-*šú* ME-*a* NU GAR-*an*

14–15. DIŠ NA *si-mat* IGI.ME-*šú* KÚR.KÚR-*ir* IGI^{II}-*šú it-ta-nap-ra-ra* ⸢NUNDUN⸣-*šú* ⸢*su-qat-su*⸣ *ú-*⸢*lap*⸣*-pat* MÚD *ina* KIR$_4$-*šú* DU-*ka* NU *par-su*[1] NA BI ⸢ḪUL⸣ DIB-*su*

16–17. [DIŠ N]A *ina a-la-ki-šú*[2] *ana* IGI-*šú* ŠUB-*ma* IGI^{II}-*šú ip-pal-ka-ma tur-ra* ⸢*la i*⸣*-da-a* [Š]U^{II}-*šú* GÌR^{II}-*šú ra-man-šú la ú-na-aš* NA BI ḪUL DIB-*su* GIN$_7$ AN.TA.ŠUB.BA *uš-tar-ri-šú*[3] (var.)

18. [DIŠ NA] GIN$_7$ (coll.) AN.TA.ŠUB.BA *ir-te-né-eḫ-ḫi-šú* ŠU^{II}-*šú u* GÌR^{II}-*šú* NÍ-*šú la ú-na-aš* NA BI ḪUL DIB-*su*

19. [DIŠ NA *ma-a*]*m-ma* IGI-*ma* TÚG-*su it-ta-na-as-suk ú-rap-pad* IGI^{II}-*šú ú-ma-ḫa-aṣ* NA BI ḪUL DIB-*su*

---

20. [DIŠ NA …]x *ḫa-ṣu-šu iš-du-ud-ma* KÚM-*em u* NÍ-*šú* NU ZU *ina* ÉN IGI^{II}-*šú iz-qup* ŠU A.LÁ ḪUL

21–22. [DIŠ GIN$_7$] Ù.SÁ DIB.DIB-*su* UB.NIGIN.NA-*šú iš-šap-pa-ka* GEŠTU^{II}-*šú* GÙ.‹DÉ›.MEŠ KA-*šú* DIB-*ma* NU DUG$_4$.DUG$_4$-*ub* ŠU A.LÁ ḪUL

23. DIŠ GIN$_7$ Ù.SÁ DIB.DIB-*su* U$_4$ DIB-*šu* GEŠTU^{II}-*šú* GÙ.DÉ.MEŠ KA-*šú* DIB-*ma* NU DUG$_4$.DUG$_4$-*ub* ŠU A.LÁ ḪUL

---

24. DIŠ A.MEŠ *ina* TU$_5$-*šú* TA ÍD *ina* E$_{11}$-*šú* ⸢NIGIN-*ma*⸣ ŠUB-⸢*ut*⸣ [MA]ŠKIM ÍD SÌG-[*s*]*u* (coll.)

25. DIŠ TA A.MEŠ *ina* E$_{11}$-*šú* AD$_6$-*šú iḫ-mi-šu-ma* NIGIN-*ma* ŠUB-*ut* MAŠKIM ÍD SÌG-[*s*]*u*

---

26. DIŠ *ip-ru-ur-ma uš-ḫa-ri-ir* GIG BI GIDIM$_7$.MEŠ *ir?-t[e?-né-du-šú]* (coll.)

27–28. DIŠ *uṣ-ṣu-ub* A.MEŠ APIN.MEŠ-*iš* KÚM *mit-ḫar* SA.MEŠ ŠU^{II}-*šú* DU-*k[a]* TA *taš-rit* GI$_6$ EN SA$_9$ EN.NUN *i-leb-bu* ŠU GIDIM$_7$

29–31. DIŠ ZI.IR ŠUB.ŠUB-*su mim-ma šá im-ma-ru ú-ṣal-la* UB.NIGIN.NA-*šú* KÚM *u* IR *u$_4$-mi-šam-ma* TUKU-*ši a-zu-za-a bi-bil* ŠÀ *ma-dam-ma* TUKU.MEŠ EN *ú-bal-lu-niš-šú* ŠÀ *i-ḫa-ḫu* U$_4$ *ú-ba-lu-niš-šú* IGI.BAR-*ma la i-lem* ŠU GIDIM$_7$ *šá ina* A SÌG-[*iṣ*]

32–34. DIŠ *tu-gu-un-šú ú-zaq-qat-su* GEŠTU^{II}-*šú* GÙ.DÉ.MEŠ SÍG SU-*šú* GUB.GUB-⸢*az*⸣ *kal* AD$_6$-*šú* GIN$_7$ *kal-ma-tum i-ba-šú-u i-nam-muš u* ŠU-*su ub-bal-ma la i-ba-aš-šú* : *la ig-gi-ig* ŠU GIDIM UD.DA LÚ GIN$_7$ ^{GIŠ}GIDRU *šá* ^{d}30 GÌR^{II}-*šú* ⸢ŠU⸣ GIDIM$_7$

35–36. DIŠ ^{GIŠ}NÍG.GIDRU *šá* ^{d}30 GAR-*su-ma* GÌR-*šú i-kap-pap u i-tar-ra-aṣ i-ram-mu-um u* ÚḪ *ina* KA-*šú* DU-*ak* GIDIM$_7$ *mur-tap-pi-du ina* EDIN DIB-*su*

Translation

1. If a [person] has a stroke affecting the face and his torso goes numb, he is sick with the effect of the stroke.[4]

2–3. If he has a ⸢stroke⸣ and then gets better (but) his temples continually afflict him and he shudders, the one who ⸢holds⸣ his head has not let go.[5]

4. If he has a stroke and his temples continually afflict him (and) he can see the one who holds his head, he will die.[6]

5–7. If he has a stroke and either his "right" side or his "left" side is affected (and) his shoulder is not released, (but) he can straighten out his fingers (and) he can lift his hand and stretch it out (and) he can bend his foot and stretch it out again (and) he is not off his food or drink, affliction by a ghost at the steppe; recovery in three (days).[7]

8. If it is difficult (for him) to bend either his hand or his foot (and) he has had a stroke, he will get well.[8]

9. If his "right" side is tense, stroke of a *rābiṣu*; he will get well.[9]

10. [If] the entire ⸢"right"⸣ side of his body is tense, stroke of a *rābiṣu* (or) he was wounded from behind.[10]

11. [If] his ⸢"left"⸣ side is tense, "hand" of Shulak.[11]

12–13. If the entire "left" side of his body is tense, he was wounded from in front (or) "hand" of Shulak, the *rābiṣu* of the lavatory; the *āšipu* should not make a prognosis as to his recovery.[12]

14–15. If a person('s) facial appearance changes (for the worse), his eyes are continually disconnected from one another, he rubs his lips and chin and blood does not stop flowing[13] from his nose, a *gallû*[14] afflicts that person.[15]

16–17. [If] as a [person] is walking,[16] he falls down and he opens his eyes wide and does not know how to turn them back, he can not move his hands and feet by himself, a *gallû* afflicts that person. It begins for him[17] like AN.TA.ŠUB.BA.[18]

18. [If] something like AN.TA.ŠUB.BA continually flows over [a person] (and) he cannot move his hands and feet by himself, a *gallû* afflicts that person.[19]

19. [If a person] sees ⌜somebody⌝ and continually throws off his garment, he wanders about (and) strikes his eyes, a *gallû* afflicts that person.[20]

---

20. [If a person] drags his [...] and he is feverish and does not know who he is (and) when (you recite) a recitation (over him), he constricts (the pupils) of his eyes, "hand" of an evil *alû*.

21–22. [If something like] a stupor continually afflicts him and his limbs are tense, his ears roar (and) his mouth is "seized" so that he cannot talk, "hand" of an evil *alû*.[21]

23. If something like a stupor continually afflicts him and, when it afflicts him, his ears roar (and) his mouth is "seized" so that he cannot talk, "hand" of an evil *alû*.[22]

---

24. If when he is bathing, when he comes up from the river, he (feels like he) is spinning and falls down, the ⌜*rābiṣu*⌝ of the river struck him.[23]

25. If when he comes up from the water, his body is paralyzed and he (feels like he) is spinning and falls down, the *rābiṣu* of the river struck him.[24]

---

26. If he is powerless and dazed, ghosts ⌜continually pursue(?)⌝ that patient.[25]

27–28. If he keeps asking for more and more water (but) his temperature is even, the blood vessels of his hands "go," (and) he groans from the beginning of the night till the middle of the watch, "hand" of ghost.[26]

29–31. If worry continually afflicts him (and) he makes supplication to whatever he sees, his limbs are hot and he sweats every day, he has a big appetite at unpredictable times, (and) until they bring him what he wants, he vomits, (but) when they bring it to him he looks at it and doesn't eat it, "hand" of a ghost who was struck in the water.[27]

32–34. If his headband seems to sting him, his ears roar, the hair of his head continually seems to stand on end, his whole body crawls as if there were lice but when he brings his hand up, there is nothing to scratch, "hand" of ghost (with) dehydration, (if) the person (bends and stretches out) his feet as in the scepter of Sîn, "hand" of ghost.[28]

35–36. If the scepter of Sîn has been placed on him so that he bends and stretches out his foot, he drones and saliva flows from his mouth, the hand of a ghost roving in the steppe afflicts him.[29]

NOTES

1. CTN 4.72 i 10′–12′ substitutes: DU-*ku la i-kal-lu-ú*
2. CTN 4.72 i 3′–9′ adds: [*ina*] ⌜E⌝.SÍR.
3. CTN 4.72 i 3′–9′ substitutes: *ir-te-ne-ḫi-šú*.
4. See Scurlock and Andersen 2005, 13.241. This entry is cited in *AMT* 77/1 i 1 as part of an introduction to treatments for stroke.
5. See Scurlock and Andersen 2005, 13.231.
6. See Scurlock and Andersen 2005, 16.70.
7. See Scurlock and Andersen 2005, 13.227, 13.285. This entry is cited in *AMT* 77/1 i 2–4 as part of an introduction to treatments for stroke.
8. See Scurlock and Andersen 2005, 13.239. This entry is cited in *AMT* 77/1 i 5 as part of an introduction to treatments for stroke.
9. See Scurlock and Andersen 2005, 13.228. This entry is cited in *AMT* 77/1 i 6 as part of an introduction to treatments for stroke.
10. See Scurlock and Andersen 2005, 13.126, 19.196. This entry is cited in *AMT* 77/1 i 7 as part of an introduction to treatments for stroke.
11. See Scurlock and Andersen 2005, 13.229. This entry is cited in *AMT* 77/1 i 8 as part of an introduction to treatments for stroke.
12. See Scurlock and Andersen 2005, 13.125, 19.195. This entry is cited in *AMT* 77/1 i 9–10 as part of an introduction to treatments for stroke.
13. CTN 4.72 i 10′–12′ substitutes: "they cannot stop the blood that flows."
14. For a justification for this reading, see Heeßel 2000, 304.
15. See Scurlock and Andersen 2005, 19.177. CTN 4.72 i 10′–14′ (Stadhouders 2011, 39–48) provides treatment for this condition.
16. CTN 4.72 i 3′–9′ adds: "[along] the street."
17. CTN 4.72 i 3′–9′ substitutes: "continually flows over him."
18. See Scurlock and Andersen 2005, 13.212. CTN 4.72 i 3′–9′ (Stadhouders 2011, 39–48) provides treatment for this condition.
19. See Scurlock and Andersen 2005, 13.213. This entry also appears in CTN 4.72 i 26′ (Stadhouders 2011, 39–48).
20. See Scurlock and Andersen 2005, 16.77, 19.26.
21. See Scurlock and Andersen 2005, 13.59, 13.273.
22. See Scurlock and Andersen 2005, 13.274, 19.306.
23. See Scurlock and Andersen 2005, 15.27. This entry also appears in Ni. 470:9–10 (Kraus 1987, 197).

24. See Scurlock and Andersen 2005, 13.41, 15.28, 19.45. This entry also appears in Ni. 470:11 (Kraus, ZA 77:197).

25. See Scurlock and Andersen 2005, 3.102.

26. See Scurlock and Andersen 2005, 3.102, 8.50.

27. See Scurlock and Andersen 2005, 15.16.

28. See Scurlock and Andersen 2005, 10.186, 15.18, 16.68.

29. See Scurlock and Andersen 2005, 15.19. A treatment for this condition appears in BAM 471 ii 21′–25′//BAM 385 i 15′–22′ (Scurlock 2006, no. 224).

DPS 28

1–3. DIŠ *šúm-ma* ŠU.GIDIM.MA *ana* AN.TA.ŠUB.BA GUR-*šú* LÚ BI ŠU DINGIR URU-*šú* GIG *ina* ŠU DINGIR URU-*šú* *KAR*-*šú* UZU A.ZA.LU.LU ŠU.SI TUR AD_6 Ì.SUMUN *lem-nu u* URUDU *ina* KUŠ MUNUSÁŠ.GÀR GÌŠ NU ZU *ina* SA PÉŠ.ÙR.RA GAG.GAG *ina* GÚ-*šú* GAR-*ma* TI.LA

4–6. DIŠ AN.TA.ŠUB.BA *ana* ŠU.GIDIM.MA GUR-*šú* SAG.ḪUL.ḪA.ZA TUKU.TUKU-*ši* ŠU d15 ŠU MAŠKIM *ana* *KAR*-*šú* ÚḪAR.ḪAR NUMUN GIŠESI TÚG MÚD MUNUS SÌG GÌR.PAD.DU A.ZA.LU.LU *ina* KUŠ MUNUSÁŠ.GÀR GÌŠ NU ZU U.ME.NI.GAG.GAG *ina* GÚ-*šú* GAR-*ma* AL.TI

7–10. DIŠ AN.TA.ŠUB.BA *ana* ŠU dINNIN GUR-*šú* ŠU NAM.ERÍM ŠU DINGIR URU-*šú* KI.MIN ŠU dINNIN URU-*šú* *ana* *KAR*-*šú* TÚG MÚD MUNUS *šá* NITA TE SIG_5 IGI AD_6 ÚEME.UR.GI_7 SÍG UR.GI_7 GI_6 NIM UR.GI_7 AMA A SÍG UGU.DUL.BI NITA *u* MUNUS *šur-ši* GIŠDÌḪ *u* GIŠ.ÚGÍR *šá* UGU KI.MAḪ KA.A.AB.BA ŠEM-dNIN.IB *ina* KUŠ MUNUSÁŠ.GÀR GÌŠ NU ZU ŠU.BI.DIDLI.ÀM

11–13. DIŠ ŠU dINNIN *ana* AN.TA.ŠUB.BA GUR-*šú* ŠU d30 : ŠU d15 *ana* *KAR*-*šú* A.RI.A NAM.LÚ.U_{18}.LU KA.A.AB.BA PÉŠ.ḪUL GIŠGI *šá* SÍG *la-aḫ-mu* *zap*$_x$-*pi* UR.GI_7 GI_6 SÍG MUNUS GI_6 SÍG KUN UR.GI_7 GI_6 *ina* SÍG MUNUSÁŠ.GÀR GÌŠ NU ZU BABBAR *u* GI_6 *ina* KUŠ ŠU.BI.DIDLI. ÀM

14–16. DIŠ ŠU dINNIN *ana* dLUGAL.ÙR.RA GUR-*šú* ŠU dUTU *ana* *KAR*-*šú* SUḪUŠ GIŠDÌḪ SUḪUŠ GIŠ.ÚGÍR SUḪUŠ Ú*u*$_5$-*ra-nu-um* NUMUN GIŠMA.NU NUMUN ÚŠAKIRA TÚG MÚD MUNUS ŠEM.dMAŠ *ina* KUŠ MUNUSÁŠ.GÀR GÌŠ NU ZU ŠU.BI.DIDLI.ÀM

17–18. DIŠ ^{d}LUGAL.ÙR.RA *ana* AN.TA.ŠUB.BA GUR-*šú ana* ŠU ^{d}INNIN GUR-*šú* ŠU ^{d}15 *ana KAR-šú* GÌŠ BAL.GI^{KU_6} NUMUN ^{Ú}*u_5-ra-nu-um* ŠEM-^{d}NIN.IB NITA *u* MUNUS *ina* KUŠ ŠU.BI.DIDLI.ÀM

---

19. DIŠ ^{d}LUGAL.ÙR.RA A.RI.A ^{d}ŠUL.PA.È.A *ana* AN.TA.ŠUB.BA GUR-*šú* ŠU DINGIR-*šú* (var. C substitutes: DINGIR URU-*šú*) *ana KAR-šú* KI.MIN

---

20. DIŠ ^{d}LUGAL.ÙR.RA *ana* ŠU ^{d}INNIN GUR-*šú* A.RI.A ^{d}ŠUL.PA.È.A *ana* ŠU.GIDIM.MA GUR-*šú* NU *i-ke-šír*

---

21. *šum$_4$-ma* SAG.ḪUL.ḪA.ZA GIG-*ma ki-ma* GUD GÌR IGI.IGI IGI.LÁ GIG BI NU *i-ke-šir*
22. DIŠ GIG GÍD.DA GIG-*ma ki-ma* ANŠE.KUR.RA IGI.LÁ GIG BI NU *ke-šir*
23. DIŠ KI.MIN UDU IGI.LÁ GIG BI GUR.GUR-*šú* : GAM
24. DIŠ KI.MIN UR.GI$_7$ IGI.LÁ GIG BI GUR.GUR-*šú* GAM
25. DIŠ KI.MIN ŠAḪ IGI.LÁ GIG.BI NU ZI-*aḫ*
26. DIŠ KI.MIN UR.MAḪ IGI.LÁ *ana dar* KI.SIKIL.LÍL.LÁ GUR-*šú*
27. DIŠ KI.MIN UR.BAR.RA IGI.LÁ *ana dar* KI.SIKIL.LÍL.LÁ GUR-*šú*
28. DIŠ KI.MIN DÀRA IGI.LÁ GIG BI AL.TI
29. DIŠ KI.MIN MAŠ.DÀ IGI.LÁ GIG BI AL.TI
30. DIŠ KI.MIN GUD IGI.LÁ *i-la-bir-šum-ma ana na-šar* GIG GUR-*šú*
31. DIŠ KI.MIN ANŠE IGI.LÁ *i-la-bir-šum-ma ana na-šar* GIG GUR-*šú*
32. DIŠ KI.MIN ŠAḪ.GIŠ.GI IGI.LÁ ÉN ŠUB.ŠUB-*šum-ma* AL.TI
33. DIŠ KI.MIN *ana* ŠU.DINGIR.RA GUR-*šú a-ši-pu-us-su* DÙ-*uš-ma* AL.TI
34. DIŠ KI.MIN *ana* ŠU ^{d}INNIN GUR-*šú* KI.MIN
35. DIŠ KI.MIN AD$_6$.MEŠ IGI.IGI-*mar* KI.MIN
36. DIŠ KI.MIN DUMU.MUNUS-*su* IGI.IGI-*mar* NU *na-kid*
37. DIŠ KI.MIN *KAR*.KID IGI.IGI-*mar* GIG BI GÍD.DA NU *na-kid*
38. DIŠ KI.MIN ÍD IGI.IGI-*mar ana* GIG BI *i-tar*
39. DIŠ KI.MIN ḪUR.SAG IGI.IGI-*mar* GIG BI *KAR-šú*
40. DIŠ KI.MIN ^{GIŠ}TIR IGI.IGI-*mar* GIG-*su* ZI-*aḫ*
41. DIŠ KI.MIN ^{GIŠ}GI IGI.IGI-*mar* GIG-*su* ZI-*aḫ*
42. DIŠ KI.MIN ^{GIŠ}KIRI$_6$ IGI.IGI-*mar* GIG-*su* LÚGUD.D[A]
43. DIŠ KI.MIN PÚ IGI.IGI-*mar* GIG-*su i*[-...]

TRANSLATION

1–3. If "hand" of ghost turns into AN.TA.ŠUB.BA, that person is sick with "hand" of his city god; in order to save him from "hand" of his city god, you sew up the flesh of wild animals, the little finger of a corpse, old rancid oil and copper in virgin she-goat skin with *arrabu*-dormouse tendon. If you put it on his neck, he should recover.[1]

4–6. If AN.TA.ŠUB.BA turns into "hand" of ghost, and he continually has a *mukīl reš lemutti* (and) "hand" of Ishtar, "hand" of a *rābiṣu*-demon; to save him, you sew up *ḫašû*-thyme, *ušû*-ebony seed, menstrual rags (and) wild animal bone in virgin she-goat skin. If you put it on his neck, he should recover.[2]

7–10. If AN.TA.ŠUB.BA turns into "hand" of Ishtar, "hand" of curse, "hand" of the god of his city. Alternatively, "hand" of the goddess of his city; to save him, (you sew up) menstrual rags from a woman who has given birth(!) to a son,[3] eye of a corpse, *lišān kalbi*, hair of a black dog, a flea, a dragonfly, hair from a male and female ape, root of *baltu*-thorn and *ašāgu*-thorn that was growing on a grave, *imbû tamtim* (and) *nikiptu* in virgin-she-goat skin. Ditto (If you put it on his neck, he should recover).[4]

11–13. If "hand" of Ishtar turns into AN.TA.ŠUB.BA, "hand" of Sîn (var. "hand" of Ishtar); to save him, (you sew up) "human semen," *imbû tamtim*, a very hairy *ḫulû*-mouse from the canebrake, bristles of a black dog, black hair from a woman (and) hair from a black dogs' tail in skin with black and white hair from a virgin she-goat. Ditto (If you put it on his neck, he should recover).[5]

14–16. If "hand" of Ishtar turns into ^{d}LUGAL.ÙR.RA, "hand" of Shamash; to save him, (you sew up) *baltu*-thorn root, *ašāgu*-thorn root, *urânu* root, *eʾru*-tree seed, *šakirû* seed, menstrual rags (and) *nikiptu* in virgin she-goat skin. Ditto (If you put it on his neck, he should recover).[6]

17–18. If ^{d}LUGAL.ÙR.RA turns into AN.TA.ŠUB.BA (and then) turns into "hand" of Ishtar, "hand" of Ishtar; to save him, (you sew up) the penis of a *šeleppû*-tortoise, *urânu* seed, (and) male and female *nikiptu* in skin. Ditto (If you put it on his neck, he should recover).[7]

---

19. If ^{d}LUGAL.ÙR.RA or "spawn of Šulpaea" turns into AN.TA.ŠUB.BA, "hand" of his god (var. C substitutes: his city god); to save him, ditto (you do exactly the same).[8]

---

20. If ^{d}LUGAL.ÙR.RA turns into "hand" of Ishtar or "spawn of Šulpaea" turns into "hand" of ghost, he will not do well.[9]

---

21. If he is sick with a *mukīl reš lemutti* and just as an ox continually looks at (its own) feet, he looks (at his own feet), that patient will not do well.[10]
22. If he is ill with a prolonged illness and, as a consequence, he sees something like a horse, that patient will not do well.
23. If ditto (he is ill with a prolonged illness and, as a consequence), he sees something like a sheep, that illness will continually take a turn for the worse (var. he will die).
24. If ditto (he is ill with a prolonged illness and, as a consequence), he sees something like a dog, that illness will continually take a turn for the worse (and) he will die.
25. If ditto (he is ill with a prolonged illness and, as a consequence), he sees something like a pig, that illness will not be removed.
26. If ditto (he is ill with a prolonged illness and, as a consequence), he sees something like a lion, it will turn into the ... of *ardāt lilî.*
27. If ditto (he is ill with a prolonged illness and, as a consequence), he sees something like a wolf, it will turn into the ... of *ardāt lilî.*
28. If ditto (he is ill with a prolonged illness and, as a consequence), he sees something like a stag, that patient will get well.
29. If ditto (he is ill with a prolonged illness and, as a consequence), he sees something like a gazelle, that patient will get well.
30. If ditto (he is ill with a prolonged illness and, as a consequence), he sees something like an ox, (even) if it is prolonged, it will turn into a diminution of the illness.
31. If ditto (he is ill with a prolonged illness and, as a consequence), he sees something like a donkey, (even if) it is prolonged, it will turn into a diminution of the illness.
32. If ditto (he is ill with a prolonged illness and, as a consequence), he sees something like a pig of the canebrake, (if) you continually cast spells over him, he will get well.
33. If ditto (he is ill with a prolonged illness and) it turns into "hand" of god, if you treat him, he will get well.

34. If ditto (he is ill with a prolonged illness and) it turns into "hand" of Ishtar, ditto (if you treat him, he will get well).[11]
35. If ditto (he is ill with a prolonged illness and) he continually sees dead persons, ditto (if you treat him, he will get well).
36. If ditto (he is ill with a prolonged illness and) he continually sees his daughter, it is not worrisome.
37. If ditto (he is ill with a prolonged illness and) he continually sees a prostitute, it is not worrisome.
38. If ditto (he is ill with a prolonged illness and) he continually sees a river, he will have a return of that illness.
39. If ditto (he is ill with a prolonged illness and) he continually sees a mountain, his illness will carry him away.
40. If ditto (he is ill with a prolonged illness and) he continually sees a forest, his illness can be removed.
41. If ditto (he is ill with a prolonged illness and) he continually sees a canebrake, his illness can be removed.
42. If ditto (he is ill with a prolonged illness and) he continually sees a garden, his illness will be short.
43. If ditto (he is ill with a prolonged illness and) he continually sees a well, his illness [...].

Notes

1. See Scurlock and Andersen 2005, 19.65.
2. See Scurlock and Andersen 2005, 19.60.
3. Or is this a sexually experienced woman?
4. See Scurlock and Andersen 2005, 19.68.
5. See Scurlock and Andersen 2005, 19.71, 19.267.
6. See Scurlock and Andersen 2005, 19.72, 19.268.
7. See Scurlock and Andersen 2005, 19.69.
8. See Scurlock and Andersen 2005, 19.66.
9. See Scurlock and Andersen 2005, 19.62, 19.70.
10. See Scurlock and Andersen 2005, 13.225.
11. See Scurlock and Andersen 2005, 19.17.

DPS 29

DPS 28:87′ (catchline) = DPS 29:1

1–3. DIŠ ^{d}LUGAL.ÙR.RA KI.BI Ù.TU *ina* GÌR^{II}-*šú* É AD-*šú* BIR-*aḫ* *ana* NU BIR-*aḫ* É AD-*šú* GIN$_7$ ^{d}KÙ.BI *tuš-na-al-šu-ma* ḪUL.BI *i-tab-bal* GIZKIM.BI GIN$_7$ *al-du i-bak-ki i-za-ár ù im-ta-nam-ga-ag*

4–5. DIŠ *ina* MU.3.‹KÁM› ŠUB-*su uš-ta-sak*(*a*)-*pá-ma* ÚŠ *a-na* NU ÚŠ-*šu* ^{Ú}ŠAKIRA *šá ina* U$_4$.⸢30⸣.KÁM ZI SÚD *ina* A ÍD ḪE.ḪE ŠÉŠ.MEŠ-*su-ma* DIN

6–7. DIŠ *ina* MU.7.KÁM ŠUB-*su ina* MU BI ÚŠ *a-na* NU ÚŠ-*šu* DÈ AN.TA.LÙ *ina* U$_4$.30.KÁM *ina* A ÍD ḪE.ḪE ŠÉŠ-*su-ma* AL.⸢TI⸣

8–10. DIŠ *ina* MU.10.KÁM ŠUB-*su ul-tab-bar tás-níq* KUR.RA GAR-*šú ana* ZI-*ḫi* U$_4$-*um* AN.GI$_6$ ^{d}[30 …] *mi-iḫ-*⸢*rit* ^{d}30⸣ ŠUB-*šú* 3 PA.MEŠ *šá* SAḪAR.ŠUB.BA-*a* nun […] x ⸢^{GIŠ}⸣ZI.NA GIŠIMMAR EN AN.GI$_6$ *ú-nam-ma-ru ina* x […]

11–12. [DIŠ *ina* MU.15?.KÁM ŠU]B-*su* DINGIR TUKU-*ši ina* GÌR^{II}-*šú* É AD-*šú i-šár-rù* [*ana* ZI-*ḫi* o o BIL.ZA.ZA SIG]$_7$.SIG$_7$ *šá ina* UGU NÚMUN GUB-*zu ina* KUŠ *ina* SA PÉŠ.ÙR.RA GAG.GAG-*p*[*í ina* GÚ-*šú* GAR-*an-ma* TI-*uṭ*]

13–14. [DIŠ KI.MIN UZ]U NAM.LÚ.U$_{18}$.LU ^{Ú}*an-ki-nu-te* SÚD *ina* A ÍD ḪE.ḪE ŠÉ[Š-*su-ma* UZU NAM.L]Ú.U$_{18}$.LU ^{Ú}*an-ki-nu-te ina* KUŠ ÙZ *ina* SA PÉŠ.ÙR.RA GAG.GAG-*pí ina* GÚ-*šú* [GAR-*an-ma* TI-*uṭ*]

15–17. [DIŠ *ina* MU].20.KÁM ŠUB-*su* NÍG.TUKU NÍG.GA DAGAL.ME *ana* ZI-*ḫi* ^{Ú}LAL ^{Ú}LÚ.U$_1$[$_8$.LU o o NIT]A *u* MUNUS *ina* KUŠ BIL.ZA.ZA SIG$_7$.SIG$_7$ *ina* SA PÉŠ.ÙR.RA GAG.GAG-[*pí*] *ina* GÚ-*šú* ⸢GAR⸣-[*a*]*n* U$_4$.9.KÁM *ina* IM.SA$_5$ *šá* SAḪAR.ŠUB.BA MU$_4$-*šú ina* U$_4$.10.KÁM *tu-še-eṣ-ṣa-*[*šum-ma* ^{d}30 *u* ^{d}UTU NU IGI…] *ina* KAL-*šú* 7-*šú u* 7-*šú* ÍD ⸢*ib-bir*⸣-[*m*]*a* [NU GUR-*šú*]

18–19. DIŠ *ina* MU.30.KÁM ŠUB-*su ina* GÌR^{II}-*šú* É AD-*šú* BIR-*aḫ ana* ZI-*aḫ* [U$_4$].⸢9.KÁM⸣ *ina* I[M.SA$_5$ *šá* SAḪAR.ŠUB.BA M]U$_4$-*šú ina* U$_4$.10.KÁM *tu-še-ṣa-šum-ma* ^{d}30 *u* ^{d}UTU NU IGI [… *ina* K]AL?-*šú* 7-*šú u* 7-*šú* ÍD *ib-*

bir-ma [NU GUR-*šú*]

---

20. [DIŠ *ina* M]U.5[0.KÁM[1] ŠU]B-*su ina* GÌR^{II}-*šú* É AD-*šú* BIR-*aḫ* NU [*i-ke-šir*?]

---

21. [… ^{d}LUGAL].ÙR.RA *ša be-en-n*[*u* …]

22–24. [DIŠ A.RI.A ^{d}ŠU]L.PA.È.A KI.BI Ù.TU *ina* GÌR^{II}-*šú* É AD-*šú* BIR-*aḫ* [*ana* NU BIR-*aḫ*] *bal-ṭú-us-su ana* ÍD ŠUB-*šu-ma* ḪUL-*šú it-*[*tab-bal* GIZKIM.BI GI]N$_7$ *al-du la ib-ki la is-si la im-t*[*a*]-*ga-*⸢*ag*⸣ […] ^{ú}[…]

25–28. [DIŠ *ina* MU].⸢3⸣.KÁM ŠUB-*su* AD-*šú* DINGIR TUKU-*ši* LÚ.TUR BI *ina* MU BI ÚŠ *ana* ZI-*ḫi* [… ^{Ú}LÚ].U$_{18}$.LU *ina* KUŠ BIL.ZA.ZA SIG$_7$.SIG$_7$ *ina* SA PÉŠ.[ÙR.RA GAG.GAG-*pí ina* GÚ-*šú* GAR-*an* DIŠ *ina* MU.3.KÁM]-*ma* AD-*šú* ÚŠ *ana* NU ÚŠ-*šú* PÉŠ.SÌLA.G[AZ *ina* KUŠ *ina* S]A PÉ[Š].ÙR.RA GAG.GAG-*pí ina* GÚ-*šú* [GAR-*an-ma* TI-*uṭ*]

---

29. DIŠ *ina* MU.7.KÁM ‹ŠUB-*su*› DINGIR TUKU-*ši ul-tab-bar tás-níq* KUR.[RA GAR-*šú ana* ZI-*ḫi* …]

30–33. [DIŠ *ina* MU].10.KÁM ŠUB-⸢*su*⸣ DINGIR TUKU-*ši ana* [ZI-*ḫi*⸣ U$_4$.9.KÁM *ina* IM.⸢SA$_5$ *šá* S⸣[AḪAR.ŠUB.BA MU$_4$-*šú ina*] ⸢^{GIŠ}⸣NÁ NÁ-*al mam-ma* KI-*šú ul i-ta-mu i*[*na* U$_4$.10.KÁM *tu-še-eṣ-ṣa-šum-ma* ^{d}30 *u* ^{d}UTU NU IGI … *in*]*a* KAL-*šú* ⸢7-*šú u*⸣ 7-*šú* ÍD *ib-bir-ma* NU GUR-*šú* x […] x [*ina* KUŠ *ina*] SA PÉŠ.ÙR.RA GAG.GAG-*p*[*í ina* GÚ-*šú* GAR-*an-ma* TI-*uṭ*]

---

34. […] DINGIR TUKU-*ši* N[U…]

35–48′. (fragmentary lines and missing lines)

49′–51′. […] ŠUB-*su* ŠU ^{d}30 *lu* ŠU ^{d}U.GU[R …o] MA.NA UZU *ab-la* ZÚ.LUM.MA [… *ina* U$_4$.#.K]ÁM *tu-še-la-šum-ma* x[…]

52′–54′. [DIŠ *ina ṣa-l*]*a-li* ŠUB-*su* ŠU ^{d}[(15 BIL.ZA.ZA) SIG$_7$.SIG$_7$ *šá* (*ina* UGU-*ḫi* ^{Ú}*sa-am-mal-lu* ^{Ú}*uru-ul-l*)*u* GÙB-*zu* Z(É-*š*)]*u ta-pat-taḫ* ⸢A⸣.[(MEŠ-*šú* ŠÉŠ-*su* ^{Ú}*ni-kip-tu*$_4$) ^{Ú}*an-ki-*(*nu-te ina* KUŠ *ina* S)]A ⸢PÉŠ!⸣.Ù[(R.RA) GAG.GAG-*pí ina* (GÚ-*šú* GAR-*an*) (DIN-*ut*)][2]

55′–59′. (fragmentary)

60′–61′. DIŠ *ina ši-mi-tan* ŠUB-*s*[(*u* ŠU ^{d}NAM.TAR) …(UZU NAM.LÚ.U$_{19}$.LU)] *ina* KUŠ *ina* SA PÉŠ.Ù[(R.RA GAG.GAG-*pí ina* GÚ-*šú* GAR-*an*)-*ma* (DIN-*uṭ*)][3]

62′. DIŠ *ina šá-túr-ri* ŠUB-*su-ma* […]

63′–64′. DIŠ AN.TA.Š[U]B.BA *ina a-lak gi-*⌜*ri*⌝ [ŠUB-*su* ŠU (^{d}UTU) *ina* MU-*šú*] ÚŠ *ana* NU ÚŠ-*šú* ^{NA_4}*mu-ṣa* ^{NA_4}AN.BAR ^{NA_4}x [(SÚD *ina* A.MEŠ ḪE.ḪE ŠÉŠ-*su*)-*ma* DIN][4]

65′–66′. DIŠ *ina* ⌜ÍD *ṭe$_4$-bi*⌝-*šú* ŠUB-*su* ŠU DINGIR URU-*šú ina* MU-*šú* ÚŠ *ana* N[(U ÚŠ-*šú*)] SAḪAR *kib-s*[(*u* NIT)]A ⌜*u*⌝ MUNUS *ni-kip-tú* NÍTA *u* MUNUS *ina* KUŠ! *i*[*na* S(A PÉŠ.ÙR.RA GAG.GAG-*pí ina* GÚ-*šú* GAR-*an*)-*ma* (DIN)][5]

67′–69′. DIŠ *ina ṭú-ub a-la-ki-šú* ŠUB-*su lu* ŠU ^{d}AMAR.UTU *lu* Š[U …] *ana* ZI-*ḫi* ^{NA_4}ZÁLAG SÚD(!) KI Ì.GIŠ *ta-ṣap-pi* ŠÉ[(Š)-*su ni-*(*kip-tu$_4$* NITA u MUNUS)] *ina* KUŠ *ina* SA PÉŠ.ÙR.RA GAG.GAG-*pí ina* GÚ.BI [GAR-*an-ma* TI-*uṭ*][6]

70′. [x AN.TA].ŠUB.BA *u bu*[*l-ṭu* …]

71′–80′. (fragmentary)

81′–82′. [DIŠ NA *r*]*a*?-⌜ʾ-*i*⌝-[*bi* ŠU(B-*su*)] ^{Ú}KINDA SÚD KI A ÍD SÌG-*aṣ* [1-*ni*]*š* ⌜ḪE⌝.ḪE ŠÉ[(Š)]-*su-ma* TI[7]

83′–84′. [ÉN xx] DU$_8$.A *be-en-num* A.R[I].A ^{d}*Šul-pa-è-a* AN.TA.ŠUB.BA [É]N ^{d}*Šu-*⌜*lak*⌝ ÉN ME.ŠÈ.BA.DA.RI

85′–86′. [(DIŠ NA)] ⌜^{d}⌝*Šu-lak* ŠUB-*su* : DIB-*su* ^{Ú}KINDA SÚD *ina* A ÍD ḪE.ḪE [(Š)]ÉŠ.MEŠ-*su-ma* TI-*uṭ*[8]

TRANSLATION

1–3. If ^{d}LUGAL.ÙR.RA is born with him, the house of his father will be scattered at his feet; in order that the house of his father not be scattered you lay him to rest as if he were a still-born child and he will carry off the evil (with him). Its sign is that, from the moment he is born, he wails, twists and is continually rigid.[9]

4–5. If it falls on him in the third year, it will knock him flat(?)[10] so that he dies; in order for him not to die, you grind *šakirû* which was pulled up on the thirtieth of the month (and) mix (it) with water. If you repeatedly rub him gently (with it), he should recover.[11]

6–7. If it falls on him in the seventh year, he will die that same year; in order for him not to die, you mix "eclipse ashes" from the thirtieth of the month with water. If you rub him gently (with it), he should recover.[12]

8–10. If it falls on him in the tenth year, he will live long; dying of old age[13] is established for him; to remove it, on the day of an eclipse of the [moon ...], you have him fall down facing the moon. You have him [...] three branches which a person with *saḫaršubbû* [...] (and) a palm frond until the eclipse brightens. In [...][14]

11–12. [If] it ⸢falls⸣ on him [in the fifteenth year], he will obtain a personal god; at his feet, the house of his father will become rich; [to remove it], you sew up [the skin] of a ⸢green⸣ [frog] which was standing on an *elpetu*-rush in a skin with *arrabu*-dormouse tendon. [If you put it on his neck, he should recover.][15]

13–14. [Alternatively], you grind "human ⸢flesh⸣" (and) *ankinutu* (and) mix (it) with river water. You ⸢rub⸣ [him] ⸢gently⸣ (with it), [and then] you sew up "⸢human⸣ [flesh]" (and) *ankinutu* in goat skin with *arrabu*-dormouse tendon. [If you put it] on his neck, [he should recover].

15–17. [If] it falls on him [in] the twentieth [year], he will become rich (and) his possessions will be numerous; [to remove it], you sew up *ašqulālu*, ⸢*amilānu*⸣, (and) ⸢male⸣ and female [...] in the skin of a green frog with *arrabu*-dormouse tendon. You put (it) on his neck. For nine days, you cover him with *šaršerru*-clay used for *saḫaršubbû* (and) on the tenth day, you have him come out [in such a way that neither the sun nor the moon sees him. ...] If he crosses the river seven and seven times when it is in flood,[16] [it will not return to him].[17]

18–19. If it falls on him in the thirtieth year, the house of his father will be scattered at his feet; to remove it, for nine [days], you ⸢cover⸣ him with [*šaršerru*]-⸢clay⸣ used for *saḫaršubbû* (and) on the tenth day, you have him come out in such a way that neither the sun nor the moon sees him. [...] If he crosses the river seven and seven times [when it is in] ⸢flood⸣,[18] [it will not return to him].[19]

---

20. [If it] ⸢falls⸣ on him [in] the ⸢fiftieth year⸣ the house of his father will be scattered at his feet; [he will] not [do well?].[20]

---

21. [... LUGAL].ÙR.RA of ⸢*bennu*⸣ [...].

22–24. [If "spawn"] of ⸢Šulpaea⸣ is born with him, the house of his father will be scattered at his feet; [in order for it not to be scattered], you throw him alive into the river and his evil will be ⸢carried⸣ [away. Its sign is that, from] the ⸢moment⸣ he is is born, he does not wail (or) cry or stiffen up.[21]

25–28. [If] it falls on him [in] the third [year], his father will obtain a personal god; that infant will die in the same year; to remove it, [you sew up ... (and)] ⸢*amilānu*⸣ in the skin of a green frog with ⸢*arrabu*-dormouse⸣ tendon [(and) you put (it) on his neck. If in the third year] also, his father will die; in order for his father not to die, [you sew up] a *ḫulû*-shrew (and) [... in a skin with] ⸢*arrabu*-dormouse tendon⸣. [If you put] (it) on his neck, [he should recover].[22]

---

29. If it falls on him in the seventh year, he will obtain a personal god; he will live long; dying of old age [is established for him; to remove it ...].[23]

30–33. [If] it falls on him [in] the tenth [year], he will obtain a personal god; to remove it, for nine days, [you cover him] with *šaršerru*-clay [used for *saḫaršubbû*]. He should lie [in] bed (and) nobody should talk with him. ⸢On⸣ [the tenth day, you have him come out in such a way that neither the sun nor the moon sees him. ...] If he crosses the river seven and seven times ⸢when it is in⸣ flood,[24] [it will not return to him]. You sew up [... in skin with] *arrabu*-dormouse tendon. [If you put it on his neck, he should recover].[25]

---

34. [If it falls on him in the ... year], he will obtain a personal god; he will ⸢not⸣ [...].

35-48′. *(fragmentary and missing lines)*

49′–51′. [If] it falls on him [...], "hand" of Sîn or "hand" of Nergal [...#] *manû*-weight of dried meat, dates [... on the #]th day, you have him go up and [...]

52′–54′. [If] it falls on him [while he is] ⸢sleeping⸣, "hand" of [(Ishtar. You pierce the ⸢gall sac⸣ of a) green (frog), which stands (on a *samallû*-plant or an *urullu*-plant and rub him gently with its juices). You sew up (*nikiptu* and) *anki*(*nutu* in skin with)] ⸢*arrabu*-dormouse tendon⸣. [If (you put it) on (his neck, he should recover.)] [26]

55′–59′. *(fragmentary)*

60′–61′. If it falls on him in the evening, [("hand" of Namtar. You sew up) ... (and "human flesh")] in skin with ⸢*arrabu*-dormouse⸣ tendon. [If you put] (it) on his neck, [he should recover].[27]

62′. If it falls on him in the morning and [...]

63′–64′. If ⸢AN.TA.ŠUB.BA⸣ [falls on him] while he is going on a journey, ["hand" of (Shamash)]; he will die [that same year]; in order for him not to die, [(you grind)] *mūṣu*-stone, an iron bead (and) [...]-stone (and) [(mix it with water). If (you rub him gently with it), he should recover].[28]

65′–66′. If it falls on him while he is going down to the river (to swim), "hand" of the god of his city; he will die that same year; in order for him ⸢not⸣ [(to die), you sew up] dust from the tracks of a ⸢man⸣ and a woman in skin ⸢with⸣ [(*arrabu*-dormouse tendon). If (you put it on his neck, he should recover)].[29]

67′–69′. If it falls on him while he is going about wherever he pleases, either "hand" of Marduk or ⸢"hand"⸣ [of DN]; to remove it, you grind *zalāqu*-

stone (and) soak (it) in oil. You ⸢rub [him] gently⸣ (with it). You sew up [(male and female ⸢*nikiptu*⸣)] in skin with *arrabu*-dormouse tendon. [If you put] (it) on his neck, [he should recover].[30]

70′. [(So many … for) AN.TA].ŠUB.BA and ⸢treatments⸣ […]

71′–80′. *(fragmentary)*

81′–82′. [If] the ⸢trembler⸣ [⸢falls⸣ on a person], you grind KINDA. You stir (it) into river water (and) mix (it) ⸢together⸣. If you ⸢rub him gently⸣ (with it), he should recover.[31]

83′–84′. [Recitation] to make […] let up; for *bennu*, "spawn" of Šulpaea, AN.TA.ŠUB.BA; ⸢recitation⸣ for Shulak; ME.ŠÈ.BA.DA.RI

85′–86′. [If] Shulak falls on [(a person)] variant: afflicts him, you grind KINDA. You mix (it) with river water. If you ⸢rub him gently⸣ (with it), he should recover.

Notes

1. The number is restored from Arnaud 1987, 695:3; see Heeßel 2000, 335.
2. Restored from parallel BM 56605 obv. 6-11, after Heeßel 2000, 117–30
3. Restored from parallel BM 56605 obv. 32-34 after Heeßel 2000, 117–30
4. Restored from the similar BM 56605 obv. 44-45 after Heeßel 2000, 117–30.
5. Restored from the parallel BM 56605 obv. 12,14-15 after Heeßel 2000, 117–30.
6. Restored from the parallel BM 56605 obv. 26-28 after Heeßel 2000, 117–30.
7. Restored from the parallel BM 56605 obv. 35-37 after Heeßel 2000, 117–30.
8. Restored from the parallel BM 56605 obv. 46-47 after Heeßel 2000, 117–30.
9. See Scurlock and Andersen 2005, 13.261.
10. Augmenting Heeßel 2000, 318.
11. See Scurlock and Andersen 2005, 19.73.
12. See Scurlock and Andersen 2005, 19.73. A similar entry appears in BM 56605 obv. 16–17 (Heeßel 2000, 117–30).
13. Literally: "arrival (in due course of time) at the (Netherworld) mountain." see Scurlock and Andersen 2005, 19.73 and p. 753 n. 68.
14. See Scurlock and Andersen 2005, 19.74.
15. The entry appears also in BM 56605 obv. 18–20 (Heeßel 2000, 117–30).
16. Literally: "at its strong(est)."
17. See Scurlock and Andersen 2005, 19.74, 20.4
18. Literally: "at its strong(est)."
19. See Scurlock and Andersen 2005, 19.75.
20. See Scurlock and Andersen 2005, 19.75.

21. See Scurlock and Andersen 2005, 13.247. The entry also appears in Arnaud 1987, 695:4 and KUB 37.87:7′–9′.
22. See Scurlock and Andersen 2005, 13.248, 20.1.
23. See Scurlock and Andersen 2005, 13.249.
24. Literally: "at its strong(est)."
25. See Scurlock and Andersen 2005, 13.250.
26. Restored from parallel BM 56605 obv. 6–11, after Heeßel 2000, 117–30.
27. Restored from parallel BM 56605 obv. 32–34 after Heeßel 2000, 117–30.
28. See Scurlock and Andersen 2005, 19.76. A similar entry appears in BM 56605 obv. 44–45 (Heeßel 2000, 117–30).
29. See Scurlock and Andersen 2005, 19.78. A similar entry appears in BM 56605 obv. 12, 14–15 (Heeßel 2000, 117–30).
30. See Scurlock and Andersen 2005, 19.77. A similar entry appears in BM 56605 obv. 26–28 (Heeßel 2000, 117–30).
31. Heeßel suggests connecting these lines with BM 56605 obv. 35-37 (Heeßel 2000, 117–30).

DPS 30

DPS 29:87′ (catchline) = DPS 30:1

1–4. DIŠ GIG-*ma* KA-*šú* BAD.BAD-*te* ŠU^{II}-*šú* GÌR^{II}-*šú* *i-par-ru-ra* ŠU DINGIR *mu-un-*[*ni*]-*ši* ^{d}ÀLAD *šá-né-e* ^{d}*A-nim* DIŠ *ina* ŠU DINGIR *mu-un-ni-ši* *KAR*-[*šú*] SÌG *pú-ḫat-ti* SI DÀRA.MAŠ ^{Ú}*an-ki-nu-te* 1-*niš* SÚD *šum-ma* NITA 9-*šú* *šum-ma* MUNUS 7-*šú* ŠÉŠ.MEŠ-*su-ma* TI

This is restored from CTN 4.72 vi 1′–8′ (Stadhouders 2011, 39–51) which can be positively identified as the incipit of DPS 30 from the catalogue (see Heeßel 2000, 15). Presumably, the other entries in col. vi originally belonged to DPS 30, since CTN 4.72 col. i is drawn from DPS 27 and the remainder of the text presumably from DPS 28–29. Since, however, the DPS 27 references are not in order, it seemed hazardous to assign the DPS 30 citations of CTN 4.72 col. vi specific line numbers. There exists also a piece of the end of what is certainly DPS 30, but it is very fragmentary.

Translation

1–4. If (he) is sick and he continually opens his mouth, and his hands and his feet become powerless, "⸢weakening⸣ hand of god" (or) a *šedû* deputized by Anu; if (you want) to save [him] from the "weakening hand of god," you grind together hair(!) from a female lamb, gazelle horn (and) *ankinutu*. If you repeatedly rub him (with it) nine times if it is a man and seven times if it is a woman, he(/she) should recover.[1]

NOTES

1. See Scurlock and Andersen 2005, 19.370. For the remainder of what was probably also on this tablet and in this order, see 19.371–372.

E. ENTERIC FEVER: DPS 31–32

DPS 31

1–2. [DIŠ NA UD.DA TAB-*s*]*u-ma ina* U_4-*mi-šú-ma* $ŠED_7$ NA BI U_4.3.KÁM GIG [*ana* GIG-*s*]*u* NU GÍD.DA Ì KÚM *u* KAŠ.SAG ŠÉŠ.MEŠ-*su-ma* DIN

3–5. [DIŠ KI.MIN MÚD] *ina* KIR_4-*šú ina* U_4-*mi-šú-ma uš-tar-ru-nim-ma* DU-*ku* NA BI U_4.7.K[ÁM] GIG [*ana* GIG-*s*]*u* NU GÍD.DA *ana* UDUN ^{LÚ}KÚRUN.NA x ti ku GUB-*su-ma* [EN ...] ŠUB?-*ú* GUB-*su ù* Ì KÚM ŠÉŠ.MEŠ-*su-ma* DIN

6–8. DIŠ ⌜KI.MIN *i*⌝-*tar-rak i-sa-kip-šú ù* KÚM *ṣar-ḫa* TUKU-*ši* NA BI U_4.14. KÁM GIG *ana* GIG-*su* NU GÍD.DA *ana* A.MEŠ $ŠED_7$.MEŠ ŠUB-*šú-ma* EN Š[À]-⌜*šu*⌝ *uš-ta-nàr-ra-bu* GUB-*su ù* Ì KÚM ŠÉŠ,MEŠ-*su-ma* DIN

9–11. DIŠ ⌜KI⌝.MIN MÚD *ina* KIR_4-*šú ina* U_4-*mi-šu-ma uš-tar-ru-nim-ma* DU-*ku* NA BI U_4.25.KÁM GIG *ana* GIG-*su* NU GÍD.DA Ì ^{ŠEM}GÚR. GÚR ^{ŠEM}AZ ŠEM-^{d}NIN.IB Ì ^{GIŠ}ERIN *ana* SAG.DU-*šu* DUB-*ak* Ì ^{Ú}*áp-ru-šú* SU-*šu* ŠÉŠ.ŠÉŠ-*ma* DIN

12–14. [(DIŠ) KI].⌜MIN *za*⌝-*mar* KÚM-*em za-mar* $ŠED_7$ *li-ʾ-ba* TUKU-*ši u* IR NU TUKU NA BI ITI.1.KÁM GIG [*ana* GI]G-*su* NU GÍD.DA Ì KÚM ŠÉŠ-*su* ‹(*ina* TÚG)› MU_4.MU_4-*su* IZI ‹(*ana* IGI-*šu*)› *ta-šar-rap-ma* [KÚM-*m*]*a* GU_7 KÚM-*ma* NAG U_4.3.KÁM *šu-ḫi-šu-ma* TI-*uṭ*[1]

---

15. [DIŠ KI.MIN ... -*m*]*a ina* U_4-[*mi-šú-ma* ... NA B]I U_4.14.K[ÁM] ⌜GIG *ana* GIG-*su*⌝ [NU GÍD.DA ...]

(gap)

16′–18′. (fragmentary)

19′–22′. DIŠ KI.MIN IR *ma-gal* TUKU.TUKU-*ši u* IR-*s*[*u* (GIN₇ A.MEŠ ... *ut-ta-na-tak* NA BI GIG *là-zi* DIB-*su*) ...] GIG A.MEŠ-*šú ḫi-iq* KAŠ ^{Ú}*su-pa-lu* [...] *ina* IM.ŠU.RIN.NA *kal-la* U_4-*me te-se-ker* [...] *la-am* ^{d}UTU È TU_5-*šú* NAG-*šú u* [...]

23′–24′. DIŠ KI.MIN IR *ma-gal* TUKU.TUKU-*ši* NA.BI U[$_4$.x.KÁM GIG] *ana* GIG-*su* NU GÍD.DA DÈ NAM.TAR? [...]

25′–27′. [DIŠ K]I.MIN *pa-nu-šu* GIN$_7$ *šá* KAŠ NAG *ma-gal* S[A$_5$ ...] GIG NA BI GIG U$_4$.21 GIG *ana* G[IG-*su* NU GÍD.DA ...] *kab-ru-ti ḫi-iq* KAŠ.SAG NAG-*šú-m*[*a* ...]

28′–29′. DIŠ KI.MIN ⸢Ù⸣.BU.BU.UL *šá* GIN$_7$ *a-ši-i* x [...] *ana* GIG-*su* NU GÍD.DA DÈ *ur-ba-ti ina* Ì [...]

30′–31′. DIŠ KI.MIN Ù.BU.BU.UL *šá* GIN$_7$ *a-ši-i* IGI [...] *ana* GIG-*su* NU GÍD.DA DÈ *ur-ba-tú* DÈ ^{GIŠ}E[RIN ...]

32′–34′. DIŠ UD.DA TAB-*su-ma* SU-*šu i-raš-ši-šum-ma e-ki-*[*ik* ...] *ana* GIG-*su* NU GÍD.DA ^{ŠEM}GÚR.GÚR *ka-man-t*[*ú*? ...] ^{Ú}GAMUN^{SAR} 1-*niš* SÚD *ina* Ì [...]

35′–39′. DIŠ KI.MIN U$_4$-*mi-šam-ma ana* GIZKIM-*šú i-ḫi-it-ṭ*[*a-áš-šú u ú-maš-šar-šú*] *e-nu-ma i-ḫi-it-ṭa-áš-šú* KÚM *ṣar-*⸢*ḫa*⸣ [TUKU-*ši* SA.MEŠ-*šú* GU$_7$.MEŠ-*šú*][2] IR ŠUB-*su-ma ina-aḫ* NA BI U$_4$.21.K[ÁM GIG *ana* GIG-*su* NU GÍD.DA] Ú.KUR.RA^{SAR} ḪÁD.DU SÚD *ana* Ì [...] *tuš-bat ina še-rim la-am* ^{d}UTU [È ...]

40′. (fragmentary)

41″–42″. (fragmentary)

43″–45″. [DIŠ KI.MIN ...]-*ši ma-gal ra-ʾi-ba* TUKU-*ši* [... NA BI U$_4$].52.KÁM GIG *ana* GIG-*su* [N]U GÍD.D[A ... L]Ú.U$_{18}$.LU 1-*niš i-lem-ma* [...]

46″–49″. [DIŠ KI.MIN NINDA] ⸢*u*⸣ [K]AŠ *la*(!) *i-maḫ-*[*ḫar ḫ*]*i-ši-iḫ-ti* ŠÀ TUKU-*ma* NU [... N]A BI U$_4$.44.KÁM G[IG *ana* GI]G-*su* NU GÍD.DA 1/3 *qa* ⸢x⸣ [...] 1/3 *qa* Ì.GIŠ 1/3 *qa* Ì.[NUN.NA] 1 *qa* KAŠ.SAG 1 *qa* SUM^{SAR} ⸢1-*niš* SÚD⸣ *ana* IGI MUL.ÙZ *tuš-ba*[*t ba*]-*lu pa-tan* NAG-*šú-ma* TI-*uṭ*

50″–51″. DIŠ KI.MIN *ka-la* U_4-*mi u* GI_6 *i-le-eb-bu* NA BI U_4.21.KÁM GIG *ana* GIG-*su* NU GÍD.DA URUDU *ḫu-luḫ-ḫa* KI.A.^{d}ÍD ÚḪ.^{d}ÍD *ina* KUŠ GAG.GAG-*pí ina* GÚ-*šú* GAR-*an-ma* DIN-*uṭ*

52″–56″. ⸢DIŠ KI⸣.MIN *ka-la* U_4-*mi u* GI_6 *i-le-eb-bu-ma la i-ṣal-lal* [NINDA] *u* KAŠ (coll.) *la i-maḫ-ḫar* GURUN GU_7 *u* A NAG NA BI ITI.1.KÁM GIG [*ana*] GIG-*su* NU GÍD.DA *al-la-an-ka-niš ina* Ì ^{GIŠ}ERIN ŠÉŠ-*su ni-kip-tú* [MUN] *eme-sal-lim* SÍG ^{MUNUS}ÁŠ.GÀR GÌŠ NU.ZU SÍG MUNUS. $SILA_4$ GÌŠ NU.ZU [*ina* KU]Š GAG.GAG-*pí ina* GÚ-*šú* GAR-*an-ma* AL.TI-⸢*uṭ*⸣

Translation

1–2. [If *ṣētu* burns a person] and on the day (you see the patient), he has chills, that person has been sick for three days; [in order that] ⸢his⸣ [illness] not be prolonged, if you repeatedly rub him gently with hot oil and first quality beer, he should recover.[3]

3-5. [If ditto (*ṣētu* burns a person)] (and) on the day (you see the patient) [blood] continually begins to flow from his nose, that person has been sick for seven days; [in order for] ⸢his⸣ [illness] not to be prolonged, you have him stand at a […] brewer's oven and then you have him stand [until] he produces [sweat(?)]. Then, if you repeatedly rub him gently with hot oil, he should recover.[4]

6–8. If ditto (*ṣētu* burns a person and) it throbs (and) knocks him down and he has a burning fever, that person has been sick for fourteen days; in order for his illness not to be prolonged, you put him down into cold water and you have him stand until his ⸢midsection⸣ is caused to continually tremble. Then, if you repeatedly rub him gently with hot oil, he should recover.[5]

9–11. If ditto (*ṣētu* burns a person and) on the day (you see the patient) blood continually begins to flow from his nose, that person has been sick for twenty-five days; in order for his illness not to be prolonged, you pour *kukru* oil, *asu*-myrtle, *nikiptu* (and) *erēnu*-cedar oil over his head. If you repeatedly gently rub his body with *aprušu* oil, he should recover.[6]

12–14. [(If)] ⸢ditto⸣ (*ṣētu* burns a person and) sometimes he is hot, sometimes he is cold, he has *liʾbu* but he does not have sweat, that person has been sick for a month; in order for his illness not to be prolonged, you rub him gently with hot oil and dress him ‹(with a garment)›. You light a fire ‹(before him)› and he should eat [hot things] (and) drink hot things. If you keep him apart[7] for three days, he should recover.[8]

---

15. [If ditto (*ṣētu* burns a person)] (and) on the day [(you see the patient) ...] ⸢that⸣ [person] has been sick for fourteen days; in order for his illness [not to be prolonged ...]

(gap)

16′–18′. *(fragmentary)*

19′–22′. If ditto (*ṣētu* "gets" a person and) he has a great deal of sweat and [(he drips sweat like ... water, a persistent illness afflicts that person)]; he has been sick [for x days]. ‹In order for his illness not to be prolonged›, you bake his drinking water, *ḫīqu*-beer, *supālu* (and) [...] for an entire day in an oven. [...] Before the sun rises you bathe him (with it) and have him drink (it) and [...].[9]

23′–24′. If ditto (*ṣētu* "gets" a person and) he has a lot of sweat, that person [has been sick for x days]; in order that his illness not be prolonged, [you mix] ashes of *pillû* [with oil and rub him gently with it].

25′–27′. [If] ⸢ditto⸣ (*ṣētu* "gets" a person and) his face is very ⸢red⸣ like one who drinks beer [...] that person is sick with an illness of twenty-one days; in order for [his] ⸢illness⸣ [not to be prolonged], ⸢if⸣ you have him drink fatty [...] (mixed) with *ḫīqu* made from first quality beer, [he should recover].[10]

28′–29′. If ditto (*ṣētu* "gets" a person) and [he has] *bubuʾtu* which are like those of *ašû*, [he has been sick for # days], in order for his illness not to be prolonged, [you mix] ashes of *urbātu*-rush with oil [and rub him gently with it].

30′–31′. If ditto (*ṣētu* "gets" a person and) [he has] *bubuʾtu* which are like (those of) *ašû*, [that person has been sick for # days]; in order that his illness not be prolonged, [you mix] ashes of *urbātu*-rush, ashes of ⸢*erēnu*⸣-cedar [(and) ... with oil and rub him gently with it].

32′–34′. If *ṣētu* burns him so that his skin is reddish and he scratches, [that person has been sick for # days]; in order that his illness not be prolonged, you grind together *kukru*, *kamantu*-henna(?), [...] (and) *kamūnu*-cumin. [You mix it] with oil [and rub him gently with it].[11]

35′–39′. If ditto (*ṣētu* burns him and) daily, at the expected time, it comes [over him and leaves him] (and) when it comes over him, [he has] burning fever [and his muscles continually hurt him] (and) sweat comes out on him and then he finds relief, that person [has been sick] for twenty-one days; [in order for his illness not to be prolonged], you dry (and) grind *ninû*-mint. [You pour? (it)] into oil. You let (it) sit out overnight [under the stars]. In the morning, before the sun [rises ...].[12]

40′. *(fragmentary)*

41″–42″. *(fragmentary)*

43″–45″. [If ditto (*ṣētu* burns him and) ...] (and) he has a lot of trembling [... that person] has been sick for fifty-two [days]; in order for his illness ⸢not⸣ to be prolonged, he should eat [...] and "human" [...] together and [...][13]

46″–49″. [If ditto (*ṣētu* burns him and)] (his insides) will not accept [bread] or ⸢beer⸣, he has (food) ⸢cravings⸣ but then does not [... that per]son has been ⸢sick⸣ for forty-four days; [in order for] his ⸢illness⸣ not to be prolonged, you grind together 1/3 *qû*-measure of [...], 1/3 *qû*-measure of oil, 1/3 *qû*-measure of ⸢ghee⸣, 1 *qû*-measure of first quality beer (and) 1 *qû*-measure of *šūmu*-garlic. You let (it) sit out overnight under the goat star. If you have him drink (it) on an ⸢empty⸣ stomach, he should recover.[14]

50″–51″. If ditto (*ṣētu* burns him and) he groans all day and all night, that person has been sick for twenty-one days; in order for his illness not to be prolonged, you sew up copper, *ḫuluḫḫu* (= white *anzaḫḫu*)-frit, *kibrītu*-sulphur (and) *ruʾtītu*-sulphur in a leather bag. If you put (it) on his neck, he should recover.[15]

52″–56″. If ditto (*ṣētu* burns him and) groans all day and all night so that he cannot sleep, (his insides) do not accept [bread] and beer (but) he can eat fruit and drink water, that person has been sick for a month; in order for his illness not to be prolonged, you rub him gently with *allankaniš* (mixed) with *erēnu*-cedar oil. You sew up *nikiptu*, *emesallim*-[salt], hair of a virgin she-goat (and) hair of a virgin lamb [in] a ⌜leather bag⌝. If you put (it) on his neck, he should recover.[16]

NOTES

1. Restored from BAM 66 obv. 10–12.
2. Restorations are based on DPS 16:81′–82′; see Heeßel, 2000, 350.
3. See Scurlock and Andersen 2005, 3.144. Heeßel 2000 suggests a parallel with BAM 66 obv. 1–3.
4. See Scurlock and Andersen 2005, 3.146.
5. See Scurlock and Andersen 2005, 3.147.
6. Heeßel suggests a parallel with BAM 66 obv. 4–6 and/or 7–9.
7. Augmenting Heeßel 2000, 342.
8. See Scurlock and Andersen 2005, 3.18, 3.152. This entry appears also in BAM 66 obv. 10–12.
9. See Scurlock and Andersen 2005, 3.122. This entry appears also in BAM 66 obv. 24–28.
10. See Scurlock and Andersen 2005, 3.149.
11. See Scurlock and Andersen 2005, 3.128.
12. See Scurlock and Andersen 2005, 3.148.
13. See Scurlock and Andersen 2005, 3.156.
14. See Scurlock and Andersen 2005, 3.154.
15. See Scurlock and Andersen 2005, 3.150.
16. See Scurlock and Andersen 2005, 3.153, 6.59.

DPS 32

DPS 31:57′ (catchline) = DPS 32:1

1. [DIŠ NA IM *i*]*š-biṭ-su-ma ma-gal e-em* [...][1]

TRANSLATION

1. [If “wind”] ⌜blasts⌝ him and he is very hot [...]

NOTE

1. A treatment for this condition was originally given in BAM 146:56′.

F. SKIN: DPS 33–34

DPS 33

1. [DIŠ GIG] GAR-*šú* GIN$_7$ *um-me-di a-šu-ú* MU.N[I]
2. [DIŠ G]IG GAR-*šú* GIN$_7$ *um-me-di i-raš-ši-šum-ma ug-gag* IGI GIG A ŠUB [...] *a-šu-ú* MU.N[I]
3. [DIŠ G]IG GAR-*šú* GIN$_7$ *um-me-di u* È-*su e-mid* SU-*šú i-raš-ši-šum-ma* EN x[...]x TE GIG *ug-dal-lab a-šu-ú* MU.N[I]
4. [DIŠ *pa*]-*nu-šú u* IGI^{II}-*šú* MÚ.MEŠ-*ḫa di-ig-la ka-bit u* DIRI *a-šu-ú* MU.N[I]
5. [DIŠ *p*]*a-nu-šú* MÚ.MEŠ-*ḫu di-gíl-šú ma-ṭi* SU-*šú bir-di ma-lu u* ŠÀ-*šú* [D]IB-*su a-šu-ú* MU.NI
6. [DIŠ] GIG GAR-*šú* GIN$_7$ *ni-šik* UḪ-*ma*[1] *pa-gar-šú* DIRI *a-šu-ú m*[*ut-ta*]*p-ri-šú* MU.NI
7. [DIŠ] GIG GAR-*šú* GIN$_7$ *ter-ke-e-ti kal* SU LÚ DIRI *kul-la-ri* MU.NI
8. [DIŠ] ⸢GIG GAR⸣-*šú* GI$_6$ *ri-šik i-raš-ši-šum-ma uk-kak kul-la-ri* MU.NI
9. [DIŠ GIG GA]R-*šú* IGI.MEŠ-*šú šag-gu*$_5$ *i-ta-ti-*⸢*šú*⸣ *um-me-di* DIRI *u i-*[...]-*un kul-la-ár a-ši-i* MU.NI
10. [DIŠ GIG GA]R-*šú* GIN$_7$ *um-me-di* MURUB$_4$.MEŠ-*šú* NIGIN-*mi ek-*[*ke-t*]*um* MU.NI
11. [DIŠ GIG GA]R-*šú* GIN$_7$ BAR KU$_6$ SU-*šú* DIRI *u a-dan-na* TUKU *ri-*[*šik-t*]*um* MU.NI
12. [DIŠ GIG GA]R-*šú* GIN$_7$ TAB KÚM-*ma* xx [...] GIG *ri-*[*šu-t*]*um* MU.NI
13. [DIŠ GIG G]AR-*šú* GIN$_7$ TAB KÚM-*ma* du x A NU *ú-kal* G[IG ...] TUKU *gir-giš-šum* MU.NI
14. [DIŠ G]IG GAR-*šú* GIN$_7$ TAB KÚM-*ma* A *ú-kal* [*bu*]-*bu-ʾ-tum* MU.NI
15. [DIŠ] GIG GAR-*šú* GIN$_7$ TAB KÚM-*ma* A NU *ú-kal* Ù.BU.[BU].UL TUR.MEŠ DIRI *i-ši-tum* MU.[NI]
16. DIŠ GIG GAR-*šú* GIN$_7$ TAB KÚM-*ma um-me-di* DIRI *ri-šu-tam* TUKU *ni-piš-tum* MU.[NI]
17. DIŠ GIG GAR-*šú* GIN$_7$ *um-me-di u* DIŠ[2] È-*su* SAMAG DIB-*bat ni-piš-tum* MU.NI
18. DIŠ GIG GAR-*šú* GIN$_7$ *um-me-di ig-gig*[3] *i-na* [...] A DU.MEŠ *ru-ṭib-tum* MU.[NI]
19. DIŠ GIG GAR-*šú* SA$_5$ BABBAR GU$_7$-*šú u* A *ú-*[*k*]*al ru-ṭib-tum* MU.[NI]

20. DIŠ GIG GAR-*šú* GI$_6$ *ḫa-ra-su* MU.[NI]
21. DIŠ SU LÚ *bir-di* DIRI UZU.MEŠ-*šú ú-zaq-qa-t*[*u-š*]*ú u ri-šu-tum* ŠUB.ŠUB-*su ḫa-ra-su* M[U.NI]
22. DIŠ GIG *ina* GÌR NA *lu ina* ŠIR! LÚ E$_{11}$-*ma* ⌈*i-raš*⌉-*ši-šum-ma ug-gag ru-ṭib-tum* M[U.NI]
23. DIŠ GIG GAR-*šú* SA$_5$ *e-em* MÚ-*iḫ u* DU-*ak sa-ma-nu* [MU.NI]
24. DIŠ GIG GAR-*šú* SA$_5$ LÚ KÚM.KÚM-*im u i-ta-nar-rù sa-ma-nu* [MU.NI]
25. DIŠ GIG GAR-*šú da-an* TAB x-*ma ina* IGI-*ka la i-na-aš mid-ru*[4] KI.MIN *sa-ma-nu* [MU.NI]
26. DIŠ GIG GAR-*šú* GIN$_7$ Ù.[BU].BU.UL *pa-gar-šú* SA$_5$ *ši-biṭ* IM MU.[NI]
27. DIŠ GIG GAR-⌈*šú*⌉ GIN$_7$ ⌈UTU⌉ SA$_5$ [GU$_7$-*šú*] x.MEŠ *ka-li-šú-nu* DIB *pi-en-du$_4$* M[U.NI][5]
28. DIŠ GIG GAR-*šú* GIN$_7$ NA$_4$.ZÚ TA (coll.) GÚ-*su* NIGIN-*me šá-da-nu* M[U.NI]
29. DIŠ GIG GAR-*šú ana* TAG *da-an ti-ik-pi* SA$_5$.MEŠ DIRI *šá-da-nu* M[U.NI]
30. DIŠ GIG GAR-*šú ana* TAG *da-an* KÚM-*im ṣa-ri-iḫ ṭu*-⌈*ù-lim*⌉ (coll.) ÍL-*šú* NINDA *u* KAŠ LAL-*ṭi šá-da-nu* MU.NI TAG ŠU ^{d}[…]
31. DIŠ GIG GAR-*šú* GIN$_7$ NA$_4$ *da-an qer-bé-nu-um-ma* GAL *qer-bé-nu-um-ma* DU-*ak* ÍL-*šú* ⌈ZI!⌉-*a* [*u*] DU.ME[Š GUB-*za*] *la i-le-e*ʾ-*e šá-da-nu* MU.NI TAG ^{d}AMAR.UTU *u* [^{d}NIN.IB][6]
32. DIŠ GIG GAR-*šú* GIN$_7$ NA$_4$ *da-an lu ina* GÚ-*šú lu ina su*-⌈*ḫa*⌉-*ti-šú lu ina ri-bi-ti-šú* GAR *ana* U$_4$.3.KAM [GAM …] MU.[NI]
33. DIŠ GIG GAR-*šú* GIN$_7$ KUD-*is* UDU.NÍTA MÚD *ṣar-ḫa* ⌈*ú-š*[*e*]-*ṣi* GI.DÙ.A *gul lu*⌉ *su ana* TI-*šú* x e xx […]
34. DIŠ GIG GAR-*šú ina ši-mi-ti* ŠUB-*su-ma la ú-ta-ša*[*r-m*]*a šim-ma-tum ka-la pag-ri-šú ṣa-ba-tu* […]
35. DIŠ GIG GAR-*šú* GIN$_7$ *la i-du-ú di-ik-šá* TUKU A.ZU x x ki ú la i? di? a *ḫa-a-at* x x […]
36. DIŠ *ina la-ku-ti-‹šú› la-biš$_X$-ma* GIN$_7$ *iḫ*-[*z*]*a ep-qé-nu* MU.NI[7]
37. DIŠ *ina la-ku-t*[*i*]-*šú la-biš$_X$-ma* GIN$_7$ *iḫ-za-ma u zi-iz* [*ep-qu*] MU.NI[8]
38. DIŠ GIG GAR-*šú* GIN$_7$ ^{IM}⌈*ṭe$_4$*⌉-*ru-ti-šú* NIGIN.ME? *u ti-ik-ka-šú* DIB [*kir-ba-nu*] MU.NI
39. DIŠ GIG GAR-*šú da-an pa-an* UZU.MEŠ-*šú* GAR *u* [KÚ]M.KÚM-*im kir*-⌈*ba*⌉-*nu* MU.NI
40. DIŠ GIG GAR-*šú kup-pu-ut ù* UGU-*šú ḫu-un-du-ud zi-iq-tum* MU.NI
41. [DIŠ GIG] GAR-*šú* GIN$_7$ *i-ba*-⌈*rim-ma*⌉ KIR$_4$-*šú* BABBAR [Š]UB *zi-iq-tum* MU.NI

42. [DIŠ GIG] GAR-*šú* SA$_5$ BABBAR TUR *u* GU$_7$-*šú zi-iq-tum* [MU].NI

43–44. (fragmentary)

45. [DIŠ *ina la-ku*]-*ti-šú la-biš*$_X$-*ma* SA$_5$ *u* GU$_7$-*š*[*ú*] ⌈*u* ÍL.MEŠ⌉-*šú* KÚM TUKU.MEŠ x x [... MU].NI

46. [DIŠ *ina la-ku*]-*ti-šú la-biš*$_X$-*ma* GU$_7$-*šú u i*-⌈*be*⌉-*la ina* šu bu ʾ ḫu [... MU].NI

47. [DIŠ *ina la-ku*]-*ti-šú la-biš*$_X$-*ma* NU GU$_7$-*šu a-ba-bu* [(x) MU].NI

48. [...] na bi? ʾ ma NU GU$_7$-*šu a-ba-bu* [(x) MU].NI

49. [...] NU GU$_7$-*šu ù* DU.DU!-*ak* KI.MIN GUR.GUR-*ar i*-x [... MU].NI

50. [DIŠ GIG GAR-*šú*] *ina* ŠÀ-*šú* GIN$_7$ A *šur*!-*de-e-tu*$_4$ DU.MEŠ GI[G *l*]*a-az-za* [... MU.N]I

51. (fragmentary)

52. [DIŠ *ina la-ku-t*]*i-šú* [*l*]*a-biš*$_X$-*ma ur-ra u* GI$_6$ GU$_7$-*šú-ma la i-ṣal-lal a-bi-ik-tum* M[U.NI]

53. [DIŠ *ina la-ku-t*]*i-šú la- biš*$_X$-*ma* GIN$_7$ x šaḫ ma? *u* ÍL-*šú* KÚM TU[KU].MEŠ *mi-iq-tum* MU.NI AŠ A.ZU IGI

54. [...]-*šu ana* MAŠ.GÁN-*šú* GUR-*ma* A *ú-kal mi-iq-tum* MU.NI A.ZU IGI

55. [... -*š*]*u*? *ana* MAŠ.GÁN-*šú* GUR-*ma* NU T[I] GIG BI IN.GA[R].E ^{d}*Ba-ú ina* KI *ul*?-*lum* KI.MIN *ina* ^{GIŠ}NÁ [...]

56. DIŠ GIG GAR-*šú* GIN$_7$ *ṣe-e-tim-ma sa-ḫi-ip ina sa-ḫi-pi-šú* IGI.MEŠ-*šú* GI$_6$ ŠUB-*ú gal-lu-ú* MU.NI[9]

57. [...] x ÚŠ.BABBAR *ú-kal* x [...]-*šú* MU.NI

58. [DIŠ GIG GAR-*šú* SA$_5$ BAB]BAR ÚŠ.BABBAR È-*ma* x [...] *šàḫ-šàḫ-ḫu* MU.NI

59. [DIŠ GIG GAR-*šú* SA$_5$ BABBAR G]U$_7$-*šú* A NU TUKU *ana* TAG *i*-[*rap-pu*]-*uš ni-lu-gu*$_4$ MU.NI

60. [DIŠ GIG GAR]-*šú* TAG-*su-ma i-rap-pu*-[*uš*] È-*su* GÚ.ZAL M[U.NI]

61. [DIŠ *ina ša-nu*]-*ti-šú* [*ina*] MURUB$_4$ *u* UZU.ÚR *il-la-a* x x x [... GÚ.Z]AL? MU.NI

62. [DIŠ...] bi il bi ir qer bi [...] x *sim-ma* GIG *ki-ṣir-tú* GIG [...] MU.NI

63. [DIŠ...] nu ne di nir SA$_5$ GAR [...] NE *sik-ka-tum* MU.NI

64. [DIŠ...]-*šú ṣa-bit u* GI$_6$ *sàg-ba-ni* M[U.NI]

65. [DIŠ...] x u i sag su bi x iš *ṣi-in-na*-[*aḫ*]-*ti-r*[*u* MU.NI]

66. [DIŠ...] ud TUKU *u* IR *ú*-[*k*]*al ṣi-in-na-aḫ-ti*-[*ru* MU.NI]

67–68. [DIŠ...] A.MEŠ *u* DU-*ak ṣi-rip-tum* [MU.NI] : [... *ṣ*]*i-rip-tu*[*m* MU.NI]

69–70. (fragmentary)

71–74. (fragmentary mentioning SAḪAR.ŠUB.BA)

75–79. (fragmentary mentioning "hand" of Išum, Ishtar, and Ishhara)

80. [DIŠ TA SAG.DU-*šú* EN GÌR^{II}-*šú* …] *pa-gar-šú* DIRI *ma-gal* BABBAR KI.MIN [*na*]-*gi-il* ŠU ^{d}30 N[U …]

81. [DIŠ…] *ina* ÚNU-*šú* È [ŠU] ^{d}*É*-[*a*]

82. [DIŠ…] *ina kir-ri-šú u* MURUB$_4$-*t*[*i*? …] x NU […]

83. [DIŠ…] *ina* SAG ŠÀ-*šú* È ⸢IGI⸣.[ME]Š-*šú* KÚR.KÚR-*ru* ŠU ^{d}*Iš-ḫ*[*a-ra*]

84. [DIŠ[…*ina ša-pu*]-*la-šú u še-pit* ŠIR-*šú* È IGI.MEŠ-*šú* KÚR.KÚR-*ru u* SA$_5$ ŠU ^{d}*Iš-tár-r*[*i-šú*]

85. [DIŠ…] ŠÀ-*šú* SÍG GI$_6$ È-⸢*a*⸣ x […]

86. [DIŠ…] ŠÀ-*šú* SÍG BABBAR È-*a* NU x

---

87. [DIŠ KA-*šú bu-bu-*ʾ]-*ta* DIRI *u il-la-tu-šu il-*⸢*la*⸣-*ka bu-*ʾ-*šá-nu* MU.[NI]

88. [DIŠ LÚ.TUR *il-la-tu-š*]*ú* MÚD *ú-kal-la bu-*ʾ-*šá-nu* MU.[NI][10]

89. [DIŠ LÚ.TUR ŠÀ.MEŠ-*šú*] *eb-ṭú* ⸢*u*⸣ KA-*šú k*[*a-b*]*it bu-*ʾ-*šá-nu* MU.[NI][11]

90. [DIŠ LÚ.TUR UGU-*šú* GABA-*s*]*u u šá-šal-la-šú* KÚM.MEŠ *bu-*ʾ-*šá-nu* MU.[NI][12]

91. [DIŠ LÚ.TUR KÚM *la ḫa-aḫ*]-*ḫaš u* ŠÀ.MEŠ-*šú eb-ṭú bu-*ʾ-*šá-nu* MU.[NI][13]

92. [DIŠ SU-*šu* SIG$_7$ IGI].MEŠ-*šú* SIG$_7$ *šiḫ-ḫat* UZU TUKU.MEŠ *a-mur-*[*ri-q*]*a-nu* M[U.NI]

93. [DIŠ IGI.MEŠ-*šú* SI]G$_7$ ŠÀ IGI^{II}-*šú* SIG$_7$ *u* SUḪUŠ EME-*šú* GI$_6$ [*a*]*ḫ-ḫ*[*a-zu* MU.NI]

94. [DIŠ SAG.DU-*su t*]*i-ik-ka-šú u ša-pu-la-šú* 1-*niš* GU$_7$.MEŠ-[*š*]*ú šá-aš-*[*šá-ṭu* MU.NI]

95. [DIŠ GÚ-*su* MUR]UB$_4$-*šú* ŠU^{II}-*šú u* GÌR^{II}-*šú aš-ṭa šá-aš-*[*šá-ṭu* MU.NI]

96. [DIŠ GÚ-*su i*]-*zu-ur-ma* IGI^{II}-*šú gal-ta-at pi-qa la pi-qa i-par-ru-ud* KI.MIN *i-gal*!-⸢*lu-ut šá*⸣-*a*[*š-šá-ṭu* MU.NI]

97. [DIŠ TA SA.G]Ú-*ni-šú* EN *eq-bi-šú* SA.MEŠ-*šú šag-gu*$_5$ *šu-*ʾ-*ra-šú kaṣ-ra u i*[*s-sa-š*]*ú ḫe-sa-a* [*šá-aš-šá-ṭu* MU.NI]

98. [DIŠ SA.M]EŠ ^{UZU}ÚR-*šú* 1-*niš* GU$_7$.MEŠ-*šú* ZI-*a u* DU.MEŠ-*ka la i-le-*ʾ*-e* SA.GAL [MU.NI]

99. [DIŠ ^{UZU}]ÚR-*šú* TA *giš-ši-šú* EN *ki-ṣal-li-šú* GU$_7$-*šú* ZI-*bi u* DU-[*a*]*k maš-ka-d*[*ù* MU.NI]

100. [DIŠ TA] ^{UZU}GIŠ.KUN-*šú* EN ŠU.SI.MEŠ GÌR^{II}-*šú* SA.MEŠ-*šú* GU$_7$.MEŠ-*šú maš-ka-d*[*ù* MU.NI]

101. [DIŠ TA *giš*]-*ši-šú* EN *pi-ṭir ki-ṣil-li-šú* GU$_7$.MEŠ-*šú ḫi-ṭám* NU TUKU *ki-iṣ-ṣa-t*[*um* MU.NI]

102. ⸢DIŠ⸣ TA *giš-ši-šú* EN ŠU.SI.⸢MEŠ GÌR^{II}-*šú* SA⸣.MEŠ-*šú it-te-nen-ṣi-l*[*a-šú k*]*i-*⸢*iṣ-ṣat*⸣ UD.D[A MU.NI]

---

103. *sa-ma-nu* [ŠU] ^{d}*Gu-la* [*a*]-*šu-ú* ŠU ^{d}[*Gu-la*]
104. *ṣi-i-tum* ŠU ^{d}*Gu-la* x [...] ŠU ^{d}[*Gu-la*]
105. *ṣar-i-šu* ŠU ^{d}*Gu-la š*[*a-da-n*]*u* ŠU ^{d}*G*[*u-la*]
106. *ṣi-in-na-aḫ-ti-ri* ŠU ^{d}*Gu-la u ša-*[*da*]*-nu* ŠU ^{d}NIN.[IB]
107. *ta-kal-tu*$_4$ ŠU ^{d}NIN.IB *aḫ-ḫ*[*a-z*]*u* ŠU ^{d}[NIN.IB]
108. *di-ik-šú* ŠU ^{d}AMAR.UTU *u* [...] x ta ra i [...]
109. xx-*aḫ-ḫi-iz* ŠU ^{d}AMAR.UTU *um-me-di* [Š]U ^{d}*É*-[*a*]
110. [...] ŠU ^{d}UTU *gir-giš-šum* ŠU ^{d}UTU
111. [...] ŠU ^{d}UTU *ek-ke-tum* ŠU ^{d}UTU
112. [...] ŠU ^{d}UTU *qu-lip-tum* ŠU ^{d}UTU
113. [...] ŠU ^{d}UTU Ù.BU.BU.U[L] BABBAR ŠU ^{d}UTU TI-*uṭ*
114. [Ù.BU.BU.UL GI$_6$] ŠU ^{d}*Iš-tar* TAG-*it* NAM.TAR NU DIN-*uṭ* ŠU ^{d}UTU Ù.BU.B[U.U]L [S]A$_5$ ŠU ^{d}30 KI.MIN
115. [GÌR 15-*šú* ... Š]U ^{d}UTU GÌR 150-*šú i*[*ḫ* ...] ŠU ^{d}[*I*]*š-tar*
116. [...] ŠU ^{d}30 *a-na* EGIR-*šú i*[*ḫ* ...] ŠU ^{d}[...]-*šú*
117. [...] ^{d}*Iš-tar bu-up-pa-ni-šu i*[*m-qut*] ŠU ^{d}[...]
118. [...] *u* ŠÀ.MEŠ-*šú it-te-nen-bi-ṭu* UZU.MEŠ-*šú* [... Š]U [...]
119. [...] UZU.MEŠ-*šú i-šaḫ-ḫu-ḫu* [Š]U [...]
120. [...] AN.TA GU$_7$-*šú-ma la i-ṣal-lal* Š[U ^{d}*Šul-p*]*a-è-a*
121. [...] AN.TA GU$_7$-*šú-ma la i-ṣal-lal* ŠU [^{d}*I*]*štar*

122–123. (fragmentary)

Translation

1. [If] the nature of the [sore] is that it is clustered, it is called *ašû*.[14]
2. [If] the nature of the ⸢sore⸣ is that it is clustered, (his skin) is reddish and he scratches (and) the top of the sore produces fluid [...], it is called *ašû*.[15]
3. [If] the nature of the ⸢sore⸣ is that it is clustered and what comes out of it clings (to it),[16] his skin is reddish and the side of the sore has been scraped until [it bleeds], ⸢it⸣ is called *ašû*.[17]
4. [If] his ⸢face⸣ and his eyes are swollen (and) his sight is difficult and (his eyes) drift downstream,[18] ⸢it⸣ is called *ašû*.[19]
5. [If] his ⸢face⸣ is swollen, his eyesight is diminished, his body is full of *birdu* and his abdomen ⸢afflicts⸣ him, it is called *ašû*.[20]

6. [If] the nature of the sore is that it is just like the bite of a louse[21] and his body is full (of them), it is called ⸢"fleeting"⸣ *ašû*.[22]
7. [If] the nature of the sore is that it is like dark spots and the person's entire body is full (of them), it is called *kullaru*.[23]
8. [If] the appearance of the sore is dark (and) dry (and his skin) is reddish and he scratches, it is called *kullaru*.[24]
9. [If] the ⸢nature⸣ of the [sore] is that its surface is stiff, the area around it is full of clusters (and) [...], it is called the *kullaru* of *ašû*.[25]
10. [If] the ⸢nature⸣ of the [sore] is that it is clustered (and) it goes round the hips, its name is ⸢*ekketu*⸣.[26]
11. [If] the ⸢nature⸣ of the [sore] is that his body is full of what look like fish scales and it has a predictable course, it is called ⸢*rišiktu*⸣.[27]
12. [If] the ⸢nature⸣ of the [sore] is that it is hot like a burn and [...], the sore is called ⸢*rišûtu*⸣.[28]
13. [If] the ⸢nature⸣ of the [sore] is that it is hot like a burn [...] does not contain fluid and the ⸢sore⸣ has a [...], its name is *girgišu*.[29]
14. [If] the nature of the ⸢sore⸣ is that it is hot like a burn and contains fluid, it is called ⸢*bubuʾtu*⸣.[30]
15. [If] the nature of the sore is that it is hot like a burn and does not contain fluid (and) is full of little ⸢*bubuʾtu*⸣, [it] is called *išītu*.[31]
16. If the nature of the sore is that it is hot like a burn and is full of clusters (and) has redness, [it] is called *nipištu*.[32]
17. If the nature of the sore is that it is clustered and if an *umṣatu* blocks its exit, it is called *nipištu*.[33]
18. If the nature of the sore is that it is clustered, he scratches (and) fluid flows from [...], [it] is called *ruṭibtu*.[34]
19. If the nature of the sore is that it is red (or) white, it hurts him and it contains fluid, [it] is called *ruṭibtu*.[35]
20. If the appearance of the sore is black, [it] is called *ḫarasu*.[36]
21. If a person's body is full of *birdu* and his flesh ⸢stings him⸣ and redness continually falls on him, [it] ⸢is called⸣ *ḫarasu*.[37]
22. If a sore comes out in a person's foot or on his testicle and (his skin) is reddish and he scratches, [it] ⸢is called⸣ *ruṭibtu*.[38]
23. If the nature of the sore is that it is red, hot, swollen and flows, [it is called] *samānu*.[39]
24. If the nature of the sore is that it is red (and) the person continually gets feverish and continually vomits, [it is called] *samānu*.[40]
25. If the nature of the sore is that it is hard, it burns [...] and does not respond to you(r treatment), [it is called] a *midru*[41] (or) alternatively *samānu*.[42]

26. If the appearance of the sore is like a *bubu'tu* (and) his body is red, [it] is called "wind blasting."[43]
27. If the appearance of the sore is that it is as red as the sun(?), [it hurts him] (and) it holds all of the [...], [it] ⌈is called⌉ *pindû*.[44]
28. If the nature of his sore is that it is like obsidian (and) goes around his neck, [it] ⌈is called⌉ *šadānu*.[45]
29. If the nature of his sore is that it is hard to the touch (and) he is full of red spots, [it] ⌈is called⌉ *šadānu*.[46]
30. If the nature of the sore is that it is hard to the touch, he burns with fever, his spleen is very puffed up, (and) his appetite for bread and beer is diminished, its name is *šadānu*; "touch" of "hand" of [...][47]
31. If the nature of his sore is that it is hard as a rock, as it grows down inside, it continually goes down inside (and) he is not able to lift (his foot), to get up [and] walk [(or) to stand], it is called *šadānu*; "touch" of Marduk and [Ninurta].[48]
32. If the nature of his sore is that it is hard as a rock (and) it is located either on his neck or on his armpit or on his abdomen (and he has been sick) for three days, [he will die]; [it] is called [...][49]
33. If the nature of the sore is that it produces hot blood like a sheep with its throat cut [...], to cure him [...][50]
34. If the nature of the sore is that it falls on him in the evening and will not ⌈let up and⌉ numbness [will not stop] afflicting his whole body. [...]
35. If the nature of the sore is like something he does not know (how he got), and he has a needling pain [...]
36. If he is clothed (with it) while a suckling child and it is like a mounting (for jewelry), it is called *epqēnu*.
37. If he is clothed (with it) while a suckling child and it is like a mounting (for jewelry) and also divided, it is called [*epqu*].[51]
38. If the nature of the sore is that it is surrounded by what looks like its silt and it afflicts his neck, it is called [*kirbānu*].[52]
39. If the nature of the sore is that it is hard, it is placed on the surface of his flesh and he is ⌈continually gets hot⌉, it is called *kirbānu*.[53]
40. If the nature of the sore is that it is compact and its tip[54] is deeply incised, it is called *ziqtu*.[55]
41. [If] the nature of the [sore] is that it is like an *ibāru*-lesion and its tip is ⌈dotted⌉ with white, it is called *ziqtu*.[56]
42. [If] the nature of the [sore] is that it is red, white, (and) small[57] and it hurts him, it [is called] *ziqtu*.[58]

43–44. *(fragmentary)*

45. If he is clothed (with it) [while] a ⸢suckling child⸣ and it is red and hurts ⸢him⸣ and it is continually puffed up (and) continually hot, it [is called ...]
46. If he is clothed (with it) [while] a ⸢suckling child⸣ and it hurts him and it bursts/is extinguished [...], it [is called ...].
47. If he is clothed (with it) [while] a ⸢suckling child⸣ and it does not hurt him, it [is called] *abābu*(?).
48. If [...] and it does not hurt him, it [is called] *abābu*(?).
49. [If ...] it does not hurt him but it continually flows; alternatively, it keeps coming back [...], it [is called ...]
50. [If the nature of the sore] is that what looks like canal overflow water flows from inside it (and it is) a ⸢persistent sore, it⸣ [is called ...][59]
51. *(fragmentary)*
52. If he is [... while] a ⸢suckling child⸣ and it hurts him day and night so that he cannot sleep, [it] ⸢is called⸣ *abiktu*.
53. If he is [... while] a ⸢suckling child⸣ and it is like [...] and it is puffed up (and) it continually ⸢has⸣ heat, it is called *miqtu*; the *asû* should look at it.
54. [If...] it returns to its place (i.e., the swelling goes down) and yet it (still) contains fluid, it is called *miqtu*; the *asû* should look at it.
55. [If...] it returns to its place (i.e., the swelling goes down) and yet he does not ⸢get well⸣, Bau put that sore (there) on the ground or, alternatively in the bed [...].
56. If the nature of the sore is that it is like a growth and it is coated and in its coating, the entire surface is unevenly colored with black, it is called "the ghoul."[60]
57. [If ...] it contains pus [...], it is called [...].
58. [If the nature of the sore is that it is red (or)] ⸢white⸣ (and) produces pus [...], it is called "the calumniater."[61]
59. [If the nature of the sore is that it is red (or) white (and)] it ⸢hurts⸣ him, there is no fluid (in it) (and) it ⸢grows larger⸣ to the touch, it is called *nilugu*.[62]
60. [If the nature of the sore is that](if) he touches it, it ⸢grows larger⸣, what it produces ⸢is called⸣ *guzallu* ("the scoundrel").[63]
61. [If] it comes ⸢once again⸣ up to the hip region or thighs [...], [what it produces] is called ⸢"the scoundrel"⸣.[64]
62. [If...] he is ill with a sickness of thick sputum; it is called [...].
63. [If...] has a red [...], it is called *sikkatu*.
64. [If ...] its [...] is linked and it is dark, [it] ⸢is called⸣ *sagbānu*.
65–66. [If..., it is called] ⸢*ṣinnaḫ tiri*⸣. [If ...] and he ⸢holds⸣ sweat, [it is called] ⸢*ṣinnaḫ tiri*⸣.

67–68. [If …] fluid and it flows, [it is called] *ṣiriptu*. [If … it is called] ⸢*ṣiriptu*⸣.

69–70. *(fragmentary)*

71–74. *(fragmentary mentioning SAḪAR.ŠUB.BA)*

75–79. *(fragmentary mentioning "hand" of Ishum, Ishtar, and Ishhara)*

80. [If from his head to his feet], his body is full [of …] (and) he/it is very white; alternatively, ⸢whitish⸣, "hand" of Sîn; he will ⸢not⸣ […].

81. [If …] erupts on the middle of his cheek, ["hand"] of ⸢Ea⸣.[65]

82. [If … erupts] on his throat and the middle of […], he will not […]

83. [If …] erupts on his epigastrium (and) his face continually changes (for the worse), "hand" of ⸢Ishhara⸣.[66]

84. [If …] erupts [on] his ⸢inguinal region⸣ or the base of his testicle (and) his face continually changes (for the worse) and it is red, "hand" of [his personal] goddess.

85. [If …] (and) a black hair grows out of it, [he/it will …].[67]

86. [If …] (and) a white hair grows out of it, he/it will not […].[68]

---

87. [If his mouth] is full of ⸢*bubuʾtu*⸣ and his saliva flows, [it] is called *buʾšānu*.[69]

88. [If an infant's spittle] contains blood, [it] is called *buʾšānu*.[70]

89. [If an infant's insides] are cramped and his mouth ⸢(feels) heavy⸣, [it] is called *buʾšānu*.[71]

90. [If an infant's skull, his breast], and his upper back are feverish, [it] is called *buʾšānu*.[72]

91. [If an infant has] a lukewarm [temperature] and his insides are cramped, *buʾšānu* afflicts him.[73]

92. [If a person's body is yellow, his face] is ⸢yellow⸣ and his eyes are yellow (and) he has wasting of the flesh, it is called *amurriqānu*.[74]

93. [If his face] is ⸢yellow⸣ and the inner part of his eyes is yellow (and) the base of the tongue is black, [it is called] ⸢*aḫḫāzu*⸣.[75]

94. [If his head], his ⸢neck⸣ and his inguinal regions all continually hurt ⸢him⸣ at the same time, [it is called] ⸢*šaššaṭu*⸣.[76]

95. [If his neck], his ⸢hip region⸣, his hands and his feet are stiff, [it is called] ⸢*šaššaṭu*⸣.[77]

96. [If he] twists [his neck] and his eye jerks (and) he shudders or jerks incessantly, [it is called] ⸢*šaššaṭu*⸣.[78]

97. [If] his muscles are stiff [from] his ⸢neck muscles⸣ to his heel, his eyebrows are knitted and ⸢his jaws⸣ are pressured, [it is called *šaššaṭu*].[79]

98. [If the muscles] of his thigh all hurt at once (and) he cannot stand up or walk about, [it is called] *sagallu*.[80]
99. [If] his thigh hurts him from his hip sockets to his ankles (but) he can stand and walk, [it is called] ⸢*maškādu*⸣.[81]
100. [If from] his coccyx to his toes his muscles continually hurt him, [it is called] ⸢*maškādu*⸣.[82]
101. [If from] his ⸢hip sockets⸣ to the opening of his ankles it continually hurts him, it is of no consequence; [it is called] ⸢"gnawing"⸣.[83]
102. If from his hip sockets to his toes, his muscles are continually ⸢sluggish⸣, [it is called] the ⸢"gnawing"⸣ of *ṣētu*.[84]

---

103. *Samānu* is "[hand]" of Gula; ⸢*ašû*⸣ is "hand" of [Gula].
104. Growths are "hand" of Gula; […] are "hand" of [Gula].[85]
105. Proliferating (sores) are "hand" of Gula; ⸢*šadānu*⸣ is "hand" of ⸢Gula⸣.[86]
106. Diarrhea is "hand" of Gula and ⸢*šadānu*⸣ is "hand" of ⸢Ninurta⸣.[87]
107. The liver: "hand" of Ninurta; ⸢*aḫḫāzu*⸣, "hand" of [Ninurta].[88]
108. Needling pain is "hand" of Marduk; […].[89]
109. ⸢"contagious"⸣(?) is "hand" of Marduk; *ummedu* is "⸢hand⸣" of E[a].[90]
110. […] is "hand" of Shamash; *girgišu* is "hand" of Shamash.[91]
111. […] is "hand" of Shamash; *ekketu* is "hand" of Shamash.[92]
112. […] is "hand" of Shamash; scales are "hand" of Shamash.[93]
113. […] is "hand" of Shamash; white *bubuʾtu* are "hand" of Shamash; he will get well.[94]
114. [Black *bubuʾtu*] : "hand" of Ishtar; "touch" of (his) personal death demon; he will not get well. ⸢Red *bubuʾtu*⸣ : "hand" of Sîn; ditto (he will get well).[95]
115. [His "right" foot …] ⸢"hand"⸣ of Shamash. His "left" foot […], "hand" of Ishtar.
116. […], "hand" of Sîn; he […] on his back, "hand" of his […].
117. [… "hand"] of Ishtar; he ⸢falls⸣ on his front side, "hand" of […]
118. […] and his insides are continually cramped, his flesh […], ⸢"hand"⸣ of […].
119. […] his flesh wastes away, ⸢"hand"⸣ of […].
120. [If] his upper […] hurts him so badly that he cannot sleep, ⸢"hand"⸣ of ⸢Šulpaea⸣.
121. [If] his upper […] hurts him so badly that he cannot sleep, "hand" of Ishtar.

122–123. *(fragmentary)*

Notes

1. Augmenting Heeßel 2000, 353.
2. Correcting Heeßel 2000, 354.
3. Correcting Heeßel 2000, 354.
4. Differently Heeßel 2000, 354.
5. After a suggestion by Geller 2007, 11–12.
6. Restorations are based in BAM 409:33′–36′.
7. Augmenting Heeßel 2000, 355.
8. Augmenting Heeßel 2000, 355.
9. Reading follows K 3526 rev. 6–7.
10. Restored from DPS 40:99.
11. Restored from DPS 40:97.
12. Restored from DPS 40:100.
13. Restored from DPS 40:101.
14. See Scurlock and Andersen 2005, 10.89. Beckman and Foster 1988, no. 18:11′–12′ originally contained a treatment for this condition.
15. See Scurlock and Andersen 2005, 10.90.
16. Differently Heeßel 2000, 353.
17. See Scurlock and Andersen 2005, 10.91.
18. After Heeßel 2000, 359, 366, reading DIRI = *neqelpû* and interpreting it as a reference to horizontal nystagmus.
19. See Scurlock and Andersen 2005, 9.31, 10.96. The treatment for this condition is given in *AMT* 84/6:5′–7′//*RA* 53.1–18 rev. 8–9.
20. See Scurlock and Andersen 2005, 10.92. The treatment for this condition is given in *AMT* 84/6:8′–10′.
21. More or less with von Weiher, SpTU 4.81,84 and augmenting Heeßel 2000, 359.
22. See Scurlock and Andersen 2005, 10.101.
23. See Scurlock and Andersen 2005, 10.64.
24. See Scurlock and Andersen 2005, 10.65.
25. See Scurlock and Andersen 2005, 10.94.
26. See Scurlock and Andersen 2005, 10.34.
27. Heeßel 2000, 353, 367 restores *ri*-[*šu*]-*tum* and, on this basis translates *rišûtu* thereafter as "scales" (359, 360). However, fish scales seem more appropriate to dryness (*rišiktu*) than to redness (*rišûtu*). See Scurlock and Andersen 2005, 10.2.
28. See Scurlock and Andersen 2005, 10.10.
29. See Scurlock and Andersen 2005, 10.142.
30. See Scurlock and Andersen 2005, 4.11, 10.77.
31. See Scurlock and Andersen 2005, 10.173.
32. See Scurlock and Andersen 2005, 10.181. A treatment for this condition appears in *RA* 53.1–18 rev. 10–11.
33. See Scurlock and Andersen 2005, 10.182.
34. See Scurlock and Andersen 2005, 10.5.
35. See Scurlock and Andersen 2005, 10.6.
36. See Scurlock and Andersen 2005, 3.280, 10.74. This entry is cited in BAM 409 obv. 18′.
37. See Scurlock and Andersen 2005, 3.281, 10.75. A treatment for this condition appears in BAM 409 obv. 19′–25′.

38. See Scurlock and Andersen 2005, 3.257, 10.7. Treatments for this condition appear in *AMT* 74/1 ii 32–iii 12.

39. See Scurlock and Andersen 2005, 3.172.

40. See Scurlock and Andersen 2005, 3.173.

41. Heeßel 2000, 354, 360 interprets these signs as MÚD ŠUB: "it produces blood."

42. See Scurlock and Andersen 2005, 3.192.

43. See Scurlock and Andersen 2005, 4.12, 10.17. A treatment for this condition appears in BAM 580 vi 8′–10′.

44. Note that *pindû* is also the name of a stone which is described as being granulated like mottled barley or cucumber seeds (*CAD* A/2, 451 s.v. *ašnan*). See Scurlock and Andersen 2005, 10.126.

45. See Scurlock and Andersen 2005, 3.228.

46. See Scurlock and Andersen 2005, 3.229.

47. A treatment for this condition is given in BAM 409 obv. 26′–32′. Heeßel 2000, 368 tentatively suggests restoring Ningeštinanna. However, the sign which precedes the NA on BAM 409 obv. 28′ does not look at all like a GEŠTIN. Instead, it appears to be a RIN suggesting a restoration of either "curse" (NAM.RIN.NA), or more probably a plant medicine: "turmeric" (KUR.GI.RIN.NA). See Scurlock and Andersen 2005, 3.225.

48. See Scurlock and Andersen 2005, 3.226, 19.100, 19.114. Treatments for this condition are given in BAM 409 obv. 33′–rev. 9.

49. See Scurlock and Andersen 2005, 3.227.

50. See Scurlock and Andersen 2005, 14.21.

51. This and the previous entry describe the lesions of SAḪAR.ŠUB.BA, one of a number of ancient diagnostic categories that grouped diseases with similar lesions, and that has long been equated with leprosy. The description of the lesions as "like mountings," that is, with elevated margins and concave centers, specifically points to the milder tubeculoid form of the disease (see chapter 7, text 3). The "divided" of the second entry presumably refers to central healing of the lesions. Leprosy is one of those diseases that present in childhood and is frequently described in ancient texts as "clothing" its victim.

52. See Scurlock and Andersen 2005, 3.240, 10.146. This entry is cited in BAM 583 i 3′–4′.

53. See Scurlock and Andersen 2005, 3.240, 10.146. A treatment for this condition is given in BAM 583 i 4′–6′.

54. Heeßel 2000, 361, 369 mistakes this passage as referring to the skull or nose of the patient.

55. See Scurlock and Andersen 2005, 10.108. The entry is cited in *AMT* 30/2:9′.

56. See Scurlock and Andersen 2005, 10.108. The entry is cited in *AMT* 30/2:10′.

57. Heeßel 2000, 361, 369 reads the "white" and the "small" together as *ut-tur* and interprets this as "exceedingly." The entry is cited in *AMT* 30/2:11′. This and the preceding lines form an introduction to treatments for this condition in *AMT* 30/2:12′–15′.

58. See Scurlock and Andersen 2005, 10.108.

59. See Scurlock and Andersen 2005, 3.178.

60. See Scurlock and Andersen 2005, 3.176.

61. See Scurlock and Andersen 2005, 3.177. A treatment for this condition is given in BAM 580 iii 31'–32′.

62. Pace Heeßel 2000, 370, this has nothing to do with "ox fat." See Scurlock and Andersen 2005, 3.276. A treatment for this condition is given in BAM 417 obv. 25–27.

63. See Scurlock and Andersen 2005, 3.278.

64. See BAM 417 rev. 9′–14′.

65. See Scurlock and Andersen 2005, 19.245.

66. See Scurlock and Andersen 2005, 19.290.

67. See Scurlock and Andersen 2005, 10.125.

68. See Scurlock and Andersen 2005, 10.125.

69. See Scurlock and Andersen 2005, 3.64, 4.17, 10.81, 18.47. The entry appears also in DPS 7:36′.

70. See Scurlock and Andersen 2005, 17.157. The entry appears also in DPS 40:99.

71. See Scurlock and Andersen 2005, 17.157. The entry appears also in DPS 40:97.

72. See Scurlock and Andersen 2005, 17.157. The entry appears also in DPS 40:100

73. See Scurlock and Andersen 2005, 17.157. The entry appears also in DPS 40:101.

74. See Scurlock and Andersen 2005, 6.121. The entry also appears in DPS 18:24. It is cited in therapeutic text BAM 578 iii 7 as an introduction to a series of simple treatments apparently drawn from pharmacological texts (iii 8–15) followed by more complex treatments for this condition.

75. See Scurlock and Andersen 2005, 6.117. The entry also appears in DPS 9:13. This entry is cited in therapeutic text BAM 578 iv 26 as an introduction to treatments for this condition.

76. See Scurlock and Andersen 2005, 3.198. This entry appears also in DPS 3:40.

77. See Scurlock and Andersen 2005, 3.199. This entry also appears in DPS 10:10. A treatment for this condition is given in BAM 129 iv 3′–5′.

78. See Scurlock and Andersen 2005, 3.197, 13.68, 13.107. This entry also appears in DPS 10:11. Treatments for this condition with similar symptoms are given in BAM 129 iv 6′–13′ and BAM 131 obv. 9–15//CT 23.5–14 iv 18–23//*AMT* 4/5:5′–8′.

79. See Scurlock and Andersen 2005, 3.196. This entry also appears in DPS 10:27 and Arnaud 1987, 694 obv. 6′.

80. See Scurlock and Andersen 2005, 11.58. This entry appears also in DPS 14:172′. It is cited in *AMT* 42/6 obv. 1 and CT 23.1–2:1 as a sort of introduction to treatments for *sagallu*.

81. See Scurlock and Andersen 2005, 11.59. This entry also appears in DPS 14:170′–171′.

82. See Scurlock and Andersen 2005, 11.60. This entry appears also in DPS 12:126″.

83. The entry also appears in DPS 14:229′.

84. See Scurlock and Andersen 2005, 3.129. This entry appears also in DPS 14:30–31, Arnaud 1987, 694 obv. 5′ and StBoT 36.48 D 2:13′.

85. See Scurlock and Andersen 2005, 19.98.

86. See Scurlock and Andersen 2005, 19.98.

87. See Scurlock and Andersen 2005, 19.99

88. See Scurlock and Andersen 2005, 19.99, 19.365.

89. See Scurlock and Andersen 2005, 19.101.

90. See Scurlock and Andersen 2005, 19.91, 19.246.

91. See Scurlock and Andersen 2005, 10.144, 19.103.

92. See Scurlock and Andersen 2005, 19.103.

93. See Scurlock and Andersen 2005, 19.103.

94. See Scurlock and Andersen 2005, 19.105.

95. See Scurlock and Andersen 2005, 19.105.

DPS 34

DPS 33:124 (catchline) = DPS 34:1

1. DIŠ NA *ana sin-niš-ti* ŠÀ-*šú* NU ÍL-*šú* MUNUS BI ŠÀ-[*šú* ...][1]

Translation

1. If a person cannot get an erection for a woman, that woman [his] erection [to obtain, ...]

Note

1. Restored from the catalogue; see Heeßel 2000, 374 ad 124.

G. OBSTETRICS AND GYNECOLOGY: DPS 36–37, 39

DPS 36

1. *šúm-ma* TU PEŠ$_4$-*ma* UGU SAG.KI-*šá* SIG$_7$ *šà*-ŠÀ-*šà* NITA : *i-kar-ri-iṣ*
2. DIŠ TU *mu-úḫ* SAG.KI-*šá* BABBAR *na-mir šà*-ŠÀ-*šà* MUNUS : *i-šar-ru*
3. DIŠ GI$_6$ *šà*-ŠÀ-*šà* MUNUS : SILIM-*im*
4. DIŠ SA$_5$ *šà*-ŠÀ-*šà* NITA : ÚŠ
5. DIŠ GÙN.A : *ba-ru-um šà*-ŠÀ-*šà* NÁ
6. DIŠ *uṭ-ṭe-ṭì* DIRI *šà*-ŠÀ-*šà* NITA : NÍG.TUKU
7. DIŠ *uṭ-ṭe-ṭì* SA$_5$.MEŠ DIRI *šà*-ŠÀ-*šà*(coll.) *i*$_{11}$-*šár-rù*
8. DIŠ *pár-sat šà*-ŠÀ-*šà* NITA
9. DIŠ TU SA SAG.KI-*ša* SA$_5$ *šà*-ŠÀ-*šà* NITA
10. DIŠ BABBAR *šà*-ŠÀ-*šà* MUNUS
11. DIŠ (TU SA SAG.KI-*šá*) KI.TA-*nu* ZAG *te-bi šà*-ŠÀ-*šà* MUNUS
12. DIŠ KI.TA-*nu* GÙB *te-bi šà*-ŠÀ-*šà* NITA
13. DIŠ TU S[A].MEŠ SAG.KI-*ša* SA$_5$ DIDLI *šà*-ŠÀ-*šà* NITA
14. DIŠ SAG.KI-*ša* BABBAR DIDLI *šà*-ŠÀ-*šà* ⸢MUNUS⸣
15. DIŠ TU K[A-*š*]*á ṣa-pir* : *za-qir* AŠ *šà*-ŠÀ-*šà* NITA [x]
16. DIŠ TU S[AG] KA *šá* ZAG ZI-*ma u* GI$_6$ *šà*-ŠÀ-*šà* Ú[Š]
17. DIŠ *šá* GÙB ZI-*ma u* GI$_6$ *šà*-ŠÀ-*šà* ÚŠ : TI
18. [DIŠ T[U x K]A *šá* KI.TA-*nu* 15 SA$_5$ *šà*-ŠÀ-*šà* ÚŠ
19. [DIŠ] KI.TA-*nu* 150 SA$_5$ *šà*-ŠÀ-*šà* NITA
20. [DIŠ] KI.TA-*nu* 15 GÙN.A *šà*-ŠÀ-*šà* DIN
21. [DIŠ] KI.TA-*nu* 150 GÙN.A *šà*-ŠÀ-*šà* DIN
22. ⸢DIŠ⸣ KI.TA-*nu* 15 ZI-*bi šà*-ŠÀ-*šà* NITA
23. DIŠ KI.TA-*nu* 150 ZI-*bi šà*-ŠÀ-*šà* MUNUS
24. DIŠ TU SAMAG.MEŠ-*šú uq-tal-la-pa u* IGI.MEŠ-*šú* SIG$_7$ *šà*-ŠÀ-*šà* NITA
25. DIŠ *u* IGI.MEŠ-*šú* SA$_5$ *šà*-ŠÀ-*šà* MUNUS
26. DIŠ TU *ap-pa* UBUR-*šá zi-i-ir*$_9$ *šà*-ŠÀ-*šà* NU SI.SA
27. DIŠ *pa-ṭi-ir*$_9$ *šà*-ŠÀ-*šà* SI.SA
28. DIŠ GI$_6$ NITA PEŠ$_4$-*at*
29. DIŠ SA$_5$ MUNUS PEŠ$_4$-*at*
30. DIŠ BABBAR NU SI.SÁ PEŠ$_4$-*at*
31. DIŠ MÚD! SA$_5$ NITA PEŠ$_4$-*at*

32. DIŠ SIG$_7$ *šà*-ŠÀ-*šà* ŠUB
33. DIŠ SAMAG.MEŠ BABBAR.MEŠ DIRI SI.SÁ PEŠ$_4$-*át*
34. DIŠ SAMAG.MEŠ SA$_5$.MEŠ DIRI NU SI.SÁ PEŠ$_4$-*át*
35. DIŠ SAMAG.MEŠ GI$_6$.MEŠ DIRI NITA PEŠ$_4$-*át*
36. DIŠ 3 BÙR-*šu* *šà*-ŠÀ-*šà* ÚKU
37. DIŠ 4 BÙR-*šu* *šà*-ŠÀ-*šà* ÚKU
38. DIŠ 5 BÙR-*šu* *šà*-ŠÀ-*šà* ÚŠ
39. DIŠ 6 BÙR-*šu* *šà*-ŠÀ-*šà* NU SI.SÁ
40. DIŠ 7 BÙR-*šu* *šà*-ŠÀ-*šà* TI-*uṭ*
41. DIŠ 8 BÙR-*šu* *šà*-ŠÀ-*šà* TI-*uṭ*
42. DIŠ 9 BÙR-*šu* DUMU.MEŠ-*šá* *ina* IGI-*šá* *ú-na-ka-ru* : GIN.ME
43. DIŠ 10 BÙR-*šu* DUMU.MEŠ-*šá* *ú-šal-lam*
44. DIŠ 14 BÙR-*šu* DUMU.MEŠ-*šá* NU *ú-šal-lam*
45. DIŠ 15 BÙR-*šu* *ù* URUxKEŠDA-*šú-nu* SA$_5$ NITA PEŠ$_4$-*at*
46. DIŠ 15 BÙR-*šu* *ù* MIN GI$_6$ *šà*-ŠÀ-*šà* MUNUS

46A. ⸢DIŠ⸣ 16 [BÙR-*š*]*u* [...]
46B. [DIŠ] 17 [BÙR-*š*]*u* [...]
46C. [DIŠ 18 BÙR-*š*]*u* [...]
46D. [DIŠ 19 BÙR-*š*]*u* [...]
46E. [DIŠ 2]0 [BÙR-*š*]*u* [...]

47. DIŠ 5 BÙR-*šu* *ù* MIN SA$_5$ *šà*-ŠÀ-*šà* NITA
48. DIŠ 5 BÙR-*šu* *ù* MIN GI$_6$ *šà*-ŠÀ-*šà* MUNUS
49. DIŠ TU SA UBUR-*šá* *šú-šú-ru* MUNUS PEŠ$_4$-*at*
50. DIŠ GU.MEŠ DIB.DIB NITA PEŠ$_4$-*at*
51. DIŠ SA$_5$ NÍTA PEŠ$_4$-*at*
51. DIŠ TU *mu-úḫ* UBUR-*šá* SA.MEŠ SA$_5$.MEŠ *pur-ru-ku* MUNUS PEŠ$_4$-*at*
53. DIŠ GI$_6$.MEŠ *pur-ru-ku* NITA PEŠ$_4$-*at*
54. DIŠ BABBAR.MEŠ *pur-ru-ku* NU SI.SÁ PEŠ$_4$-*at*
55. DIŠ SIG$_7$.MEŠ *pur-ru-ku* *šà*-ŠÀ-*šà* NU SI.SÁ
56. DIŠ TU *ina* SAG ŠÀ-*ša* SA.MEŠ SIG$_7$.MEŠ ŠUB-*ú* *šà*-ŠÀ-*šà* SI.SÁ
57. DIŠ TU ŠÀ.MEŠ-*ša* *pat-tal* NITA PEŠ-*at*
58. DIŠ *zaq-ru* : *na-šal-lu-lu-nim* MU PA PEŠ-*at*
59. DIŠ TU ŠÀ.MEŠ-*ša* *ana im-ši-ša na-šal-lu-lu-nim* MU DIN PEŠ-*at*
60. DIŠ *ana im-ši-ša zaq-ru* : *ana* ZUM ŠÀ MU DIN PEŠ-*at*
61. DIŠ *ana im-ši-ša* GAR-*nu suk-ku-ku* Ù.TU
62. DIŠ *ana im-ši-ša* ŠUB-*ú* ŠU.BI.DIL.ÀM
63. DIŠ *ana im-ši-ša zaq-ru-ú* NITA PEŠ-*at*
64. DIŠ *ana im-ši-ša* AN.TA *za-aq-ru* MUNUS PEŠ-*at*
65. DIŠ *ana im-ši-ša* KI.TA *za-aq-ru* : *saḫ-ru* NITA PEŠ-*at*

66. DIŠ *eb-ṭù* NITA PEŠ-*at*
67. DIŠ *nap-ḫu* MUNUS PEŠ-*at*
68. DIŠ *ma-ʾ-du* MUNUS PEŠ-*at*
69. DIŠ SIG_7 ŠUB-*ú šà*-ŠÀ-*šà ú-šak-lal*
70. DIŠ GIN_7 *ap-pi-šá za-qip* MUNUS PEŠ-*at*
71. DIŠ *ma-ʾ-du* GÌR DIDLI-*ša u* ZI.IN.GI DIDLI-*šá nu-up-pu-ḫa* ZAG *u* GÙB ZUKUM-*as* MAŠ.TAB.BA PEŠ-*at*
72. DIŠ TU $ŠU^{II}$-*šá* ŠÀ.ME-*šá ú-kal-la* NITA PEŠ-*at*
73. DIŠ TU SA.MEŠ-*šá ana* SAG ŠÀ-*šá zaq-ru* MUNUS PEŠ-*at*
74. DIŠ *ana im-ši-šá zaq-ru* NITA PEŠ-*at*
75. DIŠ *ma-ʾ-du* MUNUS PEŠ-*at*
76. DIŠ TU ŠÀ.MEŠ-*ša nap-ḫu* NITA PEŠ-*at*
77. DIŠ TU IGI.MEŠ-*šá ik-ki-ru ina šà*-ŠÀ-*šà* ÚŠ
78. DIŠ TU IGI.MEŠ-*šá ne-e-ḫu ina šà*-ŠÀ-*šà ú-šal-lam*
79. DIŠ TU KUŠ.TAB IGI-*šá ma-lu-ú šà*-ŠÀ-*šà* GAM
80. DIŠ TU KUŠ.TAB IGI-*šá* DIRI-*ú* IGI DIDLI-*šá tur-ru-pa qá-du šà*-ŠÀ-*šà* GAM
81. DIŠ TU *ip-ta-na-ar-ru ul ú-šal-lam*
82. DIŠ TU MÚD *ina* KA-*šú* DU-*ku ina* $PEŠ_4$-*šú* NU DIN
83. DIŠ TU MÚD.BABBAR *ina* KA-*šú* ŠUB.ŠUB-*a qá-du šà*-ŠÀ-*šà* GAM
84. DIŠ TU $GÌR^{II}$-*šá u* $ŠU^{II}$-*šú it-te-nen-ṣi-la* 21 PA.AN
85. DIŠ TU SAG *a-bu-un-na-ti-šá pa-ši-ir šá*-ŠÀ-*šà ú-šal-lam*
86. DIŠ *zi-ir₉ pa-ši-ir šá*-ŠÀ-*šà* NU DIN
87. DIŠ TU *ina* KA-*šá ša* ZAG MÚD DU *šà*-ŠÀ-*šà* GAM
88. DIŠ TU *ina* KA-*šá ša* GÙB MÚD DU *šà*-ŠÀ-*šà* GAM
89. DIŠ TU $I[GI]^{II}$-*šá* BAL.BAL.MEŠ *ar-na-ab-ba* ÍL *šà*-ŠÀ-*šà* GAM
90. DIŠ TU SA *k*[*i*]-*ṣil-li-šá* ZAG ZI-*b*[*i*] MUNUS $PEŠ_4$-*at*
91. DIŠ GÙB ZI-*b*[*i*] NITA $PEŠ_4$-*at*
92. DIŠ TU SA *ki*-[*ṣil-li*]-*šá* ZAG *u* GÙB ZI-[*bi*] [M]AŠ.TAB.BA NU SI.SÁ $PEŠ_4$-*at*
93. DIŠ TU SA *ki-ṣil-li-šá* MÚD DIRI.MEŠ NITA $PEŠ_4$-*at*
94. DIŠ TU *ina* ŠÀ *ma-ru-uš-ti-šá* ZAG ZUKUM-*as* NÁ $PEŠ_4$-*at*
95. DIŠ GÙB ZUKUM-*as* MUNUS $PEŠ_4$-*at*
96. DIŠ TU ZAG ZUKUM-*as u* GÌR-*šá* DUGUD-*at* NITA *u* MUNUS $PEŠ_4$-*at*
97 DIŠ GÙB ZUKUM-*as u* KI.MIN MUNUS $PEŠ_4$-*at*
98. DIŠ ZAG *u* GÙB ZUKUM-*as* MAŠ.TAB.BA $PEŠ_4$-*at*
99. DIŠ TU $GÌR^{II}$-*šá* TUR.MEŠ *e-ra-at u mu-šal-li-mat*
100. DIŠ TU $ŠÀ.SUR_{11}$-*sa sa-a-mu* NITA *ir-ḫi*

101. DIŠ TU ŠÀ.SUR$_{11}$-*sa pe-lu-ú* NITA *ir-ḫi*
102. DIŠ TU ŠÀ.SUR$_{11}$-*sa nam-ru* NU SI.SÁ *ir-ḫi*
103. DIŠ ⸢TU *m*⸣*i-ra-a pal-ḫat ina šà*-ŠÀ-*šà i-šal-lim*
104. DIŠ T[U *mi*]*-ra-a še-la-at ina šà*-ŠÀ-*šà* ÚŠ
105. DIŠ T[U …]-*šá i-ta-na-aš-šá-šu šà*-ŠÀ-*šà* ÚŠ
106. DIŠ T[U PEŠ$_4$-*ma š*]*a* 5 ITI 3 U$_4$-*mi iq-ri-bu-niš-šú* NAM.TI.[LA]
107. DIŠ TU ⸢PEŠ$_4$-*ma ša*⸣ ITI 4 U$_4$-*mi* KI.MIN [N]AM.TI.[LA]
108. DIŠ TU ⸢PEŠ$_4$⸣-*ma ša* ITI 5 U$_4$-*mi* KI.MIN *ša na-aḫ-šá-ti* G[IG] (coll.)
109. DIŠ TU ⸢PEŠ$_4$⸣-*ma ša* ITI 6 U$_4$-*mi* KI.MIN KI.MIN
110. DIŠ TU PEŠ$_4$-*ma ša* ITI 7 U$_4$-*mi* KI.MIN NAM.TI.[LA]
111. DIŠ TU PEŠ$_4$-*ma ša* ITI 8 U$_4$-*mi* KI.MIN ḪUL *a-bi* NAM.ÉRIM DIB-*su*
112. DIŠ TU PEŠ$_4$-*ma ša* ITI 9 U$_4$-*mi* KI.MIN BA.ÚŠ
113. DIŠ TU PEŠ$_4$-*ma ša* ITI 10 U$_4$-*mi* KI.MIN TI.LA

---

114. DIŠ MUNUS 2 UŠ.ME Ù.TU KUR *su-un-qam* IGI-*mar*
115. DIŠ MUNUS 2 SAL.ME Ù.TU É.BI *ana* IGI-*šú* DU-*ak*

---

116. DIŠ MUNUS PEŠ$_4$ GIG-*ma* 1 UŠ 54-ÀM MU.ŠID.BI *ṭup-pi* IGI-*ú* BE-*ma* TU PEŠ$_4$-*ma*

Translation

1. If a woman of childbearing age is pregnant and the top of her forehead is greenish, her fetus is male (var. it will be fully formed).[1]
2. If the top of the forehead of a woman of childbearing age is white (and) shines, her fetus is female (var. it will become rich [i.e., fat]).[2]
3. If it is dark, her fetus is female (var. it will be healthy).[3]
4. If it is reddish, her fetus is male (var. it will die).[4]
5. If it is multicolored, the child in her womb will lie down.[5]
6. If it is full of "grains," her fetus is male (var. richness [plenty of fat]).[6]
7. If it is full of red "grains," her fetus will become rich (i.e., fat).[7]
8. If she is past (normal child-bearing age), her fetus is male.[8]
9. If a muscle of a woman of childbearing age's forehead is reddish, her fetus is male.
10. If it is white, her fetus is female.
11 If it (the blood vessel of a woman of childbearing age's temple), the lower one to the "right" pulsates, her fetus is female.[9]
12 If the lower one to the "left" pulsates, her fetus is male.[10]

13 If the ⸢muscles⸣ of a woman of childbearing age's temple are reddish, her fetus is male.[11]

14 If (the muscles of a woman of childbearing age)'s temple are white, her fetus is female.[12]

15 If a woman of childbearing age's ⸢"tip"⸣ twitches (var. protrudes), her fetus is male; [it will live/die].[13]

16 If the ⸢head⸣ of a woman of childbearing age's "tip" rises to the "right" and is dark, her fetus will ⸢die⸣.

17 If it rises to the "left" and is dark, her fetus will die (var. will live).

18 [If the base?] of a ⸢woman of childbearing age's "tip"⸣ is reddish from below to the "right," her fetus will die.

19 [If it] is reddish from below to the "left," her fetus is male.

20 [If] it is multicolored from below to the "right," her fetus will live.

21 [If] it is multicolored from below to the "left," her fetus will live.

22 If it rises from below to the "right," her fetus is male.[14]

23 If it rises from below to the "left," her fetus is female.[15]

24 If a woman of childbearing age's *umṣātu*-lesions look peeled and her face is yellowish, her fetus is male.

25 If (a woman of childbearing age's *umṣātu*-lesions look peeled) and her face is reddish, her fetus is female.

26 If the tip of a woman of childbearing age's breast is twisted (shut), her fetus will not do well.[16]

27 If it is open, her fetus will do well.[17]

28 If it (the tip of a woman of childbearing age's breast) is dark, she is pregnant with a male.[18]

29 If it is reddish, she is pregnant with a female.[19]

30 If it is white, she is pregnant with fetus which will not do well.

31 If it is blood-red, she is pregnant with a male.[20]

32 If it is yellow/tan, she will abort her fetus.

33 If it is full of white *umṣatu*-lesions, the delivery will be easy.[21]

34 If it is full of reddish *umṣatu*-lesions, the delivery will not be easy.[22]

35 If it is full of dark *umṣatu*'s, she is pregnant with a male.

36 If it has three dimples, her fetus will be poor (i.e., thin).

37 If it has four dimples, her fetus will be poor (i.e., thin).

38 If it has five dimples, her fetus will die.

39 If it has six dimples, her fetus will not do well.

40 If it has seven dimples, her fetus will live.

41 If it has eight dimples, her fetus will live.

42 If it has nine dimples, her children will become hostile to her (var. will go away).
43 If it has ten dimples, she will bring her children to term.
44 If it has fourteen dimples, she will not bring her children to term.
45 If it has fifteen dimples and their ... are reddish, she is pregnant with a male.
46a If it has fifteen dimples and their ... are dark, her fetus is female.
46b If it has sixteen [dimples ...]
46c [If] it has seventeen [dimples ...]
46d [If] it [has eighteen dimples ...]
46e [If] it [has nineteen dimples ...]
46f [If] it [has] ⸢twenty⸣ [dimples ...]
47 If it has five dimples and their ditto ([...]) are reddish, her fetus is male.
48 If it has five dimples and their ditto ([...]) are dark, her fetus is female.
49 If the muscle(s)/blood vessel(s) of the breast of a woman of childbearing age run in a straight line, she is pregnant with a female.[23]
50 If they are held by threads, she is pregnant with a male.[24]
51 If they are red, she is pregnant with a male.[25]
52 If on top of the breast of a woman of childbearing age red muscles/blood vessels cross, she is pregnant with a female.
53 If dark ones cross, she is pregnant with a male.
54 If white ones cross, she is pregnant with a fetus which will not do well.
55 If yellow/tan ones cross, her fetus will not do well.
56 If on the epigastrium of a woman of childbearing age, the muscles are unevenly colored with yellow/tan, her fetus will do well.[26]
57 If a woman of childbearing age's insides feel balled up(?), she is pregnant with a male.[27]
58 If they are protruding (var. slither), she is pregnant with ...
59 If a woman of childbearing age's insides slither towards her hypograstric region, she is pregnant with ...
60 If they protrude towards her hypograstric region (var. towards her womb?), she is pregnant with ...
61 If they are packed into her hypograstric region, she will give birth to a deaf/retarded child.[28]
62 If they are poured into her hypograstric region, ditto (she will give birth to a deaf/retarded child).[29]
63 If they protrude towards her hypogastric region, she is pregnant with a male.

64 If they protrude from above towards her hypogastric region, she is pregnant with a female.

65 If they protrude (var. are turned) from below towards her hypogastric region, she is pregnant with a male.

66 If they are cramped, she is pregnant with a male.[30]

67 If they are bloated, she is pregnant with a female.[31]

68 If they are large (lit. numerous), she is pregnant with a female.[32]

69 If it (the abdomen of a woman of childbearing age) is unevenly colored with yellow/tan, she will completely form her fetus.[33]

70 If it is as pointed as her nose, she is pregnant with a female.

71 If they (the insides of a woman of childbearing age) are large, both her feet and both her ankles are swollen, (and) she steps to "right" and "left," she is pregnant with twins.[34]

72 If a woman of childbearing age holds her insides with her hands, she is pregnant with a male.[35]

73 If the muscles of a woman of childbearing age protrude towards her epigastrium, she is pregnant with a female.[36]

74 If they protrude towards her hypogastric region, she is pregnant with a male.[37]

75 If they are large, she is pregnant with a female.

76 If the insides of a woman of childbearing age are bloated, she is pregnant with a male.[38]

77 If the face of a woman of childbearing age changes (for the worse), she will die as a result of her being with child.[39]

78 If the face of a woman of childbearing age is calm, she will bring the fetus to term as a result of her being with child.[40]

79 If the face of a woman of childbearing age is full of (patches of what looks like) oxhide treated with depilatories, her fetus will die.[41]

80 If the face of a woman of childbearing age is full of (patches of what looks like) oxhide treated with depilatories (and) both her eyes are spotted, she will die together with her fetus.[42]

81 If a woman of childbearing age continually vomits, she will not bring (her fetus) to term.[43]

82 If (in) a woman of childbearing age, dark blood flows from (the womb)'s mouth, she will not get well from her pregnancy.[44]

83 If (in) a woman of childbearing age pus is continually produced from her (womb)'s mouth, she will die together with her fetus.[45]

84 If the hands and feet of a woman of childbearing age are continually sluggish, twenty-one (possible) prognoses.

85 If the head of the navel of a woman of childbearing age is unraveled, she will bring her fetus to term.[46]

86 If it is twisted loose, her fetus will not live.[47]

87 If (in) a woman of childbearing age, dark blood flows from her (womb)'s mouth to the "right," her fetus will die.

88 If (in) a woman of childbearing age, dark blood flows from her (womb)'s mouth to the "left," her fetus will die.

89 If a woman of childbearing age continually rolls her ⸢eyes⸣, she carries a hare (malformed child-with a hare lip?); her fetus will die.[48]

90 If the blood vessel of a woman of childbearing age's "right" ⸢ankle⸣ pulsates, she is pregnant with a female.[49]

91 If the (blood vessel of a woman of childbearing age's) "left" (ankle) pulsates, she is pregnant with a male.[50]

92 If the blood vessel of a woman of childbearing age's "right" and "left" ⸢ankles⸣ pulsate, she is pregnant with twins who will not do well.

93 If the blood vessel of a woman of childbearing age's ankle is continually full of blood, she is pregnant with a male.[51]

94 If a woman of childbearing age in the midst of her difficulty steps to the "right," she is pregnant with a child which lies down.[52]

95 If ditto (a woman of childbearing age in the midst of her difficulty) steps to the "left," she is pregnant with a female.[53]

96 If a woman of childbearing age steps to the "right" and her foot feels heavy, she is pregnant with a male or a female.[54]

97 If she steps to the "left" and ditto (her foot feels heavy), she is pregnant with a female.[55]

98 If she steps to the "right" and "left," she is pregnant with twins.

99 If the feet of a woman of childbearing age (seem) small, she is pregnant and is one who will bring her children to term.

100 If a woman of childbearing age's womb(?)is red, she was impregnated with a male.[56]

101 If a woman of childbearing age's womb(?)is bright red, she was impregnated with a male.[57]

102 If a woman of childbearing age's womb(?)[58] is shining, she was impregnated with a child which will not do well.[59]

103 If a woman of childbearing age is properly respectful of pregnancy, she will get well from her being with child.[60]

104 If a ⸢woman of childbearing age⸣ is careless of ⸢pregnancy⸣, she will die from her being with child.[61]

105 If a woman of ⸢childbearing⸣ age's [stomach] is continually upset, her fetus will die.[62]

106 If a woman of ⸢childbearing age⸣ [is pregnant and] ⸢at⸣ five months (and) three days they approach her, life.[63]

107 If a woman of childbearing age is pregnant and at (five) months (and) four days ditto (they approach her), life.

108 If a woman of childbearing age is pregnant and at (five) months (and) five days ditto (they approach her), she ⸢will be sick⸣ with menstrual bleeding.[64]

109 If a woman of childbearing age is pregnant and at (five) months (and) six days ditto (they approach her), ditto (she will be sick with menstrual bleeding).

110 If a woman of childbearing age is pregnant and at (five) months (and) seven days ditto (they approach her), life.[65]

111 If a woman of childbearing age is pregnant and at (five) months (and) eight days ditto (they approach her), father's evil; a curse will afflict her.[66]

112 If a woman of childbearing age is pregnant and at (five) months (and) nine days ditto (they approach her), she will die.[67]

113 If a woman of childbearing age is pregnant and at (five) months (and) ten days ditto (they approach her), life.

114–115 *(omens concerning the birth of twins)*

---

116 *(colophon)*

Notes

1. See Scurlock and Andersen 2005, 12.91, 12.108.
2. See Scurlock and Andersen 2005, 12.92, 12.107.
3. See Scurlock and Andersen 2005, 12.104.
4. See Scurlock and Andersen 2005, 12.105.
5. See Scurlock and Andersen 2005, 12.114.
6. See Scurlock and Andersen 2005, 10.154, 12.101, 12.109
7. See Scurlock and Andersen 2005, 10.155.
8. See Scurlock and Andersen 2005, 12.106.
9. See Scurlock and Andersen 2005, 12.79.
10. See Scurlock and Andersen 2005, 12.79.
11. See Scurlock and Andersen 2005, 12.87.
12. See Scurlock and Andersen 2005, 12.88.
13. See Scurlock and Andersen 2005, 12.95.
14. See Scurlock and Andersen 2005, 12.81.
15. See Scurlock and Andersen 2005, 12.81.
16. See Scurlock and Andersen 2005, 12.27.

17. See Scurlock and Andersen 2005, 12.28.
18. See Scurlock and Andersen 2005, 12.90.
19. See Scurlock and Andersen 2005, 12.89.
20. See Scurlock and Andersen 2005, 12.90.
21. See Scurlock and Andersen 2005, 10.120.
22. See Scurlock and Andersen 2005, 10.121.
23. See Scurlock and Andersen 2005, 12.77.
24. See Scurlock and Andersen 2005, 12.78.
25. See Scurlock and Andersen 2005, 12.78
26. See Scurlock and Andersen 2005, 12.93.
27. See Scurlock and Andersen 2005, 12.97.
28. See Scurlock and Andersen 2005, 12.111.
29. See Scurlock and Andersen 2005, 12.112.
30. See Scurlock and Andersen 2005, 12.99.
31. See Scurlock and Andersen 2005, 12.100.
32. See Scurlock and Andersen 2005, 12.103.
33. See Scurlock and Andersen 2005, 12.94.
34. See Scurlock and Andersen 2005, 12.110.
35. See Scurlock and Andersen 2005, 12.96.
36. See Scurlock and Andersen 2005, 12.82.
37. See Scurlock and Andersen 2005, 112.83.
38. See Scurlock and Andersen 2005, 12.98.
39. See Scurlock and Andersen 2005, 12.25.
40. See Scurlock and Andersen 2005, 12.26.
41. See Scurlock and Andersen 2005, 12.65.
42. See Scurlock and Andersen 2005, 12.66.
43. See Scurlock and Andersen 2005, 12.55, 17.5.
44. See Scurlock and Andersen 2005, 12.47.
45. See Scurlock and Andersen 2005, 12.48.
46. See Scurlock and Andersen 2005, 12.29.
47. See Scurlock and Andersen 2005, 12.30.
48. See Scurlock and Andersen 2005, 12.115, 17.63.
49. See Scurlock and Andersen 2005, 12.80.
50. See Scurlock and Andersen 2005, 12.80.
51. See Scurlock and Andersen 2005, 12.102.
52. See Scurlock and Andersen 2005, 12.113.
53. See Scurlock and Andersen 2005, 12.84.
54. See Scurlock and Andersen 2005, 12.85.
55. See Scurlock and Andersen 2005, 12.86.
56. See Scurlock and Andersen 2005, 12.2.
57. See Scurlock and Andersen 2005, 12.2.
58. This seems preferable to Stol's (2000, 200–201) interpretation of this as some sort of textile inserted into the womb. Suppositories of whatever material are usually described as such.
59. See Scurlock and Andersen 2005, 12.3.
60. See Scurlock and Andersen 2005, 12.23.
61. See Scurlock and Andersen 2005, 12.24.
62. See Scurlock and Andersen 2005, 12.56.
63. See Scurlock and Andersen 2005, 12.40.
64. See Scurlock and Andersen 2005, 12.41.

65. See Scurlock and Andersen 2005, 12.39.
66. See Scurlock and Andersen 2005, 12.42.
67. See Scurlock and Andersen 2005, 12.43.

DPS 37

DPS 36:116 (catchline) = DPS 37:1

1. DIŠ MUNUS.PEŠ$_4$ GIG-*ma šum-ma šá* ITI.3.KÁM *ir-tu-bu-niš-ši* : *iq-ru-bu-niš-ši* MUNUS BI AL.TI
2. *šum-ma šá* ITI.4.KÁM *ir-tu-bu-niš-ši* MUNUS BI AL.TI.
3. *šum-ma šá* ITI.5.KÁM *ir-tu-bu-niš-ši* MUNUS BI *na-*ʾ*-da-át*
4. *šum-ma šá* ITI.6.KÁM *ir-tu-bu-niš-ši* MUNUS BI *na-*ʾ*-da-át*
5. *šum-ma šá* ITI.7.KÁM *ir-tu-bu-niš-ši* MUNUS BI AL.TI
6. *šum-ma šá* ITI.8.KÁM *ir-tu-bu-niš-ši* MUNUS BI TI-*uṭ* : *ma-mit* AD-*šú* DIB-*si*
7. *šum-ma šá* ITI.9.KÁM ITI.10.KÁM *ir-tu-bu-niš-ši* MUNUS BI NU ‹‹NIN›› DIN : NU Ù.TU

8–9. DIŠ MUNUS GIG-*ma* AD$_6$-*šú* KÚM ÚḪ TUKU MURUB$_4$ ŠU-*šá šá* 150 *ku-uṣ-ṣu* UL$_4$.GAL *ba-li-il* : ŠUB-*ma* KÚM UL$_4$.GAL *la i-bal-lal* BA.ÚŠ

10. DIŠ MUNUS GIG-*ma ú-ru-uḫ-šá bé-e-er ana* U$_4$.2.KÁM *ana* U$_4$.3.KÁM BA.ÚŠ
11. DIŠ MUNUS GIG-*ma* ŠU^{II}-*šá ina* SAG.DU-*šá* GAR-*na-ma la ur-ra-da-ni* ŠU EN.ÙR KI.MIN MAŠKIM ÙR SÌG-*aṣ* ÚŠ
12. DIŠ MUNUS GIG-*ma* DIB-*sa ina* GI$_6$ DIB.DIB-*si* DIB-*it* LÍL.LÁ.EN.NA
13. DIŠ MUNUS GIG-*ma* DIB-*sa ina* AN.ÚSAN DIB.DIB-*si u* TÚG-*sa* ŠUB.ŠUB-*di* DIB-*it* LÍL.LÁ.EN.NA
14. DIŠ MUNUS GIG-*sà ina* GI$_6$ DIB.DIB-*si* DIB-*it* LÍL.LÁ.EN.NA
15. DIŠ MUNUS *ina* GIG-*šá* LUḪ.LUḪ-*ut* bad ina su un meš-šá bad-ši
16. DIŠ MUNUS *ina* GIG-*šá* ŠU^{II}-*šá ú-na-aš-šak* ŠU.MEŠ *lu-*ʾ*-a-ti* TAG-*ši*
17. DIŠ MUNUS *ina* GIG-*šá* ŠÀ-*bi ku-ri i-qab-bi* ŠU ^{d}15 AL.TI
18. DIŠ MUNUS *ina* GI$_6$ GIG-*ma ina šèr-ti it-te-bi* GIG-*sà i-sa-dir-ši* BA.ÚŠ
19. DIŠ MUN[US *ina* MURU]B$_4$-*šá* SÌG-*át* SAG ŠÀ-*šá* IM *li-qí* : ŠÀ-*šá* IM *ṣa-bit* BA.ÚŠ
20. DIŠ MU[NUS *ina bal-ṭ*]*ú-ti-šá ú-šam-šá u ina* GIG-*šá ú-šam-šá* DUMU DINGIR-*šú* TE-*ši*
21. DIŠ MUN[US o o o o]x *lu* ŠU^{II}-*šá lu* GÌR^{II}-*šá ú-ṣa-*⸢*bi-ta*⸣*-ši* DUMU DINGIR-*šú* TE-*ši* : DIŠ KI.NÁ-*šá* ŠUB.ŠUB-*ši* É-*sà* ⸢BIR⸣

22–29 and rev. 1. (too broken to make sense)

TRANSLATION

1. If a pregnant woman is ill and if when she is in the third month they continue to approach her, that woman will live.[1]
2. If when she is in the fourth month they continue, that woman will live.[2]
3. If when she is in the fifth month they continue, that woman is a cause for worry.[3]
4. If when she is in the sixth month they continue, that woman is a cause for worry.[4]
5. If when she is in the seventh month they continue, that woman will get well.[5]
6. If when she is in the eighth month they continue, that woman will get well (var. the curse of her father will afflict her).[6]
7. If when she is in the ninth or tenth month they continue, that woman will not get well (var. she will not give birth).[7]

8–9. If a woman is ill and her body has a burning fever[8] (var. she has collapsed and is feverish) (and) the middle of her "left" hand is very mixed with cold (var. falls and is not very mixed with fever), she will die.

10. If a woman is ill and her head hair is fine (lit. select and she has been sick) for two or three days, she will die.[9]
11. If a woman is ill and her hands are placed on her head and she does not bring them down, it is "hand" of the lord of the roof (LUGAL.ÙR.RA). Alternatively, the *rābiṣu* of the roof has struck her; she will die.[10]
12. If a woman is ill and her affliction always afflicts her during the night, it is an affliction of *lilû*.[11]
13. If a woman is ill and her affliction always afflicts her in the evening and she continually takes her clothes off, it is an affliction of *lilû*.[12]
14. If a woman's illness always afflicts her during the night, it is an affliction of *lilû*.
15. If a woman continually jerks in her illness ...
16. If a woman during her illness chews on her hands, dirty hands have touched her.
17. If a woman during her illness says: "My abdomen is (too) short," "hand" of Ishtar; she will get well.[13]
18. If a woman is sick in the night and gets up in the morning (and) her illness (afflicts) her time after time, she will die.
19. If a ⸢woman⸣ was wounded on her ⸢hip region⸣ (and) her epigastrium takes up "wind" (variant: "wind" afflicts her abdomen), she will die.

20. If a ⸢woman⸣ is kept up all night [when] she is ⸢healthy⸣ and when she is sick, the son of her god has approached her (sexually).[14]

21. If a ⸢woman⸣ [...] (and) either her hands or her feet continually afflict her, the son of her god has approached her (sexually). If the bed continually throws her off, her household will be scattered.[15]

22–29 and rev. 1 *(too broken to translate)*

NOTES

1. See Scurlock and Andersen 2005, 12.31.
2. See Scurlock and Andersen 2005, 12.32.
3. See Scurlock and Andersen 2005, 12.34.
4. See Scurlock and Andersen 2005, 12.35.
5. See Scurlock and Andersen 2005, 12.36.
6. See Scurlock and Andersen 2005, 12.37.
7. See Scurlock and Andersen 2005, 12.38.
8. See above, DPS 3:70.
9. See Scurlock and Andersen 2005, 19.42.
10. See Scurlock and Andersen 2005, 19.42.
11. See Scurlock and Andersen 2005, 12.69.
12. See Scurlock and Andersen 2005, 12.70, 16.58, 19.18.
13. See Scurlock and Andersen 2005, 12.68, 19.16.
14. See Scurlock and Andersen 2005, 16.28.
15. See Scurlock and Andersen 2005, 16.29.

DPS 39

1.[1] DIŠ MUNUS *ḫa-ri-iš-ti i-di-ip u i-geš-šú* BA.ÚŠ

TRANSLATION

1. If a woman in confinement inflates (with wind) and vomits (without having eaten),[2] she will die.

NOTES

1. The line is cited from the commentary SpTU 1.40 obv. 1. For the argument that this line represents the incipit of DPS 39, see Hunger, SpTU 1, 48–49.

2. See Scurlock and Andersen 2005, 122.

H. PEDIATRICS: DPS 40

DPS 40

1. DIŠ LÚ.TUR *la-ʾ-ḫu ki-ma al-du ṣir-ti i-ni-qu ina* ŠÀ-*šú la i-bi-ma i-tab-bak*
2. *ù* UZU.MEŠ-*šú im-ta-ṭu-ú ki-ši-id e-pe-ru*
3. DIŠ LÚ.TUR *ki-ša-da-nu-uš-šú tuš-qa-lal-šu-ma la i-gal-lut u i-di-šú la i-tar-ra-aṣ ki-šid* SAḪAR
4. DIŠ LÚ.TUR ITI.3.KÁM *šu-nu-uq-ma* UZU.MEŠ-*šú im-ta-ṭu-ú* $ŠU^{II}$-*šú u* $GÌR^{II}$-*šú it-ta-naq-na-an-na ki-šid* SAḪAR
5. DIŠ LÚ.TUR UZU.MEŠ-*šú ur-qá it-ta-du-ú* KÚM *la ú-kal* $SAG.KI^{II}$-*šú ma-aq-*ta_5 *ap-pi-šú ma-gal i-si-ir ú-pa-ṭi la i-šu* [BI.LU][1] *ṣab-tu-šú*
6. DIŠ LÚ.TUR *ina bal-ṭu-ti-šú* UZU.MEŠ-*šú ḫab-ṣu mur-ṣu* DIB-*su-ma* UZU.MEŠ-*šú im-taq-tu* U_4.3.KÁM U_4.4.KÁM
7. KÚM TUKU ŠÀ.MEŠ-*šú eb-ṭu ir-ru-šú i-šá-ru mi-iḫ-ru* DIB-*su*
8. DIŠ LÚ.TUR ITI.1.KÁM ITI.2.KÁM ITI.3.KÁM *mur-ṣu* DIB-*su-ma* U_4 *u* GI_6 *ú-šam-šá* UZU.MEŠ *im-taq-tu*
9. ŠÀ.MEŠ-*šú eb-ṭú ir-ru-šú i-šá-ru u uḫ-ta-taš-ši-il mi-iḫ-ru* DIB-*su*
10. DIŠ LÚ.TUR SAG.DU-*su* KÚM *ú-kal pa-gar-šú* KÚM *la ḫa-aḫ-ḫa-aš* IR *la i-ši* $ŠU^{II}$-*šú u* $GÌR^{II}$-*šú* ŠA *em-ma*
11. *il-la-tu-šú* DU-*ka u ú-sar-ra-aḫ ma-la* GU_7 *ina* ŠÀ-*šú la ina-aḫ-ma i-tab-ba-ka*
12. LÚ.TUR.BI ZÚ.MEŠ-*šú* È.MEŠ-*ni* U_4.15.KÁM : U_4.20.KÁM *dan-nat* IGI-*ma* DIN!
13. DIŠ LÚ.TUR *it-ta-na-as-la-ʾ-ma* A.MEŠ *ana* UGU ŠÀ-*šú* DUB-*ak-ma* ŠÀ-*šú la ú-šel-la-a* ŠÀ-*šú še-bir*
14. DIŠ LÚ.TUR *tu-la-a i-kal-ma la i-šeb-bi u ma-gal ú-šar-ra-aḫ* ŠÀ-*šú še-bir*
15. DIŠ LÚ.TUR ŠÀ.MEŠ-*šú* MÚ.MEŠ-*ḫu tu-lu-ú* ÍL-*šum-ma* NU GU_7 LÚ.TUR BI $^{MUNUS}UŠ_{11}$.ZU *ḫi-rat-su*
16. DIŠ LÚ.TUR *ina ṣa-la-li-šú i-né-e* KI.MIN *la ina-aḫ-ma u ip-ta-nar-ru-ud ina ki-rim-me* AMA-*šú šu-ul-ḫu kiš-pi ep-šú-šú*
17. DIŠ LÚ.TUR *ina ṣa-la-li-šú ip-ta-nar-ru-ud u ib-ta-nak-ki ina ki-rim-me* AMA-*šú šul-ḫu kiš-pi ep-šú-šú*

18. DIŠ LÚ.TUR ITI.3.KÁM *tu-la-a i-niq-ma* ŠU^{II}-*šú u* GÌR^{II}-*šú it-ta-naq-na-an-na*
19. UZU.MEŠ-*šú i-ma-aṭ-ṭu-ú ul-tu* ŠÀ AMA-*šú šu-ul-ḫu kiš-pi ep-šú-šú*
20. DIŠ LÚ.TUR *ina* UBUR AMA-*šú* LÙ.LÙ-*aḫ* LÍL.LÍL-*a*ʾ KI.MIN *i-bak-ki u* KÚM DIB.DIB-*su ik-ri-bu* DIB.ME-*šú*
21. DIŠ LÚ.TUR MU.1.KÁM MU.2.KÁM MU.3.KÁM MU.4.KÁM *šu-ub-bu-uṣ-ma te-ba-a ù ú-zu-uz-za*
22. *la i-le-*ʾ*-e* NINDA *a-ka-la la*(coll.) *i-le-*ʾ*-e* KA-*šú ṣu-ub-bu-ut-ma da-ba-ba*
23. *la i-le-*ʾ*-e re-ḫu-ut* ^{d}*Šùl-pa-è-a* NU SI.SÁ
24. DIŠ LÚ.TUR *ina* UBUR AMA-*šú ig-da-na-al-lut ib-ta-nak-ki* KI.MIN LÙ.LÙ-*aḫ ina bir-ki* AMA-*šú*
25. *i-šaḫ-ḫi-iṭ-ma ma-gal i-bak-ki* DUMU.MUNUS ^{d}*A-nim ḫi-rat-su*
26. DIŠ LÚ.TUR *ki-ma al-du* U_4.2.KÁM U_4.3.KÁM DU-*ma* GA *la i-maḫ-ḫar mi-iq-tu ki-ma* ŠU DINGIR.RA
27. ŠUB.ŠUB-*su* ŠU ^{d}15 *ik-ki-im-tum* TAG-*šú* BA.ÚŠ
28. DIŠ LÚ.TUR *ib-ta-nak-ki u* GÙ.GÙ-*si ek-ke-em-tum* ŠU ^{d}15 DUMU. MUNUS ^{d}*A-nim*
29. DIŠ LÚ.TUR UZU.MEŠ-*šú* SIG_7 ŠUB-*ú* ŠÀ.MEŠ-*šú eb-ṭu* ŠU^{II}-*šú* GÌR-*šú nap-ḫa li-*ʾ*-ba ma-gal* TUKU *ḫa-še-e* GIG ŠU DINGIR TI
30. DIŠ LÚ.TUR ŠÀ.MEŠ-*šú* MÚ.MÚ.MEŠ-*ḫu u ib-ta-nak-ki* ŠU *er-ṣe-ti* KI.MIN ŠU DUMU.MUNUS ^{d}*A-nim* : ŠU DINGIR TI
31. DIŠ LÚ.TUR *mit-ḫar-riš em-ma u* SAG ŠÀ-*šú za-qir* ŠU ^{d}*Kù-bi*
32. DIŠ LÚ.TUR SA.MEŠ ŠÀ-*šú* SA_5 *u* SIG_7 ŠUB-*ú* ŠU ^{d}*Kù-bi*
33. DIŠ LÚ.TUR ŠÀ.MEŠ-*šú eb-ṭú-ma* SIG_7 ŠUB-*ú* ŠU ^{d}*Kù-bi*
34. DIŠ LÚ.TUR *ik-ta-na-aṣ-ṣa u* ZÚ.MEŠ-*šú i-gaṣ-ṣa-aṣ* GIG-*su ir-ri-ik ṣi-bit* ^{d}*Kù-bi*
35. DIŠ LÚ.TUR *ig-da-na-al-lut u* LÙ.LÙ ŠU ^{d}30 AL.TI
36. DIŠ LÚ.TUR *ina te-ni-qí-šú* UZU.MEŠ *i-šaḫ-ḫu-ḫu u mu-še-niq-ta-šú* UBUR SIG-*at* UBUR ÍL-*šum-ma* NU GU_7
37. UBUR *šú-ú mur-ra i-šú ana* UBUR *eš-ši tu-na-kar-šú-ma* TI
38. DIŠ LÚ.TUR *a-šu-ú u sa-ma-ni* DIB-*su ana tu-la-a eš-šá tu-na-kar-šú-ma u* ÉN ŠUB.ŠUB-*šum-ma* TI
39. DIŠ LÚ.TUR *su-a-la* GIG IM.KAL.GUG DIRI *ina* LÀL *u* Ì.NUN.NA ḪE.ḪE *ba-lu pa-tan ú-na-ṣab*
40. *šúm-ma la-šu-ú šú-ú ina ap-pat* UBUR AMA-*šú* GAR-*ma* KI GA *i-niq-ma* DIN-⸢*uṭ*⸣
41. DIŠ LÚ.TUR *šap-pu ul-tu*[2] GÚ-*šú* EN GÚ.MURGU-*šú kàs-lu-šu* DU_8. MEŠ BA.ÚŠ

42. DIŠ LÚ.TUR *ina ni-kip-ti* ^{d}30 ŠÀ.MEŠ-*šú pur-ru-du u qa-tu-um-ma i-qat-ti ana* TI-*šú ni-kip-ti* TUR-*ár*
43. ^{ŠEM}ḪAB ^{ŠEM}GÚR.GÚR ^{ŠEM}LI Ú.KUR.RA Ú.ḪUR.SAG SIG$_7$-*su-ma* SÚD *ina* Ì ^{ŠEM}BULUḪ ḪI.ḪI ŠÉŠ.ME-*su-ma* DIN
44. DIŠ LÚ.TUR *ši-bit* SAG.DU-*šú paṭ-rat-ma mu-uḫ-ḫa-šu i-rap-pu-uš u* NU *i-ṣa-lal* U$_4$.7.KÁM U$_4$.8.KÁM GIG-*ma* DIN
45. DIŠ LÚ.TUR *ši-bit* SAG.DU-*šú paṭ-rat-ma mu-uḫ-ḫa-šu i-rap-pu-uš* BA.ÚŠ
46. DIŠ LÚ.TUR *ig-da-na-al-lut u* LÙ.LÙ-*aḫ ib-ta-nak-ki ip-ta-nar-ru-ud* ŠU^{II}-*šú u* GÌR^{II}-*šú* ÍL.ÍL-*ši* SÌG ^{d}30 *na-ag-mar-ti* TUKU-*ši*
47. DIŠ LÚ.TUR *ig-da-na-al-lut* LÙ.LÙ-*aḫ u* MUD.MUD-*ud* ŠU ^{d}30 *u* ^{d}15
48. DIŠ LÚ.TUR *ma-la* GU$_7$ *i-ḫa-ḫu* KI.MIN *iṣ-ṣa-na-aḫ* ŠU^{II}-*šú u* GÌR^{II}-*šú it-te-ṣi-la-šú qí-bit* KA *ana* ^{d}30 TUKU-*ši*
49. DIŠ LÚ.TUR ŠUB-*tu* ŠUB-*su-ma ib-lu-uṭ* LÍL-*šú ú-ra-ak-ma* BA.ÚŠ
50. DIŠ LÚ.TUR *i-mi-iš-ti* : APIN-*tim* ŠÀ-*bi i-šu* KA-*šú* BAD.BAD-*te ma-la* GU$_7$ *ut-ta-nar-ru* ŠU DINGIR.MAḪ : ŠU DINGIR TI
51. DIŠ LÚ.TUR *um-ma li-ʾ-ba ú-kal u ik-ta-na-aṣ-ṣa ṣi-bit* ^{d}DÌM.ME : ŠU DUMU.MUNUS ^{d}*A-nim*
52. DIŠ LÚ.TUR KÚM-*im i-kaṣ-ṣa u* A.MEŠ *ana* NAG-*e ma-gal* APIN.MEŠ-*iš ṣi-bit* ^{d}DÌM.ME : ŠU DUMU.MUNUS ^{d}*A-nim*
53. DIŠ LÚ.TUR ŠÀ-*šú i-mim* ŠED$_7$ *u* A.MEŠ *ana* NAG-*e ma-gal i-te-ner-reš-ma i-šat-ti* ŠU ^{d}DÌM.ME
54. DIŠ LÚ.TUR IM KA-*šú šá* 15 ŠED$_7$-*ma šá* 2,30 KÚM-*im* ŠU ^{d}DÌM.ME
55. DIŠ LÚ.TUR *i-šá-as-si i-gal-lut* LÙ.LÙ-*aḫ ib-ta-nak-ki u* MUD.MUD-*ud ṣir-tú ma-la* NAG *ut-ta-nar-ra* ŠU ^{d}30 *u* ^{d}15
56. DIŠ LÚ.TUR ŠU^{II}-*šú u* GÌR^{II}-*šú it-ta-na-an-pa-ḫa* IGI^{II}-*šú uz-za-na-qap* ^{GIŠ}GIDRU ^{d}30 *u* ^{d}15
57. DIŠ LÚ.TUR *um-ma-šú mit-ḫar-ma tu-kul-ti qin-na-ti-šú u* GEŠTU^{II}-*šú ka-ṣa-a* ^{GIŠ}GIDRU DUMU *šip-ri šá* ^{d}30
58. DIŠ LÚ.TUR GIN$_7$ DIB-*it* ^{d}DÌM.ME *u$_4$-mi-šam-ma* DIB.DIB-*su* ŠU ^{d}DÌM.ME
59. DIŠ LÚ.TUR SU-*šú* KÚM NU TUKU *u* IR *ma-gal* TUKU ŠU ^{d}DÌM.ME.LAGAB : DIŠ LÚ.TUR (*ḫe-p*[*i* …])
60. DIŠ LÚ.TUR *tu-la-a i-niq-ma mi-iq-tum* ŠUB-*su* ŠU ^{d}[15 : ^{d}30][3]
61. DIŠ LÚ.TUR UZU.MEŠ-*šú* GI$_6$.MEŠ : ŠUB-*tu u ap-pa-šú us-sà-na-ar di-im-tum ina* IGI^{II}-*šú* DU-*ak* BI.LU (*ḫe-pi*) […]
62. DIŠ LÚ.TUR ŠU.SI-*šú* GAL-*tum* ‹*ana*› ŠÀ-*šú* (var. ŠÀ ŠU^{II}-*šú*) *tur-rat u ma-diš iṣ-ṣi-ni-iḫ* UZU.MEŠ-*šú mur-ṣa i-šu-ú šiḫ-ḫat* UZU TUKU-*ši ina* ŠÀ-*bi* ÚŠ

63. DIŠ LÚ.TUR ŠÀ.MEŠ-*šú* *it-te-nin-mi-ru* IGI^{II}-*šú* DUGUD-*šú* ŠU DINGIR DIN
64. DIŠ LÚ.TUR ŠÀ.MEŠ-*šú* MÚ.MÚ-*ḫu u ib-ta-nak-ki* ŠU DINGIR DIN
65. DIŠ LÚ.TUR ŠÀ.MEŠ-*šú* MÚ.MEŠ-*ḫu* ŠU DINGIR DIN
66. DIŠ LÚ.TUR ŠÀ.MEŠ-*šú it-te-nin-bi-ṭu* ŠU DINGIR DIN
67. DIŠ LÚ.TUR UGU [K]IR$_4$-*šú* ⸢IR⸣ DU-*ak* SA$_5$ *u* SIG$_7$ ŠU DINGIR DIN
68. DIŠ LÚ.TUR ⸢*pa-ru*⸣-*ta ma-li* ŠU DINGIR DIN
69. DIŠ LÚ.TUR *pa-ru-ta sa-li-iḫ*[4] *u liq* KA-*šú* ⸢*i-ta*!-*nab-bal*⸣-*šú* ŠU DINGIR [DIN]
70. DIŠ LÚ.TUR ⸢*pa-ru*⸣-*ta sa-li-iḫ* ŠU [DINGIR DIN]
71. DIŠ LÚ.TUR IGI^{II}-*šú e-ṭa-ma-a* ŠU ^{d}NIN.GEŠTIN.NA : DIŠ LÚ.TUR IGI^{II}-[*šú*] ⸢*i-tan*⸣-*na-bal-la* [o]
72. DIŠ LÚ.TUR ŠÀ.MEŠ-*šú suk-ku-ru* ŠU ^{d}*Da-mu* : DIŠ LÚ.TUR [...] ŠU [...]
73. DIŠ LÚ.TUR UBUR ÍL-*šum-ma* NU GU$_7$ ŠÀ.MEŠ-*šú še-eb-*[*ru*]
74. DIŠ LÚ.TUR UBUR ÍL-*šum-ma* NU GU$_7$ ŠÀ.MEŠ-*šú it-te-nen-*[...]
75. [DIŠ LÚ.T]UR UZU.MEŠ-*šú* SIG$_7$ ŠUB-*ú* ŠÀ.MEŠ-*šú it-te-nen-*[...]
76. [DIŠ] LÚ.TUR UZU.MEŠ-*šú* SIG$_7$ ŠUB-*ú* ŠU ^{d}*Gu-la*
77. DIŠ LÚ.TUR ŠÀ.MEŠ-*šú* SIG$_7$ ŠUB-*ú* [ŠU ^{d}*Gu-la*]
78. DIŠ LÚ.TUR SAG ŠÀ-*šú za-qir* ŠU ⸢^{d}⸣*Gu-la*
79. DIŠ LÚ.TUR KÚM TUKU *u* ŠÀ.MEŠ-*šú eb-ṭu* ŠU [^{d}*Gu-la*]
80. DIŠ LÚ.TUR KÚM NU TUKU *u* ŠÀ.MEŠ-*šú eb-ṭu* ŠU [^{d}*Gu-la*]
81. DIŠ LÚ.TUR *ru-šu-ud* ŠU [^{d}*Gu-la*]
82. DIŠ LÚ.TUR *it-ta-na-as-ḫur it-ta-na-as-la-ʾ* ŠU [^{d}*Gu-la*]
83. DIŠ LÚ.TUR LÙ.LÙ-*aḫ* ŠU ^{d}[*Gu-la*]
84. DIŠ LÚ.TUR *iš-ta-na-ad-da-ad u* Á^{II}-*šú* GUR?-*ra* ŠU ^{d}[*Gu-la*]
85. DIŠ LÚ.TUR UZU.ME-*šú za-mar i-šaḫ-ḫu-ḫu za-mar i-šal-li-mu* ŠU ^{d}*G*[*u-la*]
86. DIŠ LÚ.TUR SA$_5$ *u* SIG$_7$ ŠU ^{d}*Gu*[-*la*]
87. DIŠ LÚ.TUR BABBAR *u* GI$_6$ ŠU ^{d}*Gu*[-*la*]
88. DIŠ LÚ.TUR *i-ba-aḫ-ḫi ù i-kab-bir* ŠU ^{d}*Gu-la*
89. DIŠ LÚ.TUR KÚM TUKU *u* UZU.MEŠ-*šú i-maṭ-ṭu-ú* ŠU ^{d}*Gu-la*
90. DIŠ LÚ.TUR KÚM *ṣa-ri-iḫ* ŠU ^{d}*Gu-la*
91. DIŠ LÚ.TUR *ur-us-su ḫa-niq* ŠU ^{d}*Gu-la*
92. DIŠ LÚ.TUR *ú-nap-paq u* UZU.MEŠ-*šú* SIG$_7$ ŠU ^{d}*Gu-la*
93. DIŠ LÚ.TUR *ú-nap-paq* UBUR NU NAG *u* SU-*šú* SIG$_7$ ŠU ^{d}*Gu-la*
94. DIŠ LÚ.TUR *ú-nap-paq* UBUR NU NAG ŠU ^{d}*Gu-la*
95. DIŠ LÚ.TUR ŠÀ.MEŠ-*šú eb-ṭu u* DÚR-*šú ḫa-niq* ŠU ^{d}*Gu-la*

96. DIŠ LÚ.TUR ŠÀ.MEŠ-*šú eb-ṭú u* SU-*šú* SIG_7 *bu-ʾ-šá-nu* DIB-*su* ŠU ᵈ*Gu-la*
97. DIŠ LÚ.TUR ŠÀ.MEŠ-*šú eb-ṭú u* KA-*šú ka-bit bu-ʾ-šá-nu* DIB-*su*
98. DIŠ LÚ.TUR *il-la-tu-šú* DU.MEŠ-*ka bu-ʾ-šá-nu* DIB-*su*
99. DIŠ LÚ.TUR *il-la-tu-šú* MÚD *ú-kal-la bu-ʾ-šá-nu* DIB-*su*
100. DIŠ LÚ.TUR UGU-*šú* GABA-*šú u šá-šal-la-šú* KÚM.MEŠ *bu-ʾ-šá-nu* DIB-*su*
101. DIŠ LÚ.TUR KÚM *la ḫa-aḫ-ḫa-aš u* ŠÀ.MEŠ *eb-ṭú bu-ʾ-šá-nu* DIB-*su*
102. DIŠ LÚ.TUR *ina* UBUR AMA-*šú* ÍR.MEŠ *ir-ru-šú* ZÉ *ú-kal-lu* BA.ÚŠ

---

103. DIŠ LÚ.TUR *ina* UBUR AMA-*šú* LÙ.LÙ-*aḫ ik-ri-bu ṣab-tu-šú*
104. DIŠ LÚ.TUR UBUR ÍL-*šum-ma* NAG-*ma ú-šar-ra-aḫ ik-ri-bu* DIB.MEŠ-*šú*
105. DIŠ LÚ.TUR UBUR ÍL-*šum-ma* NU GU_7 *u* ŠÀ.MEŠ-*šú nap-ḫu ik-ri-bu ṣab-tu-šú*
106. DIŠ LÚ.TUR KÚM NU TUKU ŠÀ.MEŠ-*šú eb-ṭu u i-bak-ki ṣi-bit* DUMU.MUNUS ᵈ*A-nim*
107. DIŠ LÚ.TUR *i-bak-ki u im-ta-nag-ga-ag* DUMU.MUNUS ᵈ*A-nim* DIB-*su*
108. DIŠ LÚ.TUR U_4-*ma u mu-šu i-bak-ki* DUMU.MUNUS ᵈ*A-nim* DIB-*su*
109. DIŠ LÚ.TUR *i-lab-bu-ma* UBUR ÍL-*šum-ma* NU GU_7 *ik-ri-bu* DIB-*šú*
110. DIŠ LÚ.TUR ITU.1.KÁM ITI.2.KÁM *šu-nu-uq-ma* ŠUB-*tu* ŠUB-*su-ma* $ŠU^{II}$-*šú u* $GÌR^{II}$-*šú am-šá* ŠU.DINGIR.RA-*ku* KI-*šú a-lid ina* GÌR-*šú lu* AD-*šú lu* AMA-*šú* ÚŠ
111. DIŠ LÚ.TUR ŠUB-*tu* ŠUB-*su-ma* $ŠU^{II}$-*šú u* $GÌR^{II}$-*šú am-šá* IGI^{II}-*šú maḫ-ḫa ina* GÌR-*šú* É AD-*šú* BIR-*aḫ*
112. DIŠ LÚ.TUR *ina* KI.NÁ-*šú ina* NU ZU-*ú is-si-ma* ŠU ᵈ*Iš-tar*
113. DIŠ LÚ.TUR *ina* KI.NÁ-*šú is-si-ma mim-ma šá i-mu-ru i-qab-bi* ŠU ᵈ15 *ik-ri-bu* DIB.ME-*šú*
114. DIŠ LÚ.TUR *ik-kil-la-šú e-sír ú-pa-ṭi* NU *i-šu* BI.LU *ṣab-tu-šú*
115. DIŠ LÚ.TUR *pa-gar-šú* KÚM *la ḫa-ḫaš* SAG.DU-*su* KÚM TUKU UBUR GU_7-*ma ma-gal ú-sar-ra-aḫ* ZÚ.MEŠ-*šú* È.ME-*ni* U_4.14.KÁM : U_4.20.KÁM SAL.KALAG.GA IGI-*ma* DIN
116. DIŠ LÚ.TUR KÚM NU TUKU SAG.DU-*su* KÚM ZÚ.MEŠ-*šú* È.MEŠ-*ni* U_4.21.KÁM SAL.KALAG.GA IGI-*ma* DIN
117. DIŠ LÚ.TUR UGU-*šú* KÚM.KÚM-*im* ŠU ᵈ*Nusku*
118. DIŠ LÚ.TUR *ú-nap-paq u* SU-*šú* SIG_7 ŠU ᵈ*Gu-la*
119. DIŠ LÚ.TUR *ú-nap-paq* KÚM DIB.DIB-*su* UBUR *muṭ-ṭu* NAM.ÉRIM DIB-*su*

120. DIŠ LÚ.TUR KÚM NU TUKU IGI^{II}-*šú bal-ṣa* ŠU^{II}-*šú u* GÌR^{II}-*šú i-ra-ʾu-ba* ŠU ^{d}30 DIN
121. DIŠ LÚ.TUR KÚM NU TUKU *u i-ra-ʾ-ub* ŠU ^{d}30
122. DIŠ LÚ.TUR KÚM NU TUKU *ra-ʾ-i-ba* DIB.DIB-*su* ŠU ^{d}30
123. DIŠ LÚ.TUR *ma-la* GU_7 *i-ḫa-*⸢*ḫu*⸣ KI.MIN *is-sà-na-ḫur* ŠU^{II}-*šú u* GÌR^{II}-*šú it-te-nen-ṣi-la-šú qí-bít* KA *ana* ^{d}30 TUKU

TRANSLATION

1–2. If an infant as soon as he is born sucks the teat (but) does not get fat from it but pours (it) out and his flesh diminishes, he was "gotten" by the dust.[5]

3. If you suspend an infant by his neck and he does not jerk and does not stretch out his arms, he was "gotten" by the dust.[6]

4. If an infant has been suckled for three months and his flesh diminishes (and) his hands and his feet are continually contorted (var. C: are continually ⸢rigid⸣), he was "gotten" by the dust.[7]

5. If an infant's flesh is unevenly colored with yellow, he does not "hold" fever, (the blood vessels of) his temples have collapsed (and) he rubs his nose in a downward direction[8] a lot (but) does not have snot, [*buʾšānu*][9] afflicts him.[10]

6–7. If when an infant is healthy, his flesh is plentiful (but) when illness afflicts him, his flesh has collapsed, he has a fever for three or four days, his insides are cramped and his bowels are loose, *meḫru*[11] afflicts him.

8–9. If an illness afflicts an infant of one, two (and then) three months so that it keeps him awake day and night, his flesh has collapsed, his insides are cramped, his bowels are loose[12] and he is completely crushed, *meḫru* afflicts him.[13]

10–12. If the infant's head holds fever (and) his body (holds) a lukewarm temperature (and) he does not sweat (but) his hands and feet are hot, his saliva flows and he drools, whatever he eats does not rest easy in his stomach and he then pours (it) out, that infant's teeth are coming out. He may suffer for fifteen or twenty days, but he get well.[14]

13. If an infant is continually ill and if you pour water onto his abdomen, it does not pool[15] in his abdomen, his abdomen has been seriously injured.[16]

14. If an infant feeds from the breast and is not sated but drools a lot, his abdomen has been seriously injured.

15. If an infant's insides are continually bloated (and) when you raise a breast to him, he will not feed, a sorceress has "married" that infant.

16. If an infant turns round in his sleep; alternatively, if he is not quiet and continually shudders, sorcerous *šulḫu* has been performed against him in his mother's arms.
17. If an infant continually shudders in his sleep and he continually wails, sorcerous *šulḫu* has been performed against him in his mother's arms.
18–19. If an infant sucks the breast for three months and his hands and his feet are continually contorted (and) his flesh diminishes, sorcerous *šulḫu* has been performed against him from (within) the womb of his mother.[17]
20. If an infant is continually restless at the breast of his mother (and) is continually sick; alternatively, (if) he wails and fever continually afflicts him, a(n unfulfilled) vow afflicts him.[18]
21–23. If a child of one, two, three, (and then) four years writhes in contortion so that he is unable to get up and stand, he is unable to eat bread (and) his mouth is "seized" so that he is unable to talk, "spawn" of Šulpaea; he will not straighten up.[19]
24–25. If an infant continually jerks at the breast of his mother (and) continually wails; alternatively, (if) he is continually restless, he jumps in the knees of his mother and wails a lot, the daughter of Anu has "married" him.
26–27. If an infant as soon as he is born (and after) two or three days pass, (his stomach) will not accept the milk and a falling spell continually falls on him as in "hand" of god, "hand" of Ishtar. The thieving one has touched him; he will die.[20]
28. If an infant continually wails and screams, the thieving one, "hand" of Ishtar, daughter of Anu.[21]
29. If an infant's flesh is unevenly colored with yellow, his insides are cramped, his hands (and) feet are swollen, he has lots of *liʾbu* and the lungs are sick, "hand" of god; he will get well.[22]
30. If an infant's insides are continually bloated and he continually wails, "hand" of the Netherworld; alternatively, "hand" of the daughter of Anu, (var. "hand" of god); he will get well.
31. If an infant is equally hot (all over) and his epigastrium protrudes, "hand" of Kubu.[23]
32. If the muscles of an infant's abdomen are unevenly colored with red and yellow, "hand" of Kubu.[24]
33. If an infant's insides are cramped and he is unevenly colored with yellow, "hand" of Kubu.[25]
34. If an infant is continually cold and he gnashes his teeth, his illness will be prolonged; affliction by Kubu.[26]

35. If an infant continually jerks and is restless, "hand" of Sîn; he will get well.[27]

36–37. If an infant's flesh wastes away while he is nursing and his wet nurse's breast is weak and if you raise the breast to him he will not eat, that breast has a bitter taste. If you move him to a new breast, he should recover.[28]

38. If *ašû* or *samānu* seizes an infant, if you move him to a new breast and also continually say a recitation over him, he should recover.[29]

39–40. If an infant is sick with a *suʾālu*-cough, you moisten *kalgukku*-clay with honey and mix (it) with ghee. He should suck it up on an empty stomach. If he is unweaned(?), you put (it) on the breast of his mother and if he sucks (it) with the milk, he should recover.

41. If the transverse processes of a bent-over[30] infant's neck including his spine are open, he will die.[31]

42–43. If an infant's chest and abdomen flutter as a result of goring (*nikiptu*) by Sîn and likewise it is (about to) perish, to cure him, you grind *nikiptu* which you have charred, *ṭūru*-aromatic, *kukru*, *burāšu*-juniper, *nīnû*-mint and fresh *azupīru*. You mix them with *baluḫḫu*-aromatic oil. If you repeatedly rub him gently with it, he should recover.[32]

44. If the seam of the infant's head is open and his forehead is getting wider and he cannot sleep, if he is sick for (only) seven or eight days, he will get well (var. B: he will die).[33]

45. If the seam of the infant's head is open and his forehead is getting wider, he will die.[34]

46. If an infant continually jerks and is restless, he continually wails, he continually shudders, he continually raises his hands and his feet, blow of Sîn; it will finish him off.[35]

47. If an infant continually jerks, is restless and shudders, "hand" of Sîn or Ishtar.[36]

48. If an infant vomits as much as he eats; alternatively, (if) he has diarrhea (and) his hands and his feet become sluggish on him, there is a(n unfulfilled) promise to Sîn.[37]

49. If a falling spell falls on an infant and he gets well, if his illness is prolonged, he will die.[38]

50. If an infant has intestinal colic, he continually opens his mouth and as much as he eats (his insides) continually return, "hand" of Dingirmaḫ (var. "hand of god"); he will get well.[39]

51. If fever and *liʾbu* grips an infant and he is continually cold, affliction by Lamashtu (var. "hand" of the daughter of Anu).[40]

52. If an infant is hot and then cold and he asks for a lot of water to drink, affliction by Lamashtu (var. "hand" of the daughter of Anu).
53. If an infant's abdomen gets hot (and) gets cold and he asks for a lot of water to drink and drinks it, "hand" of Lamashtu.[41]
54. If the air of an infant's "right" nostril gets cold and that of the "left" gets hot,[42] "hand" of Lamashtu.
55. If an infant screams, jerks, is restless, continually wails and continually shudders (and) and as much as he drinks from the breast (his insides) continually return, "hand" of Sîn or Ishtar.[43]
56. If an infant's hand and feet are continually swollen (and) he continually constricts (the pupils of) his eyes, scepter of Sîn or Ishtar.[44]
57. If an infant's temperature is even but the seat(?) of his buttocks and his ears are cold, the scepter, messenger of Sîn.
58. If something continually afflicts an infant daily like affliction by Lamashtu, "hand" of Lamashtu.[45]
59. If an infant's body does not have fever but it has a lot of sweat, "hand" of *aḫḫāzu*. If an infant [...].
60. If an infant sucks the breast and then a falling spell falls on him, "hand" of [Ishtar (var. Sîn)].[46]
61. If an infant's flesh is dark (var. looks bruised) and he continually rubs his nose in a downward direction (and) tears flow from his eyes, *buʾšānu* [afflicts him ...].[47]
62. If an infant's thumb is turned inwards[48] (var. B: towards his hands) and he laughs a great deal, his flesh has a sick (look and) he has wasting away of the flesh, he will die of it.[49]
63. If an infant's insides are continually colicky (and) his eyes (feel) heavy, "hand" of god; he will get well.[50]
64. If an infant's insides are continually bloated and he continually wails, "hand" of god; he will get well.[51]
65. If an infant's insides are continually bloated, "hand" of god; he will get well.[52]
66. If an infant's insides are continually cramped, "hand" of god; he will get well.[53]
67. If sweat flows over an infant's nose (and) he flushes and turns pale, "hand" of god; he will get well. [54]
68. If an infant is full of vomiting, "hand" of god; he will get well. [55]
69. If an infant is sick with vomiting[56] and his palate continually dries up, "hand" of god; [he will get well].[57]
70. If an infant is sick with vomiting, "hand" [of god; he will get well]. [58]

71. If an infant's eyes make oscillating movements, "hand" of Ningešti-nanna.[59] If an infant's eyes continually dry out [...].
72. If an infant's insides are blocked off, "hand" of Damu.[60] If an infant's [...], "hand" of [...].
73. If you raise the breast to an infant and he will not eat, his intestines ⌈have been seriously injured⌉.[61]
74. If you raise the breast to an infant and he will not eat (and) his insides are continually [...].
75. [If] an ⌈infant's⌉ flesh is unevenly colored with yellow (and) his insides are continually [...].
76. [If] an infant's flesh is unevenly colored with yellow, "hand" of Gula.[62]
77. If an infant's abdomen is unevenly colored with yellow, ["hand" of Gula].
78. If an infant's epigastrium protrudes, "hand" of Gula.[63]
79. If an infant has a fever and his insides are cramped, "hand" of [Gula].[64]
80. If an infant does not have a fever and his insides are cramped, "hand" of [Gula].
81. If an infant is firmly planted, "hand" of [Gula].
82. If an infant is repeatedly[65] (and) continually sick, "hand" of [Gula].[66]
83. If an infant is continually restless, "hand" of [Gula].
84. If an infant continually stretches and his arms are turned(?), "hand" of [Gula].
85. If an infant's flesh sometimes wastes away and sometimes is healthy, "hand" of ⌈Gula⌉.[67]
86. If an infant flushes and turns pale, "hand" of ⌈Gula⌉.
87. If an infant turns white and black, "hand" of ⌈Gula⌉.[68]
88. If an infant gets thin and gets fat, "hand" of Gula.[69]
89. If an infant has a fever and his flesh diminishes, "hand" of Gula.[70]
90. If an infant burns with fever, "hand" of Gula.
91. If an infant's larynx is constricted, "hand" of Gula.[71]
92. If an infant chokes and his flesh is yellow, "hand" of Gula.[72]
93. If an infant chokes (and) will not drink from the breast and his body is yellow, "hand" of Gula.[73]
94. If an infant chokes (and) will not drink from the breast, "hand" of Gula.[74]
95. If an infant's insides are cramped and his anus is constricted, "hand" of Gula.
96. If an infant's insides are cramped, his body is yellow (and) *buʾšānu* afflicts him, "hand" of Gula.[75]
97. If an infant's insides are cramped and his mouth (feels) heavy, *buʾšānu* afflicts him.[76]

98. If an infant's spittle continually flows, *bu'šānu* afflicts him.[77]
99. If an infant's spittle contains blood, *bu'šānu* afflicts him.[78]
100. If an infant's skull, his breast, and his upper back are feverish, *bu'šānu* afflicts him.[79]
101. If an infant has a lukewarm temperature and his insides are cramped, *bu'šānu* afflicts him.[80]
102. If an infant continually wails at the breast of his mother (and) his intestines contain bile, he will die.[81]

---

103. If an infant is continually restless at the breast of his mother, (unfulfilled) vows afflict him.[82]
104. If (when) you raise the breast to an infant, he drinks and then drools, (unfulfilled) vows afflict him.[83]
105. If (when) you raise the breast to an infant, he will not eat and his insides are bloated, (unfulfilled) vows afflict him.[84]
106. If an infant does not have a fever (but) his insides are cramped and he wails, affliction by the daughter of Anu.[85]
107. If an infant wails and is continually rigid, the daughter of Anu afflicts him.[86]
108. If an infant wails day and night, the daughter of Anu afflicts him.[87]
109. If an infant groans and (if) you raise the breast to him he will not eat, a(n unfulfilled) vow afflicts him.[88]
110. If the infant is breast-fed for one or two months and then falling spell(s) fall upon him and his hands and his feet are immobilized, "hand" of god was born with him; either his father or his mother will die at/by his foot.[89]
111. If falling spells fall on an infant and his hands and feet are immobilized (and) his eyes are "soaked," the house of his father will be scattered at/by his foot.[90]
112. If an infant screams in his bed without knowing (it), "hand" of Ishtar.[91]
113. If an infant screams in his bed and says whatever he sees, "hand" of Ishtar; a(n unfulfilled) vow afflicts him.[92]
114. If an infant's cry is stifled (but) he does not have snot, *bu'šānu* afflicts him.[93]
115. If an infant's body (has) lukewarm temperature (and) his head has fever, he eats (from) the breast and then drools a lot, his teeth are coming out. He may suffer for fourteen or twenty days, but he will get well.[94]
116. If the infant does not have a fever (but) his head is feverish, his teeth are coming out. He may suffer for twenty-one days, but he will get well.[95]
117. If an infant's skull continually gets feverish, "hand" of Nusku.[96]

118. If an infant chokes and his body is yellow, "hand" of Gula.
119. If an infant chokes, fever continually afflicts him (and) his appetite for the breast is diminished, a curse afflicts him.[97]
120. If an infant does not have a fever, his eyes are dilated (and) his hands and his feet tremble, "hand" of Sîn; he will get well.[98]
121. If an infant does not have a fever but he trembles, "hand" of Sîn.[99]
122. If an infant does not have a fever (but) trembling continually afflicts him, "hand" of Sîn.[100]
123. If an infant coughs up as much as he eats; alternatively, (if as much as he eats) continually returns (to his mouth and) his hands and his feet are continually sluggish, there exists a verbal promise (of a gift) to Sîn (which has not been given).

NOTES

1. Restoration is based on the commentary, SpTU 1.41:5
2. The reading follows *CAD* Š/1, 480 s.v. *šappultu*.
3. The restoration is based on K 3628+4009:5′.
4. *CAD* Š/1, 272 unaccountably reads *ša-li*.
5. The commentary SpTU 1.41:3–5 explains this as meaning that the patient has, figuratively speaking, been thrown to the earth. See Scurlock and Andersen 2005, 17.146.
6. See Scurlock and Andersen 2005, 13.281.
7. See Scurlock and Andersen 2005, 13.183.
8. The verb implies a downward motion; see *CAD* S, 227–29.
9. The restoration is based on the commentary, SpTU 1.41:5 which has : BI.LU : *bu-šá-nu*.
10. See Scurlock and Andersen 2005, 19.331.
11. The commentary, SpTU 1.41:6 explains that this is because Lamashtu has "married" him.
12. I.e., he has diarrhea.
13. See Scurlock and Andersen 2005, 3.120.
14. See Scurlock and Andersen 2005, 17.147.
15. The translation assumes that this is a verb related to the commonly attested noun *šēlu*/*šīlu*: "hole, depression."
16. See Scurlock and Andersen 2005, 17.164
17. See Scurlock and Andersen 2005, 13.184.
18. See Scurlock and Andersen 2005, 19.357.
19. See Scurlock and Andersen 2005, 13.244.
20. See Scurlock and Andersen 2005, 13.178.
21. This entry is cited in K 3628 + 4009 + Sm. 1315 obv. 6 (ch. 13, text 1) with footnote (obv. 10) as an introduction to treatments for "hand" of Ishtar (obv. 11–16).
22. See Scurlock and Andersen 2005, 4.23, 19.96
23. See Scurlock and Andersen 2005, 19.336, 20.100. This entry appears also in DPS 13:156.
24. See Scurlock and Andersen 2005, 19.336, 20.100.
25. See Scurlock and Andersen 2005, 19.336, 20.100.

26. See Scurlock and Andersen 2005, 19.336, 20.100.
27. See Scurlock and Andersen 2005, 13.179, 19.47.
28. See Scurlock and Andersen 2005, 6.49, 7.13, 17.143.
29. See Scurlock and Andersen 2005, 17.144.
30. The translation is based on the assumption that the Akkadian is related to the Hebrew *šafouf*.
31. See Scurlock and Andersen 2005, 17.70.
32. See Scurlock and Andersen 2005, 8.79
33. See Scurlock and Andersen 2005, 17.151.
34. See Scurlock and Andersen 2005, 17.152.
35. Literally, "he will have a finishing off." See Scurlock and Andersen 2005, 13.181, 19.48.
36. See Scurlock and Andersen 2005, 13.67, 19.50
37. See Scurlock and Andersen 2005, 3.107, 19.53.
38. See Scurlock and Andersen 2005, 13.176.
39. See Scurlock and Andersen 2005, 6.58, 19.344, 19.354.
40. See Scurlock and Andersen 2005, 3.16, 19.224.
41. See Scurlock and Andersen 2005, 19.229.
42. To note is that core body temperature is not the same on the right as on the left side of the body. Modern thermometers pick this up as a matter of course but it would have been noticed in the pre-thermometer age only when core body temperature was elevated.
43. See Scurlock and Andersen 2005, 19.52.
44. See Scurlock and Andersen 2005, 4.24, 19.51, 19.95.
45. See Scurlock and Andersen 2005, 19.228.
46. See Scurlock and Andersen 2005, 13.177. This entry is cited in K 3628 + 4009 + Sm. 1315 obv. 7 (ch. 13, text 1) with footnote (obv. 10) as an introduction to treatments for "hand" of Ishtar (obv. 11-16).
47. See Scurlock and Andersen 2005, 19.332.
48. See *CAD* Ṣ, 65.
49. See Scurlock and Andersen 2005, 17.167.
50. See Scurlock and Andersen 2005, 17.161.
51. See Scurlock and Andersen 2005, 17.161.
52. See Scurlock and Andersen 2005, 17.161.
53. See Scurlock and Andersen 2005, 17.161
54. See Scurlock and Andersen 2005, 19.355.
55. See Scurlock and Andersen 2005, 19.356.
56. *CAD* Š/1, 272's translation is based on an erroneous reading.
57. See Scurlock and Andersen 2005, 19.356.
58. See Scurlock and Andersen 2005, 19.356.
59. See Scurlock and Andersen 2005, 13.109
60. See Scurlock and Andersen 2005, 17.120.
61. See Scurlock and Andersen 2005, 17.163.
62. See Scurlock and Andersen 2005, 19.320.
63. See Scurlock and Andersen 2005, 19.323.
64. See Scurlock and Andersen 2005, 19.327.
65. The N-stem of *saḫāru* in hendiadys with another verb implies that you "turn right around" and do something (often contrary to what you were doing before; for references, see *CAD* S, 53–54). In this case, the infant seems to get better and then "turns right around" and gets sick again.

66. See Scurlock and Andersen 2005, 19.319, 20.99.
67. See Scurlock and Andersen 2005, 19.325.
68. See Scurlock and Andersen 2005, 19.322.
69. See Scurlock and Andersen 2005, 19.326.
70. See Scurlock and Andersen 2005, 19.324.
71. See Scurlock and Andersen 2005, 0.3, 19.333.
72. See Scurlock and Andersen 2005, 0.3.
73. See Scurlock and Andersen 2005, 0.3, 19.334.
74. See Scurlock and Andersen 2005, 0.3.
75. See Scurlock and Andersen 2005, 19.330.
76. See Scurlock and Andersen 2005, 17.157. This entry appears also in DPS 33:89.
77. See Scurlock and Andersen 2005, 17.157. This entry appears also in DPS 33:88.
78. See Scurlock and Andersen 2005, 17.157. This entry appears also in DPS 33:90.
79. See Scurlock and Andersen 2005, 17.157. This entry appears also in DPS 33:91.
80. See Scurlock and Andersen 2005, 17.157.
81. See Scurlock and Andersen 2005, 17.162.
82. See Scurlock and Andersen 2005, 19.358.
83. See Scurlock and Andersen 2005, 19.358.
84. See Scurlock and Andersen 2005, 19.358.
85. See Scurlock and Andersen 2005, 19.54.
86. See Scurlock and Andersen 2005, 19.54.
87. See Scurlock and Andersen 2005, 19.54.
88. See Scurlock and Andersen 2005, 19.359.
89. See Scurlock and Andersen 2005, 13.221.
90. See Scurlock and Andersen 2005, 13.39. For the expression, see Stol, *Epilepsy*, p. 89.
91. See Scurlock and Andersen 2005, 17.165, 19.10. This entry is cited in K 3628 + 4009 + Sm. 1315 obv. 8 (ch. 13, text 1) with footnote (obv. 10) as an introduction to treatments for "hand" of Ishtar (obv. 11-16).
92. See Scurlock and Andersen 2005, 17.166, 19.10. This entry is cited in K 3628 + 4009 + Sm. 1315 obv. 9 (ch. 13, text 1) with footnote (obv. 10) as an introduction to treatments for "hand" of Ishtar (obv. 11-16).
93. See Scurlock and Andersen 2005, 17.158.
94. See Scurlock and Andersen 2005, 17.148.
95. See Scurlock and Andersen 2005, 17.149.
96. See Scurlock and Andersen 2005, 19.346. This entry appears also in DPS 3:10.
97. See Scurlock and Andersen 2005, 6.52.
98. See Scurlock and Andersen 2005, 13.95, 13.180, 19.49.
99. See Scurlock and Andersen 2005, 19.49.
100. See Scurlock and Andersen 2005, 19.49.

2

PHARMACOLOGY

A. VADEMECUM (PHARMACIST'S COMPANION)

Pharmacological knowledge was kept "in order not to be forgotten" in a number of forms including vademecum texts (pharmacist's companion); two dedicated series with descriptions and uses of medicinal plants and stones: *Šammu šikinšu* ("the nature of plants") and *Abnu šikinšu* ("the nature of stones"); and the ancient plant glossary, URU.AN.NA. Vademecum texts are laid out in a chart format, and give the name of each plant to be discussed, its primary use, and the method of preparation. Organization is by usage. These texts were presumably primarily designed so that the pharmacist presented with a patient with an easily or already diagnosed problem knew what plants needed to be administered. Since the fewer the plants that were employed, the lower the cost, this would allow for the least expensive possible relief for the patient's condition. The physician would also have found this a handy reference work for recommending simple treatments to indigent patients.

TEXT 1: BAM 1 (= *KAR* 203) i 17–67

BAM 1 is one of the longest and best preserved of the vademeca and has a colophon that indicates that the text belonged to an *asû*. Sections of BAM 1 appear verbatim in a number of other vademecum texts and are cited both in medical commentaries and in therapeutic texts. For details, see appendix 2.

BAM 1 is also the most carefully organized of the vademeca. Col. i deals with diseases that produce symptoms relating to the head and mouth as outlined in the medical commentary SpTU 1.43:7–19. What is included in some form or other are SpTU 1.43:9 (dental problems), 12 (Lamashtu), 15 (*maškādu*), 17 (*ašû*), and 19 (burning of *ṣētu*).

The opening sections of BAM 1 (i 1–16) deal with dental problems (= SpTU 1.43:9) and appear in chapter 5, text 7. The remaining sections of BAM 1 i deal with "hand" of curse (17), the genito-urinary tract (18–29), the gall bladder (30–34), intestinal problems (35), problems with the muscles (36–39, 47–48), unhappiness and feelings of social isolation (59–61), and a variety of different types of fever (40–46, 49–58, 62–67).[1] These entries may be understood with the help of SpTU 1.43, which puts together as a category three fevers with a propensity for producing a severe frontal headache and/or hair loss and/or lesions on the face, namely Lamashtu (12), *ašû* (17), and burning of *ṣētu* (19). Lamashtu (typhoid)[2] was classified by the ancient physician as a *li'bu*-fever that affected the gall bladder (= BAM 1 i 30–34, 43). *Ašû* (= BAM 1 i 62–67) is an ancient disease category that included pox diseases.[3] *Ṣētu* (= BAM 1 i 42, 49–58) was what premodern physicians called enteric fever.[4] It affects the stomach (= BAM 1 i 35) and urinary tract (= BAM 1 i 21–29) and may be complicated by what the ancient physician called "curse" (pneumonia[5] = BAM 1 i 17). Muscle aches (= BAM 1 i 47–48), unhappiness and feelings of social isolation (= BAM 1 i 59–61) are common in all fevers.

More puzzling is the inclusion of references to two muscle problems, *maškādu* and *šimmatu* (= BAM 1 i 36–39; cf. SpTU 1.43:15).[6] However, ancient medical texts use the same term for blood vessels (involved in fever) and muscles, namely SA.MEŠ. Also, both fever and muscle problems were frequently treated with salves, as here almost invariably. The section on constriction (= BAM 1 i 21–29; cf. SpTU 1.43:26) seems also to have naturally attracted female sterility, which can result from urinary tract infections (= BAM 1 i 18–20; cf. SpTU 1.43:31).

BAM 1 column ii is also reflected in medical commentary SpTU 1.43 with BAM 1 ii 21–45 corresponding to SpTU 1.43:20–25 (lung conditions). This is followed in BAM 1 ii 46–64 by a section on liver conditions. Column iii 1–19 deals with DÚR.GIG or other problems with the anus. The rest of the text gives miscellaneous plant uses, and ends with bad omens drawn from plants (iii 40 on).

Striking in BAM 1, as always in Mesopotamian medicine, is the inclusion of "magical" elements. For example, the potion for "hand" of curse is to be taken on the day of the disappearance of the moon (17), evil eye is combated (60–61), and there are amulets (36–37, 39, 66) mixed in with the potions (17–18, 21–35, 49, 57–59, 67), aliments (59), suppositories (19–20), washes (21–23, 53), salves (21–23, 37–38, 40–52, 54–58, 60–63), and fumigants (64–65). The inclusion of these elements is, however, no reason not to take this text seriously. So, for example, *kamantu*-henna(?) seed, used for regulating female fertility (18) is, I have argued,[7] *Lawsonia inermis* (henna) which would indeed have been useful for this purpose. The Vademecum BAM 1 is fully edited and discussed in Attia and Buisson 2012.

1–16. (see chapter 5, text 7)

---

17. ⸢Ú⸣ŠE.KAK ^{GIŠ}ŠINIG Ú ŠU.^{d}NAM.ÉRIM BÚR *ina* U_4.NÁ.A NAG

18.	⌜Ú⌝NUMUN ÁB.DUḪ	Ú NUMUN TUKU	SÚD *ina* KAŠ SAG NAG
19–20	⌜Ú⌝NUMUN *at-kám*	Ú NUMUN TUKU	SÚD KI ZÍD ŠE.SA.A *ina šur-šúm-me* KAŠ / ḪE.ḪE *ina* GAL_4.LA-*šá* GAR
21.	ÚILLU NU.LUḪ.ḪA	Ú *ḫi-niq* BUN	*ina* KAŠ NAG *ina* Ì+GIŠ EŠ MUD *ana* GÌŠ-*šú* MÚ
22.	Ú.ŠEMŠEŠ	Ú *ḫi-niq* BUN	ŠU.BI.DILI.ÀM
23.	ÚILLU ŠEMBULUḪ	Ú KI.MIN	ŠU.BI.DILI.ÀM
24.	ÚŠE.KAK GIŠDÌḪ	Ú KI.MIN	SÚD *ina* KAŠ.SAG NAG
25.	Ú*imḫur-lim*	Ú KI.MIN	SÚD *ina* GEŠTIN NAG
26.	Ú*a-su-pi-ru* SIG_7	Ú KI.MIN	SÚD *ina* KAŠ.SAG NAG
27.	Ú*al-la-an-ka-niš*	Ú KI.MIN	SÚD *ina* KAŠ.SAG NAG
28.	ÚSUMSAR	Ú KI.MIN	SÚD *ina* Ì+GIŠ *u* KAŠ. SAG NAG
29.	Ú*ḫa-šá-a-nu*	Ú KI.MIN	SÚD *ina* Ì+GIŠ *u* KAŠ. SAG NAG
30.	⌜Ú⌝*ṣi-bu-ru*	Ú ZÉ	SÚD *ina* KAŠ.SAG NAG
31.	⌜Ú⌝*it-tu*	Ú ZÉ	SÚD *lu ina* KAŠ.SAG *lu ina* GEŠTIN NAG
32.	[(Ú)]*me*-[(*er*)]-*zi-nu*	Ú ZÉ	KI.MIN
33.	[(ÚUZU.DIR)].KUR.RA	Ú ZÉ	KI.MIN
34.	⌜Ú⌝[(*tu-lal*)] [(PA GIŠ)]ŠINIG ‹‹AN›› BAR MUŠ	Ú ZÉ	KI.MIN
35.	Ú*pu-ru-p*[(*u-ḫu*)]	Ú *sa*!-*ḫu*! GIG	SÚD *ina* KAŠ.SAG NAG[8]

36.	^{Ú}SUḪUŠ KUR.GI.RÍN.[(NA	[(Ú *maš-k*)]*a-di* ZI	SÍG ÙZ NIG[(IN)] *ina* GÚ NA GAR-*nu*
37.	^{Ú}NÍG.PA [SIPA	Ú] KI.MIN	⌜SÍG NIGIN SÚD⌝ [*ina*] Ì+GIŠ EŠ
38.	^{Ú}SUḪUŠ $^{\text{Ú.GIŠ}}$GÍR SUḪUŠ [^{GIŠ}DÌḪ	Ú K]I.MIN	*ina* Ì+GIŠ EŠ.MEŠ
39.	^{Ú}ILLU ^{GIŠ}ŠINI[G]	[Ú *šim-m*]*a-ti*[9]	SÍG ÙZ NIGIN *ina* GÚ NA GAR-*nu*
40.	^{Ú}PA ^{GIŠ}ŠE.NÁ.A	⌜Ú⌝ [DI]B *šá-da-ni*	SÚD *ina* Ì+GIŠ ŠÉŠ[10]
41.	^{Ú}GEŠTU ^{GIŠ}DÌḪ KAL	Ú KI.MIN	SÚD *ina* Ì+GIŠ ŠÉŠ
42.	^{Ú}PA $^{\text{GIŠ.Ú}}$GÍR	⌜Ú⌝ UD.DA	SÚD *ina* Ì+GIŠ ŠÉŠ
43.	^{Ú}NI.NE	⌜Ú⌝ *li-ʾi-bi*	SÚD *ina* Ì+GIŠ ŠÉŠ
44.	^{Ú}*ku-si-bu*	⌜Ú⌝ *ḫa-am-me*	SÚD *ina* Ì+GIŠ ŠÉŠ
45.	^{Ú}*ṣa-da-nu*	Ú [*u*]*m-ma-ṭí*	SÚD *ina* Ì+GIŠ ŠÉŠ
46.	Ú.KUR.RA^{SAR}	Ú [DI]B *aš-ri*[11]	SÚD *ina* Ì+GIŠ ŠÉŠ
47.	^{Ú}*a-su-pi-ru* SIG$_7$	Ú *qi*[*n*]-*na-ti*	SÚD *ina* Ì+GIŠ ŠÉŠ
48.	^{Ú}GA[MU]N^{SAR}	Ú KI.MIN	SÚD *ina* Ì+GIŠ ŠÉŠ
49.	^{Ú}*ṣa-ṣu-um-tú*	Ú TAB UD.DA	*ina* KAŠ SAG NAG *ina* Ì+GIŠ EŠ.MEŠ
50.	^{Ú}ŠÈ.MÁ.LAḪ$_4$	Ú TAB UD.DA	SÚD *ina* Ì+GIŠ ŠÉŠ
51.	^{Ú}*ap-ru-ša*	Ú TAB UD.DA	SÚD *ina* Ì+GIŠ ŠÉŠ
52.	^{Ú}PA ^{GIŠ}GEŠTIN.GÍR	Ú TAB [U]D.DA	SÚD *ina* Ì+GIŠ ŠÉŠ
53.	^{Ú}MI.PÀR	Ú TAB [U]D.DA	A.MEŠ ŠUB *se-ker* NA RA

54.	^{Ú}ḪAR.ḪAR ^{Ú}SUM^{SAR}	Ú TAB [U]D.DA	*ina* LÀL Ì+GIŠ ŠÉŠ
55.	^{Ú}*a-ra-rù-ú*	Ú TAB UD.[D]A	KI.MIN
56.	^{Ú}*šu-uq-da-nu*	Ú TAB UD.⸢DA⸣	SÚD *ina* Ì+GIŠ ŠÉŠ
57.	*ú-pi-ṣir*	Ú TAB UD.⸢DA⸣	*ina* KAŠ.SAG NAG KI.MIN
58.	^{Ú}*imḫur-lim*	Ú TAB UD.⸢DA⸣	SÚD *ina* KAŠ.SAG NAG KI.MIN

59.	^{Ú}*a-zal-lu-ú*	Ú SAG.PA.LAGAB	NU *pa-tan* GU$_7$ *u* NAG[12]
60.	^{Ú}NUMUN *a-zal-le-e*	Ú IGI ḪUL-*te*	*ana* NA NU TE *ina* Ì+GIŠ *dáp-ra-ni* EŠ
61.	^{Ú}NUMUN *al-lum-zi*	Ú KI.MIN	KI.MIN

62.	^{Ú}ÁB.DUḪ	Ú *a-ši-i*	SÚD *ina* Ì+GIŠ ŠÉŠ
63.	⸢^{Ú}⸣NUMUN ^{GIŠ}ESI	Ú *a-ši-i*	SÚD *ina* Ì+GIŠ ŠÉŠ
64.	⸢^{Ú}⸣KUR.KUR	Ú *a-ši-i*	NA *qut-tu-ru*
65.	[^{Ú}]*iš-bab-tum*	Ú *a-ši-i*	NA *qut-tu-ru*
66.	[^{Ú}]⸢I⸣LLU ^{ŠEM}BULUḪ	Ú *a-ši-i*	SÍG NIGIN *ina* GÚ NA GAR-*nu*
67.	$^{\text{[Ú.Š]EM}}$GÚR.GÚR	Ú *a-ši-i mu-tap-re-eš*	SÚD *ina* KAŠ SAG NAG

Translation

1–16. See chapter 5, text 7.

---

17. *Bīnu*-tamarisk shoot is a plant to dispel "hand" of curse. It is to be given to drink on the day of the disappearance of the moon.

---

18. *Kamantu* seed is a plant to have seed.[13] It is to be ground (and) given to drink (mixed) with first quality beer.

19–20. *Atkam* seed is a plant to have seed. It is to be ground, mixed with roasted grain flour in beer dregs (and) placed in her vagina.

---

21. *Nuḫurtu* resin is a plant for constriction of the urethra. It is to be given to drink (mixed) with beer, rubbed gently on (mixed) with oil (and) blown into his penis (via) a tube.

---

22. Myrrh is a plant for constriction of the urethra.[14] Ditto (It is to be given to drink mixed with beer, rubbed gently on mixed with oil and blown into his penis via a tube.)[15]
23. *Baluḫḫu*-aromatic resin is a plant ditto (for constriction of the urethra). Ditto (It is to be given to drink mixed with beer, rubbed gently on mixed with oil and blown into his penis via a tube).[16]
24. *Baltu*-thorn shoot is a plant ditto (for constriction of the urethra). It is to be ground (and) given to drink (mixed) with first quality beer.
25. *Imḫur-lim* is a plant ditto (for constriction of the urethra). It is to be ground (and) given to drink (mixed) with wine.[17]
26. Fresh *azupīru* is a plant ditto (for constriction of the urethra). It is to be ground (and) given to drink (mixed) with first quality beer.
27. *Allānkaniš*-oak is a plant ditto (for constriction of the urethra). It is to be ground (and) given to drink (mixed) with first quality beer.
28. *Šūmu*-garlic is a plant ditto (for constriction of the urethra). It is to be ground (and) given to drink (mixed) with oil and first quality beer.
29. *Ḫašānu* is a plant ditto (for constriction of the urethra). It is to be ground (and) given to drink (mixed) with oil and first quality beer.

---

30. *Ṣiburu*-aloe is a plant for the gall bladder. It is to be ground and given to drink (mixed) with first quality beer.
31. *Ittu* is a plant for the gall bladder. It is to be ground and given to drink (mixed) either with first quality beer or wine.
32. *Merzinu* is a plant for the gall bladder. Ditto (It is to be ground and given to drink mixed either with first quality beer or wine).
33. *Kamūn šadê*-fungus[18] is a plant for the gall bladder. Ditto (It is to be ground and given to drink mixed either with first quality beer or wine).
34. *Tullal*, *bīnu*-tamarisk leaves (and) snake skin(!) are plants for the gall bladder. Ditto (It is to be ground and given to drink mixed either with first quality beer or wine).

---

35. *Purupuḫu* is a plant for "sick intestines"/being sick with *saḫḫu*.[19] It is to be ground and given to drink (mixed) with first quality beer.
36. *Kurkānu*-turmeric root is a plant for removing *maškādu*. It is to be wrapped in goat wool (and) placed on the person's neck.

---

37. *Ḫaṭṭi* [*rēʾi*] is a plant ditto (for removing *maškādu*). It is to be wrapped in wool (or) ground and rubbed gently on (mixed) [with] oil.

---

38. *Ašāgu*-thorn root and [*baltu*-thorn] root are [plants] ⌈ditto (for removing *maškādu*)⌉. They are to be gently rubbed repeatedly on (mixed) with oil.

---

39. *Bīnu*-tamarisk resin is a [plant] for ⌈numbness⌉. It is to be wrapped in goat hair (and) placed on the person's neck.

---

40. *Šūnû*-chaste tree leaf is a plant for ⌈affliction⌉ by *šadānu*. It is to be ground (and) rubbed gently on (mixed) with oil.

---

41. Large *baltu*-thorn "ear" is a plant ditto (for affliction by *šadānu*). It is to be ground (and) rubbed gently on (mixed) with oil.

---

42. *Ašāgu* leaf is a plant for *ṣētu*. It is to be ground (and) rubbed gently on (mixed) with oil.

---

43. *Šūšu*-licorice[20] is a plant for *liʾbu*-fever. It is to be ground (and) rubbed gently on (mixed) with oil.

---

44. *Kusību* is a plant for *ḫammu*-fever. It is to be ground (and) rubbed gently on (mixed) with oil.

---

45. *Ṣadānu* is a plant for *ummaṭu*-fever. It is to be ground (and) rubbed gently on (mixed) with oil.

---

46. *Nīnû*-mint is a plant for ⌈affliction⌉ of *ašru*. It is to be ground (and) rubbed gently on (mixed) with oil.

---

47. Fresh *azupīru* is a plant for the buttocks. It is to be ground (and) rubbed gently on (mixed) with oil.

---

48. *Kamunu*-cumin is a plant ditto (for the buttocks). It is to be ground (and) rubbed gently on (mixed) with oil.

---

49. *Ṣaṣuntu* is a plant for burning of *ṣētu*. It is to be given to drink (mixed) with first quality beer (and) repeatedly rubbed gently on (mixed) with oil.
50. *Zê malaḫi* is a plant for burning of *ṣētu*. It is to be ground (and) rubbed gently on (mixed) with oil.
51. *Aprušu* is a plant for burning of *ṣētu*. It is to be ground (and) rubbed gently on (mixed) with oil.

52. *Amurdinnu* leaf is a plant for burning of ⸢*ṣētu*⸣. It is to be ground (and) rubbed gently on (mixed) with oil.

---

53. *Lipāru*-tree is a plant for burning of ⸢*ṣētu*⸣. It is to be poured into water, baked (and) used to bathe the person.
54. *Ḫašû*-thyme (and) *šūmu*-garlic are plants for burning of *ṣētu*. They are to be rubbed gently on (mixed) with honey (and) oil.
55. *Ararû* is a plant for burning of *ṣētu*. (It is to be rubbed gently on mixed with honey and oil).
56. *Šuqdānu* is a plant for burning of *ṣētu*. It is to be ground (and) rubbed gently on (mixed) with oil.
57. *Upinzir* is a "plant"[21] for burning of *ṣētu*. It is to be given to drink (mixed) with first quality beer ditto (and ground and rubbed gently on mixed with oil).
58. *Imḫur-lim* is a plant for burning of ⸢*ṣētu*⸣. It is to be given to drink (mixed) with first quality beer ditto (and ground and rubbed gently on mixed with oil).

---

59. *Azallû* is a plant for depression. It is to be given to eat or drink on an empty stomach.
60. *Azallû* seed is a plant to prevent evil eye from approaching a person. It is to be rubbed gently on (mixed) with *daprānu*-juniper oil.
61. *Allumzu* seed is a plant ditto (to prevent evil eye from approaching a person). Ditto (It is to be rubbed gently on mixed with *daprānu*-juniper oil).

---

62. *Kamantu* is a plant for *ašû*. It is to be ground (and) rubbed gently on (mixed) with oil.
63. *Ušû*-tree seed is a plant for *ašû*. It is to be ground (and) rubbed gently on (mixed) with oil.
64. *Atāʾišu* is a plant for *ašû*. It is used to fumigate the person.
65. *Išbabtu* is a plant for *ašû*. It is used to fumigate the person.
66. *Baluḫḫu* resin is a plant for *ašû*. It is to be wrapped in wool (and) placed on the person's neck.
67. *Kukru* is a plant for fleeting *ašû*. It is ground (and) given to drink (mixed) with first quality beer.

B. *ŠAMMU ŠIKINŠU* ("THE NATURE OF PLANTS")

Šammu šikinšu ("the nature of plants"), known to us by its ancient name, is the most important pharmacological series. Its entries begin with the appearance of the plant, described in terms of a system of taxonomy that compares the plant to be described to other plants with distinctive characteristics. This classification system also provides the principle of organization, as may be seen most clearly in *STT* 93, which groups entries around specific plants or plant groups with similar leaves, gourds, etc. The description is followed by the name of the plant, the primary use for which it was appropriate, and the method of preparation. This pharmacological series is closely related to the Vademecum texts and to Uruanna. Indeed, BAM 379 begins with *Šammu šikinšu* but, by ii 51′, it has shifted to a Vademecum. For an edition of this series, see Stadhouders 2011 and 2012.

TEXT 2: SPTU 3.106 OBV. i

[(Ú GAR-*šú* GIN$_7$ Ú.KUR.RA ^{Ú}*k*)*am*-(*ka-du* MU.NI)]
[(*ana* GIG *šá* ⸢IR⸣ ŠUB-*ú*[22] SIG$_5$ SÚD *ana* IGI GIG ŠUB-*di*)]
[(Ú GAR-*šú* GIN$_7$ ^{Ú}GÁNA.ZI *ù* SA$_5$ ^{Ú}*a-zal-lá* MU.NI)]
[(*ana* GAZ ŠÀ SIG$_5$ SÚD *ina* Ì.GIŠ Š)ÉŠ]

1′. [(Ú GAR-*šú* GIN$_7$)]⸢^{GIŠ}⸣*su-p*[(*a-li* NUMUN!-*šú* SA$_5$[coll.] ^{Ú}*el-li-bu* MU.NI)]

2′. [*ana ri-mu-t*]*i* ‹(*ù*)› *šim-ma-t*[(*i* ZI-*ḫi* SIG$_5$ SÚD *ina* Ì.GIŠ Š)É(Š)-*su*]

3′. [(Ú GAR-*šú* GI)]N$_7$ ^{Ú}*duḫ-ni* [(^{Ú}*a-nu-nu-ti*) M(U-*šú*)]

4′. *ana* GEŠTU^{II} *šá* MÚD.BABBAR ŠUB-*a* SIG$_5$ S[(ÚD *ina* Ì *ana* ŠÀ) GEŠTU^{II}-(*šú* ŠU)[B!? (sign ku)]

5′. [(Ú)] GAR-*šú* GIN$_7$ ^{GIŠ}Ù.SUḪ$_5$ *ti-ri-in-na-ti* [(*zu-ʾ-un* ^{Ú}*ud-da-šu* MU.NI *ana* DÚR SIG)][23]

6′. Ú GAR-*šú* GIN$_7$ ZAG.ḪI.LI‹$^{(SAR)}$› NUMUN-*šu* NUMUN ZAG. ḪI.LI[$^{(SAR)}$]

7′. [(^{Ú}*saḫ-la-nu* MU.NI)] *ana* ŠÀ SI.SÁ SIG$_5$ SÚD *ina* ⸢A⸣.[(MEŠ NU) *pa-tan* NAG]

8′. Ú GAR-*šú* GIN$_7$ *ú-pat*! ‹$^{(GIŠ)}$›.^{Ú}GÍR NUMUN-*šu* GIN$_7$ NUMUN ḪI.IS^{SAR} ^{Ú}*mat-qu* MU.N[(I *ana* ŠÀ SI.SÁ KI.MIN)]

9′. Ú GAR-*šú* GIN$_7$ ‹$^{(Ú)}$›ÚKUŠ.LAL ‹(*u*)› È-*su ru-uš-šat* ^{Ú}*imḫur-lim* MU.NI *ana* GIG D[(Ù.A.BI SIG$_5$)]

10′. Ú GAR-*šú* GIN$_7$ Ú.^{d}UTU NUMUN-*šú* GIN$_7$ *ši-gu-uš-ti* ^{Ú}*imḫur*-20 [(MU. NI)]

11′. *ana* GIG *la-az-zi* SIG$_5$ ḪÁD.DU SÚD *ana* IGI GI[(G ŠUB-*di*)]

12′. Ú GAR-*šú* GIN$_7$ ^{Ú}*ti-gi-il-le-e* NUMUN-*šu* GIN$_7$ *ši-gu-uš-ti* ^{Ú}AŠ.TÁL.TÁL [(MU.NI)]
13′. Ú GAR-*šú* GIN$_7$ *ši-kin za-ap-pi šid!-da* SA$_5$ ^{Ú}*el-kul-la* MU.NI *ana* IGI^{II} *šá qú*-[(⸢*qa?-ni?*⸣ ŠUB)]
14′. Ú GAR-*šú* GIN$_7$ *ši-kin* ^{GIŠ}*piš-ri* GI$_6$ *ù* UGU-*šu* ZU ^{Ú}*as*-[(*saḫ-pi* MU.NI)]
15′. *ana* DIB GIDIM ZI-⸢*ḫi*⸣ S[IG$_5$ … (*ina* GÚ-*šú* GAR-*an*)]
16′. Ú GAR-*šú* GIN$_7$ ‹‹GIŠ›› *ši-kin* ^{GIŠ}ḪAŠḪUR *ina ni-síḫ* A.AB.[(BA *a-šar šam*-⸢*mu*⸣) *u* ^{GIŠ}(GI)]
17′. NU GÁL.MEŠ *ina* IGI A.MEŠ È *ina* UGU-*ḫi-šú* [*as-*(*qú-du ra-bi-iṣ*)]
18′. ^{Ú}LAL MU.NI *ana* GIG *šu-ru-pé-e* TAB UD.DA *u* UŠ[$_{11}$ (BÚR SIG$_5$)][24]

19′. Ú GAR-*šú* GIN$_7$ *ši-kin* ^{Ú}EME.UR.GI$_7$ MIN Ú GAR-*šú* GIN$_7$ ^{Ú}LU.ÚB^{SAR}[25] ⸢*ù*⸣ [(IGI.MEŠ)]
20′. *iš-te-né-ʾe ina* A.ŠÀ *mi-ik-ri* È *e-ma* ZI-*šú šu-ru*-⸢*us*⸣-[*s*(*u*)]
21′. *ik-kap-pap* ^{Ú}*lid-da*-[*na-nu*] (*ḫi-pí eš-šú*) x […]

22′. Ú GAR-*šú* GIN$_7$ ^{Ú}LU.ÚB^{SAR} NUMUN-*šú* GIN$_7$ NUMUN ^{Ú}ŠE.LÚ^{SAR} ^{Ú}*sis-sin*-[ŠÀ MU.NI] (*ḫi-pí*) NUMUN-*šú ana* ŠÀ SI.SÁ SIG$_5$ S[ÚD]
23′. *ina* A.MEŠ NU *pa-tan* NAG

Translation

(There are at least four missing lines at the beginning of the text:)

– The plant that resembles *ninû*-mint is called *kamkādu*. It is good for putting on top of a sore that produces "sweat."[26] You grind (it and) pour (it) on top of the sore.[27]

– The plant that resembles *kanašû* but is red/brown is called *azallû*.[28] It is good for crushing sensation in the chest.[29] You grind (it and) ⸢rub (it) gently on⸣ (mixed) with oil.

1′–2′. The plant that resembles *supālu* (but) whose seed is red is called *ellibu*.[30] It is good for removing ⸢limpness⸣ and numbness. You grind (it and) ⸢rub him gently⸣ with it (mixed) with oil.

3′–4′. The plant that resembles *duḫnu*-millet is called *anunūtu*. It is good for ears that produce pus. You grind (it and) pour (it) into his [ears] (mixed) with oil.

5′. The plant that is studded with cones like an *ašuḫu*-fir is called *uddašu*. It is good for the anus.[31]

6′–7′. The plant that resembles *saḫlû*[32] (and) whose seed is like (that of) *saḫlû* is called *saḫlānu*. It is good for producing a bowel movement. You grind (it and) [have him drink it] ⸢on an empty stomach⸣ (mixed) with water.

8′. The plant that resembles the "snot" of *ašāgu*-thorn (but) whose seed is like the seed of *ḫassu* is called *matqu*. (It is good) for producing a bowel movement. Ditto (You grind it and have him drink it on an empty stomach mixed with water).[33]

9′. The plant that resembles LAL-gourd but the part that comes out of it is russet[34] is called *imḫur-lim*. It is good for every sort of illness.

10′–11′. The plant that resembles "sunflower" (but) whose seed is like (that of) *šigguštu* is called *imḫur-ešra*.[35] It is good for a persistent sore. You grind (it and) pour it on the sore.

12′. The plant that resembles *tigillû*-gourd (but) whose seed is like (that of) *šigguštu* is called *ardadillu*.

13′. The plant that has what look like bristles, which is elongated, (and) red is called *elkulla*. It is [good] for pouring into eyes with *quqānu*-worm.[36]

14′–15′. The plant that is black like *pišru*-wood but its upper part is strong[37] is called *assaḫpi*. It ⸢is good⸣ for removing affliction by a ghost. You [...] (and) put it on his neck.

16′–18′. The plant that is shaped like a *ḫašḫuru*-apple (and which) comes out on the surface of the water at the outlet(?) to the sea where there are no (other) plants or reeds (and) which ⸢*asqudu*-snakes⸣ lie on is called *ašqulālu*.[38] It is good for diseases with ice cold chills, burning of *ṣētu* and loosening *kišpu*.[39]

19′–21′. The plant that resembles *lišān kalbi* is the same.[40] The plant which resembles[41] *laptu*-vegetable but which continually seeks out the front side[42] (and which) comes up in irrigated fields (and which) when you pull it up, ⸢its⸣ root bends [is called][43] ⸢*liddanānu*⸣ [...].

22′–23′. The plant that resembles *laptu*-vegetable (but) whose seed is like the seed of *kisibirru*-coriander [is called] ⸢*sisinni libbi*⸣. Its seed is good for producing a bowel movement. You ⸢grind⸣ (it and) have him drink (it) on an empty stomach (mixed) with water.[44]

C. *ABNU ŠIKINŠU* ("THE NATURE OF STONES")

The most usual use in ancient Mesopotamian medicine of stones was in combination with other stones, either ground up to provide an abrasive substrate to ensure the better absorption of salves or, more typically, strung on colored wool and worn as necklaces or bracelets for a variety of personal problems, including strictly medical ones. A selection of thereapeutic texts deal specifically with the issue of which stones to use in which combination for what problem (see chapter 15, texts 1–2). The series *Abnu šikinšu* ("the nature of stones") was primarily intended as a reference work that allowed the practicioner to recognize the stones he needed. Organization is by stone, beginning with the most common (lapis and carnelian), which are described and listed with all their varieties. For an edition of the series as a whole, as well as numerous stone lists, see Schuster-Brandis 2008, 17–47.

TEXT 3: BAM 378 ii–iii AND *STT* 108: 1–3, 13–35, 47–48

Although fragmentary, enough survives of this text to recognize that cols ii–iii duplicate the obverse of *STT* 108//STT 109. As rare good fortune would have it, *STT* 108//STT 109 allows the partial restoration of the missing lines at the beginning of BAM 378, col. ii, as well as the end of col. ii and the beginning of col. iii of this text.

STT 108

1. NA_4 GAR-*šú* [(G)]IN$_7$ [...^{N}]^{A_4}ZA.GÌN MU.[NI]
2. NA_4 GAR-*šú* [(G)]IN$_7$ [...^{NA}]^{_4}ZA.G[ÌN] MU.[NI]
3. ^{NA_4}ZA.⌜GÌN⌝ [(BABBAR) *tuk-ku*]-*up* [^{NA_4}]ZA.GÌN.[AN(ŠE!.E)]DIN.NA MU.[NI]

BAM 378 ii 0′–15′

0′. [(^{NA_4}ZA.GÌN SIG$_7$) *tuk-ku*-(*up*)]
1′. ^{NA_4}ZA.GÌN *M*[(*ar*-[*ḫ*]*a-ši* MU).NI]

2′. NA_4 GAR-*šú* GIN$_7$ [(*ed-di-ti*)]
3′. ^{NA_4}GUG MU.N[I]
4′. ^{NA_4}GUG GI$_6$ *tak-pat*
5′. ^{NA_4}GUG *Me-luḫ-ḫi* MU.NI[45]
6′. ^{NA_4}GUG GAZI^{SAR} *tuk-ku-pat*
7′. ^{NA_4}GUG GAZI^{SAR} MU.NI
8′. ^{NA_4}GUG SIG$_7$ *tak-pat*

9′. ^{NA_4}GUG *Mar-ḫa-ši* MU.N[I][46]

10′. NA_4 GAR-*šú* GIN_7 *si-ḫi-ir ta-bar-r*[*i*]
11′. BABBAR *ka-rík* $^{NA[(_4)]}$MUŠ.GÍR [(MU.NI)]
12′. NA_4 GAR-*šú* SA_5 BABBAR [(*ud*)]-⸢*du*⸣-[(*uḫ*)]
13′. ^{NA_4}MUŠ.GÍ[R (MU.NI)]
14′. ^{NA_4}MUŠ.GÍR [(*sa-di-*⸢*ru-šú*⸣)]
15′. *ma-du* $^{N[(A_4}$MUŠ.G)ÍR NÍTA (MU.NI)]

STT 108

13. [(^{N})^{A_4}MU(Š)].GÍR GIN_7 *ka-ra-áš* [(⸢ŠU⸣)].SI ^{NA_4}MUŠ.GÍR *za-qa-ni* MU.NI

---

14. [(NA_4 GAR)]-*šú* GIN_7 ^{NA_4}NÍR ^{NA_4}MUŠ.GÍR ^{NA_4}*lu-lu$_4$-da-ni-tum* MU.[NI]
15. [(NA_4 GAR)]-*šú* SA_5 BABBAR *u* GI_6 [*ud-d*]*u-uḫ* ^{NA_4}*lu-lu$_4$-da-ni-tum* MU.NI

---

16. NA_4 GAR-⸢*šú*⸣ BABBAR *u* GI_6 [*e-di*]-*iḫ* ^{NA_4}NÍR MU.NI
17. NA_4 GAR-*šú* [G]I_6-*m*[(*a*)] 1 [BABBAR] ⸢*e*⸣-*di-iḫ* ^{NA_4}BABBAR.DIL MU.NI
18. NA_4 GAR-*šú* ⸢G⸣I_6-*ma* 2 BABBAR *e-di-iḫ* ^{NA_4}BABBAR.MIN_5 MU.NI
19. ^{NA_4}NÍR *sa-di-ru-šú ma-ʾ-du* ^{NA_4}⸢NÍR⸣ PA.MUŠEN.NA MU.[NI]
20. ^{NA_4}NÍR *sa-di-ru-šú ma-*⸢*ʾ*⸣*-du* ^{NA_4}N[Í]R.ZIZ MU.[NI]

---

21. NA_4 GAR-*šú* GIN_7 TÚG.BA ^{GIŠ}[GI]ŠIMMAR ^{NA_4}⸢A⸣.LAL.LUM MU.[NI]
22. NA_4 GAR-*šú* BABBAR GI_6 SIG_7 *ud*-[*d*]*u-u*[*ḫ*] ⸢^{NA_4}*mar-ḫal-lum* MU⸣.[NI]
23. NA_4 GAR-*šú* GIN ^{d}TIR.AN.NA ^{NA_4}*ma*[*r*]-⸢*ḫal*⸣-[*lum* MU.NI]

---

24. NA_4 GAR-*šú* GIN_7 *ir-ri* KU_6[47] ^{NA_4}NÍR *ma-dal-lum* [MU.NI]
25. NA_4 GAR-*šú* ^{NA_4}ZÚ BABBAR ^{NA_4}ZÚ GI_6 ^{NA_4}ZÚ SIG_7 ^{NA_4}⸢*ar*⸣-*za-lum* [MU.NI]
26. NA_4 GAR-*šú* [G]IN_7 *kap-pi raq-raq-qí*^{MUŠEN} ^{NA_4}*ár*-[*z*]*a-lum* [MU.NI]

---

27. NA_4 GAR-*šú* GIN_7 *ú-*⸢*ru-ut*⸣ KU_6 ^{NA_4}IGI.Z[A]G.GÁ [MU.NI]
28. NA_4 GAR-*šú* GIN_7 *i-ni* KU_6 ^{NA_4}IGI.KU_6 [MU.NI]
29. NA_4 GAR-*šú* GIN_7 KÙ.SIG_{17}-*ma* Ì ⸢*ma-ḫir*⸣ ^{NA_4}IGI.KU_6 [MU.NI]

30. NA$_4$ GAR-*šú* GIN$_7$ *i-ni* ⸢Š⸣AḪ ^{NA_4}IGI.ŠAḪ [MU.NI]
31. NA$_4$ GAR-*šú* GIN$_7$ *i-ni* [M]UŠ ^{NA_4}IGI.MUŠ [MU.NI]
32. NA$_4$ GAR-*šú* GIN$_7$ KUŠ MUŠ ^{NA_4}MUŠ [MU.NI][48]

---

33. NA$_4$ GAR-*šú* GIN$_7$ MÚD GU$_4$ *la ba-áš-li* ^{NA_4}*sa-a-bu* [MU].⸢NI⸣
34. NA$_4$ GAR-*šú* GIN$_7$ *ṭu-ḫi-ti* GU$_4$ ^{NA_4}*sa-a-b*⸢*u* M⸣U.NI
35. NA$_4$ GAR-*šú* GIN$_7$ ^{NA_4}*sa-bi-ma* AN.BAR *tuk-kup* ^{NA_4}*it-ta-*[*mir*] MU.NI

BAM 378 iii 1′–19′

1′. NA$_4$ GAR-[(*šú* GIN$_7$ *ṭi-ru-ut* ÍD-*ma*)]
2′. ^{NA_4}ZÁLAG *tuk-kup* ^{NA}[$_4$(IM.⸢MA⸣).AN].NA MU-*šú*
3′. NA$_4$ GAR-*šú* GIN$_7$ *ši-kin ti-nu-rim-ma*
4′. ^{NA_4}ZÁLAG *tuk-kup* ^{NA_4}[*š*]*u-u* MU-*šú*
5′. NA$_4$ GAR-*šú* GIN$_7$ KUŠ SA.A ⸢^{NA_4}⸣TÉŠ MU-*šú*
6′. NA$_4$ GAR-*šú* GIN$_7$ KUŠ UR.MAḪ
7′. ^{NA_4}*u$_5$-rí-zu* MU-⸢*šú*⸣

8′. NA$_4$ GAR-*šú* GIN$_7$ IGI TU.KUR$_4^{MUŠEN}$
9′. ^{NA_4}KI.ÁG.GÁ MU.NI
10′. [(NA$_4$)] GAR-*šú* GIN$_7$ LAG MUN *sà-pi*
11′. [$^{(NA_4)}$]MUD MU-*šú*[49]
12′. [(NA$_4$ GA)]R-*šú* GIN$_7$ SA.SAL BIL.ZA.ZA
13′. [(^{NA_4}*k*)]*ur-ga-ra-nu* MU.NI
14′. [(NA$_4$ GAR)]-*šú* GIN$_7$ TÚG *eš-še-bé-e*
15′. ⸢NA$_4$⸣ [(*nu*)-*ú*]-*ra* MU.NI
16′. NA$_4$ [(GAR-*šú* GIN)]$_7$ GÚ BAL.GI.KU$_6$
17′. ^{NA_4}[(*ḫal*)-*tu*] MU-*šú*
18′. NA$_4$ [(GAR-*šú* GIN$_7$ U$_4$-*me na-mi*)]*r* ^{NA_4}ZÁLAG MU-*šú*
19′. NA$_4$ [GAR-(*šú* GIN$_7$ ⸢IZI⸣ KI.A.^{d}ÍD ^{NA})]$_4$AN.[(ZA)Ḫ MU-*šú*]

STT 108

47. [NA$_4$ GAR-*šú* (GIN$_7$ AN.ZAḪ-⸢*ma*⸣ GI$_6$)] ^{NA_4}[*kut-p*]*u-ú* [MU.NI]
48. [NA$_4$ GAR-*šú* GIN$_7$ ... ^{NA_4}EN.GI].ŠA$_6$ MU.[NI]

TRANSLATION

STT 108

1. The stone that resembles […] is called lapis.
2. The stone that resembles […] is called lapis.
3. Lapis which is ⸢speckled⸣ with white is called *sirrimānu*.[50]

BAM 378 ii 0′–15′

0′–1′. Lapis which is ⸢speckled⸣ with yellow/green is called *Marḫaši* lapis.

2′–3′. The stone that resembles the berry of the *eddetu*-box-thorn is called carnelian.
4′–5′. Carnelian which is spotted with black is called *Meluḫḫan* carnelian.[51]
6′–7′. Carnelian which is speckled with *kasû*-colored (purple) spots is called *kasû* carnelian.
8′–9′. Carnelian which is spotted with yellow/green is called *Marḫaši* carnelian.[52]

10′–11′. The stone that resembles a ball of red-dyed wool intertwined[53] with white is called *muššaru*-stone.
12′–13′. The stone that is red (and) ⸢covered⸣ with white streaks is called ⸢*muššaru*-stone⸣.
14′–15′. *Muššaru*-stone with many striations is called [male][54] ⸢*muššaru*-stone⸣.

STT 108

13. *Muššaru*-stone which resembles the belly of (one's) finger[55] is called *zaqānu muššaru*-stone.

---

14. The stone that resembles *ḫulālu*-stone (and) *muššaru*-stone is called *luludānītu*-stone.
15. The stone that is red (and) ⸢covered⸣ with white and black streaks is called *luludānītu*-stone.

---

16. The stone that is white and ⸢covered⸣ with black streaks is called *ḫulālu*-stone.

17. The stone that is ⌜black⌝ and has one [white] streak is called *pappardilu*-stone.[56]
18. The stone that is ⌜black⌝ and has two white streaks[57] is called *papparminu*-stone.
19. *Ḫulālu*-stone with many striations is called bird-wing *ḫulālu*-stone.
20. *Ḫulālu*-stone with many striations is (also) called *sāsu*-stone.

---

21. The stone that resembles ⌜palm⌝ bark is called *alallu*-stone.
22. The stone that is white (and) covered with black (and) yellow/green streaks is called *marḫallu*-stone.
23. The stone that resembles the rainbow [is called] ⌜*marḫallu*-stone⌝.

---

24. The stone that resembles fish intestines [is called] *madallu-ḫulālu*-stone.
25. The stone that resembles white, black (and) green obsidian [is called] ⌜*arzallu*⌝-stone.
26. The stone that ⌜resembles⌝ a stork's wing [is called] ⌜*arzallu*⌝-stone.

---

27. The stone that resembles fish roe [is called] *egizaggû*-stone.
28. The stone that resembles the eye of a fish [is called] fish-eye stone
29. The stone that resembles gold but it absorbs[58] oil [is called] fish-eye stone.
30. The stone that resembles the eye of a pig [is called] pig-eye stone.
31. The stone that resembles the eye of a snake [is called] snake-eye stone.
32. The stone that resembles the skin of a snake [is called] snake stone. [59]

---

33. The stone that resembles unboiled ox blood is [called] *sābu*-stone.
34. The stone that resembles ox's bran[60] is ⌜called⌝ *sābu*-stone.
35. The stone that resembles *sābu*-stone but is speckled with iron is called ⌜*ittamir*⌝-stone.

BAM 378 iii 1′–19′

1′–2′. The stone that resembles river silt but is spotted with *zalāqu*-stone pebbles is called *immanakku*-stone.

3′–4′. The stone that resembles oven slag but is spotted with *zalāqu*-stone pebbles is called ⌜*šû*⌝-stone.

5′. The stone that resembles cat skin is called *aban bašti*-stone.

6′–7′. The stone that resembles lion skin is called *urīzu*-stone.

8′–9′. The stone that resembles the eye of a dove is called love stone.

10′–11′. The stone that is brittle[61] as a lump of salt is called blood-red stone.[62]
12′–13′. The stone that resembles a frog's back is called *kurgarrānu*-stone.
14′–15′. The stone that resembles the crest (lit. "garment") of an *eššebû*-bird is called light stone.
16′–17′. The stone that resembles the neck of a *šeleppû*-tortoise is called *ḫaltu*-stone.
18′. The stone that shines like the day is called *zalāqu*-stone.
19′. The stone that resembles sulphur fire is called *anzaḫḫu*-frit.

STT 108

47. [The stone that] resembles *anzaḫḫu*-frit but is black is called [*kutpû*]-frit.[63]
48. [The stone that resembles ...] is called *engissû*-stone.

D. URU.AN.NA, AN ANCIENT PLANT GLOSSARY

This series was intended as a sort of plant glossary, and contains such information as what Sumerogram indicates what plant (17, 45–46, 49–50), what the names of Mesopotamian plants were in other languages (24, 28, 42), and what other plant or plants resembled the given plant (21–23, 43–44) or could be substituted for it (47–48, 51). Of particular usefulness is the decoding of what are referred to as *Deckname*, that is, unhelpful (18–20, 25), strange (26–27), and even nasty-sounding (29–30) names that are actually just popular names for a plant along the lines of "crow foot," "dog tongue," and "Queen Anne's lace."[64] In the transliteration below, the colon separates material belonging in the left column from that in the right.

TEXT 4: CT 14.21–22 vii–viii 17–30

17. [(Ú ÚKUŠ.GÍL : Ú) *i*]*r-ru-u*
18. [(Ú *šá-mu* SIG_7 : Ú *i*)]*r-ru-u*
19. [(Ú *na-at*)-*til-l*(*a* : Ú) *i*]*r-ru-u*[65]
20. [(Ú NAM.TI.LA : Ú) *i*]*r-ru-u*
21. [(Ú IGI.LIM : Ú) *ir*]-*ru-u*
22. [(Ú *im-ḫu-‹ur›-li-mu* : Ú) *ir*]-*ru-u*
23. [(Ú *im-ḫur-lim* KUR : Ú) *ir-r*]*u-u*

24. Ú ⸢*a*⸣-[(*zu-mu* : Ú KI.MIN)]
25. Ú *šá-mu* ⸢ŠEŠ⸣ [(: Ú KI.MIN)]
26. Ì.UDU UR.MAḪ : Ú ⸢*ir*⸣-[*ru-u*]
27. Ì.UDU UR.MAḪ *šá ina me-lul-ti* G[AZ] ‹:› ⸢Ú⸣ MIN
28. Ú *bu-la-lu* : Ú MIN [(*ina Šú*)]-*ba-ri*
29. Ì.UDU UR.GI$_7$ GI$_6$ *šá ina mit-ḫu-*⸢*ṣi*⸣ [GAZ] ‹:› Ì.UDU! Ú ÚKUŠ.GÍL
30. Ì.UDU NAM.LÚ.U$_{18}$.LU [: Ì.U]DU Ú ÚKUŠ.GÍL

TRANSLATION

17. ÚKUŠ.GÍL is (the Sumerogram for) *irrû.*
18. The "green plant" is (a name for) *irrû.*
19. *Nattilu* (Akk. for "Life plant") is (a name for) *irrû.*
20. "Life plant" is (a name for) *irrû.*
21. IGI.LIM (Sum. for *imḫur-lim*) is (similar to) *irrû.*[66]
22. *Imḫur-lim* is (similar to) *irrû.*
23. Wild *imḫur-lim* is (similar to) *irrû.*
24. *Azumu* is (a name for) ditto (*irrû*).
25. The "bitter plant" is (a name for) ditto (*irrû*).
26. "Lion fat" is (a name for) *irrû.*
27. "Fat of a lion that was killed in sport" is (a name for) ditto (*irrû*).
28. *Bulālu* is (a name for) ditto (*irrû*) in Subarean.
29. "Fat of a black dog that [was killed] in a fight" is (a name for) *irrû* "fat."
30. "Human fat" is (a name for) *irrû* "fat."

TEXT 5: CT 14.22 vii–viii 42–51

42. Ú *a-du-ma-tú* : Ú *ka-na-šú-u ina* KUR ŠEŠ-*tum*
43. Ú *ka-na-šu-u* : *tam-šil* ^{d}NAM.TAR
44. PA.MEŠ-*šú* TUR.MEŠ SAL.MEŠ *ka-zi-ri* TUKU-⸢*a*⸣
45. GÁNA.ZI^{SAR} : Ú *ka-na-šu-u*
46. NUMUN GÁNA.ZI^{SAR} : NUMUN Ú MIN

---

47. Ú GÁNA.ZI-*ú* : Ú *šar-ma-du*
48. GA.MUL GÁNA.ZI : Ú *šar-ma-du*
49. Ú GURU$_5$.⸢UŠ⸣ : *a-šar-ma-du*
50. Ú BAR GURU$_5$.UŠ : Ú MIN
51. Ú *ka-su-u* : Ú MIN

TRANSLATION

42. *Adumatu* is (the name for) *kanāšu* in this country.
43–44. *Kanašû* is similar to *pillû* (except that) its leaves are small (and) thin (and) have a curly fringe.
45. GÁNA.ZI^{SAR} is (the Sumerogram for) *kanašû*.
46. The seed of GÁNA.ZI^{SAR} is the seed of ditto (*kanašû*).

---

47. *Kanašû*-leek is (a substitute for) *šarmadu*.
48. *Kamullu* (and) *kanāšu*-leek are (a substitute for) ditto (*šarmadu*).
49. GURU$_5$.UŠ is (the Sumerogram for) *šarmadu*.
50. The peel of GURU$_5$.UŠ is (the peel of) ditto (*šarmadu*).
51. *Kasû* is (a substitute for) ditto (*šarmadu*).

NOTES

1. For *šadānu* and *li'bu*, see Scurlock and Andersen 2005, 73–74, 29–32.
2. See Scurlock and Andersen 2005, 483–85.
3. See Scurlock and Andersen 2005, 224–26.
4. See Scurlock and Andersen 2005, 53–61.
5. See Scurlock and Andersen 2005, 43–44.
6. See Scurlock and Andersen 2005, 257–58, 289–90.
7. See Scurlock 2007, 517–20.
8. BAM 423 i 8′ gives a variant form of the plant name. Our text has Ú *ir-ri* GIG. However, *RA* 13.37:23 has: ^{Ú}*pu-ru-pu-ḫu* Ú *sa-ḫu* GIG SÚD [*ina*] KAŠ.SAG [NAG]. See n. 19.
9. Restored on the basis of BAM 423 i 12′–13′, which follows a treatment for *maškādu* with a treatment for *šimmatu*.
10. BAM 423 i 31′ has GIG *šá-d*[*a-ni*].
11. See *CAD* A/2, 460a and Ebeling's copy of *KAR* 203.
12. The plant appears again in BAM 1 iii 35 as a preventative for depression.
13. What is meant is that the patient will have offspring.
14. In *AMT* 31/1+59/1 (= BAM 7 pl. 1–2) i 19, myrrh is ground, mixed with oil and blown into the urethra via a bronze tube. It is accompanied by a potion of *nuṣābu* mixed with *ḫīqu*-beer.
15. This and the following line have ŠU.BI.DIDLI.ÀM to indicate that the preparation is the same. Elsewhere, the text simply has KI.MIN. We may perhaps presume from this that our text was copied from different sources.
16. The potion appears in *AMT* 31/1+59/1 (= BAM 7 pl. 1–2) i 32b, where it is specified that it is to be given on an empty stomach. The wash appears in *AMT* 31/1+59/1 (= BAM 7 pl. 1–2) i 22, where *baluḫḫu*-aromatic resin is boiled in pressed-out oil, filtered, and poured into the urethra via a bronze tube.
17. In *AMT* 31/1+59/1 (= BAM 7 pl. 1–2) i 30b, *imḫur-lim* is mixed with beer instead of

wine.

18. Stol (forthcoming), suggests that the fungi in question are specifically truffles.

19. *RA* 13.37:23 has an entry which is identical to BAM 1 i 35 except that the copy has *sa-ḫu* instead of *ir-ri*. Since IR and SA are very similar and ḪU and RI are very similar, it seems probable that one of the two copies is in error.

20. For the reading, which is based on *RA* 17.179 Sm. 22:13, see *CAD* Š/3, 386.

21. This is probably, to judge from its inclusion in lexical lists in the insect section and specification into "crawling" and "flying" forms, actually an insect. See Scurlock, *NABU* 1995, no. 110. *CAD* P, 452–53 reads this as *pizzir* and, apparently following Civil 2006, 55–61, takes it to mean "cobweb." However, a cobweb is not an insect, and it neither crawls nor flies.

22. The vademeca, BAM 380:11 and *STT* 92 iii 27′ have: ^{Ú}*kam-ka-du* Ú GIG *ša* A ŠUB. ŠUB-*u*.

23. *KADP* 33 rev. 5′–7′ adds: SIG$_7$-*su* TI-*qí* 1-*šú* 2-*šú* 3-*šú ana* DÚR-⌈*šú*⌉ GAR-*an* ⌈GUR⌉-*ma* EN MÚD.MEŠ ⌈È⌉ [*šá*]-*ni-iš* GUR-*ma* GAR-*an*.

24. *STT* 93:79′–81′ adds: [ḪÁD.A] SÚD *ina* Ì+GIŠ ŠÉŠ.⌈MEŠ⌉.

25. *STT* 93: 92′ adds PA^{MEŠ}-*šú* TUR^{MEŠ}.

26. The vademeca, BAM 380:11 and *STT* 92 iii 27′ have: "*kamkādu* is a plant for a sore which continually produces liquid." An exudate is meant.

27. The vademecum, BAM 1 ii 54 lists the plant as a treatment for "cockspur." See Scurlock and Andersen 2005, 65.

28. Uruanna II 5 (apud *CAD* A/II, 524b) also characterizes the plant as "multi-colored" *kanašû*. Both Uruanna (II 2) and the medical commentary BRM 4.32:19 have the plant being used for (forgetting) worries as also in the vademecum BAM 1 i 59 (see above).

29. See Scurlock and Andersen 2005, 168–69.

30. Uruanna I 401a (apud *CAD* E, 102a) has the fruit rather than the seed as red.

31. *KADP* 33 rev. 5′–7′ gives the full treatment: "You take it fresh (and) put it once, twice, three times into his anus. You keep putting (it) in until the blood comes out. ⌈Alternatively⌉, you (just) put it in repeatedly.

32. For the translation of *saḫlû* as "cress," see Stol 1983–84, 24–32.

33. In Uruanna text *KADP* 4:43 (*CAD* A/2, 267a) it is noted that there is a "sweet" (*matqu*) *arīḫu*. In the vademecum BAM 380:63//BAM 381 iv 18//STT 92 iv 3′, *arīḫu* (root) is used to produce a bowel movement in a potion mixed with beer.

34. *STT* 93:58′–59′, 62′ add that this plant goes along the ground like *irrû*-coloquinth, its tendrils are like those of *qiššû*-cucumber, its branches are open, its seed is like that of *ḫuratu*-madder, it is red/brown and its root is bitter.

35. The medical commentary BRM 4.32:7 adds that the plant resembles the "sheen of Ishtar" (a double scribal pun for *maštakal* tendrils).

36. See Scurlock and Andersen 2005, 81–82.

37. ZU = *leʾu*: "to be strong (enough to)."

38. Uruanna II 40, apud *CAD* A/2, 452–53, says that *ašqulālu* resembles *kasû*; it is yellow/green and comes out on the surface of the water. Similarly, BRM 4.32:18–19. *STT* 93:82′, 84′, 85′–86′ add that the plant is yellow/green as a *ḫallūru*-chickpea with a yellow/green and black fruit, resembles *ankinutu* and does not have a root.

39. *STT* 93: 79′–81′ gives the full treatment: "[You dry] (and) grind (it and) repeatedly rub (it) gently on (mixed) with oil."

40. Uruanna III 427 (apud *CAD* L, 182b) has *liddanānu* as the plant which resembles *lišan kalbi*.

41. *STT* 93:92′ adds that it has small leaves.

42. That is, the plant turns to face the sunlight.

43. There is nothing in the text except an indication that the tablet from which this was copied had recently been broken (*ḫīpu eššu*).

44. In the vademecum, BAM 380:62//BAM 381 iv 17//STT 92 iv 2′, the plant is also used in a potion to produce a bowel movement but mixed with beer.

45. This is actually an incorrect entry which we may correct from *STT* 108:6//STT 109:8 which has: $^{\mathrm{NA_4}}$GUG [(BABBAR)] *tak-pat* $^{\mathrm{NA_4}}$G[(U)]G ME.LUḪ.ḪA [(MU).NI] and from *STT* 108:8//STT 109:6 which has: $^{\mathrm{NA_4}}$GUG [(G)]I$_6$ [*t*(*a*)]*k-p*[(*at*)] $^{\mathrm{NA_4}}$⸢GUG GAZI⸣^{S}[^{AR} MU.NI].

46. *STT* 109:10 adds: $^{\mathrm{NA_4}}$G[U]G ⸢ZÚ⸣ *tak-p*[*at*] $^{\mathrm{NA_4}}$G[U]G ⸢ZÚ⸣ M[U-*šú*].

47. Since there is apparently no such thing as a *sarru*-fish, this reading seems preferable.

48. *STT* 109: 34 adds: [NA$_4$ GAR-*šú* G]IN$_7$ GAZI^{SAR} ^{Ú}GÍR^{SAR} [… MU.NI]

49. *STT* 109:42–45 adds: [N]A$_4$ ⸢GAR-*šú*⸣ GIN$_7$ SUḪUŠ ^{Ú}⸢GA.RAŠ⸣[^{SAR} … MU.NI N]A$_4$ GAR-*šú* GIN$_7$ *šá-šal-li* [… MU.NI N]A$_4$ GAR-*šú* GIN$_7$ *šá-šal-li zi-né*-[*e* … MU.NI N]A$_4$ GAR-*šú* GIN$_7$ *šá-šal-li ir-re-e* […]

50. This literally means: "wild-ass-like." Presumably the coats of wild asses were spotted with white like the stone.

51. This is actually an incorrect entry which we may correct from *STT* 108:6//STT 109:8 which has: "Carnelian which is spotted with white is called *Meluḫḫan* carnelian." and *STT* 108:8//STT 109:6 which has: "Carnelian which is spotted with black is called *kasû* carnelian."

52. *STT* 109:10 adds: ⸢Carnelian which is spotted⸣ with obsidian ⸢is called⸣ obsidian ⸢carnelian⸣.

53. See *CAD* K, 199 and Schuster-Brandis 2008, 34.

54. The "male" *muššaru*-stone is the only other variety known, and it makes sense that a stone with an unusually large number of striations would be "male."

55. With Schuster-Brandis 2008, 26, 34, 41. Landsberger 1967, 153 restored [*a*]-*si* and translated "bear's bed." If the traces may be trusted, Schuster's reading is to be preferred.

56. Lexical texts and the Agum Kakrime inscription mention *pappardilu-* and *papparminu-* stone as varieties of *ḫulālu*-stone. See *CAD* P, 110–11.

57. On lines 17 and 18, see Schuster-Brandis 2008, 26, 34–35.

58. The reference is probably to what we call "fool's gold" (iron pyrites) which is like the genuine article except that it is very shiny.

59. *STT* 109:34 adds: [The stone which] ⸢resembles⸣ *kasû* and *ašāgu* [is called …].

60. The interpretation follows Landsberger 1967, 153.

61. The term is also used of hair in protein malnutrition. See Scurlock and Andersen 2005, 156, 708 n. 4.

62. *STT* 109:42′–45′ adds: The ⸢stone⸣ which resembles the root of a *karāšu*-leek [is called …]. The ⸢stone⸣ which resembles the back of [… is called …]. The ⸢stone⸣ which resembles the back of a palm leaf [is called …]. The ⸢stone⸣ which resembles the back of *irrû*-coloquinth [is called …].

63. The restoration follows Schuster-Brandis 2008, 28, 36, 43. *CAD* A/2, 151b has *nūru*-stone. According to BAM 194 vii 5′–6′, the stone that was like *anzaḫḫu*-frit, but black, was good for sore eyes. See Schuster-Brandis 2008, 33.

64. For more details, see Scurlock 2005, 309–10.

65. See *CAD* I–J, 182.

66. *STT* 93:58′–59′ (*Šammu šikinšu*) indicates that the two plants resembled one another in appearance.

3

THE THERAPEUTIC SERIES

A. UGU CATALOG

In order to be able to treat his patients with symptoms or symptoms complexes diagnosed by means of the Diagnostic Series, the ancient physician needed to be able to find the known treatments matching his diagnosis among the thousands that were available. For this purpose, a reference work was generated, known to us as UGU, an abbreviation of its ancient title, which was also the incipit (first line) of the first tablet.

Although much is missing, the general outlines and parts of the original composition can be reconstructed using the UGU Catalog, copies of individual UGU tablets identified by incipit, contents and/or colophon as belonging to the series, and the UGU Extract Series.[1] Isolated treatments also appear in tablets extracted by the *āšipu* for a specific patient or set of patients. The existence of these isolated extract tablets demonstrates that UGU was in active use by practicing physicians.

This Therapeutic Series arranged treatments by subject matter, and was organized in head to toe (literally "toenail") order. It thus echoed the arrangement of tablets 3–14 (the first subsection) of the Diagnostic Series, and was almost certainly meant as a companion piece to it.[2] For more on this subject, see above, part 1, ch. 1. As luck would have it, one of the incipits listed in the UGU Catalog (9c16′+9d12′ = CT 23.1–2:1) appears also in the Diagnostic Series (DPS 14:172′).

TEXT 1: BECKMAN AND FOSTER 1988, NO. 9

This unfortunately very fragmentary text is precious evidence for the production in Assyria of a "new edition" of the therapeutic texts comparable to the "new edition" of the diagnostic texts produced by the Middle Babylonian scholar, Esagil-kin-apli.[3] When complete, this text listed several newly edited tablet series including UGU. Within UGU, each individual tablet had its incipit (first line) recorded. The tablets were listed by subseries (*sādiru*), each of which was named after the incipit of the first tablet in the subseries. This was followed by an inventory of the contents, after which the scribe proceeded on to the next subseries. It is hard to tell just how much of the text is missing but, to judge from what is preserved, there must have been something on the order of forty-eight tablets in the series as a whole.[4]

FRAGMENT 9A

obv.

1. [...] x x (label)

---

2. [(DIŠ NA UGU-*šú* KÚM *ú-kal*) (= BAM 480 i 1 [tablet 1]) : (DIŠ NA SAG.KI.DIB)].⸢BA⸣ TUKU.TUKU-⸢*ši*⸣ (= BAM 482 i 1 [tablet 2])
3. [(DIŠ SAG.KI.DIB.BA ŠU.GIDIM.MA *ina* SU NA Z)]AL[5]-*ma* NU [(DU$_8$)] (= *AMT* 102/1 i 1–2 [tablet 3])
4. [(DIŠ NA SAG.DU-*su* GIG.MEŠ KUR)-*du* (TAB UD.D)]A ⸢DIRI-*ú*⸣ (= CT 23.50 obv. 1 [tablet 4]; *AMT* 105/1 iv 26 [tablet 3 catchline])
5. [(DIŠ NA MURUB$_4$ SAG.DU-*šú* GÍR.GÍR-*su* UGU-*šú*) o o]-*te* ŠÉŠ (= CT 23.50 rev. 5′ [tablet 4 catchline])

---

6. [NÍGIN 5 DUB.MEŠ DIŠ NA UGU-*šú* KÚM *ú-kal* EN ...] ri *kibši*
7. [(DIŠ NA)] ⸢*a*⸣-*šu-u* DIB-*su*[6]

---

8. [DIŠ NA GEŠTU$^{II.MEŠ}$-*šú* GÙ.(DÉ.A *u neš-mu$_4$-šu* L)]ÁL ‹‹:›› DUGUD[7]
9. [DIŠ NA GEŠTU$^{II.MEŠ}$-*šú* MÚD.BABBAR] ⸢ŠUB⸣-*a*

---

10. [NÍGIN 2 DUB.MEŠ DIŠ NA GEŠTU$^{II.MEŠ}$-*šú* GÙ].⸢DÉ.A⸣ *u neš*!-*mu$_4$-šu* ⸢LÁL⸣-*a*

---

11. [EN DIŠ NA GEŠ(TU ZAG-*šú*)] GÙ.GÙ-*si*[8]

---

12. [(DIŠ NA IGI^{II}-*šú* GIG.MEŠ):[9] (DIŠ NA IGI)]^{II}-*šú* *m*[(*ur-din-ni* DIRI)] (= BAM 515 i 1 [tablet 2]; BAM 510 iv 47 [tablet 1 catchline])
13. [(DIŠ NA IGI.MEŠ-*šú* LÙ.LÙ)] (= BAM 516 i 1 [tablet 3]; BAM 515 iv 45′ [tablet 2 catchline])

TRANSLATION

(obv. 1) [...]
(obv. 2–5) (The first tablet is called): "If fever grips the crown of a person's

head."[10] (The second tablet is called): "If a person continually has an 'affliction of the temples.'"[11] (The third tablet is called): "If headache (and) 'hand' of ghost will not let up from a person's body and will not go away (in the face of bandages, salves and recitations)."[12] (The fourth tablet is called): "If lesions reach a person's head (and) he is full of the burning of *ṣētu* (enteric fever)."[13] (The fifth tablet is called): "If the middle of his head continually stings him, you gently rub the top of his head [(with) ...]."

(obv. 6–7) [Total of five tablets of (the subseries called): "If fever grips the top of a person's head," including ...], *kibšu*-fungus[14] (and) "If *ašû* afflicts a person."[15]

(obv. 8–9) [(The first tablet is called): "If a person's ears] ⸢roar⸣ and his hearing is diminished (variant: heavy)." [(The second tablet is called): "If a person's ears] produce [pus]."

(obv. 10) [Total of two tablets of (the subseries called): "If a person's ears] ⸢roar⸣ and his hearing is diminished."

(obv. 11) [This is including "If a person's] "right" ⸢ear⸣ continually rings."[16]

(obv. 12–13) (The first tablet is called): "If a person's eyes are sick/sore." (The second tablet is called): "If a person's eyes are full of *murdinnu*."[17] (The third tablet is called): "If a person's eyes are continually troubled."

The main exemplar of tablet 1 of the first subseries of UGU, whose incipit also gave its name to the entire series, is BAM 480. This tablet has been substantially reconstructed, and appears as chapter 3, text 2. BAM 482 represents tablet 2, as may be seen from the catchline of tablet 1 (BAM 480 iv 50′), which matches BAM 482's incipit (BAM 482 i 1) and from the fact that its own colophon so identifies it (BAM 482 iv 52′). The main exemplar of tablet 3 is *AMT* 102/–105/1 as is known from the catchline of tablet 2 (BAM 482 iv 51′) which matches *AMT* 102–105/1's incipit (*AMT* 102/1 i 1–2) and its own colophon (*AMT* 105/1 iv 26–27). CT 23.50 represents tablet 4 as may be seen from the catchline of tablet 3 (*AMT* 105/1 iv 26 which matches CT 23.50's incipit (CT 23.50:1) and its own colophon (CT 23.50 rev. 6′). Tablet 5 in known only from its incipit, which appears as the catchline of tablet 4 (CT 23.50 rev. 5′). However, the section on the contents of the first subseries (9a 6–7) indicates that *ašû* was a major subject matter covered in the subseries. If so, then it seems likely that BAM 494 is part of tablet 5, as indeed F. Köcher suggested.[18]

Tablet 1 of the second subseries of UGU is probably represented by BAM 503 (chapter 5, text 3), whose incipit is lost but which begins with a number of treatments for roaring in the ears. The citation of BAM 506 in 9a 11 confirms that the ear tablets were part of the UGU series, constituting a separate subseries placed after the head and before the eyes.

The main exemplars of tablets 1–3 of the third subseries of UGU are BAM 510, 515, and 516, respectively. We know from BAM 515's fragmentary colophon (BAM 515 iv 46′) that it is the second tablet in a series dealing with the eyes. The incipit of BAM 515 i 1 is cited as the catchline of BAM 510 (iv 47). This tells us that BAM 510 represents the first and BAM 515 the second tablet of the eye subseries. We know that BAM 516 is the third tablet because its incipit (BAM 516 i 1) is the same as the catchline of tablet 2 (BAM 515 iv 45′).

We have thus so far in fragment 9a seen three subseries, one with five tablets devoted to the head, one with two tablets devoted to the ears, and one with three tablets devoted to the eyes for a total of ten tablets. The summary section for the eye subseries is lost in a lacuna. Fragment 9b picks up with the incipits of the fourth subseries.

FRAGMENT 9B

obv.

1′. [(MÚD *ina* KIRI$_4$ TAR-*si*) : DIŠ NA] x te x […][19]
2′. [… *a-na*] *pa-šá-r*[*i*]

3′. [NÍGIN 2 DUB.MEŠ (MÚ)]D ‹*ina*› KIRI$_4$ TAR-[(*si*) …]

4′. [(DIŠ NA ZÚ.MEŠ-*šú* GIG) (= BAM 538 i 1 [tablet 1]) : (DIŠ NA)] ⸢*gi-mir*⸣ ZÚ.ME-*šú* [(*i-na-áš*)] (=BAM 538 iv 50′ [tablet 1 catchline]; BAM 543 i 1 [tablet 2])[20]

5′. [NÍGIN 2 DUB.MEŠ DIŠ NA ZÚ.MEŠ-*šú* GIG] ⸢EN⸣ ZÚ-*šú* GIG (KA-*šú*) DUGUD-*šú* ZÚ-*šú na-ši*
6′. [ÉN … ME]Š TA *a-pí i-ip-lu-su la-ʾu šá-aš-šu-u*
7′. […] *šá* LÚ.TUR

8′. [(DIŠ NA KA-*šú* DUGUD) (= BAM 547 iv 14′ (subseries title) :] DIŠ NA GABA-*su* GIG-*at* (= BAM 547 iv 13′ [tablet 1 catchline])[21]
9′. [(DIŠ NA GABA-*su* SAG ŠÀ-*šú*)] *u* MAŠ.SÌLA.MEŠ-*šú* GU$_7$.MEŠ-*šú* (= *AMT* 48/4 rev. 13′ [tablet 2 catchline]; *AMT* 49/4 obv. 1 [tablet 3])[22]
10′. [(DIŠ NA KÚM-*im ú-ga-na*)-*aḫ*] (= *AMT* 49/4 rev. 10′ [tablet 3 catchline]): DIŠ NA *su-a-lam* GIG (=*AMT* 49/1[+]51/5 iv 11′ [tablet 4 catchline]; *AMT* 80/1 i 1//BAM 548 i 1 [tablet 5])
11′. [(DIŠ NA *su-a-lam ḫa-ḫa*)] *u ki-ṣir-te* GIG (= BAM 548 iv 14′ [tablet 5 catchline])

12′. [NÍGIN 6 DUB.MEŠ DIŠ NA KA-*šú* DUGUD EN K]A-*šú* DUGUD ḪAR.MEŠ *ši-i-qi ù* LÚ.TUR *su-alu* GIG

13′. [(DIŠ NA *su-a-lam* GIG *ana ki-is* ŠÀ GUR)-*š*]*ú* (= BAM 574 i 1 [tablet 1]) : DIŠ NA ŠÀ-*šú* GIG (= BAM 574 iv 51 [tablet 1 catchline]; BAM 575 i 1 [tablet 2])

14′. ‹DIŠ NA SAG ŠÀ-*šú* GU$_7$-*šú ina ge-ši-šu* ZÉ *im-ta-na-ʾ* NA BI *qer-be-na* GIG:› (= BAM 575 iv 54 [tablet 2 catchline]; BAM 578 i 1 [tablet 3]) (DIŠ NA UD.DA KUR-*id* ZI SAG.KI GI)]G (= BAM 578 iv 47 [tablet 3 catchline]; *AMT* 14/7 i 1 [tablet 4]) : DIŠ NA ŠÀ-*šú* KÚM DIB-*it* (= BAM 579 i 1 [tablet 5]) ‹: DIŠ NA SAG ŠÀ-*šú na-ši* MURUB$_4$.MEŠ-*šú mi-na-tu-šú* GU$_7$.MEŠ-*šú*› (= BAM 579 iv 44 [tablet 5 catchline]; *AMT* 43/6 obv.1 [tablet 6])

15′. [NÍGIN 4 DUB.MEŠ DIŠ NA *su-a-lam* GIG *ana ki-is* Š]À GUR-*šú* EN IM *iš-biṭ-su-ma*

16′. [(DIŠ N)]A! Ú NAG-*ma la i-ár-ru*[23]

17′. [(DIŠ NA KAŠ.SAG)] NAG-*ma* SUḪUŠ.MEŠ-*šú pa-al-qa*[24]

18′. [… *mu*]*ṭ-ṭi-ta u* ŠÀ GIG *ki-is* ŠÀ

19′. [… DIR]I *ù nik-mat* IM *u* UD.DA![25]

20′. [DIŠ NA *ki*]-*is* ŠÀ *ù di-kiš* GABA TUKU-*ši*

21′. [DIŠ N(A NAM.ÉRIM)] *šaḫ-ḫi-ḫu* GIG[26]

22′. traces

TRANSLATION

(obv. 1′–2′) (The first tablet is called): “In order to stop blood (from flowing) from the nose.” (The second tablet is called): [“If … to] dispel (it). ”

(obv. 3′) [Total of two tablets of (the subseries called)]: “In order to stop blood (from flowing) from the nose.”

(obv. 4′) (The first tablet is called): “If a person’s teeth are sick/sore.” (The second tablet is called): “If all of a person’s teeth move.”[27]

(obv. 5′–7′) [Total of two tablets of (the subseries called): “If a person’s teeth are sick/sore.”] It includes his tooth being sick/sore, (his nose/mouth feeling) heavy (and) his tooth moving [(as well as) the recitation: “The […] from the pit[28] looked at[29] that baby,” (which was intended) for an infant.[30]

(obv. 8′–11′) (The first tablet is called): “If a person’s nose/mouth (feels) heavy."[31] (The second tablet is called): "If a person's breast is sore."[32] (The third tablet is called): "If a person's breast, his upper abdomen (epigastrium), (and) his shoulders continually hurt him."[33] (The fourth tablet is called): "If a person is feverish (and) *guḫḫu*-coughs."[34] (The fifth tablet is called): "If a person is sick with *suʾālu*-cough."[35] (The sixth tablet is called): "If a person is sick with *suʾālu*-cough, *ḫaḫḫu* (bloody phlegm), and "thick sputum" (in the lungs)."[36]

(obv. 12′) [Total of six tablets of (the subseries called): "If a person's nose/mouth (feels) heavy," including] his ⸢nose/mouth⸣ (feeling) heavy, "sick lungs," *šīqu* (colored sputum)[37] and an infant sick with *suʾālu*-cough.

(obv. 13′–14′) (The first tablet is called): "If a person is sick with *suʾālu*-cough and it turns into *kīs libbi*.[38] (The second tablet is called): "If a person's stomach is sick" ‹(The third tablet is called): "If a person's upper abdomen (epigastrium) hurts him and, when he belches, he continually produces bile, that person has "sick insides."›[39] (The fourth tablet is called): If *ṣētu* 'gets' a person (and) he is sick with pulsating of the temples." (The fifth tablet is called): "If a person's inside is afflicted by fever."[40] ‹(The sixth tablet is called): "If a person's upper abdomen (epigastrium) is puffed up (and) his hips (and) limbs continually hurt him."›[41]

(obv. 15′–19′) [Total of four tablets of (the subseries called): "If a person is sick with *suʾālu*-cough] (and) it turns [into] ⸢*kīs libbi*⸣, including: "If wind blasts him,"[42] "If a person drinks a plant and does not vomit (but) is distended,"[43] "If a person drinks fine beer and, as a consequence, he is unsteady on his foundations,"[44] […], ⸢loss of appetite⸣ and "sick insides," *kīs libbi*, being ⸢full⸣ of […], and stopped-up "wind" plus *ṣētu* (enteric fever).[45]

(obv. 20′–21′) [(The first tablet is called): "If a person] has ⸢*kīs libbi*⸣ and stabbing pain[46] in the breast. [(The second tablet is called): "If] a ⸢person⸣ is sick with a wasting curse.[47]

The fourth subseries of UGU is known only from the fragmentary BAM 530, which preserves the colophon of one of the tablets. To judge from their contents, BAM 524–526 will presumably have belonged to this very poorly preserved series.

Tablet 1 of the fifth subseries of UGU is represented by BAM 538, as we know from its incipit (BAM 538 i 1), and by the fact that it is identified as tablet 1 by its colophon (BAM 538 iv 50′). Tablet 2 may be identified in BAM 543 whose colophon indicates that it belonged to this subseries (BAM 543 iv 60′) and whose incipit (BAM 543 i 1) matches the catchline of tablet 1 (BAM 538 iv 50′).

Tablet 1 of the sixth subseries of UGU is represented by BAM 547, as may be seen from its colophon (BAM 547 iv 14′) and from BAM 543 iv 59′ (the catchline) which indicates that this subseries immediately followed the fifth (teeth) subseries. Tablet 2 is represented by *AMT* 48/4 whose colophon identifies it as belonging to this series (*AMT* 48/4 rev. 14′) and whose catchline (*AMT* 48/4 rev. 13′) matches the incipit of *AMT* 49/4 obv. 1 (tablet 3). We know that *AMT* 49/4 was a copy of tablet 3 since its colophon tells us so (*AMT* 49/4 rev. 11′). The incipit of tablet 4 is cited in the colophon of tablet 3 (*AMT* 49/4 rev. 10′). We know that *AMT* 49/1(+)51/5 is a copy of tablet 4, even though the incipit is lost, since its colophon indicates that it belonged to this series (*AMT* 49/1[+]51/5 iv 12′) and since its catchline (*AMT* 49/1[+]51/5 iv 11′) matches the incipit of *AMT* 80/1 i 1//BAM 548 i 1 (tablet 5). Tablet 5 is identified as such by its colophon (BAM 548 iv 13′). Tablet 6 in known only from its incipit, which appears as the catchline of tablet 5 (BAM 548 iv 14′). However, this incipit indicates that thick sputum (*kiṣirtu*) was one of the subject matters covered in the subseries. If so, then it seems likely that BAM 554–556 are part of tablet 6, as indeed F. Köcher suggested.[48]

The main exemplar of tablet 1 of the seventh subseries of UGU is BAM 574, as may be seen from the fact that its incipit (BAM 574 i 1) matches the name of the series of which it is the first tablet according to its colophon (BAM 574 iv 52). Tablet 2 is represented by BAM 575 as may be seen from the fact that the catchline of tablet 1 (BAM 574 iv 51) matches its incipit (BAM 575 i 1) and that its colophon indicates that it is tablet 2 of this subseries (BAM 575 iv 55). If there were any doubt, two of its symptom descriptions are cited among the contents of the subseries (9b 16′–17′). The main exemplar of tablet 3, which does not appear to have been included in this catalog, is BAM 578, as may be seen from the fact that the catchline of tablet 2 (BAM 575 iv 54) matches its incipit (BAM 578 i 1). Tablet 4 is represented by *AMT* 14/7, as may be seen from the fact that the catchline of tablet 3 (BAM 578 iv 47) matches its incipit (*AMT* 14/7 i 1). The main exemplar of tablet 5 is BAM 579, whose colophon confirms that it is a part of the series (BAM 579 iv 45) and the citation of whose incipit (BAM 579 i 1) in 9b 14′ places it after tablet 4. The main exemplar of tablet 6, which was certainly never cited in the UGU catalog, was *AMT* 43/6 whose incipit (*AMT* 43/6 obv. 1) matches the catchline of tablet 5 (BAM 579 iv 44).

It would appear that one (and probably two) more tablets are attested from the medical corpus from Nineveh than are registered in the UGU catalog. This would seem to indicate that there was a significant difference between the Nineveh recension (represented by BAM 574, 575, 578, 14/7, BAM 579, and *AMT* 43/6, all of which were found in Kuyuncik or have Assurbanipal palace colophons) and the Assur recension which is probably represented by the UGU catalog.[49]

In fragment 9b, we have seen three subseries, one with two tablets devoted to the nose, one with two tablets devoted to the teeth, one with six tablets devoted to the nose, throat and lungs and one with four/six tablets devoted to the stomach, liver, and gall bladder for a total of 14/16 tablets, and a grand total so far of 24/26 tablets. Fragment 9b ends with the incipits of the eighth subseries. Fragment 9c+d picks up with the summary section.

FRAGMENT 9C+D

obv.

1′. NÍGIN ⸢2⸣ [DUB.MEŠ DIŠ NA *ki-is* ŠÀ *ù di-kiš* GABA TUKU-*ši* EN …]

2′. LÁL-*ṭí* […]

3′. DIŠ NA GID[IM DIB-*su-ma* SA(G ŠÀ-*šú na-ši*) : …][50]

4′. DIŠ NA NINDA x […]

5′+1′. DIŠ NA ZI x […] x

6′+2′. NÍGIN!(text: EN) 8 DUB.ME[Š …] da […]

7′+3′. EN ÉN *ú-ša-*[*an-ni na-mir-tú*[51] … *ina* KI.NÁ-*š*]*ú re-ḫu-su* [DU-*ak*][52]

8′+4′. DIŠ NA ÉLLAG-*su* G[(U$_7$-*šú*)[53] : DIŠ NA (*mi-na-tu-šú* DUB.DUB Á^{II}-*šú* ‹*kin-ṣa-a-šú ù bir-ka-šú*›)] ⸢MÚ⸣.MEŠ-*ḫu* (= *AMT* 31/1 i 1 [tablet 2])

9′+5′. DIŠ NA *lu* ÉLLAG-*su* [GU$_7$-*šú* (*lu* KÀŠ).MEŠ-*šú* DIB.DIB ÉLLAG].ME ⸢GIG⸣ (= *AMT* 58/3 i 1–2 [tablet 3])

10′+6′. NÍGIN 3 DUB.MEŠ DIŠ [NA ÉLLAG-*su* GU$_7$-*šú* …] *šá mu-ṣi*

11′+7′. DIŠ NA *ina la si-*[(*ma-ni-šú* MURUB$_4$^{II}-*šú* GU$_7$.MEŠ-*šú*) (= *AMT* 43/1 i 1//BAM 168:70//BAM 95:16 [tablet 1])[54] : DIŠ *ina d*(*i-kiš* DÚR.GIG ŠÀ)].⸢ME⸣ NA KÚM UD.DA EN.TE.NA IM *u ša-ra* APIN NU ÍL (= *AMT* 43/2:11′ [tablet 1 catchline])

12′+8′. DIŠ NA *li-*[*diš* … : (DIŠ NA KI.NÁ)]-*ma šit-ta-šú* UGU-*šú* DÙG.GA (*AMT* 40/5 iv 29′ [tablet 3 catchline]; *AMT* 47/1+ i 1 [tablet 4])[55]

13′+9′. DIŠ NA DÚR.[(GIG)] GIG-*ma* (= *AMT* 47/1+ iv 13′ [tablet 4 catchline]; *AMT* 58/2:1 [tablet 5])

14′+10′ NÍGIN 5 D[UB.MEŠ DIŠ NA *ina la si-ma-ni-šú*] MURUB$_4$^{II}-*šú* GU$_7$.MEŠ-*šú šá* DÚR.GIG.GA.KÁM

15′+11′. EN DIŠ N[A …] x x UD.DA $BURU_8$ DIRI-*ú*

16′+12′. DIŠ x [… $MURUB_4$: (DIŠ SA.MEŠ UZU)].ÚR.MÉŠ-*šu* 1-*niš* GU_7.MEŠ-*šú* (= CT 23.1–2:1 [tablet 2])[56] : DIŠ NA *bur-ka-šú mun-ga* DIRI

13′. [DIŠ …]-*su là-a* ÍL

14′. [NÍGIN 4 DUB.MEŠ DIŠ …] $MURUB_4$ EN *maš-kad* SA.GAL *šá-aš-šá-ṭa*

15′. [… *ki*]-*is-sa-tum* GÌR^{II}-*šú* GIG.MEŠ DIRI-*ú*[57]

16′. [(GIG-*šú ib-lu-uṭ*)]-*ma* IGI GIG-*šú* BABBAR ŠUB[58] *a-si-da* $^{ŠU.SI}$U KUN ÚR[59]

17′. [NIGIN 48 DUB.MEŠ DIŠ NA UGU-*šú* KÚM *ú-kal* TA] UGU EN *ṣu-up-ri sa-di-ru-šá* SUR.GIBIL *ṣab-tu*

TRANSLATION

(obv. 1′–2′) [Total of two tablets of (the subseries called): "If a person] has *kīs libbi* and stabbing pain in the breast," including … "If …] is diminished."

(obv. 3′-5′+9d 1′) (The first tablet is called): "If a ⸢ghost⸣ [afflicts] a person [so that] his ⸢upper abdomen (epigastrium)⸣ is puffed up." […] (The third/fourth tablet is called): " If a person […] bread […]." […] (The sixth/seventh tablet is called): "If a person […]."

(obv. 6′–7′+9d 2′–3′) Total of eight tablets of (the subseries called): ["If a ghost afflicts a person so that his upper abdomen (epigastrium) is puffed up," including …], including the recitation: "I ⸢have altered⸣ [the brightness" … (and cases where)] his semen [flows in] ⸢his⸣ [bed].[60]

(obv. 8′–9′+9d 4′–5′) (The first tablet is called): "If a person's kidney hurts him."[61] [(The second tablet is called): "If a person]'s limbs are continually tense[62] (and) his arms, ‹legs and knees› are continually swollen." (The third tablet is called): If either a person's kidney [hurts him] or [he continually retains his] urine, he has 'sick [kidneys].'"

(obv. 10′+9d 6′) Total of three tablets of (the subseries called): "If [a person's kidney hurts him …]." It is for *mūṣu*.[63]

(obv. 11′–13′+9d 7′–9′) (The first tablet is called): "If a person's hips continually hurt him before (the age when) this would be expected." [(The second tablet is called): "If as a result] of the ⸢stabbing pain⸣ of DÚR.GIG, a person's insides are feverish (and he has) *ṣētu*-fever, cold, "clay" and wind (and) desire (but) lack of performance." (The third tablet is called): "If a person […]." (The fourth tablet is called): "If a person goes to sleep and his sleep is pleasing to him."[64] (The fifth tablet is called): "If a person is sick with DÚR.GIG so that ...."

(obv. 14′–15′+9d 10′–11′) Total of five ⸢tablets⸣ of [(the subseries called): "If a person]'s hips continually hurt him [before (the age when) this would be expected]." It is for DÚR.GIG,[65] including "If a person ... is full of *ṣētu* (and) vomiting.

(obv. 16′+9d 12′–13′) (The first tablet is called): "If [(you want) a lotion? for the] hips." (The second tablet is called): "If the muscles of a person's thighs all continually hurt him at once."[66] (The third tablet is called): "If a person's knees are full of *mungu*."[67] (The fourth tablet is called): "[If a person] cannot lift his [...]."

(obv. 14′–16′) [Total of four tablets of (the subseries called): "[If (you want) a lotion(?) for] the hips," including *maškādu*,[68] *sagallu*,[69] *šaššaṭu*,[70] [...], gnawing pain, his feet are full of sores, "If his sore heals and subsequently the surface of his sore is dotted with white,," (problems with) the heels, toes, tail-bone (and) thigh.

(obv. 17′) [Total of forty-eight tablets of the series "If fever grips the top of a person's head" from the top of the head to the (toe)nails. Its subseries have been newly edited.[71]

Of the eighth subseries, little is known. The material is probably somewhere in the numerous tablets dealing with lungs and internal organs. Our best clue is that the incipit (and presumably the first section) of the second tablet is quoted in BAM 156 obv. 1(–24), which also cites other passages from the UGU series.

The ninth subseries is known only from very fragmentary incipits with the exception of tablet 8 which is represented by K 3661, as we know from the fact that its colophon (K 3661 iv 18′) informs us that it was the eighth tablet in a series and that the catchline (K 3661 iv 17′) preserves the full version of the incipit of the tenth subseries.[72] The only clue as to the identity of the remaining seven tablets is to be found in the summary of the contents of the ninth subseries. As luck would have it, the recitation that is mentioned in fragment 9c:7′+d:3′, if properly restored, is quite rare, and known only from ennumerations of amulets directed against divine anger. This recitation is primarily known from SpTU 2.22+ ii 34–42 and BM 56148+ i 39–46,[73] but this or a similar recitation is cited by incipit in *STT* 95:39–40, 91, which makes it probable that *STT* 95 (part 3, ch. 15, text 2) either represents or contains material excerpted from one of the missing tablets. The end of fragment 9c:7′+d:3′ refers to a treatment that appears in *STT* 95:16–28 and which is duplicated by BAM 205:19′–21′ and *STT* 280 ii 1–3. These texts refer to urethritis and impotence and, like K 3661, they contain witchcraft material without seeming to belong to the standard witchcraft series.[74] This might suggest that we are again dealing with material from the UGU series. In any case, a discussion of urethritis and impotence would lead naturally to the urinary tract problems that follow in the tenth subseries.

In the tenth subseries, one tablet may be identified with certainty, and that is tablet 3, whose incipit in the catalog matches *AMT* 58/3+K 2960+*AMT* 62/1[75] i 1–2. One might not be sure, since this incipit is very fragmentary, but the catchline (*AMT* 58/3+K 2960+*AMT* 62/1 iv 31′) is the incipit of the first tablet of the following subseries. Tablet 2 is probably represented by *AMT* 31/1+59/1, 60/1(+) 66/7,[76] whose incipit (*AMT* 31/1 i 1) has been used to restore the UGU catalog. It is a large, multicolumn tablet devoted entirely to urinary tract problems, and cannot be either tablet 1 or tablet 3. As for tablet 1, the most promising piece is *AMT* 65/6+*AMT* 66/11+K 11230+Sm 126.[77]

In the eleventh subseries, tablet 1 is represented by *AMT* 43/1+43/2+57/6(+) 53/9(+)84/7+56/3,[78] as may be seen from the fact that its incipit (*AMT* 43/1 i 1) matches the incipit of tablet 1 in the UGU catalog. Tablet 2's incipit may be restored by combining the catchline of tablet 1 (*AMT* 43/2:11′) with the incipit of tablet 2 as preserved in the catalog.[79] The main exemplar of tablet 3 is *AMT* 40/5,[80] as may be seen from the fact that the colophon (*AMT* 40/5 iv 30′) identifies it as part of the series and the catchline (*AMT* 40/5 iv 29′) is identical with the incipit of *AMT* 47/1+.[81] We know that *AMT* 47/1+ is tablet 4 because its colophon indicates this (*AMT* 47/1+ iv 14′), and because its incipit (*AMT* 47/1+ i 1) matches the incipit of the fourth tablet in the UGU catalog. Tablet 5 is represented by *AMT* 58/2,[82] as may be seen from the fact that its incipit (*AMT* 58/2:1) matches the catchline of tablet 4 (*AMT* 47/1+ iv 13′) and the incipit of tablet 5 given in the UGU catalog.

In subseries twelve, tablet 1 seems to have had something to do with the hips. It is possibly represented by BAM 81, since *maškādu* is mentioned as one of the subject matters covered in the subseries (9d 14′). Tablet 2 is represented by CT 23.1–14 whose incipit (CT 32.1–2:1) matches the incipit of tablet 2 in the UGU catalog and by *AMT* 51/4 + 32/5 + 43/3 whose last line (iv 25′//BAM 131 rev. 9′) indicates that the first line of tablet 3 in the catalog was "after" its last line. The subject matter of this tablet was *sagallu*, which is mentioned among the contents. tablets 3 and 4 are possibly represented by BAM 32 and *AMT* 73/1 + 15/3 + 18/5, since the inventory of contents indicates that they were included in the series (9d:15′–16′).

In fragment 9c+d, we have seen five subseries, one with two tablets devoted to internal problems, one with eight tablets of unknown content, one with three tablets devoted to the urinary tract, one with five tablets devoted to DÚR.GIG, and one with four tablets devoted to the legs and feet, for a total of twenty-two tablets, and a final grand total of 46/48 tablets distributed among twelve subseries.

B. UGU TABLETS

TEXT 2: BAM 480

This text is the best preserved of the known tablets of the UGU series and also the first tablet in the first subseries. It is probably not an accident that we have so many sources for reconstruction, since it is a general rule with long compositions of any kind that there are more copies extant of the opening sections, for the simple reason that copies could not be xeroxed but had to be written out laboriously by hand and beginning at the beginning. Of interest in this tablet is the recitation in iii 52–54, where a star is asked to bring justice to the patient. Witches always, and ghosts and demons sometimes, produced medical symptoms unjustly, that is to say, the patient had done nothing to deserve being sick. It thus made sense to arraign the problem causer in a divine court and demand that something be done about the situation. What is unusual is the choice of a star as judge.

The text in general gives a good cross section of the types of recitations to be found in medical texts. Many are in "Sumerian," a no longer living language but an important part of the scribal training process, much as Latin was (and in Barcelona still is) in European Universities. The "Sumerian" is essentially academic and in many cases back-translated from Akkadian or, in any case, written by a person whose native language was Akkadian. So, when Sumerian failed the scribe, he simply turned Akkadian into faux Sumerian and forged ahead. For example, BAM 480 iii 36–37 uses I.DI (Akkadian *idu*: "side") in place of the usual BAR.ŠÈ. Just to make things more complicated, a magic circle is created by pronouncing the Akkadian for "depart!" first forwards (*ṣi*) and then backwards (*iṣ*), and this right in the midst of the Sumerian!

Where such recitations are fragmentary and/or without Akkadian "translation," they are often simply incomprehensible. Then, there are the "Subarean" recitations, perhaps actually Hurrian or better "Hurrian" treated in the same manner as the "Sumerian."[83] So, for example, BAM 480 iii 42–44, which mixes all three languages together! Most enjoyable for the translator are the Akkadian recitations although some of them (as BAM 480 iii 65–68)[84] are very close to nonsense. The purpose served by these recitations was communication with spirits who, as in many other cultures (including our own) are best approached in old, and dead languages or older forms of living ones (viz. Latin, Old Slavonic,

King James English, biblical Hebrew, classical Arabic, Sanskrit, etc). BAM 480 is edited in Worthington 2005 and 2007.

i

1. DIŠ NA UGU-*šú* KÚM *ú-kal* SA ZI SAG.KI TUKU-*ma* IGI^{II}-*šú i*-BÀR
2. IGI^{II}-*šú bir-ra-ta*$_5$ *i-pi-ta*$_5$ *i-ši-ta*$_5$ *mur-din-na qù-qa-na a-šá-a*
3. *ù* ÉR ŠUB.ŠUB-*a* 1/3 *qa* ZAG.ḪI.LI *bu-ṭu-ta*$_5$ *ina* ^{NA_4}UR$_5$ ÀRA-*en* SIM
4. SAG-*ka ú-kal ina* ŠÀ 1/3 *qa* TI-*qí ina* A GAZI^{SAR} SILA$_{11}$-*aš* ‹(SAG. DU-*su*)› SAR-*ab* LAL-*ma* U$_4$.3.KÁM* NU DU$_8$

---

5. 1/3 *qa saḫ-lé-e* 1/3 *qa* ZÍD ŠE.SA.A *ina* A GAZI^{SAR} SILA$_{11}$-*aš* ‹(SAG. DU-*su*)› SAR-*ab* LAL-*ma* U$_4$.3.KÁM* NU DU$_8$

---

6. *saḫ-lé-e* ÀRA-*tì* ^{ŠEM}GÚR.GÚR NAGA.SI *ina* KAŠ SILA$_{11}$-*aš* KI.MIN

---

7. ^{ŠEM}ŠEŠ MUN *eme-sal-lim mál-ma-liš* ḪE.ḪE *ina* Ì.NUN SÚD IGI^{II}-*šú t*[*e-qí*][85]

---

8. 1/3 *qa* ZAG.ḪI.LI ‹(*te-ʾ-né-te*)› 1/3 *qa* ŠIKA IM.ŠU.RIN.NA ‹(SUMUN)› 10 GÍN *ḫi-qa-t*[*i*[86] (GAZ *tuš-ta-bal*)]
9. *ina* A GAZI^{SAR} SILA$_{11}$-*aš* ‹(SAG.DU-*su*)› SAR-*ab* LAL-*ma* ⸢U$_4$.3⸣. [(K)ÁM* (NU DU$_8$)]

---

10. EGIR *na-aṣ-ma-da-ti an-na-ti* 10 GÍN ZAG.ḪI.LI *šá* KA ‹$^{(NA_4)}$›*ur-ṣi* [(*šá ḫul-qu ana* ŠÀ NU ŠUB-*ú*)]
11. MUN A.GEŠTIN.NA NU TAG.TAG *ina* NINDA ‹(ZÍZ.AN.NA KÚM)› *es-sip-ma* GU$_7$ 5 G[(ÍN ZAG.ḪI.LI ÀRA-*tì*)]
12. *ina* ‹(1/2 *qa*)› KAŠ.SAG SÌG-*aṣ-ma* NAG-*šú* [(*ú-za-ka-ma i-par-ra* LÁL. MEŠ *saḫ-le-e šá* IGI^{II})]

---

13. U$_4$.1.KÁM AN.ZAḪ S[(ÚD) …]

---

14. 10 GÍN GURUN ^{GIŠ}MAŠ.ḪUŠ [… ^{Ú}Z(A.BA.LAM)] 1/3 *q*[(*a*[87] ⸢Ú⸣) …]
15. GAZ SIM *ina* A GA[ZI^{SAR} SILA$_{11}$-*aš*] ⸢SAR-*ab*⸣ LAL-*ma* U$_4$.3.[KÁM NU DU$_8$]

---

16. ^{ŠEM}BI.⸢ZI⸣.[DA …] *ina* Ì.UDU UR.MAḪ SÚD [IGI^{II} *te-qí*]

---

17. […GÍ]N ^{Ú}ZA.BA.LAM 1/3 *qa* […]

18. GAZ SI[M *ina* A GAZI^{SAR} SI]LA$_{11}$-*aš* SAR-*ab* LAL-*ma* U$_4$.[3.KÁM NU DU$_8$]

---

19. 10 GÍN ZÍD DUḪ.ŠE.GIŠ.Ì Ḫ[ÁD.DU] ⸢GAZ⸣ SIM *ina* A GA[ZI^{SAR} ...]

---

20. 10 GÍN ZÍD DUḪ.ŠE.GIŠ.Ì ḪÁD.DU [...]
21. U$_4$.1.KÁM* GABA-*su* LAL SAG.DU-*s*[*u* ...]
22. *ana* SAG.DU-*šú* DUB-*ak ina* ⸢É⸣ [...]

---

23. 1 GÍN U$_5$ ARGAB^{MUŠEN} 1/2 GÍ[N ...]

---

24. 1/3 *qa* NUMUN BABBAR.ḪI^{SAR} 1/3 *qa* NUMUN LU.[ÚB^{SAR}? ...]

---

25. 1/3 *qa* ZÌ.KUM 1[0 G]ÍN ⸢BAR⸣ $^{\text{GI[Š?}}$NU?.ÚR?.MA? ...]

26–28. [...]
29. IM x [...]

---

30. 1/3 *qa* PA ^{GIŠ}P[(ÈŠ *ša i+na* ITU.BÁRA.ZAG.GAR KUD PA) ... *ina* KAŠ SILA$_{11}$-*aš*]
31. GUR-*ma* ḪÁD.A G[AZ SIM *ina* A GAZI^{SAR} SILA$_{11}$-*aš*[88] (SAG-*su tu-gal-lab* LAL) ...]

---

32. 1/3 *qa* ^{Ú}ḪAB 1/3 *qa* NU[(MUN ^{Ú}KI.^{d}IM) ... (SAG-*su tu-gal-lab* LAL-*su-ma*) ...]

---

33. NAGA.SI [...]

---

34. 1/3 [*qa* ...]
35–39. [...]
40′. [...] SÚD *te*-[*qí*]

41′. [...] SAR-*ab* LAL-*ma* K[I.MIN]

42′. [... GUR-*ma* ḪÁD].A[89] GAZ SIM *ina* A GAZI^{SAR} SILA$_{11}$-*aš* SAR-*ab* LAL-*ma* K[I.MIN]

43′. [...*ina* A GAZI$^{\text{SA(R}}$ SILA$_{11}$ *ina* Ì.UDU GÌR.PAD)].DA GÍD.DA SÚD MAR

44′. [… *sa*]-*a-qí* MAŠ.DÀ[90] SÚD *te-qí*

45′. [… (*ina* A GAZI^{SAR} SILA$_{11}$-*aš ina* ŠURUN GU$_{4}$ ŠEG$_{6}$-*šal*) *ina* … SIL]A$_{11}$-*aš* SAR-*ab* LAL-*ma* U$_{4}$.3.KÁM NU DU$_{8}$

46′. […] LUḪ [… SA]R-*ab* LAL-*ma* KI.MIN

47′. [… (L)]ÀL KUR-*i šu-ḫat* KÙ.SIG$_{17}$ SÚD MAR

48′. […]x *ina* A GAZI^{SAR} SILA$_{11}$-*aš* SAR-*ab* LAL-*ma* U$_{4}$.3.KÁM NU DU$_{8}$

49′. […] ⸢:⸣ *ina šur-šum-mi* KAŠ ŠEG$_{6}$.GÁ SILA$_{11}$-*aš* SAR-*ab* LAL-*ma* U$_{4}$.3.KÁM NU DU$_{8}$

50′. […]x *du-muq-ši-na ta-tab-bal ina* LÀL SÚD *te-qí*

51′. [… *du-muq-ši*]-*na* GAZ SIM *ina* A GAZI^{SAR} SILA$_{11}$-*aš* SAR-*ab* LAL-*ma* U$_{4}$.3.KÁM NU ⸢DU$_{8}$⸣

52′. […]x GAZ SIM *ina* A GAZI^{SAR} SILA$_{11}$-*aš* SAR-*ab* LAL-*ma* U$_{4}$.3.KÁM NU DU$_{8}$

53′. U$_{5}$ [ARGAB^{MU}]^{ŠEN} *ina* LÀL SÚD *te-qí*

54′. 1/3 *qa* PA ^{GIŠ}M[(Á.ER)]EŠ.MÁ.RA ‹(ḪÁD.DU)› GAZ SIM *ina* A GAZI^{SA}[^{R} SILA$_{11}$-*aš* ‹(SAG-*su*)› S]AR-*ab* LAL-[(*ma*)] U$_{4}$.3.KÁM NU DU$_{8}$

55′. IM.BABBAR *ba-aš-la ina* Ì *sír-di* SILA$_{11}$-*aš* SAR-*ab* LAL-*ma* KI.MIN

56′. Š[IKA] Ì.GU.LA *ša kib-šam* TUKU-*ú ina* Ì SAḪAR.[URUDU …] SÚD *te-qí*

57′. ^{Ú}ZA.BA.LAM *saḫ-lé-e* GAZ [(S)]IM *ina šur-šum-mi* KAŠ S[AG SILA$_{11}$-*aš* S]AR-*ab* LAL-*ma* U$_{4}$.3.KÁM NU DU$_{8}$[91]

58′. ^{Ú}*ḫal-tap-pa-nam* ^{GIŠ}MAŠ.ḪUŠ GAZ [SI]M *ina šur-šum-mi* KAŠ.KUR[UN.N]A SILA$_{11}$-*aš* SAR-*ab* LAL-*ma* U$_{4}$.3.KÁM NU DU$_{8}$

59′. ^{ŠEM}LI ^{ŠEM}GÚR.GÚR ^{ŠEM}BULUḪ ZAG.ḪI.L[I N]AGA.SI SÚ[D LU]Ḫ-*si ina* GA SILA$_{11}$-*aš* SAR-*ab* LAL-*ma* U$_4$.3.KÁM NU DU$_8$

60′. SAḪAR.URUDU [*ina* L]ÀL SÚD *te-qí*

61′. 1/3 *qa* ZAG.ḪI.LI 1/3 *qa* KAŠ.⸢Ú⸣.[SA …] SILA$_{11}$-*aš* SAR-*ab* LAL-*ma* U$_4$.3.KÁM NU DU$_8$

62′. 1/3 *qa* ZAG.ḪI.L[I … S]ILA$_{11}$-*aš* SAR-*ab* LAL-*ma* U$_4$.3.KÁM NU DU$_8$

63′. KUG.GAN AN.Z[AḪ … S]ÚD MAR

64′. 1/3 *qa* ZÍD GÚ.[… LAL-*m*]*a* U$_4$.3.KÁM NU DU$_8$

---

ii

1. GAZ[I^{SAR}] BÍL-*lu* GAZ SIM *ina šur-šum-mi* KAŠ SILA$_{11}$-*aš* SAR-*ab* LAL-*ma* U$_4$.3.KÁM NU DU$_8$

---

2. NUMUN [^{Ú}]EME.UR.GI$_7$ SIG$_7$-*su tu-ḫás-sà* A-*šú ana* ^{DUG}BUR.ZI SUR-*at* EN ḪÁD.DU GAR-*an*
3. U$_4$-[*m*]*a i-tab-lu ina* Ì SAḪAR.URUDU SÚD MAR

---

4. ⸢Ú⸣ BABBAR U$_5$ ARGAB^{MUŠEN} Ì.UDU ^{ŠEM}GIG ŠEM.GAM.MA NUMUN ^{Ú}SI.SÁ *ka-mun* ^{GIŠ}ŠINIG NUMUN Ú.IN.NU.UŠ
5. [^{Ú}(E)ME.(U)R)].GI$_7$ PA ^{GIŠ}ŠINIG MUN.EME.SAL.LIM Ú.KUR.RA ^{Ú}GAMUN.GI$_6$ *ma-la ni-iš* IGI^{II}-*ka* ŠU.TI
6. [(*t*)]*a-pa-aṣ ina* Ì SÚD IGI^{II}-*šú ina* NAGA.SI LUḪ-*si* EN ÉR TAR-*su te-qí* U$_4$-*ma* LAL-*šú te-qí* EGIR-*šú*
7. [DÍLIM.A.B]ÁR NU DU$_8$-*šú* A ^{GIŠ}ŠE.NÁ.A ŠEG$_6$-*šal ana* ^{DUG}GAN. SAR *te-sip ina* UL *tuš-bat ina še-rim* SAG.DU-*su*
8. [(Š)]ÉŠ A ^{GIŠ}ŠE.NÁ.A ŠEG$_6$.GÁ *ana* SAG.DU-*šú tu-qar-ra-ár* SAG. DU-*su* SUD ^{Ú}SÍG.GA.RÍG.AG.A^{SAR}[92]
9. [*ina # q*]*a* Ì.GIŠ *ana* SAG.DU-*šú* DUB *ina* É *šá ta-ra-nam* TUKU-*ú* TUŠ-*šú* U$_4$.3.KÁM *an-nam* DÙ.DÙ-*uš*

---

10. [DIŠ NA UG]U-*šú* KÚM.KÚM-*im* IM.BABBAR NAGA.SI IN.DAR *kib-rit* GÌR.PAD.DA NAGA.SI Ì.ḪUL *u* Ì.KU$_6$
11. [1-*niš*] ḪE.ḪE *ina* DÈ $^{\text{GIŠ.Ú}}$GÍR SAG.DU-*su tu-qat-tar*

---

12. [DIŠ NA SAG.DU-*s*]*u* KÚM TUKU-*ma* IGI^{II}-*šú i-bar-ru-ra* MÚD *ú-kal-la* 1/3 *qa* ZAG.ḪI.LI GAZ SIM
13. [*i*]*na* ⸢A⸣ [GAZI^{S}]^{AR} SILA$_{11}$-*aš* SAG.DU-*su* SAR-*ab* LAL-*ma* U$_{4}$.3.KÁM NU DU$_{8}$

---

14. 1/3 *qa* ⸢ZAG.ḪI⸣.[LI] 1/3 *qa* ZÌ.KUM *ina* A.GEŠTIN.NA SILA$_{11}$-*aš* SAG.DU-*su* SAR-*ab* LAL-*ma* U$_{4}$.3.KÁM NU DU$_{8}$

---

15. 1/3 *qa* PA ^{GIŠ}PÈŠ *ina* GA [SILA$_{11}$-*aš* SAR-*ab* KI.MIN] 1/3 *qa* ^{Ú}ḪAB *ina* GA SILA$_{11}$-*aš* SAR-*ab* KI.MIN

---

16. 1/3 *qa* ^{Ú}U$_{5}$.[ARGAB^{MUŠEN} …] *ina* GA SILA$_{11}$-*aš* SAR-*ab* KI.MIN

---

17. 1/3 *qa* ^{Ú}*ṣa-da-n*[*u* … *in*]*a* GA SILA$_{11}$-*aš* SAR-*ab* KI.MIN

---

18. ^{Ú}*sa-ma-nam* […] SILA$_{11}$-*aš* SAR-*ab* KI.MIN

---

19. [(DIŠ N)]A UGU-*šú* UD.DA TAB-[(*ma* IGI^{II}-*šú i-bar-ru-ra*) … (DUḪ ŠEG$_{6}$.GÁ)] ^{ŠEM}LI ^{ŠEM}GÚR.GÚR[93]
20. [(^{ŠE})]^{M}BULUḪ *saḫ-lé-e* DUḪ.Š[(E.GIŠ.Ì ^{Ú}*si-ḫu ina* GA SILA$_{11}$-*aš*)] SAR-*ab* KI.MIN

---

21. [DIŠ NA U]GU-*šú* UD.DA TAB-*ma* [IGI^{II}-*šú i-bar-r*]*u-ra ù* MÚD DIRI-*a* […] ⸢^{Ú}⸣NU.LUḪ.ḪA
22. […]x *saḫ-lé-e* ^{GIŠ}M[Á.ERIŠ].⸢MÁ⸣.RA 1-*niš* GAZ SIM *ina* KAŠ.Ú.SA ḪE.ḪE S[AR-*ab*] LAL-*id*

---

23. [1/3 (*qa*) ZAG.Ḫ]I.LI 1/3 *qa* ZÍD ^{GIŠ}E[(R)]IN 1/3 *qa* ^{ŠEM}LI 1/3 *qa* [(^{ŠEM}MAN.D)]U! 1/3 *qa* ^{GIŠ}*si-ḫu* 1/2 *q*[*a* ^{GIŠ}*ar-ga*]*n-nu*
24. [(^{Ú}*ba-ri-rat*) 1 (*qa* DUḪ.Š)]E.GIŠ.Ì ZÍD [(GÚ)].GAL Z[(ÍD MUN)]U$_{6}$ KAŠ.Ú.SA ŠEG$_{6}$.GÁ [… *ṭe-n*]*e-ti*
25. [(SAG-*ka ú-kal ina* ŠÀ 2 *q*)]*a* ŠU.TI *ina* A GAZI^{SAR} SILA$_{11}$-*aš* SAR-*ab* [KI.MI]N

---

26. [DIŠ NA UD.DA TAB-*ma* UGU-*šú* G]ÍR.GÍR-*su* SÍG SAG.DU-*šú* GUB.GUB-*za* ^{GIŠ}GÚR.GÚR ^{GI}[^{Š}LI]
27. […] SÚD *ina* ^{URUDU}ŠEN.TUR *tu-ba-ḫar* SAG.DU-*su* […]

---

28. […]x Ì.NUN.NA *ina* IZI ŠEG$_6$-*šal* […]

29. [… ^{Š}]^{EM}MUG ^{ŠEM}ŠEŠ KAŠ *ṭi-ṭi* Ì.NUN.NA *ina* IZI ŠEG$_6$[…]

30. [… *ki*]*b-rit* GÌR.PAD.DU LÚ.U$_{18}$.LU GÌR.PAD.DU AN[ŠE? …]
31. [… *in*]*a* DÈ $^{GIŠ.Ú}$GÍR SAG.DU-*su* [*tu-qat-tar*]

32. [ÉN …] GI I.BÍ Ì I.BÍ ḪÉ.[EN…]
33. [… U]B.BI ḪÉ.⸢EN⸣.x[…]
34. [… MU.U]N.NA.MUL.LA [TU$_6$ ÉN]

35. [KA.INIM.MA DIŠ NA UD.DA TAB-*ma* UGU]-*šú ú*-⸢*zaq-qat*⸣-[*su*]

36. […]x ŠID-*nu* UGU […]

37. [ÉN …]x UḪ.ME KÙ.GA […]
38. […]x GI$_4$.GI$_4$ […]

39. [KA.INIM.MA DIŠ NA UGU-*šu u li*]*q*!? KA-*šu* KÚM [*ú-kal*]

40. [… *an*]*a* MURUB$_4$ UG[U-*šú*] ŠID-[*nu*]

41. […]x ^{Ú}KUR.[…]
42. [… LAL]-*ma* U$_4$.3.KÁM NU [DU$_8$]

43. DIŠ K[I.MIN … A GAZ]I^{SAR} SILA$_{11}$-*aš* LÁL-*su-ma* [TI]

44. DIŠ KI.MIN ^{Ú}[…]x *su-pa-lam ina* KAŠ *ta-là*-[*aš* KI.MIN]

45. DIŠ KI.MIN *saḫ-lé-e* [… *ni-ki*]*p-ta*$_5$ ZÍD ŠE.SA.A 1-*niš* GAZ SIM *ina* KAŠ […]

46. DIŠ KI.MIN 1/3 *qa saḫ*-[*lé-e* … SI]LA$_{11}$-*aš* SAR-*ab* [LAL]

47. DIŠ KI.MIN 1/2 *qa* […] SILA$_{11}$-*aš* SAR-*ab* [LAL]

48. DIŠ KI.MIN 1/3 *q*[*a* … G]AZ SIM *ina* A GAZI^{SAR} SILA$_{11}$-*aš* SAR-*ab* [LAL]

49. DIŠ KI.MIN $^{\text{Š[EM}}$ ...] *ina* A GAZI^{SAR} SILA$_{11}$-*aš* [LAL]

50. DIŠ KI.MIN [...] *ina* KAŠ SILA$_{11}$-*aš* SAR-*ab* [LAL]

51. [... *ina*] A GAZI^{SAR} SILA$_{11}$-*aš* SAR-*ab* [LAL]

52. [...] *ina* A GAZI^{SAR} SILA$_{11}$-*aš* SAR-*ab* [LAL]
53. [...] *ina* A GAZI^{SAR} SILA$_{11}$-*aš* SAR-*ab* [LAL]

54. [...] *ina šur-šum-mi* KAŠ SILA$_{11}$-*aš* SAR-*ab* [LAL]

55. [... IR-*šu t*]*u-šam-maṭ ina* A GAZI^{SAR} LUḪ-*si* 1/3 *qa* ^{GIŠ}MAŠ.Ḫ[UŠ ...]
56. [... GA]Z SIM *ina* A GAZI^{SAR} SILA$_{11}$-*aš* SAG.DU-*su u* GABA-*su* LAL-*i*[*d*]

57. DIŠ K[I.MIN ... Z]Ì.KUM ḪE.ḪE *ina* A GAZI^{SAR} SILA$_{11}$-*aš* LAL-*id*

58. DIŠ K[I.MIN ... Z]Ì.KUM *ina* A GAZI^{SAR} *ta-là-aš* SAR-*ab* LAL-*ma* U$_4$.3.KÁM NU DU$_8$

59. DIŠ K[I.MIN ... ^{GIŠ}Ḫ A.L]U.ÚB 2 SÌLA.TA.ÀM ḪE.ḪE *ina* A GAZI^{SAR} *u* KAŠ SILA$_{11}$-*aš* KI.MIN

60. DIŠ K[I.MIN ...] $^{\text{⸢Ú⸣}}$*su-pa-lu ina* Ì *sír-di u* A GAZI^{SAR} SILA$_{11}$-*aš* KI.MIN

61. DIŠ NA [SAG.DU]-*su* KÚM.KÚM-*im* SAR-*ab* ZÍD ZÍZ.AN.NA *ina* A GAZI^{SAR} SILA$_{11}$-*aš* U$_4$.15.KÁM LÁL

62. DIŠ K[(I.MIN IM.)]GÚ UD.DA SÁ.SÁ GAZ SIM *ina* A GAZI^{SAR} SILA$_{11}$-*aš* U$_4$.3.KÁM : U$_4$.5.KÁM LÁL
63. DIŠ [*ina ši-b*]*it* SAG!.DU-*šú* [:] MURUB$_4$ SAG.DU-*šú ú-na*!-*maš tu-uz-za rib-ki ina* A GAZI^{SAR} SILA$_{11}$-*aš* ‹*ina*› Ì EŠ.MEŠ LAL

64. [*ana* KÚM S]AG.DU *šu-uṭ-bi-i* ŠIKA [I]M.ŠU.RIN.NA ZÌ.KUM *ina* A GAZI^{SAR} SILA$_{11}$-*aš* SAG.DU-*su* LAL

65. [DIŠ KI.MIN (*saḫ-l*)]*é-e bu-ṭu-ta*$_5$ ZÍD ŠE.SA.A *ina* A GAZI^{SAR} SILA$_{11}$-*aš* LAL : DIŠ KI.MIN *saḫ-lé-e* ^{ŠEM}LI *ina* A GAZI^{SAR} SILA$_{11}$-*aš* LAL

---

66. [...] ḪÁD.DU GAZ SIM *ina* A GAZI^{SAR} SILA$_{11}$-*aš* LAL

---

67. [DIŠ KI.MIN DÈ *ṣar-b*]*a-te*[94] *ina* A GAZI^{SAR} SILA$_{11}$-*aš* LAL : DIŠ KI.MIN [(^{Ú}*ḫal*)]-*tap-pa-nam* GURUN ^{GIŠ}MAŠ.ḪUŠ *ina* A GAZI^{SAR} SILA$_{11}$-*aš* LAL

---

68. [(DIŠ KI.MIN ^{Ú}GEŠTIN.KA$_{5}$)].A ḪÁD.A SÚD *ina* A GAZI^{SAR} SILA$_{11}$-*aš* LAL [: DIŠ KI.MIN] ^{Ú}MÁ.EREŠ.MÁ.RA *ina* A GAZI^{SAR} SILA$_{11}$-*aš* LAL

---

69. [...] ^{Ú}ZA.B[A.LAM ...] *ina* A GAZI^{SAR} SILA$_{11}$-*aš* LAL

---

iii

1. [...] DÈ *ṣar-ba-te ina* A GAZI^{SAR} SILA$_{11}$-*aš* LAL

---

2. [... ^{Š}]^{EM}GÚR.GÚR *ina* A GAZI^{SAR} SILA$_{11}$-*aš* LAL

---

3. [... ZÌ.KU]M ḪE.ḪE *ina* A GAZI^{SAR} SILA$_{11}$-*aš* LAL

---

4. [...] ZÌ.KUM ḪE.ḪE *ina* A GAZI^{SAR} SILA$_{11}$-*aš* LAL

---

5. [... *ina* A GAZI^{SA}]^{R} SILA$_{11}$-*aš* LAL : DIŠ KI.MIN *qí-lip še-el-li-bi-nu ina* A GAZI^{SAR} SILA$_{11}$-*aš* LAL

---

6. [... DÈ *ṣa*]*r-ba-te ina* A GAZI^{SAR} SILA$_{11}$-*aš* LAL

---

7. [...] *ina* A GAZI^{SAR} SILA$_{11}$-*aš* LAL

8–21. (see chapter 6, text 6)

---

22. DIŠ NA SAG.DU-*su* KÚM-*ma* S[ÍG] SAG.DU-*šú i-šaḫ-ḫu-uḫ ana* KÚM SAG.DU [ZI-*ḫi*]
23. *u* SÍG GIN-*ta*$_{5}$ GUB-*zi* ^{Ú}[(*ak-ta*)]*m* ^{Ú}*ši-ma-ḫa* Ú.BABBAR 1-*niš* SÚD *ina* A ḪE.ḪE SAG.DU-*su te-sir*
24. U$_{4}$.2.KÁM* *ina* SAG.DU-*šú i-mit-tì* ⸢x x⸣ SAG.DU-*su* LUḪ-*si* NUMUN ^{GIŠ}*bi-ni* ^{Ú}*kám-ka-da*
25. ^{Ú}NÍG.GÁN.GÁN ^{Ú}NÍG.GIDRU ŠIKA N[(UNUZ GA.NU^{MU})]^{ŠEN} 1-*niš* SÚD *ina* Ì ḪE.ḪE SAG.DU-*su* ŠÉŠ-*aš*

---

26. ÉN MÚNŠUB AL.DÚB.B[(A)] MÚNŠUB AL.KALAG.GA
27. MÚNŠUB AL.KÉŠ.DA.KÉŠ.DA[95] MÚNŠUB NÍG.GUB.BA TU$_6$ ÉN

---

28. KA.INIM.MA SÍG SAG.D[(U)] NÍG.GUB.BA KÉŠ.DA.KÁM[96]

---

29. DÙ.DÙ.BI ^{NA_4}DU$_8$.ŠI.A ^{NA_4}GUG ^{NA_4}ZA.GÌN ^{NA}[$_4$(NÍR)] ^{NA_4}BAB[(AR.MIN$_5$)] ^{NA_4}IGI.KU$_6$ ^{NA_4}ŠUBA
30. ^{NA_4}ŠUBA Á.ZI.DA ^{NA_4}ŠUBA Á.GÙB.B[(U ^{NA_4}KUR-*nu* DIB ^{NA})]$_4$MUŠ.GÍR ^{NA_4}AŠ.GÌ.GÌ ^{NA_4}UGU.AŠ.GÌ.GÌ
31. 13 *ni-bi an-nu-ti ina* SÍG.ḪÉ.ME.DA È-*ak* [(*ina* SÍG KEŠD)]A-*ma* SÍG GIN-*ta*$_5$ *ik-kal-la*

---

32. ÉN *at-ta ba-ra-an-gi zi-ba-an-*[(*gi* : *ba-te-gi-ra*)] *zi-im-ba-ra uz-mi-ya-aš*
33. *pa-at-ri un-da-kur-ra ḫé-e*[*n-n*]*a ḫ*[(*é-min na-pa-ri*)*-š*]*á* TU$_6$ ÉN

---

34. KÌD.KÌD.BI 7 *ḫa-ru-bé-e šá* IM.SI.SÁ TI-*qí ina* DÈ *ur-ba-te tur-ár ina* Ì ḪE.ḪE ÉN 7-*šú*
35. ŠID-*nu* 3-*šú* ŠÉŠ-*su* 3-*šú ta-ḫal-l*[*a*]*-su e-nu-ma ta-ḫal-la-ṣu-šú* ÉN 3-*šú ana* UGU SAG.DU-*šú* ŠID-*nu*

---

36. ÉN I.BI.GI I.BI.G[I(M ḪÉ.EN.ZÁLAG).G]E SAG.KI *ṣi* SAG.KI *ṣi* ḪÉ.EN.ZÁLAG.GE SAG.KI *iṣ* SAG.KI *iṣ*
37. ḪÉ.EN.ZÁLAG.G[E (⸢ŠE⸣.ER.ZI ḪÉ.⸢EN⸣.ZÁLAG).G]E MA.AL.LÁ I.DI MU.RA.AN.GUB ḪUL.BI ḪUL.ḪUL ‹(TU$_6$)› ÉN

---

38. KÌD.KÌD.[BI ...] SAG.DU ÍGIRA^{MUŠEN} SAG.DU BURU$_5$.ḪABRUD.DA NÍTA ^{GIŠ}U$_4$.ḪI.IN ^{GIŠ}GIŠIMMAR
39. [...] ÉN 3-*šú ana* ŠÀ ŠID-*nu* EŠ.MEŠ-*su-ma* SÍG GIN-*ta*$_5$ *ik-kal-la lu šá* NÍTA *lu* [*šá* MUNUS]

---

40. [ÉN ...Š]U.GI LIL ŠU.GE.E.NE ŠU.GI

---

41. [KÌD.KÌD.BI 7 *ḫa-ru-b*]*é-e šá* IM.SI.SÁ TI *ina* IZI *tur-ár ina* Ì ^{GIŠ}ŠUR.MÌN MÚD ^{GIŠ}ERIN ḪE.ḪE EŠ.MEŠ-*su-ma* SI.SÁ-*im*

---

42. [(ÉN MU.UL.LU)] ḪUL.A *šá* GÁL-*ma* DINGIR *ṣi-ir-ta*
43. [(*ma-ni-ir-ra-an*)]*-ni-ḫa ba-re-eš-ma ni-ir-ra-an-ni ḫal-ḫal-la-ta* LA.GU.GIM.MA TI.LA.ŠÈ

44. [o o o (*ma-ki*)]-*pi-du-ru-na-aš ḫu-ri-na-aḫ mu-un-di-ḫu-na ḫa-at-tu-uk* TU$_6$ ÉN

---

45. [KA.INIM.M]A SÍG KÉŠ.DA.KÁM

46–47. Erased

---

48. DIŠ NA SÍG TE.MEŠ-*šú ma-gal i-šaḫ-ḫu-uḫ* NA.BI DINGIR-*šú* ^{d}EŠ$_4$.DAR-*šú* KI-*šú ze-nu-u*

---

49. KÌD.KÌD.BI *ana* IGI MUL *maḫ*-⸢*re*⸣-*e* KEŠDA KEŠDA ZÚ.LUM.MA ZÌ.EŠA DUB-*aq* NINDA.Ì.DÉ.A LÀL Ì.⸢NUN.NA⸣ GAR-*an*
50. UDU.SIZKUR DÙ-*uš* UZU.ZAG UZU.ME.[ḪÉ U]ZU.KA.NE *tu-ṭaḫ-ḫa* KAŠ BAL-*qí* ^{GIŠ}ŠITA ^{GIŠ}⸢MÁ.EREŠ⸣^{leš}).MÁ-*le-e*
51. U$_5$ ARGAB^{MUŠEN} ^{Ú}*imḫur*-20 [^{Ú}ŠÈ.M]Á.LAḪ$_4$ KI Ì ḪE.ḪE *ina* IGI MUL GAR-*an* ÉN *an-ni-ta*$_5$ 3-*šú* ŠID-*nu*

---

52. *at-ta* MUL *mu-nam-mir* ⸢x x x x x x⸣ *qí-rib* AN-*e ḫa-iṭ* UB.MEŠ
53. *ana-ku* NENNI A NENNI *ina* GI$_6$ *an-né-e* IGI-*ka kám-sa-ku di-ni di-in* EŠ.BAR-*a-a* TAR-*us*
54. Ú.ḪI.A ŠEŠ.MEŠ *lip-si-su lum-ni* Á.GÚ.ZI.GA U$_4$-*ma* TE.MEŠ-*šú ta-kar*

---

55. DIŠ KI.MIN ^{GIŠ}ŠITA ^{GIŠ}LÚ-*a-nu* ^{Ú}*eli-kul-la* ^{Ú}*kur-ka-na-a* 1 [...⸣ ⸢SÍG ^{MUNUS}ÁŠ.GÀR⸣ GÌŠ.NU.ZU *ina* GÚ-*šú* GAR-*an*

---

56. 6 KA.INIM.⸢MA⸣ SÍG KÉŠ.DA.KÁM*

57–iv 8. See chapter 7, text 6.

---

iv
9. DIŠ NA SAG.DU-*su it-te-ni-ba-aš-šum* [^{NA_4}... ^{NA_4}MU]Š.GÍR ^{NA_4}DAG.GAZ ^{NA_4}GUG *mar-ḫa-ši*
10. ^{NA_4}ZÚ GI$_6$ ^{NA_4}NÍR ^{NA_4}AN.ZA.[GU]L.⸢ME⸣ [^{NA_4}A]MAŠ.PA.È 8 NA$_4$.MEŠ
11. *an-nu-ti ina* SÍG.ḪÉ.ME.DA SÍG.BABBAR NU.NU [...] SAG.KI^{II}-*šú tara-kás-ma ina-eš*

---

12. DIŠ NA ⸢SAG.DU-*su*⸣ [... GEŠTU^{II}-*šú i-ta*]-*na-az-za* ^{ŠEM}GÚR.GÚR ^{Š}[^{EM}L]I ^{ŠEM}MAN.DU ŠEM.SAL ^{ŠEM}BAL

13. [… ^{GIŠ}E]RIN.SUMUN ^{GIŠ}*si-ḫu* ^{GIŠ}*ár-*[*ga*]*-nu* ^{Ú}*ba-ri-ra-tú* GI.DÙG

---

14. […] *ina* Ì.UDU ÉLLAG UDU.NÍTA *šá* MUN NU ŠUB-*u ina* MÚD $^{\text{GI[Š}}$E]RIN SÚD *ina* KUŠ SUR-*ri* SAG.DU-*su* LAL

---

15. […]x *tum* ^{ŠEM}BULUḪ ^{Ú}*kur-ka-nu-u* [# *q*]*u-ta-ru šá* SAG.DU

---

16. [(*nap-šal-tu* SAG)].DU KI.A.^{d}ÍD BABBAR *u* GI$_6$ *ni-kip-ta* NÍTA *u* MUNUS $^{\text{NA}_4}$*mu-*⸢*ṣa*⸣ [($^{\text{NA}_4}$ZÁLAG $^{\text{NA}_4}$AN.ZAḪ K)]A.⸢A.AB.BA⸣
17. [(NUMUN ^{GIŠ}*bi-n*)]*i* SI DÀRA.MAŠ *gul-gul* NAM.LÚ.U$_{18}$.LU Ú.ḪI.A *an-nu-ti* TÉŠ.BI [(SÚD *ina* Ì *u* MÚD ^{GIŠ}ERIN ḪE.ḪE-*ma*)]
18. SAG.KI.MEŠ-*šú* [(*tu-lap-pat*)]

---

19. [(*qù-taru* SA)]G.DU ^{Ú}KUR.KUR KI.A.^{d}ÍD ^{Ú}*kur-ka-nam ni-*⸢*kip-ta*⸣ [(NÍTA *u* MUNUS)]
20. [(1-*niš tu*)]*-daq-qaq ina* MÚD ^{GIŠ}ERIN ḪE.ḪE *ina* DÈ *tu-*⸢*qat-tar-šu*⸣

---

21. [DIŠ NA SAG.D]U-*su* GIG ^{Ú}*ṣa-ṣu-um-ta*$_5$ ^{Ú}MUR.DÙ.DÙ *ú-*[*p*]*i-mu-un-zir*
22. […]x-*su* 1-*niš* SÚD *ina* A GAZI^{SAR} SILA$_{11}$-*aš* SAG.DU-*su* SAR-*ab* LAL-*ma* U$_4$.3.KÁM NU DU$_8$

---

23. [(DIŠ NA SAG.DU-*s*)]*u* DUGUD ^{ŠEM}GÚR.GÚR ^{ŠEM}LI ^{Ú}KUR.KUR ^{ŠEM}ŠEŠ ‹(Ú.KUR.RA 1-*niš* SÚD)› [(KI IL)]LU ^{ŠEM}BULUḪ
24. [(KI Ì.UDU) ÉLL]AG GU$_4$ ḪE.ḪE *ina* KUŠ ‹(EDIN)› SUR-*ri* SAR[-*ab* U$_4$].⸢5⸣.KÁM LÁL[97]

---

25. […] 15 *u* 150 3.TA.ÀM *te-*[… *ina* A.GAZI$^{\text{S]AR}}$ SILA$_{11}$-*aš* Ì ŠÉŠ LAL

---

26. [(DIŠ NA *ina* LÍL-*šú* KÚM *ana* SAG.DU-*šú ip-pu-uš-ma* SAG.DU-*su* DUGUD-*m*)]*a ina* ZI-*šú* SAG.DU-*su*
27. [(*ana* IGI-*šú* GÍD.DA-*su ana* DIN-*šú* ^{ŠEM}LI ^{Ú}*mar-gu-ṣa* ŠEM.ŠEŠ ^{Ú}*ur-nu-qa ina* ^{NA})]$_4$ZAG.ḪI.LI SÚD
28. [(*ana* ŠÀ Ì.SUMUN ŠUB SAG.DU-*su* EŠ.ME-*ma* KÚM SAG.D)]U-*šú i-be-li*[98]

---

29. [DIŠ (MIN ^{ŠEM}GÚR.GÚR ^{ŠEM}LI NUMUN ^{Ú}ÁB.DUḪ SÚD *ina* Ì.SUMUN ḪE.ḪE)] SAG.DU-*su* EŠ.MEŠ

---

30. DIŠ NA [...] im ḪÁD.A GAZ
31. SIM KI [...]x-*ma* U$_4$.3.KÁM* NU DU$_8$

---

32. DIŠ NA SAG.D[(U-*su pa-nu-šú* IGI^{II}-*šú* G)Ì(R^{II}-*šú* NUNDUN-*šú* MÚ.MEŠ-*ḫu* SA)G.DU-*su* (*ana* IGI)]-⸢*šú*⸣ GÍD.DA-*su*
33. ŠU^{II}-*šú u* GÌR^{II}-*šú* [(GU$_7$-*šú mi-na-tu-šú tab-ka* SU-*šú šim*)-*m*(*a*)]-*ta*$_5$ TUKU *ana* T[(I-*šú* ^{Š})]^{EM}GÚR.GÚR
34. ^{ŠEM}LI [(^{Ú}KUR.KUR NUMUN ^{Ú}ÁB.DUḪ) *s*(*aḫ-lé-e* ÀR-*tì* PA)] ^{GIŠ}ÍLDAG GAZI^{S}[(^{AR} ZÍ)]D.ŠE.SA.A
35. KAŠ!.Ú.SA S[(IG$_5$ ŠEM.^{d}MAŠ ^{ŠEM}SI.SÁ 1-*niš* GAZ SIM *ina*)] A GAZI^{SAR} SILA$_{11}$-*aš*
36. SAG.DU-*s*[(*u* SAR-⸢*ab*⸣ Ì.GIŠ *šú-ši* SAG.DU-*su* ŠÉŠ LÁL-*m*)]*a* U$_4$.7.KÁM NU DU$_8$

---

37. DIŠ KI.MIN ^{Ú}[...] MEŠ-*ma ina-eš*

---

38. DIŠ NA MURUB$_4$ SAG.[(DU-*šú ú-zaq-qa*-⸢*su*⸣ *bir-ka-šu* DUGUD *ú-ta-b*)*a-ka e*]-*ta-na-aḫ* GAZ ŠÀ
39. TUKU.MEŠ-*ši* É[LL(AG-*šu e-ta-na-ba*)*l* ... (⸢*i*⸣-*ṣa-nam-mu ik-ka-šu*)] *ik-ta-ner-ru*
40. *ana* GIG x[... (⸢GI.DÙG⸣ ^{Ú}KUR.KUR) ... (⸢^{GIŠ}ŠE.NÁ⸣).A KAŠ.(⸢Ú.SA *ina*⸣)] A GAZI^{SAR}
41. ZÍD ŠE.S[A.A ... (^{Ú}NÍG.GIDRU) *ina* (⸢U$_4$ ḪÁD.A GAZ SIM *ina* A GAZI^{SAR}⸣ SILA$_{11}$-*aš* LAL)]-*id*

42–47. (missing)
48′. [...]x ^{GIŠ}ŠINIG NUMUN ^{Ú}x[...]
49′. [... (*lu-ú ina* K)]AŠ.SAG *lu ina* GEŠTIN NAG

50′. [(DIŠ NA SAG.K)]I.DIB.BA TUKU.TUKU NUMUN ^{Ú}⸢ÚKUŠ⸣.GÍL

Translation

(i 1–4) If fever grips the crown[99] of a person's head, he experiences pulsating of the temporal blood vessels and his eyes flutter[100] (and) his eyes (have) dimness, cloudiness, confusion of vision, *amurdinnu*, *quqānu*-worms (or) are confused or continually tear, you mill-grind 1/3 *qû*-measure of *saḫlû*-cress[101] (and) *buṭuttu*-cereal with a millstone (and) sift (it) while he waits for you. You take 1/3 *qû*-measure of it (and) make it into a dough with *kasû* juice. You shave ‹(his head)›. You bandage him (with it) and do not take (it) off for three days.

(i 5) You make 1/3 *qû*-measure of *saḫlû*-cress (and) 1/3 *qû*-measure of roasted grain flour into a dough with *kasû* juice. You shave ‹(his head)›. You bandage him (with it) and do not take (it) off for three days.

(i 6) You make mill ground *saḫlû*-cress, *kukru* (and) *uḫḫūlu qarnānu* into a dough with beer. Ditto (You shave his head. You bandage him (with it) and do not take (it) off for three days).

(i 7) You mix myrrh and *emesallim*-salt in equal proportions. You grind (it) in ghee (and) ⸢daub⸣ his eyes (with it).

(i 8–9) You crush and mix 1/3 *qû*-measure of ‹(ground)› *saḫlû*-cress, 1/3 *qû*-measure of fragments from an ‹(old)› oven (and) 10 shekels of *ḫīqu*-beer (variant: 4 shekels of gypsum). You make (it) into a dough with *kasû* juice. You shave ‹(his head)›. You bandage him (with it) and do not take (it) off for three days.

(i 10–12) After these bandages, he should gather 10 shekels of *saḫlû*-cress from the mouth of a millstone on which something dropped[102] has not fallen (and which) salt (and) vinegar have not touched[103] into ‹ hot emmer › bread and then eat (it). You whisk 5 shekels of ground *saḫlû*-cress into ‹(1/2 *qû*)›-measure of first quality beer and then have him drink (it). He should clear (his throat) and vomit. (These are) *saḫlû*-cress bandages for the eyes.

(i 13) For one day, you grind *anzaḫḫu*-frit. [...]

(i 14–15) You crush (and) sift 10 shekels of *kalbānu* fruit, [...], *supālu* (and) 1/3 *qû* of [...]. [You make it into a dough] with ⸢*kasû*⸣ juice. You shave ‹ his head ›. You bandage (him with it) and [do not take it off] for three days.

(i 16) You grind ⸢kohl⸣ (and) [...] in "lion fat" (and) [daub his eyes (with it)].

(i 17–18) You crush (and) ⸢sift⸣ x ⸢shekels⸣ of *supālu*, 1/3 *qû* of [... and ...]. You ⸢make it into a dough⸣ [with *kasû* juice]. You shave ‹(his head)›. You bandage (him with it) and [do not take it off for three] days.

(i 19) You crush (and sift) 10 shekels of ⸢dried⸣ powdered sesame residue. [You make it into a dough] with ⸢*kasû*⸣ juice. [...]

(i 20–22) [You ...] 10 shekels of dried powdered sesame residue. You bandage his chest for one day. [You ...] his head. You pour [...] over his head. [He should stay] in the [...] house. [...]

(i 23) [You ...] one shekel of *rikibti arkabi*,[104] 1/2 ⸢shekel⸣ of [...]

(i 24) [You ...] 1/3 *qû* of *pappar*ḫ*u*-purslane seed, 1/3 *qû* of ⸢*laptu*-turnip⸣ seed [...]

(i 25) [You ...] 1/3 *qû* of *isqūqu*-flour, ⸢10 shekels⸣ of ⸢pomegranate(?)⸣ rind [...]

(i 26–29) *(too fragmentary for translation)*

(i 30–31) [You make] 1/3 *qû* of *ṭittu*-fig leaves which were picked in Nisannu (and) [...] leaves [into a dough with beer]. You redry, ⸢crush⸣ [(and) sift (it). You make (it) into a dough with *kasû* juice]. You shave his head (and) bandage (him with it). [...]

(i 32) [You ...] 1/3 *qû* of *šammi buʾšāni* (and) 1/3 *qû* of *qutru* seed. You shave his head. You bandage (him with it) [and do not take it off for three days].

(i 33) [You ...] *uḫḫūlu qarnānu* [...]

(i 34) [You ...] 1/3 [*qû* of ...]

(i 35–39) *(lost)*

(i 40′) You grind [...] (and) you [daub (it) on]

(i 41′) [...] You shave (his head). You bandage (him with it) and ⸢ditto⸣ (do not take it off for three days).

(i 42′) [...] You ⸢redry⸣, crush (and) sift (it). You make (it) into a dough with *kasû* juice . You shave (his head). You bandage (him with it) and ⸢ditto⸣ (do not take it off for three days).

(i 43′) [...] You make (it) into a dough [with *kasû* juice]. You grind (it) in marrow from the long bone (of a wether and) daub (it) on.

(i 44′) You grind [... (and)] ⸢pickled meat⸣[105] from a gazelle (and) daub (it) on.

(i 45′) [...] You make (it) into a dough with *kasû* juice. You boil it in ox dung. ⸢You make (it) into a dough⸣ [with ...]. You shave (his head). You bandage (him with it) and do not take (it) off for three days.

(i 46′) [...] You wash [...]. ⸢You shave (his head)⸣. You bandage him (with it) and ditto (do not take it off for three days).

(i 47′) You grind [...], wild honey (and) gold patina (and) daub (it) on.

(i 48′) [...] You make (it) into a dough with *kasû* juice. You shave (his head). You bandage (him with it) and do not take (it) off for three days.

(i 49′) [...] You boil (it) in [...] or beer dregs (and) make (it) into a dough. You shave (his head). You bandage (him with it) and do not take (it) off for three days.

(i 50′) [...] You dry their best parts. You grind (it) in honey (and) daub (it) on.

(i 51′) [...] You crush (and) sift ⸢their⸣ [best parts?]. You make (it) into a dough with *kasû* juice. You shave (his head). You bandage (him with it) and do not take (it) off for three days.

(i 52′) You crush (and) sift [...] and [...]. You make (it) into a dough with *kasû* juice. You shave (him). You bandage (him with it) and do not take (it) off for three days.

(i 53′) You grind *rikibti* ⸢*arkabi*⸣ in honey (and) daub (it) on.

(i 54′) You ‹(dry)›, crush (and) sift 1/3 *qû* of *mirišmaru* leaves. [You make it into a dough] with *kasû* juice. ⸢You shave ‹(his head)›⸣. You bandage (him with it) and do not take (it) off for three days.

(i 55′) You make cooked *gaṣṣu*-gypsum into a dough with olive oil. You shave (his head). You bandage him (with it) and ditto (do not take it off for three days).

(i 56′) You grind a ⸢potsherd⸣ of moldy *igulû* oil in oil impregnated with ⸢"copper dust"⸣ and [...] (and) daub (it) on.

(i 57′) You crush (and) sift *supālu* (and) *saḫlû*-cress. ⸢You make (it) into a dough⸣ with ⸢first quality⸣ beer dregs. ⸢You shave (his head)⸣. You bandage (him with it) and do not take (it) off for three days.

(i 58′) You crush (and) ⸢sift⸣ *ḫaltappānu* (and) *kalbānu*. You make (it) into a dough with dregs of ⸢*kurunnu*⸣ beer. You shave (his head). You bandage (him with it) and do not take it off for three days.

(i 59′) ⸢You grind (and) wash⸣ *burāšu*-juniper, *kukru*, *baluḫḫu*-aromatic, *saḫlû*-cress, *uḫḫūlu qarnānu* (and) [...]. You make (it) into a dough with milk. You shave (his head). You bandage (him with it) and do not take (it) off for three days.

(i 60′) You grind "copper dust" [in] ⸢honey⸣ (and) daub (it) on.

(i 61′) You make 1/3 *qû* of *saḫlû*-cress, 1/3 *qû* of beerwort and [...] into a dough [with ...]. You shave (his head). You bandage (him with it) and do not take (it) off for three days.

(i 62′) ⸢You make⸣ 1/3 *qû* of *saḫlû*-cress and [...] ⸢into a dough⸣ [with ...]. You shave (his head). You bandage (him with it) and do not take (it) off for three days.

(i 63′) ⸢You grind⸣ *lulû*-antimony, ⸢*anzaḫḫu*-frit⸣ and [...] (and) daub (it) on.

(i 64′) [You ...] 1/3 *qû* of ⸢*ḫallūru*-chickpea/*kakku*-lentil⸣ flour. [...] [You bandage (him with it)] ⸢and⸣ do not take (it) off for three days.

(ii 1) You crush (and) sift roasted[106] *kasû*. You make (it) into a dough with beer dregs. You shave (his head). You bandage (him with it) and do not take (it) off for three days.

(ii 2–3) You crush/mince fresh *lišān kalbi* seed. You press out its juices into a *pursītu*-vessel. You set (it) aside until it has dried out. ⸢When⸣ it has dried out, you grind (it) in oil impregnated with "copper dust" (and) daub (it) on.

(ii 4–9) You take as much as looks right to you of "white plant," *rikibti arkabi*, "fat" of *kanaktu*-aromatic, *ṣumlalû*, *šurdunû* seed, *kamunu*-fungus from a *bīnu*-tamarisk, *maštakal* seed, *lišān kalbi*, *bīnu*-tamarisk leaves, *emesallim* salt, *ninû*-mint (and) *zību*. You pulverize (it and) grind (it) in oil. You wash his eyes with *uḫḫūlu qarnānu* until the tears stop. You daub (it) on. When you bandage him, you daub (it) on. Afterwards, you do not release him (from application of) a ⌜lead spoon⌝. You boil *šūnû*-chastetree infusion. You decant (it) into a porous *kannu*-vessel. You let (it) sit out overnight under the stars. In the morning, you gently rub his head (with it). You put the boiled *šūnû*-tree infusion on his head (and) sprinkle his head (with it). You pour "carded wool"-plant (cotton) over his head (mixed) [with #] ⌜*qû*⌝ oil. You have him sit in a house with an awning. You do this repeatedly for three days.

(ii 10–11) [If a person's] ⌜crown of the head⌝ is continually hot, you mix [together] *gaṣṣu*-gypsum, indar-type(?) *uḫḫūlu qarnānu*, *kibrītu*-sulphur, bone, *uḫḫūlu qarnānu*, rancid oil and fish oil. You fumigate his head (with it) over *ašāgu*-thorn coals.

(ii 12–13) [If a person's head] has fever so that his eyes become dimmed and bloodshot, you crush (and) sift 1/3 *qû* of *saḫlû*-cress. You make (it) into a dough with ⌜*kasû*⌝ juice. You shave his head. You bandage (him with it) and do not take (it) off for three days.

(ii 14) You make 1/3 *qû* of ⌜*saḫlû*⌝-cress and 1/3 *qû* of *isqūqu*-flour into a dough with vinegar. You shave his head. You bandage (him with it) and do not take (it) off for three days.

(ii 15) [You make] 1/3 *qû* of *tittu*-fig leaves [into a dough] with milk. [You shave (his head). Ditto (You bandage him with it and do not take it off for three days.)] You make 1/3 *qû* of *šammi bušāni* into a dough with milk. You shave (his head). Ditto (You bandage him with it and do not take it off for three days.)

(ii 16) You make 1/3 *qû* of ⌜*rikibti arkabi*(?)⌝ into a dough with milk. You shave (his head). Ditto (You bandage him with it and do not take it off for three days.)

(ii 17) You make 1/3 *qû* of ⌜*ṣadānu*⌝ into a dough ⌜with⌝ milk. You shave (his head). Ditto (You bandage him with it and do not take it off for three days.)

(ii 18) You make *samānu* into a dough [with ...]. You shave (his head). Ditto (You bandage him with it and do not take it off for three days.)

(ii 19–20) If a person's crown of the head is burned by *ṣētu* so that his eyes become dimmed [and bloodshot], you make boiled residue, *burāšu*-juniper, *kukru* (variant: *ṣumlalû*), *baluḫḫu*-aromatic, *saḫlû*-cress, sesame residue (and) *sīḫu*-wormwood into a dough with milk. You shave (his head). Ditto (You bandage him with it and do not take it off for three days.)

(ii 21–22) [If a person]'s ⌜crown of the head⌝ is burned by *ṣētu* so that [his eyes] ⌜become dimmed⌝ and bloodshot, you crush together (and) sift [...], *nuḫurtu*, [...], *saḫlû*-cress (and) *mirišmarû*. You mix (it) with beerwort. ⌜You shave⸣ (his head). You bandage (him with it).

(ii 23–25) You take 2 *qû* out of (a mixture of) [1/3] *qû* of ⸢*saḫlû*-cress⸣, 1/3 *qû* of *erēnu*-cedar flour, 1/3 *qû* of *burāšu*-juniper, 1/3 *qû* of *su᾿ādu*, 1/3 *qû* of *sīḫu*-wormwood, 1/2 *qû* (each) of ⸢*argannu*⸣ (and) *barirātu*, [1] *qû* (each) of sesame residue, *ḫallūru*-chickpea flour, malt flour (and) boiled beerwort—[the flours are to be] ⸢mill-ground⸣ while (the patient) waits for you. You make (it) into a dough with *kasû* juice. You shave (his head). ⸢Ditto⸣ (You bandage him with it).

(ii 26–27) [If a person is burned by *ṣētu* so that the crown of his head] continually stings him (and) the hair of his head (seems) continually to stand on end, you grind *kukru*, ⸢*burāšu*-juniper⸣ (and) […]. You heat (it) up in a *tamgussu*-vessel (and) [bandage] his head (with it).

(ii 28) You boil […] (and) ghee over a fire. […]

(ii 29) You boil […] *ballukku*-aromatic, myrrh, *ṭīṭu*-beer (and) ghee over a fire. […]

(ii 30–31) [You fumigate] his head with […], ⸢sulphur⸣, "lone plant" (= "human bone"), ⸢donkey⸣ bone (and) […] over *ašāgu*-thorn coals.

(ii 32–34) *fragmentary Sumerian recitation*

(ii 35–36) [Recitation for cases where a person is burned by *ṣētu* so that the crown of] his [head] stings [him …]. You recite […] the crown of the head […].

(ii 37–38) *fragmentary Sumerian recitation*

(ii 39–40) [Recitation for cases where the crown of his head and] his ⸢palate(?)⸣ [holds] fever. You recite (it) ⸢over⸣ the middle of ⸢the crown of⸣ [his] ⸢head⸣.

(ii 41–42) […] [You bandage him with it] and do not [take it off] for three days.

(ii 43) ⸢Alternatively⸣, you make […] into a dough [with] ⸢*kasû*⸣ [juice]. If you bandage (him with it), [he should recover].

(ii 44) Alternatively, ⸢you make⸣ […] and *supālu*-plant ⸢into a dough⸣ with beer. [Ditto (If you bandage him with it, he should recover)].

(ii 45) Alternatively, you crush together (and) sift *saḫlû*-cress, […], ⸢*nikiptu*⸣ (and) roasted grain flour. [You make it into a dough] with beer. [Ditto (If you bandage [him with it], he should recover)].

(ii 46) Alternatively, ⸢you make⸣ 1/3 *qû* of *saḫlû*-cress [and …] ⸢into a dough⸣ [with …]. You shave (his head and) [bandage him with it].

(ii 47) Alternatively, you make 1/2 *qû* of […] into a dough [with …]. You shave (his head and) [bandage him with it].

(ii 48) Alternatively, you make 1/3 *qû* of […] into a dough with *kasû* juice. You shave (his head and) [bandage him with it].

(ii 49) Alternatively, you make […] into a dough with *kasû* juice. You shave (his head and) [bandage him with it].

(ii 50) Alternatively, you make […] into a dough with beer (and) [bandage him with it].

(ii 51) [If …], you make […] into a dough with *kasû* juice. You shave (his head and) [bandage him with it].

(ii 52–54) [If …], you make […] into a dough with *kasû* juice. You shave (his head and) [bandage him with it]. [Alternatively], you make […] into a dough with *kasû* juice. You shave (his head and) [bandage him with it]. [Alternatively], you make […] into a dough with beer dregs. You shave (his head and) [bandage him with it].

(ii 55–56) [If …], you wipe off [his sweat];[107] you wash (his head) with *kasû* juice. [You crush] (and) sift 1/3 *qû* of ⸢*kalbānu*⸣ (and) […]. You make (it) into a dough with *kasû* juice. You bandage his head and breast (with it).

(ii 57) ⸢Alternatively⸣, you mix [… with] ⸢*isqūqu*-flour⸣. You make (it) into a dough with *kasû* juice (and) you bandage (him with it).

(ii 58) ⸢Alternatively⸣, you make ⸢*isqūqu*-flour⸣ into a dough with *kasû* juice. You shave (his head). You bandage (him with it) and do not take (it) off for three days.

(ii 59) ⸢Alternatively⸣, you mix 2 *qû* each of […] (and) ⸢*ḫaluppu*-tree⸣ […]. You make (it) into a dough with *kasû* juice and beer. Ditto (You shave his head. You bandage him with it and do not take it off for three days).

(ii 60) ⸢Alternatively⸣, you make […] (and) *supālu* into a dough with olive oil and *kasû* juice. Ditto (You shave his head. You bandage him with it and do not take it off for three days).

(ii 61) If a person's [head] is continually feverish, you shave him. You make emmer flour into a dough with *kasû* juice. You bandage (him with it) for fifteen days.

(ii 62–63) Alternatively, you crush (and) sift riverbank silt which is all dried out. You make it into a dough with *kasû* juice and bandage him with it for three days (variant: five days). If he moves (even) a fine cloth [from] the ⸢top⸣ (variant: middle) of his head,[108] you make a dough out of a decoction with *kasû* juice.[109] You repeatedly rub him gently ‹with› oil (and) bandage (him with it).

(ii 64) [To] make [the fever in] the ⸢head⸣ go down, you make a fragment of an ‹old› oven (and) *isqūqu*-flour into a dough with *kasû* juice (and) bandage his head (with it).

(ii 65) [Alternatively], you make *saḫlû*-cress, *buṭuttu*-cereal and roasted grain flour into a dough with *kasû* juice (and) bandage (him with it). Alternatively, you make *saḫlû*-cress and *burāšu*-juniper into a dough with *kasû* juice (and) bandage (him with it).

(ii 66) You dry, crush (and) sift [...]. You make (it) into a dough with *kasû* juice (and) bandage (him with it).

(ii 67) [Alternatively], you make ⸢*ṣarbātu*-poplar⸣ [ashes] (variant: *qutrātu*) into a dough with *kasû* juice (and) bandage (him with it). Alternatively, you make *ḫaltappānu* (and) *kalbānu* fruit into a dough with *kasû* juice (and) bandage (him with it).

(ii 68) Alternatively, you dry (and) grind "fox grape." You make (it) into a dough with *kasû* juice (and) bandage (him with it). [Alternatively], you make *mirišmaru* into a dough with *kasû* juice (and) bandage (him with it).

(ii 69) [Alternatively], you make ⸢*supālu*⸣ (and) [...] into a dough with *kasû* juice (and) bandage (him with it).

(iii 1) [Alternatively], you make [...] (and) *ṣarbātu*-poplar ashes into a dough with *kasû* juice (and) bandage (him with it).

(iii 2) [Alternatively], you make [...] (and) *kukru* into a dough with *kasû* juice (and) bandage (him with it).

(iii 3) [Alternatively], you mix [... with] ⸢*isqūqu*-flour⸣. You make (it) into a dough with *kasû* juice (and) bandage (him with it).

(iii 4) [Alternatively], you mix [... with] *isqūqu*-flour. You make (it) into a dough with *kasû* juice (and) bandage (him with it).

(iii 5) [Alternatively], you make [...] into a dough [with] ⸢*kasû*⸣ [juice] (and) bandage (him with it). Alternatively, you make *šallapānu* peel into a dough with *kasû* juice (and) bandage (him with it).

(iii 6) [Alternatively], you make ⸢*ṣarbātu*-poplar⸣ [ashes (and) ...] into a dough with *kasû* juice (and) bandage (him with it).

(iii 7) [Alternatively], you make [...] into a dough with *kasû* juice (and) bandage (him with it).

(iii 8–21) *(see chapter 6, text 6)*

(iii 22–25) If a person's head is feverish and the ⸢hair⸣ of his head falls out, to [remove] the fever of his head and to make the hair that is going stand firm, you grind together *aktam*, *šimāḫu* (and) "white plant." You mix (it) with water. You plaster his head (with it). (He keeps it) on his head for two days to the right of [...]. You wash his head. You grind together *bīnu*-tamarisk seed, *kamkadu*, *egemgīru*, *ḫaṭṭi* (*rēʾi* and) a fragment of ostrich shell. You mix (it) with oil. You rub (it) gently on his head.

(iii 26–27) Recitation: Hair which is mighty, hair which is strong, hair which is bound fast, hair which stands firm. Spell and Recitation.

(iii 28) Recitation to bind fast[110] the hair of the head and to make it stand firm.

(iii 29–31) Its ritual: You thread these thirteen stones onto red-dyed wool: *dūšû*-stone, carnelian, lapis, *ḫulālu*-stone, *papparminu*-stone, "fish-eye stone," *šubû*-stone, right-sided *šubû*-stone, left-sided *šubû*-stone, magnetic hematite, *muššaru*-stone, *ašgikû*-stone (and) UGU-*ašgikû*-stone. If you bind (it) into the hair, the hair that is going should be prevented (from doing so).

(iii 32–33) Recitation: *atta barangi zibangi bategira zimbara uzmiyaš patri undakurra* ⌜*ḫenna*⌝ *ḫemin* ⌜*naparišá*⌝. Spell and Recitation.

(iii 34–35) Its ritual: You take seven *ḫarubu*-carob pods growing on the north side (of the tree). You char (them) over *urpatu*-rush coals (and) mix (it) with oil. You recite the recitation seven times. You rub him gently (with it) three times (and) comb (his hair) three times. When you comb it, you recite the recitation three times over his head.

(iii 36–37) Like smoke, like smoke, let it clear away. Depart from the temples! Depart from the temples! Let it clear away. Traped ("depart" pronounced backwards) from the temples! Traped ("depart" pronounced backwards) from the temples! Let the sheen[111] clear away. Let it clear away. It will diminish for me. It will stand aside[112] for me. Its evil shall be rubbed away.[113] Spell and Recitation.

(iii 38–39) [It's] ritual: [You ...] the head of an *igirû*-heron, the head of a male *ḫurri*-bird, a datepalm frond (and) [...]. You recite the recitation three times over it. If you repeatedly rub him gently (with it), the hair that is going should be prevented (from doing so). (This is good) either for a man or [for a woman].

(iii 40) *Fragmentary Sumerian recitation.*

(iii 41) [It's ritual]: You take [seven] ⌜*ḫarubu*-carob pods⌝ growing on the north side. You char (them) with fire (and) mix (it) with *šurmēnu*-cypress oil and *erēnu*-cedar resin. If you repeatedly rub him gently (with it), (the hair) should stay straight.

(iii 42–44) Oh star, august divinity, the evil which exists and *manirranniḫa barešma nirrani*, [may] the *ḫalḫallatu*-drum, like kiln slag, [bring it] to an end. *Makipidurnaš ḫurinaḫ mundiḫuna ḫattuk*. Spell and Recitation.

(iii 45) ⌜Recitation⌝ to bind fast the hair.

(iii 46–47) *Erased*

(iii 48) If the hair of a person's cheeks falls out a lot, that person's god (and) goddess are angry with him.

(iii 49–51) Its ritual: You set up an offering arrangement before the first star (to appear). You scatter dates (and) *sasqû*-flour. You set out *mersu*-confection made with honey (and) ghee. You perform a sacrifice (and) bring near the shoulder, ⌜caul fat⌝ (and) (some of the) roasted ⌜meat⌝. You pour out a libation of beer. You mix the "weapon" of *mirišmarû*, *rikibti arkabi*, *imḫur-ešra* (and) [*zê*] *malāḫi* with oil. You put (it) before the star (and) recite this recitation three times before the star.

(iii 52–54) "You, star that brightens [...] within the heavens, surveyor of the regions, I am so-and-so, son of son of so-and-so. On this night, I kneel before you. Judge my case, apply the law to my situation. May these plants undo my evil." You firmly rub his cheeks (with it) daily in the morning.

(iii 55) If ditto (for loss of cheek hair), you [...] the "weapon" of *amilānu*, *elikulla* (and) *kurkānu*-turmeric ⸢together⸣. [You ...] (it) [in] the hair of a virgin she-goat (and) put (it) on his neck.

(iii 56) Six recitations to bind fast the hair.

(iii 57–iv 8) *(see chapter 7, text 6)*

(iv 9–11) If a person's head (seems to) be pulsating, you twine together red-dyed wool (and) white wool (and) [thread] these eight stones on it: [...], ⸢*muššaru*-stone⸣, a small block of stone, Marḫaši carnelian, black obsidian, *ḫulālu*-chalcedony, ⸢AN.ZA.GUL.ME⸣-stone and ⸢*amašpû*-stone⸣. If you bind (it) on his temples, he should recover.

(iv 12–14) If a person's head [... and his ears continually] buzz, you [...] *kukru*, *burāšu*-juniper, *su'ādu*, *šimešallu*-aromatic, *balukku*-aromatic, [...], ⸢*šupuḫru*-cedar⸣, *sīḫu*-wormwood, ⸢*argānu*⸣, *barirātu* (and) "sweet reed." You grind (it) in fat from the unsalted kidney of a wether (and) in *erēnu*-cedar resin. You massage (it) into leather (and) bandage his head (with it).

(iv 15) [...], *baluḫḫu*-aromatic (and) *kurkānu*-turmeric: [#] ⸢fumigants⸣ for the head.

(iv 16–18) Salve for the head. You grind together these plants: white and black *kibrītu*-sulphur, male and female *nikiptu*, *mūṣu*-stone, *zalaqqu*-stone, *anzaḫḫu*-frit, *imbû tamtim*, *bīnu*-tamarisk seed, stag horn (and) human skull. You mix (it) with oil (and) *erēnu*-cedar resin and you smear his temples (with it).

(iv 19–20) Fumigant for the head. You finely crush together *atā'išu*, *kibrītu*-sulphur, *kurkānu*-turmeric (and) male and female *nikiptu*. You mix (it) with *erēnu*-cedar resin (and) fumigate him (with it) over coals.

(iv 21–22) [If a person's] ⸢head⸣ is sick/sore, you grind together *ṣaṣumtu*, *murdudû*, *upinzir*-insect (and) [...]. You make (it) into a dough with *kasû* juice. You shave his head, bandage (his head with it) and do not take (it) off for three days.

(iv 23–24) If a person's head (feels) heavy, you ‹(grind together)› *kukru*, *burāšu*-juniper, *atā'išu*, myrrh (and) ‹(*ninû*-mint)›. You mix (it) with *baluḫḫu*-aromatic resin (and) with fat from the ⸢kidney⸣ of an ox (and) massage (it) into ‹(waterproof)› leather. You shave (his head and) bandage (him with it) for five [days].[114]

(iv 25) […] right and left, three times […]. You make […] into a dough [with ⸢*kasû*⸣ [juice]. You gently rub (him with) oil (and) bandage (him with it).

(iv 26–28) If during the course of a person's illness, fever affects his head so that his head (feels like it) is so heavy that when he tries to stand, his head (seems to) draw him forward, to cure him, you grind *burāšu*-juniper, *margūṣu*, myrrh (and) *urnuqqu* in a mortar. You pour (it) into used grease. If you gently rub his head repeatedly (with it), the fever in his head should be extinguished.

(iv 29) ⸢Alternatively,⸣ you grind *kukru*, *burāšu*-juniper (and) *kamantu*-henna(?) seed. You mix (it) with used grease (and) gently rub his head repeatedly (with it).

(iv 30–31) If a person […], you dry, crush (and) sift […]. [You mix it] with […]. [You …] and do not take (it) off for three days.

(iv 32–36) If a person's head, his face, his eyes, his ⸢feet⸣, (and) his lips are swollen, his ⸢head⸣ (feels like it) draws him forward, his hands and his feet hurt him, his limbs are tense, (and) his body continually has ⸢numbness⸣,[115] to cure him, you crush and sift together *kukru*, *burāšu*-juniper, *atāʾišu*, *kamantu*-henna(?) seed, mill ground *saḫlû*-cress, *adāru*-poplar leaves, *kasû*, roasted grain flour, winnowed beerwort, *nikiptu*, (and) *šurdunû*. You make (it) into a dough with *kasû* juice. You shave his head. You rub his head with *šūšu*-licorice oil. You bandage (him with the dough) and do not take (it) off for seven days.

(iv 37) Alternatively, if you repeatedly […] with […], he should recover.

(iv 38–41) If the middle of a person's head stings him, his knees feel heavy (and) are continually ⸢tense⸣, [he] is continually tired, he continually has a crushing sensation in the chest, he continually changes the side of his ⸢kidney (lower back)⸣ (he sleeps on) […], he is continually thirsty, he is continually short of breath, in order for the illness not to […], you sun dry "sweet reed," *atāʾišu*, […], *šūnû*-chastetree, beerwort (mixed) with *kasû* juice, roasted grain flour, […] (and) *ḫaṭṭi reʾi*. You crush (and) sift (it). You make (it) into a dough with *kasû* juice (and) bandage (him with it).

(iv 42–47) *missing*

(iv 48′–49′. […] *bīnu*-tamarisk, […]. You have him drink (it mixed) either with first quality beer or with wine.

(iv 50′) If a person continually has a headache, *irrû* seed … (catchline)

C. UGU EXTRACT SERIES

The UGU series was sufficiently long and complicated that even ancient physicians found it cumbersome to use. This is presumably why the scribes of Uruk generated what was apparently essentially an abridged edition, with numbered *pirsu*-tablets arranged in sequence. So, for example, SpTU 1.44 and 46 represent the ninth and tenth tablets in this extract series. In addition, we have a number of *nisḫu*-tablets from Assur that contain a mixed bag of treatments. Of these, some seem to have been drawn primarily, if not exclusively, from the UGU series, not necessarily in any particular order. BAM 3, a text of this type, is published in Worthington 2006, 18–48. The first three columns are drawn from the first subseries, but with considerable dancing around. We begin at the beginning with a duplicate of the opening sections of BAM 480 (tablet 1), then off to skin problems (tablets 4–5), then back to BAM 480, then off to more skin problems, then back to BAM 480, off to yet more skin problems, then back to BAM 480 and finally on to BAM 482 and *AMT* 102/1 (tablets 2–3) before a final look at BAM 480. By iv 12, we have moved on to the second subseries (on the ears) and the catchline at the end indicates that the next extract tablet dealt with the third subseries (on the eyes). At least the subseries are in the correct order. Not so with other excerpt texts from Assur. BAM 152 col. i is drawn from the first subseries, col. ii from the eleventh, iii belongs somewhere in 7–9 range, and col. iv is from the twelfth. What does seem often to happen is that the excerpt text starts out with a citation from the beginning of a tablet. This is apparently the case with text 3.

TEXT 3: BAM 156

The first line is a citation of the incipit of the second tablet of the eighth subseries of UGU, and lines 1–24 probably all belong together.[116] Lines 25–31 are parallel to BAM 494 iii 24′–28′, which would place this section and the following lines down to 40 in the fifth tablet of the first subseries. Lines 41–47 duplicate BAM 480 iv 16–20, which makes them a citation of the first tablet of the first subseries. Finally, lines 48–50 appear to cite the first tablet of the third subseries.

1. [DIŠ N]A NAM.ÉRIM *šaḫ*-[*ḫi*]-*ḫu* GIG *mim-mu-u i-lem-mu*
2. *i*[*na*] ŠÀ-*šú la i-na-aḫ bal-ṭam*!-*ma*[117] *ana* DÚR-*šú ú-tab-bak*
3. NINDA NU GU$_7$ NA.BI GÍD-*ma* ÚŠ *ana maš-taq-ti-šú u bul-lu-ṭí-šú*
4. A NÍG.ÀR.RA A P[(Ú A)] ÍD A *a-gal-pe-e ḫi-iq* KAŠ

5. 1.T[A].ÀM D[UG o DIR]I-*ma ana* A NÍG.ÀR.RA GAZI^{SAR} *ana* A PÚ
6. ŠEM.ḪI.A [*ana* A Í]D ŠE.KAK ^{GIŠ}DÌḪ ŠE.KAK $^{\text{GIŠ.Ú}}$GÍR
7. *ana* A *a-g*[*al-*(*pe*)]*-e* ^{Ú}*ṣa-ṣu-un-tú* ^{GIŠ}ŠE.NA.A
8. *ana ḫi-i*[(*q* KA)]Š ^{ŠEM}MAN.DI GI.DÙG ŠUB ‹(*šum*$_{4}$*-ma* KAŠ LÚ.KÚRUN.NA ÚŠ)› *ina* UDUN ^{LÚ}KÚRUN.NA
9. BAD-*ki*[*r* (E)]$_{11}$*-ma* KÚM-*su-nu tu-še-eṣ-ṣi*
10. *t*[(*a*)]*-šá-ḫal* Ì.NUN EŠ.MEŠ-*su ina* ŠÀ RA-*su*

---

11. DIŠ KI.MIN ŠÀ ^{ŠEM}GIG ^{ŠEM}ŠEŠ ^{ŠEM}BULUḪ LAGAB ŠE.MUNU$_{7}$
12. *sik-ka-tu* GAZI^{SAR} KAŠ.ÚS.SA NUMUN ^{Ú}ÚKUŠ.GÍL Ú.ḪI.A
13. ŠEŠ 1-*niš* SÚD *ina* KAŠ ŠEG$_{6}$*-šal* Ì Ì.NUN *ana* ŠÀ ŠUB KÚM-*su*
14. *ana* DÚR-*šú* DUB-*ma* DIN

---

15. DIŠ KI.MIN ^{Ú}GEŠTIN.KA$_{5}$.A ZÍD GIG NUMUN GADA 1-*niš* ⸢SÚD⸣
16. [(*ana* ŠÀ) KAŠ (*tara-bak ina*) … (DIRI.DIRI)] LAL-*ti*

---

17. ^{GIŠ}*si-ḫu* ^{GIŠ}*ár-gan-nu* ^{GIŠ}LUM.ḪA ^{GIŠ}*šú-šú* ^{GIŠ}ŠE.NA.A
18. GAZI^{SAR} ^{Ú}*ak-tam* 7 Ú.ḪI.A *tir-ma-ak-tú* NAM.RÍN

---

19. ^{GIŠ}*al-la-nu* KA *tam-tim* ^{Ú}*a-zal-lá* ^{ŠEM}ŠEŠ 1-*niš* SÚD *ina* Ì.NUN
20. LÀL *u* DUḪ.LÀL 1-*niš* ḪE.ḪE EŠ-*su nap-šal-ti* NAM.RÍN

---

21. ^{ŠEM}GÚR.GÚR ^{ŠEM}LI ^{Ú}KUR.KUR ^{Ú}*tar-muš*$_{8}$ ^{Ú}*imḫur-lim* ^{Ú}*imḫur*-20
22. ^{ŠEM}ŠEŠ NA$_{4}$ *gab-i* ILLU LI.TAR ^{Ú}ḪAB ^{Ú}*ak-tam*
23. *saḫ-lí-i ni-nu-ú* GAZI^{SAR} 14 Ú.ḪI.A ŠEŠ 1-*niš* SÚD
24. *ina* KAŠ *ba-lu pa-tan* NAG.MEŠ-*ma ina-eš maš-qit* NAM.RÍM

---

25. DIŠ NA SAG.DU-*su ku-ra-ru* DIB-*it* ŠÈ-^{d}NISABA
26. ḪÁD.A SÚD LAL *ina še-rim ku-ra-ar-šú* SAR-*ab*
27. *laq-laq-ta-šú ta-ta-bal ina* KAŠ LUḪ-*si*
28. KU.KU ^{GIŠ}TÚG MAR-*rù* LAL *in*[(*a* I)]GI KI.NÁ-*šú* DU$_{8}$*-šú-ma*
29. *tu-šá-kal ina* KAŠ LUḪ-*si* KU.KU ^{GIŠ}*e-lam-ma-ki*
30. KU.KU ^{GIŠ}TÚG KU.KU ^{GIŠ}*kal-mar-ḫi* ŠÈ-^{d}NISABA
31. GAZI^{SAR} BÍL-*ti* MAR!-*rù* LAL

---

32. DIŠ KI.MIN KÀŠ ÁB SAG.DU-*su te-sír* A NAGA.SI
33. A GAZI^{SAR} LUḪ-*si* SAG.DU-*su* SAR-*ab*
34. NUMUN ^{GIŠ}ŠE.NA.A NUMUN ^{GIŠ}[(N)]AM.TAR NUMUN ^{GIŠ}*qut-ri* ^{Ú}ÁB.DUḪ

35. [(PA)] ⸢^{Ú}⸣TÁL.TÁL ⸢^{GIŠ}⸣x[o] ⸢^{Ú}*ru*⸣-*uš-ru-šu* ^{Ú}*ṣa-ṣu-um-tu*
36. ^{Ú}KUR.GI.ÉRIN.NA ^{Ú}*te-gi-la-a* ⸢^{Ú}MÁ⸣.EREŠ.MÁ.LÁ
37. ^{Ú}MAŠ.ḪUŠ 11 Ú.MEŠ ḪÁD.A GAZ SIM *ina* A GAZI$^{\text{SA[R]}}$
38. SILA$_{11}$-*aš* GUR-*ma* ḪÁD.A GAZ SIM *ina* KAŠ.SAG *u* A.GEŠTIN.NA ḪE.ḪE
39. SAG.DU-*su* LAL-*ma* U$_{4}$.3.KÁM NU DU$_{8}$

---

40. DIŠ KI.MIN ^{Ú}GAMUN.GI$_{6}$ *kib-rit* SÚD *ina* Ì EŠ.MEŠ DIN

---

41. *nap-šal-tu* SAG.DU KI.A.^{d}ÍD BABBAR GI$_{6}$ *ni-kip-tú* NITA *u* MUNUS
42. $^{\text{NA}_4}$*mu-ṣa* $^{\text{NA}_4}$ZÁLAG $^{\text{NA}_4}$AN.ZAḪ KA *tam-tim* NUMUN ^{GIŠ}*bi-ni*
43. *gul-gul* NAM.LÚ.U$_{18}$.LU SI DÀRA.MAŠ Ú.MEŠ ŠEŠ 1-*niš* SÚD
44. *ina* Ì *u* MÚD ^{GIŠ}*ere-ini* ḪE.ḪE-*ma* SAG.KI.MEŠ-*šú tu-lap-pat*

---

45. *qù-taru* SAG.DU ^{Ú}KUR.KUR *kib-rit* ^{Ú}*kur-ka-nam*
46. *ni-kip-tu* NÍTA *u* MUNUS 1-*niš tu-daq-qaq*
47. [(*ina* MU)]D ^{GIŠ} *ere-ini* ḪE.ḪE-*ma ina* DÈ SAR-*šú*

---

48. [DIŠ NA] IGI^{II}-*šú* GIG *saḫ-lé-e bu-tú-tú ina šur-šum-me* KAŠ
49. [SILA$_{11}$-*aš*] IGI^{II}-*šú* LAL-*ma* DIN

---

50. [DIŠ KI].MIN ZÌ.ŠE.SA.A *ina* A GAZI^{SAR} *tara-bak* LAL

Translation

(1–10) [If a] ⸢person⸣ is sick with a ⸢wasting⸣ curse, everything he eats does not rest easy in his stomach but he pours (it) raw into his anus (and) he cannot eat bread, if it is prolonged, that person will die. For his splitting off and to cure him,[118] ⸢you fill⸣ one [bowl] each with groat water, well water, river water, inundation basin[119] water (and) *ḫīqu* beer. You pour *kasû* into the groat water. (You pour) *labanātu*-incense into the well water. (You pour) *baltu*-thorn shoots (and) *ašāgu*-thorn shoots into the ⸢river⸣ [water]. You pour *ṣaṣuntu* (and) *šūnû*-chastetree into the inundation basin water. (You pour) *suʾādu* (and) "sweet reed" into the *ḫīqu* beer. ‹(If you use *kurunnu*-beer, he will die.)›[120] You bake (them) in a brewer's oven. You take (them) out and filter (them) while they are still hot. You repeatedly rub him with ghee (and) bathe him with them.

(11–14) Alternatively, you grind together these plants: *kanaktu*-aromatic pith, myrrh, *baluḫḫu*-aromatic, malt lumps, *sikkatu*-yeast, *kasû*, beerwort (and)

irrû seed. You boil (it) in beer. You pour oil (and) ghee into it and if you pour (it) into his anus while it is still hot, he should recover.

(15–16) Alternatively, you grind together "fox grape," wheat flour (and) flax seed. You decoct (it)[121] in [beer ... until] it is softened. (This is) a bandage.

(17–18) *Sīḫu*-wormwood, *argānu*-tree, *barirātu*, *šūšu*-licorice, *šūnû*-chaste-tree, *kasû* (and) *aktam* are seven plants, a bath for a curse.

(19–20) You grind together *allānu*-oak, *imbû tamtim*, *azallû* (and) myrrh. You mix (it) together with ghee, honey (and) wax (and) gently rub him (with it). (This is) a salve for a curse.

(21–24) You grind together these fourteen plants: *kukru*, *burāšu*-juniper, *atā'išu*, *tarmuš*, *imḫur-lim*, *imḫur-ešra*, myrrh, alum, *abukkatu* resin, *šammi bu'šāni*, *aktam*, *saḫlû*-cress, *nīnû*-mint (and) *kasû*. If you have him repeatedly drink (it mixed) with beer on an empty stomach, he should recover. It is a potion (to loosen) a curse.[122]

(25–31) If *kurāru* afflicts a person's head, you dry (and) grind chaff (and) bandage (him with it). In the morning, you shave his *kurāru* (and) remove its detritus. You wash (it) with beer. You daub on powdered *taskarinnu*-tree (and) bandage (him). Before he goes to bed, you take (the bandage) off and polish (the *kurāru*).[123] You wash (it) with beer. You daub on powdered *elammaku*-tree, powdered *taskarinnu*-tree, powdered *kalmarḫu*-tree, chaff (and) roasted *kasû* (and) bandage (him).

(32–39) Alternatively, you plaster his head with cow urine. You wash (it) with *uḫḫūlu qarnānu* infusion (i.e. liquid soap) (and) *kasû* juice. You shave his head. You dry, crush (and) sift (these) eleven plants: *šūnû*-chastetree seed, *pillû* seed, *qutru* seed, *kamantu*-henna(?), *urânu* leaves, [...], *rušruššu*, *ṣaṣumtu*, *kurkānu*-turmeric, *tigilû*, *mirišmara* (and) *kalbānu*. You make (it) into a dough with *kasû* juice. You redry, crush (and) sift (it). You mix (it) with first quality beer and vinegar. You bandage his head (with it) and do not take (it) off for three days.

(40) Alternatively, you grind *zibû* (and) *kibrītu*-sulphur (and) repeatedly rub (him) gently (with it mixed) with oil. He should recover.

(41–44) For a head salve, you grind together these plants: white (and) black *kibrītu*-sulphur, male and female *nikiptu*, *mūṣu*-stone, *zalāqu*-stone, *anzaḫḫu*-frit, *imbû tamtim*, *bīnu*-tamarisk seed, human skull (and) stag horn. You mix (it) with oil and *erēnu*-cedar resin and you smear his temples (with it).

(45–47) Fumigant for the head. You crush together *atā'išu*, *kibrītu*-sulphur, *kurkānu*-turmeric (and) male and female *nikiptu* finely. You mix (it) with *erēnu*-cedar resin and fumigate him (with it) over coals.

(48–49) [If a person]'s eyes are sore, [you make a dough] of *saḫlû-cress* (and) *buṭuttu*-cereal with beer dregs. If you bandage his eyes (with it), he should recover.

(50) ⌜Alternatively⌝, you decoct roasted grain flour in *kasû* juice (and) bandage (him with it).

NOTES

1. For a discussion of reconstruction efforts to date (without the benefit of the UGU catalogue), see Heeßel 2011c, 31–35.

2. So already Köcher 1978, 20.

3. For this interpretation of SUR.GIBIL, see Stol 2007b, 241–42.

4. A colophon on a fragmentary text from Uruk (SpTU 1.48 rev. 7′) gives 45? as the number of tablets in the series as a whole. A nose count of the minimum number of tablets which will have been listed in the catalog, however, yields 48. These figures can be reconciled by assuming that a third row of wedges at the top of the "45" is now invisible due to effacing of the tablet.

5. *AMT* 102/1 has *šum-ma* (for DIŠ) and *il-ta-za-az-ma* (for ZAL) but there is not enough room for all of this here.

6. Restored from the UGU extract BAM 3 i 37.

7. Since the name of a subseries is always the incipit of the first tablet, line 8 may be restored from line 10.

8. Restored from BAM 506:8′.

9. Restored from the UGU extract Heeßel and Al-Rawi 2003, 223 ii 15′. 10. See Scurlock and Andersen 2005, 9.9.

11. See Scurlock and Andersen 2005, 13.145.

12. See Scurlock and Andersen 2005, 13.155.

13. For *ṣētu*, see Scurlock and Andersen 2005, 53–61.

14. For *kibšu*, see Scurlock and Andersen 2005, 234–35.

15. For *ašû*, see Scurlock and Andersen 2005, 224–26.

16. For ringing ears, see Scurlock and Andersen 2005, 205–6.

17. For *murdinnu*, see Scurlock and Andersen 2005, 190.

18. BAM vol. 5, xxix.

19. Restored from line 3′, BAM 530 iv 2′ and BAM 524 ii 4′.

20. BAM 543 i 1 adds: *u ri-šu-tú* [TUKU-*ši*].

21. BAM 547 iv 13′ adds: NINDA *u* A *ina* GABA-*šú* GUB.MEŠ-*zu ḫa-aḫ-ḫa* TUKU.MEŠ.

22. *AMT* 49/4 obv. 2 adds: ḪAR.MEŠ GIG.

23. Restored from BAM 575 iii 42.

24. Restored from BAM 575 iii 49 which adds: *di-ig-la ma-a-ṭi*.

25. See Scurlock 2006, no. 191a.

26. Restored from excerpt tablet BAM 156 obv. 1.

27. For moving teeth, see Scurlock and Andersen 2005, 419–20. BAM 543 i 1 adds: "and (the gums) [have] redness." See Scurlock and Andersen 2005, 18.6.

28. An *apû* was a pit which gave access from the upper to the Netherworld. For references, see *CAD* A/2, 201a.

29. The use of the G-stem form of *palāsu* suggests considerable antiquity for this recitation; see *CAD* P, 52–58.

30. Presumably, whatever it was that looked at the child is responsible for the teething problems that it is experiencing.

31. See Scurlock and Andersen 2005, 9.118.

32. BAM 547 iv 13′ adds: "bread and water stick in his chest (and) he continually has *ḫaḫḫu* (bloody sputum)." See Scurlock and Andersen 2005, 3.74.

33. *AMT* 49/4 obv. 2 adds: "sick lungs." See Scurlock and Andersen 2005, 3.89.

34. For *guḫḫu*-cough, see Scurlock and Andersen 2005, 178–79.

35. For *suʾālu*-cough, see Scurlock and Andersen 2005, 178.

36. See Scurlock and Andersen 2005, 8.73.

37. For *šīqu*, see Scurlock and Andersen 2005, 42 with n. 84.

38. For *kīs libbi*, see Scurlock and Andersen 2005, 131–32.

39. Cf. Scurlock and Andersen 2005, 6.110.

40. For "internal fever," see Scurlock and Andersen 2005, 129–30.

41. See Scurlock and Andersen 2005, 6.37.

42. For "wind blasting," see Scurlock and Andersen 2005, 91–92, 203.

43. See Scurlock and Andersen 2005, 6.34.

44. BAM 575 iii 49 adds: "his eyesight is diminished." See Scurlock and Andersen 2005, 15.13.

45. See Scurlock and Andersen 2005, 53–61.

46. See Scurlock and Andersen 2005, 288–89.

47. For the full citation, see Scurlock and Andersen 2005, 6.71, 7.14, 7.21.

48. BAM vol. 6, xxiii–xxiv.

49. Beckman and Foster 1988, 1–2.

50. Restored from K 3661 iv 18′//*AMT* 44/7 iv 2′ (AMD 8/1 text 7.5). Abusch and Schwemer (2011, 128 ad 17′–18′) quote a suggestion made to them by N. Heeßel that this line is to be restored after *AMT* 43/6 whose incipit (*AMT* 43/6 obv. 1) matches the catchline of tablet 5 of the *suʾālu* subseries (BAM 579 iv 44). This is, however, hardly possible since *AMT* 43/6 represents the sixth tablet of the seventh subseries whereas this would be the eighth tablet of the ninth subseries of UGU.

51. As suggested by Geller, BAM VII, 247.

52. Restored from BAM 205:19′–21′//*STT* 95:16–18//*STT* 280 ii 1–3. For the rest of the associated symptoms, see Scurlock and Andersen 2005, 4.7.

53. Restored from BAM 396 i 23′//*AMT* 66/7 iii 18. This is considerably abbreviated; for the full citation, see Scurlock and Andersen 2005, 5.54

54. For the full citation, see Scurlock and Andersen 2005, 6.187.

55. For the full citation, see Scurlock and Andersen 2005, 13.210.

56. For the full citation, see Scurlock and Andersen 2005, 11.58.

57. See *AMT* 74/1 ii 24.

58. Restored from BAM 32:16′–18′.

59. See *AMT* 75/1 iv 17, 19, 23.

60. See Scurlock and Andersen 2005, 102–3.

61. See Scurlock and Andersen 2005, 5.54.

62. For *šapāku* as "tense," see Scurlock and Andersen 2005, 293.

63. See Scurlock and Andersen 2005, 103.

64. See Scurlock and Andersen 2005, 13.210.

65. See Scurlock and Andersen 2005, 150–53.

66. See Scurlock and Andersen 2005, 11.58.

67. For *mungu*, see Scurlock and Andersen 2005, 249–50.

68. For *maškādu*, see Scurlock and Andersen 2005, 257–58.

69. For *sagallu*, see ibid.

70. For *šaššaṭu*, see Scurlock and Andersen 2005, 66–68.

71. For this interpretation of SUR.GIBIL, see Stol 2007b, 241–42.
72. See Abusch and Schwemer, AMD 8/1 text 7.5.
73. See Schuster-Brandis 2008, 311 and Reiner 1995, 129 n. 604.
74. See AMD 8/1, 101.
75. See BAM VII, no. 9 text J.
76. See BAM VII, nos. 2 text B and 8 text H, respectively.
77. See BAM VII, no. 16 text Q.
78. See BAM VII, no. 22 text W.
79. Note that BAM VII, 142 miscombines the incipit of tablet 2 with the incipit of tablet 3 from the catalog.
80. See BAM VII, no. 23 text X.
81. See BAM VII, no. 24 text Y.
82. See BAM VII, no. 25 text Z.
83. See Prechel and Richter 2001 333–72.
84. See chapter 7, text 6.
85. BAM 3 i 11 has MAR.ME-*ma* DIN-*uṭ*.
86. BAM 3 i 12 substitutes 4 GÍN IM.BABBAR for 10 GÍN *ḫiqati*.
87. Here apparently begins the indirect join-piece K 13417, which Köcher copied as part of BAM 480 i, but placed 3 lines too high. Worthington (2005, 6) noticed that it was incorrectly placed, but did not attempt to place it.
88. The procedure is restored from lines i 42′ and iii 13.
89. The procedure is restored from lines i 31 and iii 13.
90. Pace Worthington (2005, 3). A reading *u* $\check{S}E_{10}$ is completely out of the question—different types of excrement have different names in Akkadian as in Arabic, and what gazelles leave behind is *never* referred to as $\check{S}E_{10}$, any more than human excrement would be referred to as A.GAR.GAR.
91. BAM 12: 41′–42′ replaces ^{Ú}ZA.BA.LAM with $^{Ú!}$NIGIN^{SAR}. These are equivalents; see Uruanna I 434, apud *CAD* S, 391.
92. KEŠDA is rarely, if ever, used for tying on bandages; in any case, SAR is a common determinative for plants that have to be grown in gardens.
93. BAM 3 i 20–22 replaces ^{ŠEM}GÚR.GÚR with ^{ŠEM}GAM.MA.
94. BAM 3 ii 40 replaces DÈ *ṣarbate* with *qut-ra-ta*$_5$.
95. The sign as copied is a SAR, but this is not clearly distinguished from EZEN in late texts.
96. OECT 11.71: 8′ has: KA.INIM.MA SÍG SAG.DU NÍG.GUB ŠU.DU$_8$.A.KÁM. ŠU.DU$_8$.A is often, in Old Babylonian inscriptions, written for ŠU.DÙ.A = *kamû*: "to hold fast," which confirms the reading of KÉŠ.DA = *rakasu*: "to bind." See Borger, 1957, 4–5.
97. BAM 3 ii 43–46 adds: SAG.DU-*su* SAR-*ab rib-ki ina* A GAZI^{SAR} KÚM ŠID LAL-*id*.
98. The reading of the verb follows *CAD* B, 73a; *AHw* 208a reads *i-tel-li* from Gt of *elû*.
99. The term UGU refers to the upper part of the head and its contents, which ancient Mesoptamians recognized as the seat of cognition. See Westenholz and Sigrist 2006, 1–10.
100. After a suggestion by Stol 1993, 94.
101. For the translation of *saḫlû* as "cress," see Stol 1983–84, 24–32.
102. Literally: "lost."
103. When you make mustard, you grind the seeds with salt and vinegar. In this case, not only were the salt and vinegar to be left out, but a new millstone was to be employed to ensure that there were no traces of salt or vinegar in the ground seeds. (Allergy sufferers recognize this problem, and may have to avoid purchasing items made on machinery which was previously used to process the allergen.) Both salt and vinegar strengthen purgatives. In this case, they

wanted him to vomit up what was draining out of his sinuses, but not too violently.

104. Pace *CAD* R, 344–45, this is certainly not "bat guano." Akk. *rikibtu* means "musk," and there are any number of plant and animal substances that share the smell and some of the properties of real musk.

105. The term *sāqu* is used to describe a part of an animal's body, but is also a synonym for pickled meat (*muddulu*). Presumably, the cut in question was typically used for pickling, like our ham.

106. Pace Worthington 2005, line 65, "fresh" is invariably written SIG_7 and "you take" is invariably TI-*qí*.

107. See *CAD* Š/1, 309 s.v. *šamāṭu* mng. 1d′.

108. The patient feels so hot that he refuses to have even a sheet over him.

109. See *AHw* 933b and *CAD* R, s.v. *rabāku*. Heeßel 2011c, 46 n. 112 follows Goltz in disputing Landsberger's identification in favor of "making a paste." The argument is that boiling and filtering (as one would do in preparing a decoction) are separately mentioned and that, therefore, *rabāku* must be something else. However, grinding plants and mixing them with oil or fat, i.e., making a paste, is also separately mentioned and cannot, by the same logic, be what is meant. A *ribku* can be solid, since, in this and a number of other passages (for references, see *CAD* R, 321), you make a *ribku* into a dough using a hot liquid. Alternatively, it can be a liquid as in BAM 106 obv. 1–10 (chapter 6, text 4) where a *ribku* is baked and then filtered, hardly possible with a solid. A survey of currently available references suggests that what was contemplated was indeed a decoction, made by crushing plants and cooking them in boiling liquid. The resulting decoction could be left as a liquid or, by the simple expedient of adding flour and continuing to cook the mixture, a virtually solid substance could be obtained.

110. Stol, apud Worthington 2005, 27 ad 160′ suggests reading MÚ.DA and interprets this as "grow back."

111. The reference is apparently to a shiny bald spot.

112. The correct expression would be BAR.ŠÈ but our scribe has substituted a pseudo-Sumerogram I.DI (from Akkadian *idu*, "side").

113. The phrase gains its power from the fact that the verb *lapātu*: "to rub/smear" (a reference to the salve) uses the same Sumerogram as *lemnu*: "evil."

114. BAM 3 ii 43–46 adds: You shave his head. You make a dough out of a decoction with hot *kasû* juice (and) bandage him with it.

115. See Scurlock and Andersen 2005, 5.39.

116. See above Beckman and Foster 1988, no. 9b: 21′.

117. Alternatively, one could read, with Maul (2011, 146) BAL *mim-ma-ma*. In that case. the food would turn round and every bit of it end up pouring out of the anus. In either case, it is passing through essentially undigested.

118. See Scurlock and Andersen 2005, 6.71, 7.14, 7.21.

119. For this interpretation, based on an improved reading, see Herrero 1975, 51 ad ii 2.

120. This warning appears only in Herrero 1975, 41–53 ii 5.

121. See above, n. 109.

122. The parallels use this for *ṣētu* (enteric fever)" as well as for "curse."

123. See Deller 1990.

4

MEDICAL TEXT COMMENTARIES

A. THERAPEUTIC SERIES COMMENTARY

Text commentaries in general formed an advanced stage of the pedagogic process also attested in the Hippocratic corpus. Writing such commentaries was the manner in which a student could fully demonstrate the extent of his knowledge, as is explicitly stated in the colophon to text 4: "Commentary (based on) oral tradition and questions from the mouth of an expert in it." It is also noteworthy that, not only are all commentaries unique, but we actually possess three different commentaries on the same exact original text.[1] Moreover, this particular format really separated the poor student, whose commentary carefully belabored the obvious and skipped over the difficult parts, from the truly expert who could not only explain all difficult and rare words but also grasp the deeper meanings which lay behind apparently ordinary phrases.

For the late periods at least, when school days were over, scholars continued to use the commentary format to tease ever deeper meanings from the material at hand, much in the way that contemporary Jewish scholars of the Hellenistic age were using this format to expand knowledge of the law or to engage in philosophical speculations (so, for example, Philo of Alexandria's Genesis commentary).

TEXT 1: SpTU 1.47

SpTU 1.47[2] is a commentary on SpTU 1.46, an extract tablet from the UGU series. For the most part, SpTU 1.47 confines itself to explaining rare or obscure words, not always with the best of success (9–10). Occasionally, however, the ancient commentator ventured a bit further afield, providing the interesting information that goat leather was used because the *rābiṣu*-demon had the face of a goat (13–14) and that the toilet demon's attacks were due to a lack of sanitation (2b–5), which is why well water was used in the treatment (14–15). Typical of many commentaries is the search for deeper meanings through creative retranslation. In this case, the sanitation issue is derived from taking the demon Shulak's name apart into syllables, so *Šu-la-ku*, then treating the syllables as if they were actual Sumerian or Pseudo-Sumerian words, so ŠU LA KÙ, yielding: "Unclean Hands."

1. DIŠ NA EME-*šú eb-ṭe-et-ma* : *e-bé-ṭu* : *na-pa-ḫu*
2. *e-bé-ṭu* : *ra-bu-ú* : MAŠKIM *mu-sa-a-ti* : ^{d}*Šu-lak*
3. *a-na* É *mu-sa-a-tú* NU KU$_4$-*ub* : ^{d}*Šu-lak* SÌG-*su*
4. ^{d}*Šu-lak šá* E-*ú* : ŠU : *qa-tum* : LA : *la-a* : KÙ : *el-lu*
5. *ana* É *mu-sa-a-tú* KU$_4$-*ub* ŠU^{II}-*šú* NU KÙ *ana* UGU *qa-bi*
6. *lu-ur-pa-ni ki-ma* ^{NA_4}ZA.GÌN-*ma* ZÁLAG *ta-kip šá-niš lu-ur-pa-ni* : IM.GÁ.LU
7. *mi-šit-tú* : *ma-šá-du* : *ma-ḫa-ṣu* : *mi-šit-tú* : *šá in-šu-ú*
8. *šá* TAR-*šú im-ta-šid mi-šit-tú* : IGI-*šú i-ṣa-par* : BAR : *ṣa-pa-ru*
9. BAR : *za-a-ru* : *ur*-GA-*at-tú la it-ta-na-a-a-al*
10. *ur*-^{qa}GA-*at-tú* : *bu-uš-qí-it-tú* : *muš-šu-da* : *muš-šu-ʾu*
11. *áš-šú maš-maš-ú-tu ki-i qa-bu-ú* : Ì.UDU ^{ŠEM}GIG *šá* Ì.GIŠ *ú-kal-lu*
12. ^{ŠEM}GIG SÚD EN Ì.GIŠ È-*a* : Ì.UDU *e-riš-ti* : Ì.UDU *ku-ri-tum*
13. *ina* KUŠ ÙZ *šip-ki* : *šip-ki* : *ṭu-ub-bu* : MAŠKIM KA LÚ *uṣ-ṣab-b*[*i-it*]
14. MAŠKIM : *pa-ni* ÙZ *šá-kin* : A PÚ *šá* E-*ú* : *ina* ŠÀ *šá* MAŠKIM *mu-sa-*⸢*a*⸣-[*ti*]
15. ^{d}*Šu-lak* : *lu-ú* ^{d}*Šu-lak šá mu-sa-a-*[*ti*]
16. *ina* KUŠ ⸢ŠI⸣-*pí* :[3] *ina* KUŠ *ta-šap-pi* : ŠI : [*šá-pu-ú*]
17. AL.ÚS.SA : *ši-iq* : *ṭa-ba-a-tú* […]
18. GURUN Ú.KUR.RA : NUMUN Ú.KUR.RA : SAG.DU […]
19. *šá* MUL.SIM.MAḪ : ^{d}*Dil-bat* : SIM *s*[*i-nu-un-tú*]
20. […] NUNDUN : ^{d}NIN x […]
21. traces only

rev.

1′–6′. colophon

Translation

1–2a. "If a person's tongue is cramped (enlarged) (so that it fills his mouth)."[4] "To cramp" means "to swell." "To cramp" means "to get bigger."

2b–5. "The *rābiṣu* of the toilet" is Shulak.[5] He should not go into the toilet. (Otherwise) Shulak will strike him. What is said of Shulak is that ŠU means "hand," LA means "not" and KÙ means "clean." He went into the toilet, (so) his hands are unclean. This is what is said about it.

6. *Lurpānu*[6] looks like lapis lazuli but spotted with sparkles. Secondly, *lurpānu* is (like) *kalû*-paste.

7–10. "Stroke" is from "to cause a stroke" which means "to strike." He who has forgotten what was decided for/apportioned to him has had a stroke.

"His eye flutters." BAR means "to flutter." BAR (also) means to "to twist."

"He is continually wakeful[7] and cannot sleep." *ur*-^{qa}GA-*at-tú* means "greenery" (oops!).[8]

"To massage" means "to rub."[9]

11–14a. ("You do his medical treatment") because this is a medical treatment, as it says.

"Fat of *kanaktu*-aromatic which contains oil." You grind the *kanaktu*-aromatic until the oil comes out.

Erištu-fat means marrow from the short-bone (of sheep or goats).

"In *šipku* goat leather." *Šipku* means "submerged."[10] (The treatment is for cases where) a *rābiṣu*-demon ⸢has seized⸣ a person's mouth. (Goat leather is used because) a *rābiṣu*-demon has the face of a goat.[11]

14b–15. When it says "well water,"[12] it is because it involves the *rābiṣu* of the ⸢toilet⸣. That is Shulak or Shulak of the ⸢toilet⸣.

16. "You ŠI (it) in a leather bag" means "You sew (it) up in a leather bag." ŠI means ["to sew up"].

17–18a. AL.ÚS.SA means *šiqqu*-garum.[13] Vinegar [...].

Nīnû "fruit" means *Nīnû* seed.

18b–19. "The head [...] of the Dove (Southern Fish of Pisces)" is Venus. SIM means ⸢"dove"⸣.

B. PRACTICAL INDIVIDUAL TEXT COMMENTARY

TEXT 2: BRM 4.32 AND TCL 6.34 i

TCL 6.34 i 1′–9′

TCL 6.34 provided treatments in cols. i–ii for epilepsy, col. iii for a crushing sensation in the chest,[14] and column iv for fever.[15] The ritual in TCL 6.34 i 2′–3′ requires an adult male goat to have a specified recitation recited three times into each ear and then be slaughtered. Various parts of the goat are then to be used in a variety of ways (aliment, potion, salve, and fumigant). Without the commentary in BRM 4.32 lines 4b–5a, TCL 6.34 i 4′–5′ would have been impenetrable. It is, however, clear that the actual text on which BRM 4.32 was commenting was not an exact duplicate of TCL 6.34. So, the latter text does not have "Hand" of ghost among the symptoms; neither does it have either A.RI.A NAM.LÚ.U_{18}.

LU or MÚD *ka-mi-i*, using instead these medicaments' real names. Moreover, the original of BRM 4.32 apparently had its plants in a different order from that of TCL 6.34 i 5′–8′, and had TÚG.NÍG.DÁRA.ŠU.LAL and ZÍD ŠE.MUŠ$_5$ in place of the gold and silver [beads].

1′. [DIŠ AN.T]A.ŠUB.BA ^{d}LUGAL.ÙR.RA ŠU ^{d}INNIN.NA ‹ŠU.GIDIM.MA›
2′. [UGU] LÚ GÁL-*ši ana* ZI-*ḫi* DÙ.DÙ.BI MÁŠ.ZU TI-*qí*
3′. [*ana*] GEŠTU^{II}-*šú šá* 15 *u* 150-*šú* ÉN *lem-nu* MIN[16] ‹(3-*šú*)› ŠID-*nu* KUD-*is*
4′. ⸢*ina*⸣ *ši-lip* GÍR *ši-i ta-*ʾ*a šá ḫu-pat* SAG.DU *u* GÚ
5′. A.MEŠ GI$_6$ IGI^{II}-*šú* TI-*qí* Ì.ḪUL Ì.KU$_6$ MÚD ^{GIŠ}ERIN
6′. ^{Ú}IN$_6$.ÚŠ (variant: A.RI.A LÚ.U$_{18/19}$.LU) NUMUN ^{Ú}IN$_6$.ÚŠ MÚD MUŠEN *qa-di-i* (variant: MÚD *ka-mi-i*) ‹(1-*niš* ḪE.ḪE)› KUŠ ^{d}*Ku-ši*
7′. [NA$_4$.MEŠ?] ^{d}*Ku-ši* KÙ.SIG$_{17}$ KÙ.BABBAR.MEŠ ^{Ú}*tar-muš* ^{Ú}*imḫur-lim* ^{Ú}*imḫur-ešra*
8′. [(*ana* ŠÀ ‹MÚD MÁŠ.ZU› ŠUB-*di*)] GU$_7$-*šú* NAG-*šú* ŠÉŠ-*su u ina* DÈ SAR-*šú-ma* DIN-*uṭ*
9′. [...] KÙ.GUR *šá* MÁŠ.ZU

TRANSLATION

(1′–9′) [If] ⸢AN.TA.ŠUB.BA⸣ ^{d}LUGAL.ÙR.RA, "Hand" of a god, "Hand" of a goddess ‹or "Hand" of a ghost› is [upon] a person, the ritual to remove (them) is: You take an adult male goat. You recite the recitation: "Evil, evil" ‹(three times)› into its right and left ears. You slaughter (it). Sliding in that dagger, you take, in the depths of the socket of head and neck, the liquid from the pupil of its eye. ‹(You mix together)› naptha, fish oil, *erēnu*-cedar resin, *maštakal*, *maštakal* seed (and) owl blood. You pour (this plus) Kušu's hide, Kušu's [beads of] gold (and) silver, *tarmuš*, *imḫur-lim*, (and) *imḫur-ešra* into the blood of the adult male goat. If you have him eat (it), drink (it), rub him gently (with it, and) fumigate him (with it) over coals, he should recover. Fumigant with an adult male goat.

BRM 4.32

BRM 4.32 is a commentary which partially duplicates TCL 6.34, col. i. The author was certainly a practicing physician, since he provides the symptoms distinguishing various syndromes in lines 1b–4a. It is, from every perspective, one of the most useful of the preserved commentaries since it concentrates on translation and explanation for difficult terms and is surprisingly free of esotericisms.

Our ancient commentator provides many useful plant equivalents, quoting in several cases from preserved sections of URU.AN.NA (e.g., 6, 19, 20) and *Šammu šikinšu* (e.g., 7, 18–19). The only entry that presents any real difficulties is line 28, which reads, if translated literally: ⸢"Caterpillar"⸣ means "dormouse" or "effeminate of Subartu." This apparently bizarre entry may be readily decoded by appreciating that any number of lexical equivalencies refer to the substitutability of one item for another in one of the omen series, in this case *Šumma Alu*. What this tells us, then, is that "If a black dormouse is seen in a person's house (CT 40 29 [80-7-19, 85] obv. 2) has the same predicted outcome as "If a black caterpillar is seen in a person's house" or "If a black effeminate of Subartu is seen in a person's house."

Arguably the most interesting piece of new information appears in lines 8c–10a, which read: "Kušu's hide" means the hide of the black ox which is over the *bīnu*-tamarisk planted in the Western city gate for Kušu. The "tendrils of Kušu" means the tendrils of the *bīnu*-tamarisk on which the hide of a black ox is placed for Kušu. Kušu is lexically identified as one of the *asakku*-demons and sons of Anu who were defeated by Ninurta.[17] A cultic commentary[18] also equates him with the *mašḫultuppu*. This latter was a scapegoat which was a sort of stuffed animal made and set up to draw evils off from patients. This particular example involves an oxhide placed over a tamarisk shoot planted in the Western city gate as part of the celebration of Ninurta's *akītu*. The idea was apparently that the victorious Ninurta flayed his enemy's hide and draped it onto a tamarisk-bush, a manly deed which was ritually reenacted with a view to using the result for prophylactic purposes, as with advent candles in our own folk tradition.

1. SI DÀRA.MAŠ : *qar-nu a-a-lu* : SI : *qar-nu* : DÀRA.MAŠ : *a-a-lu* : DIŠ : *šum-mu* : AN.TA.ŠUB.BA : *mar-ṣa uḫ-tan-naq ù* ÚḪ-*su* ŠUB.ŠUB-*a* AN.TA.ŠUB.BA
2. ^{d}LUGAL.ÙR.RA : IGI^{II} 15-*šú u* 150-*šú i-kap-pi-iṣ* ^{d}LUGAL.ÙR.RA : ŠU.DINGIR.RA : DINGIR.MEŠ *i-nam-zar šil-lat i-qab-bi šá im-mar i-maḫ-ḫaṣ* ŠU.DINGIR.RA : ŠU ^{d}INNIN.NA :
3. *ḫu-uṣ-ṣi* GAZ ŠÀ TUKU.TUKU-*ši ù* INIM.MEŠ-*šú im-ta-na-áš-ši* ŠU ^{d}INNIN.NA : ŠU.GIDIM.MA GEŠTU$^{II.MEŠ}$-*šú* GÙ.DÉ.MEŠ *ma-gal iṭ-ṭè-né-pi šin-na-šú ana ma-ka-le-e*
4. *la ú-qar-ra-ba-ma* ŠU.GIDIM.MA : DÙ.DÙ.BI : *e-pu-uš-ta-šú* : *nap-šar-šú* : *ú-ru-di-su* : *ta-a* : *a-par* : *ḫu-up-‹pat›* IGI : *šup-lu* IGI : *šup-lu* : *a-par šá* SAG.DU
5. *u* ‹‹x›› GÚ[19] : Ì.ḪUL : *nap-ṭu* : Ì.KU$_6$: *šam-ni nu-ú-nu* : A.RI.A NAM.

LÚ.U$_{18}$.LU : ^{Ú}*maš-ta-kal* : *áš-šú* Ú A.RI.A : ^{Ú}*maš-ta-kal šá-niš* A.RI.A *re-ḫu-tú* :

6. TÚG.NÍG.DÁRA : *ú-la-pi* : ŠU.LÁL : *lu-up-pu-ut-tum* : TÚG.NÍG. DÁRA.ŠU.LÁL : UZU KA$_5$.A[20] : ^{Ú}*tar-muš* : *ki-ma* SUḪUŠ ^{Ú}*si-il-qa* : ^{Ú}*imḫur-lim ki-ma* GÌR.PAD.DU NAM.LÚ.U$_{18}$.LU

7. ^{Ú}*imḫur-ešra ki-ma šá-ru-ru* ^{d}15 *šá-niš* ^{Ú}*imḫur-ešra ki-ma* Ú-^{d}UTU NUMUN-*šú ki-ma ši-gu-uš-ti* [21]: MÚD *ka-mi-i* : MÚD LÚ *ga-ar-ba-nu áš-šú ka-mu-ú* :

8. LÚ *ga-ar-ba-nu šá-niš* MÚD *qa-du-ú*^{MUŠEN} : 1-*niš* : *ki-ma* : *iš-ten it-ti a-ḫa-meš* ḪE.ḪE : ḪE.ḪE : *ba-la-lu* : ZÍD ŠE.MUŠ$_5$ *ši-gu-šú qé-me up-pu-lu* : KUŠ ^{d}*Ku-ši* :

9. KUŠ GU$_4$ *ṣal-mu šá ina* KÁ.GAL URU *šá* IM.MAR.TU *ina* UGU-*ḫi* ^{GIŠ}ŠINIG *ana* ^{d}*Ku-ši in-ne-ep-pu-uš* : *til-lat* : ^{d}*Ku-ši* : *til-lat šá* ^{GIŠ}ŠINIG *šá* KUŠ GU$_4$ *ṣal-mu ana* ^{d}*Ku-ši*

10. *ina* UGU *šak-na* : MÁŠ.ZU : *ki-iz-zu* : MÁŠ : *ú-ri-ṣa* : ZU : *e-du-ú* : ^{Ú}MA. LAGAB : *tu-na-as-su-ma* : *ki-ma ba-aṣ-ṣa* ^{Ú}TILLA *ki-ma* ^{GIŠ}ŠINIG *u* SA$_5$:

11. ^{Ú}LÚ.^{d}*A-nu* : *ki-ma ḫal-la e-ri-bi* : Ú DILI : *ki-ma ḫal-la* TU^{MUŠEN} : ŠEM.^{d}MAŠ NITA *ki-ma qu-lip-tú* ^{GIŠ}ŠINIG *ka-ṣar u* SA$_5$ *ni-kip-tú* SAL *ki-ma qu-lip-tú* ^{GIŠ}ŠINIG

12. *raq-qa-qu u a-ru-qu* : KI.A.^{d}ÍD ÚḪ.^{d}ÍD : KI.A.^{d}ÍD *a-ru-uq-tum* : KI.A.^{d}ÍD A.GAR.GAR.^{d}ÍD : KI.A.^{d}ÍD *ṣa-li-in-du* :

13. KI.A.^{d}ÍD BA.BA.ZA.^{d}ÍD : KI.A.^{d}ÍD *pe-ṣi-tum* : MUN.EME.SAL-*lim* : MUN *šá* ŠÀ-*bi* ÍD : ILLU ^{ŠEM}BULUḪ *ḫi-i-lu šá a-na* ^{LÚ}*a-su-tum in-ne-ep-pu-uš* : ILLU LI.DUR

14. *ki-ma e-pi-ri a-sur-re-e* : ^{ŠEM}ḪAB : *ṭu-ri* : *in-za-ru-ú* : *ḫi-biš-ti* : ^{ŠEM}GÚR. GÚR *šá ḫúp-pe-e* ŠÀ-*bu-ú* ^{ŠEM}BULUG *šem-meš-la* ŠEM LÙ.LÙ : ŠEM. MUG ŠEM.SAL

15. *ḫi-biš-ti šá ina* ŠÚ ^{d}UTU E-*u* ŠEM.ḪI.A : *ú-ru-ú* : *la-ba-na-tum* : ^{GĪŠ}ERIN.SUMUN : *šu-pu-uḫ-ru* : ^{GĪŠ}ERIN.SUMUN *šá-niš bal-ṭi-it-tum šá* ŠÀ ^{GĪŠ}ERIN : MUN *A-ma-nu* Ù.MU.UN : *A-ma-nu*

16. [Ù.M]U.UN *da-mu áš-šú* MUN *sa-mat šá* ^{KUR}*Ma-da-a-a* : IM.SA$_5$: *šèr-šèr-ri* : ^{Ú}*kur-ka-nu-ú ki-ma su-ḫa-tum gul-lu-ub* ^{Ú}*kur-ka-nu-ú šá šá-di-i*

17. [^{Ú}*pi-ri*]-*za-aḫ*[22] : ^{Ú}*kur-ka-nu-ú šá ma-a-tú* ^{Ú}*sa-pal-gi-na* : Ì.GIŠ BUR : Ì.GIŠ BÁRA : *bi-ʾ-il-ti* : BUR : *bi-ʾ-il-ti šá-niš* Ì.NUN.NA *šal-šiš* Ì *ḫal-ṣa re-bi-iš*

18. [… TU].⌈RA.KILIB⌉.BA : *nap-ḫar mur-ṣu* : ^{Ú}LAL : *ki-ma* ^{GIŠ}ḪAŠḪUR *ina ni-síḫ tam-tim a-šar šam-mu u* ^{GIŠ}GI *la ba-šu-ú ina* IGI A.MEŠ È *ina* UGU-*ḫi-šú*

19. [*as-qú-du ra-bi-iṣ*[23] ...] x *al-la-an šar-ri* : ^{Ú}*a-zal-lá* : *ki-ma* ^{Ú}*ka-na-šu-ú u* SA$_5$[24] : ^{Ú}*a-zal-lá* : Ú *ni-is-sat ma-še-e* : ^{Ú}KUR.KUR :
20. [...] ⸢x⸣ zi *e-ri-bi* : ⸢x⸣ ku : ⸢x⸣ pan-du *gul-gul* NAM.LÚ.U$_{18}$.LU : ^{GIŠ}ŠINIG : UZU NAM.LÚ.U$_{18}$.LU
21. [...] *šá ap-pa-ri* : *sik-kat* : *pa-ʾ-ṣa!-nu šá* ^{LÚ}LUNGA *sim-di šá* ŠE.BAR *u* GAZI^{SAR} 1-*niš* ḪE.ḪE-*ma*
22. [...] SUḪUŠ ^{GIŠ}ŠINIG ḪÁD.DU-*ú šá-niš ka-mun* ^{GIŠ}ŠINIG : NA$_4$ *gab-ú*[25] : NA$_4$ *gab-ú*
23. [...] x ⸢*pa*⸣-*gu-ú* : *ú-qu-pi šá ap-pi-ta-šú ana* IGI-*šú qa-pa-at* : *qa-pu* :
24. [...] x *Šu-ba-ri* : ^{Ú}ḪAR.ḪUM.BA.ŠIR *šam-mu ḫi-níq-tum* : ^{Ú}*eli-kul-la*
25. [...] ^{Ú}*ar-za-ni-ik-ka-tú* : ^{Ú}*ku-uk-ka-ni-tum*
26. [...] *lu-lu-ú* : ^{Ú}KU$_6$: *šam-mu nu-ú-nu ka-a-a-an*
27. [...] x SAR : ^{Ú}*šu-up-pa-tum* : ^{Ú}*ur-ba-nu*
28. [... *bur-ti*] ⸢*šam-ḫat*⸣ : *ar-ra-bi* : *ú-la-lu*! *šá* ^{KUR}SU.BIR$_4^{\text{KI}}$[26]
29. [...]⸢x x *qa-an-nu-um ki-ma zap-pi*⸣ ŠAḪ

30–32. Colophon

TRANSLATION

1a. SI DÀRA.MAŠ means "stag horn": SI means "horn." DÀRA.MAŠ means "stag."[27]

1b–4a.[28] DIŠ means "if."

AN.TA.ŠUB.BA—(when) the patient is continually choked and repeatedly lets his spittle fall, it is AN.TA.ŠUB.BA.[29]

^{d}LUGAL.ÙR.RA—(when) he lets his right eye and his left eye droop, it is ^{d}LUGAL.ÙR.RA.[30]

"Hand" of a god—(when) he curses the gods, speaks blashphemy (and) strikes whatever he sees, it is "hand" of a god.[31]

"Hand" of a goddess—(when) he continually has a crushing sensation in the chest and continually forgets his words, it is "hand" of a goddess.[32]

"Hand" of ghost—when his ears roar, (his face) continually smoothes out, (and) he cannot get his teeth close enough together to be able to eat, it is "hand" of ghost.[33]

4b–5a. DÙ.DÙ.BI means "its ritual."

napšaršu means "its windpipe." *taʾa* means "(the stuff) in the depths."[34] The eye socket is the hole for the eye; the hole is in the depths of head and neck.

5b–10b.[35] Ì.ḪUL means "naphtha"

Ì.KU$_6$ means "fish oil"

A.RI.A NAM.LÚ.U$_{18}$.LU (really) means the plant *maštakal* because the plant A.RI.A is *maštakal* (and) secondly A.RI.A (means) "semen."

TÚG.NÍG.DÁRA means "rag." ŠU.LAL means "soiled." TÚG.NÍG. DÁRA.ŠU.LAL (really) means "fox flesh."

Tarmuš is like *silqu*-vegetable root.

Imḫur-lim is like "human bone."

Imḫur-ešra is like "sheen of Ishtar." Secondly, *imḫur-ešra* is like "sunflower." Its seed is like (that of) *šiguštu*.

The "blood of a prisoner" means the "blood of a leper" because "prisoner" means "leper." Secondly, it is the blood of an owl.[36]

1-*niš* means "like one" or "to ḪE.ḪE with one another." ḪE.ḪE means "to mix."

ZÍD ŠE.MUŠ$_5$ is *šeguššu*, flour made from late (barley).

"Kušu's hide"[37] means the hide of the black ox which is over the *bīnu*-tamarisk planted in the Western city gate for Kušu. The "tendrils of Kušu" means the tendrils of the *bīnu*-tamarisk on which the hide of a black ox is placed for Kušu.

MÁŠ.ZU means "adult male goat." MÁŠ means "goat" (and) ZU means "to know (as in sexually experienced).

10c–18a.[38] MA.LAGAB (is a plant which) if you try to remove it, it (comes to pieces) like sand.

urṭû is like *bīnu*-tamarisk but red.

amēlānu is like the thigh of a crow.

"Lone plant" is like the thigh of a pigeon.

Male *nikiptu* (has bark) knotted like *bīnu*-tamarisk bark but it is red. Female *nikiptu* (has bark) thin and yellow like *bīnu*-tamarisk bark.

Ruʾtītu-sulphur is yellow sulphur. *Agargarītu*-sulphur is black sulphur. *Papasītu*-sulphur is white sulphur.

Emesallim-salt is salt from the river.

Baluḫḫu-aromatic resin is a resin made for the practice of pharmacology.

Abukkatu resin is like the dust from the damp course of a wall.

ŠEMḪAB is *ṭūru*-aromatic.

Inzarû is/looks like a cutting of *kukru*-aromatic with a hole in it.

Balukku-aromatic (and) *šimeššalû*. It (*balukku*-aromatic) is a cloudy aromatic; also (written) ŠEM.MUG. (The remaining reading, ŠEM. BAL means "substitute aromatic" and it usage indicates that the aromatic which it is a "substitute for" is myrrh).

Šimeššalû is a cutting which sprouts(!—the text has E for È) at sunset.

ŠEM.ḪI.A is *urû* (or) *labanātu*-incense.

^{GIŠ}ERIN.SUMUN is *šupuḫru*-cedar. Secondly, ^{GIŠ}ERIN.SUMUN is the worm that lives in (old) cedars.

Amānim-salt—UMUN (spelled syllabically) means Amanus ("red"); ⌜UMUN⌝ means "blood red." It is called that because it is the red salt of Media.

IM.SA$_5$ ("red clay") is *šeršerru*-paste.

Kurkānu-turmeric resembles a shaved armpit. Wild *kurkānu*-turmeric (is called) ⌜*pirizaḫ*⌝; cultivated *kurkānu*-turmeric (is called) *sapalginu*.

Pūru-oil is pressed-out oil. It is an alabastron; (that is,) a *pūru*-vessel is an alabastron. Secondly, it (the oil) is ghee. Thirdly, it is pressed-out oil. Fourthly, it is [...].

18b–27a. ⌜TU.RA.KILIB.BA⌝ means "the summa of illness."

Ašqulālu resembles a *ḫašḫuru*-apple (and) comes out on the surface of the water at the outlet(?) to the sea where there are no (other) plants or reeds (and) [*asqudu*-snakes lie on it].

[...] is "royal/false" *allānu*-oak.[39]

Azallû resembles a *kanāšu*-leek but it is red. *Azallû* is a plant for forgetting troubles.

Atāʾišu [...].

[...] crow's [...]

[...]

"Human skull" is (actually) *bīnu*-tamarisk.

"Human flesh" is (actually) [...] of the reed swamp.

Sikkatu is brewers' mash. You mix together barley groats and *kasû* and [...]

[...] is *bīnu*-tamarisk root. Secondly it is *bīnu*-tamarisk galls[40] which are equivalent to alum.[41] Alum means [...].

[...]

Pagû-ape is an *uqupu*-ape whose snout rises (*qapû*) towards his face. *Qapû* means ["to rise"].

[... in] Subarean.

Ḫarmunu is a plant for stricture.

Elikulla [is a plant for ...]

[...]

Arzanikkatu is (the same as) *kukkanitu*.

[...]
[KÙ.GAN] is *lulû*-antimony.
ÚKU$_6$ is (literally) "fish plant."
"Continuously" means [...]. [The original presumably required oil to be rubbed gently on continuously].

27b–29. [...]
Šuppatu-rush is papyrus.
[...]
⸢Caterpillar⸣ is (for the purposes of Šumma Alu omens equivalent to) a dormouse or an effeminate of Subartu.
[...]
[...] (with a fringe) like pig bristles.

C. ESOTERIC INDIVIDUAL TEXT COMMENTARIES

TEXT 3 (GHOSTS): SpTU 1.49

Like all too many commentaries, the texts to which SpTU 1.49 is a commentary are uncertain or lost. Fortunately, the opening lines always give a general idea of the contents. Even so, however, as is typical with esoteric commentaries, whole sections are virtually incomprehensible and broken sections virtually hopeless to restore. Nonetheless, they still contain much of interest.

Lines 1–3 are a nice example of the lexicography involved in making a commentary. We learn that "blood of a black snake" actually means the "blood of a *kušû*-tortoise and that *purunzaḫu* is a foreign (probably Hurrian) word for "frog."

Lines 23–32 are fine examples of deeper meanings whereby the god Enlil, lord of the Netherworld and of ghosts, is enlisted to help in treatment. So, the use of a raven's egg invoked the constellation Corvus, which is associated with him. Another ingredient was apparently some part of a goose. The Sumerogram for "goose," KUR.GI was taken apart and creatively retranslated as "given birth in/by the mountain," which provided another connection with Enlil, the great mountain.

Lines 33–37 are the most interesting part of this text. The symptom of roaring or ringing ears was typically laid at the door of ghosts. What our ancient commentator tells us is that the noise was thought to be a ghost actually whispering into the patient's ear. He derived this from the fact that the word for "ghost" (*e-ṭem-mu*) could be turned into Sumerian E and DIMA which allowed as retranslation as "sayer of orders." Most ingeniously, he also took a rare Sumerogram for ghost, GIDIM$_2$, and split it up into two separate signs, BAR and BÙR, translating the result as "ghost that opens the ears."

1. DIŠ NA ŠU.GIDIM.MA DIB-*s*[*u-ma*] MÚD MUŠ GI$_6$
2. MÚD *ku-*⸢*šu*⸣*-ú*$^{\mathrm{KU_6}}$: BIL.[ZA].Z[A …] ^{d}15 E-[*ú*]
3. BIL.ZA.ZA : *mu-ṣa-ʾi-*[*r*]*a-ni* : *pu-ru-un-z*[*a-ḫu*]

4–22. (not enough preserved to make connected sense)

rev.

23. *š*[*á*] KUR.S[U.BI]R$_4$^{KI} *šu-ú i-qab-bu-ú* […]
24. *a-na* 20 KÙŠ *ku-dúr-ru ú-kad-dar* : ḪUR […]
25. UR : *na-ka-su* : ŠAB : *na-ka-su* […]
26. *ta-ma-ḫi-ir* GAZ[I^{S}]^{AR} : *me-e* GAZI^{SAR} : NÍND[A :]
27. *il-lu-ru* : ⸢GURUN⸣ : NUNUZ *ḫa-aḫ-ḫu-ru š*[*á*] ⸢E-*ú*⸣
28. *ina* ŠÀ-*šá* MUL.U[G]A^{MUŠEN} : ^{d}EN.LÍL : ^{d}EN.LÍL EN KI-*tim*
29. *u* GIDIM *šu-ú* : [KUR].GI^{MUŠEN} : KUR : *šá-du-ú*
30. GI : *a-la-du* [: ^{d}]KUR.GAL : ^{d}EN.LÍL *šá-du-ú ra-bu-ú*
31. *ḫi-biš-tum* : GÚR.GÚR [*šá ḫú*]*p-pe-e iq-ta-bu-ni*
32. ^{ŠEM}GÚG.GÚG : *ḫi-*[*bi*]*š-tum* : ^{ŠEM}GÚR.GÚR
33. DIŠ NA *ina* DIB-*it* ŠU.[GIDI]M.MA GEŠTU^{II}-*šú i-šag-gu-ma*
34. GEŠTU^{II}-*šú iš-ta-n*[*a-as*]*-sa-a* : ŠU.GIDIM.MA
35. $^{\text{gi-di-im}}$GÍDIM : GIDI[M *pe*]*-tu-ú* GEŠTU^{II} : BAR : *pe-tu-ú*
36. BÙR$^{\text{bu-ur}}$: *uz-nu* : *e-*[*ṭ*]*em-me* : *qa-bu-ú ṭè-e-me*
37. E : *qa-bu-ú* : K[A$^{\text{di-i}}$]$^{\mathrm{m_4\text{-}ma}}$ḪI : *ṭè-e-me*
38. GIDIM *mur-tap-pi-du* : [*e*]*-ṭem-mu se-gu-ú*
39. *šá e-ṭem-ma-šú la paq-*[*du*] : DIB$^{\text{di-íb}}$RA.AḪ : *ra-pa-du*
40. DIB.RA.AḪ : *ri-pit-tú*

41–43. Colophon

TRANSLATION

1–3. "If a ghost afflicts a person."
"Blood of a black snake" means the blood of a *kušû*-tortoise.
The ⸢frog⸣ is said to be the [husband?] of Ishtar. BIL.ZA.ZA means "frog," also *purunzaḫu*.

4–22. *(fragmentary with references to ghosts, Damu, son of Gula, goddess of healing and the goddess Ishtar)*

23–32. They say it is ⸢from Subartu⸣. […]
"At 20 cubits he makes a boundary." It means a drawing (ḪUR): [ḪU means …]; UR means "to cut." The Sumerogram for "to cut" is ŠAB:

[…].

"You gather *kasû*." That means *kasû* juice.

⸢NÍNDA⸣ [is] *illuru-berry*. That is a fruit.

"The egg of a *ḫaḫḫuru*-raven." What is said about it is that Corvus is Enlil. Enlil is the lord of the Netherworld and of ghost(s).

⸢"Goose"⸣ (KUR.GI). KUR means "mountain" (and) GI means "to give birth." [d]KUR.GAL is Enlil, the great mountain.

"Broken pieces" means *kukru* [which] they say to ⸢crumble⸣. Kukkuk-aromatic broken in pieces is *kukru*-aromatic.

33–37. "If as a result of affliction by 'hand' of ⸢ghost⸣, a person's ears roar (or) his ears continually ⸢ring⸣." This is "hand" of ghost. GIDIM$_2$ means "⸢ghost that opens⸣ the ears." (This is because GIDIM$_2$ = BAR + BÙR and) BAR means "to open" (and) BÙR means "ear." *Eṭemmu* means "sayer of orders" because E means "to say" (and) DIMA (KA.ḪI) means "orders."

38–40. "Roaming ghost" means a ⸢ghost⸣ that moves about, one whose ghost is not ⸢entrusted⸣ (with funerary offerings). DIB.RA.AḪ means "to roam." DIB.RA.AḪ means "unrest."

TEXT 4 (DIFFICULT CHILDBIRTH): CIVIL 1974, NO. 2

Civil 1974, no. 2 is probably the best example of an esoteric commentary, since it is based on a known text, which is largely preserved, and which appears as chapter 12, text 7. From this exemplar we can best appreciate what such commentaries have to offer us.

Lines 1–6a are a commentary on BAM 248 i 5ff., which seem originally, to judge from the traces, from this commentary, and from the Akkadian version of AUAM 73.3094: 12–23,[42] to have had:

"Like a boat (for carrying) cedar, it (her boat) is full of cedar. Like a boat (for carrying) cedar fragrance, it (her boat) is full of cedar fragrance. Like a boat which is overlaid (perhaps a hearing error for 'loaded') with red carnelian, it (her boat) is full of carnelian. Like a boat which is overlaid with lapis lazuli, it (her boat) is full of lapis lazuli; (yet) she knows not if it is carnelian; she knows not if it is lapis(!)."[43]

What is interesting is the way in which a perfectly ordinary sentence in Sumerian that describes the uncertainty about the sex of the unborn child is creatively retranslated to make a comment on the situation at hand. This and other references to the uncleanliness of childbirth[44] and its offensiveness to the gods suggest the presence in Mesopotamia of some sort of cleansing ceremony after childbirth similar to what is prescribed in Lev 12.

Lines 6b-7 are apparently apropos of a phrase such as that preserved in BAM 248 i 49, i 60 or iii 44 in which it is wished of the baby: "May he come out like a snake; may he slither out like a little snake." In this context, both an intervening Belet-ili (BAM 248 i 65) and the physician could be interpreted as a "snake charmer."

Lines 8–14a indicate the presence in the broken portion of the beginning of BAM 248 of something similar to AUAM 73.3094:41-59[45] which has:

"Go, my son! When [you have taken] in hand a reed of the 'small marsh' of Eridu, pour into it the fat of a pure cow (and) the cream of a mother cow. Mix (it) together with dust from a crossroads[46] [(and) oil] and [...]."

"Break (the reed) over his (the child's) umbilical cord and then [if] it is a boy, make him look at a weapon; [if] it is a ⸢girl⸣, make her look at [spindle] and *kirissu*-clasp. [Let the infant] come out [into the light] of the sun (i.e. be born alive)."[47]

The ancient commentator creatively retranslated the Sumerian to have the ingredients used in the ritual indicate a successful outcome.[48] So the "reed from a small marsh" becomes: "The infant will come out of the woman." "Dust from a crossroads" becomes: "The little one/seed comes straight out." Akkadian could be similarly treated by the simple expedient of taking it apart into the constituent signs so "oil" (*šá-am-nu*) becomes "The woman creates the seed." An ointment filled reed was used to cut the umbilical cord in order to avoid infection.[49] The *kirissu* was a symbol of womanhood given to female children at birth to fix their gender.

Lines 14b–15a are a commentary on BAM 248 i 36, a label which says:

"[Recitation for a woman] who is having difficulty giving birth." The ancient physician was quite correct that an overly narrow birth canal was a source of great risk to the mother.

Lines 15b–27 are a commentary on BAM 248 i 37–50 which has:

"[The cow of Sîn] took in [the semen] and so made clouds; the waterskin was full (i.e. her udders filled with milk). The earth was plowed up with her horn. [With her tail, she made the whirlwind pass along.] Sîn [took] the road; [before] Enlil, [he cries (and) his tears come. Why] does ⸢Sîn⸣ cry, the pure-in-rite's tears [come]? [...] Because of my cow which has not yet given birth, [because of my she-goat which has not yet] ⸢been opened⸣.[50]

The boat is ⸢detained⸣ [at the quay] of difficulty ('narrows'); the *magurru*-boat is held back [at the quay] of hardship. [Whom should I] ⸢send to merciful⸣ Marduk? May the boat be loosed [from the quay] of difficulty; may the *magurru*-boat be freed [from the quay] of hardship. [Come out to me] ⸢like⸣ a snake;

slither out to me like a little snake. May the [...] relax so that the infant may fall to the earth and see the sunlight.

The comment on "The earth was ploughed up (*ṭe-ra-at*) with her horn" is a classic example of the lengths to which ancient commentators would go to tease a deeper layer of meaning out of their texts. "Piercing" or "ploughing up" is something the moon does with its "horns." So is "to embrace" (*edēru*). The Sumerogram for "to embrace" is GÚ.DA.RI, the last part of which (DA.RÍ) is the Sumerogram for "to last" (*darû*). It so happens that "to last" is homophonous with the verb "to pierce" (*ṭerû*). So we begin with a distraught cow "ploughing up" the earth and, when we are done, the moongod is "embracing" his cow.

The comment on "pure in rites" is on much more secure ancient lexical ground. The idea that the moon god's crying over his cow was a reference to an eclipse meshes very well with entries in astronomical texts in which the full moon is said to "cry in the Ekur."[51] Similarly, the ancient commentator had no trouble finding an appropriate quote in the literature for Sîn's association with cows. The appropriateness of the baby snake resides not simply in the fact that snakes lay their eggs easily but, as the ancient commentator explains, "little snake" means "The seed jumps out."

Lines 26b–27a are a commentary on BAM 248 i 51, the Sumerian version of the Akkadian label given in BAM 248 i 36.

Lines 27b–30a are a commentary on BAM 248 i 54–61 which has:

"[...] having difficulty [....] having difficulty. ⸢Come⸣(?) [...] Fly! Come(?) [...] Let it come out. [...] "(Who is it), Naḫundi; (who is it), Narundi?" Run(!) like a gazelle; slither like a snake. I am [Asalluhi]. May [...] see him."

Naḫundi and Narundi are brother and sister Elamite gods.[52] As the commentary reveals, "Run like a gazelle" is deliberately misspelled so as to take advantage of similar sounding words which indicate a successful birth. The comment on "like a gazelle" takes advantage of the fact that Sumerian signs have more than one reading (and meaning). Creatively retranslated, "run like a gazelle" turns into "Be plucked out! See (the light)! Come forth! Be Born!"

Lines 30b–32a are a commentary on BAM 248 i 68-69 which has: "You whisk *pūru*-oil into [...]. [If you massage her with it in a] down[wards direction], she should give birth straight away."

Here, the ancient commentator cleverly turns a rare word for the oil being used to massage the pregnant woman into "no," taken as an antonym for "yes," signaling the divine decision for the baby to be born.

Lines 32b–37a have no preserved referrent, which is lost in a lacuna. There seems to have been some sort of ritual involving a *šiltāḫu*-arrow. One possibility is an anti-infertility ritual.[53] This possibility is reinforced by the fact that the ancient commentator's creative retranslation of the Sumerograms for the arrow and the Arrow constellation yield: "The woman will have seed; she will get pregnant and give birth easily to a live child."

Alternatively, this weapon was to be given to a male child whose birth was hoped for in order to fix his gender. The practice of giving gendered objects to babies was to ensure that the goddess Ishtar did not play one of her little tricks and produce a child who was one sex and thought of him/herself as the other gender.

Lines 37b–46a parallel BAM 248 ii 14–iii 5 of which only the last part is preserved as follows:

> "[…] Her loincloths are loosened […] Stand beside her, Marduk. Entrust life, the spell of life. (With) this storm am I surrounded; reach me.
>
> May the boat be safe in […]. May the *magurru*-boat go aright in […]. May her massive mooring rope be loosened, and may her locked gate be opened. (May) the mooring rope of the boat (be moored) to the quay of health, the mooring rope of the *magurru*-boat to the quay of life. May the limbs be relaxed; may the sinews be slackened. May the sealed places be loosened; may the offspring come out, a separate body, a human creature. May he come out promptly and see the light of the sun.
>
> Like a hailstone (which can never go back to the heavens), may the (foetus) not be able to return to what is behind him. Like one who has fallen from a wall, may he not be able to turn his breast. Like a leaky drainpipe (which cannot hold water), may none of the (mother's) waters remain.
>
> When Asalluhi heard this, he became exceedingly concerned for her life. At the command of Ea, he exalted his name. He cast the incantation of life (and) the spell of health. He loosed (her) mooring rope; he undid [her] ⌈knotting⌉. The locked gates [were] ⌈opened⌉. The ⌈limbs⌉ were relaxed; [the sinews slackened]. The sealed places were loosened; [the offspring came out], a ⌈separate⌉ body, a [human] creature. He came out[54] promptly and saw [the light of the sun].
>
> Like a hailstone, he did not return [backwards]. Like one who had fallen from a wall, he did not turn [his breast]. Like a leaky drainpipe, none [of her waters] remained. The incantation of Asalluhi, the secret of ⌈Eridu⌉, the true yes of Ea, the renowned spell which Mami requested for health('s sake and which) ⌈king⌉ [Ea] gave to help make the foetus come out straight away."

Lines 37b–40a indicate that there was originally yet another version of the Cow of Sîn here. In this case, as also in BAM 248 iii 54-iv 1, the cow speaks in the first person, and we learn that her name is Egiziniti and that she was black with a white spot on her head, described rather poetically as a clearing in the forest.

As the ancient commentator explains, the appropriateness of the shell metaphor was not simply that there was something in the shell which was removed or that the Sumerian word for the shell was the same as the word for a pregnant woman, itself a little word picture with the sign for "son" inside the sign for "insides," but that the word, creatively retranslated, means "The seed will come forth from the storeroom."

The comment on "loincloths" is interesting in that it reveals that ancient philologists, like their modern counterparts, were able to discern the meaning of rare words from context, in this case, a citation from the Gilgamesh Epic. Of course, if possible, it was desirable to predict the birth of a male child in one's retranslations.

The connection between "entrusting life" and a term for cloth manufacture is obscure. Among modern Arabs, "weaving" is a euphemism for sexual intercourse, so a piece of cloth, the product of weaving, would be an appropriate metaphor for a child. Is it possible that the stamped cloth of this passage represented a fully formed foetus, and therefore a live birth?

Lines 46b–51 are a commentary on BAM 248 iii 7–9 which has:

"You mix hailstone, dust from the parapet of an abandoned wall (and) dust from a leaky drainpipe with *pūru*-oil. If you massage (her) in a downward direction, that woman should give birth straight away."

In the able hands of the ancient commentator, "hail stone from heaven" becomes: She will create/give birth to seed (i.e. male heirs)." "Dust from a fallen wall" actually means: "Her bonds will open; the little one will come straight out."

1. ÉN MUNUS Ù.TU.UD.DA.A.NI : *e-lip-pi šá uq-na-a za-na-at*
2. *za-na* : *ma-lu-ú* : GUG NU.ZU Ù GUG NU.ZU : *lu-ʾ-at-ma*
3. *a-na ni-qí-i ul na-ṭa-at* : *pu-uḫ-tum ši-i* : GUG : *el-lum*
4. NU : *la-ʾ* : ZU : *na-ṭu-u* : *a-ma-ra* : *a-na ni-qí-i ul na-ṭa-at*
5. *šá* E-*u* : SIZKUR : *ni-qu-ú* : SIZKUR : *ṣu-le-e um-ma lu-ʾ-at-ma*
6. *a-na šu-le-e ul am-ra-at* : NA.GI.RI *um-ma* ^{d}GAŠAN.DINGIR
7. *iš-ta-na-as-si* : $^{na-gi-ri}$KA×AD.KÙ *šá ka-ga-ak-ku* AD.KÙ I.GUB : *a-ši-pu*
8. GI ÈN.BAR.BÀN.DA ŠU U.ME.TI : GI : *sin-niš-tim* : BAR : *a-ṣu-u* : BÀN.DA
9. *še-er-ri* : *ṣa-aḫ-ri* : SAḪAR SIL.LA : SAḪAR : *e-pe-ri* : SA.ḪAR *u ṣa-ḫar iš-ten-ma*
10. SILA.LAM$_4$.MA : SI : *e-še-ri šá a-la-ku* : LA : *la-a* : *ṣa-ḫar* : AM.MA : *ze-ri*
11. *šá-am-nu* : $^{ni-ig}$ŠÁ *sin-niš-tim* : AM : *ze-ri* : NU : *ba-nu-u šá-niš* ^{i}NI
12. *šá-am-nu* : I : *a-ṣu-u šá* NUMUN : *e-li* LI.DUR-*šú ḫe-pi-ma aš-šum* GI
13. *na-ki-is ab-bu-un-na-ti* : *ab-bu-un-na-tú ri-ik-si šá* LÚ *ši-i*
14. ^{GIŠ}KI.RI.IS KÉŠ : *ki-ri-is-su* : É *ú-ba-nu* : *šup-šuq-tùm-ma* : *šup-šu-qa*
15. *ka-a-šú šá-niš dan-na-ti* : *ina qar-ni-šú qaq-qar ṭe-ra-at* : *da-ru-u* ‹:› SAG.

ÚS

16. *šá-niš ṭe-ra-at* : *ḫi-iṣ-ni-it* : *da-ru-u* : *ḫa-ṣa-nu* ŠÀ-*bu-u* GÚ.DA.RI[55]

17. *na-an-du-ra* : *e-lal* : *e-de-ri* : *el-la-me-e* : AGA *taš-ri-iḫ-ti*

18. ŠÀ-*bu-u* É.LAM$_{4}$.MA : É *er-bi šá-niš* SI É.GAR$_{8}$.BI TIL.LA : *el-lam-mu-u*

19. *šá nu-ú-ru la-ni-šu ú-qat-ta-a* : SI : *nu-ú-rum* : É.GAR$_{8}$: *la-a-nu*

20. BI : *šu-u* : TIL : *qa-tu-u áš-šú* ^{d}30 *šá* AN.TA.LÙ *gam-mar-ti i-šak-kan*

21. *aš-šum* ÁB-*ia la a-lit-ti áš-šú* ^{d}30 EN *la-a-tum el-le-e-ti*

22. ZI ^{d}NIN.DAR.A SIPA AB.LU-*lu-ú-a* ḪÉ.PÀ : *niš* ^{d}MIN SIPA

23. *ú-tul-la-a-tú lu-ú ta-ma-at* : ^{d}NIN.DAR.A : ^{d}30 : *ni-šil-pa-a*

24. *ni-šal-pú-u* : *e-te-qu* : *ni-šal-pú-u* : *a-la-ka* : GIR$_{5}$.GIR$_{5}$: *na-ḫal-ṣu-u*

25. GIR$_{5}$.GIR$_{5}$: *na-šal-pú-u* : $^{ni-ra-aḫ}$ ^{d}GUD : *ni-ra-ḫu* : AN : *ze-ri*

26. GUD : *šá-ḫa-ṭu* : KA.INIM.MA ‹‹:›› MUNUS LA.RA.AḪ.A.KÁM : LA.RA.AḪ : *pu-uš-qa*

27. *dan-na-ti* : *Na-ḫu-un-di* : ^{d}30 : *Na-ru-un-di* : ^{d}UTU

28. *na-am-li-su ki-ma ṣa-bi-tum* : ZÉ : *ma-la-su* : ZÉ : *ba-qa-mu*

29. *šá-niš na-am-li-su* ŠÀ-*bu-u nap-lu-su* : *a-ma-ra* : *ki-ma* MAŠ.DÀ

30. MAŠ$^{ba-ar}$: *a-ṣu-u šá* NUMUN : $^{du-u}$DÀ : *lil-li-du* : *ul-la* : *an-na*

31. *an-na* : *qí-bi-ti šá-niš* UL.LA : *ul-la* Ì$^{i-ʾ-u}$: *šá-am-nu* : Ì BUR

32. Ì *kan-nu šá* LÚ.Ì.ŠUR *šá-niš* BUR : *bi-ʾ-il-ti* : ^{URUDU}KAK.U$_{4}$.TAG.E

33. MUL.MUL : *mul-mul* : *šil-ta-ḫu* : MUL.MUL : *ze-ri*

34. ^{GI}MUL.MUL : *ze-ri šá-niš* GI : *sin-niš-ti* : URUDU : *e-ru-u*

35. *a-na a-re-e* : $^{du-u}$KAK : *lil-li-du* : $^{za-al}$U$_{4}$: *nu-úr* : TAG.GA

36. *e-ze-bi šá-niš* $^{du-u}$KAK : *lil-li-du* : SI : *e-še-ri šá a-la-ku aš-šum*

37. ^{MUL}KAK.SI.SÁ : *e-gi-zi-ni-ti* : GEME$_{2}$ ^{d}30 : *ina* SAG.DU.MU *na-ma-ra*[56]

38. *na-ma-ra* : KASKAL^{II} *šá* ^{GIŠ}GI *u* ^{GIŠ}TIR : *šá* ŠÀ *iš-qil-la-tum li-kal-lim nu-ú-rum*

39. *ana* MUNUS PEŠ$_{4}$ *iq-ta-bi* : ^{NA_4}PEŠ$_{4}$: *ṣi-il-la-tum* : NA$_{4}$: *a-ṣu-u šá ze-rum*

40. A : *ma-ra* : ŠÀ : ŠÀ-*bi* : *uš-šu-rat ḫur-da-at-su* : *ḫur-da-tú* : *ú-ru-u*

41. *šá sin-niš-ti* ŠÀ-*bu-u qa-at-ka šu-ta-am-ṣa-am-ma lu-pu-ut ḫur-da-at-na*

42. *šá-niš ḫur-da-ti* : *qim-ma-ti* : *šal-šiš ḫur-da-ti* : *ḫur-ri-da-du*

43. *da-du* : *ma-ra* : *ina kit-tab-ri-šú* : *ina i-di-šú* : *kit-tab-ri* : *i-di* : ŠE : *i-di*

44. ŠE : *kit-tab-ra* : *qí-ip nap-šá-a-tum* : *qa-a-pa* : *na-da-nu*

45. TÚG $^{tu-un}$DÚB : *ka-ma-du* : *ik-kud it-ta-ʾ-id* : *ta-an-qí-tum*

46. *ḫi-is-sa-tum* : *it-mu-du* : *še-mu-ú* : *ab-nu ti-ik-ku* AN-*e* : *ab-nu*

47. AB : *ba-nu-u šá a-la-du* : NU : *ze-rum* : U.GU$_{4}$: *ti-ik-ku* : U : *ba-nu-u*

48. GU : *a-la-du* : AN : AN-*e* : AN : *ze-ri* : SAḪAR BÀD ŠUB-*tú*

49. BÀD : *du-ú-ru* : KÉŠ : *ri-ik-si* : BAD : *pe-tu-u*
50. ŠUB-*tú šá* E-*u áš-šú* SI.A : *qa-a-pa šá* É.GAR$_8$: SI : *e-še-ri šá a-lak*
51. A : *ṣa-ḫar* : SAḪAR GÁ *šur-di-i* : $^{\text{ma-a}}$GÁ : *pi-sa-an-nu* : GÁ : *a-la-ku*

---

52. *ṣa-a-ti šu-ut* KA *u maš-ʾ-al-ti ša* KA *um-ma-nu šá* ŠÀ

Translation

1–6a. Spell for a woman who is in the process of giving birth.

"Boat which is overlaid with lapis lazuli." "To overlay" means "to be full."

"She does not know whether it is carnelian (GUG NU.ZU) or lapis lazuli(!—Text: carnelian)." This means that she is unclean and so not suited for the sacrifice. It (GUG) is an antonym.[57] GUG means "clean," NU means "not" (and) ZU means "to be suited" or "to select." When it says she is not suited to the sacrifice:[58] the Sumerian for "sacrifice" is SIZKUR; SIZKUR (also) means "prayer" So that is to say she is unclean and so not selected for prayers.

6b–7. NA.GI.RI is to say "Belet-ili continually cries." The sign KA×AD.KÙ read NA.GI.RI (NIGRU: "snake charmer") is a KA-sign with AD.KÙ standing (inside). It means *āšipu*.

8–14a. "When you take in hand a reed from a small marsh" (GI ÈN.BAR.BÀN. DA): GI means "woman"; BAR means "to come out"; BÀN.DA means "infant" or "small one."

"Dust from a (cross)roads": SAḪAR means "dust"; "dust" (SA.ḪAR) and "little one" (*ṣa-ḫar*) are the same thing.

"Crossroads" (SILA.LAM$_4$.MA): SI means "to come straight out (said) of going"; LA means "not" or "little one"; AM.MA means "seed."

"Oil" (*ša-am-nu*): ŠÁ (read NÍG) means "woman" AM means "seed"; NU means "to create."

Moreover, NI (read Ì) is "oil" and I means "to come out (said) of seed."

"Break (the reed) over his (the child's) umbilical cord and then (if it is a boy, etc.)." That is because the reed is what cuts the umbilical cord. The umbilical cord is what binds a person (to his/her mother).

GIŠ.$^{\text{ki-ri-is}}$KÉŠ is a *kirissu*-clasp or "finger house" (thimble).

14b–15a. "Having difficulty (giving birth) means "to be made (too) narrow (to give birth)" or "to be delayed (giving birth)." Moreover, it means "difficulty/danger."

15b–26a. "The earth was ploughed up (*ṭe-ra-at*) with her horn": *Darû* means "longlasting." Moreover, *ṭerât* means "she was protected." "To last" means "to protect" because GÚ.DA.RI means "to embrace one another." "(The moon) hangs" means "to embrace."[59]

"Pure in rites" means "crown of glory" (11th-15th of the month)[60] because É.LAM$_4$.MA means "house of four." Moreover, SI É.GAR$_8$.BI TIL.LA is the Sumerogram for "pure in rites" and means "the one who brings the light of his appearance to an end": SI means "light"; É.GAR$_8$ means "appearance"; BI means "his"; TIL means "to bring to an end" because Sîn establishes a total eclipse.

"Because of my cow which has not yet given birth": Sîn is the lord of pure cows. "May they be sworn by ^{d}NIN.DAR.A the shepherd (and) herdsman (Bilingual Sumerian, then Akkadian)."[61] ^{d}NIN.DAR.A is Sîn.

"Slither out to me" : "to slither" means "to pass by"; "to slither" means "to go." The Sumerogram for "to slip" is GIR$_5$.GIR$_5$ and GIR$_5$.GIR$_5$ means "to slither."

The Sumerogram for "little snake" is ^{d}GUD read ^{d}NIRAḪ: AN (^{d}) means "seed"; GUD means "to jump out."

26b–27a. "Recitation for a woman who is having difficulty giving birth" (LA.RA.AḪ): LA.RA.AḪ means "narrow place" or "difficulty."[62]

27b–30a. Naḫundi is Sîn; Narundi is Shamash.

"Be plucked out (*namlisu* from *malāsu*: "to pluck," a calque on *lasāmu*: "to run") like a gazelle": The Sumerogram for "to pluck" is ZÉ which (also) means "to shear." Moreover, it is *namlisu* because (it sounds like) *naplusu* (which) means "to see (the light, i.e. be born safely)."

"Like a gazelle (MAŠ.DÀ)": MAŠ read BAR means "to come forth, (said) of seed"; DÀ read DÙ means "let them give birth."

30b–32a. "No" (*ul-la*) means "yes"; "yes" means "word" (i.e., a divine decision). Secondly, UL.LA is the Sumerogram for *ulû*-oil. NI read Ì means "oil."

Pūru-oil (Ì BUR) is oil from the *kannu*-bowl of the oil-presser. Secondly, BUR means "stinking."

32b–37a. ^{URUDU}KAK.U$_4$.TAG.E or MUL.MUL is a *mulmullu*- or *šiltāḫu*-arrow: MUL.MUL (also) means "seed." A reed *mulmullu*-arrow (^{GI}MUL.MUL) means seed. Moreover, GI means "woman."[63]

URUDU means "copper" (which is a homophone) of "to get pregnant"; KAK read DÙ means "let them give birth"; U$_4$ read ZAL(AG) means "light"; TAG.GA means "to escape."

Moreover, KAK read DÙ means "let them give birth" and SI(.SÁ) means "to come straight out, (said) of "to go," because the Arrow constellation (Sirius) is ^{MUL}KAK.SI.SÁ.

37b–46a. Egiziniti is (otherwise known as) $GEME_2$ d30.

"On my head there is a clearing": "clearing" means a path through a canebrake or forest.

"May what is inside the *išqillatu*-shell (^{NA_4}$PEŠ_4$) see the light" is what he says to the pregnant woman (MUNUS $PEŠ_4$). ^{NA_4}$PEŠ_4$ means "storeroom"; NA_4 means "to come forth, (said) of seed." ($PEŠ_4$ is ŠÀ×A): A means "son"; ŠÀ means "inside."

"Her loincloths are loosened": "loincloth" means "a woman's genitals" because (in Gilgamesh VI 69[64] Ishtar says): "Put out your hand and touch our loincloths." Moreover, "loincloths" mean "nest." Thirdly, "loincloths (*ḫurdātu*)" (sounds like) *ḫur-ri-da-du*[65] (and) *da-du* means "son."

ina kit-tab-ri-šú means "beside him"; *kittabru* means "side." The Sumerogram for "side" is ŠE which is also the Sumerogram for *kittabru*.[66]

"Entrust life": "to entrust" means "to give."

TÚG DÚB read TUN means "to stamp (cloth)."[67]

"He became exceedingly concerned": "worry" means "grief"; "to lean oneself (near)" means "to hear.[68]

(46b-51) "Hail stone from heaven": "stone" (*ab-nu*): AB means "to create, (said) of giving birth"; NU means "seed"

The Sumerian for hail is U.GU_4: U means "to create"; GU means "to give birth."

The Sumerian for "heaven" is AN; AN (also) means "seed."

"Dust from a fallen wall": the Sumerian for wall is BÀD (this sign consists of a KÉŠ-sign with a BAD-sign drawn inside it); KÉŠ means "bond"; BAD means "to open."

When it says "fallen" that is because Sumerian SI.A means "to buckle (said) of a wall"; SI means "to come straight out (said) of going"; A means "little one."

"Dust from a leaky drainpipe": the Sumerian for drainpipe is GÁ (read MA); GÁ (also) means "to go."

---

52 Commentary (based on) oral tradition and questions from the mouth of an expert in it.[69]

NOTES

1. On this point, see also George 1991, 139–40 and Geller 2010, 139–40.
2. There were also commentaries to various tablets to the Diagnostic Series as, for example, *STT* 403, which comments on tablet 3.

3. The ancient commentator interpreted this as ŠI-*pí*, which is an otherwise unattested Sumerogram. Alternatively, as suggested in Farber 1979, 303, what the original text being commented on had was an imperative form of *šapû* (so *ši-pí*). This would be very unusual in Mesopotamian medical texts, but the commentary is Hellenistic in date, and Latin texts commonly use the imperative when giving directions, so it is vaguely possible.

4. The citation is of SpTU 1.46:1. See Scurlock and Andersen 2005, 18.33.

5. The toilet demon appears in SpTU 1.46:8.

6. This mineral appears in SpTU 1.46:10. With Köcher 1995, 211b, *lurpani* is to be equated with the *illurpani* of MSL 7 140:319, as the association of both with *kalû*-paste demonstrates. Pace *CAD* I–J, 87–88, however, *illurpani* has nothing to do with the *illuru* berry and is certainly not rouge.

7. Literally: "he fixes (his eyes)." At this point, the original text was corrupt and should have had *ur-ta-na-at-ti* as in *AMT* 76/5:11+*AMT* 79/4:2′.

8. Our commentator was grasping at straws here. See Frahm 2011, 173 n. 468.

9. This is a discussion of SpTU 1.46.16–19, which reads: "If a person has a stroke affecting the face (and) his eye flutters, day and night he is continually wakeful and cannot sleep, (and) he cannot stop rubbing his eyes with honey and ghee." See Scurlock and Andersen 2005, 13.233.

10. The reference is to the process of manufacture.

11. This comments on BAM 523 iii 3′–8′. See Scurlock and Andersen 2005, 13.234.

12. As in SpTU 1.46:28,32,34.

13. As in *AMT* 78/1 + iii 17.

14. TCL 6.34 iii 3–16 duplicates BAM 388 i 3–18 (= chapter 8, text 1).

15. TCL 6.34 iv 1′–14′ duplicates BAM 179:1′–12′.

16. For the recitation, see Köcher 1966, 20 ad line 35.

17. Lambert 1983, 382, quoting PBS 10/4 no. 12 rev. "II" 6.

18. CBS 6060:48 (Livingstone 1986, 178).

19. See *CAD* Š/3, 324b.

20. This is quoted from URU.AN.NA (CT 37.26 i 17).

21. This is quoted from SpTU 3.106 i 10′ (*Šammu šikinšu*). See above, chapter 2, text 2.

22. Restored from Hg. D 247; see *CAD* K, 560b s.v. *kurkānû* lexical section.

23. Restored from *STT* 93:79′–80′ and BAM 379 i 40′–42′//SpTU 3.106 i 16′–18′ (*Šammu šikinšu*). See pchapter 2, text 2.

24. See Uruanna II 7f, apud *CAD* A/2, 524b s.v. *azallû*, lexical section.

25. See Uruanna III 50, apud *CAD* B, 241b s.v. *bīnu* A, mng. c 9′.

26. Restored from CT 41.43 (BM 54595):8. See *CAD* A/2, 302b s.v. *arrabu*, lexical section.

27. TCL 6.34 ii 2 has SI DÀRA.MAŠ as one of 14 "plants" for a fumigant for AN.TA. ŠUB.BA(?).

28. This section is a commentary on TCL 6.34 i 1′–2′.

29. See Scurlock and Andersen 2005, 317–18.

30. See Scurlock and Andersen 2005, 19.40.

31. See Scurlock and Andersen 2005, 19.38.

32. See Scurlock and Andersen 2005, 19.13.

33. See Scurlock and Andersen 2005, 13.100.

34. For the reading of this passage, see *CAD* T, 300–301. *apar* is here assumed to be an adverb from *apru*: "hole"; cf. *ašar* from *ašru*.

35. This section is the commentary to TCL 6.34 i 5′–8′.

36. For the use of blood in the treatment of epileptics, see Stol 1993, 105.

37. This passage is to be dissociated from the *tu*$_9$-*limu* of 11N–T4:10 (pace Civil 1974, 336–37).

38. The next treatment is essentially lost, but was apparently an enema for *napḫar murṣi* more or less containing the enumerated plants mixed with the *pūru*-oil.

39. See *CAD* A/1, 354b s.v. *allānu*, mng. 1a.

40. See Streck 2004, 285–86.

41. See Uruanna III 50, apud *CAD* B, 241b s.v. *bīnu* A, mng. c 9′.

42. See Cohen 1976,136.

43. For a reconstruction of the text, see Veldhuis 1989, 241.

44. See *CAD* M/2, 239–40 s.v. *musukku*.

45. See Cohen 1976, 138.

46. This has been collated by Finkel 1980, 48 n. 25.

47. For a reconstruction of the text, see Veldhuis 1989, 241–42.

48. For a discussion of exegetical scribal word games with specific reference to this passage, see Maul 1997, 253–67.

49. See Scurlock 1991, 149.

50. The text is restored from the similar VS 17.34:1–10 (van Dijk 1972, 343–44); see Veldhuis, 1989, 243.

51. See Civil 1974, 334 ad line 17.

52. See Civil 1974, 334 ad line 27.

53. See *CAD* Š/2, 450a s.v. *šiltāḫu* mng 5′c.

54. The text incorrectly repeats the precative of BAM 248 ii 69.

55. UET 6/3.897 obv. 1′ picks up with *šá-ni-iš ṭe-*[*ra-at*].

56. UET 6/3.897 rev. 1′ picks up with *na-ma-ri* [...].

57. See Civil 1974, 333 ad line 2. Cavigneaux 1987, 252 prefers a more literal: "substitution."

58. Cavigneaux 1982, 236 n. 22 points out that GUG is the Sumerogram for *guqqû*, a monthly offering and that the relevance of SIZKUR is that it means both "sacrifice" and prayer" and since it does double duty, so too must GUG.

59. For an alternative interpretation of these lines, see George 1991, 155.

60. See Civil 1974, 334 ad line 17.

61. This is a citation of an ancient text. See Civil 1974, 334 ad lines 22–23.

62. This section is paralleled by UET 6/3.897 obv. 1′–8′. Cavigneaux 1982, 236 n. 22 argues that this represents a case of analogic reasoning. I would agree, but reconstruct the chain of logic in an inverse direction, so: ŠE = *idu*, ŠE = *kittabru*, ergo *idu* = *kittabru*.

63. These sections are paralleled by UET 6/3.897 obv. 9′–13′.

64. See Civil 1974, 335 ad line 41.

65. See Civil 1974, 335 ad line 42.

66. This section is paralleled by UET 6/3.897 rev. 1′–9′.

67. See Civil 1974, 335 ad lines 44–45

68. See Civil 1974, 335–36 ad lines 45–46.

69. Note also Civil 1974, 329, no. 3:28–29.

PART 2

THERAPEUTICS

5

EYES, EARS, NOSE, AND MOUTH

A. EYE TREATMENTS

Ancient Mesopotamian eyes were treated for loss of vision, dryness, tearing, abnormal redness and bleeding, conjunctivitis, flashes, night blindness, corneal opacities, and glaucoma. For more on this subject, see Fincke 2000 and Scurlock and Andersen 2005, 185–202. Treatments consisted of daubs, drops, plasters, washes, salves and bandages. There were also, even more rarely, potions, pills and aliments—in the case of night blindness, the patient was to eat a piece of liver. The pharmacist could be applied to for eye ointments which were called "spoons," apparently because a tiny lead spoon was used to apply them. Surgery with a barbers' razor is also attested for corneal opacities. For more on treatments in general, see Herrero 1984 and Böck 2009, 105–28.

TEXT 1: SPTU 2.50

SpTU 2.50 consists primarily of daubs for dimness (1–21), plus a bandage for tearing (22–23), eye drops for troubled eyes (24), and a salve for eyesight (27–28). There is also an out-of-place treatment for the mouth (25–26). Of these treatments, four (1–14, 27–28) are daubs or salves formulated in such a way as to suggest that they originated with or were intended to be taken to the pharmacist to be filled, whereas the remaining six (15–26) must have been intended, from the beginning, for the use of the physician. For more on this subject, see the introduction to this volume.

Of particular interest is the fact that lines 1–4 use ground stones in the daub. The most likely reason for this is to serve as an abrasive ensuring that the plant is able to penetrate the skin of the area surrounding the eye.

Lines 5–9 give the actual dosage for an individual patient, with the exact quantity of each plant required measured in carats, presumably using a jewellers' scale. This practice is an apparent innovation of late texts as also BM 78963, for which see below.[1] Neo-Assyrian texts rarely give information about dosages, although physicians clearly recognized the importance of not overdosing a patient. The usual practice was to give either just a listing of plants, animal and/or mineral substances without any quantities or with quantities too large for individual use. These large quantities may either have been meant to be made up as a preparation or, alternatively, the mention of amounts was just to indicate the proportion of plants, animal, and/or mineral substances to be used. The absence of dosages in recorded treatments is no indication that there was no oral tradition on the subject, as may readily be demonstrated by the fact that we have identical treatments with and without amounts specified. So, for example, lines 15–17 give dosages which are nowhere to be found in the duplicate.[2]

Lines 10–14, in addition to giving dosages, also indicate differing treatments for different seasons of the year. This treatment is also interesting in that it claims to have been tested and to be very old, dating back to Hammurabi of Babylon, no less.[3] Presumably the lawgiver was remembered as having had eye troubles. The combination of *rikibti arkabi*,[4] "white plant" and *emesallim*-salt (often with other medicaments added) is not infrequently encountered in eye daubs, suggesting that it is indeed of some antiquity.

Lines 27–28 give instructions for an ointment which was meant to be stored (in a box) and used regularly by the patient.

1. ^{NA_4}ZA.GÌN ^{NA_4}AŠ.GÌ.GÌ ^{NA_4}UGU.AŠ.GÌ.GÌ ^{NA_4}ŠEM.BI.ZI.DA IM.SIG$_7$.SIG$_7$
2. [^{NA_4}*šír*]-⸢*šir*$_{10}$⸣-*ma-tu*$_4$ *mál*!-*ma-liš ina ši-ri-su* ŠEG$_6$-*šal* EGIR *ina* GA ŠEG$_6$-*šal*
3. ⸢IM.SIG$_7$.SIG$_7$⸣ ^{NA_4}*šír-šir*$_{10}$-*mat* ŠUM-*aḫ* ^{Ú}ḪAB EGIR *gab-bi-šú-nu*
4. ŠUM-*aḫ ina* Ì.EGIR *u* DUḪ.LÀL *tu-la-ma te-qit la-tík-tu*$_4$ *šá bir-rat*

---

5. 2 *gír-e* IM.SIG$_7$.SIG$_7$ 2 *gír-e kur-ru-ku-um-mu gír-ú* Ú BABBAR
6. *gír-ú* KA *tam-tim* 1-*niš* ŠUM-*aḫ ina* MÚD BURU$_5$.ḪABRUD.DA^{MUŠEN} NITA *u* MUNUS
7. *ta-si-iḫ-ḫu te-qit šá bir-rat* IGI^{II} KI.MIN *ta-bi-lu* IGI^{II}-*šú* MAR
8. *ina* U$_4$-*mu* 4-*šú* GA *ina* KÚM-*mi-šú a-na* IGI^{II}-*šú* ŠUB-*di* EGIR GA
9. ^{NA_4}*as-ḫar ta-bi-lu* IGI^{II}-*šú* MAR

---

10. 1/2 GÍN U$_5$.ARGAB^{MUŠEN} 1/2 GÍN Ú.BABBAR 15 ŠE MUN *eme-sal-lim*
11. ^{Ú}ḪAB *ina* GISSU ḪÁD.DU *tu-lam šum*$_4$-*ma* KÚM.MEŠ *ina* Ì *ḫal-ṣa*
12. *šum*$_4$-*ma* EN.TE.NA *ina* Ì.NUN SÚD MAR MAR-*tú šá* ^{m}*Ḫa-mu-ra-pí*
13. *la-tík-tú e-nu-ma* DÙ-*šú* KAŠ ^{LÚ}KURUN.NA *la i-ši*
14. *li-te-qí ina* GI$_6$.GI$_6$ *li-šib*

---

15. DIŠ NA IGI^{II}-*šú i-bar-ru-ra* 1/2 GÍN Ú.BABBAR 2 GÍN

U_5.ARGAB^{MUŠEN}

16. 15 ŠE $^{\text{NA}_4}$*gab-ú* 15 ŠE MUN *eme-sal-lim bit-qa* Ì.UDU ^{ŠEM}GIG

17. [1]-*niš ina* Ì *gu-un-nu* SÚD IGI^{II}-*šú* MAR

---

18. [DIŠ NA] IGI^{II}-*šú i-bar-ru-ra u* ÍR *ú-kal-la* Ú.BABBAR LÀL

19. KUR.RA *ina* Ì SÚD MAR

---

20. DIŠ NA IGI^{II}-*šú i-bar-ru-ra* ^{ŠEM}ŠEŠ Ú.BABBAR U_5.ARGAB^{MUŠEN}

21. *ina* Ì.NUN.NA SÚD IGI^{II}-*šú* MAR

---

22. DIŠ NA IGI^{II}-*šú* ÍR *ú-kal-la saḫ-le*$_{10}$ *ṭe*$_4$*-né-e-tú ina* GA SILA_{11}-*aš*

23. IGI^{II}-*šú* LAL-*id*

---

24. DIŠ NA IGI^{II}-*šú* LÙ.LÙ-*ḫa* LÀL Ì.NUN.NA Ì.SAG : *ḫal-ṣa* 1-*niš* ‹‹x›› KÚM.KÚM-*am ta-šá-ḫal ana* IGI^{II}-*šú* ŠUB

---

25. DIŠ NA EME-*šú* GIG IM.KAL.LA.GUG URUDU.SUMUN *ina* Ì.NUN. NA ḪE.ḪE

26. ŠÉŠ-*su ša* KA *lat-ku*

---

27. A.BÁR *ina* A.MEŠ ŠE.GIG.BA *ta-sal-laq* SÚD *ina qup-pat šá* GI ŠUB-*šú*

28. *a-na* DAGAL EŠ IGI^{II} SIG_5

TRANSLATION

(1–4) You boil lapis lazuli, *ašgikû*-stone, UGU-*ašgikû*-stone, *guḫlu*-kohl, *da᾿mātu*-clay and ⌜*šeršermātu*-clay⌝ in equal quantitities in *širīšu*-beer. Afterwards, you boil (it) in milk. You integrate(?) in more *da᾿mātu*-clay and *šeršermātu*-clay. You integrate(?) in *šammi bu᾿šāni* after all of the rest of them. You soften (it) in leftover oil and wax and (daub it on). This is a tested daub for dimness.

(5–9) You integrate(?) together 2 carats of *da᾿mātu*-clay, 2 carats of *kurukummu*, a carat of "white plant" (and) a carat of *imbû tamtim*. You wet(?) (it) with the blood of a male and female *ḫurri*-bird. Daub for dimness in the eyes. Alternatively, you daub (it) dry onto his eyes. Four times a day, you let still hot milk fall into his eyes. After the milk, you daub dry *asḫar*-kohl onto his eyes.

(10–14) You soften 1/2 shekel of *rikibti arkabi*, 1/2 shekel of "white plant," 15 grains of *emesallim* salt (and) *šammi bu᾿šāni* which you have dried in the shade. If it is summer, you grind (it) in pressed-out oil (and) if it is winter in ghee (and) daub (it) on. This is the tested daub of Hammurabi.[5] If when you do it, he does not have any *kurunnu*-beer, he should daub (it) on (and) sit in the shade.

(15–17) If a person's eyes become dimmed,[6] you grind 1/2 shekel "white plant," 2 shekels *rikibti arkabi*, 15 grains of alum, 15 grains of *emesallim*-salt, (and) 1/8 shekel of *kanaktu* "fat" together in *gunnu* oil and daub it on his eyes.

(18–19) If a person's eyes become dimmed and contain tears, you grind "white plant" (and) wild honey in oil (and) daub (it) on.

(20–21) If a person's eyes become dimmed, you grind myrrh, "white plant," (and) *rikibti arkabi* in ghee (and) daub (it) on his eyes.

(22–23) If a person's eyes contain tears, you make mill-ground *saḫlû*-cress into a dough with milk (and) bandage his eyes (with it).

(24) If a person's eyes are continually troubled, you heat honey, ghee (and) first quality/pressed-out oil together (and) filter (it). You let (it) fall into his eyes.

(25–26) If a person's mouth/tongue is sore, you mix *kalgukku*-clay (and) old copper with ghee (and) rub him gently (with it). This is a tested treatment for the mouth.

(27–28) You boil lead in wheat infusion (and) grind (it). You pour (it) into a reed box. It is good to rub gently sideways on the eyes for the eyesight.

TEXT 2: BAM 159 iv 0′–v 9

BAM 159 is a very eclectic mix of treatments, with one of the more interesting selections in the corpus. The remainder of this text is discussed or treated in chapter 5 as text 8, chapter 9 as texts 3–6, 8, chapter 10 as text 3 and chapter 11, text 2. This particular section consists of a plaster (iv 0′–1′) for the eyes, a daub (iv 2′–7′) and a bandage (iv 8′–10′) for infected eyes, a bandage (iv 11′–15′) for irritated eyes, another version of Hammurabi's eye daub (iv 16′–22′), a series of daubs (iv 23′–30′) for dimness, a bandage (v 3–4) and a daub (v 5–6) for tearing and a daub (iv 7–9) for red eyes. Of these, at least one (iv 0′–1′) appears to have been available at the pharmacist's.

Lines iv 2′–7′ is a treatment for corneal opacities, possibly due to adenovirus infection. For details, see Scurlock and Andersen 2005, 9.68. In addition to the eye daub, a dough is allowed to cool on the patient's shaved head. A number of ancient treatments, this among them, state explicitly that they have been tested. Lines iv 16′–22′ have the ingredients weighed out in the scales before Shamash, which served two purposes: to ensure accurate measurement and to enlist the assistance of the god of justice in the cure. Lines v 7–9 are unusual in allowing the plant to steep for three days before grinding.

iv

0′. [(Ú BABBAR NA$_4$ *ga-bi-i* MUN *eme-sal-lim*)]
1′. [(3 Ú)] *ṭe-pu šá* IGI$^{[(II)]}$

2′. DIŠ NA IGI^{II}-*šú* GIG-*ma* U$_4$.MEŠ *ma-ʾ-du-te* NU BAD-*te*
3′. *ina* KÚM SAG.DU-*šú* IGI^{II}-*šú* GISSU DIRI
4′. SAG.DU-*su* SAR.SAR *ina* U$_4$-*me* 3-*šú* NÍG.SILAG.GÁ
5′. *tu-kaṣ-ṣa* NUMUN ^{Ú}IN.NU.UŠ *tur-ár*
6′. *ina* Ì.NUN DÍLIM A.BÁR SÚD IGI^{II}-*šú*
7′. MAR.MEŠ-*ma bul-ṭu lat-ku*

8′. [DIŠ N]A IGI^{II}-*šú* MÚ.MEŠ-*ma u* IM *le-qa-a*
9′. [(ZÍD ^{Š})]^{EM}GÚR.GÚR ZÍD GAZI^{SAR} BÍL.MEŠ ZÍD.ŠE.SA.A
10′. [(*ina* KAŠ)].SAG *tara-bak* IGI^{II}-*šú* LAL

11′. DIŠ N[A IGI]^{II}-*šú* IM *ud-du-pa-a-ma a-pá-a*
12′. *a-š*[(*a-a*)] *u* ÍR ŠUB.ŠUB-*a* ZÍD GÚ.GAL ZÍD GÚ.TUR
13′. ZÍD ^{Ú}[...].A ZÍD ŠE.SA.A ZÍD GAZI^{SAR} ZÍD ^{ŠEM}GÚR.GÚR
14′. ZÍD ^{ŠEM}LI ZÍD ^{ŠEM}MAN.DU 1-*niš* ḪE.ḪE
15′. *ina* A GAZI^{SAR} *tara-bak* SAG.KI^{II}-*šú* IGI^{II}-*šú* LAL-*ma* TI

16′. DIŠ NA IGI^{II}-*šú a-pa-a a-šá-a u* ÍR ŠUB.ŠUB-*a na-ṭa-la*
17′. *mu-uṭ-ṭu ana* TI-*šú* ^{ŠEM}ŠEŠ Ú.BABBAR U$_5$.ARGAB^{MUŠEN}
18′. MUN *eme-sal-lim* ^{ŠEM}GÚR.GÚR Ú *a-ši-i* Ú.KUR.RA
19′. 7 Ú.ḪI.A ŠEŠ IGI.4.GÁL.LA.TA.ÀM *ina* IGI ^{d}UTU
20′. *ina* GIŠ.RÍN LAL-*al ina* LÀL SÚD IGI^{II}-*šú* MAR
21′. *mìn-da ta-bi-la tu-ṭep-pi-ma ina-eš*
22′. *te-qit* IGI$^{II.MEŠ}$ *šá* ^{m}*Ḫa-am-mu-ra-pí lat-ku*

23′. DIŠ NA IGI^{II}-*šú* ⸢ÍR⸣ *bir-ra-ta*$_5$ *a-šá-a* [ÍR] ⸢*lu-ḫa-a*⸣
24′. TUKU.MEŠ-*a* 1 GÍN U$_5$.ARGAB^{MUŠEN} 1/2 [GÍN] ⸢Ú.BABBAR⸣
25′. 15 ŠE ^{MUN}*eme-sal-lim ina* Ì.NUN SÚD [IGI^{II}-*šú*] MAR

26′. DIŠ NA IGI^{II}-*šú i-bar-ru-ra* ^{ŠEM}ŠEŠ ⸢Ú⸣.BABBAR
27′. U$_5$.ARGAB^{MUŠEN} *ina* Ì.NUN SÚD IGI^{II}-*šú* MAR

28′. DIŠ NA IGI^{II}-*šú bar-ra u* ÍR *ú-kal-la*
29′. Ú.BABBAR L[(ÀL.KUR.R)]A *ina* Ì.NUN SÚD IGI^{II}-*šú* MAR

30′. 3 *te-qit* IGI^{II} [...]

---

v

1. [...]x *ri-šu saḫ-lé-e* ^{Ú}[o o]
2. *ina* KAŠ SILA$_{11}$-*aš* [LAL]

---

3. DIŠ NA IGI^{II}-*šú* ÍR *lu-ḫa-a* ŠUB.MEŠ
4. *saḫ-lé-e* KAŠ.Ú.SA *ina* A.MEŠ SILA$_{11}$-*aš* LAL

---

5. DIŠ *a-na* ÍR TAR-*si* KAL.KU$_7$.KU$_7$ *kib-r*[*it*]
6. *ina* Ì.UDU GÌR.PAD.DU GÍD.DA UDU.NÍTA SÚD M[(AR)]

---

7. DIŠ NA IGI^{II}-*šú a-šá-a bir-ra-ta*$_5$ *u ri-šu-t*[*a*$_5$]
8. *ú-kal-la* NUMUN ^{Ú}SI.SÁ *ina* A.MEŠ U$_4$.3.KÁM
9. *tara-muk i-ḫar-ra-aṣ-ma ina* A.MEŠ DUL! SÚD MAR

TRANSLATION

(iv 0′–1′) "White plant," alum and *emesallim*-salt: three plants (for) a plaster for the eyes.

(iv 2′–7′) If a person's eyes are so sore that he does not open them for many days (and) during a fever in his head his eyes fill with opaque spots,[7] you repeatedly shave his head. You let a dough cool on his head three times a day. You char *maštakal* seed. You grind (it) in ghee with a lead spoon (and) daub (it) repeatedly on his eyes. (This is) a tested treatment.

(iv 8′–10′) [If] a ⸢person's⸣ eyes are continually swollen and take up "clay," you decoct[8] *kukru* flour, roasted *kasû* flour and roasted grain flour in first quality beer (and) bandage his eyes (with it).

(iv 11′–15′) If a ⸢person's eyes⸣ have been blown into by the wind so that they are clouded, confused and continually shed tears,[9] you mix together *ḫallūru*-chickpea flour, *kakku*-lentil flour, [...] flour, roasted grain flour, *kasû* flour, *kukru* flour, *burāšu*-juniper flour (and) *su'ādu* flour. You decoct[10] (it) in *kasû* juice and, if you bandage his forehead and eyes (with it), he should recover.

(iv 16′–22′) If a person's eyes are clouded, confused, and continually shed tears (and) the eyesight is diminished,[11] to cure him, before Shamash you weigh out 1/4 shekel each of these seven plants in the scales: myrrh, "white plant," *rikibti arkabi*, *emesallim* salt, *kukru*, *šammi aší* (and) *nīnû*-mint. You grind (them) in honey (and) daub (them) on his eyes. Alternatively, if you daub a measured amount on dry, he should recover. (This is) the tested eye daub of Hammurabi.

(iv 23′–25′) If a person's eyes continually have tears, dimness, confusion of vision and dirty [tears], you grind 1 shekel of *rikibti arkabi*, 1/2 [shekel] of "white plant" (and) 15 grains of *emesallim*-salt in ghee (and) daub (it) on [his eyes].

(iv 26′–27′) If a person's eyes become dimmed,[12] you grind myrrh, "white plant" and *rikibti arkabi* in ghee (and) daub (it) on his eyes.

(iv 28′–29′) If a person's eyes are dimmed and contain tears,[13] you grind "white plant" (and) wild honey in ghee (and) daub (it) on his eyes.

(iv 30′) (The preceding treatments are) three daubs for the eyes for [dimness of the eyes].

(v 1–2) [If ...], you make *saḫlû*-cress (and) [...] into a dough with beer [and bandage him with it].

(v 3–4) If a person's eyes continually shed dirty tears,[14] you make *saḫlû*-cress (and) beerwort into a dough with water (and) bandage (him with it).

(v 5–6) If you want to keep away tears, you grind *kalgukku*-clay and ⌜*kibrītu*-sulphur⌝ in marrow from the long bone of a wether and daub (his eyes with it).

(v 7–9) If a person's eyes contain confusion of vision, dimness and redness,[15] you decoct[16] *šurdunû* seed for three days in water. He should cut (it) up and then cover (it) with water. You grind (it and) daub (it) on.

B. EAR TREATMENTS

Ancient Mesopotamian ears were treated for trauma, shingles, otitis externa, otitis media, tinnitus, and Menière's syndrome. For more details, see Scurlock and Andersen 2005, 202–6. Treatments consisted of tampons, washes, powders and drops, fumigants, and, more rarely, bandages, salves, and potions. Accompanying many treatments were instructions to eat hot things, meaning not simply heated but hot in the sense of spicy, as in mustard. There was also the ancient equivalent of a Q-tip (as in BAM 503 i 11′–16′, iv 20–22).

TEXT 3: BAM 503

BAM 503 probably represents Tablet 1 of the second sub-series of UGU (see chapter 3, text 1). It begins with three fragmentary treatments for a family ghost (i 1′–16′) and continues with fumigants (i 17′–18′, 28′–37′), washes (i 19′, 26′–27′, 40′) and tampons (i 20′–25′, 38′–39′, i 41′–ii 15) for ghost roaring or ringing in the ears. The remainder of the text lists tampons (ii 53′–60′, 63′–66′, iii 1–17, 42′–63′, 68′–78′, iv 3–10, 13–17, 29–31, 44), washes (ii 58′–66′, iii

19–21, 42′–44′, iii 48′–iv 10, iv 16–17, 27–28, 32–35, 40–43, 45–46) or earbaths (iii 79′–iv 2), drops (ii 72′, iii 1–15, 39′–41′, iv 18–19, 42–43, 45–46) or powders (ii 54′–57′, 67′–71′, iii 1–18, 37′–38′, iv 11–12, 25–26, 29–31), fumigants (ii 67′–71′, iii 19–21, 24–25, 35′–36′, iv 38–39), potions (iii 52′–56′, 72′–78′, iv 36–37), aliments (i 7′–10′, ii 58′–60′, iii 57′–60′, 68′–78′, iv 3–6, 9–10) and, rarely, bandages (i 63′–66′), and salves (iv 18–19) for ear infections. Of these treatments, only four (BAM 503 i 31′–37′), all fumigants for ghost roaring in the ears, are formulated in such a way as to suggest that they originate with the pharmacist, whereas the remaining treatments must have been intended, from the beginning, for the use of the physician.

Of special interest are the curious recitations which accompany tampons used to treat ghost roaring in the ears (i 20′–23′, i 41′–ii 18, ii 22′–36′) and which are, on occasion actually whispered into the patients' ears as the only treatment (ii 16–18, 22′–36′). For more on this type of therapy for tinnitus, see Scurlock and Stevens 2007, 1–12.

In lines ii 54′–57′ and iv 29–31, a medicated tampon containing pomegranate juice is to be left in the ears for several days. This was expected to loosen up the pus, which was then allowed to run out and be wiped off. When the pus stopped, alum was blown into the ears via a reed straw. Pus could also be loosened up by fumigation, as in lines ii 67′–71′.

Lines ii 58′–60′ accompany a medicated tampon with a wash poured over the head (cf. iii 48′–63′, 68′–71′). They also require the patient to eat emmer bread with *saḫlû*-cress mustard (cf. iii 57′–60′, iv 5–6). Similarly, the treatments in lines iii 68′–78′, iv 3–4 recommend eating hot things and iv 9–10 a plant. The bandage of lines ii 63′–66′ and the potions of iii 52′–56′, 72′–78′ and iv 36–37 seem to have served a similar purpose of encouraging suppuration.

Lines iii 48′–iv 2 are fine examples of patients taking advantage of medical conditions to gain good luck for themselves by seeking out the sanctuaries of specified gods, at the sanctuaries' expense, no less! (iii 75′–78′). However auspicious particular illnesses were, however, the patient still got treatment for his condition, as is preserved in lines iii 64′–67′, 72′–78′.

Lines iii 72′–74′ are unusual in having a rolled linen cloth in place of the usual tuft of wool in the tampon. Lines iv 18–19 use transdermal medication rubbed in with the assistance of frit, as with eye salves. Lines iv 25–26 ensure that all of the medication gets into the ear canal by the simple expedient of grasping the outer parts of the ears. Lines iv 38–39 use a turban to get the full benefit from a fumigant.

i

1′. [N]A BI GIDIM I[M.RI.A-*šú* DIB-*su* …]

2′. ^{ŠEM}ŠE.LI BABBAR ^{ŠE}[M …]

3′. ^{Ú}*tar-muš* ^{GIŠ}*si-ḫa* [...]
4′. *ina* A ŠEM.ḪI.A *šá-šu-nu* [...]
5′. *ta-lal uš-šá sír-da* x[...]
6′. Ì ^{ŠEM}ŠEŠ *ana* SAG.KI-[*šú* ŠUB-*di*...]

7′. DIŠ KI.MIN ^{GIŠ}ERIN ^{GIŠ}ŠUR.MÌN G[I.DÙG.GA ...]
8′. 8 Ú.ḪI.A ŠEŠ TÉŠ.BI *ina* KAŠ S[AG ...]
9′. KI.A.^{d}ÍD *ku-up-ri* ^{d}Í[D ... *taq-ti-ru*]
10′. *tu-qat-tar-šú ḫi-ib-ṣa ša* x [...]

11′. DIŠ NA *ina* DIB-*it* ŠU.GIDIM.MA GEŠTU [...]
12′. ŠEM.^{d}MAŠ *zap-pi* ANŠE.KUR.RA TÚ[G.NÍG.DÁRA.ŠU.LÁL ...]
13′. MÚD MUŠ ^{Ú}KI.SÌ.KI A.RI.⸢A⸣ [...]
14′. ŠU.SI.MEŠ-*šú ina* GEŠTU^{II}-*šú i-ret-ti-m*[*a* ...]
15′. *a-šar* TAB.BA *ši-i* ^{d}*É-a tas-*[*li-ti* ...]
16′. EGIR-*šú* KA *sa-par-ti* SI GUD [...]

17′. DIŠ NA GIDIM DIB-*su-ma* GEŠTU^{II}-*šú i-š*[(*ag-gu-ma*) ^{ŠE}(^{M}BAL GI.DÙG.GA ⸢^{ŠEM}⸣GÚR.GÚR)]
18′. GAZI^{SAR} *zap-pi* ANŠE.KUR.⸢RA⸣[(PAP 5 Ú.MEŠ *qu*$_5$*-taru*$_5$ *ša* GEŠTU^{II} *lat-ku*)]

19′. [...] *ina* MUD GEŠ[TU^{II}-*šú* ...]

20′. DIŠ NA ŠU.GIDIM.MA DIB-*su-ma* GEŠTU^{II}-*šú i-šag-gu-ma* ^{ŠEM}ŠEŠ ^{N}[($^{\text{A}_4}$AŠ.GÌ.GÌ $^{\text{NA}_4}$ÈŠ.ME.KÁM)]
21′. SÚD *ina* ^{SÍG}ÀKA NIGIN-*mi ina* MÚD ^{GIŠ}ERIN SUD ÉN PEŠ.DU$_8$ *ib-ni* ŠI[D-*nu*]

22′. ÉN PEŠ.DU$_8$ *ib-ni* ^{d}*É-a* IM.MA.AN.NA.AN.KI.A NA$_4$ *li-iz-zur-šú* NA$_4$ *li-iš-*⸢*kip-šú* NA$_4$ *liš*⸣*-p*[*i-šú*]
23′. NA$_4$ *li-pa-sis-su* TU$_6$ ÉN : ÉN *an-ni-tú* 3-*šú ana* UGU *líp-pi* ŠID-*nu ana* ŠÀ GEŠTU^{II}-*šú* GAR-*an*

24′. DIŠ KI.MIN ^{ŠEM}GÚR.GÚR ^{Ú}ḪAR.ḪAR ^{Ú}KUR.KUR ^{Ú}*ak-tam* ^{Ú}*imḫur-lim* ^{Ú}*imḫur*-20 ^{Ú}*tar-muš* ZAG.ḪI.LI SÚD
25′. *ina* Ì ^{GIŠ}ERIN ḪE.ḪE *ina* ^{SÍG}ÀKA NIGIN-*mi ana* ŠÀ GEŠTU^{II}-*šú* GAR-*ma ina-eš* : DIŠ KI.MIN GI.DÙG *ina* Ì+GIŠ SÚD *ana* ŠÀ GEŠTU^{II}-*šú* GAR-*an*

26′. DIŠ KI.MIN ^{ŠEM}ŠEŠ $^{\text{NA}_4}$ÁŠ.GI$_4$.GI$_4$ $^{\text{NA}_4}$ZA.GÌN $^{\text{NA}_4}$SIG$_7$.SIG$_7$ 1-*niš* SÚD

27′. *ina* Ì ^{GIŠ}ERIN ḪE.ḪE *ana* ŠÀ GEŠTU^{II}-*šú* ŠUB UZU^{II}-*šú* ŠÉŠ

28′. DIŠ NA *ina* DIB-*it* ŠU.GIDIM.MA GEŠTU^{II}-*šú i-šag-gu-ma* NUMUN *ú-ra-a-nu* NUMUN ^{GIŠ}MA.NU

29′. *ni-kip-tú* NÍTA *u* MUNUS *záp-pi* ANŠE.KUR.RA TÚG.NÍG.DÁRA.ŠU.LÁL *ina* DÈ GEŠTU^{II}-*šú tu-qat-tar*

30′. DIŠ NA *ina* DIB-*it* ŠU.GIDIM.MA GEŠTU^{II}-*šú i-šag-gu-ma* SUḪUŠ ^{GIŠ}MA.NU *ni-kip-tú* TÚG.NÍG.DÁRA.ŠU.LÁL *ina* DÈ ŠÀ GEŠTU^{II}-*šú* SAR

31′. ^{ŠEM}GÚR.GÚR ^{ŠEM}LI ^{ŠEM}ŠEŠ ^{GIŠ}ERIN GI DÙG.GA ^{ŠEM}MUG ‹(^{ŠEM}MAN.DU)› GAZI^{SAR} ^{IM}KAL.GUG

32′. 8 (variant: 9) Ú.ḪI.A *qu$_5$-taru ša* GEŠTU^{II} *ina* DÈ ‹$^{\text{GIŠ.Ú}}$(GÍR)› ŠÀ GEŠTU^{II}-*šú* SAR

33′. $^{\text{NA}_4}$*mu-ṣú* SI DÀRA.MAŠ GÌR.PAD.DU NAM.LÚ.U$_{18}$.LU KA *tam-ti$_4$* GÌR.PAD.DU UGU.DUL.BI

34′. Ú.KUR.RA *ina* [D]È ŠÀ GEŠTU^{II}-*šú tu-qat-tar*

35′. *kib-ri-tú* ^{Ú}KU$_6$ SUḪUŠ ^{GIŠ}⸢MA.NU⸣ *a-za-pi* ANŠE.KUR.RA TÚG.NÍG.DÁRA.ŠU.LÁL *ina* DÈ $^{\text{GIŠ.Ú}}$GÍR ŠÀ GEŠTU^{II}-*šú tu-qat-tar*

36′. SI DÀRA.MAŠ NA$_4$ *ga-bi-i* ⸢Ú⸣.[KUR.R]A *saḫ-lé-e* KA *tam-ti$_4$ kib-ri-tú*

37′. GÌR.PAD.DU NAM.LÚ.U$_1$[$_8$.LU] *ina* DÈ $^{\text{GIŠ.Ú}}$GÍR ŠÀ GEŠTU^{II}-*šú* SAR

38′. DIŠ NA GEŠTU^{II}-*šú i-šag-gu-ma* MÚ[D ^{GIŠ}ERIN] *a-ra-an-di* ^{ŠEM}GÚR.GÚR *ina* ^{SÍG}ÀKA NIGIN-*mi*

39′. *ana* ŠÀ A.MEŠ ŠUB-*di ina* IZI ŠE[G$_6$]-*šal ana* ŠÀ GEŠTU^{II}-*šú* GAR-*ma* TI

40′. DIŠ NA GEŠTU^{II}-*šú i-šag-gu-ma* MÚD ^{GIŠ}E[R]IN KI A ^{GIŠ}NU.ÚR.MA ḪE.ḪE-*ma ana* ŠÀ GEŠTU^{II}-*šú* ŠUB-*ma* TI

41′. ⸢ÉN⸣ *in-da-ra-aḫ ta-ra-a*[*ḫ-t*]*i šu-maš in-da-ra-aḫ ta-ra-aḫ-ti*

42′. [*ti*]*r-ki-bi in-da-ra-a*[*ḫ ta-r*]*a-aḫ-ti tir-ki-ba-su-tú* TU$_6$ ÉN

---

ii

1. ÉN ŠU.BI [IN.DU$_8$ GÌR.BI IN.DU$_8$ *bu*]*r-še bur-na bur-na-an-na su-ri-iḫ su-ri-iḫ*.E.NE
2. *su-ri-iḫ* D[U$_8$ (*ni-ik-ri-iḫ*) *s*]*u-ri-iḫ ta-aḫ-ta-aḫ* TU$_6$ ÉN

---

3. 2 KA.INIM.M[A] DIŠ NA GEŠTU^{II}-[*šú*] *i-šag-gu-ma*

---

4. DÙ.DÙ.BI ^{ŠEM}[ŠEŠ …] $^{\text{NA}_4}$ÁŠ.GI[$_4$.GI$_4$ … *in*]*a* MÚD ^{GIŠ}ERIN ḪE.ḪE
5. ÉN 3-*šú ana* ŠÀ ŠI[D-*nu ina*] ^{SÍG}ÀKA N[IGIN-*mi ana* Š]À GEŠTU^{II}-*šú* GAR-*an*

---

6. ÉN SI IN.DU$_8$ *i*[*b-ni* ^{d}*É-a* IM.MA.A]N.NA.AN.KI.A ⸢*ib*⸣-[*ni du-up-ni gú-ús*]-*sa* TU$_6$ ÉN

---

7. ⸢1⸣ KA.INI[M.MA] DIŠ NA GEŠTU^{II}-*šú i-šag-gu-ma*

---

8. [D]Ù.DÙ.BI ^{ŠEM}[ŠEŠ] $^{\text{NA}_4}$ÁŠ.GI$_4$.GI$_4$ *ni-kip-tú ina* Ì ḪE.ḪE *ina* UL *tuš-bat* ÉN 3-*šú*
9. [*ana* Š]À ŠID-*nu* ⸢^{SÍG}ÀKA⸣ [NIGIN *ana* ŠÀ GEŠTU^{II}]-*šú* GAR-*an* ÉN ŠA.RA.ZU ŠA.RA.ŠAG$_5$.GA.KÁM.A
10. [UR.SA]G ^{d}NIN.I[B] ŠA.RA.ŠAG$_5$.GA.KÁM.A
11. [EN] ^{d}NIN.IB ŠA.RA.ŠAG$_5$.GA.KÁM.A
12. [LUGAL] ^{d}NIN.IB [ME.EN] NAM.BA.TE.GÁ.E.NE TU$_6$ ÉN

---

13. [1] KA.INIM.MA DIŠ NA GEŠTU^{II}-*šú i-*[*ša*]*g-gu-ma*

---

14. [DÙ.DÙ.B]I $^{\text{NA}_4}$*èš-me-k*[*án* o]x ^{ŠEM}ŠEŠ ^{Ú}*úr-nu-u* TÉŠ.[B]I SÚD *ina* MÚD ^{GIŠ}ERIN ḪE.ḪE
15. [ÉN 3-*šú*] *ana* ŠÀ ŠID-*nu* [*ina*] ^{SÍG}ÀKA NIGIN-*mi ana* ŠÀ GEŠTU^{II}-*šú* GAR-*an*

---

16. [(ÉN *na-p*)]*i-ir-še-ri-iš* [(*pa-ta-ar*)]-*ri zu-ga*[-(*l*)]*i-ir-ri pa-at-ḫal-li pa-tar-ri*
17. [(*su-ma-áš p*)]*a-at-r*[(*i pa-ku-un*)]-*di ra-ta-*[(*aš i*)]*k-ki-ri-ri ša-ra-aš* TU$_6$ ÉN

---

18. [KA.INIM.MA DIŠ NA GEŠTU^{II}-*šú i-šag-g*]*u-ma* 3-*šú* [*ana* ŠÀ GEŠTU ZA]G-*šú* 3-*šú ana* ŠÀ GEŠTU GÙB-*šú* MÚ

Gap

22′. [(ÉN NÍG.È NÍG.È NÍG.NAM.MA UŠ).BU]

23′. [(KI.A.DÍM.MA.BI A.RI.A AN.NA.K)E_4]

24′. [(SIG$_7$ ALAM.BI GAR.AN.GIN$_7$ ŠU NU.TE.G)Á]

25′. [(ḪUR.SAG.GIN$_7$ GUL.GUL SIG$_7$ ALAM.BI ZI.IR.ZI.IR.E).DÈ]

26′. [GAR (UDUG ḪAR.RA.AN GAR UDUG KASKAL.ÀM)]

27′. NÍG.NÍ.ZU ⸢MU.UN.ŠI.IN⸣.[(GIN.NA NÍG.NÍ.ZU MU.UN.ŠI.IN.GIN.NA)]

28′. [(^{d}NIN.IB LUGAL.^{GIŠ}TUKUL.KE_4 GA)]BA.ZU ḪÉ.EN.⸢GÁ⸣.[GÁ]

29′. [(ḪUL.DÚB ZI.AN.NA ḪÉ.P)À Z]I KI.A. ḪÉ.PÀ

30′. [(KA.INIM.MA DIŠ NA GEŠTU^{I})^{L}-*šú i-šag-gu-ma* (3-*šú a-na* GEŠTU) Z]AG-*šú* 3-*šú ana* ŠÀ GEŠTU GÙB-*šú* ŠID[17]

31′. [(ÉN *ḫu-ḫu-un-ti ib-ni-a-ti ib-ni-ir*)]-*ra šá-na-an*

32′. [(*ak-ka-li-ir-ri su-gar-ri šá-at-ri ku-uk-t*)]*i ḫu-ma-at-ri su-ma-aš* TU$_6$ ÉN

33′. [(KA.INIM.MA GEŠTU^{II}-*šú i-šag-gu-ma ana* ŠÀ GEŠT)]U ZAG-*šú li-iḫ-šú*

34′. [(ÉN *a-me-am-ma-an ku-um-ma-am-ma su-um-ma-a*)]*t-ri ki-ri-ri ku-uk-ti*

35′. [(*ra-šá-na ku-uk-ti ḫu-un-di ḫu*)]-*ma-an* TU$_6$ ÉN

36′. [KA.INIM.MA (GEŠTU^{II}-*šú i-šag-gu-ma ana* ŠÀ GEŠTU G)]ÙB-*šú li-iḫ-šú*

37′. […] ^{Ú}*kur-ka-na-a*

Gap

53′. [(DIŠ NA GEŠTU^{II}-*šú* GU$_7$.MEŠ-*šú neš-ma-a ḫe-e-si* Ì+GIŠ ^{GIŠ}*du*)]*p-ra-an* SÍG.ÀKA SUD 1-*tum* 2-*šú* [(*u*)] 3-*šú ana* ŠÀ GEŠTU^{II}-*šú* GAR-*an*

54′. DIŠ N[(A GIG-*ma* GIG-*su*)] ⸢*ana*⸣ ŠÀ GEŠTU^{II}-*šú* [(*ip*)]-*pu-uš-ma neš-ma-a* DUGUD 1 GÍN A ^{GIŠ}NU.ÚR.⸢MA⸣

55′. 2 [(GÍN A)] ^{ŠEM}[(GIG)] : Ì ^{ŠEM}[GIG] ḪE.ḪE SÍG.ÀKA SUD *ana* ŠÀ GEŠTU^{II}-*šú* GAR-*an* U$_4$.3.KÁM *an-nam* DÙ-⸢*uš*⸣

56′. *ina* [(U$_4$.4.K)]ÁM MÚD.BABBAR *šá* ŠÀ [(GEŠTU^{II}-*šú*)] E$_{11}$-*ma ta-kap-par* GIN$_7$ MÚD.BABBAR *it-tag-ma*-[(*ru*)]

57′. IM.SAḪAR.NA$_4$.KUR.RA SÚD *ina* GI.SAG.KUD *ana* ŠÀ GEŠTU^{II}-*šú*

MÚ-*a*[(*ḫ*)]

58′. DIŠ [N]A KÚM *ana* ŠÀ GEŠTU^{II}-*šú i-pu-uš-ma neš-mu-šú* DUGUD *ù lu* IR *ú-kal* Ì+GIŠ ^{GIŠ}*dup-r*[*a-na*]

59′. Ì+GIŠ GI.DÙG.GA *ana* SAG.DU-*šú* ŠUB-*di* SÍG.ÀKA SUD 1-*šú* 2-*šú* 3-*šú ana* ŠÀ GEŠTU^{II}-*šú* GAR

60′. *neš-mu-šú* BAD-*te saḫ-lé-e šá mim-ma ana* ŠÀ NU ŠUB *ina* NINDA.ZÍZ.AN.NA GU$_7$

61′. DIŠ NA *ina si-li-ʾ-ti-šú* KÚM *ana* ŠÀ GEŠTU^{II}-*šú ip-pu-uš-ma* GEŠTU^{II}-*šú* DUGUD Ì KUR.GI^{M}[(^{UŠEN})]

62′. *ana* ŠÀ GEŠTU^{II}-*šú* ŠUB-*ma neš-mu-šú i-qal-líl* SUḪUŠ ^{G}[^{I}(^{Š}N)]AM.TAR NÍTA *tu-pa-aṣ ana* ŠÀ GEŠTU^{II}-*šú* ŠUB-*ma ina-*[(*eš*)]

63′. DIŠ NA ‹(ŠÀ)› GEŠTU^{II}-*šú* GIN$_7$ GAR ŠU.GIDIM.MA GU$_7$.MEŠ ⸢*ù* SÌG⸣.MEŠ-*šú* Ì+GIŠ ^{ŠEM}GIG Ì+GIŠ GI.DÙG.G[A]

64′. Ì+GIŠ ^{ŠEM}LI *a-ḫe-e tu-raq-qa* 1-*niš* ḪE.ḪE *ana* ŠÀ GEŠTU^{II}-*šú* ŠUB LAG ^{MUN}*eme-sal-lim*

65′. ^{SÍG}⸢ÀKA NIGIN⸣ *ana* ŠÀ GEŠTU^{II}-*šú* GAR KAŠ.Ú.SA SIG$_5$ ZÍD GÚ.GAL ZÍD GÚ.TUR ZÍD ZÍZ.ÀM

66′. ZÍD GAZI^{SAR} ZÍD ^{GIŠ}*ere-*⸢*ni*⸣ *ina* KAŠ *tara-bak* ‹(LAL)› TI-*uṭ*

67′. DIŠ NA GEŠTU^{II}-*šú* GI[G-*ma* ŠÀ GEŠ]TU^{II}-*šú bi-ʾ-iš* SÌG.MEŠ-*su* GÍR.GÍR-*s*[*u* […] ú ra x

68′. GU$_7$-*šú-ma la* N[Á-*lal* ^{Š}]^{EM}LI ^{ŠEM}GÚR.GÚR ^{ŠEM}GÍR ^{ŠEM}BAL [GAZI]^{SAR} IM.KAL.L[A]

69′. IM.KAL.GUG [1-*niš* GAZ] SIM *ina* DÈ ⸢^{GIŠ}⸣$^{.Ú}$GÍR ŠÀ GEŠTU^{II}-*šú* SAR-*ár*

70′. [… U$_4$.3].KÁM *an-nam* ⸢DÙ-*uš*⸣-*ma ina* U$_4$.4.KÁM ŠÀ GEŠTU^{II}-*šú ta-kap-pár-ma*

71′. [GIN$_7$ ÚŠ.BABBAR *i*]*t-tag-ma-ru* IM.SAḪAR.NA$_4$.KUR.RA SÚD *ina* ^{GI}SAG.KUD *ana* ⸢ŠÀ⸣ GEŠTU^{II}-*šú* MÚ-*aḫ*

72′. [DIŠ NA *ina*] GEŠTU^{II}-*šú* MÚD BABBAR DU-*ak* MÚD ÉLLAG GUD *u* MÚD ^{GIŠ}ERIN 1-*niš* ḪE.ḪE *ana* ŠÀ GEŠTU^{II}-*šú* BI.IZ

---

iii

1. […] *ana* ŠÀ GEŠTU^{II}-*šú* BI.IZ A ^{GIŠ}[…]

2. [… *ana* ŠÀ GEŠTU^{II}-*šú*] BI.IZ A [^{GIŠ}N]U.ÚR.⸢MA⸣ *ina* [Ì ^{GIŠ}ER]IN

ḪE.ḪE

3. [*ana* ŠÀ GEŠTU^{II}-*šú* B]I.IZ *kam-ka-*⸢*ma*⸣ *šá kim-ṣi* AN[ŠE …] *šá* ⸢GÚ⸣. MÚRGU ANŠE *ina* Ì ^{GIŠ}ERIN ḪE.ḪE
4. [^{SÍG}ÀKA] ⸢NIGIN-*mi*⸣ *ana* ŠÀ GEŠTU^{II}-*šú* GAR-*an* Ì ^{ŠEM}BULUḪ $^{Š[E]M}$[L]I ZÉ BIL.ZA.ZA *ana* ŠÀ GEŠTU^{II}-*šú* BI.IZ
5. […] an Ì-*šú ina* Ì KUR.GI^{MUŠEN} ḪE.ḪE *ana* ŠÀ GEŠTU^{II}-*šú* BI.IZ
6. […]x *ina* ZÌ.KUM ḪE.ḪE *ana* ŠÀ GEŠTU^{II}-*šú* GAR
7. [… *t*]*u-daq-qaq ina* [GI.S]AG.KUD *ana* ŠÀ GEŠTU^{II}-*šú* MÚ-*aḫ* GAZI^{SAR} *ki-ma* ŠE.SA.A *ta-qàl-lu*
8. [… *ana* Š]À GEŠTU^{II}-*šú* MÚ-*a*[*ḫ* …] ^{GIŠ}MI.PÀR *tur-ár* SÚD *ana* ŠÀ GEŠTU^{II}-*šú* MÚ-*aḫ tu-ru-u*ʾ*-a*
9. [*ta-ša-a*]*s-si lu* bu […] *tu-pa-ṣa* A-*šú ana* ŠÀ GEŠTU^{II}-*šú* BI.IZ *kám-ka-ma šá kìn-ṣi* ANŠE
10. […] *šá kal-bi* 1-*niš* ḪE.ḪE [*ana* ŠÀ GEŠTU]^{II}-*šú* GAR-*an-*⸢*ma*⸣ NAGA.SI KUG.GAN N[Í]TA *u* MUNUS SÍG.ÀKA NIGIN
11. [*ana* ŠÀ GEŠ]TU^{II}-*šú* GAR-*an* SUM.[ŠIR.DIDLI].SAR *tu-ḫa-sa ana* ŠÀ ⸢GEŠTU⸣^{II}-*šú tu-na-tak*

---

12. [DIŠ *ina* G]EŠTU^{II}-*šú* MÚD.BABBAR *i-ṣar-ru-ur* [A (^{GIŠ}NU)].ÚR.MA *ana* ŠÀ GEŠTU^{II}-*šú* BI.IZ ⸢Ú⸣ BABBAR SÚD
13. [*ina* G]I.SAG.KUD *ana* ŠÀ GEŠTU^{II}-*šú* MÚ-*a*[*ḫ* (Ì)] ^{GIŠ}ERIN Ì ^{ŠEM}M[UG? G]AMUN^{SAR} SÚD
14. [(*ina* Ì).N]UN ḪE.ḪE SÍG.ÀKA NIGIN-*mi ana* Š[(À GEŠTU^{II}-*šú*)] GAR : GAMUN.GI$_6$ [^{Š}]^{EM}ŠEŠ Ì.KU$_6$
15. [(Ú.KUR)].RA 1-*niš* ḪE.ḪE *ana* ŠÀ GEŠTU^{II}-*šú* GAR-*an* (variant: BI.IZ) [(ZÉ ŠAḪ *ina*)] ZÌ.KUM ḪE.ḪE [SÍG.ÀKA NIGI]N-*mi ana* ŠÀ GEŠTU^{II}-*šú* GAR-*an*
16. [^{GIŠ}NU].ÚR.MA ḪÁD.A SÚD *ana* ŠÀ GEŠTU^{II}-*šú* MÚ-*a*[*ḫ* … ER]IN ^{ŠEM}[… ZÉ BIL].ZA.ZA *tur-ár* SÚD
17. [*ana* ŠÀ GE]ŠTU^{II}-*šú* MÚ Ì ^{GIŠ}ŠUR.MÌN SÍG.ÀKA SU[D *ana* ŠÀ GEŠTU^{II}-*šú* GAR Ú].KUR.RA K[A…SÚD *ana* Š]À GEŠTU^{II}-*šú* GAR-*an*
18. [IZI *ta*]-*ša-rap* ‹‹x›› Ú BABBAR *ta-bi-lam ana* ŠÀ [GEŠTU^{II}-*šú* GAR-*an* IM.SAḪA]R.NA$_4$.[KUR.RA SÚD *ana* ŠÀ] GEŠTU^{II}-*šú* MÚ-*aḫ*
19. [PA ^{GIŠ}]*bi-ni* PA ^{GIŠ}Ù.⸢SUḪ$_5$⸣ *ina* ⸢DÈ⸣ […] KUR.GI^{MUŠEN}
20. [… ZÉ] BIL.ZA.ZA
21. [… GEŠTU]^{II}-*šú* GAR-*an*

---

22. [… ^{GIŠ}NU].ÚR.MA

23. […] GAR-*an*

---

24. […ḪA]R!.ḪAR
25. […] SAR

(gap)
31′. *ina* […]
32′. x […]
33′. *kám*-[…]
34′. Ú […]

35′. DIŠ GEŠTU^{II} x[…] ^{ŠEM}GÚR.[GÚR/GAM.MA …]
36′. A ^{GIŠ}NU.[ÚR.MA …] ar *ina* DÈ ^{GIŠ}ŠINIG *ta-sa-r*[*aq-ma* TI]

37′. DIŠ ‹KI.MIN› KUG.GAN SÚD *ana* ŠÀ GEŠTU^{II}-*šú ta-sa-*[*raq-ma* TI]

38′. DIŠ KI.MIN GAZI^{SAR} GIN$_7$ ŠE.SA.A *ta-qal-lu* SÚD *ana* ŠÀ GEŠTU^{II}-*šú* *ta-*[*sa-raq-ma* TI]

39′. DIŠ NA MÚD BABBAR *ina* ŠÀ GEŠTU^{II}-*šú* DU-*ak* ⸢A⸣ ^{GIŠ}NU.ÚR.MA Ì+GIŠ BÁRA.GA Ì ^{GIŠ}ERIN x[…]
40′. Ì ^{ŠEM}BULUḪ ^{ŠEM}LI Z[É B]IL.ZA.ZA SIG$_7$ *ana* ŠÀ GEŠTU^{II}-*šú* BI.IZ *še-mi* […]
41′. MÚD NIM 1-*niš* ḪE.ḪE *ana* ŠÀ GEŠTU […]

42′. DIŠ NA *ina* ŠÀ GEŠTU-*šú lu* A.MEŠ *lu* MÚD *lu* MÚD.BABBAR DU-*ak* ŠÀ GEŠTU^{II}-*šú ta-kap-p*[*ár* …]
43′. *ina* GI.SAG.KUD DUB ŠÀ GEŠTU^{II}-*šú* LUḪ-*si* MIN-*ma* A.GEŠTIN.NA BIL.LÁ *ana* ŠÀ GEŠ[TU^{II}-*šú* …]
44′. ⸢x x⸣ SÚD *ina* LÀL ḪE.ḪE *ana* ŠÀ GEŠTU^{II}-*šú* DUB SÍG.ÀKA NIGIN LÀL KUR x[…]

45′. DIŠ KI.MIN NUMUN ^{Ú}NU.LUḪ.ḪA SÍG.⸢ÀKA⸣ [NIGIN-*mi ana* Š]À GEŠTU^{II}-*šú* GAR-*an*
46′. DIŠ KI.MIN NUMUN ^{ŠEM}GÚR.GÚR SÚD [SÍG.ÀKA NIGIN] *ana* ŠÀ GEŠTU^{II}-*šú* GAR-*an*
47′. DIŠ KI.MIN GAZI^{SAR} *qa-lu-te* SÚD [SÍG.ÀKA NIGIN] *ana* ŠÀ GEŠTU^{II}-*šú* GAR-*an*

48′. DIŠ NA GEŠTU ZAG-*šú ina* KÚM [... NA BI *aš*]-*rat* ^{d}UTU : ^{d}30 KIN-*ma* ‹(: ^{d}*Í-gì-gì*)›
49′. DUG$_4$.GA *u* GIŠ.TUKU GAR [(^{MUN})*e*]*me-sal-lim ina* Ì+GIŠ ŠUR.MÌN
50′. ⸢Ì+GIŠ ^{ŠEM}GIG⸣ [SÚD ^{SÍG}ÀKA NIGIN-*mi ana* ŠÀ GEŠTU^{II}-*šú* (GAR-*an* Ì.BUR)] *el-lam ana* SAG.DU-*šú* ŠUB-*di*
51′. [... U$_4$.(⸢7⸣.KÁM)] GUR.GUR-*šum-ma* TI

52′. [DIŠ NA GEŠTU GÙB-*šú ina* KÚM ...] x NA BI *aš-rat* ^{d}NIN.IB KIN-*ma*
53′. [...]x ^{MUN}*eme-sal-lim* [*ina* Ì.GIŠ ... Ì.GIŠ] ⸢^{ŠEM}⸣GIG
54′. [^{SÍG}ÀKA NIGIN-*m*(*i ana* ŠÀ GEŠTU^{II}-*šú*) GAR-*an* Ì.BU]R *el-lam ana* [SAG.DU-*šú* ŠUB]-*di*
55′. [... ^{ŠE}]^{M}LI [... *ina* UL *tuš*-(*bat* NAG.MEŠ KAŠ ^{LÚ}KURUN.NA NAG. MEŠ)]
56′. [U$_4$.7.KÁM GUR].GUR-*šum-ma* TI

57′. [...]-*šú* NA BI *aš-rat* ^{d}UTU KIN-*ma*
58′. [... ^{ŠEM}L]I SÚD SÍG.ÀKA NIGIN-*mi ana* ŠÀ GEŠTU^{II}-*šú* GAR-*an*
59′. [Ì.BUR *el-lam ana* SAG.DU-*šú* ŠUB-*di saḫ-lé-e*] *ina* NINDA.ZÍZ.ÀM GU$_7$ MIN
60′. [U$_4$.7.KAM] GUR.GUR-*šú-ma* TI

61′. [...] KIN-*ma* 7 ITI ŠAG$_5$.GA IGI-*mar*
62′. [...SÚD SÍG.ÀKA NIGIN-*mi ana* ŠÀ GEŠTU]^{II}-*šú* GAR Ì.BUR *el-lam ana* SAG.DU-*šú* ŠUB-*di*
63′. [...] U$_4$.7.KÁM GUR.GUR-*šum-ma* TI-*uṭ*

64′. [DIŠ ... NA BI G]IG UD.DA GIG NA BI ZI.GA
65′. [...] SIG$_5$ IGI-*mar ana* TI-*šú*
66′. [...] Ì+GIŠ ŠUR.MÌN *ana* SAG.DU-*šú* ŠUB-*di*
67′. [... KÁ]M GUR.GUR-*šum-ma* TI-*u*[*ṭ*]

68′. [... *qe*]*r-bi-nu* [...]
69′. [... U$_4$].9.KÁM A.ESIR! *šú*-⸢*šum*⸣ [...]
70′. [...] Ì+GIŠ ^{ŠEM}GIG ^{SÍG}[À]KA [...]
71′. [... Š]UB?-*di bu-úḫ-ra* x[...]

72′. [DIŠ NA GEŠTU ZAG-*šú*] IR *ana qer-bi-nu ip-ḫur*-[*ma* ...] x x x x x x NE GÁL-*šú* NA BI
73′. [*aš-rat* DN K]IN-*ma* SIG$_5$ IGI-*mar ana* TI-*šú* GADA *ta-ṣap-pir* Ì+GIŠ

ŠUR.MÌN Ì+GIŠ ERIN SUD *ana* ŠÀ GEŠTU^{II}-*šú* GAR-*an*

74′. [...] *ana* SAG.DU-*šú* ŠUB *an-nu-u* K[ÚM]? GU$_7$ MIN ^{Ú}ḪAR.ḪAR *ina* KAŠ NAG MIN U$_4$.7.KÁM GUR.GUR-*šum-ma* TI

75′. [DIŠ NA GEŠTU] GÙB-*šú* IR *ana qer-bi-nu ip-ḫur-*⸢*ma*⸣ MÚD.BABBAR ŠUB-*ni* NA BI *aš-rat* ^{d}EŠ$_4$.DAR KIN-*ma* SIG$_5$ IGI-*mar*

76′. [...]x *ša-šú ḫal-qam* IGI-*mar ana* TI-*šú* Ì+GIŠ ^{GIŠ}ERIN Ì+GIŠ Ì+GIŠ ^{GIŠ}ŠUR.MÌN Ì+GIŠ ^{ŠEM}BA[L]

77′. [Ì+GIŠ GI].DÙG.GA Ì+GIŠ ^{ŠEM}GIG SÍG.ḪÉ.ME.DA SUD *ana* ŠÀ GEŠTU-*šú* GAR Ì+GIŠ ^{ŠEM}GIG *ana* S[AG.DU-*šú*]

78′. [ŠUB] *bu-úḫ-ra* GU$_7$ MIN KAŠ NAG MIN U$_4$.7.KÁM GU[R.GUR-*šum-ma* TI-*uṭ*]

79′. [DIŠ NA GEŠTU]-*šú* GÙ.GÙ-*si* IM *ḫa-sat* ⸢*lu*?⸣ MÚD.BABBAR DÙ-*ni aš-rat* ^{d}[...]

iv

1. [...]

2. A ^{GIŠ}NU.ÚR.MA ⸢SIG$_7$.SIG$_7$⸣ RA-*su* Ì+GIŠ SUD [...] ⸢SÚD⸣ *ana* SAG.KI.MEŠ-*šú* ŠUB DÙG [IGI-*mar*]

---

3. DIŠ KI.MIN MUN SÚD SÍG.ÀKA NIGIN Ì+GIŠ ŠUR.MÌN SUD *ana* ŠÀ GEŠTU^{II}-*šú* GAR-*an* Ì+GIŠ ŠUR.MÌN *ana* SAG.K[I.MEŠ-*šú* ŠUB]

4. *baḫ-ra* GU$_7$ *u* NAG U$_4$.3.KÁM *an-nam* DÙ-*uš-ma* DÙG [IGI-*mar*]

---

5. DIŠ KI.MIN ^{ŠEM}LI SÚD SÍG.ÀKA NIGIN *ana* ŠÀ GEŠTU^{II}-*šú* GAR-*an* Ì ILLU ^{ŠEM}BULUḪ *ana* SA[G.KI.MEŠ-*šú* ŠUB]

6. ⸢*saḫ-lé*⸣-*e* KI NINDA.ZÍZ.ÀM GU$_7$.MEŠ 3 U$_4$-*mi an-nam* DÙ.DÙ-*ma* [...]

---

7. [DIŠ KI.MIN] ⸢Ì⸣ ^{GIŠ}ERIN.NA SÍG.GA.RÍG.AK.A SUD ⸢*ana* ŠÀ⸣ [GEŠTU^{II}-*šú* GAR-*an* ...]

8. [...] *ana* SAG.KI.MEŠ-*šú* ŠUB.ŠUB-*ma* [...]

---

9. [DIŠ KI.MIN Ì] ^{GIŠ}ERIN Ì+GIŠ ŠUR.MÌN SÍG.GA.RÍG.AK.A S[UD ...]

10. [*ana* SAG.K]I.MEŠ-*šú* ŠUB.MEŠ ^{Ú}ḪAR.ḪAR GU[$_7$ ...]

---

11. [(DIŠ NA GEŠ)]TU ZAG-*šú* DUGUD SUM.ŠIR.DIDLI[(^{SAR} *tu-pa-ṣa* *ana* ŠÀ GEŠTU-*šú* GAR-*an*)]

---

12. [(PA ^{GIŠ})]ŠINIG SIG$_{7}$-*su* SÚD *ina* ZÌ.K[(UM ḪE.ḪE *ana* ŠÀ GEŠTU-*šú* GAR-*an*)]

---

13. $^{\text{[(GIŠ)]}}$ERIN.‹(SUMUN)› ^{ŠEM}LI GAMUN GI$_{6}$ SUM[(^{SAR} SÚD *ina* Ì.NUN ḪE.ḪE)] ‹(^{SÍG}ÀKA [SUD])›
14. *ana* ŠÀ GEŠTU-*šú* GAR-*an* Ì+GIŠ [(⸢ŠUR.MÌN⸣ ^{SÍG}ÀKA SUD *ana* ŠÀ GEŠTU-*šú*) GAR-*an*

---

15. ^{ŠEM}ḪAB Ì.ŠAḪ PA ^{GIŠ}MAŠ.ḪUŠ ‹(BURU$_{5}$.ḪABRUD.DA)› SÍG ^{MUNUS}[(SILA$_{4}$ SÍG ^{MUNUS}ÁŠ.GÀR GÌŠ NU ZU *ta-zák* ^{SÍG}ÀKA NIGIN-*mi ana* ŠÀ GEŠTU-*šú*) GAR-*an*]

---

16. Ì+GIŠ *dup-ra-na* ^{SÍ}[(^{G}ÀKA SUD *ana* ŠÀ GEŠTU-*šú*) GAR-*an*]
17. MÚD ^{d}NIN.KILIM.EDIN.NA KI [(Ì ^{GIŠ}ERIN Ì ^{GIŠ}ŠUR.MÌN ḪE.ḪE *ana* ŠÀ) GEŠTU-*šú* DUB]

---

18. A ^{GIŠ}NU.ÚR.MA AN.ZAḪ.GI$_{6}$ [(*tu-daq-qaq ana*) … (MAR *ḫa-si-sa-ti-šú* ŠÉŠ)]
19. BURU$_{5}$.ḪABRUD.DA NITA SAG.DU-*s*[(*u* KUD-*is* ⸢MÚD.MEŠ KÚM?⸣) *ana* ŠÀ GEŠTU-*šú tu-na-tak*]

---

20. DIŠ NA GEŠTU GÙB-*šú* DUGUD ^{ŠEM}ŠEŠ : ^{ŠEM}GIG SÚD […]
21. LÀL KUR *ina* Ì.UDU UR.[MAḪ …]

---

22. EGIR-*šú* DÍLIM A.BÁR [o o] Ì+GIŠ x[…]

---

23. Ì+GIŠ ERIN ŠE.MU[Š$_{5}$ …]

---

24. *si-ik-ti* ^{GIŠ}*šu-šu*[*m* …]

---

25. *ḫa-si-sa-šú* DIB-*at* ZÍ[D …]x x
26. ZÍD *bu-ṭu-tú* LAL […]x ŠUB

---

27. Ì+GIŠ *ina* KA-*ka ana* ŠÀ GEŠTU [… DU]B-*ak*
28. *kám-ma ša* AŠGAB […] MÚ-*aḫ*

---

29. DIŠ NA GEŠTU^{II}-*šú* DUGUD 1 GÍN A ^{GI}[(^{Š}NU.ÚR.MA 1 GÍN A ^{ŠEM}GIG *ina* SÍG.ÀKA SUD *ana*)] ŠÀ GEŠTU-*šú* GAR
30. 3 U$_{4}$-*me an-na-a* DÙ.DÙ-*uš* [(*ina* U$_{4}$.4.KÁM)] ‹(MÚD BABBAR *šá* ŠÀ)›

[(GEŠTU^{II})]-*šú* ‹(E_{11}-*m*)*a*› *ta-kap-pár*

31. IM.SAḪAR.NA_4.KUR.RA SÚD ‹(*ina* ^{GI}SAG.KUD)› [(*ana* ŠÀ)] GEŠTU^{II}-*šú* MÚ-*aḫ*

---

32. ^{GIŠ}*šu-ru-uš* ^{GIŠ}NAM.TAL N[ÍTA…]-*šú* ŠU.TI
33. SIG_7-*su* SÚD A-*šú* x[… *neš-m*]*u-šú* BAD-*te*

---

34. ^{ŠEM}ḪAB Ì.ŠAḪ KA.A.AB.[BA … ^{MUNUS}ÁŠ.G]ÀR GÌŠ.NU.ZU
35. *tur-ár* SÚD [… *ana* Š]À GEŠTU^{II}-⸢*šú*⸣ ŠUB

---

36. SUM.SIKIL PA ^{GIŠ}MA[… *k*]*i-ma an-nam i-te-*⸢*ep*⸣*-šu*
37. ZAG.ḪI.LI *šá*?[…] *ina* KAŠ NAG-*ma*

---

38. ^{TÚG}BAR.SI x […] ^{TÚG}DUL-*šú*
39. x x […] 3.KÁM SAR.SAR-*ma* TI

---

40. […] ŠÀ GEŠTU^{II}-*šú* ŠUB-*di*
41. [… *a*]*na* ŠÀ GEŠTU^{II}-*šú* ŠUB-*di*

---

42. [… *ana*] ŠÀ GEŠTU^{II}-*šú* ŠUB-*di*
43. [… ḪE].ḪE *ana* ŠÀ GEŠTU^{II}-*šú tu-na-tak*

---

44. […]x *ana* ŠÀ GEŠTU^{II}-*šú* GAR-*an*

---

45. [… ŠÀ] GEŠTU^{II}-*šú tu-na-tak*
46. […] *ana* ŠÀ GEŠTU^{II}-*šú* ŠUB

---

47 […]x

TRANSLATION

(i 1′–6′) […] a ⸢family⸣ ghost [afflicts] that ⸢person. [You …] these aromatics: *kikkirānu*-juniper berries, […], *tarmuš*, *sīḫu*-wormwood, (and) […] in water. […] You hang […]. You […] *uššu*-rush, *sirdu*-olive (and) […]. You pour] myrrh oil on [his] forehead. […]

(i 7′–10′) Alternatively, [you …] these eight plants: *erēnu*-cedar, *šurmēnu*-cypress, ⸢"sweet reed"⸣, (and) […] together in beer (and) […] *Kibrītu*-sulphur, bitumen from the ⸢river⸣ (and) [… are the fumigants]. You fumigate him (with them). [You have him eat] a *ḫibṣu*-preparation made with [*saḫlû*-cress …]

(i 11′–16′) If, as a result of affliction by "hand" of ghost, a person['s] ears [... , you ...] *nikiptu*, horse bristle, [...] ⌜*sikillu*⌝ (= "soiled rag"), [...], "snake blood," (snake's) nest, ⌜*maštakal*⌝ (= "[human] semen") [...] He sticks his fingers in his ears and [...] As soon as (the trouble) starts,[18] [he says]: Ea [accept? my] ⌜prayer⌝? [...] Afterwards, the very tip of an ox horn [...]

(i 17′–18′) If a ghost afflicts a person so that his ears roar, *ballukku*-aromatic, "sweet reed," *kukru*, *kasû*, (and) horse hair: total of five plants. A tested fumigant for the ears.

(i 19′) [... You blow (it into) his] ⌜ears⌝ via a straw.

(i 20′–21′) If "hand" of ghost afflicts a person so that his ears roar, you grind myrrh, *ašgikû*-stone (and) *ešmekku*-stone. You wrap (it) in a tuft of wool. You sprinkle (it) with *erēnu*-cedar resin. You ⌜recite⌝ the recitation "PEŠ.DU$_8$ *ib-ni*."

(i 22′–23′) Recitation: "Ea created the PEŠ.DU$_8$ long ago in heaven and earth. May the stone curse it. May the stone overturn it. May the stone lace [it] up. May the stone efface it" : spell (and) recitation. You recite this recitation three times over the tampon. You put (it) into his ears.

(i 24′–25′) Alternatively, you grind *kukru*, *ḫašû*-thyme, *atāʾišu*, *aktam*, *imḫur-lim*, *imḫur-ešra*, *tarmuš*, (and) *saḫlû*-cress. You mix (it) with *erēnu*-cedar oil. You wrap (it) in a tuft of wool. If you put (it) into his ears, he should recover. Alternatively, you grind "sweet reed" in oil (and) put (it) into his ears.

(i 26′–27′) Alternatively, you grind together myrrh, *ašgikû*-stone, lapis lazuli, (and) "green-green"-stone. You mix (it) with *erēnu*-cedar oil. You pour (it) into his ears. You rub (it) on his (temporal) muscles/blood vessels.[19]

(i 28′–29′) If, as a result of affliction by "hand" of ghost, a person's ears roar, you fumigate his ears with *urânu* seed, *eʾru*-tree seed, male and female *nikiptu*, horse hair, (and) *sikillu* (= "soiled rag") over coals.[20]

(i 30′) If, as a result of affliction by "hand" of ghost, a person's ears roar, you fumigate the inside of his ears with *eʾru*-tree root, *nikiptu*, (and) *sikillu* (= "soiled rag"). You fumigate the inside of his ears (with them) over ⌜coals⌝.

(i 31′–32′) *Kukru*, *burāšu*-juniper, myrrh, *erēnu*-cedar, "sweet reed," *ballukku*, ‹(*suʾādu*)›, *kasû*, (and) *kalgukku*-clay are eight (variant: nine) plants, fumigants for the ears. You fumigate the inside of his ears (with them) over ‹(*ašāgu*-thorn)› coals.

(i 33′–34′) You fumigate the inside of his ears (with) *mūṣu*-stone, stag horn, "lone plant" (= "human bone"),[21] *imbû tâmti*, ape bone, (and) *nīnû*-mint over coals.

(i 35′) You fumigate the inside of his ears (with) *kibrītu*-sulphur, *šimru*, *eʾru*-tree root, horse hair, (and) *sikillu* (= "soiled rag") over *ašāgu*-thorn coals.

(i 36′–37′) You fumigate the inside of his ears (with) stag horn, alum, ⌈*nīnû*-mint⌉, *saḫlû*-cress, *imbû tâmti*, *kibrītu*-sulphur, (and) "lone plant" (= ⌈"human bone"⌉) over *ašāgu*-thorn coals.

(i 38′–39′) If a person's ears roar, [22] you wrap [*erēnu*-cedar] resin, *arantu*-grass, (and) *kukru* in a tuft of wool. You drop (it) into water (and) boil (it) over a fire. If you put (it) into his ears, he should recover.

(i 40′) If a person's ears roar, you mix ⌈*erēnu*-cedar⌉ resin with *nurmû*-pomegranate juice and, if you pour (it) into the inside of his ears, he should recover.

(i 41′–ii 5) Recitation: "*Indaraḫ* ⌈*taraḫti*⌉ *šumaš, indaraḫ taraḫti* ⌈*tirkibi*⌉, ⌈*indaraḫ*⌉ ⌈*taraḫti*⌉ *tirkibasutu*": spell (and) recitation. § Recitation: "[It loosened] its hand; [it loosened its foot]. ⌈*Burše*⌉ *burna burnanna, suriḫ* of *suriḫ*'s, ⌈it loosened⌉ the *suriḫ, nikriḫ* ⌈*suriḫ*⌉ *taḫtaḫ*": spell (and) recitation. § Two recitations (for cases) where a person['s] ears roar. § Its ritual: [You ...] ⌈myrrh⌉, [...] (and) ⌈*ašgikû*⌉-stone. You mix (it) ⌈with⌉ *erēnu*-cedar resin. You ⌈recite⌉ the recitation three times over (it). You ⌈wrap⌉ (it) [in] a tuft of wool (and) put (it) ⌈into⌉ his ears.

(ii 6–9a) Recitation: "The horn loosened it. [Ea] ⌈created⌉ (it). [Long ago, in] ⌈heaven⌉ and earth, ⌈he created⌉ (it). [You (horn) knock down its ...]": spell (and) recitation. § A ⌈recitation⌉ (for cases) where a person's ears roar. § Its ⌈ritual⌉: you mix [myrrh], *ašgikû*-stone, (and) *nikiptu* in oil. You put (it) out overnight under the stars. You recite the recitation three times ⌈over⌉ (it). [You wrap it in] a tuft of wool (and) put (it) [into] his [ears].

(ii 9b–15) Recitation: "(Since) you truly know, since you are truly good, ⌈hero Ninurta⌉, since you are truly good, [lord] Ninurta, since you are truly good, [king] Ninurta, may they (the ghosts) never approach": spell (and) recitation. § [One] recitation (for cases) where a person's ears ⌈roar⌉. § ⌈Its⌉ [ritual]: you grind ⌈together⌉ *ešmekku*-stone, [...], myrrh, (and) *urnû*-mint. You mix (it) with *erēnu*-cedar resin. You recite [the recitation three times] over it. You wrap (it) [in] a tuft of wool (and) put (it) into his ears.

(ii 16–18) Recitation: "*Napiršeriš*[23] *patarri zugalirri patḫalli patarri sumaš patri, pakundi rataš ikkiriri šaraš*": spell (and) recitation. § [Recitation (for cases) where a person's ears] ⌈roar⌉. You say/sing (it) three times [into] his ⌈"right"⌉ [ear] (and) three times into his "left" ear.[24]

(gap)

(ii 22′–30′) Recitation: "Watchful watcher who tracks down everything, whatever was created in the earth (or) the spawn of heaven, for (it) not to approach his (the patient's) shape or form (any more than one could approach) heaven, for him to utterly to destroy (them) just as (he destroyed) the mountain, to completely remove(?) them from his (the patient's) shape or form, [putting] the ghost/demon on the path(?), putting the ghost/demon on the road—when you go there by yourself, when you go there by yourself, Ninurta, king of the weapon, let it (the weapon) be put before you to smash the evil. May it swear by heaven. May it swear ⌜by⌝ earth." § Recitation (for cases) where a person's ears roar. You recite (it) three times into his "right" ear (and) three times into his "left" ear.

(ii 31′–33′) Recitation: "*Ḫuḫunti ibniati ibnirra šanan akkalirri sugarri šatri kukti ḫumatri sumaš*": spell (and) recitation. § Recitation (for cases) where his ears roar. A whispered prayer into his "right" ear.

(ii 34′–36′) Recitation: "*Amiamman kummamma summatri kiriri kukti rašana kukti ḫundi ḫumman*": spell (and) recitation. § [Recitation] (for cases) where his ears roar. A whispered prayer into his "left" ear.

(ii 37′) [...] *kurkānu*-turmeric [...]

(gap)

(ii 53′) If a person's ears continually hurt him (and) his hearing feels pressured, you sprinkle *daprānu*-juniper oil on a tuft of wool. You insert (it) once, twice and three times into his ears.

(ii 54′–57′) If fever spreads into a person's ears so that his hearing is heavy, you sprinkle 1 shekel of *nurmû*-pomegranate juice (and) 2 shekels of infusion of *kanaktu*-aromatic (variant: [*kanaktu*]-aromatic oil) on a tuft of wool (and) insert (it) into his ears. You do this for three days. On the fourth day, if the pus which is in his ears comes out, you wipe (it) off. When the pus has finished, you grind alum (and) blow (it) into his ears via a reed straw.

(ii 58′–60′) If fever spreads into a ⌜person's⌝ ears so that his hearing (feels) heavy or (his ears) contain sweat,[25] you pour ⌜*daprānu*⌝-juniper oil (and) "sweet reed" oil over his head. You sprinkle a tuft of wool (with it and) insert (it) once, twice and three times into his ears. His hearing should open up. You have him eat *saḫlû*-cress upon which nothing has been allowed to fall in emmer bread.

(ii 61′–62′) If during the course of a person's illness,[26] fever spreads into his ears so that his ears feel heavy, if you pour *kurkû*-goose fat into his ears, his hearing should lighten up. You pulverize male *pillû* root. If you pour (it) into his ears, he should recover.

(ii 63′–66′) If ‹(the insides of)› a person's ears continually hurt him and continually give him a jabbing pain like an attack of "hand" of ghost,[27] you press out separately oil of *kanaktu*-aromatic, oil of "sweet reed," (and) oil of *burāšu*-juniper. You mix (them) together. You pour (it) into his ears. You wrap a lump of *emesalim*-salt ‹in› a tuft of wool and put (it) into his ears. You decoct[28] winnowed beerwort, *ḫallūru*-pea flour, *kakku*-pea flour, emmer flour, *kasû* flour, (and) *erēnu*-cedar flour in beer. ‹(You bandage him with it)›. He should recover.

(ii 67′–71′) If a person's ears are ⌜sore⌝ [and the inside of] his ⌜ears⌝ stinks (and) continually gives him a jabbing pain, continually stings him (and) [...] (and) it hurts him so that he cannot ⌜sleep⌝, [you crush together] and sift *burāšu*-juniper, *kukru*, *asu*-myrtle, *balukku*-aromatic, [*kasû*], *kalû*-clay (and) *kal*-

gukku-clay. You fumigate the inside of his ears (with it) over *ašāgu*-thorn coals. You do this for [three days] and, on the fourth day, you wipe off the inside of his ears. [When the pus] has finished, you grind alum (and) blow (it) into his ears via a reed straw.

(ii 72′) [If] pus flows [from a person]'s ears, you mix together blood from the kidney of an ox and *erēnu*-cedar resin (and) drip (it) into his ears.

(iii 1–11) (For pus flowing from the ears), you drip [...] into his ears. You drip [...] infusion (and) [...] into his ears]. You mix *nurmû*-pomegranate juice with ⸢*erēnu*-cedar⸣ [oil] (and) ⸢drip⸣ (it) [into his ears]. You mix *kamkamu*-glue(?) made from ⸢donkey⸣ shins (and) [...] from the spine of a donkey with *erēnu*-cedar oil. You wrap (it) in [a tuft of wool] (and) insert (it) into his ears. You drip *baluḫḫu*-aromatic oil, ⸢*burāšu*-juniper⸣ (oil) (and) frog bile into his ears. [...] You mix its oil/fat with goose fat (and) drip (it) into his ears. You mix [...] with *isqūqu*-flour (and) put (it) into his ears. You finely crush [...] (and) blow (it) into his ears with a ⸢reed straw⸣. You roast *kasû* as if it were roasted grain flour [and grind it]. You blow (it) [into] his ears. You char (and) grind [...] (and) *līparu*-tree and blow (it) into his ears. ⸢You shout⸣ a *turuʾa*-shout.[29] You pulverize [...] (so *AHw*)/You pulverize *turuʾa*-plant [with the ...] of a ⸢ram's⸣ horn (so *CAD*). You drip its liquid into his ears. You mix together *kamkamu*-glue(?) made from donkey shins and [...] from a dog. You put (it) [into] his ⸢ears⸣. You wrap *uḫḫūlu qarnānu* (and) male and female *lulû*-mineral in a tuft of wool (and) insert (it) [into] his ⸢ears⸣. You crush/mince *turû*-garlic (and) drip (it) into his ears.

(iii 12–21) [If] pus drips [from a person's] ⸢ears⸣, you drip *nurmû*-pomegranate [juice] into his ears. You grind "white plant" (and) blow (it) into his ears [via] a ⸢reed⸣ straw.) You grind *erēnu*-cedar oil, ⸢*ballukku*⸣(?)-aromatic oil (and) *kamunu*-cumin. You mix (it) with ghee, wrap (it) in a tuft of wool (and) insert (it) into his ears. Alternatively, you mix together *zibû*, myrrh, fish oil, (and) *nīnû*-mint and put (variant: drip) (it) into his ears. You mix pig gall with *isqūqu*-flour. You ⸢wrap⸣ (it) [in a tuft of wool] (and) insert (it) into his ears. You dry (and) grind ⸢*nurmû*⸣-pomegranate (and) blow (it) into his ears. You grind ⸢*erēnu*⸣-cedar, [...]-aromatic (and) ⸢frog⸣ [bile] which you have charred. You blow (it) [into] his ⸢ears⸣. You ⸢sprinkle⸣ *šurmēnu*-cypress oil on a tuft of wool [and insert it into his ears. You grind] ⸢*nīnû*-mint⸣ (and) insert (it) ⸢into⸣ his ears. You ⸢ignite⸣ [a fire]. You put "white plant" dried (in the fire) into [his ears. You grind] ⸢alum⸣ (and) blow (it) [into] his ears. [You fumigate him with] *bīnu*-tamarisk [leaves] (and) *ašûḫu*-pine[30] leaves over coals. [You mix] goose [fat], [...] (and) frog [bile and blow it into his ears. You ...] (and) put (it) [into] his ⸢ears⸣.

(iii 22–23) [If ...], [you ...] [...], *nurmû*-pomegranate juice and [...]. You put (it) [into his ears].

(iii 24–25) You fumigate (him) with […], ⸢*ḫašû*⸣-thyme and [… over coals].

(iii 31′–34′) *Too fragmentary for translation.*

(iii 35′–36′) If the ears […], [if] you ⸢strew⸣ *kukru*/*ṣumlalû*, […], *nurmû*-pomegranate infusion (and) […] on *bīnu*-tamarisk coals, [he should recover].

(iii 37′) Alternatively, you grind *lulû*-mineral. [If] you ⸢strew⸣ it into his ears, [he should recover].

(iii 38′) Alternatively, you roast *kasû* as if it were roasted grain flour (and) grind (it). [If] you [strew] (it) into his ears, [he should recover].

(iii 39′–41′) If pus flows from a person's ears, [31] you drip *nurmû*-pomegranate juice, pressed-out oil, *erēnu*-cedar oil, […], *baluḫḫu*-aromatic oil, *burāšu*-juniper (oil) (and) ⸢gall⸣ of a green ⸢frog⸣ into his ears. [His] hearing [should show improvement]. You mix […] and "fly blood" together (and) […] (it) into his ears.

(iii 42′–44′) If either liquid or blood or pus flows from a person's ear,[32] you ⸢wipe off⸣ the insides of his ears. You pour [… into his ears] via a reed straw. You wash out the insides of his ears. You do this again and then [you pour] wine vinegar into [his] ⸢ears⸣. You grind […] (and) mix (it) with honey. You pour (it) into his ears. You wrap (it) in a tuft of wool, [sprinkle it] with wild honey [and insert it into his ears].

(iii 45′–47′) Alternatively, [you wrap] *nuḫurtu* in a tuft of wool (and) insert (it) into his ears. Alternatively, you grind *kukru* seed. [You wrap it in a tuft of wool] (and) insert (it) into his ears. Alternatively, you grind roasted *kasû*. [You wrap it in a tuft of wool] (and) insert (it) into his ears.

(iii 48′–51′) If a person's "right" ear […] as a result of a fever, if [that person] seeks out ⸢the sanctuary⸣ of Shamash or Sîn (variant: the Igigi), people will listen to what he says. [You grind] *emesallim*-salt in *šurmēnu*-cypress oil (and) *kanaktu*-aromatic oil. [You wrap (it) in a tuft of wool] (and) insert (it) [into his ears]. You pour pure *pūru*-oil over his head. […]. If you do this repeatedly for seven [days], he should recover.

(iii 52′–56′) [If a person's "left" ear … as a result of a fever], if that person seeks out the sanctuary of Ninurta, […].[33] [You grind] *emesallim*-salt [in … oil] (and) *kanaktu*-aromatic [oil]. You ⸢wrap⸣ (it) [in a tuft of wool] (and) [insert (it)] into his ears. You ⸢pour⸣ pure ⸢*pūru*-oil⸣ over [his head]. [You …] […], *burāšu*-juniper (and) […]. You ⸢leave (it) out overnight⸣ [under the stars] (and) have him drink (it) repeatedly. You have him repeatedly drink *kurunnu*-beer. If you do this repeatedly [for seven days], he should recover.

(iii 57′–60′) [If …], if that person seeks out the sanctuary of Shamash, […]. You grind […] (and) ⸢*burāšu*-juniper⸣. You wrap (it) in a tuft of wool (and) insert (it) into his ears. [You pour pure *pūru*-oil over his head]. You have him eat [*saḫlû*-cress] in emmer bread twice (a day). If you do this repeatedly [for seven days], he should recover.

(iii 61′–63′) [If ...], if [that person] seeks out [the sanctuary of ...], he will experience improvement for seven months. [You grind ... You wrap (it) in a tuft of wool] (and) insert (it) [into] his ⸢ears⸣. You pour pure *pūru*-oil over his head. [...] If you do this repeatedly for seven days, he should recover.

(iii 64′–67′) [If ... that person] is sick with an ⸢illness⸣ of *ṣētu*, that person [...] losses [...]; he will experience improvement. To cure him, you pour [...] (and) *šurmēnu*-cypress oil over his head. If you do this repeatedly [for # days], he should recover.

(iii 68′–71′) [...] ⸢within⸣ [...] nine [days] [You ...] bitumen, *šūšu*-licorice (and) [...]. [You sprinkle] a tuft of wool [with] *kanaktu*-aromatic oil. [...] You pour [*pūru*-oil over his head. You have him eat] hot things [...]

(iii 72′–74′) [If a person's "right" ear] collects sweat on the inside (and) [produces pus],[34] he will have [...]. If that person ⸢seeks out⸣ [the sanctuary of DN], he will have good fortune. To cure him, you roll a linen cloth, sprinkle (it) with *šurmēnu*-cypress oil (and) *erēnu*-cedar oil (and) insert (it) into his ears. You pour [...] over his head. You have him eat ⸢hot things⸣ twice (a day and) drink *ḫašû*-thyme (mixed) with beer twice (a day). If you have him do this repeatedly for seven days, he should recover.

(iii 75′–78′) [If a person's] "left" [ear] collects sweat on the inside (and) produces pus, if that person seeks out the sanctuary of Ishtar, he will have good fortune but that [sanctuary] will experience a loss. To cure him, you sprinkle red-dyed wool with *erēnu*-cedar oil, oil, *šurmēnu*-cypress oil, *balukku*-aromatic oil, "sweet [reed" oil] (and) *kanaktu*-aromatic oil (and) insert (it) into his ears. [You pour] *kanaktu*-aromatic oil over [his] ⸢head⸣. You have him eat hot things twice (a day). You have him drink beer twice (a day). [If you have him do this repeatedly] for seven days, [he should recover].

(iii 79′–iv 2) [If a person's ears] continually ring (and) are pressured with "clay" or pus comes out, [if he seeks out] the sanctuary of DN, [he will have good fortune]. You bathe (his ears) [with] green *nurmû*-pomegranate juice (and) sprinkle (them) with oil. You grind [...] (and) pour (it) over his temples. [He should exprience] improvement.

(iv 3–4) Alternatively, you grind salt, wrap (it) in a tuft of wool, sprinkle (it) with *šurmēnu*-cypress oil (and) insert (it) into his ears. [You pour] *šurmēnu*-cypress oil over his temples. You have him eat and drink hot things. If you do this for three days, [he should experience] improvement.

(iv 5–6) Alternatively, you grind *burāšu*-juniper, wrap (it) in a tuft of wool (and) insert (it) into his ears. [You pour] *baluḫḫu*-aromatic resin oil over [his] ⸢temples⸣. You have him repeatedly eat *saḫlû*-cress with emmer bread. If you do this repeatedly for three days, [he should experience improvement].

(iv 7–8) [Alternatively], you sprinkle carded wool with *erēnu*-cedar oil (and) [insert (it) into his ears]. If you repeatedly pour [...] over his temples, [...]

(iv 9–10) [Alternatively], you ⸢sprinkle⸣ carded wool with *erēnu*-cedar [oil] (and) *šurmēnu*-cypress oil (and) [insert (it) into his ears]. You repeatedly pour [... over] his ⸢temples⸣. You have him eat *ḫašû*-thyme [...]

(iv 11) If a person's "right" ear feels heavy, you pulverize *turû*-garlic (and) put (it) into his ears.

(iv 12) You grind fresh *bīnu*-tamarisk leaves. You mix (it) with *isqūqu*-flour (and) put (it) into his ears.

(iv 13–14) You grind *erēnu*-cedar (variant: *šupuḫru*-cedar), *burāšu*-juniper, *zibû* (and) *šūmu*-garlic. You mix (it) with ghee. ‹You [sprinkle] (it) on a tuft of wool› (and) insert (it) into his ears. You sprinkle *šurmēnu*-cypress oil on a tuft of wool and [insert (it)] into his ear.

(iv 15) You grind *ṭūru*-aromatic, pig fat, *kalbānu* (leaves), ‹(*ḫurri*-bird)›, hair from a female lamb (and) hair from a virgin she-goat. You wrap (it) in a tuft of wool (and) [insert (it)] into his ears.

(iv 16–17) You sprinkle *daprānu*-juniper oil on a tuft of wool (and) [insert (it)] into his ear. You mix the blood of a mongoose with *erēnu*-cedar oil (and) *šurmēnu*-cypress oil (and) [pour (it)] into [his ear].

(iv 18–19) You finely crush *nurmû*-pomegranate juice (and) black *anzaḫḫu*-frit. [...] You daub (it) on (and) gently rub the outsides of his ears (with it). You cut off the head of a male *ḫurri*-bird. [You drip] its blood while still hot [into his ears].

(iv 20–22) If a person's "left" ear feels heavy, you grind myrrh (variant: *kanaktu*) and [... You ...] wild honey with ⸢lion⸣ "fat" [...] Afterwards, a lead spoon [...] oil [...]

(iv 23) [You ...] *erēnu*-cedar, *šegūšu*-flour [...]

(iv 24) You [...] powdered *šūšu*-licorice [...]

(iv 25–26) You grasp the outer parts of his ears. You weigh out powdered [...] (and) powdered *buṭuttu*-cereal. [...] You pour (it) [into his ears].

(iv 27–28) [You blow] oil into [his] ears with your mouth. You pour [... into his ears]. You blow tanner's *kammu* [into his ears with ...]

(iv 29–31) If a person's ears feel heavy, you sprinkle 1 shekel of *nurmû*-pomegranate juice (and) 1 shekel of infusion of *kanaktu*-aromatic on a tuft of wool (and) insert (it) into his ears. You repeatedly do this for three days. On the fourth day, ‹(if the pus which is in)› his ears ‹(comes out)›, you wipe (it) off. You grind alum (and) blow (it) into his ears ‹(via a reed straw)›.

(iv 32–33) (For heavy ears), you take the [...] of fresh *pillû* root and grind (it). [You pour?] its juices [into his ear]. His ⸢hearing⸣ should open up.

(iv 34–35) You char (and) grind *ṭūru*-aromatic, pig fat, *imbû tamtim*, [...] (and) [hair] from a virgin ⸢she-goat⸣. [...] You pour (it) [into] his ears.

(iv 36–37) [You ...] *Šamaškillu*-onion (and) *eʾru*/fig[35] leaves. When you have done this, [you ...] *saḫlû*-cress. If he drinks (it mixed) with beer, etc.[36]

(iv 38–39) A turban [...] his cover [...] If you repeatedly fumigate him for three [days], he should recover.

(iv 40–41) [...] You pour (it) into his ears. [...] You pour (it) into his ears.

(iv 42–43) [...] You pour (it) into his ears. [...] You ⌜mix⌝ (it and) drip (it) into his ears.

(iv 44) [...] You insert (it) into his ears.

(iv 45–46) [...] You drip (it) [into] his ears. [...] You pour (it) into his ears.

C. EAR AND NOSE TREATMENTS

Ancient Mesopotamian noses were treated for pain and bleeding. Treatments for nosebleeds consisted of washes and daubs or tampons.

TEXT 4: *AMT* 105/1 iv 7–20

AMT 105/1 iv 7–20 represents the last column of UGU Subseries 1, Tablet 3.[37] This section lists two washes with aliments (iv 7–13) for ear infections and two treatments (iv 14–20) for hurting nostrils. Of special interest in the ear treatments is that they are contemplated for the fifth and sixth months, presumably part of a series that included all of the months and provided a more detailed version of the usual different treatments for summer and winter.

The patient with a hurting nose is treated by the simple expedient of creating pain and tingling on the opposite side of the body, thus obscuring the unsolicited discomfort. One has, however, to feel sorry for the gecko and the worm that were sacrificed for this purpose.

iv

7. DIŠ NA GEŠTU ZAG-*šú* TAG-*su* IM DIRI-*at u* MÚ.MEŠ U_4.8.KÁM* : U_4.9.KÁM* *ša* ITI.NE
8. ^{GIŠ}NU.ÚR.MA $KU_7.KU_7$ *šá ina* UGU GIŠ-*šá zaq-pat* A.MEŠ-*šá*(coll.) *ta-še-ṣa-ʾ*
9. Ì.DÙG.GA *ana* ŠÀ GEŠTU-*šú* ŠUB Ì ^{ŠEM}BAL *ana* SAG.DU-*šú* ŠUB *síl-qet* KÚM GU_7.MEŠ

---

10. [DIŠ N]A GEŠTU GÙB-*šú* TAG-*su* IM DIRI-*at u* MÚ.MEŠ U_4.15.KÁM* *ša* ITI.KIN
11. [Ì.U]DU KUR.GI^{MUŠEN} $ŠEG_6$-*šal bàḫ-ru-us-su ana* ŠÀ GEŠTU^{II}-*šú* ŠUB

12. UZU! KUR.GI^{MUŠEN} ŠEG$_6$-*šal* GU$_7$
13. Ì ^{GIŠ}ERIN *ana* SAG.DU-*šú* ŠUB-*di ḫi-ib-ṣa ina saḫ-lé-e* GU$_7$

---

14. [DIŠ] NA KIRI$_4$ ZAG-*šú* TAG-*su ina* U$_4$.1.KÁM* *ša* ITI.SIG$_4$ ŠU.SI GÙB-*šú* GAL 7 DÈ GAR-*an*
15. [M]UŠ.DÍM.GURUN.NA *šá* EDIN U$_5$.MEŠ *ina* UGU KIRI$_4$-*šú ú-ḫap-pa*
16. [IL]LU ^{ŠEM}BULUḪ *ana* GEŠTU GÙB-*šú* GAR-*an*

---

17. [DIŠ] NA KIRI$_4$ GÙB-*šú* TAG-*su ina* U$_4$.11.KÁM* *ša* ITI.APIN
18. [SU]M^{SAR} *ina* UGU *ú-ḫaš-šá ṭul-tú šá* ŠÀ GI
19. [*ina*] UGU KIRI$_4$-*šú ú-ḫap-pa* ŠU.SI ZAG-*šú* 7 DÈ GAR-*an*
20. [IL]LU ^{ŠEM}BULUḪ *ana* ŠÀ GEŠTU^{II}-*šú* GAR-*an*

TRANSLATION

(7–9) If a person's "right" ear[38] hurts him intensely, is full of "clay" and is continually swollen, on the eighth (variant: ninth) of Abu (the fifth month), you extract the juice of a sweet *nurmû*-pomegranate which stands up on its branch. You pour (it and) sweet oil into his ear. You pour *ballukku* oil over his head. You have him repeatedly eat hot boilings.

(10–13) [If] a ⸢person's⸣ "left" ear hurts him intensely, is full of "clay" and is swollen, on the fifteenth of Ululu (the sixth month), you boil goose ⸢fat⸣ (and) pour (it) while still hot into his ear. You boil goose flesh (and) have him eat (it). You pour *erēnu*-cedar oil over his head. You have him eat *ḫibṣu* preparation made with *saḫlû*-cress.

(14–16) [If] a person's "right" nostril hurts him intensely, on the first of Simanu (the third month), he puts seven coals on his "left" thumb. He smashes coupled steppe geckoes on his nose. He puts *baluḫḫu* ⸢resin⸣ in his "left" ear.

(17–20) [If] a person's "left" nostril hurts him intensely, on the eleventh of Araḫšamna (the eighth month), you chop up ⸢*šūmu*-garlic⸣ over it. He smashes the worm which is inside a reed on his nose. He puts seven coals on his "right" thumb. He puts *baluḫḫu* ⸢resin⸣ in his "right" ear.

TEXT 5: SpTU 1.45 REV.

The subject matter of SpTU 1.45 might seem trivial and, indeed, two of the treatments (16′–18′) are formulated in such a way as to suggest that they originated with a pharmacist, but the colophon clearly indicates that this tablet belonged to a physician. It consists of washes (16′–17′, 19′–20′) and tampons (21′–22′) for nosebleed.

rev.

1′–15′ are fragmentary and not clearly nosebleeds.

16′. [Ú BABBAR ŠEM]⌈ŠEŠ⌉ NA$_4$ ⌈*ga*⌉-*bu-u* Ú.ḪI.A *na-ḫi-*[*r*]*i* x

17′. […] KAŠ.SAG *ana* KIR$_4$-*šú ta-nam-di*

18′. […]x NA$_4$ *ga-bu-u* Ú ⌈*na*⌉-*ḫi-ri*

19′. [MÚD *šá* TA *ap*]-*pi-šú il-la-ku ana ka-le-e* Ì *ḫal-ṣa ana na-ḫi-ri-šú* ⌈*ta*⌉-*at-ta-*⌈*nam*⌉-*di*

20′. [DIŠ KI.MIN Ì *s*]*e-er-du ana na-ḫi-ri-šú* [*t*]*a-at-*⌈*ta*⌉-*na*[*m-di*]

21′. [(DIŠ KI.MIN ŠURUN)] UDU.U$_8$ ANŠE SUMUN SÍG.ÀKA NIGIN *šum$_4$-ma na-ḫir* 15-*šú ana na-ḫir* 150–*šú*

22′. [(*šum$_4$-ma na-ḫir*)] 150-*šú ana na-ḫir* 15-*šú* GAR-*an*[39]

23′. [DIŠ NA …]x-*šú ḫu-up-pa-a* (catch line)

24′–26′. colophon (belonging to an *āšipu*)

TRANSLATION

(16′–17′) ["White plant"], ⌈myrrh⌉ (and) alum are plants for the nostrils. You pour (them) into his nose [(mixed) with] first quality beer.

(18′) […] Alum is a "plant" for the nostrils.

(19′) To stop [the blood which] flows [from] his ⌈nose⌉, you repeatedly pour pressed-out oil into his nostrils.

(20′) [Alternatively], you ⌈repeatedly pour olive⌉ [oil] into his nostrils.

(21′–22′) Alternatively, you wrap old sheep, goat or donkey dung in a tuft of wool. If it is his "right" nostril,[40] you insert (it) into his "left" nostril and if it is his "left" nostril, into his "right" nostril.

D. *BU*ʾ*ŠĀNU*

This was an ancient syndrome characterized by foul odor (*bu*ʾ*šānu* literally means "stinking") and lesions or exudate which were grayish in color. There were three types of *bu*ʾ*šānu* (BI.LU in Sumerian): one which "set up its throne in the windpipe (trachea and/or bronchi)," one which "set up its throne among the teeth," and one which "set up its throne in the hard and soft palates." These three types of *bu*ʾ*šānu* appear to refer to three separate diseases: diphtheria, Vincent's angina or trench mouth, and oral infection with HSV 1. For more details, see Scurlock and Andersen 2005, 40–42. *Buʾšānu* was treated with potions, salves, mouth rubs, daubs and washes, tampons, and, more rarely, plasters, fumigants, and bandages.

TEXT 6: SpTU 1.44:16–83

The colophon of this text identifies it as the ninth tablet in an abridged edition of the UGU series. SpTU 1.44:1–15 are either fragmentary or deal with breathing difficulties not caused by *buʾšānu*. SpTU 1.44:16–83 consist of one/two bandages (16–19), eight rubs (17–23, 32–33, 35–39, 46–47, 76, 80–83), five/six daubs (17–19, 31–32, 34), three nasal tampons (20–23, 29–30, 35–39), twenty-one potions (20–28, 40–43, 51–54, 62–64), one aspirant (64), five nasal washes (29–30, 32–33, 35–39, 44–45), a fumigant (35–39), a salve (68), and two mouth plasters and a mouth wash (48–50, 77–79) for *buʾšānu*. Of these, only one (17–19) is formulated in such a way as to suggest origin as a pharmacist's preparation. Of particular interest are lines 55–79, which allow us to know exactly which type of *buʾšānu* was being treated and with which treatments. So, in lines 55–64, we have four potions and an aspirant, which were definitely for the diphtheria. To this, we may add the treatments in lines 20–33 and 35–39 on the basis of described symptoms. In lines 65–68, we have a salve that was definitely for the Vincent's angina. To this, we may add the treatments in lines 48–50 and 80–83 on the basis of the described symptoms. Finally, in lines 69–79, we have a mouth rub and plaster for the HSV 1 infection, to which we may perhaps add the two bandages and a rub from lines 16–19 on the basis of the described symptoms. Of particular interest are the magical analogies invoked in the first two recitations (55–61, 65–67): "Just as a dead person has to abandon the caravan and (just as) the aborted fetus cannot grasp the breast/drink the milk of its mother, may you never return to your attack." "Just as the son of a *nadītu* does not prosper and (just as) the aborted fetus cannot grasp the breast of its mother, [may you never] return to your attack." *Nadītu*'s were the ancient equivalent of nuns and forbidden from having children. The text cruelly contemplates them getting rid of an embarrassing and unwanted child. One might expect to have something in the treatment to cement these messages with visual reinforcement say, for example, a piece of human skull. This often happens, but not here, a good example of theory not overriding practice. Also of note is the fact that the recitations are said to be the gifts of the gods, and in particular patrons of healing like Ea and Asalluhi or Damu and Gula.

The third recitation (69–74) is a fine example of the daughters of Anu type. In these treatments, often to do with fever or burning, the daughters of Anu are sent to the rescue of the patient armed with water-filled vessels of precious metals or semi-precious stones. The water in these vessels is, of course, extra pure, which opens up for us a window into the ideas of what constituted gross impurity for ancient Mesopotamians. For more on this type of recitation, see Farber 1990, 299–321.

16. [DIŠ NA KA-(*šú* KÚM *il-la-tu-šú*)] DU-*ku bu-ʾ-šá-nu* DIB-*su* GAZI^{SAR} *ina* A.MEŠ [(*tara-bak* SAG.DU-*su* LAL)]

---

17. [^{Ú}GA(MUN.GI$_6$ Ú)].KUR.[(R)]A ^{Ú}NÍG.GÍR.NU[41] ŠIM.BI.KÙ.SIG$_{17}$ IM.SAḪAR.NA$_4$.KUR.RA Ú.[(BABBAR)]
18. [… (*ta-šá-qal* SÚD)] ⸢*ḫu*⸣*-um-bi-ṣa-a-te* [(*ša* NÍG)].SILAG.GÁ UGU ‹(*e-piš*)› KA-*šú* [(*ta-kar*)]
19. [E(N MÚD)] ⸢È⸣-*ni* Ú.ḪI.A *an-nu-t*[*i* (*ana*)] UGU KA-*šú* LAL (variant: MAR)-[(*ma ina-eš*)]

---

20. DIŠ [(NA *ap-pa*)]-*šú u* ⸢KA⸣-*šú bu-ʾ-šá-*⸢*nu*⸣ DI[(B)]-⸢*it*⸣ TÚG.⸢GADA⸣ *ta-ṣap-pir* LÀL SUD [(IM)].SAḪAR.N[(A$_4$.KUR.RA)]
21. *t*[(*u*)-*l*]*a-am ana na-ḫi-ri-šú ta-*[*sa*]*-an-niš* Ú.KUR.RA IM.SAḪA[R.NA$_4$.KUR.R]A SÚD T[(ÚG.GADA Ì+GIŠ SUD)]
22. *t*[(*u*)]*-la-a-am* KIR$_4$-*šú u* KA-*šú* EN MÚD IGI *ta-kar* U[D.3.KÁM *a*]*n-nam* DÙ-⸢*uš*⸣ [*ina* U$_4$.KÁM]
23. ^{Ú}ḪAB SIG$_7$-*su tu-ḫas-sà* A.MEŠ TI-*qé* 2 (variant: 5) GÍN Ì.GIŠ *ana* Š[À-*š*]*ú-nu* ḪE.ḪE NU *pa-tan* ‹([N]AG-*šú-ma*)› *tu-šá-ʾ-*[*ra-šu-ma ina-eš*]

---

24. Ú.BABBAR ‹(SÚD)› *ina* ‹(Ì+GIŠ *u*)› KAŠ NU *pa-tan* NAG-*šú-ma*! ⸢KI.MIN⸣! ^{Ú}*ak-tam* SÚD *ina* ‹(Ì.+GIŠ *u*)› KAŠ NU *pa-tan* N[(AG *i*)-*ár-ru-ma ina-eš*]
25. KI.MIN BAR MUŠ *tur-ár* SÚD *ina* Ì *u* KAŠ [N(AG-*ma i*)-*ár-ru-ma ina-eš*]

---

26. DIŠ NA *ap-pa-šú u* ⸢KA-*šú bu-ʾ-š*⸣*á-nu* DIB-*it-ma* ŠÀ.MEŠ-*šú nap-ḫu* ILLU LI.TAR [(SÚD) *ina* (Ì *u* KAŠ) NAG]

---

27. Ú.⸢KUR.RA⸣ [(SÚ)]D *ina* Ì *u* KAŠ NAG-*ma ina-eš* IM.KAL.G[U]G SÚD *ina* Ì *u* KAŠ NA[(G)-*ma ina-eš*]
28. [(IM.SAḪAR)].NA$_4$.KUR.RA ‹(S)ÚD› *ina* LÀL Ì *u* KAŠ NA[G-*ma ina-eš*]

---

29. DIŠ [(KA)]-*šú bu-ʾ-šá-nu* DIB-*ma na-ḫi-ra-šú* GU$_7$.MEŠ-*šú* GIG.MEŠ

DIRI.MEŠ TÚG.GA[(DA *ta-ṣap-pir na*)*-ḫi-ra-šú ta-sa-an-niš*]

30. IM.SAḪAR.NA$_4$.KUR.RA *tu-la-am ana* [(K)]A ḪAR-*š*[*ú?*] DIM$_4$-*ma ina* GI.SAG.KUD M[(Ú-*ma* DU$_8$)]

---

31. [IM.KA(L)].⸢GUG⸣ SÚD *ta-za-ru-ma ina-eš* : BAR ^{GIŠ}NU.⸢ÚR⸣.[(MA)] SÚD *ta-za-ru-ma ina-eš* : A x[…] *ta-za-ru-ma ina-*[*eš*]

---

32. $^{\text{[ŠE]M}}$ŠEŠ SÚD *ta-za-ru-ma ina-eš* : *šum$_4$-ma ina na-ḫi-ri-šú in-né-eṣ-ṣ*[*i-in*]

33. [BAR M]UŠ *tur-ár* SÚD *na-ḫi-ri-šú tu-kap-par* 1-*šú* 2-*šú* 3-*šú ana na-ḫi-ri-šú* [ŠUB-*di* …]

---

34. DIŠ NA *na-ḫi-ri-šú um-ṣa-at ḫi-li it-tab-ši* NA$_4$ *gab-ú* ^{ŠEM}ŠEŠ Ú.BABBAR 1-*niš* [(SÚD)] *ana* UGU MAR-[(*ma ina-eš*)]

---

35. DIŠ NA BI.LU *na-ḫi-ri-šú* DIB-*tu* Ú.KUR.RA ^{Ú}*úr-né-e* GAZI^{SAR} Ú.BABBAR I[LLU (LI.DUR)]

36. IM.SAḪAR.NA$_4$.KUR.RA 1-*niš* SÚD TÚG.GADA *ta-ṣap-pir* LÀL SUD Ú.ḪI.A *an-nu-tì tu-la*[(*m ana ap-pi-šú*)]

37. [(EN)] TI.LA GAR.GAR-*an* NAGA.SI *te-bé-er* Ú.KUR.RA 1-*niš* SÚD *ina* Ì.KUR.RA ḪE.ḪE [(*ana* ŠÀ *ap-pi-šú/na-ḫi-ri-šú*)][42]

38. [*tak-t*]*a-na-ar* A ^{GIŠ}NU.ÚR.MA KÚM.MEŠ[43] *gi-na-a ana* KIR$_4$-*šú* ŠUB.ŠU[(B-*di* Ì KÚM-*ma*)]

39. [(*tu-ub-ta-n*)]*a-ḫar* Ú.KUR.RA ^{Ú}*si-i-*[(*ḫu*)] *ina* DÈ SAR-*šú* ^{Ú}*úr-né-e ina* Ì [(^{GIŠ}ERIN ḪE.ḪE)] *ana na-ḫ*[(*i-ri-šú* ŠUB.ŠUB-*di*)]

---

40. [DIŠ NA *bu-ʾ-šá*]*-nu* GIG 1 ŠE ^{ŠEM}KU$_7$.KU$_7$ 1 [ŠE] ^{ŠEM}LI 1 Š[E Ú.(KUR.RA 1 ŠE *saḫ-lé-e*)]

41. [(1 ŠE GAMUN.GI$_6$) IM.SAḪAR.N]A$_4$.KUR.RA BAR MU[(Š *tur-á*)]*r* SÚD [(*ina* Ì *u* KAŠ N)AG]

---

42. [DIŠ NA *bu-ʾ-šá-nu*] DIB-*ma* NU DU$_8$ 7 ŠE ÚKU[Š …]

43. […] 1-*niš* SÚD *ina* Ì [*u* KAŠ NAG]

---

44. [DIŠ NA (B)]I.LU *ṣab-tu* Ú.KUR.RA ^{Ú}[(*ši-ma-ḫa*)]

45. [(^{Ú}) …] ^{Ú}*úr-né-e ina* Ì ^{GIŠ}E[RIN (*ana na-ḫi-ri*)]*-šú* ŠUB-*di*]

---

46. [DIŠ N(A KA-*šú bu-ʾ-šá*)]*-nu* DIB-*it* ^{Ú}*ak-tam* SÚD *ana* KA[-*šú* ..]

---

47. [DIŠ K(I.MIN NA$_4$ *ga-bi*)]-*i* UGU KA-*šú*[44] [...]

---

48. [DIŠ NA (*bu-ʾ-šá-nu* D)]IB-⸢*su* ^{Ú}⸣*tuš-ru* NA$_4$ *gab-bu-ú* Ú.K[(UR.R)A *saḫ-l*(*é*-⸢*e*⸣? NUMUN ^{GIŠ}*a-da-ri*)]
49. [(UZU MAŠ.DÀ TAL.TAL GIŠIMMAR.T)UR?] ^{NA_4}*ḫar-pu-ṣa-ṣu*[45] $^{NA_4.SI}$*sim-kád-r*[(*u* ^{Ú}GEŠTIN.KA$_5$.A *mun-zi-qa* KA *tam-tim* ZÍ)D ...]
50. [x (Ú)ḪI.(A *mál-ma-li*)]*š* GAZ SIM ZÚ.MEŠ *en-še-e-tú šá* MÚ[D *i-ḫi-i*(*l-la ina* IGI NÁ-*šú tu-ṭap-pi*)] *ina še-e-r*[*i* (*ina* A.MEŠ Ú.KUR.RA L)UḪ-*si-ma* TI]

---

51. [(DIŠ NA)] *bu-ʾ-šá-nu* DIB-*su* 2 GÍN Ú.BABBAR *ina* KAŠ NAG : [(DIŠ)] K[(I.MIN ^{Ú}ḪAB *ina* Ì *u* KAŠ NAG)]

---

52. [(DIŠ KI.MIN) ^{Ú}]*ak-tam ina* Ì.[G(IŠ) NA]G : DIŠ KI.MIN [(Ú.KUR.RA *saḫ-lé-e ina* Ì *u* KAŠ NAG)]

---

53. [DIŠ KI.MIN] ^{Ú}*zi-ba-a ina* Ì *u* KAŠ NAG : DIŠ KI.MIN [(^{Ú}*tar-muš ina* Ì *u* KAŠ NAG)]

---

54. [DIŠ KI.MIN] NA$_4$ *gab-ú* SÚD *ina* GEŠTIN NAG : DIŠ KI.M[(IN Ú.KUR.RA *ina* ^{GIŠ}GEŠTIN) NAG]

---

55. ÉN *bu-ʾ-šá-nu da-an* DIB-*su* GIN$_7$ U[R.M(AḪ *nap-šá-ra iṣ-bat*)]
56. GIN$_7$ UR.BAR.RA *iṣ-ṣa-bat nu-ur-za iṣ-ṣ*[*a-*(*bat nu*)*-ur-ba* (*iṣ-ṣa-bat* EME)]
57. *ina* G[I].GÍD Ḫ[(A)]R.MEŠ *it-ta-di* ^{GIŠ}GU.ZA-*šú ṣ*[(*i-i bu-u*ʾ*-šá-nu ul ṣi-bit-ka*)]
58. GIN$_7$ ÚŠ *šu-ud-du-ú a-lak-ti u ni-id* ⸢ŠÀ⸣-[(*bi la iṣ-ba-tú* UBUR AMA-*šú*)[46]]
59. *at-ta e t*[(*a-t*)]*ur*[47] *ana ṣib-ti-ka* ÉN ‹(*ul*)› *ya-ut-t*[(*u-un* ÉN ^{d}*É-a u* ^{d}*Asal-lú-ḫi*)]
60. ÉN ^{d}*Da-mu u* ^{d}*Gu-la* ÉN ^{d}N[(IN.GÌRIM *be-let* ÉN)]
61. ÉN ^{d}*Gu-la be-let* TI.LA ^{d}*Gu-*[(*la ti-di-ma šá*) ... (*ki-šat-ki* TI-*e* TU$_6$ ÉN)]

---

62. KA.INIM.MA *bu-ʾ-šá-nu* DIB-*su* : DÙ.DÙ.BI ^{Ú}Ḫ[(AB ḪÁD.A SÚD *ina* Ì.GIŠ *u* KAŠ NAG-*ma ina-e*)*š*]

---

63. DIŠ KI.MIN Ú.KUR.RA *ina* Ì *u* ⸢KAŠ⸣ NAG-*ma ina-eš* : DIŠ KI.MIN [...]

64. DIŠ KI.MIN NA$_4$ *gab-ú ina* LÀL ḪE.ḪE *ú-na-ṣab* : DIŠ KI.MIN [... (NU *pa-tan* NAG-*ma ina-eš*)]

65. ÉN *da-an šá bu-ʾ-šá-nu* DIB-*su* GIN$_7$ UR.MAḪ SAG.DU *i*[(*ṣ-bat*) G(IN$_7$ UR.BAR.RA *iṣ-ṣa-bat lu-ʾu-ḫa*)]
66. *iṣ-bat* KA *iṣ-bat* EME *ina b*[(*i*)]-*rit* ZÚ.MEŠ *it-ta-di* ^{GI}[(^{Š}GU.ZA-*šú*) *ṣ*(*i-i*) *bu-ʾ*(*u-šá-a-nu*[48] *ul ṣi-bit-ka*)]
67. GIN$_7$ DUMU LUKUR *la i-bu-r*[*a* G]IN$_7$ *ni-id* ŠÀ-[(*b*)]*i la iṣ-bat*[49] U[(BUR AMA-*šú*) *at-*(*ta e ta-sa-aḫ-ra a-na ṣib-ti-ka* TU$_6$ ÉN)

68. KA.INIM.MA *bu-ʾ-šá-nu* DIB-*su* : DÙ.DÙ.BI IM.KAL.GUG [(*ina* LÀL.KUR.RA SÚD) *ina* (*ṣi-b*)*it bu-u*(*ʾ-šá-nu* ŠÉŠ-*ma ina-eš*)]

69. ÉN *bu-ʾ-šá-nu a-mir* GIN$_7$ UR.MAḪ DIŠ *la šá* UR.MAḪ *šá bu-u*[(*ʾ-šá-ni da-an* DIB-*su ki-m*)*a* (UR.BAR.RA)]
70. *nap-šá-ri iṣ-bat ki-i mìn-di-ni iṣ-ṣa-bat la-ḫe-e* ‹(*ina*)› *n*[(*u-u*)]*r-za nar-*[(*ba-ti it-ta-di* ^{GIŠ}GU.ZA-*šú man-na-*)]
71. *-mi lu-uš-pur ana* DUMU.MUNUS^{ME} ^{d}*A-nu šá* AN-*e liš-šá-nim-ma tal-li-ši-na* [(*šá* KÙ.BABBAR *u kan-du-ra-ni-ši-na šá* KÙ.SIG$_{17}$)]
72. *liḫ-ba-nim* A.MEŠ A.AB.BA[50] *tam-tim* DAGAL-*tim a-šar ur-ru-uš-ti* [(*la im-su-ú* ŠU^{II}-*šá*)]
73. *u-suk-ka-tum la im-su-u lu-ba-re-e-šú iṣ-ṣur ḫur-ri la id-*⌈*lu*⌉-*ʾu* ⌈*la ú*⌉-[(*na-as-si-su kàp-pi-šú*)]
74. *la id-lu-u*ʾ UR.GI$_7$ GI$_6$ *lid-da-a ana pi-šú-ma* ZI-*iḫ šá* KA-*šú um-mu sik-ka-tum lu*!-*ba-*⌈*ṭu*⌉ *u bu-ʾ-šá-nu* TU$_6$ ÉN[51]

75. KA.INIM.MA *bu-ʾ-šá-nu* DIB-*su ana bul-lu-ṭu šá bu-ʾ-šá-nu* DÙ.A.BI ŠID-*nu*

76. DÙ.DÙ.BI NA$_4$ *gab-ú* ^{Ú}*ni-na-a* SÚD *ina* LÀL ḪE.ḪE ÉN 7-*šú ana* ŠÀ-*bi* ŠID-*nu* KA-*šú tak-ta-na-par-*‹(*ma*)› *ina-eš*

77. DIŠ KI.MIN Ú.KUR.RA *saḫ-lé-e* NA$_4$ *ga-bi-i* GAZI^{SAR} ^{Ú}ḪAB ^{GIŠ}TAL.TAL.GIŠIMMAR *ḫar-pu-ṣa-ṣa* ŠIKA ^{GIŠ}NU.ÚR.MA
78. *u* ^{ŠEM}ŠEŠ UZU MAŠ.DÀ ^{GIŠ}GEŠTIN.ḪÁD.A ^{Ú}MAŠ.TAB.BA 12 Ú.ḪI.A ḪÁD.A GAZ SIM *ina* ZÍD ŠE.SA.A ḪE.ḪE
79. KI KA-*šú tu-ṭap-pi-ma* (*ḫe-pí eš-šu*) *ṭè-pu šá* KA LAL KA

80. DIŠ NA ZÚ.MEŠ-*šú mu-nu u bu-ʾ-šá-nu* (*ḫe-pí eš-šu*) ‹*ú-ka*›-*al ina* DAL.BA.AN.NA ZÚ.MEŠ-*šú*
81. MÚD È.MEŠ-*ni* NA_4 *gab-bu-ú* Ú.KUR.RA ^{Ú}*zi-bu-ú* 1-*niš* SÚD
82. ŠU.SI-*ka mu-šá-ṭu* NIGIN-*mi* Ì.UDU ŠAḪ! SUD x[o o o *t*]*u-lam*
83. ZÚ-*šú* EN MÚD È.MEŠ-*ni ta-kar* [... TI]-*uṭ*

Translation

(16) [If a person's mouth?] is feverish (and) his saliva flows, *buʾšānu* afflicts him. You decoct[52] *kasû* in water (and) bandage his head (with it).

(17–19) ⸢*Zibû*⸣, *nīnû-mint*, *egemgiru*,[53] *šīpu*, alum, (and) "white plant" [are 6 plants for *buʾšānu*]. You weigh (them) out (and) grind (them). You firmly rub a lump of dough on his ‹(open)› mouth [until] the blood comes out. If you bandage (variant: daub) these plants on his mouth, he should recover.

(20–23) If *buʾšānu* afflicts a person's nose and his mouth, you roll a linen cloth (and) sprinkle (it) with honey. You use (it) to ⸢soften⸣[54] alum (and) ⸢insert⸣ (it) into his nostril. You grind *nīnû*-mint (and) ⸢alum⸣. You sprinkle a linen cloth with oil (and) use (it) to soften (it). You firmly rub his nose and his mouth (with it) until the blood comes out. You do this for [three] ⸢days⸣ (and) [on the fourth day], you crush/mince fresh *šammi buʾšāni*. You take the juices (and) mix 2 (variant 5) shekels of oil ⸢with them⸣. ‹(You have him ⸢drink⸣ it)› on an empty stomach ‹(and)›, [if] you can get him to ⸢vomit⸣, [he should recover].

(24–25) ‹(You grind)› "white plant." You have him drink (it) on an empty stomach, (mixed) with ‹(oil and)› beer, etc.[55] Alternatively, you grind *aktam*. You have him drink (it) on an empty stomach, (mixed) with ‹(oil and)› beer. [If] he ⸢vomits⸣, [he should recover]. Alternatively, you char (and) grind snake skin. You have him drink (it mixed) with oil and beer and, [if] he ⸢vomits⸣, [he should recover].

(26) If *buʾšānu* afflicts a person's nose and his mouth so that his insides are bloated,[56] you grind *abukkatu* resin (and) [have him drink it mixed with] oil and beer.

(27–28) You grind *nīnû*-mint. If you have him drink (it mixed) with oil and beer, he should recover. You grind *kalgukku*-clay. [If] you have him drink (it mixed) with oil and beer, [he should recover]. You ‹(⸢grind⸣)› alum. [If] you ⸢have him drink⸣ (it mixed) with honey, oil and beer, [he should recover].

(29–30) If *buʾšānu* afflicts a person's nose/mouth so that his nostrils continually hurt him (and) are continually full of sores,[57] you roll a linen cloth (and) [insert it into his nostril]. You use (it) to soften alum. You close off the "mouth of ⸢his⸣ lungs" (his nostril) (with it) and then, if you blow (alum) in with a reed straw, it should let up.

(31–32a) You grind *kalgukku*-[clay]. If you daub (it) on, he should recover. You grind *nurmû*-pomegranate peel. If you daub (it) on, he should recover. If you daub on […] infusion, ⸢he should recover⸣. § You grind myrrh. If you daub (it) on, he should recover.

(32b–33) If it ⸢stinks⸣ inside his nostrils,[58] you char (and) grind ⸢snake⸣ [skin] and wipe off his nostils (with it). [You pour] (it) once, twice, and three times into his nostrils.

(34) If there is a suppurating nasal turbinate in his nostrils,[59] you grind together alum, myrrh (and) "white plant." If you daub (it) on it, he should recover.

(35–39) If *buʾšānu* afflicts a person's nostrils, you grind together *nīnû*-mint, *urnû*-mint, *kasû*, "white plant," *abukkatu* resin (and) alum. You roll a linen cloth (and) sprinkle (it) with honey. You use (it) to soften these plants. You repeatedly put (it) into his nose until he has recovered. You select *uḫḫūlu qarnānu* (and) grind (it) together (with) *nīnû*-mint. You mix (it) with naphtha. You repeatedly ⸢rub⸣ (it) firmly inside his nose/nostrils.[60] You repeatedly and continually pour hot *nurmû*-pomegranate juice into his nose.[61] You continually keep (it) hot with hot oil. You fumigate him with *nīnû*-mint (and) *sīḫu*-wormwood over coals. You mix *urnû*-mint with *erēnu*-cedar oil (and) repeatedly pour (it) into his nostrils.

(40–41) [If a person] is sick with ⸢*buʾšānu*⸣, you grind 1 grain of *kukru*, 1 [grain] of *burāšu*-juniper, 1 ⸢grain⸣ of *nīnû*-mint, 1 grain of *saḫlû*-cress, 1 grain of *zibû*, ⸢alum⸣ and snake skin which you have charred. ⸢You have him drink⸣ (it mixed) with oil and beer.

(42–43) [If *buʾšānu*] afflicts [a person] and will not let up, you grind together seven grains of […]-gourd (and) […]. [You have him drink (it mixed)] with oil [and beer].

(44–45) If ⸢*buʾšānu*⸣ afflicts [a person], [you pour] *nīnû*-mint, *šimāḫu*-thorn, […] and *urnû*-mint (mixed) with ⸢*erēnu*-cedar⸣ oil into [his] nostrils.

(46) [If] *buʾšānu* afflicts a ⸢person's⸣ mouth, you grind *aktam* (and) […] (it) on [his] mouth.

(47) ⸢Alternatively⸣, [you …] alum on his mouth.[62]

(48–50) [If] *buʾšānu* afflicts [a person], you crush (and) sift (these) [x] ⸢plants⸣ in equal proportions: *tušru*, alum, *nīnû*-mint, ⸢*saḫlû*-cress⸣, *addāru*-poplar seed, "gazelle flesh," ⸢dwarf⸣? palm frond, *ḫarpuṣaṣu*-mineral,[63] *sinkadru*-mineral, "fox grape," raisins, *imbû tamtim* (and) […] ⸢flour⸣. You plaster (it) onto the weak teeth which ⸢ooze blood⸣ before he goes to sleep. In the morning, [if] you ⸢wash⸣ them with *nīnû*-mint infusion, [he should recover].

(51) If *buʾšānu* afflicts a person, you have him drink 2 shekels of "white plant" (mixed) with beer. Alternatively, you have him drink *šammi buʾšāni* (mixed) with oil and beer.

(52) Alternatively, ⸢you have him drink⸣ *aktam* (mixed) with oil. Alternatively, you have him drink *nīnû*-mint (and) *saḫlû*-cress (mixed) with oil and beer.

(53) [Alternatively], you have him drink *zibû* (mixed) with oil and beer. Alternatively, you have him drink *tarmuš* (mixed) with oil and beer.

(54) [Alternatively], you grind alum (and) have him drink (it mixed) with wine. Alternatively, [you have him drink] *nīnû*-mint (mixed) with wine.

(55–61) Mighty is the affliction of *buʾšānu*. It ⸢seized⸣ the uvula like a ⸢lion⸣; (then)[64] it seized the hard palate like a wolf. It seized the ⸢soft palate⸣; it seized the tongue. It set up its throne in the windpipe (trachea and/or bronchi).[65] ⸢Go out⸣, *buʾšānu*; it is not your portion. Just as a dead person has to abandon the caravan and (just as) the aborted fetus cannot grasp the breast of its mother,[66] may you never return to your attack. The spell is not mine; it is the spell of Ea and Asalluhi, the spell of Damu and Gula, the spell of Ningirim, the mistress of spells, the spell of Gula, mistress of life. Gula—you know (it) and [... to] all of your (people) for the taking. Recitation (and) spell.

(62) Recitation for *buʾšānu* afflicting a person. Its ritual: you dry (and) grind *šammi buʾšāni*. If you have him drink (it mixed) with oil and beer, he should ⸢recover⸣.

(63) Alternatively, if you have him drink *nīnû*-mint (mixed) with oil and beer, he should recover. Alternatively, [...]

(64) Alternatively, he should suck up alum (mixed) with honey. Alternatively, if he drinks [...] on an empty stomach, he should recover.

(65–67) Mighty is the affliction of *buʾšānu*. It seized the head like a lion; (then)[67]it seized his throat ⸢like⸣ a wolf. It seized the mouth; it seized the tongue. It set up its throne among the teeth.[68] ⸢Go out⸣, *buʾšānu*; it is not your portion. Just the son of a *nadītu* does not prosper and (just as) the aborted fetus cannot grasp[69] the breast of its mother, [may you never] return to your attack. Recitation (and) spell.

(68) Recitation for *buʾšānu* afflicting a person. Its ritual: you grind *kalgukku*-clay in wild honey. If you rub it gently [on] the ⸢affliction of *buʾšānu*⸣, he should recover.

(69–74) *Buʾšānu* has the appearance of a lion; *buʾšānu*'s affliction is mightier than all but a lion.[70] It seized the uvula ⸢like⸣ a wolf; (then)[71]it seized the jaws like a tiger. It set up its throne in the hard and soft palates. "Whom should I send to the daughters of Anu?"[72] From the heavens, let them lift up their buckets of silver and their nipple vases[73] of gold. Let them draw water from the Cosmic Ocean,[74] the broad sea, a place where a woman who has recently had intercourse[75] has not washed her hands, a woman with a flow of blood has not washed her clothes, a shellduck has not roiled(?) the water,[76] not dipped its wings (and) a black dog has not roiled(?)the water. Let it fall on his mouth so that fever, *sikkatu*,[77] *lubāṭu* and *bu'šānu* may be removed from his mouth.

(75) Recitation for *bu'šānu* afflicting a person to be recited over any treatment for *bu'šānu*.

(76) Its ritual: You grind alum (and) *nīnû*-mint (and) mix (it) with honey. You recite the recitation seven times over it. ‹(If)› you repeatedly wipe off his mouth (with it), he should recover.

(77–79) Alternatively, you dry, crush, (and) sift (these) twelve plants: *nīnû*-mint, *saḫlû*-cress, alum, *kasû*, *šammi bu'šāni*, palm frond, *ḫarpuṣaṣu*-mineral,[78] a fragment of *nurmû* pomegranate, myrrh, "gazelle flesh," raisins (and) *šammi ašî* seed. You mix (it) with roasted grain flour. You plaster where his mouth is (with it) and [...]. Plaster for the mouth; bandage for the mouth.

(80–83) If *munu* and *bu'šānu* ⌈grip⌉ a person's teeth (and) blood comes out between his teeth,[79] you grind together alum, *nīnû*-mint and *zibû*. You wrap your finger with hair combings (and) sprinkle (it) with pig fat. You use it to soften [these plants]. You firmly rub his teeth (with it) until the blood comes out. [If you do this repeatedly for ... days], ⌈he should recover⌉.

E. TEETH TREATMENTS

Ancient Mesopotamian's complained of teeth having pain, coming loose, falling out (due to periodontal disease), and being attacked by the "tooth worm" (cavities). For more details, see Scurlock and Andersen 2005, chapter 18.

Treatments usually consisted of applications or plasters. A bit of wax allowed the physician to pull out a loose tooth, and rotten teeth may have been forcibly extracted. For those who would be instructed, there was the ancient equivalent of toothpaste.

TEXT 7: BAM 1 i 1–16

BAM 1 is a vademecum (pharmacist's companion), the rest of column i of which appears above in chapter 2 as text 1. Various plants are recommended for putting in the mouth next to bad teeth, either fresh (1–7, 11–14) or dried, ground, and mixed with oil to form a paste (8–10). The "tooth worm" (7) is a reference to dental caries.[80] The plant for "tooth worm" was to be picked in such a way that "the sun does not see it." In other words, it was to be picked at night before sunrise. Indeed, modern reports show that there is a diurnal variation in alkaloid content in plants.[81]

The progression in treatments from soreness (1–6) to cavities (7) to teeth falling out (8–10) or loose (11–14) shows that ancient physicians understood that poor dental hygiene could lead to pain and tooth loss. Recommendations for the ancient equivalent of a brush with toothpaste first thing in the morning (15–16) should perhaps have been listed first.

1.	[(^{Ú}NAM.TAR NÍT)]A	Ú ZÚ.GIG.GA.KE$_4$	*ana* UGU ZÚ-*šú* GAR-*nu*
2.	[(^{Ú}SUḪUŠ NAM.TAR NÍTA)]	Ú KI.MIN	KI.MIN
3.	[(^{Ú}*gul-gul-la-nu* SIG)]$_7$	Ú KI.MIN	KI.MIN
4.	[(^{Ú}*lu-lum-t*)]*um*	Ú KI.MIN	KI.MIN
5.	[(^{Ú}*ḫa-lu-la*)]-*ya*	Ú KI.MIN	KI.MIN
6.	[(^{Ú}*šur-ši* Ú)].^{d}UTU	Ú KI.MIN	KI.MIN
7.	[(^{Ú}*šur-ši*)] $^{\text{GIŠ.Ú}}$GÍR *ša ina* ZI-*ka* ^{d}UTU NU IGI.D[(U)]$_8$.A	Ú *tul*$_5$-*te*	KI.MIN
8.	^{Ú}*ku-di-me-ru*	Ú ZÚ Š[(U)]B	ḪÁD.A SÚD *ina* Ì+GIŠ ḪE.ḪE KI.MIN
9.	^{Ú}*ši-bir* ‹(SUḪUŠ)› MAḪ	Ú ZÚ Š[(U)]B	ḪÁD.A SÚD *ina* Ì+GIŠ ḪE.ḪE KI.MIN
10.	^{Ú}*šur-ši* ^{GIŠ}DÌḪ ‹(BABBAR *šá*)› *ina* ZI-*ka* ^{d}UTU NU IGI.DU$_8$.A	Ú ZÚ ŠUB	KI.MIN
11.	^{Ú}MÁ.RÍ.EREŠ.MÁ.LÁ	Ú ZÚ.MEŠ *un-nu-šá-ti*	TI *ana* UGU ZÚ.MEŠ GAR-*nu*
12.	^{Ú}SUḪUŠ *ḫal-tap-‹(pa)›-ni* ^{Ú}SUḪUŠ *al-lum-zi*	Ú KI.MIN	KI.MIN
13.	^{Ú}ILLU *šim-ṭa-te* ^{ŠEM}ŠEŠ	Ú KI.MIN	KI.MIN
14.	^{Ú}ILLU ^{ŠEM}BULUḪ	Ú KI.MIN	KI.MIN
15.	^{Ú}*mar-gu-ṣu*	Ú ZÚ.⸢ZÚ⸣ *ka-pa-ri*	NU *pa-tan* ZÚ.MEŠ-*šú ta-kap-par*[82]
16.	^{Ú}NA$_4$ *ga-bi-i* Ú.KUR.RA ^{ŠEM}ḪAB	KI.M[I]N	KI.MIN

TRANSLATION

1. Male *pillû* is a plant for a sore tooth. It is to be put on his tooth.
2. Male *pillû* root is a plant (for a sore tooth). (It is to be put on his tooth).[83]
3. Fresh *qulquliānu* is a plant (for a sore tooth). (It is to be put on his tooth).
4. *Lulumtu* is a plant (for a sore tooth). (It is to be put on his tooth).
5. *Ḫalulāya* is a plant (for a sore tooth). (It is to be put on his tooth).
6. "Sunflower" root is a plant for (a sore tooth). (It is to be put on his tooth).

---

7. *Ašāgu*-thorn root, which the sun did not see when you pulled it, is a plant for the tooth worm. It is to be put on his tooth.

---

8. *Kudimēru* is a plant for a tooth falling out. It is to be dried, ground, mixed with oil (and put on his tooth).
9. Giant-rooted *šibru* is a plant for a tooth falling out. It is to be dried, ground, mixed with oil (and put on his tooth).

---

10. White *baltu*-thorn root which the sun did not see when you pulled it is a plant for a tooth falling out. (It is to be dried, ground, mixed with oil and put on his tooth.)

---

11. *Mirišmara* is a plant for loose ("weak") teeth. It is to be taken (and) put on the teeth.
12. *Ḫaltappānu* root (and) *allumzu* root are plants (for loose teeth). (They are to be put on the teeth).[84]
13. Resin scrapings(?)[85] of myrrh is a plant (for loose teeth). (It is to be put on the teeth).
14. *Baluḫḫu* resin is a plant (for loose teeth). (It is to be put on the teeth).
15. *Margūṣu* is a plant for rubbing the teeth. You rub his teeth (with it) on an empty stomach.
16. Alum, *nīnû*-mint (and) *ṭūru*-aromatic (are plants for rubbing the teeth). (You rub his teeth with them on an empty stomach).[86]

TEXT 8: BAM 159 v 10–16

BAM 159 v 10–16 consists of physician's rub and aliment (v 10–14) and a pharmacist's powder (v 15–16) for loose teeth. Lines v 15–16 are essentially a direct quote from the vademecum BAM 1 i 12.

10. DIŠ NA *gi-mir* ZÚ.MEŠ-*šú i-na-áš u ri-šu-tú*
11. TUKU-*ši* Ú.BABBAR ^{Ú}ḪAB Ú.KUR.RA NA_4 *ga-bi-*⸢*i*⸣
12. 1-*niš* SÚD TÚG.GADA LÀL SUD *tu-lam* UGU ZÚ.MEŠ-*š*[*ú*]
13. EN MÚD È-*ni ta-kar* Ì.UDU UR.MA[Ḫ]
14. *šum*$_4$-*ma* Ì.UDU KA_5.A [(GU_7)]

---

15. SUḪUŠ ^{Ú}*ḫal-tap-pa-ni* SUḪUŠ ^{Ú}*al-lum-zi* MIN
16. [ZÚ].MEŠ-*šú* SIG!.MEŠ *ta-bi-la bi-rit* ZÚ.MEŠ [GAR]

TRANSLATION

(v 10–14) If all of a person's teeth move and (the gums) have redness,[87] you grind together "white plant," plant for *buʾšāni*, *nīnû*-mint and alum. You sprinkle a linen cloth with honey and soften (the plant mixture with it). You firmly rub (it) over his teeth until the blood comes out. He should eat either "lion fat" or "fox fat."

(v 15–16) *Ḫaltappānu* root and *allumzu* root (are plants) for loose ("weak") [teeth]. [You put it] dry between his teeth.

TEXT 9: CT 17.50

This charming recitation is a classic historiola. On the one hand it provides an etiology for how dental carries came to be which is surprisingly close to the mark (decaying food particles in the jaw) and on the other it enlists Ea in a cure. The topos of the offensive disease causer who brings down the wrath of the gods on his own head by gross misbehavior also appears with the demonness Lamashtu. The fact that the recitation is in Akkadian rather than "Subarean" or academic Sumerian as well as the formulation of the label (just "sore tooth" without "If a person has a") suggests that this treatment could have originated with a pharmacist.

1. *ul-tu* ^{d}*A-nu-um* [*ib-nu-ú* AN-*ú*]
2. AN-*ú ib-nu-ú* [*er-ṣe-tam*]
3. *er-ṣe-tum ib-nu-ú* ÍD.MEŠ
4. ÍD.MEŠ *ib-na-a a-tap-pa-ti*
5. *a-tap-pa-ti ib-na-a ru-šum-ta*
6. *ru-šum-ta ib-nu-ú tu-ul-tu*
7. *il-lik tu-ul-tu ana* IGI ^{d}UTU *i-bak-ki*
8. *ana* IGI ^{d}*É-a il-la-ka di-ma-a-ša*

9. *mi-na-a ta-at-ta-an-na a-na a-ka-li-ia*
10. *mi-na-a ta-at-ta-an-na a-na mun-zu-qí-ia*
11. *at-tan-nak-ki* ^{GIŠ}PÈŠ *ba-ši-il-ta*
12. *ar-ma-na-a* ^{GIŠ}ḪAŠḪUR
13. *ana-ku am-mi-na-an-na-a* ^{GIŠ}PÈŠ *ba-ši-il-ta*
14. *ù ar-ma-na-a* ^{GIŠ}ḪAŠḪUR
15. *šu-uk-na!-an-ni-ma ina bi-rit ši-in-ni*
16. *ù la-áš-ḫi šu-ši-ba-an-ni*
17. *ša ši-in-ni-ma lu-un-zu-qa da-mi-šu*
18. *ù ša la-áš-ḫi-*‹‹ši››*-im lu-uk-su-u*[*s*]
19. *ku-sa-se-e-šu*
20. *sik-ka-ta ri-te-ma* GÌR *ṣa-ba-at*
21. *aš-šum an-na-a taq-bi-i tu-ul-tu*
22. *lim-ḫa-aṣ-ki* ^{d}*É-a i-na dan-na-ti*
23. *ri-it-ti-šu*

---

24. KA.INIM.MA ZÚ.GIG.GA.KÁM*

---

25. KÌD.KÌD.BI KAŠ.Ú.SA LAGAB MUNU$_7$ *ù* Ì.GIŠ 1-*niš* ḪE.ḪE
26. ÉN 3-*šú ana* UGU ŠID-*nu i-na* UGU *ši-in-ni-šu* GAR-*an*

TRANSLATION

(1–23) When (the sky god) Anu [created the heavens], the heavens created [the earth]. The earth created the rivers, the rivers created the branch canals. The branch canals created the dampness, the dampness created the tooth worm. The tooth worm came, crying, before Shamash (god of justice); before Ea (god of wisdom) his tears flowed. "What will you give for me to eat? What will you give for me to suck?" "I will give you the ripe fig (and) the apricot." "What would I want with the ripe fig or the apricot? Put me among the teeth and set me in the jaw so that I may suck the blood of the tooth and chew up the chewed up (food particles collected) in the jaw."

Drive in a peg and so get hold of the foot (of the tooth).[88]

"Because you said (all this), O tooth worm, may Ea strike you with his mighty hand!"

(24) Recitation for a sore tooth.[89]

(25–26) Its ritual: You mix together *billatu*-beerwort, a lump of malt and oil. You recite the recitation three times over it. You put (it) on his tooth.

NOTES

1. Chapter 8, text 3.
2. BM 54641+BM 54826 (Fincke 2009, 84–93) obv. 19′–20′.
3. For other ascriptions of this kind, see Leichty 1988, 261–64.
4. Pace *CAD* R, 344–45, this is certainly not "bat guano." *Rikibtu* means "musk," and there are any number of plant and animal substances that share the smell and some of the properties of real musk.
5. This daub is also mentioned, inter alia, in BM 54641+BM 54826 (Fincke 2009, 84–93) rev. 2–3; BAM 159 iv 16′–22′; and BAM 382:9–11.
6. See Scurlock and Andersen 2005, 9.5.
7. See Scurlock and Andersen 2005, 9.68.
8. See chapter 3, n. 109.
9. See Scurlock and Andersen 2005, 9.48.
10. See chapter 3, n. 109.
11. See Scurlock and Andersen 2005, 9.44.
12. See Scurlock and Andersen 2005, 9.5.
13. See Scurlock and Andersen 2005, 9.45.
14. See Scurlock and Andersen 2005, 9.43. Fincke 2009, 88 suggests instead: "tears or lost things."
15. See Scurlock and Andersen 2005, 9.66.
16. See chapter 3, n. 109.
17. This recitation properly belongs to the series *Utukkū lemnūtu*. See Geller 1985, 40–43, lines 377–383.
18. Suggestion courtesy M. Stol.
19. UZU^{II} = *šīru* ("flesh")+ *ān* (dual) = *šerʾānu*: "blood vessel"/"muscle"—a particularly nice example of a scribal pun of the sort not infrequently found in BAM and in texts of Neo-Assyrian date in general. Schwemer 2009, 174 prefers to see this as a synonym for "body." I would, however, think that if they meant for the whole body to be rubbed, they would have said so in so many words.
20. For this procedure, see Stol 1998, 350. Fumigations will have been over coals, not an open fire.
21. Heeßel 2011c, 53 n. 130 identifies "human bone" as a *Deckname* for *ḫaṭṭi reʾi*, "shephard's staff" on the basis of Uruanna (q.v.). What the passage actually does is to identify "human bone" as "lone plant" and then "lone plant" as *ḫaṭṭi reʾi*. So one could conclude from this that "lone plant" is also another name for *ḫaṭṭi reʾi*, which is the actual plant. The problem is that Uruanna's equations are not always simply different names for the same plant. The idea of Uruanna was to help the user find a plant he could use when faced with unavailable (or in the case of *Deckname* and foreign names) unfamiliar plants. So the possibility always exists that any two plants which are equated are completely different plants with similar properties. In this case, the fact that "human bone" is never directly equated with *ḫaṭṭi reʾi* suggests that "lone plant" and *ḫaṭṭi reʾi* are two different plants with similar properties, and that "human bone" is a *Deckname* for "lone plant" and not *ḫaṭṭi reʾi*.
22. See Scurlock and Andersen 2005, 9.114.
23. Napir is the Elamite word for god.
24. That is, "right" and "left" from the perspective of the viewer. See Scurlock and Andersen 2005, xxii–xxiii.
25. See Scurlock and Andersen 2005, 9.104.

26. For a discussion of terms for illness, see Stol 2009b, 29–46.

27. See Scurlock and Andersen 2005, 9.106.

28. See chapter 3, n. 109.

29. Stol 2007b, 241 follows von Soden's reading of the passage and interprets this shout as a battle cry on the basis of its Hebrew cognate. He also has the patient performing the action. This is certainly a possibility, but much depends upon whether the patient or his doctor is imagined as doing battle with the problem.

30. See Stol 1979, 18, n. 68.

31. See Scurlock and Andersen 2005, 9.108.

32. See Scurlock and Andersen 2005, 9.101.

33. For this use of the enclitic *-ma* in medical texts, see Scurlock and Andersen 2005, xvi.

34. See Scurlock and Andersen 2005, 9.107.

35. This is either GIŠ.MA.[NU]: *eʾru*-tree or GIŠ.PÈŠ: "fig."

36. The hanging *-ma* which appears at the end of treatments seems to function like our "etc." See chapter 6, text 2 ad line 62.

37. See chapter 3, text 1.

38. That is, "right" and "left" from the perspective of the viewer. See Scurlock and Andersen 2005 xxii–xxiii.

39. See Farber 1979, 303.

40. That is, "right" and "left" from the perspective of the viewer. See Scurlock and Andersen 2005 xxii–xxiii.

41. BAM 543 ii 26 has ^{Ú}NÍG.GÁN.GÁN.

42. Heeßel and Al-Rawi 2003, 223 ii 42 has: ŠÀ *na-ḫi-ri-šú*; BAM 543 i 65′ has: *ana* ŠÀ *ap-pi-šú*.

43. Heeßel and Al-Rawi 2003, 223 ii 43 has: A ^{GIŠ}NU.ÚR.MA ŠEG$_6$-*šal*.

44. BM 66560 rev. 2′ has: *ana* UGU ZÚ.MEŠ-*šú*.

45. BM 66560 rev. 4′ has: [$^{\text{NA}_4}$]*mu-ṣa* SAL.

46. BAM 537 rev. 5′ and BAM 533:43 substitute *ù* ^{d}*Kù-bu la i-ni-qu ši-zib* AMA-*šú*

47. BAM 537 rev. 6′ and BAM 533:44 substitute *e ta-as-saḫ-ra*.

48. BAM 533:53 has KA.ḪAB.

49. BAM 533:55 substitutes *i-ni-qu*.

50. All duplicates substitute ^{ÍD}*Ú-la-a-a* for A.AB.BA.

51. See Farber 1990, 313–16.

52. See chapter 3, n. 109.

53. So the parallel. The main text is apparently corrupt.

54. The interpretation assumes a relationship with *lamāmu*: "to chew." See *CAD* L, 59b.

55. The hanging *-ma* which appears at the end of treatments seems to function like our "etc." See chapter 6, text 2 ad line 62.

56. See Scurlock and Andersen 2005, 3.63.

57. See Scurlock and Andersen 2005, 3.62.

58. See Scurlock and Andersen 2005, 3.62.

59. See Scurlock and Andersen 2005, 6.172, 9.124, 10.119.

60. Heeßel and Al-Rawi 2003, 223 ii 42 has: "inside his nostrils"; BAM 543 i 65′ has: "inside his nose."

61. Heeßel and Al-Rawi 2003, 223 ii 43 has: "You boil *nurmû*-pomegranate juice."

62. BM 66560 has: "on his teeth."

63. BM 66560 rev. 3′ has: "female *mūṣu*-stone."

64. The first verb is preterite, and the second perfect, implying that the second action is closer to the present than the first.

65. See Scurlock and Andersen 2005, 3.61.

66. BAM 537 rev. 5 and BAM 533:43 substitute: "and ^{d}*Kù-bu* cannot suck the milk of its mother."

67. The first verb is preterite, and the second perfect, implying that the second action is closer to the present than the first.

68. See Scurlock and Andersen 2005, 3.67.

69. BAM 533:55 substitutes "suck."

70. Literally: "If not of a lion, *bu'šānu*'s affliction is mighty."

71. The first verb is preterite, and the second perfect, implying that the second action is closer to the present than the first.

72. An awkwardly placed enclitic *–mi* at the beginning of line 71 marks this as direct speach.

73. The vessel in question had to be put in a potstand, since otherwise it went over on its side, spilling the contents. The daughters of Anu are imagined as drawing water in silver buckets of a *sūtu*-capacity (*tallu*) and then transferring it to golden vases for transport.

74. All duplicates substitute the River Ulai for the Cosmic Ocean.

75. Literally "ploughed (with a seeder plow)."

76. With Hunger, this must be from a by-form of the root *dlḫ*, or have similar meaning.

77. See Scurlock and Andersen 2005, 235–36.

78. This also appears in BM 66560 rev. 4′//SpTU 1.44:49. Heeßel (2011c, 57) suggests "frog lung," reading BIL! instead of the BU. This would, of course, mean that the same mistake was made twice. It seems more likely that we are dealing with a mineral, perhaps "female" *mūṣu*-stone as in BM 66560 rev. 3′.

79. See Scurlock and Andersen 2005, 3.69.

80. See Scurlock and Andersen 2005, 420–21.

81. See Riddle 1985, 73.

82. CTN 4.194:10 mentions that the plant is to be crushed/minced.

83. In BAM 538 ii 48′, male *pillû* root is bruised and rested together with its juices on the sore tooth for toothache.

84. BAM 159 v 15–16 has these two plants being put dry between the teeth.

85. The translation assumes that *šim-ṭa-te* is from *šamāṭu*: "to strip off."

86. In BAM 159 v 23–25, these three are to be rubbed on the base of the teeth to remove "heaviness" in the mouth.

87. See Scurlock and Andersen 2005, 18.6.

88. These are instructions for the procedure accompanying the recitation.

89. See Scurlock and Andersen 2005, 18.15.

6

FEVER

A. TREATMENTS FOR FEVER IN GENERAL

The ancient Mesopotamian physician recognized five grades of temperature (including normal), and made careful note of fever patterns. For more details, see Scurlock and Andersen 2005, 27–34. Fevers were most commonly treated with salves and bandages, but potions, fumigants, baths, and, more rarely, daubs, washes, and enemas are also attested. There were also specialized treatments for specific fevers, as for example *di'u* (text 4) and *ṣētu* (texts 5–6).

TEXT 1: BAM 147

BAM 147 consists of salves (obv. 1–20), amulets (obv. 21–24), and a potion (obv. 24) for high fever. This is followed by a ritual (obv. 25–33) for a persistent fever that seems never to want to go away. The reverse contains a daub (rev. 1′–2′), an amulet (rev. 3′–4′) and a salve (rev. 5′–16′) for biphasic fevers. This is followed by a salve and amulet for a persistent fever (rev. 17′–25′). Since medical amulets often accompany other treatments and contain the same sort of medicines used in them, it is probable that the aim of amulets was to force the medicines being administered to the patient in another form to do their job. For more on this subject, see Scurlock 2006, 59–62.

Of special interest are those treatments (obv. 16–20, rev. 5′–16′, 17′–25′) that use lizards. Lines obv. 16–20 content themselves with including the lizard among the plant medicines which are boiled to make the salve. In lines rev. 5′–16′, the freshly boiled lizard is the main ingredient, but accompanied by an odd set of dusts and a plaster which encode messages to the lizard as to what the patient wanted. The esoteric commentaries in chapter 4 give highly intellectualized decodings of the messages embedded in objects used in rituals; the texts themselves are rather more straightforward. So, the dust from shade and sunlight signifies: "The shade brings (shade) in proportion to the heat of the sunlight (The hotter the sun, the cooler the shade)," meaning that the patient wishes to be as cool as he is now hot. Dust from both doorposts betokens a wish for the illness not to approach, dust from the threshold that the illness not "marry" the patient, that is, be with him day and night for life. The dust from under a continually used reed basket meaning that the patient will not be given up on is a bit of a stretch, but dust from a tomb bringing undisturbed sleep is spot on. In lines rev. 17′–25′, the poor lizard escapes boiling but is hardly better treated. He gets to ride round the patient's neck trapped inside a hollow reed as an unusual amulet.

There is also a quite fun ritual in lines obv. 25–33 in which a figurine representing the illness is manufactured from clay rubbed onto the patient. The idea was, obviously, to transfer the fever from the patient to the figurine, which was why it was taken out into the steppe, made to face the setting sun, tied to a tree and, just for good measure, surrounded with a magic circle. Note also the precautions about looking behind or taking the same street to get home. Failure here would make the entire ritual a waste of time, since the fever would come right back into the patient. For more on this subject, see Scurlock 2002b, 209–23. Given that the sickness was not exactly a friend, it is striking, and by no means unusual in Mesopotamian rituals, that the figurine is well treated and given clothing and travel provisions before being literally bound to go away and leave the patient alone.

obv.

1. DIŠ NA KÚM *dan-nu* DIB-*su* ^{Ú}*e-li-kul-la*
2. ^{Ú}*ir-kul-la* ^{Ú}LÚ.U$_{18}$.LU ^{Ú}*an-ki-nu-te*
3. ^{Ú}*eli-kul-la* SA$_5$ KA.A.AB.BA ŠURUN-^{d}*Še-riš*
4. 1-*niš* SÚD *ina* KI.A.^{d}ÍD ḪE.ḪE Ì *ana* ŠÀ ŠUB-*ma* ḪE.ḪE-*ma*
5. ŠÉŠ-*su-ma li-ʾ-bu šá iṣ-ba-tu-šú* ZI-*aḫ*

---

6. DIŠ KI.MIN ^{Ú}*eli-kul-la* SI.DÀRA.MAŠ ^{GIŠ}ŠINIG SIG$_7$
7. KA.A.AB.BA ŠURUN-^{d}*Še-riš* 1-*niš ina* A.MEŠ SÚD
8. *ina* Ì.GIŠ ḪE.ḪE ŠÉŠ-*su*

---

9. DIŠ KI.MIN ^{Ú}*eli-kul-la el-kul-la* ^{Ú}*eli-kul-la* SA$_5$
10. ^{Ú}LÚ.U$_{18}$.LU NUMUN ^{GIŠ}ŠINIG *ni-kip-tú* NÍTA *u* MUNUS
11. KI.A.^{d}ÍD MÚD ^{GIŠ}ERIN ḪE.ḪE ŠÉŠ.MEŠ-*su-ma*
12. KÚM *dan-nu li-ʾ-bu šá* DIB-*šu in-na-saḫ*

---

13. *a-na* KÚM *dan-ni* ZI-*aḫ kur-ra šá* ^{LÚ}AŠGAB SUMUN ^{Ú}IN$_6$.ÚŠ
14. *ni-kip-tú* KA.A.AB.BA 1-*niš* SÚD *ina* Ì.GIŠ
15. ŠÉŠ.ME-*su-ma ina-eš*

---

16. DIŠ KI.MIN ^{ŠEM}GÚR.GÚR ^{ŠEM}LI Ú *a-ši-i ni-kip-tú* SÚD
17. ^{Ú}KUR.ZI ^{GIŠ}GEŠTIN.KA$_5$.A ^{Ú}GAMUN^{SAR} KI.A.^{d}ÍD
18. ^{Ú}ḪUR.SAG^{SAR} SIG$_7$-*su* EME.ŠID *ša* IZ.ZI

19. *ana* ŠÀ ŠUB-*di* ŠEG$_6$-*ma an-na-a u an-na-*[*a*]
20. *ina* IZI *ta-sal-laq-ma* ŠÉŠ.ME-*su-ma ina-eš*

---

21. DIŠ KI.MIN *iṣ piš-ri* SÍG ÙZ GÌŠ.NU.ZU NIGIN-*mi ina* GÚ-*šú* GAR-*an*

---

22. DIŠ NA *um-mi dan-ni* ZI-*ḫi* ^{Ú}*el-kul-la*
23. ^{Ú}*eli-kul-la* ^{Ú}LÚ.U$_{18}$.LU SÍG ^{MUNUS}ÁŠ.GÀR *ina* SÍG.ÀKA

---

24. DIŠ KI.MIN ^{Ú}*eli-kul-la ina* SÍG.ÀKA ^{Ú}*šu-mut-tú ina* A.MEŠ NAG

---

25. DIŠ NA KÚM *ka-a-a-ma-an* DIB-*su* IM PA$_5$ TI-*qí*
26. *ina* A PA$_5$ ḪE.ḪE SU LÚ.GIG *tu-kap-‹(par)›* NU DÙ-*uš*
27. *ina* MAŠ.SÌLA GÙB-*šú* NU *mim-ma lem-ni* SAR SÍG *pu-ti*
28. [(G)]UD.UDU.ḪI.A TI-*qí* TÚG.U$_4$.1.KÁM TÚG.GÚ.È.U$_4$.1.KÁM*
29. [(TÚG.BAR.SIG)].U$_4$.1.KÁM* *ta-maḫ-ḫaṣ* NÍG.ÀR.RA [(BAPPIR)]
30. [(MUNU$_4$ ZÍD) o (x *ina se*)]-*pí tàra-kás ina* U$_4$.GAM.MA *ana* IGI [(^{d}UTU)]
31. [(*ta-dan-šu-ma ana*)] EDIN È-*šú ana* ^{d}UTU.[(ŠÚ.A)]
32. [(IGI-*šú* GAR)-*m*(*a* KI ^{GIŠ}DÌḪ *u*)] $^{\text{GIŠ.Ú}}$GÍR *tu-*[*ra-kas-su-ma*][1]
33. [(ZÌ.SUR.RA.A NIGIN-*šú ana* EGIR-*ka* N)]U IGI.BAR [(SILA *šá-ni-tú*) ...]

---

rev.

1′. [(DIŠ KI.MIN ŠIKA *ar-sin-ni* ŠAḪ *šá*)] ⸢GÙB *tur*⸣-[(*ár*)]
2′. [(*e-ma* DIB-*šú ana* UG)]U-*šú ta-zar-ru-ma* [...]

3′. [(DIŠ KI.MIN SÍG UGU.DU)]L.BI GÌR.PAD.DU NAM.LÚ.[(U$_{18}$.LU)]
4′. [(*tur-ár* SÚD)] *ina* GÚ-*šú* [(GAR-*an*)]

5′. DIŠ KI.MIN[2] *ina* AN.BAR$_7$ SAḪAR GISSU ‹*u*› UD.DA TI-*qí si-ra*
6′. *šá sip-pí* ⸢*ana*⸣ *sip-pí* SAḪAR KUN$_4$ IGI-*ti* SAḪAR *šá* KI.TA x x -*šú*
7′. SAḪAR KI.MAḪ ^{Ú}KUR.ZI SÚD *ina* Ì.^{GIŠ}BUR ḪE.ḪE *ina* $^{\text{NA}_4}$BUR.ALGAMES
8′. *ina* IZI ŠEG$_6$-*šal* EME.ŠID TI-*qí* TI-*sa ana* ŠÀ ŠUB-*di*
9′. *tu-tar-ra-ma ta-na-suk ana* ŠÀ-*bi ki-a-am* ŠID

10′. ÉN *ki-i* UD.DA KÚM-*im* : *ki-i* GISSU *ur-ra*
11′. *ki-i sip-pí ana sip-*⸢*pí*⸣ [*a-a i*]*q-ri-bu*[3] : *bir*[4]-*ṣu a-a iq-rib-šú*
12′. GIN$_7$ KUN$_4$ *li-*[(*kab-bi*)]-*su-šu-ma ma-am-ma-an a-a ir-ši*

13′. GIN$_7$ *pi-sa-an-ni ana ur-ḫu-šú u ti-bi-šú la iz-zi-bu*
14′. GIG *a-a in-né-zíb* GIN$_7$ LÚ.ÚŠ *la in-nu-u* ÉLLAG-*su*
15′. GIG ÉLLAG-*su a-a i-ni* TU$_6$ ÉN É.NU.RU
16′. 7-*šú ana* ŠÀ ŠID-*nu-ma* ŠÉŠ-*su*

17′. A.RA.ZU ^{d}NIN.A.ZU ME.UR ḪÉ.I.I
18′. ^{d}KÙ.A.NI ŠÚ.DIB.BA UB.BI MIN MIN : *i-na ni-pi-iḫ ni-ri šá* AN
19′. ^{d}EN.LÍL.LE ^{d}*É-a* TU$_6$ ÉN

20′. KA.INIM.MA KÚM *la-az-zi* ZI

21′. DÙ.DÙ.BI Ú.KUR.RA KI.A.^{d}ÍD ^{Ú}KUR.KUR *ni-kip-tú*
22′. *tur-ár* SÚD KI Ì.GIŠ ḪE.ḪE ÉN 3-*šú ana* ŠÀ ŠID-*nu*
23′. ŠÉŠ.ŠÉŠ-*su-ma* TI-*uṭ* GI.DÙ.A TI-*qí* 7 ŠU.SI
24′. *te-še-rim* EME.ŠID TI.LA-*su* SAG.DU-*nu-uš-šá ana* ŠÀ ŠUB-*di*
25′. *ina* TÚG GI$_6$ KÁ-*šá* KEŠDA-*ma ina* GÚ-*šú* GAR-*an*

26′. ÉN KÚM *te-šu-ú* KÚM *qab-lu* EGIR-*šú* (catchline)
(colophon of Kiṣir-Nabu, the famous *āšipu* of Assur) = BAM 148 rev. 28′–33′

Translation

(obv. 1–5) If a high fever afflicts a person,[5] you grind together *elikulla*, *erkulla*, *amilānu*, *ankinutu*, red *elikulla*, *imbû tamtim* (and) "ox dung." You mix (it) with *kibrītu*-sulphur. You pour oil into it (and) mix (it) together. Then, if you rub him gently (with it), the *li'bu* which afflicts him should be removed.

(obv. 6–8) Alternatively, you grind together *elikulla*, stag horn, fresh *bīnu*-tamarisk, *imbû tamtim* (and) "ox dung" in water. You mix (it) with oil (and) rub him gently (with it).

(obv. 9–12) Alternatively, you mix together *elikulla*, *elkulla*, red *elikulla*, *amilānu*, *bīnu*-tamarisk seed, male and female *nikiptu*, *kibrītu*-sulphur (and) *erēnu*-cedar resin. If you repeatedly rub him gently (with it), the high fever (and) *li'bu* which afflicts him should be removed.

(obv. 13–15) To remove a high fever, you grind together used tanner's depilatory paste,[6] *maštakal*, *nikiptu* (and) *imbû tamtim*. If you rub (it) gently on him (mixed) with oil, he should recover.

(obv. 16–20) Alternatively, you grind *kukru*, *burāšu*-juniper, *šammi ašî* (and) *nikiptu*. You pour *samīdu*, "fox grape," *kamūnu*-cumin, *kibrītu*-sulphur, fresh *azupīru* (and) a *ṣurāru*-lizard from a wall into it (and) boil (it). You boil this and this over a fire and, if you rub him gently (with it), he should recover.

(obv. 21) Alternatively, you wrap *pišru* wood in hair from a virgin she-goat (and) put (it) on his neck.

(obv. 22–23) If you want to remove a person's high fever, (you put) *elkulla, elikulla, amilānu* (and) virgin she-goat hair in a tuft of wool.

(obv. 24) Alternatively, (you wrap), *elikulla* in a tuft of wool. You have him drink *šumuttu* (mixed) with water.

(obv. 25–33) If fever continually afflicts a person, you take clay from a canal. You mix (it) with canal water. You wipe off the body of the sick person (with it and) make a figurine. On its left shoulder, you write "Figurine of anything evil." You take hair from the forehead of oxen and sheep. You weave (it) into a makeshift garment, a makeshift cloak (and) a makeshift turban. You arrange groats, beer bread, malt (and) [...] flour on *sēpu*-bread. In the late afternoon, you sue it before Shamash. You take (it) out into the steppe region. You make (it) face the setting sun. and then you tie (it) to a *baltu*-thorn or *ašāgu*-thorn and then you surround (it) with a magic circle. You do not look behind you. [You take] another street (home from the one on which you came).

(rev. 1′–2′) Alternatively,[7] you char a fragment of the left tusk? of a pig. (If) you daub (it) on wherever it afflicts him, [...]

(rev. 3′–4′) Alternatively, you char (and) grind ape hair (and) "lone plant" (= "human bone"). You put (it) on his neck (as an amulet).

(rev. 5′–9′) Alternatively,[8] at noon, you take dust from shade and sunlight. You grind (it and) plaster from both doorposts, dust from the front threshold, dust from below ... (a drainpipe/from below a post-menopausal woman),[9] dust from a tomb (and) *samīdu* (and) mix (it) with *pūru* oil. You boil (it) over a fire in a *pūru*-vessel made from *algamešu*-stone. You take a live *ṣurāru*-lizard and throw (it) into it. You have him recite over it as follows.

(rev. 10′–16′) "The shade brings (shade) in proportion to the heat of the sunlight (The hotter the sun, the cooler the shade). Just as one door post may never approach the other, so may the sickness never approach the patient. Just as should anyone step on the threshold, (he will never obtain anybody as a wife), so may (the illness) not obtain anybody (as a wife).[10] Just as a drainpipe can never abandon[11] its runnel and its riser so may the sick person not be given up on. Just as a dead person does not change his kidney (i.e., toss and turn), so may the sick person not change his kidney: spell and recitation." You recite the É.NU.RU over it seven times and then rub him gently (with it).

(rev. 17′–19′) ^{d}Ninazu, may petition (and) oracle be exalted! Command intercession in the pure heavens! Ditto Ditto at the rising of the Yoke star of Anu, Enlil (and) Ea. Spell and Recitation.

(rev. 20′) Recitation to remove a persistent fever.

(rev. 21′–25′) Its ritual: You char (and) grind *nīnû*-mint, *kibrītu*-sulphur, *atāʾišu* (and) *nikiptu*. You mix (it) with oil. You recite the recitation three times over it. If you repeatedly rub him gently (with it), he should recover. You take any kind of reed (and) trim off seven fingers (worth). You drop a live *ṣurāru*-lizard head first into it.[12] You tie its (i.e., the reed's) mouth with a black cloth and then put (it) on his neck.

(rev. 26′) Recitation: "Fever, melée; fever, battle" (catchline)

TEXT 2: BM 42272:32–85

BM 42272 is a nice example of a mixed subject text. The first 31 lines deal with various forms of witchcraft (see chapter 14, text 1). Lines 32–85 consist of salves (32–62, 66–69, 74–75, 78–79, 84), amulets (39–48, 54–63, 66–83) and fumigants (49–53, 64–65, 70–71, 78–79) for fever.

Of particular interest is yet another lizard-based salve (32–36). In this version, you are told that the lizard is supposed to be removed and thrown away, a detail omitted in the earlier BAM 147. Lines 37–38 instruct the physician to use a hot version rather than the usual cold one if it was winter. The types of dust in lines 39–44 provide a curious cross section of city life in ancient Mesopotamia. Silly but harmless is the Plautus-esque use of horse sweat in lines 49–53. To know is that horses absolutely have to be cooled down within fifteen minutes of vigorous sweating, so the analogy with the patient ill with fever is appropriate enough. Lines 54–62 give an alternative version of rev. 5′–16′ of BAM 147 in which a second lizard is used as an amulet as in BAM 147 rev. 17′–25′.

32. DIŠ NA K[(Ú)]M DIB-*su* ^{Ú}⸢GAMUN^{SAR}⸣ ^{Ú}⸢*ka*⸣-*man-tú* ^{Ú}*kám**-*ka*-[(*d*)]*u*
33. ^{Ú}EME.UR.GI$_7$ ŠEM.^{d}MAŠ NITA *u* MUNUS ^{ŠEM}BABBAR ^{ŠEM}[(L)]I ^{Ú}ḪUR.SAG$^{\text{[SA]R}}$ ^{GIŠ}GEŠTIN.KA$_5$.A!
34. KUŠ UZU.DIR.KUR.RA 1-*niš* SÚD *ina* Ì.GIŠ ḪE.ḪE *ana* ^{URUDU}ŠEN.TUR DUB-*ak* EME.ŠID
35. TI-*sa ana* ŠÀ ŠUB-*di ina* ⸢IZI ŠEG$_6$⸣-[*š*(*al*) EN (ŠEG)]$_6$-*lu ša* ŠUB-*ú* E$_{11}$-*ma ta-na-suk*
36. *tu-kaṣ-ṣa* ÉN DINGIR-*šu* GUL.KI (i.e., ḪUL.GIG?) BA.DU$_8$ 3-*šú* ŠID-*ma* ŠÉŠ-*su-ma* DIN

---

37. DIŠ KI.MIN ^{Ú}*an-ki-nu-tú* ^{ŠEM}LI ^{ŠEM}GÚR.GÚR ŠEM.GAM.MA 1-*niš ta-zák* [(*ina* Ì.GIŠ)] ḪE.ḪE
38. ŠÉŠ-*su šum*$_4$-*ma* EN.[TE].NA KÚM-*tu* (*ḫe-pi*)

---

39. DIŠ KI.MIN SAḪAR SILA LIMMU.BA ⸢SAḪAR⸣ É.ÈŠ.TAM.MA SAḪAR É KÁ GAL (KÁ É.GAL) SAḪAR KÁ É DINGIR

40. SAḪAR KÁ É ^{LÚ}KURUN.NAM SAḪAR KÁ É ^{LÚ}MUḪALDIM SAḪAR KÁ É ^{LÚ}*ka-ṣir*
41. SAḪAR ^{GIŠ}MÁ.DIRI.GA SAḪAR *kar-ri u ni-bir* ‹(1-*niš ta-šab-ba-aš*)› *ina* Ì ḪE.ḪE *ša*![13]-*lal-la* (*ḫe-pi*)[14] *šá* ŠÀ-*šá*
42. *u* MÚD-*šá* TI ‹(*ina* SÍG.ÀKA NIGIN-*mi ana* IGI ^{d}UTU)› KEŠDA *tara-kás* (*ḫe-pi*) *ina* UGU ^{GIŠ}(*ḫe-pi*) BI ŠID-*nu* ÉN ^{d}DÌM.ME
43. DUMU AN.N[A] 7-*šú ana* IGI ^{d}UTU *ana* ŠÀ Ì.GIŠ ŠID-*nu mi-iṣ* SÍG. BABBAR[15] *ina* GÚ-*šú* GAR-*an ù* Ì.GIŠ *an-na-a*
44. ŠÉŠ-*su-ma* DIN (on the bottom edge)

---

45. DIŠ KI.MIN ^{Ú}*ṣa-ṣu-un-tú* ^{Ú}*áp-ru-šá* ^{GIŠ}GEŠTIN.KA$_5$.A ḪÁD.DU SÚD *ina* Ì.GIŠ
46. ḪE.ḪE ‹*ina*› $^{\text{NA}_4}$BUR.ALGAMES *tu-ba-ḫar-ma* ŠÉŠ-*su* ^{SÍG}ḪÉ.ME.DA SÍG UR.MAḪ
47. SÍG ^{MUNUS}ÁŠ.GÀR 1-*niš* DUR NU.NU ^{Ú}EME.UR.GI$_7$ ^{Ú}*imḫur-lim* ^{Ú}LÚ-*a-nu*
48. ^{Ú}LAL ŠURUN-^{d}ŠERIŠ KI-*šú-nu ina* DUR NIGIN-*mi ina* GÚ-*šú* [GAR-*an-m*]*a ina-eš*

---

49. DIŠ NA MIN KÚM DIB-*su ḫal*-[(*l*)]*u-la-a-a ina* Ì ŠÉŠ-*su* [(NUMUN GADA *ina*)] DÈ SAR-*šú*
50. ANŠE.KUR.RA *pu-ḫa-la ina* ^{GIŠ}GIGIR[16] *ana* GÙB LAL-*su-ma* A[NŠE. KUR.RA] *šá* GÙB
51. Ì.UDU LIBIR.RA *tu-kaṣ-ṣa tu-kaš-šad-ma* ANŠE.K[(UR.RA IR ŠUB-*di-ma*) Ì.UDU] LIBIR.[RA]
52. *ni-ma-a-ti* ^{LÚ}GIG ŠÉŠ Ì.UDU U$_4$-*um* DIB-*šú ina* [DÈ $^{\text{GIŠ.Ú}}$GÍ]R 2-[(*šú*)]
53. 3-*šú tu-qat-tar-šú a-ḫu-ú ú-qat-tar-šu-ma* TI

---

54. DIŠ KI.MIN *ina* AN.⸢BAR$_7$⸣ SAḪAR GIS⸢SU *u* UD⸣.DA TI-*qí-ma* (*ḫe-pi*)[17]

---

55. SAḪAR I.D[(I)]B IGI-*i* SAḪAR KI.TA MUNUS *šá* Ù.TU TAR-*si* SAḪAR K[(I.MAḪ)] ⸢Ú⸣[(KUR.ZI)]
56. SÚD ⸢*ina*⸣ Ì.BUR ḪE.ḪE ‹(*ina*)› $^{\text{NA}_4}$BUR $^{\text{NA}_4}$ALGAMES *ina* IZI ŠEG$_6$-*šal* EME.ŠID ⸢TI-*sa ana* ŠÀ⸣ [(Š)]UB-*di*
57. ⸢E$_{11}$⸣-[(*m*)]*a ta-na-suk ana* ŠÀ *ki-a-am* ŠID-*nu* ÉN *ki-i* UD.DA KÚM-*im*
58. *ki*-⸢*i*⸣ [(GIS)]SU *ur-a*(sic) *ki-i* ZAG TA ZAG GABA *la i*-⸢*qàr*⸣-*ru-bu mur*-⸢*ṣa*⸣
59. NENNI [(A NE)]NNI *a-a* ⸢*iq*⸣-*rib-šú ki-ma id-da* ⸢*li*⸣-*kab-bi-su ù ma-am-*

man

60. *a-a* [(*ir-š*)]*ú ki-ma pi-sa-an-na ana ur-ri*(sic)*-šú u ti-bi-šú la iz-zi-bu mur-ṣu*

61. *a-a in-ne-zíb* [(*ki-m*)]*a mi-tu la* ⸢*in*⸣*-nu-ú* ÉLLAG-*su* GIG ÉLLAG-*su*

62. *a-a i-ni* TU[($_{6}$)] ÉN ÉN 7-*šú ana* ŠÀ ŠID-*ma* ŠÉŠ-[(*su*)] EME.ŠID TI-*ma*[18]

---

63. DIŠ KI.[MIN ^{Ú}]SI.SÁ *ina* TÚG.GI$_{6}$ NIGIN-[*mi-m*]*a ina* GÚ-*šú* GAR-*ma* DIN

---

64. DIŠ KI.[MIN] Ì.UDU ÉLLAG GUD.GI$_{6}$ A.GAR.GAR M[AŠ.D]À SI DÀRA.MAŠ GÌR.PAD.DU NAM.LÚ.U$_{18}$.LU

65. NAGA.[SI] KI.A.^{d}ÍD *ina* DÈ *tu-qat-tar-šú-ma* TI

---

66. DIŠ KI.[MIN] ⸢^{Ú}⸣*imḫur-ešra* SAḪAR KI.TA MUNUS ⸢*šá*⸣ Ù.TU *par-sat* Ì+^{GIŠ}DÌḪ Ì+^{GIŠ}*bi-ni*

67. *ina* Ì.GIŠ *ina* SÍG.ÀKA

---

68. DIŠ KI.MIN *ina ša-*⸢*nim*⸣ *i-bar-ru ḫal-lu-la-a-a* NIM UR.GI$_{7}$

69. ^{Ú}EME.UR.GI$_{7}$ *ina* Ì.GIŠ *ina* KUŠ

---

70. DIŠ KI.MIN ^{Ú}*u$_{5}$-ra-an-nam* Ì+^{GIŠ}DÌḪ TÚG.NÍG.DÁRA.ŠU.LÁL *ina* GÚ-*šú* BAR.MUŠ

71. UM.ME GÍR.TAB ZAG.ḪI.LI^{SAR} TÚG.NÍG.DÁRA.ŠU.LÁL SÍG.ŠAB *ina* DÈ SAR-*šú*

---

72. DIŠ KI.MIN SÍG UGU.DUL.BI GÌR.PAD.DU NAM.LÚ.U$_{18}$.LU *ina* KUŠ *ina* GÚ-*šú* GAR-*an*

---

73. DIŠ KI.MIN *ina ša-nim i-bar-ru ina* SÍG.ÀKA

---

74. DIŠ KI.MIN GI$_{6}$ PAP.ḪAL ANŠE GI$_{6}$ PAP.ḪAL ANŠE.‹KUR.RA› *kur-ra* ⸢*šá* ^{LÚ}⸣AŠGAB *ina* KUŠ GAG.GAG

75. *u* ^{Ú}*áp-ru-šá ina* Ì.GIŠ

---

76. DIŠ KI.MIN BAR.MUŠ GÌR.PAD.DU NAM.LÚ.U$_{18}$.LU UM.ME GÍR.TAB TÚG.NÍG.DÁRA.ŠU.LÁL $^{\text{NA}_4}$*kut-pa-a*

77. $^{\text{NA}_4}$*mu-ṣa* ^{Ú}*ṣa-ṣu-un-tú ina* KUŠ

---

78. DIŠ KI.MIN SÍG ANŠE.KUR.RA SÍG UR.MAḪ SÍG UR.BAR.RA SÍG UR.GI$_7$ GI$_6$ *ina* KUŠ GAG.GAG-*pí*

79. *ina* GÚ-*šú* GAR-*an* Ú.KUR.RA *saḫ-lé-e ina* DÈ *ni-kip-tú* KA *tam-tim ina* Ì.GIŠ ŠÉŠ-*su-ma* [DIN]

---

80. DIŠ KI.MIN PÉŠ.SÌLA.GAZ Ú ^{d}DÌM.ME *ina* SÍG.ÀKA NIGIN-*mi ina* GÚ-*šú* GAR-*an*

---

81. DIŠ KI.MIN ^{GIŠ}GEŠTIN.KA$_5$.A ^{Ú}IN.NU.UŠ *ina* KUŠ

---

82. DIŠ KI.MIN UMBIN SU.UD^{MUŠEN} ^{Ú}GÌR.UGA^{MUŠEN} *šá* 7 SAG. DU.MEŠ-*šá* [*ina* KUŠ]

---

83. DIŠ KI.MIN ^{Ú}LAL ^{ŠEM}LI *ina* SÍG.ÀKA NIGIN-*mi* [*ina* GÚ-*šú* GAR-*an*]

---

84. DIŠ KI.⸢MIN⸣ PA ^{GIŠ}DÌḪ *ina* Ì.GIŠ ⸢ŠÉŠ⸣

---

85. [DIŠ NA] KÚM DIB-*su* ^{Ú}AN.KI.NU.[TE ...]

Translation

(32–36) If fever afflicts a person, you grind together *kamūnu*-cumin, *kamantu*-henna(?), *kamkādu*, *lišān kalbi*, male and female *nikiptu*, *kukru* (= "white aromatic"), ⸢*burāšu*-juniper⸣, *azupīru*, "fox grape" (and) *kamūn šadê*-fungus.[19] You mix (it) with oil (and) pour (it) into a *tamgussu*-vessel. You drop a live *ṣurāru*-lizard into it (and) boil (it) over a fire [until] ⸢it has cooked⸣. What you dropped in (i.e., the lizard), you take out and throw away. You let (the mixture) cool. You recite the recitation "The hatred(?) of his god has been loosened" three times over it and, if you rub him gently with it, he should recover.

(37–38) Alternatively, you grind together *ankinutu*, *burāšu*-juniper, *kukru* (and) *ṣumlalû*. You mix (it) with oil (and) rub him gently (with it). If it is ⸢winter⸣, you use (it) hot.

(39–44) Alternatively, ‹(you collect together)› dust from a crossroads, dust from a tavern, dust from the gate of the palace, dust from the gate of a temple, dust from the gate of the house of a brewer, dust from the house of a cook, dust from the house of a rug weaver, dust from a boat going downstream (and) dust from quays and crossings. You mix (it) with oil. [You ...] a *šalālu*-reed. You take its pith and resin. ‹(You wrap it in a tuft of wool. Before Shamash)›, you set up an offering arrangement. [You ... the oil and this amulet] on a wooden

[…]. You recite [the recitation …] times. You recite the recitation "Lamashtu, daughter of Anu" seven times before Shamash over the oil. You put a bit[20] of white wool (the amulet) on his neck and if you rub him gently with this oil, he should recover.

(45–48) Alternatively, you dry (and) grind *ṣaṣuntu*, *aprušu* (and) "fox grape" (and) mix (it) with oil. You heat (it)[21] in a *pūru*-vessel made from *algamešu*-stone and then rub him gently (with it). You twine together red-dyed wool, lion hair (and) hair of a virgin she-goat into a cord. You work *lišān kalbi*, *imḫur-lim*, *amilānu*, *ašqulalu*, and "ox dung" with them into the cord. If [you put it] on his neck, he should recover.

(49–53) If fever afflicts a person, you rub him gently with *ḫalulaya*-insect (mixed) with oil. You fumigate him with flax seed over coals. You hitch a stallion to a chariot on the left side and you cool down the ⌜horse⌝ on the left with old sheep fat. You drive (it) so that the ⌜horse⌝ sweats and then you rub the garment(?)[22] of the patient gently with the old [sheep fat]. The day it afflicts him, you fumigate him (with) the fat two or three times over ⌜*ašāgu*-thorn⌝ [coals]. If a stranger fumigates him, he should recover.

(54–62) Alternatively, at noon, you take dust from shade and sunlight. You grind (it and) plaster from both doorposts, dust from the front threshold, dust from below a post-menopausal[23] woman, dust from a tomb (and) *samīdu* (and) mix (it) with *pūru* oil. You boil it over a fire ‹(in)› a *pūru*-vessel made from *algamešu*-stone. You drop a live *ṣurāru*-lizard into it. You take (it) out and throw (it) away. You have him recite over it as follows. "The shade brings (shade) in proportion to the heat of the sunlight (The hotter the sun, the cooler the shade). Just as one door post does not approach the other, so may the sickness never approach the patient, so-and-so, son of so-and-so. Just as should anyone step on the threshold, (he will never obtain anybody as a wife), so may (the illness) not obtain anybody (as a wife).[24] Just as a drainpipe can never abandon[25] its runnel and its riser so may the sick person not be given up on. Just as a dead person does not change his kidney (i.e., toss and turn), so may the sick person not change his kidney: spell and recitation." You recite the recitation over it seven times and then rub him gently (with it). A live *ṣurāru*-lizard, etc.

(63) ⌜Alternatively⌝, you wrap *šurdunû* in a black cloth and, if you put (it) on his neck, he should recover.

(64–65) ⌜Alternatively⌝, if you fumigate him with fat from the kidney of a black ox, gazelle droppings, stag horn, "lone plant" (= "human bone"), *uḫḫūlu* [*qarnānu*] (and) *kibrītu*-sulphur over coals, he should recover.

(66–67) ⌜Alternatively⌝, you (rub him gently) with *imḫur-ešra*, dust from beneath a a post-menopausal woman, *baltu*-thorn oil (and) *bīnu*-tamarisk oil (mixed) with oil (and you wrap it) in a tuft of wool (and put it on his neck).

(68–69) If ditto (fever afflicts a person), (and) on the second (day) he feels well, you (rub him gently) with a *ḫalulaya*-cricket, a fly (i.e., flea) from a dog (and) *lišān kalbi* (mixed) with oil (and you put it on his neck) in a leather bag.

(70–71) Alternatively, (you put) *urânu*, *baltu*-thorn oil (and) *sikillu* (= "soiled rag") on his neck. You fumigate him with snake skin, scorpion stinger, *saḫlû*-cress,[26] *sikillu* (= "soiled rag") (and) bristles over coals.

(72) Alternatively, you put ape hair (and) "lone plant" (= "human bone") in a leather bag on his neck.

(73) If ditto (fever afflicts a person), (and) on the second (day) he feels well, (you wrap it) in a tuft of wool (and put it on his neck).

(74–75) Alternatively, you sew up (a tuft of) black (hair) from the thigh of a donkey, (a tuft of) black (hair) from the thigh of a horse(!) (and) tanner's depilatory paste in a leather bag and (you also rub him gently with) *aprušu* (mixed) with oil.

(76–77) Alternatively, (you put) snake skin, scorpion stinger, "lone plant" (= "human bone"), *sikillu* (= "soiled rag"), *kutpû*-mineral, *mūṣu*-stone (and) *ṣaṣuntu* in a leather bag.

(78–79) Alternatively, you sew up horse hair, lion hair, wolf hair (and) black dog hair into a leather bag (and) put (it) on his neck. (You fumigate him with) *nīnû*-mint (and) *saḫlû*-cress over *nikiptu* coals. If you rub him gently with *imbû tamtim* (mixed) with oil, [he should recover].

(80) Alternatively, you wrap a *ḫulu*-shrew (and) "plant for Lamashtu" in a tuft of wool (and) put (it) on his neck.

(81) Alternatively, (you put) "fox grape" (and) *maštakal* in a leather bag.

(82) Alternatively, [(you put)] bat(?) claw (and) seven headed "crow's foot" [in a leather bag].

(83) Alternatively, you wrap *ašqulalu* (and) *burāšu*-juniper in a tuft of wool [(and) put it on his neck].

(84) Alternatively, you rub him gently with *baltu*-thorn leaves (mixed) with oil.

(85) [If] fever afflicts [a person], *ankinutu* [...]

TEXT 3: TSUKIMOTO 1999: 199–200, LINES 1–36

Tsukimoto 1999: 199–200 is a rare example of a Middle Babylonian medical text from Emar. Beginning in line 37, the tablet contains even rarer treatments for *saḫaršubbû* (see chapter 7 text 3). Lines 1–36 consist of an *asû*'s bandage (1–7), baths (8–18), potions (16–19), salves (16–18), a fumigant (20), and an amulet (21–35) for fever.

Of particular interest is the bath of 8–15, which is extremely unusual in having the physician dig a patient-sized hole for a sauna-style up to the neck burial in medicated mud. More common, but still precious is the provision of back-up treatments (16–35) in case the main one doesn't work. The recitation in lines 27–35 invites the fever to go vegetarian or, qua fire, to burn down a forest. The facts that water flows down rather than up and that doves build a new nest every year are exploited to instruct the fever never to return. A basic distinction between ancient Mesopotamian "magic" and ancient Greek "science" is that, in the former, the analogies from nature are always, and in the latter, never or almost never, accurate.

1. Ú.MEŠ *ša* KÚM ^{Ú}SI.SI.NUN.NA SUḪUŠ ^{Ú}ḪAB *u* PA-*šu* ^{Ú}KUR.KUR.RA SUḪUŠ ^{GIŠ}MES.GÀM
2. SUḪUŠ ^{Ú}*šal-la-mi*[27] SUḪUŠ ^{GIŠ}ŠE.NA *u* NUMUN-*šú* NUMUN ^{GIŠ}ŠINIG NUMUN ^{Ú}*qú-ut-ra-ti*
3. NUMUN GADA NUMUN ^{GIŠ}ŠEM.GIG ^{Ú}*ba-ri-ra-ti zé-e* ^{DUG}SÌLA!.BUR BAR IM.ŠU.RIN
4. ŠE.GÍN IM.⸢SAḪAR⸣.[NA]$_4$.BABBAR.KUR.RA ZÍD.DA *qa-ia-a-ti* ŠE.GÍN MUN SAḪAR DAG×KIŠIM$_5$×KASKAL
5. *ša 7 aš-re-š*[*ú* SA]ḪAR *tu-ḫu-ul-la-ti* NUMUN $^{GIŠ.ŠEM}$GÚR.GÚR NUMUN ^{GIŠ}ŠEM.LI
6. ⸢NUMUN ^{GIŠ}⸣MES *mur-ra-an-nu* LAGAB×UDU UDU *zé-e* TU^{MUŠEN} ^{UZU}Ì.UDU GUD *u* KAŠ.Ú.SA
7. [*an-nu*]-⸢*ú*⸣ TÉ[Š.B]I [*i*]*t-ti* KAŠ *ḫa-am-ri ta-ḫaš-šal ta-ṣa-na-mi-id-šu-ma* TI-*uṭ*
8. [*šum*$_4$]-*ma* [LÚ] KÚM *dan-na-aš-šu qa-qa-ra ma-la* ZA *te-ḫe-er-ru*
9. [AN].ZAḪ [BABBAR/GI$_6$] *šar-šàr* ^{Ú}ḪAB *ina* ŠÀ *tu-ma-aṣ-ṣa u* ZA *ina* ŠÀ
10. [*t*]*u-uš-n*[*a-a*]*l u tu-kat-tam-šú u ki-i-me-e iš-tu* ŠÀ MIN *tu-še-la-a-šú*
11. *ina ma-ar-ḫi-ṣi tu-še-ša-ab-šu* SUḪUŠ ^{GIŠ}GEŠTIN SUḪUŠ ^{GIŠ}ḪAŠḪUR SUḪUŠ ^{GIŠ}ḪAŠḪUR.KUR.RA
12. SUḪUŠ ^{GIŠ}ḪAŠḪUR.KUR.RA SUḪUŠ×ŠE ^{GIŠ}ŠENNUR SUḪUŠ ^{GIŠ}MES.GÀM SUḪUŠ ^{GIŠ}ŠE.NA
13. SUḪUŠ ^{GIŠ}*mur-di-in-ni* SUḪUŠ ^{GIŠ}*tu-ub-li* SUḪUŠ ^{GIŠ}*šu-ur-dì* SUḪUŠ ^{GIŠ}*šu-ši*
14. ^{GIŠ}*kal-ba-a-ni* ^{GIŠ}*si*$_{20}$*-i-ḫa* ^{GIŠ}*ar-ga-an-nu-um* ^{GIŠ}*mar-gu*$_5$*-uṣ-ṣa*
15. ^{Ú}KUR.KUR.RA ^{Ú}ḪAB ^{Ú}*ba-ri-ra-ti ina* ŠÀ A.MEŠ U$_4$.7.KÁM* *ir-ta-na-ḫi-iṣ-ma* TI-*uṭ*

---

16. *ta-tu-ur-ma ina gáb-bi* ^{GIŠ}ŠEM.MEŠ *ina* KAŠ *ḫi-i-qì* U$_4$.7.KÁM* *ir-ta-*

na-ḫi-iṣ-ma TI

17. $^{\text{GIŠ.ŠEM}}$GÚR.GÚR $^{\text{GIŠ.⌈ŠEM⌉}}$LI *ina* KAŠ *ta-ma-ḫa-aṣ* NAG-*ma i-pár-ru a-di* TI-*uṭ* NAG.NAG

18. $^{\text{GIŠ.ŠEM}}$GÚR.GÚR *ina* Ì.GIŠ *tu-ša-ḫa-an-ma* ŠÉŠ.ŠÉŠ-*sú-ma* TI-*uṭ*

---

19. ^{Ú}ḪAR.ḪAR Ú.KUR.RA ^{Ú}ZAG.ḪI.LI.A *ta-mar-ra-*[*a*]*q ina* KAŠ NAG. NAG-*ma i-pa-ru* TI-*uṭ*

---

20. $^{\text{GIŠ.ŠEM}}$GÚR.GÚR $^{\text{GIŠ.ŠEM}}$LI Ú *a-še-e ina* DÈ *a-di* TI-*uṭ tu-qa-tar-šu ina* IM PAP-*šu*

---

21. URUDU.SA$_{5}$ AN.BAR $^{\text{NA}_4}$ZA.GÌN $^{\text{NA}_4}$NÍR.MUŠ.‹GÍR›-*rù* $^{\text{NA}_4}$‹GIŠ›. NU$_{11}$.GAL $^{\text{NA}_4}$ŠUBA $^{\text{NA}_4}$*šu-u* NITA

22. $^{\text{NA}_4}$*šu-u* MUNUS $^{\text{NA}_4}$*ú-ru-ti-i-ti* $^{\text{NA}_4}$NÍR.BABBAR.DIL $^{\text{NA}_4}$*ḫal-tu*$_{4}$ $^{\text{NA}_4}$ZÁLAG.GA

23. NA$_{4}$.MEŠ *an-nu-ti ina* ŠU.MEŠ-*šú* GÌR.MEŠ-*šú ta-ra-kás u* ÉN *kad-da-ri-du*$_{4}$[28]

24. *kad-da-ri-du*$_{4}$ *u* ÉN *ša* KÚM/IZI SÌ.SÌ-*ma* TI-*uṭ*

---

25. *kad-da-ri-du kad-da-ri-du èz-zu kad-da-r*[*i-d*]*u šá-gu èz-zu kad-da-ri-du*

26. SAHAR *èz-zu kad-da-ri-du kad-da-r*[*i-du èz-zu* TU$_{6}$] ÉN

---

27. *ina* U$_{4}$-*mi ina* AN-*e ib-⌈ba-ni* KI.MIN⌉ [o o o o o *i*]*š-t*[*u* AN-*e ur*]-*d*[*a-am*]

28. *i-kúl* ^{GIŠ}TIR DAGAL GU$_{7}$ AM.MA.A ^{GI}BAR *is-sú-uq* GUD *ina* ÁB.GUD.ḪI.A

29. *is-sú-uq* UDU *ina* TÙR *is-sú-uq* GURUŠ *ina* Á.MEŠ-*šú is-sú-uq* ^{MUNUS}KI.SIKIL

30. [*ina*] *tu-li-i-šá ták-sí-šu ták-ta-sí-šu ta-ṣa-bat* Á.MEŠ-*šú ta-ku-li* UZU. MEŠ-*šú*

31. *ták-sà-sí* ^{UZU}GÌR.PAD.DU-*šú am-mi-ni ta-ṣa-bat* Á.MEŠ-*šú am-mi-ni ta-ku-li* UZU.MEŠ-*šú*

32. *am-mi-ni ták-sà-sí* ^{UZU}GÌR.PAD.DU-*šú ri-dì-ma ina* GI.ŠÚ GU$_{7}$ *ka-ak-ka-a*

33. *u ka-mu-na e-li-ma ina* ḪUR.SAG GU$_{7}$ ^{GIŠ}LAM.ḪUR *u* ^{GIŠ}LAM.GAL

34. GU$_{7}$ ^{GIŠ}ÁSAL.A *a-di li-ri-šá* KÚM GIN$_{7}$ A.MEŠ *pí-šá-an-ni a-a is-sa-*SUḪUR

35. *ina* EGIR-*šá* KÚM GIN$_{7}$ *qín-ni* SIM.MAḪ^{MUŠEN} *ina qín-ni-šá a-a i-túr*

---

36. : TIL :

TRANSLATION

(1–7) Plants for fever: *sissin-libbi*, *šammi bu'šāni* root and its leaves, *atā'išu*, *šaššugu*-tree root, *šallamu* root, *šunû*-chastetree root and its seed, *bīnu*-tamarisk seed, *qutrātu* seed, flax seed, *kanaktu*-aromatic seed, *barirātu*, potter's grog, oven peelings,[29] varnish made with "white" alum, roasted grain flour, varnish made with salt, dirt from an army(?)-anthill with seven entrances, ⌈dirt⌉ from palm frond baskets, *kukru* seed, *burāšu*-juniper seed, *mēsu*-tree seed, *murrānu*-tree, sheep bladder, "dove dung," ox fat and beerwort. ⌈These⌉ you crush ⌈together⌉ with freshly fermented wine.[30] If you repeatedly bandage him (with it), he should recover.

(8–15) ⌈If⌉ a [person's] fever gets too high, you dig out a hole in the earth in proportion to his height. You spread [white/black] ⌈*anzaḫḫu*⌉-frit, *šaršarru*-paste (and) *šammi bu'šāni* in it and ⌈you have him lie down⌉ lengthwise in it and you cover him and when you have him come up from inside ditto (the hole in the earth), you have him sit in a place for bathing. If he repeatedly bathes in wine root, *ḫašḫurru*-apple root, *armannu*-apricot root, noded?[31] *šalluru*-plum root, *šaššugu*-tree root, *šunû*-chastetree root, *amurdinnu*-rose root, *tublu*-tree root, *šurdu*-tree root, *šūšu*-licorice root, *kalbānu*, *sīḫu*-wormwood, *argannu*, *markuṣṣu*, *atā'išu*, *šammi bu'šāni* (and) *barirātu* (mixed) with water for seven days, he should recover.

(16–18) (If he doesn't), you do (it) again and, if he repeatedly bathes in *labanātu*-incense (mixed) with *ḫīqu*-beer for seven days, he should recover. You whisk *kukru* (and) *burāšu*-juniper in beer. If he drinks (it), he should vomit. You should have him drink (it) repeatedly until he recovers. You heat *kukru* in oil and, if you repeatedly rub him gently (with it), he should recover.

(19) You crush *ḫašû*-thyme, *nīnû*-mint (and) *saḫlû*-cress finely. If you have him repeatedly drink (it mixed) with beer, he should vomit. He should recover.

(20) You fumigate him with *kukru*, *burāšu*-juniper (and) *šammi ašî* over coals until he recovers. You protect him from the wind.[32]

(21–24) You bind these stones: red copper, iron, lapis lazuli, *muššaru*-stone, *gišnugallu*-alabaster, *šubû*-stone, male *šû*-stone, female *šû*-stone, *ru'tītu*-sulphur, *pappardillu-ḫulālu*-stone, *ḫaltu*-stone (and) *zalāqu*-stone onto his hands and feet and, if you cast the spell *kaddaridu kaddaridu* and the spell for fever/fire, he should recover.

(25–26) *Kaddaridu*, *kaddaridu*, angry,[33] ⌈*kaddaridu*⌉, raging,[34] angry, *kaddaridu*, turn round!,[35] angry, *kaddaridu*, ⌈*kaddaridu*⌉, [angry. Spell] and recitation.

(27–35) When ditto (fever/fire) was created in heaven [...] ⌈she came down from⌉ heaven. She consumed the wide forest; she consumed the canebrake.[36] She singled out the ox from the cattle; she singled out the sheep from the sheepfold.

She singled out the young man from his comrades; she singled out the young woman (from her friends). At her breast, she bound him; she repeatedly bound him. She seized his arms; she ate his flesh; she repeatedly bound his bones. Why did you seize his arms? Why did you eat his flesh? Why did you repeatedly bind his bones? Go down and eat *kakku*-lentils and *kamunu*-cumin in the canebrake! Go up and eat *šiqdu*-almonds and *buṭuttu*-pistachios in the mountains! Eat a *ṣar-batu*-poplar, branches[37] and all! May the fever, like water in the drainpipe, not come back; may the fever, as with the nest of a dove, not return to its nest.

(36) (The fever section) is finished.

B. TREATMENTS FOR SPECIFIC FEVER CATEGORIES

TEXT 4: BAM 107 AND BAM 106 OBV. 1–10

BAM 107 contains a fragment of a triple-dose oil-based enema for *diʾu*. This was a fever category corresponding to our enteric fever, but without the dehydration characteristic of *ṣētu*. For more details, see Scurlock and Andersen 2005, 59–60. This text is a classic example of how important a task it is to locate duplicates. In BAM 107, the symptoms to be treated are not given and the procedure is lost, but both may be reconstructed from the parallels as follows:

BAM 106 OBV. 1–4

1. [DIŠ N(A ⸢ŠÀ⸣)].MEŠ-*šú* MÚ.⸢MEŠ-*ḫu ir*⸣-*ru-šú* ⸢*i-ár*⸣-[(*ru-ru* IGI. MEŠ-*šú* NIGIN.MEŠ-*du*)]
2. [SA.(MEŠ-*šú*)] *tab*!-*ku-ma* ‹(TA! GÌR^{II}-*šú*) EN› MURUB$_4$.[(MEŠ-*šú* Z)]I-*ma kin-ṣ*[(*a-a-šú* GU$_7$.MEŠ-*šú*)]
3. [*mim-m*(*a*)] GU$_7$ *u* NAG UGU-*š*[(*ú* NU D)]U-*ak* N[(A BI GIG *di-ʾu* GIG)]
4. [(⸢*šum-ma*⸣ N)]A BI TI.LA *ḫa*-[(*š*)]*i-iḫ* [(*ana* TI)]-*šú* …

BAM 107

1. ^{GIŠ}*ere-nu* ^{GIŠ}ŠUR.MÌN ^{GIŠ}*dap-ra-nu*
2. ^{ŠEM}GÍR ^{ŠEM}BAL ^{ŠEM}ŠEŠ ŠEM.SAL
3. GI DÙG.GA ^{ŠEM}BULUḪ ^{GIŠ}ERIN.SUMUN
4. ^{ŠEM}GIG ^{ŠEM}GÚR.GÚR ^{ŠEM}MAN.D[(U)]
5. ^{GIŠ}ŠE.NÁ.A ^{Ú}KUR.KUR [(Ú)] *a-ši-i*

6. ^{GIŠ}*si-ḫa* ^{GIŠ}*ár-ga-nu* ^{GIŠ}*ba-ri-ra*[*t*]
7. [(M)]UN KÙ.BAD ^{Ú}ḪAR.ḪAR ⸢^{Ú}⸣[(NU.LUḪ.ḪA)]
8. [(^{Ú}*a*)]*k-tam* 23 [(Ú.ḪI.A ŠEŠ)]

BAM 106 OBV. 9–10

9. [(*ina*) KAŠ KALAG.GA U$_4$.⸢3⸣.KÁM *tara*-[(*b*)]*ak ina* [(NINDU BAD-*ir* E$_{11}$-*ma*)]
10. [(*ta-šá-ḫal* 1 *qa*)] Ì+GIŠ *ana* ŠÀ ḪE.ḪE 1-*šú* [(2)]-*šú* 3-*šú* [(*ana* DÚR-*šú* DUB-*ma* TI-*uṭ*)]

Translation

BAM 106 obv. 1–4

(obv. 1–4) If a person's insides are continually bloated, his intestines rumble, his face seems continually to spin, his [blood vessels] are tense and pulsate from his feet ‹to› his hip region and consequently his legs continually hurt him, (and) [whatever] he eats and drinks does not agree with him, that person is sick with *diʾu*.[38] If that person wants to live, to cure him,

BAM 107

(1–8) these twenty-three plants: *erēnu*-cedar, *šurmēnu*-cypress, *daprānu*-juniper, *asû* myrtle, *balukku*-aromatic, myrrh, *šimešallu*, "sweet reed," *baluḫḫu*-aromatic, *šupuḫru*-cedar, *kanaktu*-aromatic, *kukru*, *suʾādu*, *šunû*-chastetree, *atāʾišu*, *šammi ašî*, *sīḫu*-wormwood, *argānu*, *barirātu*, KÙ.PAD salt, *ḫašû*-thyme, *nuḫurtu*, (and) *aktam*.

BAM 106 obv. 9–10

(obv. 9–10) You decoct (them)[39] for three days in strong beer. You bake (it) in an oven. You take (it) out and filter (it and) you mix 1 *qû* of oil into it. If you pour (it) one, two, (and) three times into his anus, he should recover.

TEXT 5: BAM 145 (= *KAR* 199)

BAM 145 contains a potion and salve for *ṣētu*. This is an ancient diagnosis which roughly corresponds to our "enteric fever." For more details, see Scurlock and Andersen 2005, 53–61. The colophon of BAM 145 is not preserved, but it is of the "excerpted for specific performance" type. In other words, the physician was faced with a patient displaying the appropriate symptoms, and he looked up and wrote out the requisite treatment. Of interest is the fact that the same plant medicines are administered as a potion and as a salve and that the two duplicates have slightly differing composition, since BAM 146 substitutes *ṣaṣuntu* and *burāšu*-juniper for the *samānu* of BAM 145.

1. [DIŠ NA U]D.DA TAB.⸢BA⸣-[(*ma* SÍG SAG.DU-*šú*)]
2. [(GU)]B.MEŠ IGI.MEŠ-*šú* NIGIN.MEŠ-⸢*du*⸣-*šú*-[*ma*]
3. *i-ta-na-aṣ-ra-ḫu*
4. SU-*šú ta-ni-ḫu* TUKU.TUKU-*ši*
5. KÚM *la ḫa-aḫ-ḫaš* ‹(TUKU.T[UKU])›
6. *su-a-lam* TUKU.TUKU-*ši*
7. ŠÀ-*šú e-ta-na-áš-šá-áš*
8. *il-la-tu-šú* DU!-*ku*
9. ŠÀ-*šú ig-da-na-ru-ur*
10. *re-du-ut ir-ri* GIG *u ú-šar-d*[(*a*)]
11. *e-le-nu* UZU-*šú* ŠED$_7$
12. [(*ša*)*p-l*]*a-nu* GÌR.PAD.MEŠ-*šú ṣar-ḫa*
13. [(*ina* ⸢*ṣa*⸣-*la*)]-*li-šú* ‹(*i-ni-ʾ-i*)› GI.GÍD *ḫa-še-šú*
14. [(*it*)]-⸢*ti*⸣-*ni*![40]-*is-kìr*
15. [(*ú*)]-*ga-na-aḫ*[41]
16. [(*ṣi-ri-iḫ-t*)]*i* KÚM ŠÀ TUKU.MEŠ
17. [(NA BI UD.DA.TAB.BA *ana* TI-*šú*)]
18. [(ÚGA)MUN] *ka*-⸢*ta*⸣-[*r*]*a*
19. [Ú*k*]*am-man-tú* ÚŠ[(E.L)]ILLAN
20. Ú*kám-ka-du* ÚNIM.NIM[42] ÚGEŠTIN.KA$_5$.A
21. 7 (variant: 8) Ú.MEŠ ŠEŠ 1-*niš* GAZ SIM
22. *ina* KAŠ ‹‹KAŠ›› NAG.MEŠ
23. *ina* Ì EŠ.MEŠ-*su-ma* TI

24–29 effaced colophon

Translation

(1–23) [If] ⸢*ṣētu*⸣ burns [a person] so that the hair of his head continually stands on end, his face seems continually to spin [and] he continually feels burning hot, his body is continually tired (and) ‹(he continually has)› a lukewarm temperature, he continually has *suʾālu*-cough, his stomach is continually upset, his saliva flows, his stomach turns over and over, he is sick with "flowing" of the intestines and makes (one bowel movement) ⸢follow⸣ (another), the flesh above is cold (but) his bones below (feel) burning hot, when he tries to sleep, (his breath) turns back (and) his wind pipe continually closes up, he coughs (variant: belches), (and) he continually has burning intestinal fever, that person is burned by *ṣētu*.[43]

To cure him, you crush together (and) sift these seven (variant: eight) plants: ⸢*kamūnu*⸣-cumin, *katarru*-fungus (variant: *kamūn šadê*-fungus), *kamantu*-henna(?), *lillânu* (ripe grain), *kamkādu*, *samānu*[44] (and) "fox grape." You have him repeatedly drink (it mixed) with beer. If you repeatedly rub him gently (with it mixed) with oil, he should recover.

TEXT 6: BAM 480 iii 8–21

We have already seen BAM 480 in chapter 3, text 2. Lines iii 8–21 of the first tablet of the first subseries of UGU is of a type which presents treatments for specific symptoms of a specific fever category. It consists of three-day shaved-head bandages for the headache (iii 8–16) or swollen head and hurting body (iii 17–21) of *ṣētu*.

iii

8. DIŠ [(NA SAG.DU-*šú* UD.DA TAB-*ma* SÍG)] SAG.DU-*šú i-šaḫ-ḫu-uḫ* ZI SAG.KI TUKU.TUKU
9. 1 G[(ÍN U_5 ARGAB^{MUŠEN} *ina* Ì.GIŠ SÚD)] SAG.DU-*su* SAR-*ab tu-kaṣ-ṣa* LAL-*ma* U_4.3.KÁM NU DU_8

---

10. DIŠ KI.MIN [10 G(ÍN ZÍD) ^{GIŠ}(ERIN 10 GÍN)] ZÍD ^{GIŠ}ŠUR.MÌN 10 GÍN ZÍD ^{GIŠ}MAN.DU 10 GÍN ZÍD ^{ŠEM}LI 10 GÍN ZÍD ^{ŠEM}GÚR.GÚR
11. 10 GÍN ZÍD [(GAZI^{SAR} 10 GÍN ZÍ)]D GÚ.GAL 10 GÍN ZÍD GÚ.TUR 10 GÍN BAR ZÚ.LUM.MA 10 GÍN ZAG.ḪI.LI
12. 10 GÍN KAŠ.Ú.⸢SA⸣ SIG_5 10 GÍN ZÍD $MUNU_6$ 1-*niš* ḪE.ḪE *ina* KAŠ $SILA_{11}$-*aš* GUR-*ma* ḪÁD.A GAZ SIM
13. SAG-*ka ú-kal ina* ŠÀ 1/3 *qa* TI-*qí ina* A GAZI^{SAR} $SILA_{11}$-*aš* SAR-*ab* LAL-*ma* KI.MIN

---

14. [DIŠ K]I.MIN ZAG.ḪI.LI ÀR-*tim* ^{ŠEM}GÚR.GÚR NAGA.SI 1-*niš* SÚD *ina* KAŠ $SILA_{11}$-*aš* SAR-*ab* KI.MIN

---

15. [DIŠ KI.M]IN ^{ŠEM}GÚR.GÚR ^{ŠEM}LI ŠEM.^{d}NIN.IB NUMUN ^{Ú}ÁB.DUḪ KA.A.AB.BA ^{ŠEM}ŠEŠ 1-*niš* SÚD *ina* KAŠ SILA$_{11}$-*aš* SAR-*ab* KI.MIN

---

16. [DIŠ KI.MIN ^{Š}]^{EM}GÚR.GÚR ^{ŠEM}LI ILLU ^{ŠEM}BULUḪ ZÚ.LUM Ì.UDU ÉLLAG UDU.NÍTA 1-*niš* SÚD *ina* KUŠ SUR-*ri* SAR-*ab* KI.MIN

---

17. [(DIŠ NA SAG.D)]U-*su* UD.DA TAB-*ma u* SU-*šú* GU$_7$-*šú* SAG.DU-*su* *nu-pu-uḫ* PA ^{GIŠ}MES.MÁ.GAN.NA
18. [(ḪÁD.DU GAZ S)]IM ZÍD GÚ.GAL ZÍD GÚ.TUR ZÍD ŠE IN.NU.ḪA 1-*niš ina šur-šum-mi* KAŠ SILA$_{11}$-*aš* SAR-*ab* KI.MIN

---

19. [(DIŠ KI.MIN DUḪ ŠE.GIŠ)].Ì ḪÁD.A-*ti* ^{ŠEM}GÚR.GÚR ^{ŠEM}LI ZÌ.KUM *ina šur-šum-mi* KAŠ SILA$_{11}$-*aš* SAR-*ab* KI.MIN

---

20. DIŠ KI.MIN ⸢^{Ú}⸣ḪAR.ḪAR ^{ŠEM}GÚR.GÚR ^{ŠEM}LI ZÌ.KUM KAŠ SILA$_{11}$-*aš* ⸢SAR-*ab*⸣ [KI.MIN]

---

21. DIŠ KI.MIN ^{Ú}LAL ḪÁD.A [SÚ]D *ina* A ŠED$_7$ SILA$_{11}$-*aš* SAR-*a*[*b* KI.MIN]

TRANSLATION

(iii 8–9) If *ṣētu* (enteric fever)[45] burns a person so that the hair of his head falls out (and) he continually experiences pulsating of the temples, you grind 1 shekel of *rikibti arkabi* in oil. You shave his head and let (it) cool. You bandage (him with it) and do not take (it) off for three days.

(iii 10–13) Alternatively, you mix together [10] ⸢shekels⸣ of *erēnu*-cedar flour, 10 shekels of *šurmēnu*-cypress flour, 10 shekels of *su᾿ādu* flour, 10 shekels of *burāšu*-juniper flour, 10 shekels of *kukru* flour, 10 shekels of *kasû* flour, 10 shekels of *ḫallūru*-chickpea flour, 10 shekels of *kakku*-lentil flour, 10 shekels of date rind, 10 shekels of *saḫlû*-cress, 10 shekels of winnowed beerwort (and) 10 shekels of malt flour. You make (it) into a dough with beer. You redry, crush (and) sift (it) while the patient waits. You take 1/3 *qû*-measure and make (it) into a dough with *kasû* juice. You shave (his head). You bandage (him with it) and ditto (do not take it off for three days).

(iii 14) ⸢Alternatively⸣, you grind together mill ground *saḫlû*-cress, *kukru* (and) *uḫḫūlu qarnānu*. You make (it) into a dough with beer. You shave (his head). Ditto (You bandage him with it and do not take it off for three days).

(iii 15) ⸢Alternatively⸣, you grind together *kukru*, *burāšu*-juniper, *nikiptu*, *kamantu*-henna(?) seed, *imbû tamtim* (and) myrrh. You make (it) into a dough with beer. You shave (his head). Ditto (You bandage him with it and do not take it off for three days).

(iii 16) [Alternatively], you grind together *kukru*, *burāšu*-juniper, *baluḫḫu*-aromatic resin, dates, (and) fat from the kidney of a wether. You massage (it) into leather. You shave (his head). Ditto (You bandage him with it and do not take it off for three days).

(iii 17–18) If a person's head is burned by *ṣētu* and his body hurts him (and) his head is swollen, you dry, crush (and) sift *musukkānu*-tree leaves. You make (it and) *ḫallūru*-chick pea flour, *kakku*-lentil flour (and) *inninnu*-barley flour together into a dough with beer dregs. You shave (his head). Ditto (You bandage him with it and do not take it off for three days).

(iii 19) Alternatively, you make dried sesame residue, *kukru*, *burāšu*-juniper (and) *isqūqu*-flour into a dough with beer dregs. You shave (his head). Ditto (You bandage him with it and do not take it off for three days).

(iii 20) Alternatively, you make *ḫašû*-thyme, *kukru*, *burāšu*-juniper (and) *isqūqu*-flour into a dough with beer. You shave (his head). [Ditto (You bandage him with it and do not take it off for three days)].

(iii 21) Alternatively, you dry (and) ⸢grind⸣ *ašqulālu*. You make (it) into a dough with cold water. You shave (his head). [Ditto (You bandage him with it and do not take it off for three days)].

Notes

1. BM 35512 rev. 14 has KEŠDA-*su-ma*.
2. K 2581 rev. 7′ has [DIŠ U_4.1].KÁM DIB-*su* U_4.1.KÁM *ú-maš-šar-šú*.
3. K 2581 rev. 14′ has NU KU.NU.
4. This is a mistake for "*mur*" as in the duplicates.
5. See Scurlock and Andersen 2005, 3.6, 3.13.
6. See Deller 1985, 327–30.
7. For the symptoms see next note.
8. K 2581 rev. 7′ has: "[one day] it afflicts him and one day it releases him."
9. The variants are given from the two parallels. The main text seems to have had something else. Böck 2011, 83 translates: "dust from the upper door post," but does not explain where this translation is coming from.
10. A similar superstition attends marriages in our own culture, and is why we carry the bride over the threshold.
11. *CAD* T, 390a emends(?) *iz-zi-bu* to *iz-zi-qa* and translates: "just as a basket does not groan at its lowering and raising." Unfortunately, the word being translated "lowering" (*urḫu*) means "road/path." Böck 2011, 84 takes the "basket" (*pisannu*) to be a doorpost. Unfortunately, *pisannu* is rarely used for parts of a door, and when it is, it is the socket which is being referred to. A third option, and the one taken here, is to take *pisannu* as meaning "drainpipe" which makes perfect sense in the context.

12. See *CAD* Q, 105b.

13. The text has ID, but the duplicate has *ša*.

14. The original from which the scribe was copying was broken at this point and, as usual with ancient scribes, the copyist did not try to fill in the gap but simply put "broken."

15. This is probably a mistake for *mi-el-tú*.

16. BAM 149:12′ has the horse being hitched to the *bubūtu* of the chariot. See *CAD* B, 302–3.

17. The original from which the scribe was copying was broken at this point and, as usual with ancient scribes, the copyist did not try to fill in the gap but simply put "broken." We know from BAM 147 rev. 5′–6′ that what was missing at this point was: *si-ra šá sip-pí ana sip-pí*.

18. K 2581 obv. 19′ has, instead of EME.ŠID TI-*ma* : [(EME)].ŠID TI-*su ina* GI.SAG. KUD ŠUB *ina* TÚG GI_6 KÁ-*šú* KEŠDA *ina* GÚ-*šú* GAR-[(*ma* TI)]. It is clear from this that the dangling -*ma* which occasionally appears at the end of treatments is the ancient equivalent of our "etc."

19. Stol, *RLA* forthcoming, suggests that the fungi in question are specifically truffles.

20. See *CAD* M/2, 116.

21. Since the verb is used of heating bath water and the vessel in question likely to have been delicate, it is possible that you were intended to heat the vessel by placing it in boiling water rather than putting it directly on the heat. Suggestion courtesy M. Stol.

22. Alternatively, the *ni-ma-ti* should be taken as an error for *mi-na-ti* and the phrase taken to mean that the limbs of the patient were to be rubbed. This makes good sense, but requires a bit of dyslexia on the part of the ancient scribe. Suggestion courtesy M. Stol.

23. Literally: "a woman for whom giving birth has stopped (*parāsu*)."

24. A similar superstition attends marriages in our own culture, and is why we carry the bride over the threshold.

25. The *CAD* T, 390a emends(?) *iz-zi-bu* to *iz-zi-qa* and translates: "just as a basket does not groan at its lowering and raising." Unfortunately, the word being translated "lowering" (*urḫu*) means "road/path." Böck 2011, 84 takes the "basket" (*pisannu*) to be a doorpost. Unfortunately, *pisannu* is rarely used for parts of a door, and when it is, it is the socket which is being referred to. A third option, and the one taken here, is to take *pisannu* as meaning "drainpipe" which makes perfect sense in the context.

26. For the translation of *saḫlû* as "cress," see Stol 1983–84, 24–32.

27. Tsukimoto 1999, 198 (followed by Schwemer 2011, 41) suggests also "black vulva" (GAL_4.LA GI_6) as the reading for the plant name, which is possible, but seems less likely.

28. For the recitation, see Finkel, 1999, no. 30 and Böck 2007, 62, 295–96.

29. More commonly, a fragment of an old oven is called for.

30. The translation assumes that *ḫamru* = Ugaritic *ḫmr*: "foaming (new wine)."

31. The inclusion of ŠE inside the SUḪUŠ should indicate that it has "grain." "Noded" is a suggestion of Tsukimoto 1999, 195.

32. Schwemer 2011, 42 takes this as "clay," which does not make sense in this context.

33. The interpretation assumes that this is *èz-zu* rather than AB.ZU. An angry demon is an obvious fever-causer, whereas, the cosmic ocean does not seem terribly appropriate.

34. For the suggestion that this is a rendering of *šegû*, see Tsukimoto 1999, 188.

35. The translation assumes that the mysterious IŠ/SAḪAR is a pseudo-ideogram for Akkadian *saḫar*, 3ms imperative of *saḫāru*: "to turn round."

36. The mysterious AM.MA.A ^{GI}BAR is probably pseudo-syllabic Sumerian for AMBAR, "canebrake."

37. For the suggestion, see Tsukimoto 1999, 195.

38. See Scurlock and Andersen 2005, 3.161.

39. See chapter 3, n. 109.
40. Copy *-nu-* but dupl. correctly *-ni-*.
41. BAM 146:37′ has: *ú-ga-aš-ši*.
42. BAM 146:40′–41′ has ^{Ú}*ṣa-ṣu-un-tú* and ^{ŠEM}LI instead of ^{Ú}NIM.NIM.
43. See Scurlock and Andersen 2005, 3.121.
44. BAM 146:40′–41′ has *ṣaṣuntu* and *burāšu*-juniper instead of *samānu*.
45. See Scurlock and Andersen 2005, 53–61.

SKIN AND BONES

A. SKIN ERUPTIONS ON THE HEAD

Ancient Mesopotamian patients complained of *ekketu* (itchiness),[1] *kiṣṣatu* (hairless patches), *rišiktu* (dry patches) and *rišūtu* (redness) on their heads. The ancient physician was also prepared to treat *kibšu* (favus), *kurāru/guraštu* (ringworm) and sores, not to mention the ubiquitous head lice. For more details, see Scurlock and Andersen 2005, chapter 10 and Fincke 2011b, 169–87. The most common treatments were salves, daubs and plasters. The ancient physician also shaved the head and bandaged it, or used medicated shampoo.

TEXT 1: BAM 33

BAM 33 consists of medicated shampoos (1–7, 9–18), salves (8, 15–19), and a plaster (15–18) for hairless patches, itching and redness, favus, and ringworm. Of particular interest is the specification in lines 1–8 that the plants are to be dried in the shade rather than the sun.

1. [(DIŠ NA SA)]G.DU-*su lu* PEŠ-*ta lu gi-iṣ-ṣa-tú*
2. [*lu* (*kib-š*)]*á lu-u gu-*[(*r*)]*iš-ta* DIRI
3. [*ana* T]I-*šú* KI.A.^dÍD NA[(G)]A.SI U₅ ARGAB^{MUŠEN}
4. [(*ḫaš-ḫal*)-*lat*] ^{GIŠ}PEŠ *ḫaš-ḫal-lat* ^{GIŠ}MA.N[U] ^{GIŠ}MES.MÁ.KAN.NA
5. [(BAR)] ^{GIŠ}ŠINIG ^Ú*ak-*⌈*tam*⌉ A.GAR.GAR MAŠ.DÀ
6. 9 Ú.ḪI.A *an-nu-ti* 1-*niš ina* GISSU ḪÁD.A GAZ SIM
7. *ina* KÀŠ ÁB GI₆ SAG.DU-*su* ‹(*tu-ḫap-pap-ma kib-šá gi-iṣ-ṣa-tam gu-reš-tam*)› (*ḫe-pí*)[2] TIL!-*ma* TI-*uṭ*

---

8. Ì+GIŠ ^Ú*imḫur-lim* SAG.DU-*su* ŠÉŠ.ŠÉŠ

---

9. DIŠ NA SAG.DU-*su* GIG (*ḫe-pí*) [GI]G ^{ŠEM}GIG
10. ŠEM.^dMAŠ NAGA.SI MUN A.GAR.GAR MAŠ.DÀ
11. UZU.DIR.KUR.RA DUḪ.ŠE.GIŠ.Ì (*ḫe-pí*) *an* ḪÁD.DU *ta-mar-raq*

12. *ina* KAŠ ^{LÚ}KURUN.NAM SÚD SAG.DU-*su tu-kaṣ-ṣa*
13. EGIR-*šú* ^{Ú}SULLIM^{SAR} *ina* Ì.NUN.NA ḪE.ḪE-*ma*
14. SAG.DU-*su tu-kaṣ-ṣa*

---

15. EGIR-*šú up-pu-la u* MUN [(*ina* ^{URU})]^{DU}ŠEN *ina* IZI-*ma* ŠEG$_6$-*šal*
16. *ina* Ì.NUN.NA ḪE.ḪE-*ma* SAG.D[(U-*s*)]*u tu-kaṣ-ṣa*
17. [ŠÉ(Š)].ŠÉŠ-*su gu-*[*ú-*(*r*)]*a ina* $^{\text{NA}_4}$ÀR ÀR
18. [*ta-m*]*ar-raq* SAG.DU-*su tu-tap-pa*

---

19. [DIŠ NA SAG.D]U-*su ek-ke-ta u ri-šu-ta* DIRI
(catchline = BAM 494 i 33′//BAM 3 ii 3–4)
20. colophon (belonged to an apprentice *āšipu*)

Translation

(1–7) If a person's head is full of *kibšu*, *kiṣṣatu*, (and) *gur*[*a*]*štu*, [to] ⸢cure⸣ him, you dry together in the shade, crush (and) sift these nine plants: *kibrītu*-sulphur, *uḫḫūlu qarnānu*, *rikibti arkabi*, *tittu*-fig cuttings, *eʾru*-tree cuttings, *mussukānu*-tree, *bīnu*-tamarisk bark, *aktam* (and) gazelle droppings. You (mix it) with urine from a black cow. You wash his head (with it). If ‹(the *kibšu*, *kiṣṣatu* and *gurаštu*)› is extinguished, he should recover.

(8) You repeatedly rub his head gently with *imḫur-lim* oil.

(9–14) If a person's head ‹is ⸢sick⸣ with ⸢*kurāru*⸣›, you dry (and) crush finely *kanaktu*, *nikiptu*, *uḫḫūlu qarnānu*, salt, gazelle droppings, *kamūn šadê*-fungus, sesame residue (and) [...]. You grind (it) in *kurunnu* beer. You cool his head (with it). You mix *šambaliltu*-fenugreek with ghee and cool his head (with it).

(15–18) Afterwards, you boil late barley and salt in a *tamgussu*-vessel over a fire. You mix (it) with ghee and cool his head (with it). You ⸢repeatedly⸣ rub him gently (with it). You ⸢crush⸣ reed blades ⸢finely⸣ in a mill (and) you plaster his head (with it).

(19) If a person's head is full of *ekketu* and redness, ‹(you grind *kibrītu*-sulphur and mix it with *erēnu*-cedar oil. If you gently rub him repeatedly with it, he should recover)›. *(catchline)*

TEXT 2: BAM 156:25–40

We have already seen BAM 156 (see chapter 3, text 3). This section of this UGU excerpt text consists of bandaged-over daubs (25–31), washes (25–39), a plaster (32–39), a bandage (32–39) and a salve (40) for ringworm. Of special interest in lines 25–31 is the use of irritants, debridement, and successive bandaging as treatment. Lines 32–39 prescribe both medicated shampoo and a bandage.

25. DIŠ NA SAG.DU-*su ku-ra-ru* DIB-*it* ŠÈ-^{d}NISABA
26. ḪÁD.A SÚD LAL *ina še-rim ku-ra-ar-šú* SAR-*ab*
27. *laq-laq-ta-šú ta-ta-bal ina* KAŠ LUḪ-*si*
28. KU.KU ^{GIŠ}TASKARIN MAR-*rù* LAL *in*[(*a* I)]GI KI.NÁ-*šú* DU$_8$-*šú-ma*
29. *tu-šá-kal ina* KAŠ LUḪ-*si* KU.KU ^{GIŠ}*e-lam-ma-ki*
30. KU.KU ^{GIŠ}TASKARIN KU.KU ^{GIŠ}*kal-mar-ḫi* ŠÈ-^{d}NISABA
31. GAZI^{SAR} BÍL-*ti* MAR!-*rù* LAL

---

32. DIŠ KI.MIN KÀŠ ÁB SAG.DU-*su te-sír* A NAGA.SI
33. A GAZI^{SAR} LUḪ-*si* SAG.DU-*su* SAR-*ab*
34. NUMUN ^{GIŠ}ŠE.NA.A NUMUN ^{GIŠ}[(N)]AM.TAR NUMUN ^{GIŠ}*qut-ri* ^{Ú}ÁB.DUḪ
35. [(PA)] ⸢^{Ú}⸣TÁL.TÁL ⸢^{GIŠ}⸣x[o] ⸢^{Ú}*ru*⸣-*uš-ru-šu* ^{Ú}*ṣa-ṣu-um-tu*
36. ^{Ú}KUR.GI.RÍN.NA ^{Ú}*te-gi-la-a* ⸢^{Ú}MÁ⸣.EREŠ.MÁ.LÁ
37. ^{Ú}MAŠ.ḪUŠ 11 Ú.MEŠ ḪÁD.A GAZ SIM *ina* A GAZI$^{\text{SA[R]}}$
38. SILA$_{11}$-*aš* GUR-*ma* ḪÁD.A GAZ SIM *ina* KAŠ.SAG *u* A.GEŠTIN.NA ḪE.ḪE
39. SAG.DU-*su* LAL-*ma* U$_4$.3.KÁM NU DU$_8$

---

40. DIŠ KI.MIN ^{Ú}GAMUN.GI$_6$ *kib-rit* SÚD *ina* Ì EŠ.MEŠ DIN

TRANSLATION

(25–31) If *kurāru* afflicts a person's head, you dry (and) grind chaff (and) bandage (him with it). In the morning, you shave his *kurāru* (and) remove its detritus. You wash (it) with beer. You daub on powdered *taskarinnu*-boxwood (and) bandage (him). Before he goes to bed, you take (the bandage) off and polish (the *kurāru*).[3] You wash (it) with beer. You daub on powdered *elammaku*-tree, powdered *taskarinnu*-boxwood, powdered *kalmarḫu*-tree, chaff (and) roasted *kasû* (and) bandage (him).

(32–39) Alternatively, you plaster his head with cow urine. You wash (it) with *uḫḫūlu qarnānu* infusion (i.e., liquid soap) (and) *kasû* juice. You shave his head. You dry, crush (and) sift (these) eleven plants: *šunû*-chastetree seed, *pillû* seed, *qutru* seed, *kamantu*-henna(?), *urânu* leaves, [...], *rušruššu*, *ṣaṣumtu*, *kurkānu*-turmeric, *tigilû*, *mirišmara*, (and) *kalbānu*. You make (it) into a dough with *kasû* juice. You redry, crush (and) sift (it). You mix (it) with first quality beer and vinegar. You bandage his head (with it) and do not take (it) off for three days.

(40) Alternatively, you grind *zibû* (and) *kibrītu*-sulphur (and) repeatedly rub (him) gently (with it mixed) with oil. He should recover.

B. *SAḪARŠUBBÛ*

Ancient physicians made groupings of diseases which covered the body with distinctive lesions. Of these groupings, one, *ašû*, includes the pox diseases plus measles and shingles, diseases which we now know to be viral. For more details, see Scurlock and Andersen 2005, 224–27. Another, *saḫaršubbû*, includes the lesions of Hansens' Disease (Leprosy). For more details, see Scurlock and Andersen 2005, 70–73, 231–33. *Saḫaršubbû* was treated with bandages, salves and daubs. Some treatments were unusually aggressive, the lesions being attacked with blistering agents or cut or even burned.

TEXT 3: TSUKIMOTO 1999: 199–200 LINES 37–97

The first 36 lines of this text deal with fever, and have already been discussed in chapter 6 as text 3. The remainder describes bandages (43–49, 56–57, 72–84), salves (43–49, 53–55, 58–62, 70–71), a rub (63–69), and (bandaged-over) daubs (50–52, 63–69, 72–84) for *saḫaršubbû* and a single potion (94–97) for inabililty to urinate. Of these treatments, one (72–84) is formulated in such a way as to suggest origin with a pharmacist.

Of particular interest in lines 37–42 is the fact that a recitation usually employed for numbness is to be recited prophylacticly by the physician before approaching the patient. The mention of anesthesia points to the milder tuberculoid or borderline tuberculoid forms of leprosy. The more serious *Lepromatous* leprosy is not characterized by anesthesic skin lesions, nor does it have single lesions, as described here. Its reversal reaction results in a papular rash accompanied by fever, whereas borderline tuberculoid lesions actually themselves change color and become scaly or "put down dust" (SAḪAR.ŠUB.BA). To note also is that patients with tuberculoid leprosy eventually "cure themselves" even without treatment, so the expectations of recovery for treated cases are by no means unrealistic.[4]

Lines 63–69 represents a very aggressive treatment involving cauterization. Fortunately, the lesions of tuberculoid leprosy are insensitive. Lines 72–84 are interesting in involving a multiday treatment with a backup if things don't work as expected. Lines 85–93 requires that infected bandages be burned, which shows that the physician recognized the contagious nature of the disease.

Most interesting from a comparative religions point of view is, however, the NAM.BÚR.BI with which this section ends. Like the conventional Mesopotamian versions, the basic structure is of a transfer rite in which evil influences end up rubbed off and dumped in the river with the assistance of Shamash whose participation is rewarded by sacrifice. The lapis-colored wool indicates the Netherworld as the ultimate recipient of the evil. Unusual is the sacrifice of one bird and the releasing of another, reminiscent of Lev 14:1–9, which also employs wool, if of a different color.

37. ME.ŠÈ BÁ.DA.RI I.KI.GUB BA.DA.AN.ZA.AḪ ME.TE.GUB.BA I.KI.GUB NU.GUB.BA
38. *an-nu* Ú.MÌN KI Ú.ME.EN BAR.DA I.KI Ú.ME.EN[5] UTUK ḪÚL A.LÁ ḪUL
39. GIDIM ḪUL GAL$_5$.LÁ ḪUL DINGIR ḪUL MÁŠKIM ḪUL EME ḪUL GÁL
40. BAR.ŠÈ ḪÉ.EN.DA.GU.UB ZI.AN.NA ḪÉ!.PÀD ZI.KI.A ḪÉ.PÀD ÉN[6]

---

41. *a-di-ni a-na* UGU-*ḫi* SAḪAR.ŠUB.BA NU *qè-re-bi* ÉN ME.ŠÈ BÁ.DA.RI
42. 3-*šú ana* UGU-*ḫi-šú* ŠID-*nu*

---

43. BAD ZA SAḪAR.ŠUB.BA UGU-*šú* GÁL-*ši* ZÍD.SAḪAR *ša* ŠE TI-*qí* KI ÙŠ GIN$_7$-*ma*
44. *ra-bi-ki* AL.ŠEG$_6$.GÁ KEŠDA-*ma* TA *ik-ta-ṣu-ú* DU$_8$ *si-im-ma* SAḪAR *l*[*u*? ...]
45. UGU *si-im-me* LÀL Ì ŠÉŠ-*ma*

---

46. BAD SAḪAR.ŠUB.BA *du-ug-li* KAŠ$_4$ NAM.TAR.RU *šá ina na-pa-li* ^{d}UTU NU IGI.BAR
47. *ta-sàk* TÉŠ.BI ḪE.ḪE *za-mar za-mar* KEŠDA.KEŠDA ÙŠ *tu-šab-šal*
48. *tu-up-ra ana* ŠÀ-*bi* ŠUB-*di si-im-ma* LUḪ-*si* TA *si-im-mu*
49. *e-tab-lu* ŠÉŠ

---

50. *šum$_4$-ma* LÚ SAḪAR.ŠUB.BA *ka-mu-ni* ^{Ú}*imḫur-áš-na-an ta-sàk* TÉŠ.BI ḪE.ḪE
51. *ina* UGU *si-im-me ta-zar-ru* TÚG.GADA *ina* UGU GAR-*an* Ú.MEŠ *an-nu-ti* KEŠDA.MEŠ

52. *ina še-er-ti* SUḪUŠ ^{GIŠ}NAM.TAR PA ^{GIŠ}NAM.TAR *ta-zar-ru* KEŠDA.MEŠ *i-né-eš*

---

53. BAD LÚ SAḪAR.ŠUB.BA BABBAR *ina* NÍ.TE-*šú* GÁL ^{GIŠ}Ú.GÍR MUN ZÍD.DA ŠE
54. ^{GIŠ}KÌM ZI.NA$^{?}$ NITA *u* MUNUS *tu-bal* GAZ ŠÉŠ-*ma* TI-*uṭ*

---

55. KI.MIN SIG_7 *ina* NÍ.TE-*šú* GÁL Ì A.ZA.LU.LU U_4.7.KÁM* ŠÉŠ.MEŠ

---

56. KI.MIN SA_5 *u* GI_6 *ina* NÍ.TE-*šú* GÁL Ì MUŠ Ì KU_6 ‹Ì› LÚ *ḫa-aḫ-ḫa-aš*
57. *ša* KI.MAḪ Ì MUŠ.DÍM.GAL *ša* MUŠ U_4.7.KÁM* KEŠDA.MEŠ

---

58. KI.MIN SA_5 *u* BABBAR *ina* NÍ.TE -*šú* GÁL SUḪUŠ ^{GIŠ}Ú.GÍR MUN ZÍD.DA ŠE
59. ^{GIŠ}KÌM ZI.NA NITA *u* MUNUS *tu-šab-šal* ŠÉŠ-*sú-ma* TI.LA

---

60. KI.MIN SAḪAR.ŠUB.BA SIG_7 SA_5 ŠU ^{d}30 *ana* ZI-*šú ni-il* NAM.LÚ.U_{19}.LU U_4.7.KÁM* ŠÉ[Š-*sú-ma* TI-*uṭ*]

---

61. KI.MIN SAḪAR.ŠUB.BA SA_5 BABBAR GI_6 ŠU DINGIR LÚ *ana* ZI-*šú* Ì UR.MAḪ
62. Ì MUŠ.GAL.EDIN.NA U_4.7.KÁM* ŠÉŠ-*sú-ma* TI-*uṭ*

---

63. KI.MIN SAḪAR.ŠUB.BA *im-ta-la* BAR ^{GIŠ}NU.ÚR.MA *ta-sàk ina* Ì.NUN ḪE.ḪE SAG-*ka*
64. *ú-ka-al* LÚ *šá ep-qé-nam* DIRI *ina* KUN_4 KÁ.BI *ka-a-mi tu-ul-za-as-sú-ma*
65. BAR ^{GIŠ}NU.ÚR.MA *ša-a-šú i-da-a-at sí-im-me-šu te-eq-qí*
66. *ù* SAḪAR KUN_4 TI *ina ru-ú*ʾ*-ti* 7-*šú u* 7-*šú ta-kar-ma ina* U_4-*mi-šu-ma*
67. [*ep*]-*qé-nu i-bé-el-li* TI-*uṭ* BAD *ri-gi*$_5$-*im-šá* TUKU-*ši* Ì.GIŠ *ina* IZI *tu-um-ma-am*
68. [*tu*]-*ṣar-ra-ap ta-at-ta-na-ar-šu-ma mim-ma ú-ul tu-ṭá-aḫ-ḫa*
69. ⸢LÚ⸣ BI TI-*uṭ*

---

70. KI.MIN SAḪAR.ŠUB.BA SA_5 BABBAR *u* GI_6 ŠU DINGIR LÚ *ana* ZI-*šú* Ì MUŠ Ú.GÍR *tal-ma-a*
71. Ì UR.MAḪ Ì MUŠ.GAL.EDIN U_4.7.KÁM* ŠÉŠ.ŠÉŠ-*sú-ma* TI-*uṭ*

---

72. Ú.MEŠ *ša ep-qa-an-ni ina* PA *ša* ^{GIŠ}PÈŠ *i-maḫ-ḫa-aṣ-ma* ⸢GURUN⸣

^{GIŠ}PÈŠ

73. *u* ^{GIŠ}GEŠTIN ḪÁD.DU *i-ḫaš-šal-ma i-rak-kaš-šu-nu-ti ina* U$_4$.2 GI$_6$ *i-pát-ṭar-⸢šu-nu-ti⸣*
74. *šum-ma pé-ṣú-ú ap-pu-na i-rak-kaš-šu-nu-ti ina* U$_4$.3.KÁM* *i-pát-ṭar-šu-nu-ti*
75. *šum$_4$-ma* BABBAR-*ú ap-pu-na i-rak-kaš-šu-nu-ti šum$_4$-ma pé-ṣú-ú i-ḫal-li-qu*
76. *u šum$_4$-ma pé-ṣú-šu-nu la-a ig-ga-mar* TA $^{\text{NA}_4}$ZÚ *ú-ḫap-pa-šu-nu-ti-ma*
77. IM.SAḪAR.NA$_4$.KUR.RA ^{IM}KAL.GUG$_x$[8] $^{\text{NA}_4}$*lu-ur-pa-na* ^{Ú}NAGA TÉŠ.BI
78. *ina* A.MEŠ GEŠTIN *ta-sàk* U$_4$.7.KÁM* *tar-ta-na-kàs* U$_4$.2 GI$_6$ *ú-maš-šar-ma*
79. *ina* U$_4$.2.KÁM* *i-rak-kàs* U$_4$.2.KÁM* *ú-maš-šar ina* U$_4$.2.KÁM* *i-rak-kàs šum-ma pa-ni*
80. *sí-im-mi-šu mi-it-ḫu-ru-ma sà-a-mu* ŠE.MUŠ$_5$ GUD$_4$ ^{Ú}*šar-mi-da*
81. *it-ti a-ḫa-mèš i-ḫaš-šal-ma i-za-ru-ma* TI-*uṭ šum$_4$-ma la-a i-bal-lu-uṭ*
82. MÚD EME.DIR *pa-aḫ-ḫa-a-ni šum$_4$-ma* MUŠEN *ḫur-ri* MÚD BÍL.ZA.ZA
83. KI IM.SAḪAR.RA.NA$_4$.KUR.RA *ka-la-ku-ut-ta* $^{\text{NA}_4}$*lu-ur-pa-na u* KI ^{Ú}NAGA
84. ḪE.ḪE-*ma tar-ta-na-ka-aš-šú* TI-*uṭ*

---

85. *ki-i-me-e* TI-*uṭ u mi-nu-me-e na-aṣ-ma-da-tu$_4$ ša ir-ta-na-ka-sú*
86. *ina* IZI *ú-qa-al-la-šu-nu-ti* ^{GIŠ}BANŠUR *ana* IGI ^{d}UTU *i-ra-kás*
87. [N]ÍG.NA ^{GIŠ}ŠEM.LI GAR-*an* NINDA.‹Ì›.DÉ.A LÀL Ì.NUN.NA GAR-*an* LÚ.GIG BI *ana* IGI ^{d}UTU
88. ⸢*i*⸣-*za-az* 1 MUŠEN *ḫur-ri u al-lu-ut-ta ana* IGI ^{d}UTU *ta-qa-al-lu*
89. [*u*] *iš-tu* MUŠEN *ḫur-ri ra-ma-an-šu tu-kap-pár-ma ú-maš-šar u ki-i* LÚ.GIG
90. [*ana*] IGI ^{d}UTU *tu-še-za-az* SAG.DU-*šu u* MURUB$_4$-*šu iš-tu* SÍG ZA.GÌN *ša* ^{GIŠ}KIRI$_6$
91. [*t*]*a-ra-kás ki-i-me-e* TA IGI ^{d}UTU *it-ta-ṣa-a* SÍG ZA.GÌN *šá* SAG.DU-*šú u* MURUB$_4$-*šú*
92. [*u*] *gáb-bi né-pè-ši šá ana* IGI ^{d}UTU GAR-*nu ana* ÍD ŠUB-*di* ÍD ḪUL-*šu i-ta-bíl*
93. ⸢*ù*⸣ LÚ.GIG ḪUL ŠÀ-*šú ana* IGI ^{d}UTU *i-dáb-bu-ub*

---

94. [B]AD NA *ši-na-ti-šu ana ta-ba-ku* NU *i-le-ʾ-e* LÀL.MEŠ ^{GIŠ}PÈŠ ^{GIŠ}GEŠTIN.ḪÁD.DU.A

95. $^{\text{[G]IŠ}}$ZÚ.LUM NUNUZ GA.NU$_{11}$^{MUŠEN} *el-gul-la* ^{Ú}*šu-li-li-an-na i-ya-ar* KÙ.BABBAR
96. ⌈*i*⌉-*ya-ar* KÙ.SIG$_{17}$ KI *a-ḫa-mèš* GAZ-*aq ina* KAŠ GEŠTIN NAG-*ma* TI-*uṭ*
97. ÉN *ṭá-ri-da-at* DÙ.A.BI GIG *ana* UGU-*ḫi* GIG 3-*šú* ŠID-*nu*[9]

Translation

(37–40). Where has it flown? It has escaped to the earth![10] Where[11] is it standing? It should not be standing on the earth! Heaven seven times, earth seven times, from (my) sight seven times. May the evil *utukku*-demon, the evil *alû*-demon, the evil ghost, the evil *gallû*-demon, the evil god, the evil *rabiṣu*-demon, (and) the evil tongue stand aside. By heaven may (it) swear; by earth may (it) swear.

(41–42) Before approaching (someone with) *saḫaršubbû*, you should recite the recitation ME.ŠÈ BA.DA.RI (a recitation for numbness) three times over him.[12]

(43–45) If there is *saḫaršubbû* on a person, you take *kukkušu* flour of barley. You bind (it) on him boiled like a decoction[13] with an afterbirth and, after it has cooled, you take (it) off. The sore should [shed?] "dust." You gently rub honey (and) oil on the sore.

(46–49) If it is visible(?) *saḫaršubbû*, you grind noded(?) *pillû* root which the sun did not see when you pulled (it) out. You mix (it) together (and) repeatedly bind (it) on here (and) there (wherever there is a sore). You boil a placenta (and) pour *tubru*-fruit(?) on it. You wash the sore (and) rub (it) gently on after the sore has dried.

(50–52) If a person (has) *saḫaršubbû*, you grind *kamūnu* (and) *imḫur-ašnan*[14] (and) mix (it) together. You daub (it) on the sore (and) put a linen cloth on top. You repeatedly bind these plants on. In the morning, you daub on *pillû* root (and) *pillû* leaves (and) repeatedly bind (it) on. He should recover.

(53–54) If there is white *saḫaršubbû* on a person's body,[15] you dry (and) crush *ašāgu*-thorn, salt, barley flour, *ḫilēpu*-willow, (and) male and female palm fronds.[16] If you rub (it) gently on him, he should recover.

(55) Ditto (If there is) yellow (*saḫaršubbû*) on his body, you repeatedly gently rub (him) with wild animal fat for seven days.

(56–57) Ditto (If there is) red and black (*saḫaršubbû*) on his body, for seven days you repeatedly bind on snake oil, fish oil, hot[17] "human (fat)" from a grave (and) fat of a large snake (hunting) gecko.

(58–59) Ditto (If there is) red and white (*saḫaršubbû*) on his body, you boil *ašāgu*-thorn root, salt, barley flour, *ḫilēpu*-willow (and) male and female palm fronds.[18] If you rub (it) gently on him, he should recover.

(60) Ditto (If there is) yellow (and) red *saḫaršubbû* (on his body), "hand" of Sîn.[19] To remove it, [if] ⌜you gently rub⌝ "human semen" [on him] for seven days, [he should recover].

(61–62) Ditto (If there is) red. white (and) black *saḫaršubbû* (on his body), "hand" of the person's god. To remove it, if you gently rub him with "lion fat" (and) fat of a large steppe-dwelling snake for seven days, he should recover.

(63–69) Ditto (If his body) is full of *saḫaršubbû*, you grind *nurmû*-pomegranate peel. You mix (it) with ghee while he waits for you. You have the person who is full of *epqēnu*-lesions sit on the threshold of his outer gate and you daub that *nurmû*-pomegranate peel around his sore. You also take dust from the threshold. If you rub (him) firmly (with it) seven and seven times (mixed) with saliva, on that same day, the ⌜*epqēnu*⌝ should be extinguished. He should recover. If he still has its complaint, you heat oil over a fire (and) burn (it with it). You do this repeatedly again and again and do not let anything come near (it). That [person] should recover.

(70–71) Ditto (If there is) red, white and black *saḫaršubbû* (on his body), "hand" of the person's god.[20] To remove it, if you repeatedly rub him gently (with) snake fat, giant[21] *ašāgu*-thorn, "lion fat" (and) fat of a large steppe-dwelling snake for seven days, he should recover.

(72–84) Plants for a person with *epqēnu*: he strikes (the sores) with a fig branch and then crushes (together) figs and raisins and then binds them (with it). On the second day at night, he releases them (from the bandage). If they are still white, he binds them (again and) releases them (from the bandage) on the third day. Whether the whiteness has disappeared or whether their whiteness is not yet finished, he crushes them with an obsidian knife and then you grind together alum, *kalgukku*-clay, *lurpānu*-mineral, (and) *uḫḫūlu* in vinegar. You repeatedly bind (it on him) for seven days. He releases (them from the bandage) for two nights and on the second day, he binds (them). He releases (them from the bandage) for two days. On the second day, he binds (them). If the surface of his sores is uniform and red, he crushes together cracked[22] *šigūšu*-grain (and) *šarmidu* and if he daubs (it) on, he should recover. If he does not recover, you mix *paḫḫānu*-lizard blood or (blood of) a *ḫurru*-bird (and) blood of a frog with alum, *kalakuttu*-clay, *lurpānu*-mineral and with *uḫḫūlu* and then repeatedly bind him (with it). He should recover.

(85–93) When he has recovered, he burns with fire whatever bandages he repeatedly bound on. He sets up a table before Shamash. You put out a ⌜censer⌝ burning *burāšu*-juniper. You set out *mersu*-confection (made with) honey and ghee. That patient stands before Shamash. You burn a *ḫurru*-bird and a crab before Shamash. [And] you wipe him off with (another) *ḫurru*-bird and then he releases it. And when you have the patient stand ⸢before⸣ Shamash, ⸢you⸣ bind his head and his hip region with lapis-colored wool (dyed with dye) from the garden. When he comes out from before Shamash, you throw the lapis-colored wool from his head and his hip region [and] all of the ritual paraphernalia which was placed before Shamash into the river. The river will carry off its evil. And the patient should unburden his heart before Shamash.

(94–97) ⸢If⸣ a person is unable to pour out his urine, you crush together honey, figs, raisins, dates, ostrich shell, *elkulla*. *šuliliānu*, "silver blossom," (and) "gold blossom" (*nuṣābu*) into little pieces. If he drinks (it mixed) with beer or wine, he should recover. You recite the recitation: "(I will cast for you a spell) that drives away every illness"[23] three times over the patient.

C. WOUND TREATMENTS

Infected wounds were an occupational hazard for ancient Mesopotamians of military age. If battlefield first aid failed to do the job, the physician needed to be applied to for help. For more details, see Scurlock and Andersen 2005, 62–66. Wounds were treated with bandages, salves, and daubs.

TEXT 4: BAM 32

BAM 32 contains salves (1′–4′, 7′–8′, 13′–17′), (bandaged-over) daubs (1′–12′), bandages (1′–4′, 13′–15′) for infected wounds. Without exception, they are formulated in such a way as to suggest that these treatments belonged to the purview of the physician. Of special interest in lines 1′–4′ and 13′–15′ is the alternation of hot and cold bandages. The "cockspur" of lines 7′–8′ refers to a pointing abscess. See Scurlock and Andersen 2005, 65.

1′. [o o] x x x x [(⸢ZÍD.GIG⸣)] MÚD ^{GIŠ}ERIN ŠÉŠ-*su*
2′. ^{Ú}GAMUN^{SAR} SÚD *ana* IGI GIG ‹(MAR)› NUMUN ^{Ú}KI.^{d}IM SÚD
3′. *ina* A GAZI^{SAR} ŠID-*aš lu ba-ḫír* LAL-*su ina ša-nu-ti-šú*
4′. *an-na-a-ma* ŠED$_7$-*ma* LAL-*su-ma* TI-*uṭ*

5′. *šum*$_4$-*ma* GIG *im-šid-ma* SA.MEŠ-*šú* A.MEŠ *ú-šal-la-ku*
6′. ^{Ú}*kam-ka-du* ḪÁD.DU GAZ SIM *ana* IGI GIG MAR LAL-*su-ma* DIN

7′. *šu*[(*m*$_4$-*ma* G)]IG *ḫi-dúr* MUŠEN ŠUB-*ma* IGI GIG *ṣa-bit* GAZI^{SAR} *qa-*

lu-ti

8′. *in*[*a* UGU]-*ḫi te-ḫi-tu* Ì.NUN.NA ŠÉŠ *ana* IGI GIG MAR LÁL-*su-ma* DIN

9′. ⸢DIŠ⸣ [(KI.MIN ^{Ú}*š*)]⸢*ar-ma*⸣-*da* PA ^{GIŠ}*šu-ši* PA ^{GIŠ}GEŠTIN.KA$_5$.A ^{Ú}*ur-né-e*

10′. [… (5 Ú.ḪI.A)] ⸢*an-nu-tim*⸣ TÉŠ.BI SÚD *ina* ⸢A.GEŠTIN⸣.NA

11′. [(KAŠ.SAG A GAZI^{SAR} *mál*-⸢*ma-liš*⸣ *ina* ^{URUDU}ŠEN.T)]UR ŠEG$_6$-*šal*

12′. U$_4$-⸢*ma*⸣ [(*ba-áš-la* Ú.ḪI.A)] ⸢ŠEŠ⸣ [(*ana* ŠÀ! KAŠ *tara-b*)*a*]*k* KI.MIN

13′. *šum*$_4$-*ma ina* ŠÀ GIG UZU.⸢KAK⸣.MEŠ È *re*-⸢*ḫu*⸣-*ut* NAM.LÚ.U$_{18}$.LU

14′. *pít-nim* ŠÉŠ ZÌ.KUM ZÍD.GIG *ana* IGI! DÈ *ta-šár-raq*

15′. *lu ba-ḫir* LAL-*su ina ša-nu-ti-šú an-nam* ŠED$_7$ LAL-*ma* DIN

16′. GIG-*šú ib-lu-uṭ-ma* IGI GIG-⸢*šú*⸣ [(G)]I$_6$ ŠUB!-*ú*

17′. $^{\text{NA4}}$*ás-ḫar ina ru-ti* SÚD EŠ-[*ma*] LÁL-*su-ma tuš-šir*$_4$-*šú-ma* ŠID-*nu*

18′. IGI GIG BABBAR *(catchline)*

Translation

(1′–4′) [If …], you gently rub the ⸢sore⸣ with wheat flour(?) (and) *erēnu*-cedar resin. You grind *kamunu*-cumin (and) daub (it) onto the sore. You grind *qutru* seed (and) make (it) into a dough with *kasû* juice. It should be hot when you bandage him (with it). The second time, you let this cool and, if you bandage him (with it), he should recover.

(5′–6′) If he was stricken with a wound/sore and his blood vessels make liquid flow out (of it),[24] you dry, crush (and) sift *kamkādu* (and) daub (it) onto the sore. If you bandage him, he should recover.

(7′–8′) If a sore produces a "cockspur" and it takes up a position on top of the sore,[25] (you add) roasted *kasû* ⸢to⸣ the ingredients. You gently rub on ghee. You repeatedly daub (it) onto the sore ⸢and⸣, if you bandage him, he should recover.

(9′–12′) Alternatively, you grind together these five plants: *šarmadu*, *šūšu*-licorice leaves, "fox grape" leaves, *urnû*-mint and […]. You boil (it) in vinegar, first quality beer (and) *kasû* juice in equal proportions in a *tamgussu*-vessel. When (it) has cooked, you ⸢decoct⸣[26] these plants in beer. Ditto (You repeatedly daub it onto the sore and, if you bandage him, he should recover).

(13′–15′) If *sikkatu* come out in the sore, you gently rub (him) with "semen from a strong man." You scatter *isqūqu*-flour (and) wheat flour over coals. It should be hot when you bandage him (with it). The second time, you let this cool. If you bandage him with it, he should recover.

(16′–17′) If his sore heals and subsequently the surface of his sore is dotted with black, you grind *asḫar*-mineral in spittle. You rub (him) gently (with it) [and then] you bandage him and then you release him (from the bandage) and then you make a recitation.

(18′) (If) the surface of the sore is white … (*catchline*)

TEXT 5: *AMT* 16/5 ii 1–10

AMT 16/5 ii 1–10 is a very interesting fragment of a treatment for an intractable wound. It gives alternative courses of action depending on the physician's observations of the appearance of the sore after the bandages have been removed. Lines ii 9–10 gives a very nice description of an abscess. See Scurlock and Andersen 2005, 65.

ii

1. *ina* A GAZI^{SAR} SUD *ta-là-aš* GIG MÚD MUŠ [GI_6]
2. *ana* IGI MAR LAL-*su-ma* TI

---

3. 3 KEŠDA.MEŠ ŠEŠ 15.TA.ÀM U_4-*me* LAL-[*su*]
4. *šum*$_4$-*ma ina* ŠÀ KEŠDA *maḫ-re-e la iš-ta-ri*[*k*]
5. KEŠDA *šá-na-ma* LAL-*su ina* ŠÀ KEŠDA MÚD.BABBAR-*ma* GAR ŠÀ-*bi-šú* KEŠ[DA DU_8]
6. TÚG.GADA *te-ṣe-pír* LÀL [SUD]
7. $[NA]_4$ *ga-bé-e tu-lam ana* ŠÀ GIG GAR-*an* LAL-[*su*]
8. [DIŠ Š]À-*šú* KALAG Ú BABBAR MIN DUḪ.LÀL SIG_7 [MIN]

---

9. [DIŠ N]A GIG GIN_7 *il-qí ú-ma-gag* x […]
10. […] bu ḪE.ḪE […]

TRANSLATION

(ii 1–2) […], you grind […] in *kasû* juice (and) make (it) into a dough. You daub the sore with "blood of a [black] snake." If you bandage him, he should recover.

(ii 3–8) You bandage [him] with these three bandages for fifteen days each. If it (the sore) has not produced pus[27] during the previous bindings (or if when) the bindings are put on and bandaged on him, during the binding, there is still pus inside it, [you remove] the ⸢bandage⸣. You roll a linen cloth (and) [sprinkle] (it) with honey. You soften alum (with it) and put (it) on the sore (and) bandage [him]. [If] ⸢inside⸣ it (the sore) is hard, ditto (you roll a linen cloth and sprinkle it with) "white plant." (You soften) yellow wax (with it and) [ditto (put it on the sore and bandage him)].

(ii 9–10) [If] a ⸢person's⸣ sore[28] stiffens like a leech, you mix [...].

D. SURGICAL DRAINING OF AN ABSCESS

TEXT 6: BAM 480 iii 57–iv 8

We have already seen this text above in chapter 3, text 2 and chapter 6, text 6. For a discussion of the procedure, see Scurlock and Andersen 2005, 65–66, with previous bibliography. BAM 480 iii 65–68 is one of several recitations in which color plays a prominent role. Apart from this picturesque "red" recitation and accompanying amulet, these treatments would pass muster today.

iii

57. DIŠ NA UGU-*šú* A *ú-[kal]* ŠU.SI-*ka* GAL-*ti a-šar* A.MEŠ *ú-kal-lu* TAG. TAG-*at šum-ma* UZU.GIŠ-*šú*
58. *bi-ʾ-ša[t* A.MEŠ *šá gul-gu]l-li-šú it-tar-du* BAD-*ma gul-gul-la-šú te-ser-rim A ša gul-gul-li-šú*
59. *t[u-bal* TÚG SIG A L]UḪ-*si* Ì+GIŠ SUD *ana* UGU GIG GAR-*an* KU.KU ^{GIŠ}KÍN ŠÈ BÁḪAR SÚD *ana* UGU GIG
60. [MAR U$_4$.1.KÁM* LAL DU$_8$-*m]a* TÚG SIG A LUḪ-*si* Ì+GIŠ SUD *ana* UGU GIG GAR-*an* ^{TÚG}*na-al-ti-ip-ti*
61. [... U$_4$].2.KÁM* LAL DU$_8$-*ma* TÚG SIG A LUḪ-*si* Ì+GIŠ SUD *ana* UGU GIG GAR-*an*
62. [... *-t]i* GAZI^{SAR} BÍL-*ti* KI ZÍD ŠE.SA.A ḪE.ḪE *ana* UGU GIG MAR U$_4$.1.KÁM* LAL DU$_8$-*ma*
63. [... ^{Š}]^{EM}LI GAZ KI ZÌ.KUM ḪE.ḪE *ina* A GAZI^{SAR} SILA$_{11}$-*aš* LAL IGI GIG *tu-gal-lab* EN TI.LA LÁL
64. *t[u-la]p-pat-ma šum-ma* UZU.GIŠ-*šú la bi-ʾ-šat ana li-mit* SAG.DU-*šú* KÚM NA$_4$.MEŠ GAR-*an*

---

65. ÉN *u[r-b]a-tum ur-ba-tum sa-am-tum* ZI-*am-ma ur-pa-ta* SA$_5$ *ik-tùm* IM.ŠÈG SA$_5$
66. ZI-[*m*]*a* KI-*ta*$_5$ SA$_5$-*tum ir-ḫu* A.ZI.GA SA$_5$ ZI-*ma* ÍD SA$_5$-*tum im-la* ^{LÚ}ENGAR SA$_5$

67. ^{GIŠ}[MA]R SA$_5$ ^{GIŠ}DUSU SA$_5$ ÍL-*ši*-⸢*ma*⸣ A.MEŠ SA$_5$.MEŠ *li-is-kir* ^{GIŠ}IG-*ma* SA$_5$ ^{GIŠ}SAG.KUL-*mi* SA$_5$

68. ⸢KÁ⸣-*šú-nu ed-li man-nu-um-ma šá ip-pe-et-ta-ku-nu-ši i-ri-iš ma-ra i-ri-iš ma-ra* TU$_6$ ÉN[29]

---

iv

1. KA.I[NIM.MA A.MEŠ SAG.DU] *la ik-kal-lu-ú*

---

2. DÙ.DÙ.BI *ḫal-lu-ta-na-a šá* GÌR ^{MUNUS}[ANŠE ...] NIGIN-*mi ana* ŠÀ *ḫi-pe-e-ti* GAR-*an*

3. ÉN 7-*šú* ŠID-*nu ina* TÚG *ta-pa-ti$_4$-iq* [... N]U.NU 7 KA.KEŠDA KEŠDA *e-ma* KEŠDA

4. ÉN ŠID-*nu ina* SAG.KI-*šú* K[EŠDA-*ma*] *ina-eš*

---

5. DIŠ NA SAG.DU-*su* A *ú-kal*[30] *e-le-nu da-da*-[(*ni-šú ti-ik-ki-šú*)] ⸢Ì.NUN⸣ *ḫum-ṭám* GAR-*an-ma* A-*šú ub-bal*

---

6. DIŠ NA *a-bu-ut-ta-šú* A *ú-kal kal* U[$_4$ LA]L U$_4$.7.KÁM* LAL

7. *ina* U$_4$.8.KÁM* *ab-bu-ut-ta-šú* 3-*šú te*-[*ser-rim ka-a*]-*na-am* LÁL

---

8. DIŠ NA SAG.DU-*su še-ḫa ú-kal* [Ì.NUN *ḫum*]-*ṭám* GAR-*an*

TRANSLATION

(iii 57–64) If a man's scalp ⸢contains⸣ liquid, you repeatedly touch the place where it contains liquid with your thumb. If his ear stinks, [liquid] has come down [from his] ⸢skull⸣. You open up and make an incision in his skull. You [dry up] the liquid of his skull. You ⸢wash⸣ [a thin cloth with water]. You sprinkle (it) with oil (and) put (it) on the wound. You grind powdered *kiškanû*-tree (and) potter's grog (and) [daub] (it) on the wound. [You bandage him for one day. You take it off] ⸢and⸣ you wash a thin cloth with water. You sprinkle (it) with oil (and) put (it) on the wound. You [...] a *naltiptu*-bandage (and) bandage (him) for two [days]. You take (it) off and you wash a thin cloth with water. You sprinkle (it) with oil (and) put (it) on the wound. You mix [...] (and) roasted *kasû* with roasted grain flour (and) daub (it) on the wound. You bandage (him) for one day. You take (it) off and [...]. You crush *burāšu*-juniper. You mix (it) with *isqūqu*-flour. You make (it) into a dough with *kasû* juice (and) bandage (him with it). You shave the surface of the wound. You bandage (him) until he recovers. [...] If you ⸢touch⸣ (the place where it contains liquid) and if his ear does not stink, you put hot coals around his head (to ripen the abscess).

(iii 65–68) ⸢*Urbatu*⸣, *Urbatu*. The red *urbatu* rose up and covered the red cloud. The red rain rose up ⸢and⸣ poured down on the red earth. The red flood rose up and swelled the red river. May the red farmer take up the red ⸢spade⸣ (and) the red hod so that he may dam up the red water! The door is red; the bolt is red. Who is the one who will open their locked door for you (O water)? He asks for a spade; he asks for a spade.[31]

(iv 1) Recitation so that [the waters of the head] may not be detained (i.e., to ensure complete drainage of the abscess).

(iv 2–4) Its ritual: You wrap a tuft of hair from the foot of a female [donkey] in [...] (and) put (it) on the places that have been smashed. You recite the recitation seven times. You shape (it) with a cloth. ⸢You twine⸣ [...]. You tie seven knots (in it and) whenever you tie a knot, you recite the recitation. [If] you ⸢bind⸣ (it) on his temples, he should recover.

(iv 5) If a person's head contains liquid,[32] you apply hot ghee over the muscles on the back of his neck and it will dry up his liquid.

(iv 6–7) If a person's forelock area contains liquid, you bandage (him) all ⸢day⸣ for seven days. On the eighth day, you [make an incision] three times in his forelock area (and) you bandage him ⸢continually⸣ (as above).

(iv 8) If a person's head contains delirium, you apply ⸢hot⸣ [ghee] (as above).

E. MYCETOMA

An ancient Mesopotamian syndrome which they called *muruṣ kabbarti* corresponds to our mycetoma or Madura foot. For more on this fungal infection of the foot, see Scurlock and Andersen 2005, 78–80. Mycetoma was treated with bandages, salves and daubs, washes and powders, and baths.

TEXT 7: BAM 124 i 1–ii 50

BAM 124 begins with a section containing treatments for *muruṣ kabbarti*. It consists of baths (i 1–4, ii 6–18), bandages (i 5–ii 18, ii 22, 36–39), salves (ii 19–21, 23–33) and daubs (ii 23–28, 30–33, 47, 50), powders (ii 40–43, 48–49) and washes (ii 44–46). To notice is that different plant medicines are used depending on the specific symptoms of the patient and that particularly intractable cases (ii 6–18) get both a bath and a bandage. Of special interest in lines i 19–20 is a note as to when in the course of the illness the bandage is meant to be applied. Line ii 22 is an interesting case of "Oops, I forgot to tell you." Lines ii 34–35 warn the physician of grave symptoms indicating the impossibility of cure and the impending death of the patient. The "lead spoon" of ii 50 is a pharmacist's preparation made originally for the eyes.

i

1. [DIŠ N(A GIG *ka-bar-tim* GIG-*ma ši-kìn* UZU)].MEŠ-*šú* BABBAR GI$_{6}$ ŠUB
2. [(GIG BI *ir-te-ḫi* PA ^{GIŠ}MI.PÀR P)]A GI.ZÚ.LUM.MA
3. PA ^{GIŠ}PÈŠ PA ^{GIŠ}⸢ḪAŠḪUR⸣ PA ^{G}[(^{IŠ}ŠINIG P)]A GI.ŠUL.ḪI
4. PA ^{GIŠ}ŠENNUR ‹(PA ^{GIŠ}GIŠIMMAR TUR)› *ina* A ŠUB-*di ina* ⸢NINDU⸣ BAD GÌR^{II}-*šú tara-ḫáṣ-ma*

---

5. DIŠ KI.MIN ^{GIŠ}*si-ḫu* ^{Ú}*ar-ga-nu* ^{Ú}*ba-ri-ra-tú* ^{Ú}*kám-ka-du*
6. NAGA.SI ^{Ú}*a-zal-la-a* 1-*niš* GAZ *ina* SAḪAR MUNU$_{6}$ ZÍD MUNU$_{6}$ ḪE.ḪE
7. *ina* KAŠ *ina* ^{URUDU}ŠEN.TUR *ina* GA *tara-bak ina* TÚG SUR-*ri* LAL-*id*

---

8. DIŠ NA GIG *ka-bar-ti* GIG *eq-ba-šu* MÚ.MÚ-*ḫu* SA GÌR^{II}-*šú*
9. *kab-ba-ru-ma i-tal-lu-ka la i-le-ʾi* IM.⸢BABBAR *saḫ-lé*⸣-*e*
10. NAGA.SI *pu-ut-ri* SÚD *ina* GA *ina* URUDU.ŠEN.⸢TUR⸣ [(*tara-bak ba-aḫ-ru-us-s*)]*u*
11. *ina* TÚG *te‹-ṭer-ri›* LAL U$_{4}$.3.KAM NU DU$_{8}$

---

12. DIŠ NA GIG *ka-bar-ti* GIG-*ma* SA MUD-*šu* IM DIRI-*ú*
13. *ana šu-ṣi-i* [(^{ŠEM}L)]I ^{ŠEM}GÚR.GÚR IM.BABBAR GAZI×SAR ^{Ú}ḪAR.ḪAR ŠE.SA.A
14. *ina* A SÚD [(*ina* ZÌ.K)]UM ḪE.ḪE *ina* KAŠ *ina* URUDU.ŠEN.TUR *tara-bak ina* TÚG *te‹-ṭer-ri›* LAL-*id-ma* IM È-*a*

---

15. [(DIŠ NA G)]IG *ka-bar-ti* GIG-*ma* GÌR^{II}-*šú* MÚD DIRI KUŠ ^{GIŠ}NU.ÚR.MA.A
16. [(A.GAR)].GAR MAŠ.DÀ SÚD *ina* A.MEŠ GAZI^{SAR} ‹(*ina*)› ŠEN.TUR *tara-bak* LAL-*id*

---

17. DIŠ NA GIG *ka-bar-ti* GIG PA ^{Ú}ÚKUŠ.GÍL Ì.UDU ÚKUŠ.GÍL
18. SÚD *ina* ZÌ.KUM ḪE.ḪE *ina* KAŠ *ina* ŠEN.TUR *tara-bak* LAL-*id*

---

19. ^{Ú}*si-ḫu* ^{Ú}*ar-ga-nu ka-man-du* ^{Ú}EME.UR.GI$_{7}$ $^{\text{Ú.d}}$UTU SÚD
20. *ina* Ì.UDU ḪE.ḪE LAL-*ma* U$_{4}$.1.KÁM NU DU$_{8}$ GIN$_{7}$ UZU-*šu i-ṭíb-bu* LÁL-*id*

---

21. DIŠ KI.MIN ^{ŠEM}GÚR.GÚR ^{ŠEM}LI SÚD *ina* Ì.ŠAḪ! ZÍD MUNU$_6$ ḪE.ḪE *ina* KAŠ *ina* ŠEN.TUR *tara-bak* LAL

---

22. DIŠ KI.MIN ^{Ú}*a-zal-lá* ḪÁD.DU GAZ *ina* ZÌ.KUM ḪE.ḪE *ina* A.MEŠ GAZI^{SAR}
23. *ina* URUDU.ŠEN.TUR *tara-bak* LAL U$_4$.1.KAM NU.DU$_8$

---

24. DIŠ KI.MIN ^{Ú}⸢ŠAKIR⸣ ḪÁD.DU GAZ *ina* SAḪAR MUNU$_6$ ḪE.ḪE GIN$_7$ KAM.KU.DA *tara-bak* LAL

---

25. DIŠ KI.MIN ŠÚR!.DÙ$^{\text{KU}_6}$ ḪÁD.DU GAZ *ina* A GAZI^{SAR} *tara-bak* LAL

---

26. DIŠ NA GIG *ka-bar-ti* GIG-*ma ši-kìn* GIG *e-šu-ú* ^{Ú}*kám-ka-du*
27. ^{Ú}[(GÌR)] UGA^{MUŠEN} ^{Ú}*tu-lal* ḪÁD.DU GAZ GIN$_7$ *ra-bi-ki tara-bak* LAL

---

28. DIŠ NA GIG *ka-bar-ti* GIG-*ma* SA GÌR^{II}-*šú šàg-gu* ^{Ú}*si-ḫu*
29. ^{Ú}*ar-ga-nu* ^{Ú}*ba-ri-ra-tú* PA ^{GIŠ}*šu-še* SIG$_7$ SÚD
30. *ina* ZÌ.KUM ḪE.ḪE *ina* A GAZI^{SAR} *tara-bak* LAL-*id-ma* U$_4$.1.KÁM NU DU$_8$

---

31. DIŠ NA GIG ⸢*ka*⸣-*bar-ti a-tál-lu-ka la i-le-ʾi* ^{Ú}EME.UR.GI$_7$
32. P[(A) ^{GIŠ}Š]INIG ḪÁD.DU GAZ *ina* ZÍD MUNU$_6$ ḪE.ḪE *ina* A GAZI^{SAR} *tara-bak* LAL-*id*

---

33. DIŠ NA GIG *ka-bar-ti ši-kìn* GIG-*šú* GI$_6$ PA ^{GIŠ}MI.⸢PÀR GAZ SIM⸣
34. *ina* ZÌ.KUM ḪE.ḪE *ina* A GAZI^{SAR} *tara-bak* LAL : PA ^{GIŠ}ŠINIG

---

35. ^{Ú}ḪAR.ḪAR Ú.KUR.RA *tu-daq-qaq iš-tu* ZÍD.DA
36. ḪE.ḪE *ina* A GAZI^{SAR} *tara-bak* LAL-*id*

---

37. GURUN $^{\text{GIŠ.Ú}}$GÍR SIG$_7$-*su* SÚD LAL-*id*

---

38. ^{Ú}*šu-šum* SIG$_7$-*su* SÚD LAL-*id*

---

39. ^{Ú}ÚKUŠ.GÍL SÚD LAL-*id*

---

40. GI.DÙG.GA ^{Ú}A.GUG$_4$! ḪÁD.DU GAZ ZÍD ^{GIŠ}ERIN.SUMUN
41. ZÌ.KUM *ina* A GAZI^{SAR} *tara-bak* LAL-*id*

---

42. DIŠ KI.MIN PA $^{\text{GIŠ.Ú}}$GÍR PA ^{GIŠ}DÌḪ PA ^{GIŠ}*šu-ši* PA GI.ŠUL.ḪI
43. PA ^{GIŠ}ḪAŠḪUR PA ^{GIŠ}PÈŠ PA ^{GIŠ}NU.ÚR.MA PA ^{GIŠ}GIŠIMMAR.TUR
44. ḪÁD.DU GAZ *ina* ZÍD.DA ḪE.ḪE *ina* ŠEN.TUR *tara-bak* LAL

---

45. DIŠ KI.MIN ^{Ú}IN.NU.UŠ ^{Ú}*kám-ka-du* ḪÁD.A GAZ *ina* ZÌ.KUM
46. ḪE.ḪE *ina* A.MEŠ GAZI^{SAR} *tara-bak* LAL-*id*

---

47. NUMUN ^{ŠEM}LI ^{ŠEM}GÚR.GÚR ^{ŠEM}IM.M[AN.D]U GAZ *ina* KAŠ.Ú.SA ḪE.ḪE LAL

---

48. [DIŠ KI].MIN PA ^{GIŠ}*šu-še* PA GI.ZÚ.LUM.MA PA ^{Ú}EME.UR.GI$_7$
49. [SIG]$_7$-*su-nu* GAZ *ina* ^{URUDU}ŠEN.TUR *tara-bak* SAḪAR MUNU$_6$ ZÍD.DA ḪE.ḪE LAL-*id*

---

50. [DIŠ N]A [*t*]*u-ḫar eq-bi-šu ka-bíl* IGI UZU.MEŠ-*šú* KÚR.KÚR GIG
51. [… G]A DUGUD PA ^{GIŠ}KIRI$_6$ DÙ.A.BI TI-*qí ina* NINDU BAD-*ir*
52. […*ana* ^{DUG}*nam*]-*ḫa-ri* DUB-*ak ina* ŠÀ *i-ra-ḫaṣ* EN ^{d}UTU.ŠÚ.A ŠUB-*šu*
53. […] x […] *kib*?-*šú* GIG x x *tú ma*
54. […]x x nu
55. […] x x
56. […]

ii

1. GAZ *ina* GA [*ina* URUDU].ŠEN.TUR *tara-bak baḫ-ru-su* […]

---

2. DIŠ NA GIG *ka-*[*bar-t*]*i tu-ḫar eq-bi-šu* GI[G UZU.MEŠ-*šú*]
3. GI$_6$ ŠUB x x ta x x x GÌR.PAD.DU […]
4. ^{Ú}NÍNDA Ú.^{d}UTU ^{Ú}EME.UR.GI$_7$ PA ^{GIŠ}*bi-*[*ni* …]
5. GURUN $^{\text{GIŠ.Ú}}$GÍR *ta-sàk* ḪE.ḪE *ina* KAŠ *ina* URUDU.ŠE[N.TUR *tara-bak* LAL]

---

6. DIŠ NA GIG *ka-bar-ti* GIG EN GÌR.PAD.DU *i*[*r-te-ḫi*]
7. GIG *il-ta-za-az ina* SU-*šú* NU DU$_8$ KAŠ.Ú.SA x[…]
8. ^{DUG}*nam-ḫa-ri* DUB-*ak* GÌR^{II}-*šú tara-ḫáṣ ta-sar* E[N …]
9. *ra-aḫ-ṣa na-aṣ-ma-ti* ni/ir […]
10. ^{Ú}ḪAR.ḪAR ŠE.SA.A *ina* Ì.NUN *ina* URUDU.ŠEN.TUR *tara-bak* [LAL]

---

11. DIŠ NA GIG *ka-bar-ti* GIG EN *kìn-ṣi-šú* E$_{11}$-*a ši-kìn* U[ZU]

12. *tu-ri-iḫ* IGI GIG-*šú* GI$_6$ GIG.BI *ina na-aṣ-ma-ti* [...]
13. *ul i-tel-li* LAGAB ŠURUN GUD A.GAR.GAR MAŠ.DÀ ^{GIŠ}ŠE.NU *ina* NINDU BAD-[*ir*]
14. GÌR^{II}-*šú i-ra-ḫaṣ* ^{Ú}EME UR.GI$_7$ Ú.^{d}UTU ^{GIŠ}LI ^{ŠEM}[...]
15. ^{Ú}*ana-me-rù* ^{Ú}*a-zal-la* ^{Ú}ḪAR.ḪU.BA.NU$_{11}$ ^{Ú}*am-*[*ḫa-ra*]
16. ^{Ú}*pi$_4$-za-lu-ur-tú* ^{Ú}ÁB.DUḪ ^{Ú}*kám-ka-du* [... Z]Ú.LUM
17. Ú.SIKIL ^{Ú}GEŠTIN.KA$_5$.A ^{Ú}MAŠ.ḪUŠ Ú.KUR.RA [NUMUN? ^{GIŠ}*b*]*i-nu*
18. GAZ *ina* KAŠ *ina* ŠEN.TUR *tara-bak* LAL-*id*

---

19. DIŠ NA GIG *ka-*[*bar-t*]*i* GIG-*ma* ^{Ú}*a-zal-l*[*a* ... *ina* Ì].NUN EŠ-*aš*

---

20. DIŠ KI.MIN ^{ŠEM}GÍ[R?/BAL? ^{GIŠ}GEŠTI]N.KA$_5$.A *ina* Ì.NUN ŠÉŠ-*aš*

---

21. DIŠ KI.MIN ZÍD ^{Ú}ÚKUŠ.G[ÍL] *ina* Ì.NUN ŠÉŠ-*aš*

---

22. EN LAL.MEŠ *an-na-te* LAL-*du* [EGIR-*šú ri*]-*ip*!-*ḫu ta-bi-lam*! LAL

---

23. DIŠ KI.MIN Ú.BABBAR ^{Ú}EME.UR.GI$_7$ ^{Ú}I[N.NU.U]Š ḪÁD.DU GAZ Ì+GIŠ EŠ-*aš ta-za-ru*

---

24. DIŠ KI.MIN BURU$_5$.ÍD.DA ^{ŠEM}LI ḪÁD.DU SÚD [*ina*] Ì.NUN EŠ MAR

---

25. DIŠ KI.MIN DUḪ ŠE.GIŠ.Ì GAZ IGI GIG *it-*⸢*tu-šú*⸣ EŠ MAR-*rù*

---

26. DIŠ KI.MIN PA ^{GIŠ}ÚKUŠ.[(GÍL)] ‹(ḪÁD.DU)› GAZ IGI GIG *it-tu-š*[*ú*] EŠ MAR-*rù*

---

27. DIŠ KI.MIN $^{\text{NA}_4}$PEŠ$_4$.Í[(D.DA)] GAZ IGI GIG *še-šen* EŠ [MA]R-*rù* LAL

---

28. DIŠ KI.MIN ^{GIŠ}*si-ḫa* ‹(^{Ú}*ár-zal-lá*)› [(NUMUN ^{Ú})]*áp-ru-šá* Ú.^{d}UTU GAZ *i*[*na* Ì.N]UN EŠ MAR

---

29. DIŠ KI.MIN ^{GIŠ}[(GEŠTIN.KA$_5$.A)] ⸢^{Ú}⸣*tu-lal* GAZ *ina šur-šum-me* KAŠ Ì.[NU]N ŠÉŠ-[*aš*]

---

30. DIŠ ⸢KI.MIN⸣ NA$_4$ ZÚ.L[(UM.M)]A SÚD *ina* Ì.ŠAḪ EŠ-*aš* MAR-*rù*

---

31. DIŠ KI.MIN ^{Ú}*pi$_4$-zal-lu-ur-ta* SÚD *ina* Ì+GIŠ EŠ-*aš* MAR-*rù*

---

32. DIŠ KI.MIN ^{Ú}*a-zal-la-a* ^{Ú}SIKIL GAZ ⸢Ì⸣.KUR EŠ-[*aš*] MAR-*rù*

33. DIŠ KI.MIN PA (variant: BAR) ^{GIŠ}NU.ÚR.MA *tur-ár* SÚD Ì+GIŠ.KU$_6$ E[Š-*aš*] MAR-*rù*

34. DIŠ [N]A GIG *ka-bar-ti ma-gal* NAM.ÉR[(IM DI)]B-*su i-pa-áš-še-eḫ* ‹(*ina* EGIR U$_4$-*me*)› [(BA.ÚŠ)]

35. DIŠ GIG *ka-bar-ti ru-šum-tú ib-ta-ni* BA.ÚŠ

36. DIŠ GIG *ka-bar-ti* A.GAR.GAR SIG$_7$ *ina* KÀŠ *ru-uš-še-ti ina* URUDU.ŠEN.TUR

37. *ina* ZÌ.KUM ḪE.ḪE LAL-*i*[*d*]

38. DIŠ KI.MIN ^{Ú}*úr-né-e* ^{GIŠ}*si-ḫa* ^{GIŠ}*ar-ga-nu* ^{GIŠ}LUM.[ḪA]

39. ZÍD ^{Ú}ÚKUŠ.GÍL *ina* Ì.NUN Ì.ŠAḪ *ina* ^{URUDU}ŠE[(N)].TUR *tara-bak* [(LAL)]

40. DIŠ ‹(KI.MIN)› GIG MIN ^{Ú}*i-ši-in*-A.ŠÀ *tur-ár ana* IGI ŠUB-[*di*]

41. DIŠ ‹(KI.MIN)› PA ^{GIŠ}*šu-ši* SÚD *ana* IGI ŠUB-*d*[*i*]

42. DIŠ ‹(KI.MIN)› ŠIKA ^{GIŠ}NU.ÚR.MA *ta-qal-lu ana* IGI ŠUB-*di*

43. DIŠ ‹(KI.MIN)› ŠÚR!.DÙ.KU$_6$ *ta-qal-lu ana* IGI ŠUB-*di*

44. DIŠ KI.MIN PA GI.ZÚ.LUM.MA *ta-sal-laq ana* IGI ŠUB-*di*

45. DIŠ KI.MIN PA GI.ZÚ.LUM.MA PA ^{GIŠ}*úr-zi-ni* KI.MIN

46. DIŠ KI.MIN ‹(PA)› ^{Ú}UR.TÁL.TÁL *ta-sal-laq ana* IGI *ta-tab-bak*

47. DIŠ NA *ka-bal-ta-šu* GIG SAG.DU EME.DIR *tur-ár* SÚD *ana* IGI ‹(GIG)› MAR.MEŠ

48. DIŠ KI.MIN ŠIKA ^{GIŠ}NU.ÚR.MA SÚD *ana* IGI ŠUB-*di*

49. DIŠ KI.MIN SAG.DU *ka-zi-ri ta-qa-lu ana* IGI ŠUB-*di*

50. DIŠ KI.MIN IGI GIG *ta-ka-par it-qur-ta*$_5$ *te-*[(*qí*)]

TRANSLATION

(i 1–4) [If] a ⌜person⌝ is sick with *muruṣ kabbarti* so that the appearance of his flesh is white dotted with black, that illness has penetrated.[33] You pour *lipāru*-tree leaves, *buṣinnu* leaves, *tittu*-fig leaves, *ḫašḫuru*-apple leaves, *bīnu*-tamarisk leaves, *qān šalāli* leaves *šallūru*-plum leaves (and) ‹(dwarf palm leaves)›into water. You bake (it) in an oven. If you bathe his feet (with it), etc. (he should recover).

(i 5–7) Alternatively, you crush together *sīḫu*-wormwood, *argannu*, *barirātu*, *kamkādu*, *uḫḫūlu qarnānu* (and) *azallû*. You mix (it) with malt dust (and) malt flour. You decoct (it)[34] in beer in a *tamgussu*-vessel (or) in milk. You massage (it) into a cloth (and) bandage (him with it).

(i 8–11) If a person is sick with *muruṣ kabbarti* so that his heels are swollen (and) the muscles of his feet are so thickened that he cannot walk,[35] you grind *gaṣṣu*-gypsum, *saḫlû*-cress,[36] *uḫḫūlu qarnānu* (and) a cowdung patty. You decoct (it)[37] in milk in a *tamgussu*-vessel. You massage (it) while still hot into a cloth. You bandage (him with it and) do not take (it) off for three days.

(i 12–14) If a person is sick with *muruṣ kabbarti* so that his Achilles' tendon(s) are full of "clay," to make (it) go out,[38] you grind *kukru*, *burāšu*-juniper, *gaṣṣu*-gypsum, *kasû*, *ḫašû*-thyme (and) roasted grain in water. You mix (it) with *isqūqu*-flour. You decoct (it) in beer in a *tamgussu*-vessel. You massage (it) into a cloth. If you bandage (him with it), the "clay" should go out.

(i 15–16) If a person is sick with *muruṣ kabbarti* so that his feet are full of blood, you grind *nurmû*-pomegranate skin (and) gazelle dung. You decoct (it) in *kasû* juice in a *tamgussu*-vessel. You bandage (him with it).

(i 17–18) If a person is sick with *muruṣ kabbarti*, you grind *irrû* leaves (and) *irrû* "fat." You mix (it) with *isqūqu*-flour. You decoct (it) in beer in a *tamgussu*-vessel. You massage (it) into a cloth. You bandage (him with it).

(i 19–20) You grind *sīḫu*-wormwood, *argannu*, *kamantu*-henna(?), *lišān kalbi* (and) "sunflower." You mix (it) with fat. You bandage (him with it) and do not take (it) off for one day. You bandage (him with it) as soon as his flesh looks better.

(i 21) Alternatively, you grind *kukru* (and) *burāšu*-juniper. You mix (it) with pig fat (and) malt flour. You decoct (it) in beer in a *tamgussu*-vessel. You bandage (him with it).

(i 22–23) Alternatively, you dry (and) crush *azallû*. You mix (it) with *isqūqu*-flour. You decoct (it) in *kasû* juice in a *tamgussu*-vessel. You bandage (him with it) and do not take (it) off for one day.

(i 24) Alternatively, you dry (and) crush *šakirû*. You mix (it) with malt dust. You decoct (it) till decocted. You bandage (him with it).

(i 25) Alternatively, you dry (and) crush a *šurdû*-falcon-fish. You decoct (it) in *kasû* juice (and) bandage (him with it).

(i 26–27) If a person is sick with *muruṣ kabbarti* so that the appearance of the sore is confused, you dry (and) crush *kamkādu*, "crowfoot" (and) *tullal*. You decoct (it) till decocted and bandage (him with it).

(i 28–30) If a person is sick with *muruṣ kabbarti* so that the muscles of his feet are stiff,[39] you grind *sīḫu*-wormwood, *argannu*, *barirātu* (and) fresh *šūšu*-licorice leaves. You mix (it) with *isqūqu*-flour. You decoct (it) in *kasû* juice. You bandage (him with it) and do not take (it) off for one day.

(i 31–32) If a person has *muruṣ kabbarti* (and) he cannot walk,[40] you dry (and) crush *lišān kalbi* (and) *bīnu*-tamarisk leaves. You mix (it) with malt flour. You decoct (it) in *kasû* juice (and) bandage (him with it).

(i 33–34) If a person (has) *muruṣ kabbarti* (and) the appearance of his sore is black,[41] you crush (and) sift *lipāru*-tree leaves. You mix (it) with *isqūqu*-flour. You decoct (it) in *kasû* juice (and) bandage (him with it). Alternatively, (you do this with) *bīnu*-tamarisk leaves.

(i 35–36) You finely crush *ḫašû*-thyme (and) *nīnû*-mint. You mix (it) with flour. You decoct (it) in *kasû* juice (and) bandage (him with it).

(i 37) You grind fresh *ašāgu*-thorn fruit (and) bandage (him with it).

(i 38) You grind fresh *šūšu*-licorice (and) bandage (him with it).

(i 39) You grind *irrû* (and) bandage (him with it).

(i 40–41) You dry (and) crush "sweet reed" (and) garden *elpetu*-rush. (You mix it with) *šupuḫru*-cedar flour (and) *isqūqu*-flour. You decoct (it) in *kasû* juice (and) bandage (him with it).

(i 42–44) Alternatively, you dry (and) crush *ašāgu*-thorn leaves, *baltu*-thorn leaves, *šūšu*-licorice leaves, *qān šalāli* leaves, *ḫašḫuru*-apple leaves, *tittu*-fig leaves, *nurmû*-pomegranate leaves (and) dwarf palm leaves. You mix (it) with flour. You decoct (it)[42] in a *tamgussu*-vessel (and) bandage (him with it).

(i 45–46) Alternatively, you dry (and) crush *maštakal* (and) *kamkādu*. You mix (it) with *isqūqu*-flour. You decoct (it) in *kasû* juice (and) bandage (him with it).

(i 47) You crush *burāšu*-juniper, *kukru* (and) *suʾādu*. You mix (it) with beerwort (and) bandage (him with it).

(i 48–49) ⌜Alternatively⌝, you crush [fresh] *šūšu*-licorice leaves, *buṣinnu* leaves (and) *lišān kalbi* leaves. You decoct (it) in a *tamgussu*-vessel. You mix (it) with malt dust (and) flour (and) bandage (him with it).

(i 50–ii 1) [If] a ⌜person⌝'s Achilles tendon(s) are immobilized (and) his flesh looks worse and worse, the illness [...] will be difficult. You take leaves of every sort of garden tree. You bake (it) in an oven. You pour (it) [... into] a ⸢*namḫaru*⸣-vat (and) he bathes with it. You pour (it) on him until sunset. [...] You crush [...]. You decoct (it) in milk [in] a *tamgussu*-vessel. [You bandage him with it] while it is still hot.

(ii 2–5) If a person has ⸢*muruṣ kabbarti*⸣ (and) his Achilles tendon(s) are ⸢sore⸣, [his flesh] is unevenly colored with black, [... and it penetrates as far as] the bone,[43] you grind *illūru*, "sunflower," *lišān kalbi*, ⸢*bīnu*⸣-tamarisk leaves, [...] (and) *ašāgu*-thorn fruit. You mix (them). [You decoct (it)] in beer in a ⸢*tamgussu*⸣-vessel [and bandage (him with it)].

(ii 6–10) If a person is sick with *muruṣ kabbarti* (and) it ⸢pentrates⸣ as far as the bone (and) the soreness stays continuously (and) cannot be dispelled from his body,[44] you pour beerwort (and) [... into] a *namḫaru*-vat (and) bathe his feet (with it). You [...] encircle (him with) bandages(?) ⸢when⸣ [the feet] have been bathed. You decoct [...], *ḫašû*-thyme (and) roasted grain in ghee in a *tamgussu*-vessel [and bandage (him with it)].

(ii 11–18) If a person has *muruṣ kabbarti* (and) the soreness extends as far as his shins, the appearance of [his] ⸢flesh⸣ rapidly [changes (for the worse)?], the surface of his sore looks black, (and) that illness does not let up despite the use of bandages (and) [...],[45] you bake ox dung, gazelle dung (and) *šunû*-chastetree in an oven. He bathes his feet (with it). You crush *lišān kalbi*, "sunflower," *burāšu*-juniper, [*kukru*?], *anameru*, *azallû*, *ḫarmunu*, ⸢*amḫaru*⸣, *pizallurtu*-gecko plant, *kamantu*-henna(?), *kamkādu*, date [...], *sikillu*, "fox grape," *kalbānu*, *nīnû*-mint (and) *bīnu*-tamarisk [seed]. You decoct (it) in beer in a *tamgussu*-vessel (and) bandage (him with it).

(ii 19) If a person is sick with *muruṣ* ⸢*kabbarti*⸣, etc.,[46] you rub him gently with *azallû* (and) [...] (mixed) [with] ⸢ghee⸣.

(ii 20) Alternatively, you rub him gently with ⸢*asu*⸣-myrtle[47] and ⸢"fox grape"⸣ (mixed) with ghee.

(ii 21) Alternatively, you rub him gently with powdered ⸢*irrû*⸣ (mixed) with ghee.

(ii 22) When you have bandaged (him with) these bandages, [afterwards], you bandage ⸢the swelling⸣ dry.

(ii 23) Alternatively, you dry (and) crush "white plant," *lišān kalbi* (and) ⸢*maštakal*⸣. You gently rub (him with) oil (and) daub (it on).

(ii 24) Alternatively, you dry (and) grind river shrimp (and) *burāšu*-juniper. You gently rub (him) [with] ghee (and) daub (it on).

(ii 25) Alternatively, you crush sesame residue. You gently rub (and) daub the surface of the sore with it.

(ii 26) Alternatively, you ‹(dry)› (and) crush *irrû* leaves. You gently rub (and) daub the surface of the sore with ⸢it⸣.

(ii 27) Alternatively, you crush river *biṣṣuru*-shell. You gently rub the surface of the sore with a palm frond(?) (and) ⸢daub⸣ (it) on (and) bandage (it over).

(ii 28) Alternatively, you crush *sīḫu*-wormwood, ‹(*arzallu*)›, *aprušu* seed (and) "sunflower." You gently rub (him) ⸢with ghee⸣ (and) daub (him with it).

(ii 29) Alternatively, you crush "fox grape" (and) *tullal*. You rub (him) gently (with it mixed) with beer dregs (and) ⸢ghee⸣.

(ii 30) Alternatively, you grind date stones. You gently rub (him) with pig fat (and) daub (him with it).

(ii 31) Alternatively, you grind *pizallurtu*-gecko plant. You gently rub (him) with oil (and) daub (him with it).

(ii 32) Alternatively, you crush *azallû* (and) *sikillu*. You gently rub (him) with naphtha (and) daub (him with it).

(ii 33) Alternatively, you grind *nurmû*-pomegranate leaves (variant: peel). You gently ⸢rub⸣ (him) with fish oil (and) daub (him with it).

(ii 34) If a ⸢person⸣ (has) *muruṣ kabbarti* (and) the curse greatly afflicts him, he may find relief but (later) he will die.[48]

(ii 35) If (a person has) *muruṣ kabbarti* (and) there is oozing, he will die.[49]

(ii 36–37) If (a person has) *muruṣ kabbarti*, you decoct fresh gazelle dung in red urine in a *tamgussu*-vessel. You mix (it) with *isqūqu*-four (and) bandage (him with it).

(ii 38–39) Alternatively, you decoct *urnû*-mint, *sīḫu*-wormwood, *argannu*, *barirātu* (and) powdered *irrû* in ghee (and) pig fat in a *tamgussu*-vessel (and) bandage (him with it).

(ii 40) ‹(Alternatively)›, (for) *muruṣ* ditto (*kabbarti*), you char *išin-eqli* (and) pour (it) on.

(ii 41) ‹(Alternatively)›, you grind *šūšu*-licorice leaves (and) pour (it) on.

(ii 42) ‹(Alternatively)›, you roast a fragment of *nurmû*-pomegranate (peel and) pour (it) on.

(ii 43) ‹(Alternatively)›, you roast a *šurdû*-falcon-fish (and) pour (it) on.

(ii 44) Alternatively, you boil *buṣinnu* leaves (and) pour (it) on.

(ii 45) Alternatively, you boil *buṣinnu* leaves (and) *urzinnu*-tree leaves (and) ditto (you pour it on).

(ii 46) Alternatively, you boil *uzun lalî* ‹(leaves)› (and) pour (it) on.

(ii 47) If a person's *kabbaltu* is sick/sore, you char (and) grind the head of a lizard. You daub (it) on the ‹(sore)›.

(ii 48) Alternatively, you grind a fragment of *nurmû*-pomegranate (peel and) pour (it) on.

(ii 49) Alternatively, you roast the head of a *kaṣiru*-bird (and) pour (it) on.

(ii 50) Alternatively, you wipe off the sore (and) daub on a "spoon."

F. SETTING BONES

Ancient Mesopotamians knew how to set bones, using their own version of a cast. They also attempted to avoid complications by lacing their bandages with plant medicines designed "to soothe what feels heavy, to lubricate what is *ašṭu*-stiff/*šaggu*-stiff, to stretch out what is bent, to stop the flow of pus, to straighten up what is fractured, for what jerks violently to be disconnected (and) to repair what is broken into pieces." Physicians also had to deal with stiff joints, arthritis and low back pain, using bandages, salves and plasters, potions, baths, and enemas. For more details, see Scurlock and Andersen 2005, chapter 11.

TEXT 8: BAM 124 ii 51–iv 35

BAM 124 ii 51–iv 35 consists of a medicated cast for a broken bone (ii 51–54), bandages (iii 1–13, 41–43) for stiff joints, a bandage (iii 14–15) and a daub (iii 16–17) for inflammation(?), bandages (iii 18–21) for sprains(?), a nice example of a "great powder" (iii 44–59), an amulet (iv 10–33) for *sagallu* (lower back pain), and bandages (iii 22–40) for other conditions not preserved. With the exception of the (partially) Sumerian recitation which accompanied the "great powder," these treatments are formulated in such a way as to indicate that they could have originated with a pharmacist.

Of interest in lines iii 38–40 is the remark that the "usual proportions" are to be used. We have guessed, and this indicates clearly, that the amount of various plant medicines to be used in a given treatment was a matter of oral tradition. Lines iii 44–59 give a "great powder" to be used in bandages. Winter bandages were made with beer whereas the summer variety used a plant antiseptic. The text clearly indicates that the "great powder" was used both by physicians and pharmacists. The following (partially) Sumerian recitation (iii 60–iv 9) will have been for the physician. It is a typical example of academic Sumerian gobbledygook which, when not provided with its Akkadian "translation," is often impenetrable. The relevance to context is actually rather subtle—apart from fullsome praise for Ninisinna (Gula "mistress of Isin"), the pharmacist's patron, it is requested that the patient's legal case be straightened out, an oblique reference to the desired straightening of the broken bone. The Akkadian language recitation in lines iv 10–27 gives a charming, patient's eye view, of lower back pain. Particularly interesting is that the ailment is not personified despite the fact that its behavior positively invites personification.

ii

51. [(ŠEMGÚR.GÚR GAZISAR)] ZÍD.ŠE.SA.A *šik-na-te* LAGAB MUNU$_6$

ŠÈ [(TU^{MUŠEN})]
52. [(*pu-ut-ri* A.GAR.GAR MAŠ.DÀ)] IM.BABBAR ZÍD GIG *ḫa-ḫu-*⸢*ú*⸣ [(*šá* UDUN GIBIL)]
53. [(GI.MEŠ MÚD.MEŠ *šu-luṭ* ŠEM.ḪI.A)] ⸢1-*niš*⸣ G[(AZ SIM)]
54. [(*ina* KAŠ ŠEG$_6$-*šal* LAL 14 NÍG.LAL SI.SÁ)]

---

iii
1. [(^{ŠEM}GÚR.GÚR ^{Š})]^{EM}LI ^{Ú}*ak-tam* NUMUN GADA GAZI^{SAR} L[(AGAB [variant: ZÍD] MUNU$_6$ ZÍD ^{ŠE}GIG ZÌ.KUM)]
2. ⸢KAŠ⸣.[(Ú.SA S)]IG$_5$.GA 1-*niš* SÚD : *ina* KUŠ SUR LAL 9 NÍG.LAL [(*šig-ga*$_{14}$*-ti*)]

---

3. ^{ŠEM}GÚR.[(GÚR Ì.U)]DU ÉLLAG UDU NÍTA ^{ŠEM}BULUḪ ILLU ^{ŠEM}BULUḪ IL[(LU LI.DUR)]
4. ^{GIŠ}ERI[(N SUMUN Ì.GIŠ)] ^{ŠEM}GÍR MÚD ^{GIŠ}*e-re-ni* ^{ŠEM}ḪAB
5. 9 NÍG.LAL *šig-ga*$_{14}$-[(*te*)]

---

6. Ì.UDU ÉLLAG UDU NÍTA DUḪ.LÀL ^{ŠEM}BULUḪ ILLU ^{ŠEM}[(BULUḪ)]
7. ^{ŠEM}GÚR.GÚR ILLU LI.DU[(R ^{Š})]^{EM}ŠEŠ ^{GIŠ}ERIN [(SUMUN)]
8. Ì+GIŠ ^{ŠEM}GÍR[50] ^{ŠEM}ḪAB *a*[(*n-nu*)]*-u* NÍG.LAL *šig-ga*$_{14}$*-te šá* E[(N. TE.NA)]

---

9. ^{ŠEM}GÚR.GÚR ^{ŠEM}LI ^{ŠEM}⸢ŠEŠ ^{ŠEM}⸣GAM.MA ILLU LI.[DUR ^{ŠEM}BULUḪ]
10. ILLU ⸢^{ŠEM}BULUḪ⸣ ^{ŠEM}ḪAB MÚD ^{GIŠ}ERIN x […]
11. ^{Ú}KUR.KUR 11 Ú.ḪI.A NÍG.LAL *šig-ga*$_{14}$*-te*

---

12. *ḫa-ḫu-ú šá* UDUN *i-ra šá* MUNU$_6$ LAGAB MUNU$_6$ x[…]
13. *ina* ZÌ.KUM ḪE.ḪE *ina* A GAZI^{SAR} ŠEG$_6$-*šal* LAL 4 NÍG.LAL GÚ-[(*su šig-g*)*a*$_{14}$*-te*]

---

14. ZÍD […] ZÍD LAGAB MUNU$_6$ ZÍD GAZI^{SAR} BÍL.MEŠ *ḫa-ḫu-*[*u šá* UDUN]
15. *ina* [KAŠ ŠI]D-*aš* LAL 4 NÍG.LAL *ṣir-ḫi*

---

16. ZÍD GURUN ^{GIŠ}NU.ÚR.MA ZÍD GURUN $^{\text{GIŠ.Ú}}$GÍR ZÍD NUMUN BABBAR.ḪI$^{\text{[SAR]}}$
17. ZÍD NUMUN ^{Ú}EME.UR.GI$_7$ 4 ZÍD.MEŠ *an-nu-ti ana* UGU GI[G MAR]

---

18. *saḫ-lé-e qa-lu-te* GAZI^{SAR} *si-ku-ú-ti ina* KA[(Š ŠEG$_6$-*šal*)]
19. 3 U$_4$-*me* ‹(LAL)› 3 NÍG.LAL GÌR *nu-uḫ-ḫur-*[(*ti*)]

---

20. EGIR-*šu ina* 4.KÁM U$_4$-*me* SI DÀRA.MAŠ! ^{NA_4}ZÚ.LUM.[(MA)]
21. *tur-ár* SÚD *ina* Ì.UDU ḪE.ḪE Ì.NUN EŠ-*aš* ⸢2!⸣ NÍG.LAL [(NÍG.GIG *nu-ḫur-ti*)]

---

22. ZÍD.ŠE.SA.A ZÍD GAZI^{SAR} ZÌ.KUM *ina* Ì.[…]
23. [*ina* I]ZI ŠEG$_6$-*šal* 3 NÍG.LAL […]

---

24. […G]I$_6$? ILLU ^{Š}[^{EM}BULUḪ]
25. x[…]
26. ZÍD.ŠE.⸢SA⸣.[A…]
27. ZÍD ^{ŠEM}[…]
28. ^{ŠEM}ŠEŠ […]
29. ILLU LI.T[AR …]x ba x x […]
30. Ì.UDU SUMUN DUḪ.[LÀL x] NÍG.LAL ⸢maš x⸣ […]

---

31. *saḫ-lé-e ina* A [G]AZI^{SAR} *tara-bak* ZÍD.ŠE.SA.A […]
32. ŠEM.MEŠ *u* ^{Ú}*imḫur-lim ana* IGI *ta-šap-paḫ ina* x[…]
33. Ì TAG KÚM-*su* LAL 4 NÍG.LAL GIG x[…]

---

34. ^{ŠEM}[o o *ina*] A GAZI^{SAR} *tara-bak* ZÌ.KUM ZÍD GAZI^{S}[^{AR} …]
35. *ana* IGI *t*[*a-šap*]-*paḫ* Ì TAG KÚM-*su* LAL-*id* x […]

---

36. ^{ŠEM}x [o?] ^{ŠEM}BULUḪ ILLU ^{ŠEM}BULUḪ ^{ŠEM}ḪAB [^{ŠEM}]LI x […]
37. ^{GIŠ}ER[IN o o?] LÀL Ì.UDU SUMUN 8 NÍG.LAL x x nap tu […]

---

38. ^{ŠEM}GÚR.GÚR [^{ŠEM}LI ^{Ú}]KUR.KUR ŠEM.ŠEŠ ILLU ^{ŠEM}BULUḪ ^{ŠEM}[BULUḪ]
39. *qí-lip* ZÚ.L[UM.MA x]x ka nim DUḪ.LÀL Ì.UDU ÉLLAG UDU.NÍTA *šá* ⸢150?⸣
40. MÚD ^{GIŠ}ERIN 11[+ Ú].ḪI.A *šá a-pí-iš$_6$-šat*[51] *ina* IZI *tu-šá-ḫa-an*

---

41. *ana šig-ga-ti šup-*[(*šu-ḫ*)]*i* Ú BABBAR ILLU LI.DUR ILLU ^{ŠEM}BULUḪ
42. PA ^{Ú}ÚKUŠ.GÍL N[(UMUN ^{Ú}*lap-ti*)] ^{ŠEM}ŠEŠ ^{ŠEM}GÚR.GÚR NAGA.SI
43. KI.A.^{d}ÍD A.GAR.GAR MAŠ.[(DÀ)] ‹(ZÚ.LUM.MA NI.TUK^{KI})› ZÌ.KUM DUḪ.LÀL Ì.UDU ÉLLAG NÍG.LÁL *šig-ga$_{14}$-ti*

---

44. ZÍD *šib-ri* ZÍD LAGAB.MUNU$_6$ ZÍD [ŠE.BAR.SUMUN (ZÍD)] ŠE.GUD ZÍD ŠE.MUŠ$_5$ ZÍD ŠE.NU.ḪA
45. ZÍD GIG ZÍD GÚ.GAL ZÍD GÚ.[TUR (ZÍD G)]Ú.NÍG.ÀR.RA ZÍD ŠE.SA.A
46. ZÍD ŠE *sa-ḫi-*⌈*in-di*⌉ ZÍD ZÍZ.ÀM [(Z)]ÍD *pu-ut-ri* ZÍD ŠÈ TU.MUŠEN
47. ZÍD NUMUN.GADA ZÍD GAZI^{SAR} BÍL.MEŠ [(ZÍD) ZAG.ḪI].LI BÍL-*te* ZÍD IM.BABBAR
48. ZÍD DUḪ.ŠE.GIŠ.Ì ḪÁD.DU-*ti* ZÍD ^{GI}[(^{Š}ÙR SUMUN ZÍ)]D GI.GI.SAL BÀD SUMUN
49. ZÍD ŠIKA IM.ŠU.RIN.NA SUMUN ZÍD M[(UNU$_6$ ZÍD)] *ḫa-ḫe-e šá* UDUN
50. ZÍD *di-ik-me-ni šá* ^{DUG}ÚTUL ZÍD ^{Ú}*ṣa-d*[(*a-ni* ZÍD ^{GI})]^{Š}*si-ḫi* ZÍD ‹(GIŠ)›*ar-ga-ni*
51. ZÍD ^{GIŠ}LUM.ḪA ZÍD ^{Ú}*áp-ru-še* ‹(ZÍD)› ^{Ú}*ak-tam* ZÍD ⌈A⌉.[(GAR.GAR MAŠ.DÀ)] ZÍD ^{Ú}*ṣa-ṣu-un-*[(*tu*)]
52. ZÍD ^{GIŠ}ERIN ZÍD ^{GIŠ}ŠUR.MÌN ZÍD ^{GIŠ}*dup-ra-ni* ZÍD ^{Š}[(^{EM})]GÚR.GÚR ZÍD ^{ŠEM}⌈LI⌉
53. [(ZÍ)]D ŠEM.GAM.MA ZÍD ^{ŠEM}ŠEŠ ZÍD ^{ŠEM}GÍR ZÍD ^{ŠEM}[(SAL ZÍD ^{ŠEM}MUG ZÍD ^{ŠE})]^{M}GIG
54. [(ZÍD)] GI.DÙG.GA ZÍD ^{GIŠ}MAN.DU PAP 46 ZÍD.DA.MEŠ [Ú.ḪI].A
55. [(*u* ŠE)]M.ḪI.A *si-ku* GAL-*ú na-aṣ-*[*ma-t*]*i* ‹(MAŠ.MAŠ-*ti*)› *a-*[(*s*)]*u-t*[(*i*)]
56. [(*kab-di*)] *ana šup-šu-ḫi áš-ṭa* (variant: *šag-gá*) *ana lu-ub-bu-ki saḫ-ra* [(*a-na su-up-pu-ḫi*)]
57. [(MÚD.BABBAR *a-na p*)]*a-ta-ḫi še-bir-te ana* ⌈*ke*⌉*-še-ri šá-ḫi-it-t*[(*e a-na-pá-ru-ri*)]
58. [(*bít-qa*)] *a-*[(*na ka*)]*-ṣa-ri šum$_4$-ma* EN.TE.NA *ina* KAŠ.[(SAG)]
59. [(*šum$_4$-ma* AMA.MEŠ *ina* A GAZI^{SAR} ŠID-*aš*) *in*]*a* Ì.NUN TAG.TAG LAL-*id-*[(*ma* TI-*uṭ*)]

---

60. [(ÉN A.ZU.KALAM.MA)] ⌈^{d}⌉NIN.Ì.SI.IN.NA.[K(E)]$_4$! AMA ARḪUŠ.K[(ALAM.MA ME.EN)]
61. [(AGRIG É.KUR)] ⌈NIN⌉ É.DUB.B[(A)]

iv

1. [(UŠ)UM.(GAL AN.NA)] NIN.SAG.G[(I$_6$.GA.KE$_4$)]
2. [(^{d}URAŠ DAGAL.LA)] ^{d}KUD (variant ^{d}KUR) KALAG [(BA.GAR.RA *š*)*a*]
3. [*ina* (AN-*e a*)]-⌈*ge*⌉ *nam!-ri-ri šá* ^{d}*A-n*[(*im* ^{d}EN.LÍL *u* ^{d}*É-a*)]

4. [(*iš-ku*)]-*nu-ši re-eš* ⌈BÁRA⌉ KUR.KUR [*ša* (DINGIR.MEŠ GAL.MEŠ *i-na*)]-⌈*áš*!⌉-*šú-u-ši* ‹‹*ki*››
5. [o o (*paṭ-r*)]*a Ḫu-bur* ŠE.GÁ.GÁ ^{d}*É-a za-ru-ú šá* KUR
6. [(*ul-gi-r*)]*i-tum til-la-tum* IM.MA.AN.ŠUB
7. [(Á)B *in*(*a* SI)]-*šá* U$_{8}$ *ina* SÍG.ḪI.A-*šá* ⌈^{ÍD}⌉*Ir*(!)-*ḫa-an ina kib-ri-šá*
8. [(*šá i-na-ḫ*)]*u lid-di-ma pa-áš-ḫu liš-ši*
9. [(*qí-ba-a*)]-⌈*ma*⌉ *šá* NENNI A NENNI *pa-rik-ta-šú li-šír*
10. [ÉN (*šu-u š*)]*um-šu maš-ka-du ki-nu-us-su ul maš*!-*ka-du*
11. *ki-nu-us-su šu-u šum-šu*
12. *ul-tu* MUL *šá-ma-me ur-da*
13. *ur-dam-ma ul-tu* MUL *šá-ma-mi*
14. *mi-šil im-ti šá* MUŠ *il-qí mi-šil im-ti šá* GÍR.TAB *il-qí*
15. *pa-a la* GAR-*in* GAR-*in šin-ni šin-ni la* GAR-[*i*]*n ṣa-bit* SA.MEŠ
16. ŠU.SI.MEŠ *la* GAR-*in ṣa-bit kap-pal-ti*
17. *ki-ma šar-ti qa-tan la i-du ina* UZU.MEŠ
18. *ul i-šá-a pa-na u* KÁ *iṣ-bat giš-šá kìn-ṣa ki-ṣil-la*
19. *qab-la ra-pa-áš-tu u šá-šal-li gu-ub-gu-ba pu-ḫur* SA.MEŠ
20. *ṣa-bit šá* NENNI A NENNI *pu-ḫur ka-li-šú-nu* SA.GAL
21. *ul-tú* U$_{4}$-*um i* ᵓ-*al-du ul-la-nu-um-ma* ⌈*ib*⌉-*ni-šu* DINGIR-*šu*
22. IN.DIB IN.⌈SAR IN⌉.[(DU$_{8}$ *lip-pa-ṭir liṭ-ṭa-ri*)]*d lik-ka-mi*
23. É[(N *ul y*)]*a*-⌈*ut*⌉-*tú* ÉN [(^{d}*É-a u* ^{d})]⌈*Asal*⌉-*lú-ḫi*
24. [(ÉN ^{d})]*Da-mu u* [(^{d}*Gu-l*)]*a*
25. ⌈ÉN⌉ ^{d}NIN.GÌRIMA [(EN)] ÉN
26. *šu-nu iq-bu-ni-ma ana-ku ú-šá*-[(*an-ni šap-liš lit-t*)]*a-ṣi-ma*
27. *e-liš a-a i-li* EME.ḪUL.GÁL BAR.[(ŠÈ ḪÉ.EM.TA.GUB)][52]

---

28. KA.INIM.MA ⌈SA⌉.[(GAL.LA.KÁM)]

---

29. KÌD.KÌD.BI SÍG.ÀKA ^{MUNUS}SILA$_{4}$.NIM! *u* MUNUS.SILA$_{4}$.NIM! *ina* [S(A)] MAŠ.DÀ
30. NU.NU $^{\text{NA}_4}$*šu-u* NÍTA *u* MUNUS $^{\text{NA}_4}$GUG $^{\text{NA}_4}$PA $^{\text{NA}_4}$*iá-ni-bu*
31. $^{\text{NA}_4}$ŠUBA $^{\text{NA}_4}$*zi-bitu* $^{\text{NA}_4}$*a-ba-aš-mu* $^{\text{NA}_4}$ZÁLAG $^{\text{NA}_4}$KUR-*nu* DIB.BA
32. $^{\text{NA}_4}$*kak-ku-sak-ku* $^{\text{NA}_4}$PEŠ$_{4}$.A.A[(B.B)]A È ^{Ú}*kur-ka-nam ina* SÍG.SA$_{5}$
33. [(7)] *líp-pi tál-pap ina* ⌈*giš*⌉-*ši-šu* KEŠDA-*as-ma i-šal-lim*

---

34. [ÉN *kiš*-(*pu ze-r*)]*u-tum it-ta-ṣu-ú ana ki-di* (catchline)
35. (colophon)

TRANSLATION

(ii 51–54) You crush together (and) sift *kukru*, *kasû*, roasted grain flour, riverbank silt, malt lumps (variant: flour), "dove dung," ox dung patty, gazelle dung, *gaṣṣu*-gypsum, wheat flour, slag from a new kiln, reeds, blood,[53] (and) assorted incense. You boil (it) in beer (and) bandage (him with it). Fourteen (plants): a bandage to make (limbs) go straight.

(iii 1–2) You grind together *kukru*, *burāšu*-juniper, *aktam*, flax seed, *kasû*, malt lumps, wheat flour, *isqūqu* flour (and) winnowed beerwort. You massage (it) into leather (and) bandage (him with it). Nine (plants): a bandage for stiffness.

(iii 3–5) Nine (plants): *kukru*, kidney fat from a wether, *baluḫḫu*-aromatic, *baluḫḫu*-aromatic resin, *abukkatu* resin, *šupuḫru*-cedar, *asu*-myrtle oil, *erēnu*-cedar resin, (and) *ṭūru*-aromatic are a bandage for stiffness.

(iii 6–8) These (plants): kidney fat from a wether, wax, *baluḫḫu*-aromatic, *baluḫḫu*-aromatic resin, *kukru*, *abukkatu* resin, myrrh, *šupuḫru*-cedar, *asu*-myrtle oil (and) *ṭūru*-aromatic are a bandage for stiffness due to the cold season.[54]

(iii 9–11) Eleven plants: *kukru*, *burāšu*-juniper, myrrh, *ṣumlalû*, ⌜*abukkatu*⌝ resin, [*baluḫḫu*-aromatic], *baluḫḫu*-aromatic resin, *ṭūru*-aromatic, *erēnu*-cedar resin, […], (and) *atāʾišu* are a bandage for stiffness.

(iii 12–13) You mix oven slag, malt dregs, malt lumps, (and) […] with *isqūqu*-flour. You boil (it) in *kasû* juice (and) bandage (him with it). Four (plants): a bandage for his neck for ⌜stiffness⌝.

(iii 14–15) ⌜You make⌝ […] flour, malt lump flour, roasted *kasû* flour (and) [kiln] slag ⌜into a dough⌝ with […] (and) bandage (him with it). Four (plants): a bandage for inflammation(?).

(iii 16–17) (For inflammation[?]), these four flours: flour made from the fruit of *nurmû*-pomegranate, flour made from the fruit of the *ašāgu*-thorn, flour made from the seed of *papparḫu* (and) flour made from the seed of *lišān kalbi* [you daub] on the ⌜sore spot⌝.

(iii 18–19) You boil roasted *saḫlû*-cress (and) powdered *kasû* in beer. ‹(You bandage)› (him with it) for three days. Three (plants): a bandage for a sprained(?) foot.

(iii 20–21) Afterwards, on the fourth day, you char (and) grind stag horn (and) date stones. You mix (it) with oil. You rub (him) gently with ghee (and bandage him with it). Two (plants): a bandage for sore due to a sprain(?).

(iii 22–23) [You mix] roasted grain flour, *kasû* flour, *isqūqu*-flour with […] oil. You boil (it) [over] a ⌜fire⌝. Three (plants): a bandage for […].

(iii 24–30) [#] plants: […], [*baluḫḫu*]-⌜aromatic⌝ resin, […]. roasted grain flour, […], […]-aromatic flour, […], myrrh, […], ⌜*abukkatu*⌝ resin, […], used grease (and) ⌜wax⌝, [#] plants are a bandage for …

(iii 31–33) You decoct[55] *saḫlû*-cress in *kasû* juice. You scatter roasted grain flour, [...], *libanātu*-incense and *imḫur-lim* on it. [You ... (it)] in [...]. You smear (him) with oil (and) bandage (him with it) while it is still hot. Four plants: a bandage for ...

(iii 34–35) You decoct [...] in *kasû* juice. You sprinkle *isqūqu*-flour, ⌜*kasû*⌝ flour and [...] on it. You smear (him) with oil (and) bandage (him with it) while it is still hot. [...]

(iii 36–37) Eight (plants): [...]-aromatic, *baluḫḫu*-aromatic, *baluḫḫu*-aromatic resin, *ṭūru*-aromatc, ⌜*kikkirānu*-juniper berries(?)⌝, [...], ⌜*erēnu*⌝-cedar(?), honey/wax, (and) used grease are a bandage for ...

(iii 38–40) You heat over a fire *kukru*, [*burāšu*-juniper], *atā'išu*, myrrh, *baluḫḫu*-aromatic resin, [*baluḫḫu*-aromatic, ⌜date⌝ rind, ..., wax, fat from the left kidney of a wether (and) *erēnu*-cedar resin in the usual proportions.

(iii 41–43) If you want to soothe stiffness, "white plant," *abukkatu* resin, *baluḫḫu*-aromatic resin, *irrû* leaves, *laptu*-turnip seed, myrrh, *kukru*, *uḫḫūlu qarnānu*, *kibrītu*-sulphur, gazelle droppings, ‹(*asnû*)› *isqūqu*-flour, wax (and) kidney fat are a bandage for stiffness.

(iii 44–59) Coarsely ground flour, malt lump flour, [old barley] flour, *arsuppu* flour, *šigūšu* flour, powdered straw, wheat flour, *ḫallūru*-chick pea flour. ⌜*kakku*⌝-lentil flour, *kiššēnu*-bean flour, roasted grain flour, yeasted grain flour, emmer flour, powdered ox-dung patty, "dove dung" flour, flax seed flour, roasted *kasû* flour, roasted ⌜*saḫlû*-cress⌝ flour, powdered *gaṣṣu* gypsum, powdered dried sesame residue, powdered old roof beam, powdered reed screen from an abandoned wall, powdered fragment of an old oven, malt flour, powdered kiln slag, powdered ashes from a *dīqaru*-bowl, *ṣadānu* flour, *sīḫu*-wormwood flour, *argannu* flour, *barirātu* flour, *aprušu* flour, *aktam* flour, gazelle dung flour, *ṣaṣuntu* flour, *erēnu*-cedar flour, *šurmēnu*-cypress flour, *daprānu*-juniper flour, *kukru* flour, *burāšu*-juniper flour, *ṣumlalû* flour, myrrh flour, *asû*-myrtle flour, *šimešallu* flour, *ballukku*-aromatic flour, *kanaktu*-aromatic flour, "sweet reed" flour, (and) *su'ādu*-flour, a total of fourty-six flours. (These are) [plants] and aromatics, a great powder (for) ⌜bandages⌝ of medicine and pharmacology to soothe what feels heavy, to lubricate what is *ašṭu*-stiff (variant: *šaggu*-stiff), to stretch out what is bent, to stop the flow of pus, to straighten up what is fractured,[56] for what jerks violently to be disconnected (and) to repair what is broken into pieces. If it is winter, you make it into a dough with first quality beer, if summer with *kasû* juice. You repeatedly rub him ⌜with⌝ ghee. If you bandage him with it, he should recover.

(iii 60–iv 9) Recitation: *Asû* of the land, Ninisinna, you are the merciful mother of the land, steward of the Ekur, mistress of the library, ⌜dragon⌝ of heaven, mistress of the black headed (people). She is the one (for whom) Urash (Ninurta), broad (of understanding), mighty divine judge (variant: mountain) was established (as husband). She is ⌜the one⌝ for whom Anu, Enlil, and Ea established a tiara of resplendence [in] the heavens, the backrest of the dias of the lands [which] the great gods carry for her. ... Release (the river) Hubur, pleasing to Ea, sower of the land; let it irrigate the ... vines. The ⌜cow with⌝ its horn, the ewe with its wool, the river Irhan with its bank—may he who is tired put (his burden) down and may the one at ease take (it) up. Command that the judgment against so-and-so, son of so-and-so be straightened out.

(iv 10–27) That is its name, *maškadu* is its true name. Is not *maškadu* its true name? That is its name. It came down from the star(s) of heaven. It came down from the star(s) of heaven and took half of the venom of a snake. It took half the venom of a scorpion. It does not have a mouth (but) it has teeth. It does not have (real) teeth (but) it grips the muscles. It does not have fingers (but) it grips the flat of the foot. It is thin as a hair; it cannot be recognized in the flesh. It does not have a face or mouth (but) it grips the hip socket, lower leg, ankle, hip, coccyx and lower back, the calf,[57] all of the muscles. It has gripped those of so-and-so, son of so-and-so, each and every one of them, since the day *sagallu* was born, since its god created it. May it be bound, may it be sent away, may it be released. May it be released, may it be sent away, may it be bound.[58] The spell is not mine; it is the spell of Ea and Asalluhi. It is the spell of Damu and Gula. It is the spell of Ningirimma, mistress of spell(s). They said (it) and I repeated (it). Let (the illness) go out downwards; may it not come up (again). May the evil tongue stand aside.

(iv 28) Recitation for *sagallu.*

(iv 29–33) Its ritual: you twine together a tuft of wool from a male and female spring lamb with gazelle ⌜tendon⌝. You thread (it) with male and female *šû*-stone, carnelian, coral, *ianibu*-stone, *šubû*-stone, *ṣibittu*-stone, *abašmû*-stone, *zalaqqu*-stone, magnetic hematite, *kakkusakku*-stone (and) sea *išqillatu*-shell. You wind *kurkānu*-turmeric into seven burls with red wool. If you tie (it) to his hip socket, he should recover.

(iv 34) [The recitation] "⌜Sorcery⌝ and hate magic got out to the outside" (is next). *(catchline)*

NOTES

1. For more on itching and scratching, see Stol 2007b, 235.

2. The original from which the scribe was copying was broken at this point and, as usual with ancient scribes, the copyist did not try to fill in the gap but simply put "broken."

3. See Deller 1990, no. 3.

4. See Beeson and McDermot 1975, 412–16.

5. BAM 508 iv 12 has AN IMIN KI IMIN ... IGI IMIN BAR IMIN BAR.TA IG[I IMIN].

6. For the recitation, see Finkel 1999, no. 30; Böck 2007, 64–65; Schuster-Brandis 2008, 378, 386, 388.

7. Alternatively, one could read *bu-ṣi-na*. However this is rarely written out and hardly, if ever, comes in male and female.

8. Labat's GÙG (= TAR), ruled nonexistent in MZL² no. 9 and its number assigned to another sign, is here shown to exist.

9. For the recitation, see Böck 2007, 45–46, 150–58.

10. SpTU 4.129 vi 43 has ME.ŠÈ BA.DA.RI KI.ŠÈ BA.DA.ZÁḪ

11. BAM 508 iv 11 has ME.ŠÈ GUB.BA IGI.MU N[U.GUB.BA]

12. See Scurlock and Andersen 2005, 3.222

13. See chapter 3, n. 109.

14. This is the same as *imḫur-ešra*.

15. See Scurlock and Andersen 2005, 10.133.

16. Schwemer 2011, 43 interprets this as male and female *buṣinnu* (^{GIŠ}*bu-ṣí-na*). However, sexual differentiation is otherwise unattested for *buṣinnu*, and is highly unusual for plants other than mandrake and date palms.

17. For this expression, see Scurlock and Andersen 2005, 27. The fat is hot because it is allegedly being taken from a fresh corpse. Schwemer 2011, 44 interprets this expression as *ḫarḫaru*: "scoundrel," which seems less likely. *Deckname* for plants are not usually of this type. In either case, we are dealing with a plant.

18. See above, n. 16.

19. See Scurlock and Andersen 2005, 3.219.

20. See Scurlock and Andersen 2005, 3.220.

21. *Talmu* is Hurrian for "large."

22. For the suggestion that this is GUD_4 for KUD: *šebru*, see Tsukimoto 1999, 198. *Šebru* means literally "broken," a close equivalent to English "cracked" as in "cracked wheat." This quite ancient method of preparing grain for eating requires boiling, and then sun drying, the kernels.

23. For the full text of this recitation, see Böck 2007, 45–46, 150–58

24. See Scurlock and Andersen 2005, 3.179.

25. See Scurlock and Andersen 2005, 3.186.

26. See chapter 3, n. 109.

27. See *CAD* Š/2, 48 s.v. *šarāku* B.

28. Pace *CAD* I/J, 88b, this passage has nothing to do with penises!

29. See Finkel 1998, 81 n. 10 and Collins 1999, 277–78.

30. BAM 3 ii 7–8 adds here: MURUB_4 SAG.DU-*šú u* SAG.KI^{II}.MEŠ-*šú* TAG.MEŠ-*šú*.

31. The translation of the end of the spell is after a suggestion by Worthington 2005, 21 followed by Heeßel 2011c, 50.

32. BAM 3 ii 7–8 adds here: "(and) the middle of his head (and) his temples continually hurt him intensely." See Scurlock and Andersen 2005, 3.190.

33. See Scurlock and Andersen 2005, 3.246.

34. See chapter 3, n. 109.

35. See Scurlock and Andersen 2005, 3.241.

36. For the translation of *saḫlû* as "cress," see Stol 1983–84, 24–32.

37. See chapter 3, n. 109.

38. See Scurlock and Andersen 2005, 3.251.

39. See Scurlock and Andersen 2005, 3.242.

40. See Scurlock and Andersen 2005, 3.243.

41. See Scurlock and Andersen 2005, 3.247.

42. See chapter 3, n. 109.

43. See Scurlock and Andersen 2005, 3.244.

44. See Scurlock and Andersen 2005, 3.245.

45. See Scurlock and Andersen 2005, 3.248.

46. The hanging *-ma* which appears at the end of phrases seems to function like our "etc." See chapter 6, text 2 ad line 62.

47. This could also be *ballukku*-aromatic.

48. See Scurlock and Andersen 2005, 3.252.

49. See Scurlock and Andersen 2005, 3.253.

50. Both duplicates substitute ^{ŠEM}ŠEŠ.

51. There are only a few references to this mysterious lemma. The BAM 124 context has something wrong with the feet that makes walking difficult; BAM 177:1–7 is an extract tablet (the other entry on the tablet is enteric fever); *KADP* 36 is a shelf list. This is unlikely to have anything to do with Apišaleans; more probably we are dealing with *apšitu* which would represent a Sumerian loanword for "agreed proportion."

52. This recitation is edited in Collins 1999, 243–49 as *maškadu* 8.

53. This is a key element in Yemeni cement.

54. See Scurlock and Andersen 2005, 11.9.

55. See chapter 3, n. 109.

56. See Scurlock and Andersen 2005, 11.2.

57. Literally: "alabastron-shaped (part of the body)."

58. Note that the Sumerian and Akkadian phrases form a magic circle.

8

HEART AND LUNGS

A. HEART

Ancient physicians observed the heart's rate and rhythm, observed the pulse, and treated crushing pain in the heart with salves, fumigants, and potions. There are also descriptions of what appear to be congestive heart failure. For more details, see Scurlock and Andersen 2005, 165–77.

TEXT 1: BAM 388

BAM 388 column i begins with a fumigant for stroke (i 1–2) and continues with fumigants (i 3–7) and a salve (i 8–11) for a crushing sensation in the chest. All are formatted in such a way as to suggest a pharmacist as the ultimate source. The last treatment of potions and a bath (i 12–18) is parallel to BAM 445:10–25,[1] which lists the symptoms to be treated as follows: "If a person continually has a crushing sensation in his heart, [his limbs are continually tense], his tongue is continually cramped, he ⸢bites⸣ his lips, his ears continually ring, his hands go numb, [his knees] give him a gnawing pain, his upper abdomen (epigastrium) continually ⸢protrudes⸣, his desire to go to a woman is diminished, chills keep falling on him, [he is now fat and now thin], spittle keeps falling from his mouth and [...].[2] The ancient physician's suspicion was that the patient had been poisoned. If so, it was with a cardiotoxic poison.

i

1. [... Ú.K]UR.RA ^{Ú}*kám*-gad-du*
2. [... *qù-t*]*aru šá mi-šit-tú*

---

3. [(MUŠ.DÍM.GURIN.NA U_5.MEŠ *šá* EDIN) ^{ŠE}]^{M}LI ^{GIŠ}ŠINIG
4. [(^{Ú}*kur-ka-nam*)] ^{Ú}KUR.KUR KI.A.^{d}ÍD
5. [(ŠÈ $BURU_5$.ḪABRUD.DA)] ŠE.KAK ^{GIŠ}MES *ka-mun*
6. [(^{GIŠ}ŠINIG 10 Ú.ḪI.A)] *qù-taru šá* GAZ ŠÀ

---

7. [(^{Ú}*kur-ka-nam* ^{Ú}K)]UR.KUR NAGA.SI *ina* DÈ SAR *qù-taru šá* GAZ ŠÀ

---

8. [(MÚD BU)]RU$_4$.GI$_6$^{MUŠEN} $^{\text{NA}_4}$ZÁLAG Ú DILI KA *tam-tim nu-ṣa-bu*
9. [(^{GIŠ}ŠUR.MÌN)] ^{Ú}*su-pa-lu* NIM UR.GI$_7$ *up-pat tim-bu-ut-tum*-A.ŠÀ
10. [(SAḪAR DAL)].ḪA.MUN SAḪAR.SILA.LIMMU.BA ^{Ú}NAM.LÚ.U$_{18}$.LU
11. [(^{GIŠ}ŠINI)]G 14 Ú *nap-šal-tú šá* GAZ ŠÀ-*bi*

---

12. [(1 GÍN ^{Ú}*tar-mu*)]*š* 1/2 GÍN ^{Ú}*imḫur-lim* 4-*tú* ^{Ú}*imḫur*-20 1 GÍN ^{GIŠ}ŠINIG
13. [(1 GÍN ^{Ú}IN$_6$.ÚŠ 1/2)] GÍN ^{Ú}SIKIL 1 GÍN ^{Ú}*el-kul-lum*
14. [(1/2 GÍN KA.A.AB.BA 1)] GÍN *la-pat ár-man-nu* 1 GÍN NUMUN $^{\text{‹(GIŠ)›}}$ḪA.LU.ÚB
15. [(1 GÍN ^{Ú}*úr-né*)]-⸢*e*⸣ 1 GÍN ^{Ú}ḪAR.ḪAR 1 GÍN
16. [(^{Ú}LUḪ.MAR.TU 1 G)]ÍN ^{Ú}NU.LUḪ.ḪA 4-*tú* (variant: 1/2 GÍN) ^{Ú}KUR.KUR
17. [(1 GÍN ^{ŠEM})LI # GÍN (^{GI})]^{Š}ḪAŠḪUR.^{GIŠ}GI
18. [(1/2 GÍN GI.ŠUL.ḪI 1 GÍN NUMUN ^{GIŠ}ŠINIG) # GÍN] ^{Ú}*ši* x *tum*

19–20. [… (-*šú-nu* ḪÁD.DU GAZ S)IM … (*ina še-rim ba-lu pa-t*)*an* … (NAG-*šú*) … *tu*-(*šap-ra-šú-ma* EGIR-*šú*) *ina* (A ŠEG$_6$-*šal ina*) G(EŠTIN SUR.RA NAG) … (x-x ŠUB-*di ina* U$_4$.NÁ.A TU$_5$-*šú-ma* TI)][3]

Translation

(i 1–2) […] ⸢*nīnû*-mint⸣, *kamkādu*, and […] are ⸢fumigants⸣ for stroke.

(i 3–6) Copulating *pizzalurtu*-lizards from the steppe, *burāšu*-juniper, *bīnu*-tamarisk, *kurkānu*-turmeric, *atāʾišu*, *kibrītu*-sulphur, *ḫurri*-bird excrement, *mēsu*-tree shoots, (and) *kamunu*-fungus growing on a *bīnu*-tamarisk are ten plants for a fumigant for crushing sensation in the chest.

(i 7) You fumigate him with *kurkānu*-turmeric, *atāʾišu*, (and) *uḫḫulu qarnānu* over coals. This is a fumigant for crushing sensation in the chest.

(i 8–11) Blood of a black *āribu*-crow, *zalaqqu*-stone, "lone plant," *imbû tamtim*, *nuṣābu*, *šurmēnu*-cypress, *supalu*-plant, fly (i.e., flea) from a dog, *uppatu*-insect, *timbut-eqli*-insect, dust from a duststorm, dust from a crossroads, *amilānu*, (and) *bīnu*-tamarisk are fourteen plants for a salve for crushing sensation in the chest.

(i 12–20) You dry, crush (and) ⸢sift⸣ 1 shekel of *tarmuš*, 1/2 shekel of *imḫur-lim*, 1/4 shekel of *imḫur-ešra*, 1 shekel of *bīnu*-tamarisk, 1 shekel of *maštakal*, 1/2 shekel of *sikillu*, 1 shekel of *erkulla*, 1/2 shekel of *imbû tamtim*, 1 shekel of *lapat armanni*, 1 shekel of *ḫaluppu*-tree seed, 1 shekel of *urnû*-mint, 1 shekel of *ḫašû*-thyme, 1 shekel of *šibburratu*, 1 shekel of *nuḫurtu*, 1/4 (variant:

1/2) shekel of *atāʾišu*, 1 shekel of [*burāšu*-juniper, x shekel of] "swamp apple," 1/2 shekel of *qan šalāli*-reed, 1 shekel of *bīnu*-tamarisk (and) [... You pour (it) down into ...] In the morning, you have him drink (it) on an empty stomach. You induce vomiting [with a feather] and then afterwards you boil (it) [in] water (and) have him drink (it mixed) with drawn wine. You pour (it) down [into ...]. If you bathe him (with it) on the day of the new moon, he should recover.

B. LUNGS

Ancient Mesopamian lungs were spared tobacco smoking and modern pollution, but they still suffered from pneumonia, empyema, tuberculosis, pertussis, anaerobic lung abscesses, and pulmonary edema. For details, see Scurlock and Andersen 2005, 42–48 and 177–84. The basic strategy for treating lung problems of all types was to clear the lungs, for which purpose emetic and laxative potions were generally employed. There were also bandages and baths and, more rarely, salves to loosen things up. The use of aspirants had the virtue of clearing the nasal passages as well as the lungs. In addition to the medicines, the patient might be given hot broth, typically made from pork (BAM 548 i 5–7, 12–13). Winter required special measures, as keeping the patient near a fire (BAM 548 i 5–7) or bandaging with carded wool (BM 78963: 47, cf. 17–18, 45–46).

1. COUGH

TEXT 2: BAM 548

BAM 548 represents the fifth tablet of the sixth sub-series of UGU (see chapter 3, text 1). It consists of potions (i 1–18, 25–28, iv 2′–5', 14′–15′), aliments (i 5–7, 12–13) and aspirants (i 19–24, iv 6′–12′) for *suʾālu*-cough.[4] As is clear from this text, the production of the desired vomiting of phlegm was something of an art. The tongue was held (i 14–16) to avoid premature, and a feather used (i 14–16) to ensure, eventual vomiting. Salt, which encourages vomiting, was given first to start the process (i 12–13) and honey, which discourages vomiting, to moderate the amount or to stop the process from continuing too long (i 12–13, 14–16).

Of special interest are lines i 19–24, which require the patient to aspirate a boiling plant mixture via a hollow reed and iv 6′–12′ in which the aspirant is a distillate. The procedure, as this can be reconstructed from this and similar treatments (e.g., BAM 558 iv 15–19—chapter 8, text 4) was simple, but ingenious. The plant mixture to be distilled went into a crescent-shaped *diqāru* bowl and a second, *burzigallu*, bowl with a hole bored into it was inverted over the top and sealed round the rim with a dough made from emmer flour. When the bottom bowl was put over a fire, the mixture boiled and distillate condensed onto the cool upper bowl where it was harvested by means of a straw inserted through the hole. The reed also served a secondary purpose of slapping more of the distillate onto the patient's chest.

i

1. [DIŠ NA *su-a-l*]*am* GIG *ana ša-ḫa-ṭi* ^{Ú}EME.UR.GI$_7$ [(SIG$_7$ *tu-pa-ṣa*)]
2. [...] GAZI^{SAR} *ḫaš-la-a-ti* : *qa-lu-ti ana* ŠÀ ŠUB-*di* [(ḪE.ḪE NAG-*ma*)]
3. [*lu ina* KA]-*šú lu ina* DÚR-*šú i-šaḫ-ḫa-ṭa-a*[(*m-ma* TI-*uṭ*)]

---

4. [DIŠ KI.MIN] A *u* Ì+GIŠ EME-*šú* DIB-*bat* N[(AG.NAG)]

---

5. [ZAG].ḪI.LI *ṭe-ne-tim* GAZI^{SAR} *pa-ʾ*-[(*ṣú-tim*)]
6. [GIN$_7$ *ra*]-*bi-ki tara-bak ina* Ì+GIŠ *u* LÀL GU$_7$ A UZU ŠA[(Ḫ)]
7. [(NAG)]-*šú* IZI *ana* IGI-*šú ta-šár-rap ina* DÚR-*šú ú-šeš-še-r*[(*a-am-ma* TI)]

---

8. [DIŠ N]A *su-a-lam* GIG ^{Ú}EME.UR.GI$_7$ SIG$_7$-*su* GIN$_7$ LU.ÚB[(^{SAR} ŠEG$_6$.GÁ)]
9. [*ina*] GA.KU$_7$.KU$_7$ *u* Ì *ḫal-ṣi* ḪE.ḪE NU *pa-tan* NAG-*ma* [(TI)]

---

10. [DIŠ] KI.MIN NUMUN ^{GIŠ}GI.ZÚ.LUM.MA ḪÁD.DU *ta-sàk ina* A GAZI^{SA}[(^{R} *sek-ru-ti*)]
11. [*b*]*a-aḫ-ru-te* NU *pa-tan* NAG-*ma i-ár-rù-ma* [(TI)]

---

12. DIŠ KI.MIN LAG MUN *a-sal-lim ina* KA-*šú* GAR-*ma ú-ma-raq* A-*šu* ⌜*ú*⌝-[(*al-lat*)]
13. A UZU ŠAḪ *kab-ru-te* NAG KAŠ LÀL NAG U$_4$.3.KÁM GUR.[(GUR-*šum-ma* TI)]

---

14. DIŠ KI.MIN Ú BABBAR *ina* KAŠ.SAG LÀL Ì *ḫal-ṣi* GAZ NU *pa-t*[(*an* EME-*šú* DIB-*bat*)]
15. KAŠ LÀL *baḫ-ra* NAG-*šú ina* Á *tu-šap*-[(*ra-šu-ma*)]
16. EGIR-*šu ra-bi-ki* KI LÀL *u* Ì.NUN NAG GEŠTIN DÙ[(G.GA NAG-*ma* TI)]

---

17. DIŠ NA *su-a-lum* DIB-*su da-li-la* [(*šá* ŠÀ ^{NA_4}PEŠ$_4$)]

18. *tur-ár ta-sàk ina* Ì *ḫal-ṣi* [(NAG-*ma* TI)]

---

19. DIŠ KI.MIN IM.KAL.GUG ^{GIŠ}ERIN ^{ŠEM}BAL [(NUMUN ^{Ú}SI.SÁ)]
20. GI DÙG.GA ZÌ.KUM ZAG.ḪI.LI ^{GIŠ}GÚR.GÚR ^{GIŠ}LI [(^{Ú}ÁB.DUḪ)]
21. [(ILLU ^{ŠEM}BULUḪ)] Ì.UDU ÉLLAG UDU.NÍTA *ina* ^{GIŠ}N[(ÀGA GAZ)]
22. […] x DÈ SA$_5$ TI-*q*[(*í*) … (*ḫu-ru-up-pa*)]
23. [(K)Ù.(SIG$_{17}$) *ina* UGU ŠEG$_6$]-*šal*! GI.SAG.KU[D *ta-pal-la-aš-ma*]
24. [*ana* ŠÀ GAR E$_{11}$]-⸢*ma*⸣ KA-*šú* GÍD-*m*[(*a*) …][5]

---

25. DIŠ NA [*su-a-la*]*m* GIG x[…]
26. x[…] MEŠ *ina* […]
27. 10 [… (Ì.NUN) …]
28. x[… (NAG.MEŠ-*ma*) TI]

---

iv

1′. *ša* IGI […]

2′. DIŠ NA *su-a-lam* [GI(G Ú.BABBAR SÚD)]
3′. *ina* Ì *ḫal-ṣa* [NU (*pa-tan* NAG-*ma* TI)]

4′. DIŠ KI.MIN ^{Ú}NU.LUḪ.ḪA S[Ú(D *ina* ^{GIŠ}GEŠTIN)]
5′. *ba-lu pa-tan* N[(AG-*ma* ⸢TI⸣)]

6′. *šum$_4$-ma* DÙG NU IGI.DU$_8$ ÚT[(UL ZABAR) GAR-*an*]
7′. Ú.KUR.RA GAZ SUḪUŠ ^{GIŠ}*šu-ši* […]
8′. ^{Ú}AN.DAḪ.ŠI ^{ŠEM}GÚR.GÚR ÀR-*en* SIM Ì.G[IŠ …]
9′. KAŠ *u* Ì.NUN *ana* ŠÀ ŠUB-*di* ^{DUG}BUR.ZI.GA[L NÍG.BÙR.BÙR]
10′. Á.MEŠ-*šá ina* NÍG.ŠILAG.GÁ ZÍZ.ÀM [BAD-*ḫi*][6]
11′. *ina* IZI ŠEG$_6$-*šal* GI.SAG.KUD GIN-*an ana* [KA-*šú* (*baḫ-ra* GÍD.DA-*ma*)]
12′. *a-na* ḪAR^{II}.MEŠ-*šú* [(GAZ-*ma* TI)][7]

13′. DUB.5.KÁM-*ma* DIŠ NA K[A-(*šú* DUGUD)]

14′. DIŠ NA *su-a-lam ḫa-ḫa u ki-ṣir-tú* Ḫ[AR.MEŠ GIG (*saḫ-lé-e si-ki-te*)]
15′. *ina* KAŠ.SAG *ba-lu pa-*[*tan* (NAG-*šú*)]

Colophon (Assurbanipal's library)

TRANSLATION

(i 1–3) [If a person] is sick with ⸢*suʾalu*-cough⸣, to remove it, you pulverize fresh *lišān kalbi*. You pour [...] and crushed/roasted *kasû* on it (and) mix (it). If you have him drink (it), (phlegm) will be removed [either via] his [mouth] or via his anus and he should recover.

(i 4) [If ditto (a person is sick with *suʾalu*-cough)], you have him repeatedly drink water and oil while holding his tongue.

(i 5–7) You decoct[8] ground ⸢*saḫlû*⸣-cress[9] (and) pulverized *kasû* [till] ⸢decocted⸣. You have him eat (it) with oil and honey. You have him drink pork broth. You keep a fire burning near him. If he has a bowel movement, he should recover.

(i 8–9) [If] a ⸢person⸣ is sick with *suʾalu*-cough, you boil fresh *lišān kalbi* as you would *laptu*-vegetable. You mix (it) [with] sweet milk and pressed-out oil. If you have him drink (it) on an empty stomach, he should recover.

(i 10–11) ⸢Alternatively⸣, you dry (and) grind *buṣinnu* seed. You have him drink (it) on an empty stomach in hot oven-baked *kasû* juice and, if he vomits, he should recover.

(i 12–13) Alternatively, you put a lump of *asallu* salt in his mouth and he chews (it) up (and) swallows its water. You have him drink broth made from fatty pork. You have him drink beer (and) honey. If you repeat (this procedure) for three days, he should recover.

(i 14–16) Alternatively, you crush "white plant" in first quality beer, honey (and) pressed-out oil. (You give it to him) on an empty stomach while holding his tongue. You have him drink hot honey beer. You induce vomiting with a feather and, afterwards, you have him drink a decoction[10] with honey and ghee. If you have him drink sweet wine, he should recover.

(i 17–18) If *suʾalu*-cough afflicts a person, you char (and) grind the *dālilu* inside a *biṣṣuru*-shell. If you have him drink (it mixed) with pressed-out oil, he should recover.

(i 19–24) If ditto (a person is sick with *suʾalu*-cough), you crush *kalgukku*-clay, *erēnu*-cedar, *ballukku*-aromatic, *šurdunû* seed, "sweet reed," *isqūqu*-flour, *saḫlû*-cress, *kukru*, *burāšu*-juniper, *kamantu*-henna(?), *baluḫḫu*-aromatic resin, (and) fat from the kidney of a wether with a wooden *esittu*-pestle. [You ... (it)]. You take red (hot) coals. [...] ⸢You bring⸣ a ⸢gold⸣ *ḫuruppu*-dish ⸢to a boil⸣ [over them. You hollow out] a reed straw [and put (it) in] and, ⸢if⸣ he sucks (it) [with] his mouth, [...].

(i 25–28) If a person is sick with ⸢*suʾalu*-cough⸣, [...] in [...] ten [...] ghee [...] If you have him drink (it) repeatedly, [he should recover].

(Two columns of text lost here.)

(iv 1′) *(too fragmentary for translation)*

(iv 2′–3′) If a person ⸢is sick with⸣ *su᾿alu*-cough, you grind "white plant." If you have him drink (it mixed) with pressed-out oil on an [empty] stomach, he should recover.

(iv 4′–5′) If ditto (a person is sick with *su᾿alu*-cough), ⸢you grind⸣ *nuḫurtu*. If you have him drink (it mixed) with wine on an empty stomach, he should recover.

(iv 6′–12′) If he does not experience improvement (with the previous treatments), [you put out] a copper soup bowl. You crush *nīnû*-mint. You mill grind (and) sift *šūšu*-licorice root, [...], *antaḫšum*-vegetable (and) *kukru*. You pour [...] ⸢oil⸣, [...], beer and ghee over it. [You bore a hole in] a *burzigallu* bowl (and invert it over the other bowl). [You cover] its sides with a dough made of emmer (flour). You boil (it) over a fire. You stick in a reed straw. He should suck (it) up hot into [his mouth] and, if ⸢you pound⸣ (it)] onto his lungs,[11] he should recover.

(iv 13′) Tablet 5 of the series: "If a person's ⸢mouth⸣ (feels) heavy."

(iv 14′–15′) If a person [is sick with] *su᾿ālu*-cough, *ḫaḫḫu* and thick sputum in the ⸢lungs⸣, you have him drink powdered *saḫlû*-cress in first quality beer ⸢on an empty stomach⸣.

2. SICK LUNGS

TEXT 3: BM 78963

What is particularly interesting about this late text, besides the fact that a number of the treatments (22–24, 36–41, 58–78) give the actual amounts required for an individual patient, is the degree to which apparent divergences from the subject at hand are nothing of the kind. BM 78963 begins with two potions (1–3, 4–6) for "internal fever," an ancient Mesopotamian term for fevers with symptoms relating to the chest and abdomen. It continues with potions (7–16) and mechanical means (sucking on the finger—13) to induce vomiting and then an aliment and a potion (17–18) to stop vomiting, just the sort of thing typically used to treat lung conditions. What is most fascinating is that an aliment (19) and two potions (56–57, 58–59) for ulcers are included with the treatments for the lungs. This is for the simple reason that histamine is involved in both cases, which would have meant significant overlap in the plants used in treatments. To put it differently, ulcer treatments appear in this text because they were also useful for patients with lung problems. Indeed, lines 56–57 indicate this directly.

The next forty odd lines of the text present aspirants (20–24, 36–39, 42–43, 45–46, 50–51, 53–54), *tāriḫus* (25–35), potions (36–41, 44, 48–49, 52, 55) and a bath (47) for various problems with the lungs. Noticeable in the text is the alteration of aspirants and potions, a fact which suggests that they were meant to be used together.

This is followed by a potion (60–65) to prevent premature breaking of the waters, a potion (66–68) and pills (69–72) for urinary tract problems, a potion (73–75) for all sorts, pills and a potion (76–78) for the cold season, potions (79–81) for vomiting blood, potions (82–84) for crushing sensation in the heart and a potion(?) (85–86) for fever. What these all presumably have in common is that they would have been useful for lung conditions. This is obvious with the treatments for fever and vomiting blood, but constriction of the urethra would benefit from a vasodilator which would also be useful for congested lungs. Of these treatments, those to make a person vomit (7–16), the three for ulcers (19, 56–57, 58–59), two for the lungs (42–43, 48–49), the cure-all (73–75), the treatment for cold (76–78) and the potions for crushing sensation in the heart (82–84) are formulated in such a way as to suggest that they originated with a pharmacist.

Lines 1–3 are unusual in giving practical advice—the physician is not to worry if the patient seems to be getting worse after the administration of the treatment. Drinking in thirds means that three doses are to be given. This would be once in the morning, once at noon, and once in the evening. Lines 7–10, which exploit items available at the brewery, give insights into ancient Mesopotamian sweet beers, made with berries and dates. The stale urine of line 16 will have been essentially sterile. Lines 25–31, 32–35 give interesting examples of what ancient physicians called a *tarīḫu*. What distinguished this from similar preparations called *saḫūnu* (as, for example, BAM 42:1–12) was that the latter was freshly made and taken with honey and pressed-out oil, whereas the former was always fermented for at least three and as many as seven days before use. Both types are designated as "for a man (only)," "for the king" or "secret of kingship." This was for the simple reason that juniper is an abortifacient. The "secret of kingship" is not a snide remark, but refers to tactics to ensure a minimum of conflicts between potential successors to the throne.

Lines 36–39 are a classic. The chest was to be inspected to ensure that the treatment was necessary. The stale urine, soured beer, and pressed-out oil were enough to make the patient vomit without any prodding. Indeed, the physician was supposed to get a good grip on the tongue with cloths to make sure that the mixture stayed down long enough to do its job. Afterwards, the finest sweet beer served to stop the vomiting.

Lines 45–46 describe a rare pediatric treatment. His father's turban serves as an impromptu bandage. The adult of line 47 gets the ancient equivalent of a down jacket. Lines 53–54 make explicit what we have otherwise guessed, namely, that there was an oral tradition of medicine much of which probably never made it to writing.

1. [(DIŠ NA *ṣ*)]*i-ri-iḫ-ti* ŠÀ TUKU-*ma* ⸢ŠÀ-*šú*⸣ KÚM *ú-kal mi-na-t*[(*ú-šú* DUB GABA-*su i-ka-sa-su*)]
2. [NA].BI UD.DA *ḫa-miṭ ana* DIN-*šú* 1/2 GÍN ^{Ú}*ak-tam* 4-*tú* ILLU LI.[DUR ...]
3. 2 NINDA KAŠ NAG-*ma* BURU$_8$ EGIR-*šú šal-šá-a-tú* NAG-*ma* BURU$_8$ *is-sal-l*[*a-ʾ-ma* TI]

---

4. [DIŠ K]I.MIN 1 NINDA *si-in-du* ZÍZ.ÀM 1/2 NINDA *as-né-e* 1/2 NINDA ^{ŠEM}LI *šal-šú* NINDA GA[ZI^{SAR} GAZ SIM ḪE.ḪE]
5. [*ina*] 1 *qa* KAŠ.ŠE ŠEG$_6$-*šal ta-ša$_6$-ḫal* 1 NINDA Ì.GIŠ *ḫal-ṣa* 1 NINDA LÀL [*ana* ŠÀ DUB NAG-*ma* BURU$_8$]
6. [E]GIR-*šú šal-šá-a-tú* NAG-*ma* [BURU$_8$]

---

7. [*š*]*um-ma* LÚ *ana* BURU$_8$-*šú* 1 NINDA LAGAB MUNU$_6$ 1 NINDA *mu-un-du* GAZI^{SAR} 1 NINDA *m*[*u-un-du*]
8. *as-né-*⸢*e*⸣ *ina* A ŠEG$_6$-*šal* NAG-*ma ina* KAŠ BURU$_8$ KI.MIN Ú.ME *an-nu-t*[*ú* GAZ SIM ḪE.ḪE]
9. [*ina*] 3 *q*[*a*] KAŠ ŠEG$_6$-*šal ta-ša$_6$-ḫal* 1 NINDA Ì.GIŠ *ḫal-ṣa* 1 [NINDA LÀL *ana* ŠÀ DUB NAG-*ma* BURU$_8$]
10. [EGIR]-⸢*šú*⸣ *šal-šá-a-tú* NAG-*ma* BURU$_8$ 3 Ú.ḪI.A BURU$_8$ [...]

---

11. [# *g*]*i-re-e* ILLU LI.DUR *gi-ru-ú* ^{ŠEM}LI [GAZ SIM ḪE.ḪE]
12. *ina* 2 NINDA Ì NAG-*ma* BURU$_8$ EGIR-*šú šal-šá-a-tú* NAG-*ma* BURU$_8$

---

13. Ì.GIŠ *lam-mu* 5-*šú lu-u-šú ina* ŠU.SI-[*š*]*ú ú-na-ṣab* EGIR-*šú šal-šá-a-tú* NAG-*ma* BURU$_8$

---

14. 2 NINDA LÀL 2 GÍN Ú.KUR.RA *lu* ^{Ú}GAMUN^{SAR} GAZ SIM ḪE.ḪE
15. *ina* 2 NINDA SUM^{SAR} NAG EGIR-*šú šal-šá-a-tú* NAG-*ma* BURU$_8$

---

16. KÀŠ.MEŠ SUMUN.MEŠ NAG-*ma* BURU$_8$ *ana a-mur-ri-qa-nu* SIG$_5$ ⸢*mál*⸣-*tak-tú*[12]

---

17. DIŠ BURU$_8$ TAR-*si mu-raṭ-ṭi-bu* GU$_7$-*šú* A ^{GIŠ}NU.ÚR.MA NAG-*šú šum$_4$-ma* KÚM.MEŠ ^{ŠEM}ŠEŠ NUMUN ^{Ú}*qut-ri*
18. ^{Ú}*lìb-na-tu ina* A SÚD *tak-ṣa-a-tú ina* UGU ŠÀ-*šú* LAL *u maš-qut an-ni-tú*

NAG-*šú*

---

19. 2 GÍN ^{Ú}DÚR.NU.LUḪ.ḪA *ḫi-tim tu-sal-lat it-ti* 2 NINDA LÀL *ina* IGI NÁ-*šú* GU$_7$ *šá* KA *kar-šú*

---

20. *šum-ma* LÚ GABA-*su* IM *le-qa-at-ma ú-šá-an-na-ʾ* 1 GÍN ^{Ú}DÚR. NU.LUḪ.ḪA
21. 1 GÍN LAGAB MUNU$_6$ 1/2 GÍN ZÍD ŠE.SA.A *ina* LÀL *u* Ì *ḫal-ṣa ú-na-ṣab*

---

22. *šum-ma* GABA-*su ta-ta-kal-šú šá nu-uṣ-ṣu-pu a-na nu-uṣ-ṣu-pi-šú* LÀL Ì.NUN.NA
23. Ì *ḫal-ṣa* ^{Ú}DÚR.NU.LUḪ.ḪA 4-*tú mu-un-du* GAZI^{SAR} 2 *gi-re-e* Ú.BABBAR 2 *gi-re-e* ^{Ú}*šu-un-ḫu*
24. 2 *gi-re-e* IM.KAL.GUG AN.DA‹(Ḫ)›.ŠUM SÚD-*ma ina* KAŠ *ṭa-a-bi ú-na-ṣab*

---

25. DIŠ NA *lu* ḪAR.MEŠ *lu ki-ṣir-ti* ḪAR.MEŠ *lu su-alu* GIG *ana* DIN-*šú mun-zi-qu te-bé-er*
26. *ina* A LUḪ-*si ta-šá-an-ni-ma*! LUḪ 1 GÍN ^{GIŠ}ERIN 2 GÍN ^{GIŠ}ŠUR.MÌN 1 1/2 GÍN ^{GIŠ}*dup-ra-nu*
27. 2 GÍN ^{ŠEM}GÍR 2 GÍN ^{ŠEM}MUG 2 GÍN ŠEM.SAL 4 GÍN GI.DÙG.GA 2 GÍN ŠEM.^{d}MAŠ
28. 2 GÍN ^{ŠEM}MAN.DU 1/2 GÍN ^{ŠEM}ŠEŠ 1/2 GÍN ^{ŠEM}ḪAB 4-*tú* ILLU ^{ŠEM}BULUḪ 2 GÍN *bu-uṭ-na-na*
29. 2 GÍN ^{Ú}*ḫa-šá-nu* 2 GÍN ^{Ú}*kur-ka-nu-ú* 10 GÍN ^{Ú}*qul-qul-la-nu* 16 Ú ŠEŠ. MEŠ 1-*niš ta-par-ras*
30. *a-na* 1 BÁN *mun-ziq tu-sam-maḫ ana* DUG *te-es-sip* ^{GIŠ}GEŠTIN *dan-nu* DÙG.GA *ana* ŠÀ DUB 7 U$_4$ GAR
31. *e-nu-ma il-tab-ku ina* GI.SAG.KUD GI.DÙG.GA *la pa-tan* NAG.MEŠ ^{DUG}*ta-ri-ḫu šá* Ú.ḪI.A *šá* LUGAL

---

32. 3 GÍN ^{GIŠ}*qu-un-na-bu* 3 GÍN ŠEM.SAL 3 GÍN ^{ŠEM}MUG 3 GÍN ^{ŠEM}GÍR 3 GÍN ^{ŠEM}GAM.MA
33. 3 GÍN ^{ŠEM}BULUḪ 2 GÍN ^{Ú}*ia-a-ru-ut-tú* 2 GÍN ^{GIŠ}ERIN 4 GÍN GI.DÙG. GA PAP 1/3 + 6 GÍN ŠEM
34. *ina ma-suk-tu tu-ḫa-ṣa-aṣ* ^{GIŠ}*mun-ziq ina* KAŠ ZÚ.LUM.MA LUḪ E$_{11}$-*ma* ŠEM *šu-a-tim*
35. *ana* ŠÀ ḪE.ḪE *pa-ṣu-ú ana* UGU ŠUB-*ma* 3 U$_4$ *ka-ník ina* U$_4$.3.KÁM*

BAD-*ma ana* ^{d}GAŠAN BAL

---

36. *šum-ma* LÚ *ḫa-še-e* GIG *bit-qa* ^{Ú}NAM.TAR *ina* A ^{GIŠ}NU.ÚR.MA SÚD-*ma* NAG
37. GABA-*su te-še-ʾi šá nu-ṣu-bu ú-na-ṣab* 1 NINDA KÀŠ SUMUN.MEŠ 1 NINDA KAŠ DÙG.GA *lu-um-nu* Ì *ḫal-ṣa*
38. *ana* ŠÀ *a-ḫa-meš tu-sam-maḫ* EME-*šú ina mu-ṣi-pi-e-ti ta-ṣab-bat ana* EME-*šú* ŠUB-*ma*
39. *tu-šap-riš* KAŠ.SAG ZÚ.LUM.MA DÙG.GA NAG-*šú*

---

40. DIŠ NA *em-bu-bu ḫa-še-e* GIG-*ma ú-gan-na-aḫ* KI *ru-ṭi-šú* MÚD ŠUB-*a* 1/2 NINDA A ^{GIŠ}NU.ÚR.MA
41. 15 ŠE ^{Ú}NAM.TI.LA *ina* 2 NINDA.ḪI.A Ì *ḫal-ṣa* 1-*niš* ḪE.ḪE-*ma* NAG-*šú*

---

42. 1 GÍN ^{Ú}DÚR.NU.LUḪ.ḪA 1/2 GÍN GAZI^{SAR} 1 GÍN Ú.BABBAR 1 GÍN ^{Ú}*šu-un-ḫu* 2 GÍN ^{Ú}AN.DAḪ.ŠUM
43. 5 Ú ḪAR.MEŠ GAZ SIM *ina* LÀL *u* Ì *ḫal-ṣa ú-na-ṣab*[13]

---

44. DIŠ NA *su-alu* GIG ^{Ú}AN.DAḪ.ŠUM SÚD *ina* LÀL *u* Ì *ḫal-ṣa* ḪE.ḪE NU *pa-tan* NAG.ME ^{Ú}ḪAR.ḪAR SÚD *ina* KAŠ NAG-*ma* DIN

---

45. DIŠ NA *su-alu ṭup-šu-su* GIG IM.KAL.GUG SÚD *ina* LÀL ZÚ.LUM.MA *u* Ì.NUN.NA ḪE.ḪE
46. *ina šer-ti u ka-ṣi-tú* 7-*šú u* 7-*šú tu-šá-ṣab-šú ina* GABA-*šú* TÚG.BÁRA.SIG NU DU$_8$

---

47. *šum-ma* EN.TE.NA *pu-šik-ku* LAL *ina* A ^{GIŠ}ŠE.NÁ.A RA-*ma* DIN

---

48. ^{Ú}*qiš-še-e* GAZI^{SAR} ^{Ú}ḪAR.ḪAR ^{Ú}DÚR.NU.LUḪ.ḪA ^{ŠEM}BULUḪ *mál-ma-liš* GAZ SIM
49. *ba-lu pa-tan ina* KAŠ ŠE SUMUN *lu ina* GEŠTIN 4-*tú ḫa-a-ṭu* NAG *šá su-alu ana ka-ma-a-si*

---

50. DIŠ NA *ši-qá* DIB-*su pa-ṣu-ú* GA KU$_7$.KU$_7$ Ì *ḫal-ṣa* GEŠTIN LÀL *u* Ì.NUN
51. *mál-ma-liš* ḪE.ḪE NU *pa-tan ú-na-ṣab*

---

52. DIŠ NA *ši-qá* DIB-*su šá-ʾ-i-lu* A.ŠÀ SÚD *ina* GA NAG-*ma ina-eš*

---

53. DIŠ *šit-qá* TAR-*si* ^{Ú}*zi-ba-a ta-mar-raq ina* TÚG.GADA KEŠDA *tu-še-en-ṣi-šu-ma ina-eš šu-ut* KA
54. DIŠ KI.MIN LÀL Ì.NUN.NA Ì *ḫal-ṣa* ^{ŠEM}ḪAB *tu-ma-ḫar ú-na-ṣab*

---

55. DIŠ NA *ši-i-qu lu-ḫu-ʾ* GIG GA KU$_7$.KU$_7$ NAG

---

56. 1 GÍN ^{Ú}ḪAR.ḪAR 1/2 GÍN GAZI^{SAR} 1 GÍN *šu-un-ʾu* 1 GÍN Ú.BABBAR 4 Ú KA *kar-šú tu-ga-n*[*i*]
57. *u* IM *la-qa-a-tú ba-lu pa-tan ina* KAŠ N[AG]

---

58. 6-*ʾu* ^{Ú}*tar-muš ḫum-mu-šú* ^{Ú}*imḫur-lim* 6-*ʾu* ^{Ú}*imḫur*-20 1/2 GÍN Ú.BABBAR
59. 1/2 GÍN *bit-qa* Ú.KUR.RA *bit-qa* ^{Ú}NAM.TAR 6 Ú KA *kar-šú*

---

60. 1/2 GÍN ^{Ú}*tar-muš* 1/2 GÍN ^{Ú}*imḫur-lim* 1/2 GÍN ^{Ú}*imḫur*-20 1/2 GÍN Ú.KUR.RA 1/2 GÍN NAGA.SI
61. 1/2 GÍN NA$_4$ *ga-bu-u* 1/2 GÍN ^{Ú}NAM.TAR 1/2 GÍN ^{Ú}ḪAR.ḪAR PAP 8 Ú ŠEŠ.ME
62. *mál-ma-liš* GAZ SIM *ki-ṣir-šú-nu la i-ri-iḫ-ḫa tu-daq-qaq* EN Ú *u ki-ṣir-šú-nu*
63. *tu-daq-qa-qu-ma ana* ŠÀ *a-ḫa-meš tu-sam-maḫ* 1/2 GÍN ZÍD ŠÀ LAL-*ma* 1 NINDA LÀL
64. *ina* ŠÀ 4 NINDA KAŠ ŠE SUMUN SAG.MEŠ *ta-šaḫ-ḫi* Ú *ina* ŠÀ ḪE.ḪE-*ma* Ú *me-re-e-ma* NAG *šá* KAR A.MEŠ *ana* KA DU
65. ÉN ^{d}*Gu-la* GAŠAN *šur-bu-tum* AMA *rem-ni-tum a-ši-bat* AN-*e* KÙ.MEŠ *ana* UGU ŠID-*nu*

---

66. *šum-ma* LÚ *ḫi-níq-ti* GIG ÉLLAG.ME GIG DÚR.GIG MIN TAB UD.DA MIN *um-ma* DIB.DIB-*su*
67. 2 *gi-re-e* NA$_4$ *ga-bu-ú* 2 *gi-re-e* NAGA.SI 2 *gi-re-e* Ú.KUR.RA
68. 2 *gi-re-e* MUN 2 *gi-re-e* ^{Ú}NAM.TAR *ina* UGU A SÚD-*ma* NAG

---

69. 4-*tú* $^{\text{NA}_4}$AN.ZAḪ SÚD ZÚ.LUM.MA *tu-kap-pat i-la-ʾa-tú* EGIR-*šú* KAŠ ŠE SUMUN NAG-*šú*

---

70. 2 *gi-re-e* ^{Ú}NAM.TAR 2 *gi-re-e* NAGA.SI *gi-ru-ú* ^{MUN}*eme-sal-lim*
71. *gi-ru-ú* Ú.KUR.RA *gi-ru-ú nam-ra-qu gi-ru-ú* NA$_4$ ⸢*ga-bu*⸣-*ú*
72. *ina* Ì *ḫal-ṣa* SÚD *ina* BAR ZÚ.LUM.MA NIGIN NUNDUN.ME ZI *ra-bu*

šá ŠU^{II} [*šu-ṣa*]*-a*

---

73. 4-*tú* ^{Ú}NAM.TI.LA *bit-qu* NAGA.SI *la* TAR-*su-ú bit-qa* NA$_4$ *ga-bu-ú šá ṣi-*[*tu-šú*] *sa-a-mu*
74. *bit-qu* ^{MUN}*eme-sal-lim* 4 Ú.MEŠ *an-nu-tú ina* Ì *gu-un-nu* SÚD *lu ina* ⸢LÀL *lu*⸣ *ina* ‹KAŠ› ZÚ.LUM.MA DIB-*ma* [NA]G-*šú*
75. EGIR-*šú* 3 NINDA KAŠ ŠE SUMUN *a-na* UGU NAG-*ma* DIN *maš-qut šá nap-ḫar mur-ṣu ana* GIG DÙ.A.BI SI[G$_5$]

---

76. *šul-lul-tú* 1 GÍN ^{Ú}*nam-ra-*⸢*qu* 2 *gi-re-e*⸣ NAGA.SI SÚD *ina* Ì ^{GIŠ}BUR *tu-šá-ṣa-a ku-*⸢*pa-tin*⸣
77. *tu-kap-pat* LÀL SUD-*ma i-l*[*a-ʾa*]*-ut* EGI[R-*šú*] 3 NINDA KAŠ ŠE SUMUN NAG-[*š*]*ú*
78. [*maš*]-*qut šá* EN.TE.N[A] *šá ina* ⸢*šu-bur-ri*⸣*-šú* ⸢NAG?⸣.NAG

---

79. ⸢DIŠ⸣ NA *ina* KA-*šú* MÚD BURU$_8$ ^{Ú}NU.⸢LUḪ⸣.ḪA IM.KAL.GUG *mál-ma-liš* SÚD x x x x KAŠ ŠID
80. *ina* UL *tuš-bat ina* ⸢*še-rim*⸣ NU ⸢*pa-tan* NAG⸣-*ma* BURU$_8$: DIN-*ut ana* KA DU KI.MIN ^{Ú}IN.UŠ S[ÚD … *ina*] KAŠ NAG

---

81. DIŠ KI.MIN IM.SAḪAR.N[A$_4$.KUR.RA SÚD] ⸢*ana* KAŠ ŠUB⸣ *ina* UL *tuš-bat la pa-tan* NAG *e-ma* NAG ⸢RA?⸣.RA.MEŠ

---

82. [^{G}]^{IŠ}ŠUR.MÌN KA.[A.AB.B]A $^{\text{NA}_4}$KUR-*nu* DIB ^{Ú}*u$_5$-ra-nu* ^{Ú}IN.UŠ *ki-ṣir* ^{GIŠ}⸢MA⸣.NU
83. [NU]MUN ^{GIŠ}Š[IN]IG 7 Ú.ḪI.A ŠEŠ.MEŠ *maš-qut šá* GAZ ŠÀ [*ina* KAŠ] NAG
84. [^{Ú}]*a-ra-ri-ia-a-nu* NUMUN ^{GIŠ}Š[I]NIG ^{Ú}*a-zal-lá* 3 Ú.ME *ḫu-uṣ* GAZ ŠÀ T[UKU.MEŠ-*ši i*]*na* KAŠ ⸢NAG⸣

---

85. [DIŠ N]A *li-ʾ-ba* DIB-*su* Ì ^{GIŠ}LI SÍG ŠAḪ.GI 1/2 NINDA ^{Ú}ḪAR.ḪAR 1/2 NINDA ^{Ú}NU.LUḪ.ḪA […]
86. EN 2 Ú NU AL.TIL (catchline)

Colophon

Translation

(1–3) If a person has burning internal fever and his abdomen holds fever, his ⸢limbs⸣ are tense and his chest gnaws at him, that person is burned by *ṣētu* (enteric fever), to cure him, if you have him drink 1/2 shekel of *aktam*, 1/4 shekel of ⸢*abukkatu*⸣ resin and [...] (mixed) [with] 2 NINDA of beer, he should vomit. Afterwards, if you have him drink it in thirds, he should vomit. He will appear to get worse, [but he should recover (in the end)].[14]

(4–6) [If] ⸢ditto (a person has burning internal fever)⸣, you [crush, sift and mix] 1 NINDA of emmer *sindu*-groats, 1/2 NINDA of *asnû*-dates, 1/2 NINDA of *burāšu*-juniper (and) 1/3 NINDA of *kasû*. You boil (it) [in] 1 *qû* of barley beer and filter (it). [You pour] 1 NINDA of pressed-out oil (and) 1 NINDA of honey [onto it. If you have him drink it, he should vomit]. Afterwards, if you have him drink (it) in thirds, [he should vomit].

(7–10) If you want to make a person vomit, you boil 1 NINDA of malt lumps, 1 NINDA of *mundu*-groats made with *kasû* (and) 1 NINDA of [*mundu*-groats] made with *asnû*-dates in water. If you have him drink (it mixed) with beer, he should vomit. Alternatively, [you crush, sift and mix] these plants and boil them [in] 3 ⸢*qû*⸣ of beer. [You pour] 1 NINDA pressed-out oil (and) 1 [NINDA of honey onto it. If you have him drink it, he should vomit]. ⸢Afterwards⸣, if you have him drink it in thirds, he should vomit. These are three plants to induce vomiting.

(11–12) [You crush, sift, and mix #] carats of *abukkatu* resin (and) a carat of *burāšu*-juniper. If you have him drink (it mixed) with 2 NINDA of oil, he should vomit. Afterwards, if you have him drink (it) in thirds, he should vomit.

(13) He should suck oil of *lammu*-almonds (and) 1/5 shekel of used grease on his finger. Afterwards, if you have him drink (it) in thirds, he should vomit.

(14–15) You crush, sift (and) mix 2 NINDA of honey, 2 shekels of *nīnû*-mint or *kamunu*-cumin. You have him drink (it mixed) with 2 NINDA of *šūmu*-garlic. Afterwards, if you have him drink (it) in thirds, he should vomit.

(16) If he drinks stale urine, he should vomit. It is good for *amurriqānu*; tested treatment.

(17–18) If you want to stop vomiting, you have him eat (the contents of) a *muraṭṭibu*-vessel (and) have him drink *nurmû*-pomegranate juice. If it is summer, you grind myrrh, *qutru* seed (and) *labanātu*-incense[15] in water. (If it is) winter, you bind (it) onto his abdomen and you have him drink this potion.

(19) You cut up 2 shekels (and) a *hitmu*[16] of *tiyātu*. You have him eat (it) with 2 NINDA of honey before he goes to bed. (This is) for the mouth of the stomach.

(20–21) If a person's breast takes up "clay" and it suffuses (it), he should suck up 1 shekel of *tiyātu*, 1 shekel of malt lumps (and) 1/2 shekel of roasted grain flour (mixed) with honey and pressed-out oil.

(22–24) If a person's breast hurts him, to give him to suck what is for him to suck, you grind honey, ghee, pressed-out oil, *tiyātu*, 1/4 shekel of *mundu*-groats made with *kasû*, 2 carats of "white plant," 2 carats of *šunḫu*, 2 carats of *kalgukku*-clay (and) *antaḫšum*-vegetable and he sucks (it) up (mixed) with sweet beer.

(25–31) If a person is sick with either "sick lungs" or thick sputum in the lungs or *suʾālu*-cough, to cure him, you pick over raisins (and) wash (them) in water. You wash (them) again. You chop together these sixteen plants: 1 shekel of *erēnu*-cedar, 2 shekel of *šurmēnu*-cypress, 1 1/2 shekels of *daprānu*-juniper, 2 shekels of *asu*-myrtle, 2 shekels of *ballukku*-aromatic, 2 shekels of *šimeššalû*-aromatic, 4 shekels of "sweet reed," 2 shekels of *nikiptu*, 2 shekels of *suʾādu*, 1/2 shekel of myrrh, 1/2 shekel of *ṭūru*-aromatic, 1/4 shekel of *baluḫḫu*-aromatic resin, 2 shekels of *buṭnānu*, 2 shekels of *ḫašānu*, 2 shekels of *kurkānû*-turmeric, and 10 shekels of *qulquliānu*. You mix it with 1 *sūtu* of raisins. You collect (it) in a *karpatu*-vessel (and) pour undiluted sweet wine onto it. You set (it) aside for seven days. When it is moistened, you have him drink (it) repeatedly through a "sweet reed" straw on an empty stomach. This is a *tariḫu* of plants for the king.[17]

(32–35) You pulverize 3 shekels of *qunnabu*, 3 skekels of *šimešallu*-aromatic, 3 shekels of *balukku*-aromatic, 3 skekels of *asu*-myrtle, 3 skekels of *ṣumlalû*, 3 shekels of *baluḫḫu*-aromatic, 2 shekels of *iaruttu*, 2 shekels of *erēnu*-cedar (and) 4 shekels of "sweet reed," a total of 26 shekels of aromatics in a mortar. You wash raisins in date beer. You take (them) out and mix these aromatics into them. You pour white (beer) onto it and then it is sealed for three days. On the fourth(!) day, you open (it) and pour out a libation to Bēltu (before use).

(36–39) If a person's lungs are sick, you grind 1/8 shekel of *pillû* in *nurmû*-pomegranate juice and have him drink (it). You inspect his chest (and) he sucks up what is to be sucked up. You mix together 1 NINDA of stale urine, 1 NINDA of sweet beer that has soured (and) pressed-out oil. You take hold of his tongue with *muṣiptu*-cloths (and) pour (it) onto his tongue and then you let him vomit. You have him drink first quality sweet date beer.

(40–41) If a person's windpipe is sick/sore so that he *guḫḫu*-coughs (and) he produces blood with his spittle,[18] you mix together 1/2 NINDA *nurmû*-pomegranate juice, 15 grains of ᵁNAM.TI.LA (and) 2 NINDA of pressed-out oil and you have him drink (it).

(42–43) You crush (and) sift five plants for the lungs: 1 shekel of *tiyātu*, 1/2 shekel of *kasû*, 1 shekel of "white plant," 1 shekel of *šunḫu* (and) 2 shekels of *antaḫšum*-vegetable. He sucks (it) up (mixed) with honey and pressed-out oil.

(44) If a person is sick with *suʾalu*-cough, you grind *antaḫšum*-vegetable (and) mix (it) with honey and pressed-out oil. You have him drink (it) repeatedly on an empty stomach. You grind *ḫašû*-thyme. If he drinks (it mixed) with beer, he should recover.

(45–46) If a person in his baby fat is sick with *su ʾālu*-cough,[19] you grind *kalgukku*-clay. You mix (it) with honey, dates and ghee. You have him suck (it) seven times in the morning and seven times in the cool of evening. (You wrap) a turban on his breast (and) do not take (it) off.

(47) If it is the cold season. you bandage him with carded wool. If you bathe him with *šunû*-chastetree infusion, he should recover.

(48–49) You crush (and) sift *qiššû*, *kasû*, *ḫašû*-thyme, *tiyātu*, and *baluḫḫu*-aromatic in equal proportions. You have him drink one fourth (of it) by weight (mixed) with old barley beer or wine. (This is) to finish off *su ʾālu*-cough.

(50–51) If a *šīqu* (colored phlegm) afflicts a person, you mix together white (beer), sweet milk, pressed-out oil, wine, honey, and ghee in equal proportions (and) he sucks (it) up on an empty stomach.

(52) If *šīqu* afflicts a person, you grind a *šā ʾilu*-insect of the field. If you have him drink (it mixed) with milk, he should recover.

(53–54) To keep away a "cleft," you finely crush *zibû* (and) tie (it) on in a linen cloth. If you make sure to use enough of it, he should recover. (This is) a traditional treatment. Alternatively, you mix honey, ghee, pressed-out oil (and) *ṭūru*-aromatic (and) he sucks (it) up.

(55) If a person is sick with dirty *šīqu*,[20] you have him drink sweet milk.

(56–57) 1 shekel of *ḫašû*-thyme, 1/2 shekel of *kasû*, 1 shekel of *šunḫu* (and) 1 shekel of "white plant" are four plants for the mouth of the stomach or *tugānu* or (lungs) taking up "clay." You ⌈have him drink⌉ (it mixed) with beer on an empty stomach.

(58–59) 1/6 shekel of *tarmuš*, 1/5 shekel of *imḫur-lim*, 1/6 shekel of *imḫur-ešra*, 1/2 shekel of "white plant," 5/8 shekel of *nīnû*-mint (and) 1/8 shekel of *pillû* (are) six plants for the mouth of the stomach.

(60–65) You finely crush (and) sift these eight plants in equal proportions: 1/2 shekel of *tarmuš*, 1/2 shekel of *imḫur-lim*, 1/2 shekel of *imḫur-ešra*, 1/2 shekel of *nīnû*-mint, 1/2 shekel of *uḫḫūlu qarnānu*, 1/2 shekel of alum, 1/2 shekel of *pillû* and 1/2 shekel of *ḫašû*-thyme. There should be no lumps left in it. You break (it) into tiny pieces (and) when you have broken the plants and their lumps into tiny pieces, you mix (them) thoroughly together. You weigh out 1/2 shekel of the resulting flour. Then, you mix 1 NINDA of honey into 4 NINDA of old first quality barley beer. You mix the plants into it and you have her drink the plants while pregnant to avoid having (KAR) the waters come (DU) to the mouth (of the vagina). You recite the recitation: "Gula, great mistress, merciful mother who lives in the pure heavens" over it.

(66–68) If a person is sick with constriction of the urethra (or) sick kidneys (or) DÚR.GIG (or) burning of *ṣētu* (or) if fever repeatedly afflicts him, you grind 2 carats of alum, 2 carats of *uḫḫūlu qarnānu*, 2 carats of *nīnû*-mint, 2 carats of salt (and) 2 carats of *pillû* on top of water and have him drink (it).

(69) You grind 1/4 shekel of *anzaḫḫu*-frit. You form (it) into a pill with dates (and) he swallows (it). Afterwards, you have him drink old barley beer.

(70–72) You grind 2 carats of *pillû*, 2 carats of *uḫḫūlu qarnānu*, a carat of *emesallim*-salt, a carat of *nīnû*-mint, a carat of *namruqu*, (and) a carat of alum in pressed-out oil. You wrap (it) in a piece of date rind whose edges you have cut off, as big as is ⌜available⌝.

(73–75) You grind these four plants: 1/4 shekel of "life plant," 1/8 shekel of *uḫḫūlu qarnānu* which has not been cut up, 1/8 shekel of alum whose ⌜bloom(?)⌝ is red, (and) 1/8 shekel of *emesallim*-salt in *gunnu* oil. ⌜You have him drink⌝ (it mixed) either with honey or with date ‹beer› while holding (his tongue). Afterwards, if you have him drink 3 NINDA of old barley beer on top of it, he should recover. ⌜It is good⌝ for all and every sort of illness.

(76–78) You grind 1/3 shekel of *namruqqu* (and) 2 carats of *uḫḫūlu qarnānu*. You integrate (it) with *pūru*-oil (and) form (it) into pills. You sprinkle (it) with honey and he ⌜swallows⌝ (it). ⌜Afterwards⌝, you have him drink 3 NINDA of old barley beer. (This is) a ⌜potion⌝ for the cold season (and for) what is in his anus. It should be drunk repeatedly.

(79–80) If a person vomits blood from his mouth, you grind *nuḫurtu* (and) *kalgukku*-clay in equal proportions. [...] You make (it) into a dough with beer (and) leave (it) out overnight under the stars. In the morning, if you have him drink (it) on an empty stomach, he should vomit (variant: recover). (If blood) comes to his mouth, you ⌜grind⌝ *maštakal*. [...] You have him drink (it mixed) [with] beer.

(81) If ditto (a person vomits blood from his mouth), [you grind] ⌜alum⌝ (and) pour (it) into beer. You leave (it) out overnight under the stars (and) have him drink (it) on an empty stomach. While he is drinking (it), he should bathe repeatedly.

(82–83) These seven plants: *šurmēnu*-cypress, ⌜*imbû tamtim*⌝, magnetic hematite, *urânu*, *maštakal*, a block of *eʾru*-wood, (and) ⌜*bīnu*-tamarisk seed⌝ are a potion for crushing sensation in the chest. You have him drink (it mixed) [with beer].

(84) *Arariānu*, *bīnu*-tamarisk seed, and *azallû* seed are three plants for crushing sensation in the chest. You have him drink [their] ⌜flours⌝ (mixed) with beer.

(85–86) [If] *liʾbu*-fever afflicts a ⌜person⌝, *burāšu*-juniper oil, hair from a wild boar of the canebrake, 1/2 NINDA of *ḫašû*-thyme, 1/2 NINDA of *nuḫurtu* [...] together with two (other) plants (the copy is not finished).

3. TUBERCULOSIS

TEXT 4: BAM 558

The particular interest of BAM 558 is treatments designed to "lubricate" the lungs. It contains a variety of lung problems including secondary pneumonia (i 14′–17′) and what may be descriptions of tuberculosis. There is another treatment for this disease in BM 78963:40–41 above. For more details, see Scurlock and Andersen 2005, 42–43, 47. In the preserved sections of the text, there are wet bandages (i 7′–17′, iv 3–11), potions (i 14′–22′), a salve (i 18′–22′), an aliment (i 18′–22′), baths (iv 7–14), a fumigant (iv 12–14), and a distillate daub (iv 15–19).

The typical treatment in this text is a wet bandage made using waterproof leather, usually accompanied by a potion. The most interesting variants are a back-up distillate daub (iv 15–19), for which see above, and lines iv 7–11, which describe a body soak with the dregs of winnowed beerwort.

i

1′. x [...]

2′. ⸢GI⸣ [...]
3′. Ú[...]
4′. *lu ina* x [...]

5′. ZÍD GAZI⸢SAR⸣ [...]
6′. Ú*ti-ya-*[*tú* ...]

7′. ŠEMGÚR.GÚR [...]
8′. 6 [...]
9′. [...] x [...]
10′. ÚNÍG.GÁN.GÁN Úx [... EN]
11′. ḪAR.MEŠ-*šú i-lab-bi-ku* x[...]
12′. ILLU! NU.LUḪ.ḪA ŠEMGAM.⸢MA⸣ [...]
13′. *ina* KAŠ SAG *tara-bak ina* KUŠ EDIN SUR-*ri* G[ABA-*su* LAL]

14′. DIŠ NA ḪAR.MEŠ GIG-*ma* KA-*šú bu-ša-nu* D[(IB-*it* GAZISAR BIL-*tum pu-qut-tim* ÚGEŠTIN!?.KA$_5$!?.A)]
15′. *an-nu-ḫa-ra* NUMUN ÚNÍG.GÁN.GÁN Ú.BABBAR SÚD [(*ina* Ì.GIŠ *u* KAŠ NAG-*šú*)]
16′. ŠEMGÚR.GÚR ŠEMLI GIŠMAN.DU GIŠERIN GIŠŠUR.M[ÌN ...]
17′. *qí-lip* ZÚ.LUM.MA ḪE.ḪE *ina* KUŠ EDIN SUR LAL [...]

18′. DIŠ NA ḪAR.MEŠ GIG-*ma ma-gal ip-ta-nar-ru i-*[…]
19′. 1/2 *qa* ^{GIŠ}ŠUR.MÌN 1/2 *qa* ZÍD ŠE.BAR 1/2 *qa* ZÍD.GIG 1/2 *qa* [(ZÍD ZÍZ.AN).NA) …]
20′. Ì+GIŠ *ina mu-šá-ḫi-ni* ŠEG$_6$-*šal* ZÍD ^{GIŠ}ERIN ZÍD.GIG *ana* ŠÀ ŠUB-[(*di* KÚM-*su* ŠÉ)Š …]
21′. ^{Ú}*a-ri-a-ni* SÚD *ina* KAŠ NU *pa-tan* NAG.MEŠ 1/2 [(*qa*) … (*ina* A ḪE.ḪE *ina* NINDU BAD-ir)]
22′. KI Ì.NUN.NA *ta-mar-ras* GU$_7$.MEŠ EN ḪAR.MEŠ-*šú* [*i-lab-bi-ku* …]

23′. DIŠ NA ḪAR.MEŠ-*šú* GIG-*ma i*-x […]
24′. DUḪ.ŠE.GIŠ.Ì ŠÈ TU[^{MUŠEN} …]

---

iv
1. DIŠ NA ḪAR^{II}-*šú* IM *it-pu-qa* KAŠ.Ú.SA SIG *ana* ^{DU}[^{G} …]
2. GI.DÙG ^{ŠEM}BAL LÀL Ì *ḫal-ṣa u* KAŠ.SAG *ana* ŠÀ ŠUB-*d*[*i* …]

---

3. DIŠ NA ḪAR.MEŠ-*šú* KI KAK.TI-*šú it-pu-qu ana* TI-*šú* ^{Ú}x[…]
4. NUMUN ^{Ú}*kit-ta-tur-ra* NUMUN ^{Ú}*ši-ma-ḫi* ^{ŠEM}IM.DI x[…]
5. ^{ŠEM}BAL NUMUN ^{Ú}EME.UR.GI$_7$ NUMUN ^{GIŠ}ŠE.NU GAZ SIM *ina* Ì.GI[Š …]
6. *ina* KUŠ EDIN SUR EN *i-nu-ḫa* […]

---

7. DIŠ NA ḪAR^{II}-*šú* KI KAK.TI-*šú it-pu-qu ana* TI-*šú* ^{URUDU}ŠEN.TUR [(A *u* KAŠ) DIRI ^{GIŠ}*si-ḫ*(*u* ^{GIŠ}*ár-gan-nu*!)]
8. ^{GIŠ}LUM.ḪA ^{Ú}ḪAR.ḪAR ^{Ú}*ak-tam ana* ŠÀ ŠUB-*di* ŠEG$_6$-*šal* [(*ta-šá-ḫal ina* ŠÀ RA-*su* E$_{11}$ KI)]
9. Ì+^{GIŠ}*e-re-ni* EŠ-*su é-ra*[21] *šá* KAŠ.Ú.SA SIG DU$_6$-*šú* [(EN *pit-ru-šú i-lab-bi-ku*)]
10. [(*u i*)]*r-ru-u* DU-*ak* ^{ŠEM}GÚR.GÚR ^{ŠEM}LI ^{ŠEM}BAL ZÍD.G[(I)G … (5 Ú.ME *an-nu-ti* 1-*niš* SÚD)]
11. [(*ana* ŠÀ)] ⸢KAŠ⸣ SAG GEŠTIN BÍL.LÁ ŠUB-*di* ‹*ina* › ^{URUDU}ŠE[(N. TUR *tara-bak ina* KUŠ EDIN SUR-*ri* LAL-*su-ma*)]

---

12. [DIŠ KI.MIN[22] (*ana*)] ⸢TI-*šú* ÚḪ⸣.^{d}ÍD *saḫ-lé-e* ^{ŠE}[(^{M}ḪAB KI Ì.UDU *u* KAŠ ⸢SAG⸣ ḪE.ḪE)]
13. [(*ana* IGI D)]È $^{\text{GIŠ.Ú}}$GÍR ŠUB-*di tu-qat-tar-šú* EN [(uš-) ta x [(*i-tar-ra-ak*) … *šum*$_4$-*ma*]
14. DÙG IGI.DU$_8$ *ina* A ^{GIŠ}*šu-nim* RA-*su* Ì+GIŠ ŠÉŠ-*su tu*-[…]

---

15. *šum*$_4$*-ma* DÙG NU IGI.DU$_8$ ^{DUG}ÚTUL.U$_4$.SAKAR GAR-*an* GI.DÙG.GA ^{ŠEM}BAL x[…]
16. KI KAŠ.Ú.SA SIG$_5$ *ana* ^{DUG}ÚTUL ŠUB-*di* ŠEG$_6$-*šal* ^{DUG}[BUR.ZI.GAL NÍG.BÙR.BÙR]
17. Á.MEŠ-*šá ina* NÍG.ŠILAG.GÁ ZÍZ.ÀM BAD-*ḫi* GI.SAG.KUD *ana* ŠÀ [GAR-*an* LÀL *u* Ì.NUN.NA]
18. *ana* [KA]-*šú* GAR-*an ina* GI.SAG.KUD *baḫ-ra* [*ana* ḪAR.MEŠ-*šú* SÌG-*aṣ*]
19. [EN Ḫ]AR^{II}-*šú* [DÙG IGI.D]U$_8$ 9 U$_4$-*me an-na-a* DÙ.[DÙ …]

Translation

(i 1′–6′) *Too fragmentary for translation.*

(i 7′–13′) (For …), [you …] *kukru*, […], 6 […], *egemgirû* and […]. [You have him drink (it) mixed with … until] his lungs become lubricated. You decoct[23] […], *nuḫurtu* resin, *ṣumlalû* and […] in first quality beer. You massage (it) into waterproof leather (and) [bandage his] ⸢breast⸣ (with it).

(i 14′–17′) If a person's lungs are sick and *bu ʾšānu* afflicts his nose/mouth,[24] you grind roasted *kasû*, *puquttu*-thornbush, ⸢"fox grape"⸣, *annuḫāru*-alum, *egemgirû* seed and "white plant." You have him drink (it mixed) with oil and beer. (His lungs should be lubricated). You mix *kukru*, *burāšu*-juniper, *su ʾādu*, *erēnu*-cedar, ⸢*šurmēnu*-cypress⸣, […] (and) date rind. You massage (it) into waterproof leather (and) bandage (him with it).

(i 18′–22′) If a person's lungs are sick and he repeatedly vomits a lot (and) […], you boil 1/2 *qû* of *šurmēnu*-cypress, 1/2 *qû* of barley flour, 1/2 *qû* of wheat flour, 1/2 *qû* of emmer flour, […] (and) oil in a copper kettle. You pour *erēnu*-cedar flour (and) wheat flour into it, ⸢you rub him gently⸣ (with it) while still hot (and) [bandage it over?]. You grind *ariānu* (and) have him repeatedly drink (it mixed) with beer on an empty stomach. You […] 1/2 *qû* of […], mix (it) with water, bake (it) in an oven, stir (it) with ghee (and) have him repeatedly eat (it) until his lungs [are lubricated].

(i 23′–24′) If a person's lungs are sick and he […], [you …] sesame reside, "dove dung" and […].

(two columns of text lost)

(iv 1–2) If a person's lungs are solidified with "clay,"[25] you fill a […] vessel with winnowed beerwort. You pour "sweet reed," *balukku*-aromatic, honey, pressed-out oil and first quality beer into it. […]

(iv 3–6) If a person's lungs form a solid mass with his breastbone, [26] to cure him, you crush (and) sift […], *kittaturru* seed, *šimāḫu* seed, *su ʾādu*, […], *ballukku*-aromatic, *lišān kalbi* seed (and) *šunû*-chastetree seed. [You …] (it) with oil. You massage (it) into waterproof leather. [You bandage him with it] until it relents.

(iv 7–11) If a person's lungs form a solid mass with his breastbone,[27] to cure him, [you fill] a *tamgussu*-vessel with water and beer. You pour ⌜*sīḫu*-wormwood⌝, *argānu*, *barirātu*, *ḫašû*-thyme and *aktam* into it. You boil (and) filter (it and) bathe him with it. You have him come out (and) rub him gently with *erēnu*-cedar oil. You cover him with dregs of winnowed beerwort until his chest and abdomen are lubricated and the bowels move. You grind together these five plants: *kukru*, *burāšu*-juniper, *ballukku*-aromatic, ⌜wheat⌝ flour (and) [...]. You pour first quality beer and soured wine into it. You decoct (it) in a *tamgussu*-vessel. You massage (it) into waterproof leather (and) bandage him (with it), etc.[28]

(iv 12–14) [Alternatively], to cure him, you mix *ruʾtītu*-sulphur, *saḫlû*-cress, (and) *ṭūru*-aromatic with sheep fat and first quality beer. You pour (it) onto *ašāgu*-thorn coals (and) fumigate him (with it) until [...] beats/throbs [... If] he shows improvement, you bathe him with *šunû*-chastetree infusion, rub him gently with oil (and) [fumigate him again?].

(iv 15–19) If he does not show improvement, you put out a crescent-shaped *diqāru*-bowl. You pour "sweet reed," *ballukku*-aromatic (and) [...] along with winnowed beerwort into the *diqāru*-bowl (and) bring (it) to a boil. [You bore a hole in a *burzigallu* bowl (and invert it over the other bowl)]. You cover the sides (of the upper bowl) with a dough made of emmer flour. [You insert] a reed straw into it. You put [honey and ghee] to his [mouth]. [You slap] the reed straw while it is still hot [onto his lungs until] his ⌜lungs show⌝ [improvement]. You keep doing this for nine days. [...]

4. ANAEROBIC LUNG ABSCESS

TEXT 5: BAM 55

BAM 55 contains an aliment for what appears to be an anaerobic lung abscess. For more details, see Scurlock and Andersen 2005, 48. The fragmentary treatment that follows was for *aganutillû* (edema), for which see Scurlock and Andersen 2005, 170.

1. [(DIŠ N)]A IM *ina* ŠÀ *u*[(*š-tar-ʾ-ab*)]
2. *ù i-lè-ḫi-ib* [(SU-*šú ni-i*)*p-še* DIRI]
3. GABA-*su* MAŠ.SÌLA.MEŠ-[(*šú* GU_7.MEŠ-*šú*)]
4. UZU.MEŠ-*šú* GÍR.GÍR-[(*šú ú-šam-ma-mu-šú*)]

5. UZU.MEŠ-*šú áš-ṭu* [(*u ni-ip-še* DIRI)]
6. SAG.MEŠ-*šú i-te-né-*[(*nu-ú* KÚM.MEŠ *kal* U$_4$-*me*)]
7. *ú-kal-šú ana* TI-[(*šú* ^{GIŠ}GÚR.GÚR ^{GIŠ}LI)]
8. ^{Ú}KUR.KUR ^{Ú}ḪA[(R.ḪAR ^{Ú}*úr-né-e*)]
9. PA ^{GIŠ}*bi-ni saḫ-lí-*[(*i* GAZI^{SAR} MUN *A-ma-nim*)]
10. 9 Ú.ḪI.A ŠEŠ [(1-*niš* SÚD *ina* GEŠTIN DÙG.GA)]
11. *u* KAŠ.SAG *tara-bak* [(*ina* GI$_6$ *ana* IGI UL *tuš-bat*)]
12. ^{d}UTU NU IGI.LÁ *in*[(*a še-rim* ŠEG$_6$-*šal*)]
13. *ta-šá-ḫal* ŠE[(D$_7$ 7 ŠE.MEŠ ŠE.KAK ^{Ú}ÚKUŠ.GÍL)]
14. 7 ŠE AN.ZAḪ 1-*niš* [(SÚD *ana* ŠÀ GAZ)]
15. *ina še-rim la-am* [(^{d}UTU *na-pa-ḫi* GU$_7$-*šú*)]
16. *ina* Á [(*tu-šap-ra-šú*)]
17. *šum$_4$-ma* DÙG.GA NU [(IGI-*mar ana* DÚR-*šú* DUB)]

---

18. DIŠ NA A.GA.N[U.TIL.LA …]
19. [o] x […]

TRANSLATION

(1–17) If "wind" rumbles in a person's insides or he makes a growling noise, his body [is full] of ⸢stink⸣, his breast (and) his shoulders continually hurt him, his flesh continually stings him, (and) is numb; his flesh is stiff and full of stink, he continually changes (the side of) his head (he sleeps on and) he is gripped by fever all day, to cure him,[29] you grind together these nine plants: *kukru*, *burāšu*-juniper, *atāʾišu*, *ḫašû*-thyme, *urnû*-mint, *bīnu*-tamarisk leaves, *saḫlû*-cress, *kasû*, (and) *amanim* salt. You decoct (it)[30] in sweet wine and first quality beer. At night, you leave (it) out overnight under the stars. The sun should not be allowed to see (it). In the morning, you boil (and) filter (it and) let (it) cool. You grind together 7 grains of *irrû* shoots (and) 7 grains of *anzaḫḫu*-frit (and) crush (it) into (the mixture). You have him eat (it) in the morning, before sunrise. You make him vomit with a feather. If he does not experience relief, you pour (it) into his anus.

(18–19) If a person [has] *aganutillû* […]

5. SURGICAL DRAINING OF EMPYEMA

For more on this condition of the lungs, see Scurlock and Andersen 2005, 46–47.

TEXT 6: BAM 39

BAM 39 is one of a few rare ancient Mesopotamian surgical procedures, in this case designed to drain an empyema. It has the distinction of being one of the few ancient Mesopotamian treatments to have survived humoral theory. Unfortunately, the plant antiseptic used to cleanse the wound during the procedure and on the bandage afterwards got lost in translation.[31]

BAM 39

1′. [(DIŠ NA *mu-kil* SAG ḪUL-*tim* DIB-*su* KÚ)]M *ina* [(SU-*šú*)]
2′. [(*la-zi-iz-ma u ma-gal i-le*)]-*ḫi-ib* NA BI *bit-qu*$_5$ [KÚM? (*u* IR TUKU)]
3′. [… *tu-sa*]-*ba*-ʾ-*šu-ma* 3 UZU.TI.MEŠ […]
4′. [… *ina* ^{NA_4}]ZÚ *ina* 4 UZU.TI BAD-*te* A.MEŠ *u* MÚD […]
5′. [… (5)] *qa* A GAZI^{SAR} *sik-ru-te*[32] *ta-šá-ḫal* […]
6′. […] *tu-sa-ba*-ʾ-*šu-ma tu-za-ak* GUR-[*ma* …]
7′. [… TÉ]Š.BI[33] *tu-šá-ḫa-an ana* ŠÀ-*šú* DUB-*ak* […]
8′. [(NAM.SI.SÁ A.BÁR D)]Ù-*uš ina* TÚG.GADA *ta-ša-kak ana* ŠÀ-*šú* [(GAR)-*an*]
9′. [(*rib-ku ina* A GAZI^{SAR})] ŠEG$_6$.GÁ ŠILA$_{11}$-*aš* LÁL-*su-ma* T[I-*uṭ*]

10′. […] Ú.KUR.RA Ú x[…]
11′. [… NU].LUḪ.ḪA ^{Ú}an-[…]
12′. […] x x […]

Translation

(1′–9′) If a generalized headache[34] afflicts a person (and) fever persists in his body and also he makes a loud growling noise, that person has a “cleft,” [fever?] and sweat. [You] ⸢spill⸣ […] over him and [count down] three ribs. […] You make an opening in the fourth rib[35] [with] a flint knife. Water and blood […] You filter 5 *qû* of baked[36] *kasû* juice. […] You spill (it) over him and you clear (it) away. Once again [you spill it over him and clear it away]. You heat (it) together and pour (it) in. […] You make a lead drainage instrument. You thread (it) on a linen cloth and put (it) in. You boil the decoction[37] in *kasû* juice. You make (it) into a dough. If you bandage him (with it), ⸢he should recover⸣.[38]

(10′–12′) [If … you …] *nīnû*-mint, […], ⸢*nuḫurtu*/*tiyātu*⸣, […].

Notes

1. See Abusch and Schwemer 2011, 154.
2. See Scurlock and Andersen 2005, 15.10.
3. See Abusch and Schwemer 2011, 154 (without the duplicates).
4. See Scurlock and Andersen 2005, 178–79.
5. For lines i 23–24, see the similar procedure in BAM 494 ii 16–18//BAM 498 iv 2–6.
6. Restored from the similar procedures in BAM 558 (chapter 8, text 4).
7. The similar procedure in BAM 557:6′ has HAR.MEŠ-*šú* SÌG-*aṣ*.
8. See chapter 3, n. 109.
9. For the translation of *saḫlû* as "cress," see Stol 1983–84, 24–32.
10. See chapter 3, n. 109.
11. The similar procedure in BAM 557:6′ has: "you slap (it) onto his lungs."
12. BAM 52:88 has *šu-ut* KA.
13. BAM 44:11′–12′ is very similar and adds a sixth ingredient: IM.KAL[…].
14. The same warning appears in BAM 578 i 41//BAM 159 i 36–37 (see ch. 9, text 7).
15. The ideogram typically used for this, ŠEM.ḪI.A, would seem to indicate that, like the incense used in the Temple in Jerusalem, this was a mixture.
16. A subdivision of the grain, and an amount so tiny usually only precious metals are measured with it.
17. The characteristic of *tariḫu*-preparations is that they are always allowed to sit for three to seven days before being used. "Plants for the king" or "secret of kingship" refers to treatments which should be given to women only if they are not pregnant, since they may cause abortions.
18. See Scurlock and Andersen 2005, 3.96.
19. See Scurlock and Andersen 2005, 3.97.
20. See Scurlock and Andersen 2005, 3.73.
21. M. Stol (personal communication) suggests that the word for "beer dregs" is not actually *erû* but *piṭru*. *Piṭru* (*CAD* P, 449–50) means: "fissure" or "separation" and the dregs are indeed something that has separated from the rest of the beer or wine.
22. BAM 174 obv. 17′ repeats the symptoms to be treated.
23. See chapter 3, n. 109.
24. See Scurlock and Andersen 2005, 3.86.
25. See Scurlock and Andersen 2005, 3.75.
26. See Scurlock and Andersen 2005, 3.76.
27. See Scurlock and Andersen 2005, 3.76.
28. The hanging *-ma* which appears at the end of phrases seems to function like our "etc." See chapter 6, text 2 ad line 62.
29. See Scurlock and Andersen 2005, 3.99.
30. See chapter 3, n. 109.
31. See Scurlock 2005, 312.
32. *AMT* 49/4 rev. 5 substitutes ŠEG$_6$-*šal*.
33. *AMT* 49/4 rev. 7 has 1-*niš*.
34. For this interpretation of *mukīl-rēš-lemutti*, see Scurlock and Andersen 2005, 311.
35. This is counting from the top down. Labat 1954, 246–48 argues that the ribs were counted from the bottom up. This is, however, based on the erroneous assumption that the text refers to a liver abscess. The liver at this level is very deep, and draining an abscess through the chest wall would involve going into the pleural space and lungs, a very difficult, and extremely dangerous maneuver.

36. *AMT* 49/4 rev. 5 has: "(which) you (have) boil(ed)."
37. See chapter 3, n. 109.
38. See Scurlock and Andersen 2005, 3.93.

9

GASTROINTESTINAL TRACT

A. DIGESTIVE TRACT

The ancient physician had an excellent grasp of the human gastrointestinal tract, and was able to offer treatments for various symptoms of gastrointestinal illness: nausea/vomiting, constipation, diarrhea, abdominal bloating and pain. For more details, see Scurlock and Andersen 2005, chapter 6. Among numerous treatments for unhappy stomachs, a number stand out.

1. GHOST STOMACH

One of the most interesting set of diseases attributed to a single causal agent on symptomatic grounds is the "Hand" of Ghost complex. Diseases involving some combination of severe headache, ringing in the ears, hallucinations, pain, and dehydration were likely to be laid at the door of these unhappy spirits of the dead. For details, see Scurlock and Andersen 2005, 437–39, 441, 464–65, 471–72, 489, 495–98, 500–503 and 525–27.

TEXT 1: *AMT* 76/1

AMT 76/1 consists of a pharmacist's salve (1–3) for ghost headache, followed by potions (4–29) for ghost stomach. Other texts envisage salves, baths, and enemas. Possibilities for the modern diagnoses of the illnesses producing the enumerated symptoms include cholera, Bornholm's disease, and alcoholism. A particularly noisy stomach was also likely to be blamed on a ghost. For modern physicians, this situation would be a disaster, since treatment for many diseases is specific to the presumed causal agent and misdiagnoses consequently a severe problem. Since, however, ancient Mesopotamian treatments were generated by trial and error for each symptom or set of symptoms, there was much less trouble finding the right treatment, one of the virtues of this approach.

1. [Ú.MEŠ *nap-šal*]-*ti*[1] ŠU.GIDIM.MA SAG.ḪUL.ḪA.ZA(coll.) ^{Ú}*tar-muš*

^{Ú}x[ ]

2. [NUMUN ^{GIŠ}ŠI]NIG NUMUN ^{GIŠ}MA.NU NA$_4$ *ga-bi-i* ^{Ú}KUR.KUR $^{\text{NA}_4}$*mu-ṣa* ^{Ú}[…]
3. [^{Ú}NU.L]UḪ.ḪA ^{Ú}*úr-nu-u* ^{Ú}*ti-ia-a-tú* 12 Ú.MEŠ ŠU.GIDIM.MA *u* SAG.ḪUL.⸢ḪA.ZA⸣

---

4. [DIŠ NA Š]À.MEŠ-*šú it-te-*⸢*nem*⸣*-mi-ru liq* KA-*šú i-ta-nab-b*[*al*]
5. [Á$^{\text{II.MEŠ}}$]-*šú šim-ma-tú* TUKU.MEŠ-*a i-ge-eš-šú az-zu-za-a bi-bil* ŠÀ TUKU.MEŠ
6. [IGI.DU]$_8$-*ma* UGU-*šú* NU DÙG.GA MUNUS ŠÀ-*šú ḫa-šiḫ-ma* MUNUS IGI.DU$_8$-*ma* ŠÀ-*šú* NU ÍL-*šú*
7. [ŠÀ-*šú a*]-*na da-ba-bi ša-pil* NA BI ŠU.GIDIM.MA ÚS-*šú ana* TI-*šú*
8. [^{Ú}*tar-mu*]*š$_8$* ^{Ú}*imḫur-lim* ^{Ú}*imḫur*-20 ^{Ú}KUR.KUR UMBIN UR.GI$_7$ GI$_6$
9. [^{Ú}*ú*]*r-nu-u* ^{Ú}NU.LUḪ.ḪA ^{Ú}*ti-iá-tum* ^{IM}SAḪAR.NA$_4$.KUR.RA
10. [TÉŠ.BI] GAZ SIM *lu ina* KAŠ *lu ina* GEŠTIN NAG.NAG-*ma ina-eš*

---

11. [DIŠ NA *ina*] DIB ŠU.GIDIM.MA SAG ŠÀ-*šú* KÚM-*im* KÚM ŠÀ TUKU-*ši* SAG ŠÀ-*šú*
12. [*i-k*]*a-as-sa-su* ^{Ú}*tar-muš* ^{Ú}*imḫur-lim* ^{Ú}*imḫur*-20 ^{Ú}ḪAR.ḪAR
13. [NUMU]N ^{GIŠ}ŠINIG NUMUN ^{GIŠ}MA.NU ^{Ú}*úr-nu-u* $^{\text{Ú(coll.)}}$GEŠTIN.KA$_5$.A ^{Ú}*ti-iá-tum*
14. ⸢^{Ú}⸣NU.LUḪ.ḪA *ina* KAŠ SAG *ma-al-da-ra* NAG.NAG-*ma* DIN-*uṭ*

---

15. [DI]Š NA *ina* DIB ŠU.GIDIM.MA SAG ŠÀ-*šú i-kàs-sa-su ana* TI-*šú* ^{Ú}*tar-muš$_8$* ^{Ú}*imḫur-lim*
16. ^{Ú}*imḫur*-20 ^{Ú}ḪAR.ḪAR ^{GIŠ}ŠINIG A ^{Ú}*úr-né-e* NUMUN ^{GIŠ}ŠINIG NUMUN ^{GIŠ}MA.NU *ina* KAŠ NAG.MEŠ-*šú*

---

17. DIŠ NA ŠU.GIDIM.MA DIB-*su-ma* ÚS.ÚS-*šú ana* TI-*šú* ^{Ú}*tar-muš$_8$* ^{Ú}*imḫur-lim*
18. ^{Ú}*imḫur*-20 ^{Ú}ḪAR.ḪAR ^{Ú}KUR.KUR ^{Ú}*úr-nu-u* $^{\text{Ú(coll.)}}$GEŠTIN.KA$_5$.A
19. 7 Ú.ḪI.A ŠU.GIDIM.MA *pa-šá-ri ta-sàk ina* KAŠ SAG NAG.MEŠ-*ma ina-eš*

---

20. DIŠ KI.MIN ^{Ú}*tar-muš$_8$* ^{Ú}*imḫur-lim* ^{Ú}*imḫur*-20 ^{Ú}ḪAR.ḪAR ^{Ú}KUR.KUR NUMUN ^{GIŠ}ŠINIG
21. NUMUN ^{GIŠ}MA.NU ^{Ú}*a-zal-lá* ^{Ú}NU.LUḪ.ḪA ^{Ú}ÚR.NU.LUḪ.ḪA ^{Ú}*úr-nu-u*
22. ^{IM}SAḪAR.NA$_4$.KUR.RA 12 Ú.ḪI.A ŠU.GIDIM.MA *ina* KAŠ NAG.

MEŠ-*ma ina-eš*

---

23. DIŠ KI.MIN ^{Ú}*imḫur-lim* NUMUN ^{GIŠ}ŠINIG NA$_4$ *ga-bi-i* 3 Ú.ḪI.A ŠU.GIDIM.MA *ina* KAŠ NAG.MEŠ-*ma* ⸢*ina-eš*⸣

---

24. DIŠ NA ŠU.GIDIM DIB-*su-ma* ÚS.ÚS-*šú* ^{Ú}*tar-muš*$_8$ ^{Ú}*imḫur-lim* ^{Ú}*imḫur-*20 ^{Ú}ḪAR.ḪAR ⸢x⸣
25. NUMUN ^{GIŠ}ŠINIG NUMUN ^{GIŠ}MA.NU NUMUN ^{Ú}IN.NU.UŠ NUMUN ^{Ú}*u*$_5$*-ra-n*[*u*]
26. ^{Ú}*ár-zal-lum* 10 Ú.ḪI.A ŠU.GIDIM.MA *ina* KAŠ NAG.MEŠ-*ma ina-*[*eš*]

---

27. [DIŠ KI.MIN ...] ⸢^{Ú}*imḫur-lim* ^{Ú}⸣*imḫur-*20 ^{Ú}ḪAR.ḪAR ^{Ú}KUR.KUR NUMUN ^{GIŠ}MA.[NU]
28. [...] x NA$_4$ *ga-bi-i* GÌR.PAD.DU NAM.LÚ.U$_1$[$_8$.LU]
29. [... x Ú.ḪI.A ŠU.GIDIM.MA *ina* KAŠ NA]G.MEŠ-⸢*ma*⸣ *ina-*[*eš*]

TRANSLATION

(1–3) [Plants for] a ⸢salve⸣ for "hand" of ghost and the *mukil rēš lemutti*-demon: *tarmuš*, [*imḫur-lim*], [*imḫur-ešra*], ⸢*bīnu*-tamarisk⸣ [seed], seed of *eʾru*-tree, alum, *atāʾišu*, *mūṣu*-stone, [...], ⸢*nuḫurtu*⸣, *urnû*-mint, (and) *tīyatu*: twelve plants for "hand" of ghost and the *mukil rēš lemutti*-demon.

(4–10) [If a person's] ⸢insides⸣ are continually colicky, his palate continually gets ⸢dry⸣, his [arms] are continually numb, he belches, he has plenty of appetite (for food), but when [he sees it], it does not please him; he wants a woman, but when he sees a woman, his heart does not rise in him; [his heart] is (too) depressed (for him) to speak—"hand" of ghost is pursuing that person.[2] To cure him, you crush [together] (and) sift ⸢*tarmuš*⸣, *imḫur-lim*, *imḫur-ešra*, *atāʾišu*, *ḫašû*-thyme (= "claw of a black dog"), ⸢*urnû*⸣-mint, *nuḫurtu*, *tīyatu*, (and) alum. If he continually drinks (it mixed) either with beer or wine, he should recover.

(11–14) [If, as the result of] affliction by "hand" of ghost, [a person]'s epigastrium is hot; he has internal fever (and) his upper abdomen (epigastrium) gnaws at him,[3] if you have him repeatedly drink *tarmuš*, *imḫur-lim*, *imḫur ešra*, *ḫašû*-thyme, *bīnu*-tamarisk ⸢seed⸣, seed of *eʾru*-tree, *urnû*-mint, "fox grape," *tīyatu*, (and) *nuḫurtu* (mixed) with beer, he should recover.

(15–16) If, as the result of affliction by "hand" of ghost a person's upper abdomen (epigastrium) gnaws at him,[4] to cure him, you have him drink *tarmuš*, *imḫur-lim*, *imḫur ešra*, *ḫašû*-thyme, *bīnu*-tamarisk, *urnû*-mint infusion, *bīnu*-tamarisk seed, (and) seed of *eʾru*-tree (mixed) with beer.

(17–19) If "hand" of ghost afflicts a person and continually pursues him, to cure him, you grind seven plants to clear up "hand" of ghost: *tarmuš*, *imḫur-lim*, *imḫur ešra*, *ḫašû*-thyme, *atāʾišu*, *urnû*-mint, (and) "fox grape." If he repeatedly drinks (it mixed) with beer, he should recover.

(20–22) Alternatively, if he repeatedly drinks twelve plants for "hand" of ghost: *tarmuš*, *imḫur-lim*, *imḫur ešra*, *ḫašû*-thyme, *atāʾišu*, *bīnu*-tamarisk seed, seed of *eʾru*-tree, *azallû*, *nuḫurtu*, *tīyatu*, *urnû*-mint, (and) alum (mixed) with beer, he should recover.

(23) Alternatively, if you have him repeatedly drink three plants for "hand" of ghost: *imḫur-lim*, *imḫur ešra*, *bīnu*-tamarisk seed, (and) alum (mixed) with beer, he should recover.

(24–26) If "hand" of ghost afflicts a person and continually pursues him, if you repeatedly have him drink ten plants for "hand" of ghost: *tarmuš*, *imḫur-lim*, *imḫur ešra*, *ḫašû*-thyme, *bīnu*-tamarisk seed, seed of *eʾru*-tree, seed of *maštakal*, *urânu* seed, (and) *arzallu* (mixed) with beer, he should ⸢recover⸣.

(27–29) [Alternatively], if you have him repeatedly ⸢drink⸣ [so many plants for "hand" of ghost]: [*tarmuš*], *imḫur-lim*, *imḫur ešra*, *ḫašû*-thyme, *atāʾišu*, seed of ⸢*eʾru*⸣-tree, [...], alum, "lone plant" (= "human bone"), (and [...] (mixed) [with beer], he should ⸢recover⸣.

2. ULCERS

The recognition that the symptoms of peptic ulcer are connected with constriction of the mouth of the stomach indicates that the ancient physician performed autopsies as part of his practice. For more, see Scurlock and Andersen 2005, 133–35.

TEXT 2: *STT* 96

STT 96 contains potions (1–19) and a bandage (20–28) for ulcers. Of these, one (5–8) bears the telltale signs of original pharmacist origin. The recommendation to eat or drink hot things (9–15, 20–28) once again links these treatments to those for lung conditions. The alum of lines 16–19 would serve as an antiacid. Lines 20–28 are interesting in taking the patients' wishes on the subject of bandages into consideration.

1. DIŠ NA KA *kar-še* ⸢GIG⸣-[*ma d*]*u-ga-nu* DIB.MEŠ-⸢*su*⸣ *ana* TI-*šú*

2. 1/2 GÍN ^{ŠEM}GÚR.GÚR 1/2 GÍN $^{\text{Š[E]M}}$BI‹.ZI.DA› 5/6 ^{Ú}NU.LUḪ.ḪA 2/3 ^{Ú}ḪAR.ḪAR

3. 1/3 SUḪUŠ NAM.TAR NÍTA 5 ⸢Ú⸣.ḪI.A ⸢ŠEŠ⸣ 1-*niš* SÚD *ina* GEŠTIN SUR *lu ina* KAŠ.SAG

4. NU *pa-tan* NA[G.M]EŠ-*su-ma* TI-*uṭ*

---

5. DIŠ NA ⸢*du*⸣-[*ga-nu šá l*]*a*(!) ⸢*nu*(!)-*uḫ*⸣-*ḫu*[5] TUKU-*ši* NA BI [K]A *kar-še* GIG *ana* TI-[*šú*]

6. ^{Ú}MAN.[DU] ⸢$^{\text{Ú?}}$⸣[o] ⸢^{Ú}⸣NU.LU[Ḫ].ḪA ^{Ú}ḪAR.ḪAR S[UḪUŠ] ^{GIŠ}NAM.TAR NÍTA

7. ^{Ú}*imḫur-lim* ⸢^{Ú}⸣*imḫur*-20 7 Ú ⸢KA⸣ *kar-še* ⸢GIG⸣ [*m*]*ál-la-ma-liš* ⸢*tu*⸣-*šam-ṣa*

8. 1-*niš* ⸢SÚD⸣ *ina* GEŠTIN SUR *lu* [*ina* KAŠ] SAG NAG.MEŠ-*su* TI-*uṭ*

---

9. DIŠ NA *du-ga-nu* DIB-*su* SAG ⸢ŠÀ-*šú*⸣ *ú-ṣa-rap-šú* NU *pa-tan ú-ga-áš*

10. ⸢NA BI⸣ KA *kar-še* GIG *ana* TI-*šú* ^{Ú}*tar-muš*$_8$ ^{Ú}*imḫur-lim* ^{Ú}*imḫur*-20 ^{Ú}SIKIL

11. ^{Ú}KUR.KUR ^{Ú}ḪAR.ḪAR GAZI^{SAR} SUḪUŠ ^{GIŠ}NAM.TAR NÍTA GÚ.TUR *qa-lu-a*

12. 9 Ú.ḪI.A ŠEŠ 1-*niš* SÚD *ina* KAŠ SAG ⸢NAG⸣ Ú.ḪI.A ŠEŠ *ina* IGI KI.NÁ-*šú* NAG

13. ⸢BAD GÚ⸣.TUR *qa-la-a mál-li-riš ik-ta-na-li baḫ*-[*ra*]

14. [GU$_7$ ^{Ú}]SIKIL ^{Ú}GEŠTIN!.KA$_5$.A GAZI^{SAR} ^{ŠEM}GÚR.GÚR ^{ŠEM}LI ^{ŠEM}ŠE.LI.BABBAR

15. ⸢15⸣ Ú.ḪI.A ŠEŠ *mál-ma-liš* 1-*niš* SÚD *ina* KAŠ SAG NU *pa-tan* NAG-*ma* TI-*uṭ*

---

16. DIŠ NA *tu*!-*ga-nu* GIG *ana* TI-*šú* ⸢^{Ú}⸣*ak-tam* ^{Ú}*imḫur-lim* ^{Ú}*imḫur*-20 ^{Ú}*tar-muš*

17. ^{Ú}KUR.KUR ^{Ú}DÙ-SIG ^{Ú}KUR.G[I.R]IN.NA ^{Ú}GAMUN.GI$_6$ Ú.BABBAR $^{\text{Š[EM]}}$ŠEŠ

18. IM.SAḪAR.⸢NA$_4$⸣.KUR.RA IM.KÙ.SIG[$_{17}$ I]M.SA$_5$ *é-ni-na* ILLU [LI].DUR

19. 15 ⸢Ú⸣.[ḪI].⸢A⸣ ŠEŠ 1-*niš* SÚD *ina* ⸢KAŠ SAG⸣ *ina* Ì *ḫal-ṣi* NU *pa-tan* N[AG-*ma*] ⸢TI⸣-*uṭ*

---

20. DIŠ NA KA *kar-ši* GIG SAG ŠÀ-*šú ú-ḫa-mat-su ú-ṣar-rap-su ú-zaq-qat-šú*

21. *u* GU$_7$.MEŠ-*su* ⸢NA? BI?⸣ *túga-ni u* DÚR.GIG [*ana*] ⸢TI⸣-*šú* 2/3 MA.NA

Ì.UDU

22. ÉLLAG UDU.NÍTA 2/3 MA.NA ⸢*qí*⸣-*lip* ZÚ.LUM.MA [x GÍ]N ⸢^{ŠEM}GÚR.GÚR 6 GÍN⸣ ^{ŠEM}BAL
23. 5 GÍN ^{ŠEM}ŠEŠ 5 GÍN ^{ŠEM}LI 5 GÍN [o o] 5 ⸢GÍN⸣ ^{ŠEM}ḪAB 5 GÍN
24. ⸢^{ŠEM}⸣BULUḪ 5 GÍN ILLU ^{ŠEM}BULUḪ 1-*niš* SÚD ⸢KI⸣ 1 MA.NA Ú.ḪI.A 1/2 MA 5 GÍN 4-*tú*
25. ⸢Ì.UDU⸣ ÉLLAG UDU.NÍTA 1/2 MA.NA 5 ⸢GÍN⸣ 4-*tú qí-lip* ⸢ZÚ.LUM. MA⸣ 1-*niš* ⸢*tu*⸣-*sam-maḫ*
26. [*ina* KU]Š EDIN.NA *ma-la* ŠÀ-*šú* A.RA.ME *tu*-⸢*šam*⸣-*ṣa* SAG ŠÀ-*šú*
27. [GABA-*s*]*u u* DÚR-*šú* LAL-*ma baḫ-ra* GU$_7$! *baḫ-ra* ⸢NAG⸣ U$_4$.5.KÁM ŠEŠ
28. [DÙ.DÙ-*u*]*š-ma* TI-*uṭ*

Translation

(1–4) If the mouth of a person's stomach is sick [so that] ⸢*tugānu*⸣ continually afflicts him, to cure him, you grind together these five plants: 1/2 shekel of *kukru*, 1/2 shekel of ⸢*guḫlu*-antimony⸣, 5/6 shekel of *nuḫurtu*, 2/3 shekel of *ḫašû*-thyme (and) 1/3 shekel of male *pillû* root. If you have him ⸢repeatedly drink⸣ (it mixed) with drawn wine or first-quality beer on an empty stomach, he should recover.

(5–8) If a person has ⸢*tugānu*⸣ that cannot be calmed down, that person (has) sick ⸢mouth⸣ of the stomach,[6] to cure him, ⸢*su*ʾ*ādu*⸣, […], *nuḫurtu*, *ḫašû*-thyme, male *pillû* ⸢root⸣, *imḫur-lim* (and) *imḫur-ešra* are seven plants for sick mouth of the stomach. You take them in equal proportions. You grind them together. You have him repeatedly drink (it mixed) with drawn wine or first quality [beer]. He should recover.

(9–15) If *tugānu* afflicts a person, his upper abdomen (epigastrium) burns him (and) he vomits without having eaten, that person (has) sick mouth of the stomach,[7] to cure him, you grind together these nine plants: *tarmuš*, *imḫur-lim*, *imḫur-ešra*, *sikillu*, *atā*ʾ*išu*, *ḫašû*-thyme, *kasû*, male *pillû* root, (and) roasted *kakku*-lentils. You have him drink (it mixed) with first-quality beer. You have him drink these plants before he goes to bed. If he can consistently[8] keep down the roasted *kakku*-lentils, [you have him eat] ⸢hot things⸣. You grind together these fifteen plants in equal proportions: (the previously mentioned nine plants plus) *sikillu*, "fox grape," *kasû*, *kukru*, *burāšu*-juniper, (and) *kikkirānu*-juniper berries. If you have him drink (it mixed) with first-quality beer on an empty stomach, he should recover.

(16–19) If a person is sick with *tugānu*, to cure him, you grind together these fifteen plants: *aktam*, *imḫur-lim*, *imḫur-ešra*, *tarmuš*, *atā*ʾ*išu*, *kalbānu*,

⸢*kurkānu*-turmeric⸣, *zibû*, "white plant," myrrh, alum, *šīpu*, *šaršerru*, *ininnu*-barley, (and) ⸢*abukkatu*⸣ resin. [If] ⸢you have him drink⸣ (it) on an empty stomach (mixed) with first-quality beer (and) with pressed-out oil, he should recover.

(20–28) If the mouth of a person's stomach is sick, his upper abdomen (epigastrium) burns him, burns him hotly, stings him and hurts him, that person (has) *tugānu* or DÚR.GIG,[9] [to] cure him, you grind together 2/3 *manû* of fat from the kidney of a wether, 2/3 *manû* of date rind, [6?] ⸢shekels⸣ of *kukru*, 6 shekels of *ballukku*-aromatic, 5 shekels of myrrh, 5 shekels of *burāšu*-juniper, 5 shekels of [...], 5 shekels of *ṭūru*-aromatic, 5 shekels of *baluḫḫu*-aromatic, (and) 5 shekels of *baluḫḫu*-aromatic resin. You thoroughly mix (it) together in a proportion of 1/2 *manû* 5 1/4 shekel of fat from the kidney of a wether and 1/2 *manû* 5 1/4 shekel of date rind per 1 *manû* of plants. (You massage it) [into] waterproof ⸢leather⸣ (and) use it as many times as the patient desires to bandage his epigastrium [and breast] or his anus. And then, you have him eat and drink hot things. If [you do this repeatedly] for five days, he should recover.

3. INTESTINAL WORMS

Ancient Mesopotamians had close encounters with a number of unwelcome guests. The *urbātu*-worm, if indeed what we call ascaris, will have varied in size from 10–20 cm (4–8 inches) and have made itself at home in the gastrointestinal tract, occasionally, to the patient's dismay, crawling out his anus, nose or mouth. For more details, see Scurlock and Andersen 2005, 82–83.

TEXT 3: BAM 159 ii 20–48

BAM 159 ii 20–48 is preceded by a section on the liver and gall bladder (i 21–ii 19) and followed by a section on DÚR.GIG (ii 49–iii 24, 47–56), which actually connect to each other (see below). What attracted these references to this location was presumably the bloated insides treated in the immediately preceding ii 19. This section consists of potions (ii 20–42), aliments (ii 25–27, 35) and enemas (ii 43–48) for *urbātu*-worms. With the potions and aliments, the patient was expected to "groan" and produce the worm. The enemas were lubricated with pressed-out oil.

ii

20. DIŠ NA ŠÀ.MEŠ-*šú* MÚ.MEŠ-*ḫu* IM *ina* ŠÀ-*šú uš-tar-a*ʾ*-ab*
21. ŠÀ-*šú* DIB.DIB-*su-ma rit-ta-šú ina* ŠÀ-*šú e-ta-nab-bal*[10]
22. NA BI *ur-ba-tu* GIG *ana* TI-*šú* NUMUN Ú DIDLI

23. NUMUN ^{Ú}TÁL.TÁL ^{Ú}*saḫ-la-na* 3 Ú.ḪI.A ŠEŠ
24. 1-*niš* SÚD *ina* GEŠTIN NAG-*šú* [(*ú-na-ḫa-sa*)]!-*ma* ŠUB-*a*

---

25. DIŠ NA *ur-ba-tu* GIG x[…] SUM^{SAR}
26. NU *pa-tan* GU$_7$ KAŠ ⸢KÚM⸣ x[… *tu*]-*šá-ʾ-ad-ma* NAG
27. *ú*-⸢*na-ḫa*⸣-*sa-ma* ŠUB-*a*

---

28. DIŠ MIN PA ^{GIŠ}NU.ÚR.MA *šá* IGI I[M.S]I.SÁ TI-*qí*
29. *ina* A ⸢^{GIŠ}ŠE⸣.[NÁ].⸢A⸣ *ina* NINDU BAD-*ir ina še-rim* E$_{11}$-*a*
30. *ta-šá-ḫal* ⸢ŠED$_7$⸣ [Ì].KU$_6$ ⸢A?⸣.MEŠ *ana* ŠÀ ŠUB-*di*
31. 3 U$_4$-*me* [… *tu-šap*]-*ra-šú-ma* […] ⸢MIN⸣

---

32. DIŠ MIN SUḪUŠ ^{GIŠ}*šu-ši* SÚD *ana* Š[À] Ì+GIŠ ŠUB […] ⸢MIN⸣

---

33. DIŠ MIN ^{Ú}LAG.GÁN SÚD *ina* Ì+GIŠ *u* KAŠ.SAG [NAG] MIN

---

34. DIŠ MIN SUM^{SAR} SÚD *saḫ-lé-e ta-pa-aṣ* […] NU *pa-tan* NAG MIN

---

35. DIŠ MIN GA.RAŠ^{SAR} *ú-pa-qam* GU$_7$ KAŠ ⸢KÚM⸣ [… *tu*]-*šá-ʾ-ad-ma* NAG MIN

---

36. DIŠ MIN ^{Ú}ŠE.LÚ^{SAR} SÚD *ina* LÀL […]
37. DIŠ MIN Ú.⸢KUR⸣.RA^{SAR} SÚD *ina* A.MEŠ N[AG]-⸢*ma*⸣ [ŠUB-*a*]
38. DIŠ MIN ^{Ú}ḪUR.SAG^{SAR} SÚD *ina* KAŠ NAG-*ma* ŠUB-[*a*]
39. DIŠ MIN ^{Ú}*úr-nu-u* SÚD *ina* KAŠ NAG-*ma* ŠUB-*a*
40. DIŠ MIN ^{Ú}PA ^{GIŠ}Ù.SUḪ$_5$ SÚD *ina* KAŠ NAG-*ma* ŠUB-*a*
41. DIŠ MIN SUM^{SAR} SÚD *ina* A.GEŠTIN.NA NAG-*ma* ŠUB-*a*
42. DIŠ MIN Ì.KU$_6$ NAG-*ma* ŠUB-*a*

---

43. DIŠ NA ŠÀ-*šú ur-ba-tu qu-qa-nu u pi-lu-u*
44. DIB-*it* 14 ŠE.BAR ^{Ú}*imḫur-lim* SÚD *ina* Ì+GIŠ *ḫal-ṣi*
45. GAZ *ana* DÚR-*šú* DUB-*ak-ma* TI

---

46. DIŠ NA ŠÀ-*šú ur-ba-tu* DIB-*it rit-ta-šú i-ta-nab-bal*
47. ŠEM.ḪI.A DÙ.⸢A⸣.BI-*šú-nu ina* GEŠTIN SUR *u* KAŠ *tu-la-bak* ŠEG$_6$-*šal ta-šá-ḫal*
48. 10 GÍN LÀL 1/3 *qa* Ì+GIŠ *ḫal-ṣa ana* ŠÀ ŠUB *ana* DÚR-*šú ta-ḫi-ṭa-šú*

TRANSLATION

(ii 20–24) If a person's insides are continually bloated and "wind" rumbles in his stomach, his stomach continually afflicts him, (and) he keeps bringing his hand up to his abdomen, that person is sick with *urbatu*-worms.[11] To cure him, you grind together these three plants: "lone plant" seed, *urânu* seed, (and) *saḫlānu*. You have him drink (it mixed) with wine. He should groan and produce (the worm).

(ii 25–27) If a person is sick with *urbātu*-worms, you have him eat [...] and *šūmu*-garlic on an empty stomach and [you] add enough hot beer (and) [...] and have him drink (it). He should groan and produce (the worm).

(ii 28–31) Alternatively, you take the leaves of a *nurmû*-pomegranate which faces ⸢north⸣ (and) bake (it) in [...] water. In the morning, you take (it) out, filter (it and) let (it) cool. You pour fish [oil] and water(?) into it [and have him drink it] for three days. If ⸢you have him vomit⸣, [he should groan] (and) ditto (produce the worm).

(ii 32) Alternatively, you grind *šūšu*-licorice root, pour (it) into oil [and have him drink (it)]. Ditto. (He should groan and produce the worm).

(ii 33) Alternatively, you grind *kirbān eqli* (and) [have him drink (it)] (mixed) with oil and first-quality beer. Ditto. (He should groan and produce the worm).

(ii 34) Alternatively, you grind *šūmu*-garlic (and) pulverize *saḫlû*-cress.[12] [...] You have him drink (it) on an empty stomach. Ditto. (He should groan and produce the worm).

(ii 35) Alternatively, he should carefully eat *karāšu*-leek. [You] add enough hot beer (and) [...] and have him drink (it). Ditto. (He should groan and produce the worm).

(ii 36–42) Alternatively, you grind *kisibirrītu*. [If you have him drink (it)] (mixed) with honey [he should produce the worm]. Alternatively, you grind *nīnû*-mint. ⸢If you have him drink (it)⸣ (mixed) with water [he should produce the worm]. Alternatively, you grind *azupīru*. If you have him drink (it mixed) with beer, he should produce (the worm). Alternatively, you grind *urnû*-mint. If you have him drink (it mixed) with beer, he should produce (the worm). Alternatively, you grind *ašūḫu*-tree leaves. If you have him drink (it mixed) with beer, he should produce (the worm). Alternatively, you grind *šūmu*-garlic. If you have him drink (it mixed) with vinegar, he should produce (the worm). Alternatively, if you have him drink fish oil, he should produce (the worm).

(ii 43–45) If a person's stomach is afflicted by *urbātu*-worms, *quqānu*-worms and eggs,[13] you grind fourteen grains of *imḫur-lim*. You crush (it) in pressed-out oil. If you pour (it) into his anus, he should recover.

(ii 46–48) If *urbātu*-worms afflict a person's stomach (and) he continually brings up his hand, you moisten *labanātu*-incense with drawn wine and beer. You boil (and) filter (it). You pour 10 shekels of honey and 1/3 *qû* of pressed-out oil into it. You weigh it out for his anus.[14]

4. HORSE INDIGESTION

Virtually nothing is known about veterinary science in ancient Mesopotamia. Only the odd reference to skin lesions in animals and this precious set of treatments hint at what we are missing. For more on this subject, see Stol 2011, 363–402 with special reference to this text. BAM 159 v 33–47 consists of a potion (v 33–36) and an enema (v 37–47) for indigestion in a horse. Both are formulated in such a way as to suggest that they were normally in the purview of the pharmacist, which may be why we have so few of them. We learn that enemas were administered using a leather bag and that horses got medicine poured into their nostrils. This section follows a treatment for the mouth and nostrils for *bu'šānu*. The mention of nostrils is what presumably attracted this reference to this particular location.

TEXT 4: BAM 159 v 33–47

v

33. ^{Ú}*zi-im*-KÚ.BABBAR ^{Ú}*zi-im*-KÚ.SIG$_{17}$ ^{Ú}*ár-zal-lá*
34. ^{Ú}SAR-A.ŠÀ ^{Ú}*el-lat*-A.ŠÀ ^{Ú}⸢*ka-su*⸣*-u*
35. ^{Ú}*tur-a-ni*[15] SUḪUŠ ^{Ú}*tur-a-ni* 8 Ú *ki-iṣ* ŠÀ-*bi*
36. *šá* ANŠE.KUR.RA *ina* GEŠTIN SUR *ina na-ḫir* GÙB-*šú* DUB-*aq-ma* TI

---

37. ^{GIŠ}*e-ri-nu* ^{GIŠ}ŠUR.MÌN ^{GIŠ}*dap-ra-nu* ^{ŠEM}GÍR ŠEM.SAL
38. GI.DÙG.GA ^{ŠEM}BAL ŠEM.^{d}MAŠ ^{ŠEM}MAN.DU ^{Ú}KUR.KUR
39. ^{ŠEM}GÚR.GÚR ^{ŠEM}LI ^{ŠEM}ŠE.LI.BABBAR ^{ŠEM}GAM.MA
40. ^{Ú}ḪAR.ḪAR ^{Ú}*si-ḫu* ^{GIŠ}*ár-gan-nu* ^{GIŠ}LUM.ḪA NAGA.SI
41. ^{Ú}NU.LUḪ.ḪA MUN *saḫ-lé-e* GAZI^{SAR} 23 Ú.ḪI.A ŠEŠ
42. 1/3 *qa*.TA.ÀM TI-*qí ina* KAŠ *tu*-^{LA}*lab-bak ina* GI$_6$
43. *ana* IGI MUL.ÙZ *tuš-bat ina še-rim* ŠEG$_6$-*šal ta-šá-ḫal*
44. ŠE.KAK ^{Ú}ÚKUŠ.GÍL Ú x MEŠ SÚD KI 1 *qa* LÀL
45. *u* 1 *qa* Ì+GIŠ ⸢GAZ⸣ *ana* KUŠ *maš-qí-te te-sip*
46. *ana* DÚR-*šú* DUB-*ak maš-qí-tu ša* ANŠE.KUR.RA
47. *ša* 1-*en* ANŠE.KUR.RA 4 *qa* KAŠ.SAG *ba-áš-lu*

TRANSLATION

(v 33–36) "Silver blossom," "gold blossom" (*nuṣābu*), *arzalla*, ^{Ú}SAR-A.ŠÀ, *illat eqli*, *kasû*, *turânu*, and *turânu* root are eight plants for *kīṣ libbi* in a horse.[16] If you pour it into his right nostril (mixed) with drawn wine, he should recover.

(v 37–47) You take 1/3 *qa* each of these twenty-three plants: *erēnu*-cedar, *šurmēnu*-cypress, *daprānu*-juniper, *asu*-myrtle, *šimešallu*-aromatic, "sweet reed," *ballukku*-aromatic, *nikiptu*, *su'ādu*, *atā'išu*, *kukru*, *burāšu*-juniper, *kikkirānu*-juniper berries, *ṣumlalû*, *ḫašû*-thyme, *sīḫu*-wormwood, *argannu*, *barirātu*, *uḫḫūlu qarnānu*, *nuḫurtu*, salt, *saḫlû*-cress, (and) *kasû*. You moisten (it) with beer. You let (it) sit out overnight under the goat star. In the morning, you boil (and) filter (it). You grind *irrû* shoots (and) [these?] plants. You crush (everything) with 1 *qû* of honey and 11 *qû* of oil. You decant (it) into a leather enema bag (and) pour (it) into his anus. (This is) a potion for a horse; (you use) 4 *qû* of boiled first-quality beer per horse.[17]

5. "WIND"

TEXT 5: BAM 159 v 48–vi 33

The preserved parts of BAM 159 v 48–vi 33 contain enemas (v 48–vi 15, vi 23–33) for "wind." Other texts attest the use of potions and anal suppositories, and rarely, salves, plasters, baths, and bandages for this problem. Lines vi 23–33 are unusual in having the patient rinse his anus before and flush it out after application. This section is immediately preceded by horse indigestion (v 36–47). It is followed by a miscellaneous grab bag mostly dealing with ghostly fever (vi 41–47), headache (vi 48–50) and numbness (vi 51–54).

v

48. DIŠ NA ŠÀ.MEŠ-*šú* MÚ.MEŠ-*ḫu ir-ru-šú i-ár-ru-ru ir-ru-šú*
49. GÙ.GÙ-*ú* IM *ina* ŠÀ-*šú i-li-ib-bu ina* DÚR!-*šú ú-na-kap*
50. NA BI *nik-ma-ti* GIG *ana* TI-*šú* ^{Ú}KUR.KUR ^{Ú}*ti-iá-tú*
51. ^{Ú}ÚKUŠ.GÍL ^{MUN}*eme-sal-lim* NA$_4$ *ga-bi-i* 5 Ú.ḪI.A ŠEŠ
52. *ina* A.MEŠ *tu-lab-bak ana* DÚR-*šú* DUB-*ak-ma* TI

---

vi

1. [(DIŠ NA *e-sil-ti* ŠÀ-*šú šu-šu-ri u ur-še* GAZ.MEŠ)][18]
2. [(^{ŠEM}LI ^{ŠEM}GÚR.GÚR ^{Ú}NU.LUḪ.ḪA NAGA.SI ^{Ú}NAM.T)]I.LA *mál-*

ma-liš LAL *ina* KAŠ

3. [(*u* A.GEŠTIN.NA *ina* IZI ŠEG-*šal ta*)]-*šá-ḫal* ŠED$_7$-*ma* ‹Ì.GIŠ› *ana* IGI ŠUB-*di*
4. [(*ana* DÚR-*šú* DUB-*ak*) *ú-še-eš*]-*šir*!-*ma* TI

---

5. [...] *is-kir* IM GIN$_7$ *rit-ti*
6. [... S]Á.SÁ DÚR.GIG GIG
7. [... ^{ŠEM}]LI GAZI^{SAR} NAGA.SI
8. [...]x *saḫ-lé-e* Ú.KUR.RA
9. [...] *qa* A.GEŠTIN.NA
10. [... ŠE]N.TUR ŠEG$_6$-*šal ta-šá-ḫal* ŠED$_7$
11. [... D]UB-*ma* TI

---

12. [... ME]Š-*su* 1/3 GÍN ^{GIŠ}ERIN
13. [...]x 1/3 GÍN ^{GIŠ}ERIN SUMUN
14. [...]x ^{ŠEM}GÚR.GÚR 1-*niš* GAZ
15. [... *ina* A GAZI^{SAR} DÚR-*šú i-šá*]-*ḫat ana* DÚR-*šú* DUB-*ak*

---

16. [...]x GI.DÙG ^{ŠEM}BAL
17. [...^{GIŠ}]ERIN SUMUN ^{GIŠ}ŠE.NU
18. [...]x si LUM.MA

19–23. [...]

---

24. [(DIŠ NA SAG ŠÀ-*šú* DIB.DIB-*su* ŠÀ-*šú* MÚ.MÚ.MEŠ-*ḫ*)*u*]
25. [(*u* IM *e-ri* SA.MEŠ *šá* ⸢MURGU?⸣-*šú šad-d*)*u* (MURUB$_4$.MEŠ-*šú aš-ṭ*)]*a*
26. [(*kin-ṣa-a-šú* GU$_7$.MEŠ-*šú ina pa-ni ma-ka-le-e* MÚ)].MÚ-*aḫ*
27. (*u i-šá-aq*)-*qa* (NA BI *ni-kim-tú* IM *u* UD.DA GIG *la-a*)]*m* NA BI GIG *la-az-zi*
28. [(GUR-*šú* Ú.KUR.RA ^{Ú}KUR.KUR ^{Ú}*úr*)]-*né-e* ^{ŠEM}LI
29. [(^{ŠEM}ŠE.LI ^{ŠEM}GÚR.GÚR) ^{ŠE}]^{M}BAL 7 Ú.ḪI.A ŠEŠ
30. [IGI.(4.GÁL.BI *ina* NINDU) B]AD-*ir ina še-rim* E$_{11}$-*ma*
31. [(*tu-kaṣ*)-*ṣa ina* A (GAZ)]I^{SAR} *i-šá-ḫat* EGIR-*šú*
32. [...] EGIR-*šú* Ì+GIŠ u KAŠ.SAG
33. [*k*(*a-an-nam ana* DÚR-*šú* DUB-*ak-m*)]*a i-lab-bak*

TRANSLATION

(v 48–52) If a person's insides are continually bloated, his intestines rumble, his intestines continually make a loud noise, "wind" groans in his stomach (and) "buts" into his anus, that person is sick with pent-up (wind).[19] To cure him, you moisten these five plants: *atāʾišu*, *tiyātu*, *irrû*, *emesallim*-salt, (and) alum with water. If you pour (it) into his anus, he should recover.

(vi 1–4) In order to make a person's stopped-up bowels move and to annihilate *uršu*-lesions,[20] you measure out equal quantities of *burāšu*-juniper, *kukru*, *nuḫurtu*, *uḫḫūlu qarnānu*, (and) "life plant." You boil (it) over a fire in beer and vinegar, filter (it and) let (it) cool and then you pour on ‹oil›. You pour (it) into his anus. If he ⌜has a bowel movement,⌝ he should recover.

(vi 5–11) [If ...] he is stopped up (and) [he has] "wind" [(that hurts him so badly) that he has to bring] a hand [up], he was ⌜gotten⌝ by [*ṣētu*] or is sick with DÚR.GIG. [You ...] *burāšu*-juniper, *kasû*, *uḫḫūlu qarnānu*, [...], *saḫlû*-cress, *nīnû*-mint, and [...]. You boil (it) [in #] *qû* of vinegar [in] a ⌜*tamgussu*⌝-vessel, filter (it and) let (it) cool. [...] If you pour (it) [into his anus], he should recover.

(vi 12–15) [If ...], you crush together [...] 1/3 shekel of *erēnu*-cedar, [...], 1/3 shekel of *šupuḫru*-cedar, [...] (and) *kukru*. [...] [He] ⌜rinses⌝ [his anus with *kasû* juice]. You pour (it) into his anus.

(vi 16–18) [...], "sweet reed," *ballukku*-aromatic, [...], *šupuḫru*-cedar, *šunû*-chastetree, [...]

(vi 19–22) *(lost)*

(vi 23–33) If a person's epigastrium continually afflicts him, his insides are continually bloated and he is pregnant with "wind," the muscles of his ⌜back?⌝ are drawn taut; his hips are stiff, his legs continually hurt him and, before he eats, (his stomach) repeatedly bloats and ⌜raises up⌝, it may turn into a persistent illness (with) pent-up "wind" for that person. ⌜You bake 1/4 shekel⌝ (each) of these seven plants: *nīnû*-mint, *atāʾišu*, ⌜*urnû*-mint⌝, *burāšu*-juniper, *kikkirānu*-juniper berries, *kukru*, (and) *ballukku*-aromatic in an oven. In the morning, you take (it) out (and) ⌜let (it) cool⌝. He rinses (his anus) [with] *kasû* [juice]. Afterwards, [you pour (it) into his anus]. Afterwards, if you ⌜continually⌝ pour oil and first-quality beer into his anus, it will lubricate (it).

6. DÚR.GIG

This ancient Mesopotamian disease category covered chronic conditions that blocked or retarded the passage of urine or stool. For more details, see Scurlock and Andersen 2005, 150–53.

TEXT 6: BAM 159 COLS. ii 49–iii 24, 47–56

BAM 159 ii 49–iii 24, 47–56[21] consists of an enema (ii 49–53), a special diet (iii 1–6), potions (iii 7–9, 20–22), anal suppositories (iii 10–17), a daub (iii

10–14), salves (iii 18–19, 23–24) and a bandage (iii 47–54) for what appears, from the described symptoms, to be ulcerative colitis. Of these, eight (iii 15–24, 47–56) are formulated in such a way that they could have originated with (or been intended to be filled by) a pharmacist. Leaving a decoction out overnight under the stars as in lines ii 49–53 had the practical purpose of allowing the ingredients to cold steep but was supposed to gain the benefit of astral influences, as we know from the occasional instruction to put the decoction out under a particular star, usually that associated with Gula, goddess of healing. The rolled pickled beef and fish of lines iii 1–6 are an interesting addition to what we know of the ancient Mesopotamian diet. In lines iii 10–14, the pharmacist's lead spoon joins the physician's anal suppository. Suppositories came in finger and acorn shapes.

ii
49. DIŠ NA *ina-aṭ-ma lu ni-ṭa lu* MÚD.BABBAR *lu nik-ma-tu*
50. *šá* ⸢DÚR.GIG⸣ *ú-tab-ba-ka ana* TI-*šú* ^{ŠEM}GÚR.GÚR
51. ^{ŠEM}LI NAGA.SI ^{Ú}NU.LUḪ.ḪA ^{Ú}ÚKUŠ.GÍL
52. [...] *tara-muk ina* UL *tuš-bat ina še-rim*
53. [... Ì+G]IŠ *ana* IGI ŠUB-*di ana* DÚR-*šú* DUB-*ak-ma* TI

---

iii
1. [...] GA KU$_7$.KU$_7$ GA ⸢U$_8$.UDU.ME⸣
2. Ì.N[UN] Ì+GIŠ *ḫal-ṣa* U$_4$.1.⸢KÁM⸣.TA.ÀM ⸢GU$_7$⸣.MEŠ
3. DIŠ KI.MIN *mu-du-ul* GUD NIGIN-*ra mu-du-ul* KU$_6$
4. ⸢NIGIN-*ra* U$_4$.1.KÁM⸣.TA.ÀM ⸢GU$_7$⸣.MEŠ
5. DIŠ KI.MIN *mu-du-ul* GUD NIGIN-*ra* KI Ì.NUN
6. *ba-lu pa-tan* GU$_7$.MEŠ-*ma* TI

---

7. DIŠ KI.MIN ^{Ú}ḪAR.ḪAR *ina* KAŠ NAG Ì.UDU ^{Ú}ÚKUŠ.GÍL x[...]
8. DIŠ KI.MIN Ú.BABBAR SIG$_7$-*su ina* GA ŠEG$_6$-*ma* [...]
9. DIŠ KI.MIN Ú.KUR.RA *ina* KAŠ NAG-*ma* T[I]

---

10. DIŠ NA *ina-aṭ-ma ni-ṭa ú-tab-ba-ka* NA BI
11. *nik-ma-ti šá* DÚR.GIG *ana* TI-*šú* ŠEM.ŠEŠ
12. ^{ŠEM}ŠE.LI.BABBAR SÚD *ina* Ì.UDU ḪE.ḪE NAGAR-*nu* DÙ-*uš* [...]
13. DIŠ A ^{GIŠ}ŠE.NU ŠUB.ŠUB-*šú* DÚR-*šú i-par-ru* [...]
14. Ú.KUR.RA SÚD [...] SUD *it-gur-ti* DÚR-*šú te-*[*qí* ...]

---

15. ^{ŠEM}[o o o] *ni-kip-tú šu-nu* [o o] x [o]x
16. ^{Ú}[o o *bu*]-*uṭ-ṭu-tú* 7 Ú x[... G]IG

17. SÚD *kiš-še-ni* [o o] SUD *ina* [o o o *i*]*š-šá-ḫat*

---

18. DIŠ KI.MIN ^{Ú}[o o o] SÚD [o o] ⸢Ì⸣.NUN EŠ.MEŠ
19. DIŠ KI.MIN ^{Ú}*am-ḫa-*⸢*ra*⸣ SÚD *ina* Ì+GIŠ [...]

---

20. NA$_4$ *ga-bi-i a-ḫu-sa* KI.A.^{d}ÍD
21. x x [o]x pap pi ta NAGA.SI 1-*niš tur-ár*
22. *ina* Ì+GIŠ ‹‹GIŠ›› SUD Ú.ḪI.A ⸢*ta*⸣-*ri-*⸢*ḫat*⸣-*ti ša* KUR *Ḫat-ti*

---

23. DIŠ KI.MIN Ú.KUR.RA ^{Ú}GAMUN SÚD *ina* Ì+GIŠ EŠ.MEŠ
24. DIŠ KI.MIN ^{Ú}GA-*a-nu* SÚD *ina* Ì+GIŠ EŠ.MEŠ

25–46. (see chapter 11, text 2)

47. ^{Ú}*tar-muš*$_8$ ^{Ú}[...]
48. $^{\text{NA}_4}$PEŠ$_4$.ANŠE x[...]
49. *kar-áš tam-tim* [...]
50. NUMUN ^{GIŠ}*bi-ni* NUMUN [...]
51. ^{Ú}NU.LUḪ.ḪA [...]
52. ^{Ú}*šib-bur-r*[*a-tú* ...]
53. 30 Ú NÍG.LAL DÚR.G[IG ...]
54. *lu ina* KAŠ ^{LÚ}KÚR[UN.NA ...]

---

55. ^{IM}SAḪAR.NA$_4$.KU[R.RA ...]
56. 3 Ú MÚD.MEŠ [TAR-*si*]

TRANSLATION

(ii 49–53) If a person has bloody stools and pours out bloody excrement or pus or the pent-up (wind) of DÚR.GIG, to cure him,[22] you decoct[23] *kukru*, *burāšu*-juniper, *uḫḫūlu qarnānu*, *nuḫurtu*, (and) *irrû* [in ...]. You leave (it) out overnight under the stars. In the morning, you [...]. You pour ⸢oil⸣ onto it. If you pour (it) into his anus, he should recover.

(iii 1–6) [Alternatively], he should repeatedly eat [...] sweet milk, sheep's milk, ghee (and) pressed-out oil for one day each. Alternatively, he should repeatedly eat rolled pickled beef[24] (and) rolled pickled fish for one day each. Alternatively, if you have him repeatedly eat rolled pickled beef with ghee on an empty stomach, he should recover.

(iii 7) Alternatively, you have him drink *ḫašû*-thyme (mixed) with beer. [You ...] *irrû* "fat" [...].

(iii 8) Alternatively, you boil fresh "white plant" in milk and [...]

(iii 9) Alternatively, if you have him drink *nīnû*-mint (mixed) with beer, he should ⸢recover⸣.

(iii 10–14) If a person has bloody stools and pours out bloody excrement, that person (has) the pent-up (wind) of DÚR.GIG, to cure him, you grind myrrh (and) *kikkirānu*-juniper berries. You mix (it) with sheep fat. You form an acorn-shaped suppository and [insert (it) into his anus]. You repeatedly dip (the suppository) into *šunû*-chastetree infusion; his anus should vomit. You grind [...] (and) *nīnû*-mint (and) sprinkle (it) [on the suppository]. ⸢You daub⸣ his anus with a (lead) spoon. [...]

(iii 15–17) [...], *nikiptu*, *šunû*-chastetree, [...], [...], (and) ⸢*buṭuttu*⸣ (are) seven plants for [DÚR].GIG. You grind (them). You sprinkle [on] *kiššēnu*-bean. It should be rinsed with [*kasû* juice].

(iii 18) Alternatively, you grind [...]. You repeatedly gently rub (it) gently (on him mixed) [with] ghee.

(iii 19) Alternatively, you grind *amḫara*. [You repeatedly gently rub it on him mixed] with oil.

(iii 20–22) You char together alum, alkali, *kibrītu*-sulphur, [...], [...] (and) *uḫḫūlu qarnānu*. You sprinkle (it) with oil. Plants for Hittite *tarīḫus*.[25]

(iii 23) Alternatively, you grind *nīnû*-mint (and) *kamunu*-cumin. You repeatedly gently rub (it on him mixed) with oil.

(iii 24) Alternatively, you grind *šizbānu*. You repeatedly gently rub (it on him mixed) with oil.

(iii 25–46) *(see chapter 11 text 2)*

(iii 47–54) *Tarmuš*, [...], *biṣṣur atāne*-shell, [...], *karaš tamtim*, [...], *bīnu*-tamarisk seed, [...] seed, [...], *nuḫurtu*, [...], *šibburātu*, and [...] are thirty plants for a bandage for DÚR.GIG. [...] or in *kurunnu* beer [...].

(iii 55–56) Alum, [...] (and) [...] are three plants [to prevent] bleeding.

B. LIVER AND GALL BLADDER

Ancient Mesopotamians suffered from bladder stones, cholecystitis, and ascending cholangitis. They became jaundiced and, due to excessive consumption of alcoholic beverages and/or hepatitis, they got cirrhosis and, inevitably, some died of liver failure. Two types of jaundice were recognized by ancient physicians, *aḫḫāzu* and *amurriqānu*. They differentiated them on the basis of the presence or absence of wasting. For more details, see Scurlock and Andersen 2005, 136–47.

TEXT 7: BAM 578

BAM 578 represents tablet 3 of the seventh subseries of the Nineveh recension of UGU (see chapter 3, text 1), and belongs to that part of the UGU series dealing with problems of the liver and gall bladder. It begins with a bandage, potion and bath (i 1–13) for "sick insides." This is followed by potions (i 14–26) for "sick gall bladder," potions (i 27–37, ii 11–12, ii 67–iii 3), an enema (i 46–48) and an anal suppository (i 49) for what could be ascending cholangitis, a potion (i 38–41), an enema with preparatory rinse (i 42–44), and a bandage (i 45) for what could be gall stones, emetic potions (i 50–69) for possible chronic biliary obstruction and potions (ii 13–15, 18–22, 29–66), and an enema (ii 18–19) for *pašittu* (cholecystitis). There are also an enema with a preparatory rinse (i 70–ii 1) for jaundice of any type, potions (iii 8–24, iv 1–4, 6–14, 16–25), a fumigant (iii 17), salves (iii 18–19), aliments (iii 25–26, iv 1) and bandages (iv 8–9) for *amurriqānu*-jaundice and potions (iv 26–30, 35–42), a fumigant (iv 31–32) and salves (iv 31–34) for *aḫḫāzu*-jaundice. Jaundice in the eyes could also be treated with a wash (iv 5) or a daub (iv 15). Among these treatments, there are thirteen simple potions for the gall bladder (i 20–26), which look to be excerpts from a pharmacist's vademecum.

Lines i 1–13 are interesting in that they provide a rare diagnostic bandage. The physician thoughtfully cured the blister that was produced in the process before treating the patient's problem. Lines i 27–32 accompany the potion with a warming bandage and a diet of hot things. Lines i 38–41 describe one of those treatments that seem initially to make things worse. The physician is not to worry but, just in case, he enlists the goat star, puts a magic circle round the decoction, filters it three times and administers it on a propitious day.

Lines i 46–48 are interesting in describing positional vertigo. The hurting neck, hips, shins and feet are presumably reactive arthritis. Lines i 50–52 are interesting in that they mention teeth oozing blood which is caused by vitamin K deficiency, a known concomitant of gall bladder disease. Lines i 67–69 finish off the treatment by having the patient drink fatty pork broth. If that stays down, he is in the clear.

Lines ii 29–38 are a nice example of the continuing tradition of academic Sumerian. which begins in the Old Babylonian period, from which the earliest duplicates to this recitation come. Also typical of Old Babylonian material is the description of the treatment as part of the recitation. The bile came by itself, the recitation notes, now let it go away by itself! The evisaged treatment is salt which is to be eaten by the patient and expected to produce a loose bowel movement rather graphically described as a mixture of solid waste, "wind" and stinky brown bits. Interesting to note is that the younger version of this recitation preserved in ii 45–51 has added thyme to the salt.

Lines ii 39–44 gives an imaginative description of the symptoms of *pašittu*. Lines ii 45–51 is interesting in warning that imagining a disease as an animal does not entitle you to treat it like one. In other words, you, as a physician, are to use whatever works and not to allow your theory to dictate your treatment. Lines iii 4–7 cite the diagnostic handbook for conditions under which *amurriqānu*-jaundice can and cannot be treated. Lines iv 43–46 do the same for *aḫḫāzu*-jaundice.

Line iii 20, right in the middle of a section on potions for jaundice, has a nice transfer rite, whereby the patient goes straight home on a reddish road and crosses an abandoned bridge. Similarly, he wears a red gold ring in line iv 4 and a gold bead threaded on red wool in lines iv 12–13. To be avoided, because a bad sign, was anything black (iv 1).

Line iv 16 gives a salutary warning about the dosage of an effective, if dangerous, potion for jaundice. Unusually, the exact amount of the key ingredient is given, namely, five grains. Of interest to note in lines iv 31–34 is that this treatment for *aḫḫāzu*-jaundice is very similar to one already given for *amurriqānu*-jaundice (iii 17–20). The dangerous treatment of line iv 16 is also repeated in line iv 39 for *aḫḫāzu*-jaundice. We are safe in presuming that the fifteen grains were to be administered in three five-grain batches.

i

1. DIŠ NA SAG ŠÀ-*šú* GU$_7$-*šú ina ge-ši-šu* ZÉ *im-ta-na-ʾ* NA BI *qer-be-na* GIG
2. SUM^{SAR} GA.RAŠ^{SAR} UZU GUD UZU ŠAḪ KAŠ ^{LÚ}KÚRUN.NA NU *uš-ta-maḫ-ḫar ana* TI-*šú*
3. 1/2 *qa* ZAG.ḪI.LI 1/2 *qa* ^{ŠEM}LI 1/2 *qa* ^{ŠEM}GÚR.GÚR 1/2 *qa* NUMUN GADA 1/2 *qa pa-pa-si* MUNU$_6$ 1/2 *qa* ^{ŠEM}IM.DI
4. 1/2 *qa* NUMUN ^{Ú}*qut-ra-ti* 1/2 *qa* GAZI^{SAR} 1/2 *qa* ^{GIŠ}ŠE.NU 1/2 *qa* GÚ NÍG.ÀR.RA 1/2 *qa pa-pa-si*-^{d}ÍD
5. 1/2 *qa* Ú *a-ši-i* 1/2 *qa* Ú.KUR.RA 1/2 *qa* ŠÈ TU^{MUŠEN} 1/3 *qa* NUMUN ^{Ú}ÁB.DUḪ 1/3 *qa e-riš-ti* A.ŠÀ
6. 10 GÍN ILLU ^{ŠEM}BULUḪ 10 GÍN KA.A.AB.BA 1 *qa* ZÍD GIG 1 *qa* ZÚ.LUM.MA 1 *qa* KAŠ.Ú.SA SIG
7. 1 *qa* ZÌ.KUM TÉŠ.BI GAZ SIM *ina* KAŠ GIN$_7$ *ra-bi-ki ta-rab-bak ina* TÚG.ḪI.A SUR-*ri šu-lu-uš-ti* 9 U$_4$-*me* LAL
8. *ina* 4 U$_4$-*me* DU$_8$-*ma ta-mar šúm-ma* Ù.BÚ.BÚ.UL BABBAR ŠÀ-*šú i-pa-šaḫ*
9. *šúm-ma* Ù.BÚ.BÚ.UL SA$_5$ ŠÀ-*šú* KÚM *ú-kal šúm-ma* Ù.BÚ.BÚ.UL SIG$_7$ UD.DA KUR-*id*
10. GUR.GUR-*šu šúm-ma* Ù.BÚ.BÚ.UL GI$_6$ *ú-šam-ra-su-ma* NU TI

11. *ana* Ù.BÚ.BÚ.UL *bu-le-e* ^{Ú}LAG A.ŠÀ IM.GÚ *šá* UD.DA *di-kàt*
12. GAZ SIM *ina* A GAZI^{SAR} *ta-la-áš* LAL-*id* EGIR-*šú saḫ-lé-e ina* KAŠ NAG
13. U$_4$-*ma* NAG Ú.DILI A ^{GIŠ}*šu-nu* ^{GIŠ}ŠINIG ^{Ú}*ak-tam* ^{Ú}IN$_6$.ÚŠ *ir-ta-na-ḫaṣ*

---

14. DIŠ NA ZÉ GIG SUM^{SAR} SÚD *ina* A NU *pa-tan* NAG

---

15. A.GEŠTIN.NA KALAG.GA AL.ÚS.SA GAZI^{SAR} *kab-ru-ti* NAG

---

16. KAŠ.BIR$_8$ NAG *tu-šá-ʾ-raš-šú*

---

17. GAZI^{SAR} SÚD *ina* A NAG : MUN SÚD *ina* A NU *pa-tan* NAG : MUN SÚD *ina* KAŠ NU *pa-tan* NAG

---

18. ILLU *a-bu-kàt* GAZ *ana* KAŠ.BIR$_8$ ŠUB-*di ina* UL *tuš-bat ina še-rim* LÀL Ì *ḫal-ṣa ana* ŠÀ ŠUB NAG-*ma i-ár-ru*

---

19. NUMUN GI.ZÚ.LUM.MA SÚD *ina* KAŠ NAG : ^{Ú}*nam-ruq-qa* SÚD *ina* KAŠ NAG

---

20. Ú.DILI Ú ZÉ *ina* KAŠ NAG
21. ^{Ú}*me-er-gi-ra-nu* Ú ZÉ *ina* KAŠ NAG GAZI^{SAR} Ú ZÉ *ina* KAŠ NAG
22. $^{Ú.ŠEM}$LI Ú ZÉ *ina* KAŠ NAG ^{Ú}NU.LUḪ.ḪA Ú ZÉ *ina* KAŠ NAG
23. ^{Ú}BAR ^{GIŠ}*šu-ši* Ú ZÉ *ina* KAŠ NAG PA ^{Ú}*al-la-nu* Ú ZÉ *ina* KAŠ NAG
24. ^{Ú}U$_5$.ARGAB^{MUŠEN} Ú ZÉ *ina* KAŠ NAG ^{Ú}LAG MUN Ú ZÉ *ina* KAŠ NAG
25. ^{Ú}SUM^{SAR} Ú ZÉ *ina* KAŠ NAG ^{Ú}SUḪUŠ ^{GIŠ}NAM.TAR NÍTA Ú ZÉ SÚD *ina* KAŠ NAG
26. ^{Ú}SUḪUŠ ^{GIŠ}*šu-ši* Ú ZÉ S[ÚD] *ina* Ì *u* KAŠ NAG ^{Ú}*ṣi-ba-ru* Ú ZÉ SÚD *ina* A NAG

---

27. DIŠ NA NU *pa-tan* ŠÀ-*šú ana pa-re-e e-te-né-la-a* ÚḪ *ma-gal* ŠUB.MEŠ A.MEŠ *ina* KA-*šú mal-da-riš* DU-*ku*
28. *pa-nu-šú iṣ-ṣa-nu-du* ŠÀ.MEŠ-*šú* MÚ.MÚ-*ḫu* MURUB$_4$^{II}-*šú kin-ṣa-šú* TAG.GA.MEŠ-*šú* KÚM ŠED$_7$ IR TUKU.MEŠ-*ši*
29. NINDA *u* KAŠ LAL A ŠED$_7$ *ma-gal* NAG *i-par-ru ina* DÚR-*šú* GÌŠ-*šú* SIG$_7$ *ú-tab-ba-kam šur-šu*^{MEŠ}-*šú i-te-nen-nu-u*
30. UZU.MEŠ-*šu tab-ku mìm-ma* GU$_7$-*ma* UGU-*šú ul* DÙG.GA NA BI ZÉ *saḫ-pa-su ana* TI-*šú* ^{ŠEM}GÚR.[GÚR]

31. ^{ŠEM}LI ŠEM.GAM.MA 3 Ú.ḪI.A ŠEŠ SIG$_7$-*su-nu* TI-*qí* ḪÁD.A SÚD *ina* GEŠTIN.KALAG.GA NU *pa-tan* [NAG …]
32. ⸢SI.SÁ-*ma* SAG.ŠÀ⸣-*šú* ŠÀ-*šú* LAL-⸢*id*⸣ *baḫ-ra* GU$_7$ […]x U$_4$.3.KÁM* ku x […]

---

33. DIŠ KI.MIN ^{Ú}*a-ra-ri-a-nu* SÚD *ina* KAŠ *ina* IGI [NÁ-*šú* …]

---

34. DIŠ KI.MIN ^{Ú}*saḫ-la-a-nu* SÚD *ina* GEŠTIN KALAG.GA NU *pa-tan* [NAG-*šú* …]

---

35. DIŠ KI.MIN ^{Ú}*ṣi-bu-ru* SÚD *ina* GA KU$_7$.KU$_7$ N[AG-*šú* …]

---

36. DIŠ KI.MIN ŠE.KAK ^{Ú}ÚKUŠ.GÍL SÚD *ina* GEŠTIN LÀL *u* Ì *ḫal-ṣi* NAG-*šú* K[I.MIN]
37. DIŠ KI.MIN Ú.SIG.MEŠ *šá* KUR-*e ina* GEŠTIN LÀL *u* Ì *ḫal-ṣi* NAG-*šú* KI.[MIN]

---

38. DIŠ NA NINDA GU$_7$ KAŠ NAG-*ma ú-nap-paq u* IGI.MEŠ-*šú* NIGIN.MEŠ-*du* NA BI GIG ZÉ GIG *ana* TI-*šú* ^{Ú}[(ÚKUŠ.G)]ÍL ‹(GIBIL)›
39. *šá* IM.SI.SÁ *ina* A LUḪ-*si* ^{ŠEM}BULUḪ *tu-sal-lat* ^{Ú}NU.LUḪ. ḪA *te-be-er* 3 Ú.ḪI.A ⸢ŠEŠ⸣ [(*ina* 1/2 *qa*)] KAŠ.SAG
40. *ki-ma pi-i mal-ma-liš tara-muk ana* IGI MUL.ÙZ GAR-*an* ^{GIŠ}ḪUR ⸢NIGIN⸣-*mi ina* ⸢Á⸣.[(GÚ.ZI.GA 3-*šú*)]-*nu ta-šá-ḫal*
41. NU *pa-tan* NAG-*ma i-lap-pat-su-ma is-sal-la-ʾ la ta-na-*[(*kud* TI-*uṭ ina*)] ⸢U$_4$ ŠE⸣.GA NAG-*šu*

---

42. [… ^{Ú}*imḫur*]-*lim* ^{Ú}[… *sa*]*ḫ-lé-e*[26] ^{ŠEM}BAL ^{Ú}KUR.KUR ^{GIŠ}GEŠTIN.KA$_5$.A
43. […] *ina* 3 *qa* ⸢KAŠ *ḫi-qa*⸣ x[…] *ana* 2 *qa i-tur-ru i-kàṣ-ṣa-aṣ*
44. [… *ana*] IGI ŠUB-*di pa-na* A GAZI^{SAR} *i-š*[*a*]-*ḫat* EGIR-*šú an-na-a ana* DÚR-*šú* DUB-*aq*

---

45. [DIŠ KI].MIN ^{Ú}ÚKUŠ.GÍL ḪÁD.A GAZ SIM KI ZÌ.KUM [ḪE].ḪE *ina* A GAZI^{SAR} *tara-bak ina* KUŠ SUR LAL

---

46. DIŠ NA *ina ti-bi-šú* SAG.DU-*su ana* IGI-*šú iš-ta-na-da-as-su* GÚ-*su* MURUB$_4^{\text{II}}$-*šú kin-ṣa-šú* GÌR^{II}-*šú* GU$_7^{\text{II}}$-*šú*
47. ŠÀ-*šú ya-ʾ-áš* ŠÀ-*šú ana pa-re-e i-te-né-*⸢*el-la*⸣ [I]GI.MEŠ-*šú iṣ-ṣa-nu-du-šú* NA BI ZÉ DIB-*su ana* TI-*šú*

48. $^{\text{[G]IŠ}}$ERIN ^{GIŠ}ŠUR.MÌN ^{ŠEM}GÍR GI.DÙG NAGA.SI ^{ŠEM}IM.[DI MUN *e*]*me-sal-lim ina* KAŠ *tara-bak ina* NINDU BAD-*ir ana* DÚR-*šú* DUB-*aq*

---

49. [Ø?] ⸢Ú⸣NU.LUḪ.ḪA ^{ŠEM}LI $^{\text{NA}_4}$ZÚ.LUM.MA [...] 1-*niš* ÀR.ÀR *ina* Ì.UDU ḪE.ḪE NAGAR-*nu* DÙ-*uš* Ì+GIŠ SUD *ana* DÚR-*šú* GAR

---

50. [(DIŠ NA)] GABA-*su u šá-šal-la-šú* KÚM.MEŠ ZÚ.MEŠ-⸢*šú*⸣ [(*i-ḫi-la*)] ⸢*e*⸣-*piš* KA-*šú* DUGUD NA BI ZÉ GIG *ana* TI-*šú*
51. [(^{ŠEM})]GÚR.GÚR ^{ŠEM}LI ^{ŠEM}GAM.MA MUN IL[(LU LI.TAR)] ^{Ú}KU$_6$ Ú BABBAR ^{Ú}ḪAB ^{Ú}*ak-tam*
52. [(^{GIŠ}ḪAB)] ⸢Ú⸣KUR.KUR U$_5$ ARGAB^{MUŠEN} 12 ⸢Ú⸣.[ḪI.(A ŠE)]Š ‹(1-*niš* SÚD)› *ina* KAŠ *ba-lu pa-tan* NAG-*ma* BURU$_8$

---

53. [... *sa*]*ḫ-lé-e*[27] Ú.KUR.RA *kam-mu* ILLU LI.[TAR] ⸢^{ŠEM}⸣BULUḪ ⸢^{ŠEM}LI⸣ ^{ŠEM}GÚR.GÚR ILLU ^{ŠEM}BULUḪ
54. [...] ⸢Ú⸣NU.LUḪ.ḪA DÚR-^{Ú}NU.LUḪ.ḪA [... N]AG-*ma* BURU$_8$

---

55. [...] ⸢Ú⸣KUR.KUR ^{Ú}NU.LUḪ.ḪA [...] ⸢x x x⸣
56. [... ^{Ú}G]AMUN ⸢Ú⸣[...]

---

57. [... NA]G-*ma* BURU$_8$

---

58. [... NAG-*m*]*a* BURU$_8$

---

59. [... *ina* I]ZI ŠEG$_6$-*šal* NAG-*ma* BURU$_8$

---

60. [...] ⸢Ú⸣.KUR.RA ^{ŠEM}IM.MAN.DU
61. [... *an-nu-t*]*i ina* KAŠ NAG-*ma* BURU$_8$

---

62. [... $^{\text{Š]EM}}$BULUḪ ^{Ú}NAM.TI.LA ZÚ.LUM.MA
63. [... *ina* U]L *tuš-bat ina še-rim* NU *pa-tan* NAG-*ma* BURU$_8$

---

64. [...] Ú [...] ⸢x⸣ ILLU LI.TAR 7 Ú.ḪI.A ŠEŠ *ina* KAŠ NAG-*ma* BURU$_8$

---

65. [... (Ú.BABBAR) ...]x Ú.KUR.[(RA ^{ŠEM}GÚR.GÚR NA)]GA.SI MUN ^{Ú}*imḫur-lim* ^{Ú}*imḫur*-20 ^{Ú}*tar-muš*$_8$
66. [(^{Ú}KUR.KUR NA$_4$ *ga-bi-i* ^{Ú}*ak-tam* ^{Ú}Ḫ)]AR.ḪAR 14 Ú.[ḪI.A ŠE]Š 1-*niš* SÚD *ina* KAŠ NAG-*ma* BURU$_8$

---

67. [… 10 GÍN ^{GIŠ}ER]IN SUMUN 10 GÍN AL.[ÚS.SA 10 GÍN A.GE]ŠTIN.NA KALAG.GA 10 GÍN KAŠ 10 GÍN BABBAR.ḪI^{SAR}!

68. [… ^{Ú}ḪAR].ḪAR 1 GÍN SUM^{SAR} 1/2 GÍN x[… GA]ZI^{SAR} *tuš-te-med ina* UL *tuš-bat ina še-rim*

69. […]*ina*! DÚR-*šú* SI.SÁ-*ma* TI […] A UZU *kab-ru-ti* NAG-*ma ina-eš*

---

70. [DIŠ N(A *lu-ú* ZÉ *lu-ú aḫ-ḫa*)]-⸢*za lu*⸣ *a-mur-ri-qa-nu* ⸢DIB⸣-[(*su* ^{Ú}*úr-nu*)-*u*] ⸢^{Ú}⸣KUR.KUR ^{Ú}GEŠTIN.KA$_5$.A ^{ŠEM}LI

ii

1. ^{ŠEM}⸢MUG *ina*⸣ [(3 *qa* KAŠ *ina* URUDU.ŠEN.TUR ŠEG$_6$-*šal ta-šá-ḫal* Ì.GIŠ *ana* IGI ŠUB-*di ina pa-ni* A GAZI^{SAR} DUB-*ma* KI).MIN … (*ina* DÚR-*šú* SI.SÁ-*ma* TI)]

---

2. ^{Ú}GÍR-*a-nu* ^{Ú}[…]
3. ^{Ú}*ṣa-ṣu-un-tú* ⸢^{Ú}⸣ […]
4. ^{Ú}ÚKUŠ.GÍL ^{Ú}[…] : ^{Ú}[…]
5. ŠE.KAK ^{Ú}EME.UR.GI$_7$: ŠE.KAK ^{ŠEM}LI […]
6. ŠE.KAK ^{Ú}ÚKUŠ.GÍL ^{Ú}[…]

---

7. DIŠ NA ZÉ *saḫ-ḫa*[28] DIB-*su* […]
8. ^{Ú}*tar-muš* ^{Ú}*imḫur-lim* ^{ŠEM}[…]

---

9. DIŠ NA *a-šá-a pa-šit-tú u lu-*[*ba-ṭi* GIG …]
10. Ú.KUR.RA URUDU.SUMUN 7 Ú.[ḪI.A …]

---

11. DIŠ NA ZÉ DIB-*su* Ú.KUR.RA NU *pa-tan a-ḫe-en-n*[*a* …]
12. *ina* KAŠ NAG-*ma* KAŠ.SAL.LA NAG […]

---

13. *ana a-šá-a pa-šit-tú u lu-ba-ṭi* ZI-*ḫi* Ú.BABBAR ILLU LI.TA[(R ^{Ú}*ak-tam kám-mu* 1-*niš* ḪE!?-*al ina* KAŠ NAG-*ma* TI-*u*)*ṭ*]

---

14. DIŠ NA *pa-šit-tú* DIB-*su* ^{ŠEM}GÚR.GÚR ^{Ú}ḪAR.ḪAR ^{Ú}KUR.KUR Ú.KUR.[RA …]

15. ILLU LI.TAR ^{Ú}NU.LUḪ.ḪA *kám-mu šá* ^{LÚ}AŠGAB ^{Ú}LAG.A.ŠÀ [… NAG-*ma i*]-⸢*ár-ru*⸣?

---

16. ^{Ú}ḪAR.ḪAR ^{Ú}NU.LUḪ.ḪA ILLU LI.TAR ^{ŠEM}LI ^{ŠEM}GÚR.GÚR 5 ⸢Ú⸣ […]

---

17. ^{Ú}*ak-tam* ^{Ú}KUR.KUR NAGA.SI ^{ŠEM}GÚR.GÚR ^{ŠEM}LI ILLU LI.TAR MUN ⸢x x x x x x⸣ [...] SILIM-*im*

---

18. DIŠ NA SAG.KI.DIB.BA TUKU *a-ši-a pa-šit-tum u lu-ba-ṭi* GIG *ana* TI-*šú* 15 GÍN ^{ŠEM}GÚR.GÚR 15 GÍN ^{Ú}*úr-nu-u*
19. 15 GÍN ^{Ú}KUR.KUR 1-*niš* GAZ SIM *ina* Ì KAŠ.SAG *tu-šá-ḫa-an ana* DÚR-*šú* DUB *ana ši-bi* NAG-*šú*

---

20. DIŠ NA NU *pa-tan* SAG ŠÀ-*šú i-kaṣ-ṣa-as-su* KÚM ŠÀ TUKU.MEŠ *ina ge-ši-šu* ZÉ *i-ár-rù* NA BI *pa-šit-tú*
21. *tu-ga-na* GIG *ana* TI-*šú* ^{ŠEM}GÚR.GÚR ^{ŠEM}LI ILLU LI.TAR ^{Ú}*ak-tam* ^{Ú}KUR.KUR MUN NAGA.SI TI-*su-nu*
22. *ina* KAŠ SAG *tara-muk ina* UL *tuš-bat ina še-rim* NU *pa-tan ta-šá-ḫal* NAG-*ma tu-šá-ʾ-ra-šu-ma* TI

---

23. DIŠ NA ZÉ.GIG [GIG]

---

24. ÉN ZÉ *eṭ-li* ZÉ *eṭ-li* : Z[É ...]
25. x ri *et-li* e an da li li x [...]
26. x ti ma *ga-ra-aš ga-ra-a*[*š* ...]
27. x ra ti e zib ba x x x [...]

---

28. x [...]

---

29. [ÉN É.(NU.R)]U$^{(?)}$ Z[(É$^{(?)}$.ÀM Ú.ŠIM.GIN$_7$ KI.MU.UN.DAR)]
30. [(ÙZ.DA.ÀM SAG NAM.ÍL MÁŠ ÙZ.DA.GIN$_7$ DADAG NAM.ÍL)]
31. [(MUŠ.A.GIN$_7$ EME NA.NA.E$_{11}$.DÈ MUŠ.KI.PÍL.LÁ.GIN$_7$ ZÉ NA.NA. DÚB.BÉ)]
32. [ZÉ.NÍ.ZA MU.E)].ŠE.D[(Ù.A DUG.GIN$_7$ GAZ.BA)]
33. ⸢IZI⸣.GIN$_7$ TE.NI.I[(B$^{(!)}$) IZI Ú.A.NÚMUN.GIN$_7$ NÍ.ZA TE.NI.IB)]
34. TU$_6$ DUG$_4$.GA ^{d}NI[(N.GIRIM NAM.ŠUB ERIDU^{KI}.GA)]
35. ^{d}EN.KI.KE$_4$ D[(AG AGRUN.NA.KA ḪÉ.EM.MA.AN.DU$_8$.DU$_8$.E)]
36. LAG MUN ŠU Ù.[(ME.TI NAM.ŠUB)] ⸢Ù⸣.[(ME.SÌ)]
37. KA.KA.ŠÈ Ù.[(ME.GAR ŠE$_{10}$.GIN$_7$ ḪÉ.DÚR.RE)]
38. IM$^{(!)}$(text: UḪ).GIN$_7$ GU.DU.NI.TA ḪÉ.E[(M.MA.RA.]⸢DU⸣$^{(?)}$ BU.LU. UḪ.⸢GIN$_7$[29] ḪÉ⸣.[(SI.IL.E)][30]

---

39. ÉN *mar-tu mar-tu mar-tu* ⸢*pa-šit*⸣-[*tu-ma*]
40. *mar-tu* GIN$_7$ KI.SAG.SAL^{MUŠEN} SIG$_7$ *it-ta-na-al-lak* ⸢*a-lak*?⸣-[*ta*]

41. *it-ta-na-za-az ina gi-šal-li ša* BÀD
42. *i-da-gal a-ki-lum ak-li i-da-gal šá-tu-ú ku-ru-un-ni*
43. *ki-i tak-ka-la ak-la ki-i ta-ša-ta-a ku-ru-un-ni*
44. *a-ma-qú-tak-ku-nu-šim-ma tu-ga-ša-a ki-i* GUD TU$_6$ ÉN[31]

---

45. ÉN ÙZ *ar-qá-at a-ruq* DUMU-*ša a-ruq* ^{LÚ}SIPA-*ša a-ruq na-qid-sa*
46. *ina e-qí* SIG$_7$ Ú.MEŠ SIG$_7$.MEŠ *ik-kal ina a-tap-pi a-ruq-ti* A.MEŠ SIG$_7$.MEŠ *i-šat-ti*
47. *i-suk-ši* ^{GIŠ}PA *ul ú-tir-ra pa-ni-ša* : *i*!*-suk-ši qir-ba-nam ul ú-šaq-qa-a re-ši-ša*
48. *i-suk-ši píl-li* ^{Ú}ḪAR.ḪAR *u* MUN : *mar-tu* GIN$_7$ *im-ba-ri ana šá-ḫa-ḫi it-bi*
49. ÉN *ul ia-ut-tu* ÉN ^{d}*É*-[*a* ^{d}*Asal*]-⸢*lú-ḫi* ÉN ^{d}*Da*⸣-*mu u* ^{d}*Gu-la* TU$_6$ ÉN[32]

---

50. K[A.INIM.MA *š*]*a pa-šit-ti* […] sar pa pi ra 1-*niš* SÌG-*aṣ*
51. ÉN […] x […] x x ti šá

---

52. ÉN x […] x la
53. […] *É-a* […] x dur ÉN

---

54. [DÙ.DÙ.BI …] MUN x x ti ŠUB-*di*
55. x ⸢ÉN⸣ […]x NAG-*ma ina-eš*

---

56. [K]A.INIM.MA […] ZÉ.A.KAM

---

57. I[GI.4.G]ÁL.LA ILLU LI.TAR SÚD *ina* A NAG-*šú*

---

58. 15 [ŠE G]I.ZÚ.LUM.MA SÚD *ina* 5 GÍN Ì+GIŠ *u* KAŠ NAG-*šú*

---

59. 21 ‹ŠE› ^{Ú}*nap-ruq-qa ina* 10 GÍN Ì+GIŠ *u* KAŠ NAG-*šú*

---

60. 15 ŠE ^{Ú}*imḫur-lim ina* 1/2 *qa* Ì+GIŠ *u* KAŠ NAG-*šú*

---

61. 90 ‹ŠE› ^{Ú}*sis-sin-ni* ŠÀ-*bi ina* 10 GÍN A NAG-*šú*

---

62. IGI.4.GÁL.LA ^{Ú}*ma-at-qa ina* 10 GÍN A NAG-*šú*

---

63. IGI.4.GÁL.LA ^{Ú}NAM.TI.LA *ina* 10 GÍN Ì+GIŠ NAG-*šú*

---

64. 1/2 GÍN ^{Ú}*a-ra-ri-a-nu ina* 10 GÍN A NAG-*šú*

---

65. IGI.4.GÁL.LA ^{Ú}*imḫur-*20 *ina* 10 GÍN A NAG-*šú*

---

66. IGI.4.GÁL.LA ^{Ú}*me-er-gi-ra-nu ina* 10 GÍN KAŠ [NAG-*šú*]

---

67. DIŠ NA ZÉ DIB-*su* GAZI^{SAR} SÚD *ina* KAŠ NAG-*ma i-ár-rù* : DIŠ KI.MIN *ḫi-qa* KAŠ NAG-*ma i-á*[*r-rù*]

---

68. DIŠ KI.MIN *ḫi-qa* A.GEŠTIN.NA KALAG.GA NAG-*ma i-ár-rù* : DIŠ KI.MIN ^{ŠEM}LI SÚD *ina* KAŠ NAG-*ma i-ár-rù*

---

69. DIŠ KI.MIN ^{Ú}*me-er-gi-ra-a-na* SÚD *ina* A NAG-*ma i-ár-rù* : DIŠ KI.MIN ^{Ú}*imḫur-lim* SÚD *ina* KAŠ NAG-*ma i-ár-rù*

---

70. DIŠ KI.MIN MUN *lu ina* A *lu ina* KAŠ NAG-*ma i-ár-rù* : DIŠ KI.MIN SUM^{SAR} SÚD *ina* A NAG-*ma i-ár-rù*

---

iii

1. DIŠ KI.MIN ILLU LI.TAR SÚD *ina* A NAG-*ma i-ár-rù* : DIŠ KI.MIN ILLU LI.TAR SÚD *ina* A *tara-muk ina* UL *tuš-bat* NAG-*ma i-ár-rù*

---

2. DIŠ KI.MIN ^{Ú}ÚKUŠ.GÍL ^{ŠEM}BULUḪ ^{Ú}ḪAR.ḪAR *ina* Ì *ina* UL *tuš-bat* NAG-*ma i-ár-rù*
3. DIŠ KI.MIN ^{Ú}NU.LUḪ.ḪA SUM^{SAR} *a-ḫi-na-a* SÚD *ina* KAŠ NAG-*ma i-ár-rù*

---

4. DIŠ NA IGI.[S]IG$_7$.SIG$_7$ GIG-*ma* GIG-*su ana* ŠÀ IGI^{II}-*šú* E$_{11}$-*a* ŠÀ IGI.MEŠ-*šú* GU.MEŠ SIG$_7$.MEŠ *ud-du-ḫu*
5. ŠÀ.MEŠ-*š*[*ú n*]*a-šu-u* NINDA *u* KAŠ *ú-tar-ra* NA BI IM.DÙ.A.BI GIG *ú-za-bal-ma* BA.ÚŠ

---

6. DIŠ NA [I]GI.SIG$_7$.SIG$_7$ GIG-*ma* SAG.DU-*su pa-nu-šú ka-lu* AD$_6$-*šú* SUḪUŠ EME-*šú ṣa-bit ši-pir-šú* SUMUN-*ma* BA.ÚŠ

---

7. DIŠ NA SU-*šú* SIG$_7$ *pa-nu-šú* SIG$_7$ *ši-ḫat* UZU TUKU-*a a-mur-ri-qa-nu* MU.NI

---

8. ^{ŠEM}LI SÚD *ina* KAŠ NAG ^{ŠEM}ŠE.LI SÚD *ina* KAŠ NAG ^{ŠEM}ŠEŠ SÚD

ina KAŠ NAG

9. SUḪUŠ ^{GIŠ}NAM.TAR NÍTA *šá* IM.SI.SÁ *šá* GURUN NU ÍL SÚD *ina* KAŠ NAG ^{Ú}*mur-ra-an* KUR-*i* SÚD *ina* KAŠ NAG

10. ^{Ú}*kur-ka-nam* SÚD *ina* KAŠ NAG ^{Ú}*imḫur-lim* SÚD *ina* KAŠ NAG ^{Ú}*nam-ruq-qa* SÚD *ina* KAŠ NAG

11. ^{Ú}*nam-ruq-qa* SÚD *ina* A NAG IM.SAḪAR.NA$_4$.KUR.RA SÚD *ana* A.MEŠ ŠUB *tu-zak* NAG ^{ŠEM}LI SÚD *ina* GA NAG

12. ^{ŠEM}ŠE.LI SÚD *ina* GA NAG ^{ŠEM}ŠEŠ SÚD *ina* GA NAG ^{Ú}*nam-ruq-qa* SÚD *ina* GA NAG

13. 5 ŠE KU.KU AN.ZAḪ *ina* KAŠ ŠUB *ina* UL *tuš-bat tu-zak* NAG IM.KAL.LA SÚD *ina* Ì *e-ri-ni u* KAŠ NAG

14. NUMUN ^{GIŠ}*bi-ni* ⸢Ú⸣SUMUN.DAR SÚD *ina* KAŠ NAG NUMUN ^{GIŠ}*bi-ni* SÚD *ina* KAŠ NAG

15. NUMUN ^{GIŠ}*bi-ni* SÚD *ina* [Ì *u* KA]Š ⸢NAG⸣ SUḪUŠ ^{GIŠ}*šu-ši* SÚD MIN : ^{Ú}*imḫur*-20 SÚD *ina* KAŠ NAG

16. SUḪUŠ ^{GIŠ}MA.NU SUḪUŠ ^{GIŠ}NU.[ÚR.MA *ina* A^{MEŠ} *ina* UD]UN BAD-*er* A^{MEŠ} *šu-nu-tim tu-zak tu-kaṣ-ṣa* NAG-*ma ina-eš*

17. ^{Ú}*a-ṣu-ṣu-tú* ⸢Ú⸣[*a-nu-nu*]-*tú ina qut-rin-ni tu-qat-tar-šu*

18. MÚD ^{d}NIN.KILIM.EDIN [(*šá*) *ina* UGU] ⸢Ú⸣NINNI$_5$ GUB-*zu ta-maḫ-ḫar ina* Ì EŠ.MEŠ

19. Ì SUMUN *sip-pí* KÁ.GA[L *ki-la-l*]*e-e* TI *ina* Ì EŠ.MEŠ

20. *gìr-ra-am ru-us-sà*-[(*a-a*)*m uš-t*]*e-eš-šer ti-tur-ra na-di-tú e-ti*-⸢*iq*⸣

21. ^{Ú}NÍG.PA SA$_5$ SÚD *ina* KAŠ ⸢NAG ^{ŠEM}⸣GÚR.GÚR SÚD *ina* KAŠ NAG GURUN ^{Ú}*ka-zi-ri* SÚD *ina* KA[Š NAG]

22. ^{Ú}ḪAR.ḪAR SÚD *ina* KAŠ NAG KUŠ ^{GIŠ}NU.ÚR.MA SÚD *ina* KAŠ NAG [...]x x [...]

23. SUḪUŠ ^{Ú}EME.UR.GI$_7$ SÚD *ina* KAŠ NAG IGI.6.GÁL.LA [^{Ú}*imḫur-lim* SÚD *ina* KAŠ NAG]

24. ^{Ú}*imḫur*-20 NUMUN ḪAB SÚD *ina* Ì *u* KAŠ NAG PA ^{GIŠ}NU.Ú[(R.MA PA ^{GIŠ}) ... NAG]

---

25. DIŠ NA IGI.SIG$_7$.SIG$_7$ DIRI SUḪUŠ ^{GIŠ}*šu-ši* x [o] ⸢IM⸣.[...]

26. *ina* UL *tuš-bat* GU$_7$ *ḫu-bi-bi*-[*tú* ...]

---

27. SUḪUŠ ^{GIŠ}NU.ÚR.MA x[...]

28. *šum-ma ina* x[...]

---

29. BAR ^{GIŠ}⸢NU⸣.Ú[R.MA? ...]

---

30. x x [...]

Break of about ten lines.

41′. *traces*

42′. DIŠ NA IGI.SIG$_7$.SIG$_7$ BAR ^{GI}[^{Š}...]

43′. *ta-tab-bal* Ì.UDU Ú[KUŠ? ...]

44′. MUŠ.DÍM.GURUN.N[A ...]

45′. traces

iv

1. [...]x *ina* Ì.UDU ÚKUŠ.GÍL S[ÚD ... K]AŠ NAG : DIŠ MIN UZU GUD *kab-ra* GU$_7$.MEŠ TÚG GI$_6$ NU IGI

2. [... N]AM.LÚ.U$_{18}$.LU ^{ŠEM}ŠEŠ *ina* Ì ⸢*u*⸣ KAŠ NAG : DIŠ MIN AMA.A.A ḪÁD.DU SÚD *ina* Ì *u* KAŠ ^{LÚ}KÚRUN.NA NAG-*ma* BURU$_8$

3. [DIŠ MI]N ^{Ú}*ak-tam* ILLU LI.TAR Ú.BABBAR *ina* Ì *u* KAŠ NAG : DIŠ MIN Ì.UDU ÚKUŠ.GÍL *ina* KAŠ NAG

4. [DIŠ] MIN ^{ŠEM}ŠEŠ NUMUN ^{ŠEM}LI IM.SAḪAR.NA$_4$.KUR.RA SÚD *ina* Ì *u* KAŠ NAG : DIŠ MIN ḪAR KÙ.SIG$_{17}$ ḪUŠ-*a ina* ŠU-*šú* GAR-*an*

5. [DIŠ N]A IGI^{II}-*šú* IGI.SIG$_7$.SIG$_7$ PA ^{GIŠ}NU.ÚR.MA SÚD *ina* GI.SAG.KUD *ana* ŠÀ IGI^{II}-*šú* MÚ-*aḫ*

6. [DIŠ N]A IGI.SIG$_7$.SIG$_7$ IGI.MEŠ-*šú* UZU.MEŠ-*šú* DIRI 7 MUŠ.DÍM.GURUN.NA *ri-it-ku-ba-ti*

7. [...T]I-*qí tu*-⸢*qal*⸣-*lap ina* $^{\text{NA}_4}$NA.ZAG.ḪI.LI SÚD *ina* KAŠ.Ú.SA ḪE.ḪE NAG.MEŠ-*ma ina-eš*

8. [...] ⸢x x *saḫ*⸣-*lé-e* ZÍD.ŠE.SA.A LAL-*su u* KAŠ.Ú.SA ḪE.ḪE NAG.MEŠ-*ma ina-eš*

9. [...]-*ma ina* Ì *u* KAŠ NAG-*ma ina-eš*

10. [...] ḫu ši ši [...] ⸢KAŠ⸣ NAG-*šú*

11. [...] *ta-qal-lap* x[... NA]G-*šú*

---

12. [… SIG]$_7$ DIRI ^{Ú}LAG.A.ŠÀ SÚD *ina* KAŠ NAG *an-nu-*⸢*ḫa-ra*⸣ […] *ina* KAŠ
13. […] *ina* KAŠ ŠIKA NUNUZ GÁ.NU$_{11}$^{MUŠEN} SÚD *ina* KAŠ KÙ.SIG$_{17}$ *ina* SÍG SA$_5$ *ina* ŠU^{II}-*šú* KEŠDA

---

14. DIŠ KI.MIN ⸢Ú⸣[…] ^{Ú}ŠAKIRA ^{Ú}SA$_5$ ^{Ú}LAL GAZ A.BI *ta-ṣa-ḫat ina* KAŠ NAG-*ma ina-eš*

---

15. DIŠ KI.MIN G[AZI]^{SAR} U$_5$ ARGAB^{MUŠEN} Ú.BABBAR *ina* Ì.NUN SÚD IGI^{II}-*šú te-te-né-qí-ma ši-ši-tú* ZI-*aḫ*

---

16. DIŠ NA SU-*šú* SIG$_7$ 5 ŠE AN.ZAḪ SÚD *ina* Ì *u* KAŠ NAG-*šú tu-šam-ad-ma* BA.ÚŠ

---

17. DIŠ NA IGI^{II}-*šú a-mur-ri-qa-nu* DIRI ^{Ú}ḪAB SÚD *ina* KAŠ NAG-*ma ina-eš*
18. DIŠ MIN SUḪUŠ ^{GIŠ}*šu-ši tu-bal ta-sàk ina* KAŠ *tàra-sà-an* IGI ^{d}UTU NAG-*ma ina-eš*
19. DIŠ SUḪUŠ ^{Ú}EME.UR.GI$_7$ *tu-bal ta-sàk ina* KAŠ *tàra-sà-an* NAG-*ma ina-eš*
20. DIŠ ^{Ú}*an-nu-ḫa-ra* SÚD *ina* KAŠ NAG-*ma ina-eš* : DIŠ NUNUZ GÁ.NU$_{11}$^{MUŠEN} SÚD *ina* KAŠ NAG-*ma ina-eš*
21. DIŠ SUḪUŠ ^{GIŠ}NU.ÚR.MA SÚD *ina* KAŠ *ina* MUL *tuš-bat ina* Á.GÚ.ZI.GA NAG-*šú*
22. ⸢DIŠ NUMUN GI.ZÚ⸣.LUM.MA SÚD *ina* KAŠ *ina* MUL *tuš-bat ina* Á.GÚ.ZI.GA NAG-*šú*
23. DIŠ ^{GIŠ}GEŠTIN.KA$_5$.A SÚD *ina* KAŠ NAG-*šú* : DIŠ ^{Ú}NU.LUḪ.ḪA SÚD *ina* KAŠ NAG-*šú*
24. DIŠ SUḪUŠ ^{GIŠ}NAM.TAR SÚD *ina* KAŠ NAG-*šú* : DIŠ ILLU [*a-bu*]-*ka-ti ta-sàk ina* KAŠ NAG-*šú*
25. DIŠ ^{Ú}MUŠ.DÍM.GURUN.NA GAL *ta-sàk ina* [KAŠ] *u* Ì NAG-*šú*

---

26. DIŠ NA SU-*šú* SIG$_7$ IGI-*šú* SIG$_7$ *u* GI$_6$ SUḪUŠ EME-*šú* GI$_6$ *aḫ-*[*ḫa-z*]*u* MU.NE
27. MUŠ.DÍM.GURUN.NA GAL-*ta šá* EDIN *ta-sàk ina* KAŠ NAG *aḫ-ḫa-zu šá* ŠÀ-*šú* SI.SÁ-*am*

---

28. DIŠ NA *aḫ-ḫa-za* DIRI ^{ŠEM}LI SÚD *ina* KAŠ NAG ^{ŠEM}ŠE.LI.BABBAR

IM.SAḪAR.NA$_4$.KUR.RA SÚD *ina* Ì *u* KAŠ NAG-*ma ina-eš*

29. ^{ŠEM}KU$_7$.KU$_7$ SÚD *ina* KAŠ NAG ^{Ú}*ḫa-še-e* SÚD *ina* KAŠ NAG SUḪUŠ GI.ZÚ.LUM.MA SÚD *ina* A NAG ^{ŠEM}ŠEŠ SÚD *ina* GA NAG

---

30. DIŠ NA *aḫ-ḫa-za* DIRI SUḪUŠ ^{GIŠ}*šu-še ta-sàk ina* KAŠ *tara-muk ina* UL *tuš-bat* NAG

---

31. DIŠ NA *aḫ-ḫa-za* DIRI ^{Ú}*ṣú-ṣi-im-tú* ^{Ú}*a-nu-nu-tú ina qut-ri-ni tu-qat-tar-*[*š*]*ú*

32. *u* MÚD KUN.DAR.GURUN.NA ŠÉŠ-*su-ma ina-*[*eš*]

---

33. *ru-ša-am ša si-ip-pi* KÁ.GAL *ki-lal-le-en* TI-*qí ana* Ì+GIŠ ŠUB-*di ta-ap-ta-na-*[*aš-šá-aš*]

34. *gi-ir-ra ru-us-sà-a-am uš-te-eš-še-er ti-tur-ra na-di-a-am i-t*[*e-eq*]

---

35. DIŠ NA *aḫ-ḫa-za* DIB-*su* SUḪUŠ ^{GIŠ}NAM.TAR NÍTA *šá* IGI IM.SI.SÁ TI-*qí ina* KAŠ NAG ^{Ú}ḪAR.[ḪAR ...]

36. ^{Ú}KUR.GI.RÍN.NA SÚD *ina* KAŠ ^{ŠEM}ŠE.LI.BABBAR SÚD *ina* KAŠ NAG ^{Ú}*imḫur-lim* ^{Ú}*imḫur*-20 *ina* KAŠ SUḪUŠ ^{Ú}[...]

---

37. DIŠ NA MIN IGI.SIG$_7$.SIG$_7$ ^{ŠEM}LI ^{ŠEM}ŠE[Š SÚ]D *ina* KAŠ N[AG]

---

38. DIŠ NA MIN IM.SAḪAR.NA$_4$.KUR.RA IM.SAḪAR.GI$_6$.KUR.RA 1-*niš ina* KAŠ *tara-sud tu-zak-ka* [...]

---

39. DIŠ MIN 15 ŠE.MEŠ AN.ZAḪ SÚD *ina* KAŠ *tara-sud tu-zak-ka* Ì *ḫal-ṣa ana* ŠÀ ŠUB-*di* NU *p*[*a-tan* NAG]

---

40. DIŠ NA MIN IM.KAL.LA SÚD *ina* Ì *u* KAŠ NAG NUMUN ^{GIŠ}*bi-ni ina* KAŠ NAG NUMUN ^{GIŠ}*bi-ni* [*ina* Ì NAG]

41. NUMUN ^{GIŠ}*bi-ni* SÚD *ina* Ì *u* KAŠ NAG SUḪUŠ ^{GIŠ}*šu-ši ina* Ì *u* KAŠ NAG ^{Ú}*imḫur*-20 SÚD [...]

---

42. DIŠ MIN SUḪUŠ ^{GIŠ}*šu-ši* SUḪUŠ ^{GIŠ}NU.ÚR.MA *ana* A ŠUB *ina* NINDU BAD-*ir* E$_{11}$-*a ta-šá-ḫal* ŠED$_7$ *ina* [...] NAG.MEŠ

---

43. DIŠ NA *aḫ-ḫa-zu* IGI^{II}-*šú* E$_{11}$-*a-ma* IGI^{II}-*šú* GU.MEŠ SIG$_7$.MEŠ [*u*]*d-du-ḫa*

44. ŠÀ.MEŠ-*šú na-šu-ú* NINDA *u* KAŠ *ú-tar-ra* NA BI *ú-za-bal-ma* ⸢BA.ÚŠ⸣

---

45. DIŠ NA *aḫ-ḫa-zu* GIG SAG.DU-*su pa-nu-šu* SU-*šú ka-la-šú ù* SUḪUŠ E[ME-*šú ṣa-bit*]
46. *ana* GIG *šu-a-tu* LÚA.ZU ŠU-*su* NU *ub-bal* NA BI ÚŠ NU [TI.LA]

---

47. DIŠ NA UD.DA KUR-*id* ZI SAG.KI GIG *ina lam* DUGUD-*šú ana* TI.BI *ru-uš-ša ša sip*-[*pi* …] (catchline = *AMT* 14/7:1–2)

TRANSLATION

(i 1–13) If a person's epigastrium hurts him and, when he belches, he continualy produces bile, that person (has) "sick insides." He is continually unable to keep down garlic, leeks, beef, pork or *kurunnu* beer.[33] To cure him, you crush together (and) sift 1/2 *qû*-measure of *saḫlû*-cress, 1/2 *qû*-measure of *burāšu*-juniper, 1/2 *qû*-measure of *kukru*, 1/2 *qû*-measure of flax seed, 1/2 *qû*-measure of malt gruel, 1/2 *qû*-measure of *su᾿ādu*, 1/2 *qû*-measure of *qutrātu* seed, 1/2 *qû*-measure of *kasû*, 1/2 *qû*-measure of *šunû*-chastetree, 1/2 *qû*-measure of *kiššēnu*-bean, 1/2 *qû*-measure of *pappasītu*-sulphur, 1/2 *qû*-measure of *šammi ašî*, 1/2 *qû*-measure of *nīnû*-mint, 1/2 *qû*-measure of "dove dung," 1/3 *qû*-measure of *kamantu*-henna(?) seed, 1/3 *qû*-measure of *erišti eqli*, 10 shekels of *baluḫḫu*-aromatic resin, 10 shekels *of imbû tamtim*, 1 *qû*-measure of wheat flour, 1 *qû*-measure of dates, 1 *qû*-measure of winnowed beerwort (and) 1 *qû*-measure of *isqūqu* flour. You decoct (it)[34] in beer till decocted. You massage (it) into cloth (and) bandage him (with it) for a third of nine days. On the fourth day, you take (it) off and have a look (at it). If the *bubu᾿tu*-blister is white, his stomach should calm down. If the *bubu᾿tu*-blister is red, his stomach holds fever. If the *bubu᾿tu*-blister is yellow/green, he was "gotten" by *ṣētu* (enteric fever). It will keep coming back. If the *bubu᾿tu*-blister is black, it will make him so sick that he does not recover. To extinguish the *bubu᾿tu*-blister, you crush (and) sift *kirbān eqli* (and) mud that has been "killed" by the sun. You make (it) into a dough with *kasû* juice (and) bandage (him with it). Afterwards, you have him drink *saḫlû*-cress (mixed) with beer. When he has drunk (it), he should continually bathe in "lone plant," *šunû*-chastetree infusion, *bīnu*-tamarisk, *aktam*, (and) *maštakal*.

(i 14) If a person (has) sick gall bladder, you grind *šūmu*-garlic (and) have him drink (it mixed) with water on an empty stomach.

(i 15) You have him drink undiluted vinegar, *šiqqu*-garum (and) plump *kasû*.

(i 16) You have him drink *ḫīqu*-beer (and) make him vomit.

(i 17) You grind *kasû* (and) have him drink it (mixed) with water. You grind salt (and) have him drink (it) on an empty stomach (mixed) with water. You grind salt (and) have him drink (it) on an empty stomach (mixed) with beer.

(i 18) You crush *abukkatu* resin (and) pour (it) into *ḫīqu*-beer. You leave (it) out overnight under the stars. In the morning, you pour honey (and) pressed-out oil into it. If you have him drink (it), he should vomit.

(i 19) You grind *buṣinnu* seed (and) have him drink (it mixed) with beer. You grind *namruqqu* (and) have him drink (it mixed) with beer.

(i 20–26) "Lone plant" is a plant for the gall bladder. It is to be drunk (mixed) with beer. *Mergirānu* is a plant for the gall bladder. It is to be drunk (mixed) with beer. *Kasû* is a plant for the gall bladder. It is to be drunk (mixed) with beer. *Burāšu*-juniper is a plant for the gall bladder. It is to be drunk (mixed) with beer. *Nuḫurtu* is a plant for the gall bladder. It is to be drunk (mixed) with beer. *Šūšu*-licorice peel is a plant for the gall bladder. It is to be drunk (mixed) with beer. *Allānu*-oak leaf is a plant for the gall bladder. It is to be drunk (mixed) with beer. *Rikibti arkabi* is a plant for the gall bladder. It is to be drunk (mixed) with beer. A lump of salt is a plant for the gall bladder. It is to be drunk (mixed) with beer. *Šūmu*-garlic is a plant for the gall bladder. It is to be drunk (mixed) with beer. Male *pillû* root is a plant for the gall bladder. It is to be ground (and) drunk (mixed) with beer. *Šūšu*-licorice root is a plant for the gall bladder. It is to be ⸢ground⸣ (and) drunk (mixed) with oil and beer. *Ṣibūru* is a plant for the gall bladder. It is to be ground (and) drunk (mixed) with water.

(i 27–32) If, (despite) his not having eaten, a person's stomach continually rises up to vomit, he continually produces a lot of phlegm, liquid continuously flows from his mouth, his face continually (feels like it) is spinning, his insides are continually bloated, his hips (and) his shins continually hurt him intensely, he is hot and then cold, he continually has sweat, his appetite for bread and beer is diminished, he drinks a great deal of cold water (and then) vomits, he pours yellow/green (matter) from his anus (and) his penis, his appearance continually changes (for the worse), his flesh is tense (and) whatever he eats does not agree with him, the gall bladder has turned over on that person.[35] To cure him, you take these three plants while still fresh: ⸢*kukru*⸣, *burāšu*-juniper (and) *ṣumlalû*. You dry (and) grind (them). [You have him drink (it)] on an empty stomach (mixed) with undiluted wine. He should have a bowel movement and then you bandage his ⸢epigastrium⸣ (and) his abdomen. You have him eat hot things. [...] three days [...]

(i 33) Alternatively, you grind *arariānu* (and) [have him drink (it)] (mixed) with beer before [he goes to bed].

(i 34) Alternatively, you grind *saḫlānu* (and) [have him drink (it)] on an empty stomach (mixed) with undiluted wine. [...].

(i 35) Alternatively, you grind *ṣibūru* (and) ⌜have him drink (it)⌝ (mixed) with sweet milk. [...]

(i 36–37) Alternatively, you grind *irrû* shoots (and) have him drink (it mixed) with wine, honey, and pressed-out oil. ⌜Ditto⌝ ([...]). Alternatively, you have him drink late-blooming(?) wildflowers (mixed) with wine, honey and pressed-out oil. ⌜Ditto⌝ ([...]).

(i 38–41) If a person eats bread (and) drinks beer and then chokes and his face (seems) continually to spin, that person is sick with an illness of the gall bladder,[36] to cure him, you wash *irrû* ‹(newly›)growing on the north side with water, you cut up *baluḫḫu*-aromatic (and) you select *nuḫurtu*. You decoct[37] these three plants in equal proportions in 1/2 *qû* of beer. You put (it) out under the goat star. You surround (it) with a drawing. In the morning, you filter (it) three times. If you have him drink (it) on an empty stomach, it will affect him so that he will appear to get worse. Do not worry; he should recover (in the end). You have him drink (it) [on] a propitious day.

(i 42–44) [You ...] [...], ⌜*imḫur-lim*⌝, [...], ⌜*saḫlû/urnû*⌝, *ballukku*-aromatic, *atāʾišu*, (and) "fox grape." [You boil (it)] in 3 *qû* of *ḫīqu*-beer [until] it has been reduced to 2 *qû*. He cuts up [...] and pours (it) on. Beforehand, he ⌜rinses⌝ (his anus) (with) *kasû* juice. Afterwards, you pour this into his anus.

(i 45) ⌜Alternatively⌝, you dry, crush (and) sift *irrû*. You ⌜mix⌝ (it) with *isqūqu*-flour. You decoct (it)[38] in *kasû* juice. You massage (it) into leather (and) bandage (him with it).

(i 46–48) If a person's head continually (feels like it) draws him forward when he stands up,[39] his neck, his hips, his shins (and) his feet continually hurt him, his stomach heaves, his stomach continually rises to vomit (and) his ⌜face⌝ continually (feels like it) is spinning, the gall bladder afflicts that person. To cure him, you decoct *erēnu*-cedar, *šurmēnu*-cypress, *asû* myrtle, "sweet reed," *uḫḫūlu qarnānu*, ⌜*suʾādu*⌝, (and) ⌜*emesallim*-salt⌝ in beer. You bake (it) in an oven (and) pour (it) into his anus.

(i 49) You mill grind together *nuḫurtu*, *burāšu*-juniper, date stones (and) [...]. You mix (it) with sheep fat, make (it) into an acorn-shaped suppository. You sprinkle (it) with oil (and) put (it) into his anus.

(i 50–52) If a person's breast and back are continually hot, his teeth ooze blood (and) opening his mouth is difficult, that person (has) sick gall bladder.[40] To cure him, ‹(you grind together)› these twelve plants: *kukru*, *burāšu*-juniper, *ṣumlalû*, salt, *abukkatu* resin, *šimru*, "white plant," *šammi buʾšāni*, *aktam*, *ḫurātu*-madder, *atāʾišu*, (and) *rikibti arkabi*. If you have him drink (it) on an empty stomach (mixed) with beer, he should vomit.

(i 53–54) If you have him ⌜drink⌝ [...], ⌜*saḫlû/urnû*⌝, *nīnû*-mint, *kammu*, ⌜*abukkatu*⌝ resin, *baluḫḫu*-aromatic, *burāšu*-juniper, *kukru*, *baluḫḫu*-aromatic resin, [...], *nuḫurtu*, (and) *tiyātu*, he should vomit.

(i 55–56) [...], *atāʾišu*, *nuḫurtu* [...], *kamunu*-cumin [...]

(i 57) If you have him ⌜drink⌝ [... (mixed) with ...], he should vomit.

(i 58) ⌜If⌝ [you have him drink ... (mixed) with ...], he should vomit.

(i 59) [...] You boil (it) over a ⌜fire⌝. If you have him drink (it), he should vomit.

(i 60–61) If you have him drink ⌜these⌝ [# plants: ...], *nīnû*-mint, *suʾādu*, (and) [...] (mixed) with beer, he should vomit.

(i 62–63) [You ...] *baluḫḫu*-aromatic, "life plant" (and) dates. You leave (it) out overnight [under] the ⌜stars⌝. In the morning, if you have him drink (it) on an empty stomach, he should vomit.

(i 64) If you have him drink these seven plants: [...] (and) *abukkatu* resin (mixed) with beer, he should vomit.

(i 65–66) You grind together ⌜these⌝ fourteen plants: "white plant," [...]. *nīnû*-mint, *kukru*, *uḫḫūlu qarnānu*, salt, *imḫur-lim*, *imḫur-ešra*, *tarmuš*, *atāʾišu*, alum, *aktam*, (and) *ḫašû*-thyme. If you have him drink (it mixed) with beer, he should vomit.

(i 67–69) You meld [...], [10 shekels] ⌜*šupuḫru*-cedar⌝, 10 shekels of ⌜*šiqqu*-garum⌝, [10 shekels] of undiluted ⌜vinegar⌝, 10 shekels of beer, 10 shekels of [...], [# shekels] of ⌜*ḫašû*-thyme⌝, 1 shekel of *šūmu*-garlic, 1/2 shekel of [...], (and) [# shekels] of ⌜*kasû*⌝. You leave (it) out overnight under the stars. In the morning, [you have him drink it]. If he has a bowel movement, he should recover. [Afterwards], if he drinks fatty meat broth, he should recover.

(i 70–ii 1) [If] either the gall bladder or *aḫḫāzu* or *amurriqānu* afflicts ⌜a person⌝, you boil *urnû*-mint, *atāʾišu*, "fox grape," *burāšu*-juniper (and) *ballukku*-aromatic in 3 *qû* of beer in a *tamgussu*-vessel. You filter it (and) pour oil over it. First, you pour in *kasû* juice and then ⌜ditto⌝ (you pour it into his anus. If he has a bowel movement, he should recover).

(ii 2–6) [You ...] *paṭrānu*, [...], *ṣaṣuntu*, [...], *irrû*, [...] or [...], [...] shoots of *lišān kalbi* or shoots of *burāšu*-juniper, [...], shoots of *irrû*, [...]

(ii 7–8) If gall (and) *saḫḫu* afflicts a person, [you ...] *tarmuš*, *imḫur-lim*, [...]

(ii 9–10) If a person [is sick] with nausea, *pašittu* and ⌜bouts of sweating⌝, [you ... these] seven plants: [...], *nīnû*-mint and old copper. [...]

(ii 11–12) If the gall bladder afflicts a person, [you have him drink] *nīnû*-mint by itself on an empty stomach. You have him drink [...] (mixed) with beer and then you have him drink light beer [...]

(ii 13) To remove nausea, *pašittu*, and bouts of sweating, you mix together "white plant," *abukkatu* resin, *aktam* (and) *kammu*. If you have him drink (it mixed) with beer, he should recover.

(ii 14–15) If *pašittu* afflicts a person, [you …] *kukru*, *ḫašû*-thyme, *atāʾišu*, *nīnû*-mint […], *abukkatu* resin, *nuḫurtu*, tanner's *kammu* (and) *kirbān eqli*. [If you have him drink (it) mixed with …], he should vomit(?)

(ii 16) [You ... these] five plants: *ḫašû*-thyme, *nuḫurtu*, *abukkatu* resin, *burāšu*-juniper, (and) *kukru*. […]

(ii 17) [You …] *aktam*, *atāʾišu*, *uḫḫūlu qarnānu*, *kukru*, *burāšu*-juniper, *abukkatu* resin (and) salt. [If …] he should recover.

(ii 18–19) If a person is sick with headache, nausea, *pašittu*, and bouts of sweating, to cure him, you crush together (and) sift fifteen grains of *kukru*, fifteen grains of *urnû*-mint (and) 15 shekels of *atāʾišu*. You heat (it) in oil (and) first-quality beer (and) pour (it) into his anus. You have him drink as much as he wants (of it).[41]

(ii 20–22) If, before he has eaten, a person's upper abdomen (epigastrium) gnaws at him, he continually has internal fever (and), when he belches, he vomits bile, that person is sick with *pašittu* (or) *tugānu*.[42] To cure him, you decoct fresh *kukru*, *burāšu*-juniper, *abukkatu* resin, *aktam*, *atāʾišu*, salt (and) *uḫḫūlu qarnānu* in first-quality beer. You leave (it) out overnight under the stars. In the morning, you filter (it and) have him drink (it) on an empty stomach (and) if you induce vomiting, he should recover.

(ii 23) *Label*: If a person [is sick with] sick gall bladder.

(ii 24–27) *fragmentary recitation.*

(ii 28) *Label*: […]

(ii 29–38) ⸢É.NU.RU⸣ [spell]: (In the form of) bile, it broke through the earth like a weed. (In the form of a) she-goat, it raised its head. Like a buck, it raised its pure (head). Like a water snake it sticks out (its) tongue. Like a desert snake, it spits out (its) venom. You, gall who have reared up by yourself, be smashed like a pot! Be put out like fire! Go out by yourself like a rush fire! Go out by yourself like a fire in a palm tree! It is the recitation of Ningirim, the spell of Eridu. May Enki in (his) dwelling place in the Apsû dispel (it)! When you have taken a lump of salt in your hand, when you have recited the recitation, (and) when you have put (it) in his mouth, (and) may it be excreted like shit; may it come forth from the anus like wind! May it be crumbled like *baluḫḫu*-aromatic resin!

(ii 39–44) "Bile, bile, bile, ⸢*pašittu*⸣. Bile goes about in the form of a yellow heron standing on the parapet of a wall. He sees the one who eats bread; he sees the one who drinks *kurunnu*-beer, (saying) "When you eat bread, when you drink *kurunnu*-beer, I will fall upon you and you will belch like a bull!"[43]

(ii 45–49) The she-goat is yellow; her kid is yellow; her shepherd is yellow; her chief herdsman is yellow; she eats yellow grass on the yellow ditchbank; she drinks yellow water from the yellow ditch. He threw a stick at her (but) it does not turn her back; he threw! a clod at her (but) it did not raise her head. He threw at her a mixture of *ḫašû*-thyme and salt (and) the bile began to dissolve like the mist. The recitation is not mine; it is the recitation of E[a and Asal]luḫi, the recitation of Damu and Gula.

(ii 50–51) Re[citation f]or *pašittu*.[44] [...] You whisk together [...]. [You recite] the recitation [x times over it and ...]

(ii 52–56) *fragmentary recitation and potion for the gall bladder.*

(ii 57) You grind ⸢1/4⸣ shekel of *abukkatu* resin (and) have him drink (it mixed) with water.

(ii 58) You grind fifteen grains of *buṣinnu* (and) have him drink (it mixed) with 5 shekels of oil and beer.

(ii 59) You have him drink twenty-one ‹grains› of *namruqqu* (mixed) with 10 shekels of oil and beer.

(ii 60) You have him drink fifteen grains of *imḫur-lim* (mixed) with 1/2 *qû* of oil and beer.

(ii 61) You have him drink ninety ‹grains› of date palm frond (mixed) with 10 shekels of water.

(ii 62) You have him drink 1/4 shekel of "sweet plant" (mixed) with 10 shekels of water.

(ii 63) You have him drink 1/4 shekel of "life plant" (mixed) with 10 shekels of oil.

(ii 64) You have him drink 1/2 shekel of *arariānu* (mixed) with 10 shekels of water.

(ii 65) You have him drink 1/4 shekel of *imḫur-ešra* (mixed) with 10 shekels of water.

(ii 66) [You have him drink] 1/4 shekel of *mergirānu* (mixed) with 10 shekels of beer.

(ii 67) If the gall bladder afflicts a person, you grind *kasû*. If you have him drink (it mixed) with beer, he should vomit. Alternatively, if you have him drink *ḫīqu* beer, ⸢he should vomit⸣.

(ii 68) Alternatively, if you have him drink *ḫīqu* beer (and) undiluted vinegar, he should vomit. Alternatively, you grind *burāšu*-juniper. If you have him drink (it mixed) with beer, he should vomit.

(ii 69) Alternatively, you grind *mergirānu*. If you have him drink (it mixed) with water, he should vomit. Alternatively, you grind *imḫur-lim*. If you have him drink (it mixed) with beer, he should vomit.

(ii 70) Alternatively, if you have him drink salt (mixed) either with water or beer, he should vomit. Alternatively, you grind *šūmu*-garlic. If you have him drink (it mixed) with water, he should vomit.

(iii 1) Alternatively, you grind *abukkatu* resin. If you have him drink (it mixed) with water, he should vomit. Alternatively, you grind *abukkatu* resin.

You decoct (it) in water (and) let it sit out overnight under the stars. If you have him drink (it), he should vomit.

(iii 2–3) Alternatively, you let *irrû*, *baluḫḫu*-aromatic (and) *ḫašû*-thyme sit out overnight (mixed) with oil. If you have him drink (it), he should vomit. Alternatively, you grind *nuḫurtu* (and) *šūmu*-garlic separately. If you have him drink it (mixed) with beer, he should vomit.

(iii 4–5) If a person is sick with *amurriqānu* and his illness rises to his eyes, the inside of his eyes is covered with a network of yellow threads, ⌜his⌝ insides are ⌜puffed up⌝ (and) return bread and beer (to his mouth) (and) that person is sick with any sort of "wind," if he lingers, he will die.[45]

(iii 6) If a person is sick with *amurriqānu* and his head, his face, his whole body (and) the base of his tongue are affected, if his suffering is prolonged, he will die.

(iii 7) If a person's body is yellow, his face is yellow (and) he has wasting of the flesh, it is called *amurriqānu*.[46]

(iii 8–24) You grind *burāšu*-juniper (and) have him drink (it mixed) with beer. You grind *kikkirānu*-juniper berries (and) have him drink (it mixed) with beer. You grind myrrh (and) have him drink (it mixed) with beer. You grind male *pillû* root which grows on the north side and does not bear fruit (and) have him drink (it mixed) with beer. You grind wild *murranu* (and) have him drink (it mixed) with beer. You grind *kurkānu*-turmeric (and) have him drink (it mixed) with beer. You grind *imḫur-lim* (and) have him drink (it mixed) with beer. You grind *namruqqu* (and) have him drink (it mixed) with beer. You grind *namruqqu* (and) have him drink (it mixed) with water. You grind alum (and) pour it into water. You clarify (it and) have him drink (it). You grind *burâšu*-juniper (and) have him drink (it mixed) with milk. You grind *kikkirānu*-juniper berries (and) have him drink (it mixed) with milk. You grind *namruqqu* (and) have him drink (it mixed) with milk. You grind five grains of powdered *anzaḫḫu*-frit (and) pour (it) into beer. You leave (it) out overnight under the stars. You clarify (it and) have him drink (it). You grind *kalû*-clay (and) have him drink (it mixed) with *erēnu*-cedar oil and beer. You grind *bīnu*-tamarisk seed (and) *šumuttu*-vegetable (and) have him drink (it mixed) with beer. You grind *bīnu*-tamarisk seed (and) have him drink (it mixed) with beer. You grind *bīnu*-tamarisk seed (and) have him drink (it mixed) with [oil and] ⌜beer⌝. You grind *šūšu*-licorice root (and) ditto (have him drink it mixed with oil and beer). You grind *imḫur-ešra* (and) have him drink (it mixed) with beer. You bake *eʾru*-tree root (and) ⌜*nurmû*⌝-pomegranate root [in water in] an ⌜oven⌝. You clarify those juices (and) let (it) cool. If you have him drink (it), he should recover. You fumigate him with *aṣuṣimtu* (and) ⌜*anunūtu*⌝ (mixed) with incense. You obtain the blood of an *ayaṣu*-weasel which stands [on] an *ašlu*-rush. You repeatedly rub him gently (with it mixed) with oil. You take used grease from ⌜both⌝ door posts of the main gate. You repeatedly rub him gently (with it mixed) with oil. ⸢He should go straight home⸣ on a reddish[47] road. He should cross an abandoned bridge. You grind red *ḫaṭṭi rēʾi* (and) have him drink (it mixed) with beer. You grind *kukru* (and) have him drink (it mixed) with beer. You grind *kaziru* fruit (and) [have him drink] (it mixed) with beer. You grind *ḫašû*-thyme (and) have him drink (it mixed) with beer. You grind *nurmû*-pomegranate skin (and) have him drink (it mixed) with beer. [...] You grind *lišān kalbi* root (and) have him drink (it mixed) with beer. You grind 1/6 shekel of [*imḫur-lim* (and) have him drink (it mixed) with beer]. You grind *imḫur-ešra* (and) *šammi buʾšāni*? seed (and) have him drink (it mixed) with oil and beer. [You grind] *nurmû*-pomegranate leaves (and) [...] *leaves* [(and) have him drink (it mixed) with ...]

(iii 25–26) If a person is full of *amurriqānu*, [you ...] *šūšu*-licorice root. You leave it out overnight under the stars (and) have him eat (it). [You ...] a *ḫumbibītu*-reptile [...]

(iii 27–28) [You ...] *nurmû*-pomegranate root [...] If in [...]

(iii 29) [You ...] ⸢*nurmû*-pomegranate⸣ peel [...]

(iii 30–41′) *fragmentary or lost*

(iii 42′–43′) If a person (has) *amurriqānu*, you dry [...] skin and [...]. [You ....] ⸢*irrû*?⸣ fat [...]

(iii 44′) (For *amurriqānu*), [you ...] a *pizzalurtu*-gecko [...]

(iii 45′) *lost*

(iv 1) [Alternatively (for *amurriqānu*), you ⸢grind⸣ [...] in *irrû* "fat" (and) you have him drink (it mixed) [with oil and] ⸢beer⸣. Alternatively, you have him repeatedly eat fatty beef. He should not wear a black garment.

(iv 2) [Alternatively], you have him drink *amilānu* (and) myrrh (mixed) with oil and beer. Alternatively, you dry and crush *ummi mê*.[48] If you have him drink (it mixed) with oil and *kurunnu*-beer, he should vomit.

(iv 3) ⸢Alternatively⸣, you have him drink *aktam*, *abukkatu* resin (and) "white plant" (mixed) with oil and beer. Alternatively, you have him drink *irrû* "fat" (mixed) with beer.

(iv 4) ⸢Alternatively⸣, you grind myrrh, *burāšu*-juniper seed (and) alum (and) have him drink (it mixed) with oil and beer. Alternatively, you put a ring made from red gold on his hand.

(iv 5) [If] ⸢a person's⸣ eyes are full of *amurriqānu*, you grind *nurmû*-pomegranate leaves. You blow (it) into his eyes using a reed straw.

(iv 6–7) [If a person's] face and flesh are full of *amurriqānu*, you take seven copulating [steppe dwelling] *pizzalurtu*-lizards. You skin them (and) crush them with a stone pestle. You mix (it) with beerwort. If you have him repeatedly drink (it), he should recover.

(iv 8) You bandage him with [...], *saḫlû*-cress (and) roasted grain flour and you also mix (it) with beerwort. If he drinks (it) repeatedly, he should recover.

(iv 9–10) *fragmentary*

(iv 11) You skin [...] ⸢You have him drink⸣ (it).

(iv 12–13) If [a person's eyes] are full [of *amurriqānu*], you grind *kirbān eqli* (and) have him drink (it mixed) with beer. [You grind] *annuḫaru*-alum (and have him drink it mixed) with beer. (You have him drink) [...] (mixed) with beer. You grind ostrich shell (and have him drink it mixed) with beer. You bind a gold bead (threaded) on red wool on his hands.

(iv 14) Alternatively, you crush [...], *šakirû*, "red plant" (and) *ašqulālu*. You squeeze out their juices. If you have him drink (it mixed) with beer, he should recover.

(iv 15) Alternatively, you grind ⸢*kasû*⸣, *rikibti arkabi*, (and) "white plant" in ghee (and) daub (it) repeatedly on his eyes. The membrane should be removed.[49]

(iv 16) If a person's body is yellow, you grind five grains of *anzaḫḫu*-frit (and) have him drink (it mixed) with oil and beer. If you give him too much of it, he will die.

(iv 17–25) If a person's eyes are full of *amurriqānu*,[50] you grind *šammi buʾšāni*. If you have him drink (it mixed) with beer, he should recover. Alternatively, you dry (and) grind *šūšu*-licorice root (and) soak (it) in beer. If you have him drink (it) before Shamash, he should recover. Alternatively, you dry (and) grind *lišān kalbi* root (and) soak (it) in beer. If you have him drink (it), he should recover. Alternatively, you grind *annuḫaru*-alum. If you have him drink (it mixed) with beer, he should recover. Alternatively, you grind ostrich shell. If you have him drink (it mixed) with beer, he should recover. Alternatively, you grind *nurmû*-pomegranate root. You leave it out overnight under the stars (mixed) with beer (and) have him drink it in the morning. Alternatively, you grind ⸢*buṣinnu* seed⸣. You leave (it) out overnight under the stars (mixed) with beer (and) have him drink (it) in the morning. Alternatively, you grind "fox grape" (and) have him drink (it mixed) with beer. Alternatively, you grind *nuḫurtu* (and) have him drink (it mixed) with beer. Alternatively, you grind *pillû* root and have him drink (it mixed) with beer. Alternatively, you grind ⸢*abukkatu*⸣ resin (and) have him drink (it mixed) with beer. Alternatively, you grind a large *pizzalurtu*-lizard (and) have him drink (it mixed) with [beer] and oil.

(iv 26–27) If a person's flesh is yellow, his face his yellow and black (and) the base of his tongue is black, it is called ⸢*aḫḫāzu*⸣. You grind a large steppe dwelling *pizzalurtu*-lizard (and) you have him drink (it mixed) with beer. The *aḫḫāzu* inside him should be excreted.

(iv 28–29) If a person is full of *aḫḫāzu*, you grind *burāšu*-juniper (and) have him drink (it mixed) with beer. You grind *kikkirānu*-juniper berries (and) alum. If you have him drink (it mixed) with oil and beer, he should recover. You grind *kukru* (and) have him drink (it mixed) with beer. You grind *ḫašû*-

thyme (and) have him drink (it mixed) with beer. You grind *buṣinnu* root (and) have him drink (it mixed) with water. You grind myrrh (and) have him drink (it mixed) with milk.

(iv 30) If a person is full of *aḫḫāzu*, you grind *šūšu*-licorice root (and) decoct (it) in beer. You let (it) sit out overnight under the stars (and) have him drink (it).

(iv 31–32) If a person is full of *aḫḫāzu*, you fumigate ⸢him⸣ with *aṣuṣimtu* (and) *anunūtu* (mixed) with incense and, if you rub him gently with the blood of a steppe dwelling *anduḫallatu*-lizard, ⸢he should recover⸣.

(iv 33–34) You take used grease from both door posts of the main gate. You pour (it) into oil (and) repeatedly ⸢rub him gently⸣ (with it). He should go straight home on a reddish road. ⸢He should cross⸣ an abandoned bridge.

(iv 35–36) If *aḫḫāzu* afflicts a person, you take male *pillû* root which grows on the north side (and) have him drink (it mixed) with beer. You grind ⸢*ḫašû*-thyme⸣, [...] and *kurkānû*-turmeric (and have him drink it mixed) with beer. You grind *kikkirānu*-juniper berries (and) have him drink (it mixed) with beer. (You have him drink) *imḫur-lim* (and) *imḫur-ešra* (mixed) with beer. [(You have him drink) ...] root [(mixed) with beer].

(iv 37) If ditto (*aḫḫāzu* afflicts a person) or *amurriqānu*, ⸢you grind⸣ *burāšu*-juniper (and) ⸢myrrh⸣ (and) ⸢have him drink (it)⸣ (mixed) with beer.

(iv 38) Alternatively, you soak? alum (and) black alum together in beer (and) clarify (it). [...]

(iv 39) Alternatively, you grind fifteen grains[51] of *anzaḫḫu*-frit. You soak? (it) in beer (and) clarify (it). You pour pressed-out oil into it (and) [have him drink it] ⸢on an empty stomach⸣.

(iv 40–41) Alternatively, you grind *kalû*-paste (and) have him drink (it mixed) with oil and beer. You have him drink *bīnu*-tamarisk seed (mixed) with beer. [You have him drink] *bīnu*-tamarisk seed (mixed) [with oil]. You grind *bīnu*-tamarisk seed (and) have him drink (it mixed) with oil and beer. You have him drink *šūšu*-licorice root (mixed) with oil and beer. You grind *imḫur-ešra* (and) [have him drink (it) mixed with ...].

(iv 42) Alternatively, you pour *šūšu*-licorice root (and) *nurmû*-pomegranate root into water. You bake (it) in an oven. You take (it) out, filter (it and) let (it) cool. You have him drink (it) repeatedly (mixed) with [...].

(iv 43–44) If *aḫḫāzu* rises to a person's eyes so that his eyes are ⸢covered⸣ with a network of yellow threads, his insides are puffed up (and) return bread and beer (to his mouth), if that person lingers, he will die.[52]

(iv 45–46) If a person is sick with *aḫḫāzu* (jaundice without wasting) and his head, his face, his whole body and the base of his ⸢tongue⸣ [are affected], the *asû* (pharmacist) is not to lay his hands on that patient (to treat him); that person will die; he will not [live].[53]

(iv 47) If *ṣētu* (enteric fever) has "gotten" a person (and) he is sick with a pulsating headache, before it becomes difficult for him, used grease from the doorpost … (*catchline*)

Colophon (Assurbanipal's library)

TEXT 8: BAM 159 i 21–ii 19

This section of BAM 159 follows a section (i 1–20) on genitourinary tract problems, for which see chapter 10. BAM 159 i 21–ii 19 contains anal suppositories (i 21–26) and potions (i 27–28) for what appears to be liver failure connected with ulcerative colitis (for which see above under DÚR.GIG). It then cites entries from the UGU therapeutic series dealing with the gall bladder (lines i 29–37 = BAM 578 i 38-41; lines i 38–42 = BAM 578 i 50–52). This is followed by potions (ii 1–5, 11), a bath (ii 6–10), an aliment (ii 6–10) and an amulet (ii 6–10) for jaundice. This section ends with pills washed down with date beer (ii 12–16), a potion (ii 17–18) and an anal suppository (ii 19) for bloated insides and cramped feet, probably due to edema.

Lines ii 6–10 have an accompanying amulet. Like those of BAM 578, it has red in it, plus blue and white but no black. Lines ii 12–16 are interesting in describing the manufacture of pills. To note that coloquinth (which is what we think *irrû* is) is exceedingly bitter and would indeed need the honey and date beer to get it down.

i

21. DIŠ NA TÙN ŠÀ-*šú* DIB.DIB-*su gi-na-a* MÚD *ina* KA-*šú*
22. DU-*ku* MÚ.MÚ-*aḫ u in-ne-sil* NA BI
23. DÚR.GIG *ana* TI-*šú* KUŠ UR.MAḪ *tur-ár* SÚD
24. *ina* Ì.UDU ḪE.ḪE U DÙ-*uš ana* DÚR-*šú* GAR-*ma* TI

---

25. DIŠ KI.MIN *qí-lip* ZÚ.LUM.MA SÚD *ina* Ì.UDU ḪE.ḪE U DÙ
26. *ana* DÚR-*šú* GAR-*ma* TI

---

27. DIŠ KI.MIN ^{Ú}GEŠTIN.KA$_5$.A *ina* KAŠ NAG ^{GIŠ}ŠE.NÁ.A *ina* KAŠ NAG
28. ⌈Ú⌉KUR.KUR *ina* KAŠ NAG

---

29. [(DIŠ NA NINDA G)]U$_7$ KAŠ NAG-*ma ú-nap-paq* IGI.MEŠ-*šú* NIGIN.MEŠ-*du*
30. [(NA BI GIG ZÉ GI)]G *ana* TI-*šú* ^{Ú}ÚKUŠ.GÍL GIBIL

31. [(*šá* IM.SI.SÁ) Z]I-*aḫ ina* A.MEŠ LUḪ-*si*
32. [(^{ŠEM}BULUḪ *tu-sal-lat*)] ⸢^{Ú}⸣NU.LUḪ.ḪA *te-be-er*
33. [(3 Ú.ḪI.A ŠEŠ *ina* 1/2 *qa* KAŠ).S]AG *ki pi-i*
34. [(*mál-ma-liš tara-muk ana* IGI M)]UL GI$_6$ GAR-*an*
35. ^{GIŠ}ḪUR NIGIN-*mi ina* Á.GÚ.ZI.[(GA 3)]-⸢*šú-nu*⸣ *ta-šá-ḫal*
36. NU *pa-tan* NAG *i-lap-pat-su-ma is-sa-la-ʾ*
37. *la ta-na-kud* TI-*uṭ ina* U$_4$ ŠE.GA NAG-*šú*

---

38. DIŠ NA GABA-*su u šá-šal-la-šú* KÚM.MEŠ ZÚ.MEŠ-*šú i-ḫi-la*
39. *e-piš* KA-*šú* DUGUD NA BI ZÉ GIG *ana* TI-*šú*
40. ^{ŠEM}GÚR.GÚR ^{ŠEM}LI ^{ŠEM}GAM.MA MUN ILLU LI.TAR
41. ^{Ú}KU$_6$ Ú BABBAR ^{Ú}ḪAB ^{Ú}*ak-tam* ^{GIŠ}ḪAB ^{Ú}KUR.KUR U$_5$ ARGAB^{MUŠEN}
42. [(12 Ú).ḪI].A ŠEŠ 1-*niš* SÚD *ina* KAŠ NU *pa-tan* NAG-*ma i-ár-rù*

---

43. [...] ⸢*e*⸣-*piš* KA DUGUD
44. [...] *ina* KAŠ NAG-*ma* TI

---

45. [...^{ŠE}]^{M}ŠEŠ
46. [...] SÚD
47. [...]x

ii

1. ^{IM}SAḪAR.NA$_4$.KUR.RA [*ina* KAŠ NAG ...]
2. *ina* KAŠ NAG ^{Ú}GÍR-*a-nu ina* KAŠ NAG ^{Ú}*nab-ru-qu*
3. *ina* KAŠ NAG SUḪUŠ! ^{GIŠ}*šu-še ša ina* ZI-*ka* ^{d}UTU NU IGI-*ru*
4. *tu-bal tu-pa-ṣa ina* KAŠ *tara-muk ina* UL *tuš-bat ina še-rim*
5. NU *pa-tan* NAG

---

6. DIŠ MIN SUḪUŠ! ^{GIŠ}*šu-še ta-ka-sím a-na* A.MEŠ ŠUB-*di*
7. *ina* NINDU BAD-*ir ina* ŠÀ RA-*su* : DIŠ MIN GÚ.NÍG.ÀR.RA
8. *sa-an-du-ti ina* ^{DUG}BUR.ZI.GAL *ana* IGI-*šú* GAR-*an*
9. $^{\text{NA}_4}$KÙ.SIG$_{17}$ $^{\text{NA}_4}$GUG $^{\text{NA}_4}$ZA.GÌN $^{\text{NA}_4}$*pa-ru-tú*
10. *ina* ^{SÍG}ḪÉ.MED È *ina* ŠU-*šú* KEŠDA-*ma ina-ri*

---

11. DIŠ NA *aḫ-ḫa-za* GIG ^{Ú}LAG.GÁN ^{ŠEM}LI 1-*niš* SÚD *ina* GA U$_8$ KU$_7$.KU$_7$ NAG

---

12. DIŠ NA ŠÀ.MEŠ-*šú* MÚ.MÚ-*ḫu* GÌR^{II}-*šú it-te-nen-bi-ṭa*
13. GURUN ^{Ú}*ir-re-e* ḪÁD.A SÚD *ina* NÍG.SILAG.GÁ ŠE.SA.A
14. ḪE.ḪE 7 *u* 7 *ku-pa-tin-ni* DÙ-*uš* LÀL KUR-*i*

15. *ú-ṣap-pa ú-al-lat* KAŠ ZÚ.LUM.MA NAG
16. *ina* DÚR-*šú* SI.SÁ-*ma* TI

---

17. DIŠ MIN SUḪUŠ ^{GIŠ}*šu-še ina* A *tara-muk ina* UL *tuš-bat*
18. *ta-šá-ḫal* NU *pa-tan* NAG-*ma* TI

---

19. DIŠ MIN Ì.U[D]U ^{Ú}ÚKUŠ.GÍL *ana* DÚR-*šú* GAR-*an*

TRANSLATION

(i 21–24) If a person's liver continually afflicts him, blood comes constantly from his nose/mouth, he is continually bloated and constipated, that person (has) DÚR.GIG.[54] To cure him, you char (and) grind lion skin. You mix (it) with sheep fat. You form a finger-shaped suppository. If you insert (it) into his anus, he should recover.

(i 25–26) Alternatively, you grind date rind. You mix (it) with sheep fat. You form a finger-shaped suppository. If you insert (it) into his anus, he should recover.

(i 27–28) Alternatively, you have (him) drink "fox grape" (mixed) with beer. You have (him) drink *šunû*-chastetree (mixed) with beer. You have (him) drink *atāʾišu* (mixed) with beer.

(i 29–37) If a person eats bread (and) drinks beer and then chokes and his face seems continually to spin, that person is sick with an illness of the gall bladder.[55] To cure him, ⌜you uproot⌝ *irrû* newly growing on the north side (and) wash (it) with water. You cut up *baluḫḫu*-aromatic (and) you select *nuḫurtu*. You decoct[56] these three plants in equal proportions [in] 1/2 *qû* of first-quality beer. You put (it) out under the night stars. You surround (it) with a drawing. In the morning, you filter (it) three times. You have him drink (it) on an empty stomach. It will affect him so that he will appear to get worse. Do not worry; he should recover in the end. You have him drink (it) on a propitious day.

(i 38–42) If a person's breast and back are continually hot, his teeth ooze blood and opening his mouth is difficult, that person has sick gall bladder.[57] To cure him, you grind together these twelve plants: *kukru*, *burāšu*-juniper, *ṣumlalû*, salt, *abukkatu* resin, *šimru*, "white plant," *šammi buʾšāni*, *aktam*, *ḫurātu*, *atāʾišu*, and *rikibti arkabi*. If you have him drink (it) on an empty stomach (mixed) with beer, he should vomit.

(i 43–44) [If …] (and) opening the mouth is difficult, […]. If you have him drink (it mixed) with beer.

(i 45–47) [If …], you grind […], myrrh, […]

(ii 1–5) (For *amurriqānu*?), [you have him drink] alum [(mixed) with beer]. You have him drink […] (mixed) with beer. You have him drink *patrānu* (mixed) with beer. You have him drink *namruqqu* (mixed) with beer. You dry and pulverize *šūšu*-licorice root which the sun did not see when you pulled (it) up. You decoct (it) in beer (and) leave (it) out overnight under the stars. You have him drink (it) in the morning on an empty stomach.

(ii 6–10) Alternatively, you chop *šūšu*-licorice root and pour (it) into water. You bake (it) in an oven (and) bathe him with it. Alternatively, you place *kiššēnu* groats in a *burzigallu*-vessel before him (to eat). You thread gold, carnelian, lapis (and) *parūtu*-marble on red-dyed wool. If you bind (it) on his hand, (the jaundice) should be vomited up.

(ii 11) If a person is sick with *aḫḫāzu*, you grind *kirbān eqli* (and) *burāšu*-juniper and have him drink (it) in sweet sheep's milk.

(ii 12–16) If a person's insides are continually bloated (and) his feet continually have cramps,[58] you dry (and) grind *irrû* fruit. You mix (it) with dough made from roasted wheat flour (and) make seven and seven pills. He soaks (them) in wild honey (and) swallows (them). You have him drink date beer. If he has a bowel movement, he should recover.

(ii 17–18) Alternatively, you decoct *šūšu*-licorice root in water. You leave (it) out overnight under the stars. You filter (it). If you have him drink (it) on an empty stomach, he should recover.

(ii 19) Alternatively, you put *irrû* "fat" into his anus.

C. SPLEEN

Problems with the spleen are a common concomitant of malaria. For details, see Scurlock and Andersen 2005, 135–36.

TEXT 9: BAM 77

BAM 77 consists of an aspirant (20′–27′), potions (20′–50′), aliments (20′–27′, 37′–38′, 43′–50′), and an enema (20′–27′) for hurting and/or enlarged spleen. It was Marduk who was responsible for making your spleen act up, which is why the patient is to seek out his sanctuary in lines 20′–27′. The efficacy of lizards also found ready explanation in the fact that Marduk was essentially a dragon, according to the commentary, Civil 1974, 336:12–13. Noteworthy in the treatments for splenomegaly is the use of dog spleen (30′–32′, 33′–36′, 39′–42′), essentially hormone replacement therapy.

1′. [...] NAG x [...]

2′. [… ^{Ú}]ḪAR.ḪAR ^{Ú}KUR.KUR NAGA.SI […]
3′. […] ud (*ḫe-pí*) ILLU LI.TAR MUN *e*[*me-sal-lim* …]
4′. […] NA BI NAG-*ma* […]

5′. […] ^{ŠEM}MUG ^{ŠEM}IM.MAN.DU […]
6′. […] ^{Ú}NU.LUḪ.ḪA KA x[…]
7′. [… 1]-*niš* GAZ SIM *ina* L[ÀL …]
8′. […] ⸢*ta*⸣-*šá-ḫal* x […]
9′. […] x […]
gap
19′. […]x ḪE […]

20′. [(DIŠ NA *tu-limi-šú* ⸢GU$_7$⸣-*šú* U$_4$)] *u* GI$_6$ NU NÁ *pa-gar-šú* KÚM *ú*-[*kal*]
21′. [KAŠ NAG *u* NINDA G(U$_7$) *i*]-⸢*maṭ-ṭám*⸣[59] *aš-rat* ^{d}AMAR.UTU KIN.KIN-*ma* T[(I)-*uṭ*][60]
22′. [$^{\text{(Ú)}}$…] ^{Ú}*tar-muš* $^{\text{NA}_4}$ZÚ GI$_6$ NUMUN ^{GIŠ}ŠINIG
23′. [(NA$_4$ *ga-bi-i* 1-*niš* SÚ)]D *ina* LÀL.KUR.RA ḪE.ḪE NU *pa-tan*
24′. [(*ú-na-ṣab-ma* TI) DIŠ *ga*]-*bid* GUD[61] ḪÁD.A SÚD *ina* KAŠ ^{LÚ}KÚRUN.N[A]
25′. [NAG.MEŠ *ba*]-*a-a-ri*[62] *ik-ta-na-su-u*[*s*]
26′. […]x tú Ì.UDU ÚKUŠ.GÍL *ana* ŠÀ 1 *qa* KAŠ ŠUB-*d*[*i*]
27′. […] SI.SÁ-*ma* EGIR-*šú* Ì *u* KAŠ DUB-*ak-ma* TI

28′. [DIŠ NA *tu-limi-šú*] ⸢GU$_7$⸣-*šú u* GUB.GUB-*az* LAG A.ŠÀ.G[A]
29′. ḪÁD.DU GAZ SIM *ina* A ÍD SÌG-*aṣ ba-lu pa-tan* NAG.MEŠ-*ma* TI

30′. DIŠ NA *tu-limi-šú* GUB.GUB-⸢*az*⸣ *tu-limi šá* UR.GI$_7$ ^{d}NIN.KILIM.EDIN.N[A]
31′. *ša taš-te-tum* MU.NI *tu-šab-šal* U$_4$.3.KÁM
32′. *ba-lu pa-tan* GU$_7$-*ma ù me-e i-šat-ti-ma ina-eš*

33′. DIŠ NA BI.RI-*šú* GUB.GUB-*az* BI.RI UR.GI$_7$ [G]I$_6$
34′. *in-du-ḫal-la-tú ša* EDIN [*š*]*a taš-lam-tum* MU.NE
35′. […] SUMUN.DAR SÚD *ina* MÚD-*ša* ḪE.ḪE BI.RI
36′. [… *a*]*n-nu-ti tu-šab-šal* U$_4$.3.KÁM x x x x

37′. [DIŠ KI.MIN *in*]-*du-ḫal-la-tu* ḪÁD.DU SÚD *ina* KAŠ N[A]G
38′. [*ba-a-a-ri*] *ik-ta-na-su-us*

39′. [DIŠ NA BI.RI]-*šú* GUB.GUB-*az* BI.RI UR.GI$_7$ GI$_6$
40′. [*in-du-ḫal-la-t*]*ú ša* EDIN *ša taš-lam-tu* MU.NE
41′. [… S]ÚD *ina* MÚD-*šá* ḪE.ḪE E$_{11}$-*a* ŠEG$_6$-*šal*
42′. […] *ina-eš*

43′. [… *pi-za-lu-u*]*r-ti ša* EDIN ḪÁD.A SÚD
44′. […] NAG.MEŠ *ba-a-r*[*i*]
45′. [… -*m*]*a* T[I]

46′. […]x *tu-limi an-du-ḫal-la-t*[*i*]
47′. [… *ta*]*š-lam-tum* MU.N[I]
48′. […] NU *pa-tan* N[AG]
49′. […] ÀR.RA NU *pa-tan* N[AG]
50′. [… *ik-ta-na*]-*as-su-u*[*s*]

51′. […] ^{Ú}*tar-muš* ^{Ú}*imḫur-*[*lim*]
52′. […] ^{Ú}*ḫal-tap-pa-*[*nu*]
53′. […] x […]

TRANSLATION

(1′) […] You have him drink (it) […]

(2′–4′) […] *ḫašû*-thyme, *atāʾišu*, *uḫḫūlu qarnanu* […] *abukkatu* resin, ⌜*emesallim*⌝-salt […] If you have that person drink (it) […].

(5′–9′) […] You crush ⌜together⌝ (and) sift *ballukku*-aromatic, *suʾādu* […] *nuḫurtu*, […] with ⌜honey⌝ […] You filter (it). […]

(gap)

(19′) […] You mix (it) […].

(20′–27′) If a person's spleen hurts him, he is unable to sleep day or night, his body ⌜holds⌝ fever and [the amount of beer he drinks and bread] ⌜he eats⌝ diminishes,[63] if he continually seeks out the shrine of Marduk, he should recover.[64] You grind together […], *tarmuš*, black obisidian, *bīnu*-tamarisk seed, (and) alum. You mix (it) with wild honey. If he sucks (it) on an empty stomach, he should recover. [Alternatively], you dry (and) grind (the lobe)[65] of an ox ⌜liver⌝ [and have him repeatedly drink it] (mixed) with *kurunnu*-beer. He should repeatedly chew on rawhide.[66] You pour […] (and) *irrû* "fat" into 1 *qû* of beer. […] He should have a bowel movement and afterwards, if you pour oil and beer (into his anus), he should recover.

(28′–29′) [If a person's spleen] hurts him and continually stands up,[67] you dry, crush (and) sift *kirbān eqli*. You stir (it) into river water. If you have him drink (it) repeatedly on an empty stomach, he should recover.

(30′–32′) If a person's spleen continually stands up,[68] you boil the spleen of a dog[69] (and) an *ayaṣu*-weasel of the type which is called *taštitu*. If you have him eat (it) for three days on an empty stomach and then if he drinks water, he should recover.

(33′–36′) If a person's spleen continually stands up, (you take) the spleen of a ⌈black⌉ dog (and) an *anduḫallatu*-lizard[70] from the steppe of the type called *tašlamtu*. You grind [...] (and) *šumuttu*-vegetable and mix (it) with its blood. You boil the spleen and these [...]. [You have him drink it] for three days [...]

(37′–38′) [Alternatively], you dry (and) grind an ⌈*anduḫallatu*⌉-lizard (and) have him drink (it mixed) with beer. He should repeatedly chew on [rawhide].

(39′–42′) [If a person's spleen] continually stands up, (you take) the spleen of a black dog (and) an ⌈*anduḫallatu*⌉-lizard from the steppe of the type called *tašlamtu*. You ⌈grind⌉ [...] and mix (it) with its blood. You throw (the lizard) out (and) boil (the rest). [If you have him drink it on an empty stomach], he should recover.

(43′–45′) [Alternatively], you dry (and) grind a ⌈*pizzalurtu*⌉-lizard of the steppe (and) have him repeatedly drink (it mixed) [with beer]. ⌈If⌉ [he repeatedly chews on] hide, ⌈he should recover⌉.

(46′–50′) [For standing up] of the spleen, [you ...] an *anduḫallatu*-lizard of the type called ⌈*tašlamtu*⌉. [...] You have him drink (it) on an empty stomach. ⌈You have him drink⌉ [...] on an empty stomach. ⌈He should repeatedly chew⌉ [rawhide].

(51′–53′) [...] *tarmuš*, *imḫur*-[*lim*], [...], *ḫaltappānu* [...]

Notes

1. After a suggestion by Schwemer 2009, 177.
2. See Scurlock and Andersen 2005, 3.108, 19.295.
3. See Scurlock and Andersen 2005, 6.75, 19.387.
4. See Scurlock and Andersen 2005, 13.22.
5. The reading follows *AHw*, 1366a.
6. See Scurlock and Andersen 2005, 6.101.
7. See Scurlock and Andersen 2005, 6.30, 6.98, 6.102.
8. The translation assumes that the mysterious *mál-li-riš* is a contracted form of *mala lirīšu*: "as much as he might wish."
9. See Scurlock and Andersen 2005, 6.92.
10. Alternatively, one could read *šit-ta-šú* and iterpret this and ii 46 as referring to the patient's excrement drying up. Suggestion courtesy M. Stol.
11. See Scurlock and Andersen 2005, 3.266.
12. For the translation of *saḫlû* as "cress," see Stol 1983–84, 24–32.

13. See Scurlock and Andersen 2005, 3.262.

14. A similar treatment (but for headache) appears in BAM 482 iv 7–8.

15. In *KADP* 1 iv 23, this is given as an equivalent of *labubītu*. This could either mean that DUMU.A.NI: "Its son" is the Sumerogram for *labubītu* or that *labubītu* may be substituted for the *turû*-garlic-like plant reading DUMU.A.NI as *tur-a-ní* (*turânu*).

16. See Scurlock and Andersen 2005, 6.87.

17. This is similar to BAM 579 iv 1–11, which is a treatment for a person with "sick insides."

18. The duplicates add: *um-ṣa-a-te qut-tu-pi*.

19. See Scurlock and Andersen 2005, 6.44.

20. The duplicates add: "to remove *umṣātu*-lesions." See Scurlock and Andersen 2005, 149–50.

21. For the intervening section, see chapter 11, text 2.

22. See Scurlock and Andersen 2005, 3.119, 6.179.

23. See chapter 3, n. 109.

24. Rolled pickled meat also appears in BAM 180:3′–5′.

25. See chapter 8, text 3. Either the "Hittite" version was different or the procedure was itself "Hittite."

26. A restoration of [*ú*]*r-né-e* would also be possible.

27. A restoration of [*ú*]*r-né-e* would also be possible.

28. *CAD* Q, 251a places the references under *qidḫu* but acknowledges *saḫḫu* as a possible reading.

29. It is here assumed that BU.LU.UḪ is syllabic Sumerian for BULUḪ.

30. Restored from numerous duplicates. See Michalowski 1981, 13–18.

31. See Collins 1999, 230–31: *mārtu* 1.

32. See Collins 1999, 231–32: *mārtu* 2; see also Foster 1996, 831. For a Sumerian parallel, see Michalowski 1981, 4.

33. See Scurlock and Andersen 2005, 6.26, 6.107.

34. See chapter 3, n. 109.

35. See Scurlock and Andersen 2005, 6.72, 6.109.

36. See Scurlock and Andersen 2005, 6.108.

37. See chapter 3, n. 109.

38. See chapter 3, n. 109.

39. This is a description of positional vertigo—see Scurlock and Andersen 2005, 302.

40. See Scurlock and Andersen 2005, 6.113.

41. Literally: "to satiation." See Herrero 1975, 49 n. 6.

42. See Scurlock and Andersen 2005, 6.96, 6.99, 6.110.

43. See Scurlock and Andersen 2005, 6.111.

44. For a discussion of this text, see Scurlock 2005, 312–13.

45. See Scurlock and Andersen 2005, 6.122.

46. See Scurlock and Andersen 2005, 6.120.

47. This ritual exploits the fact that the word for "used grease" is very similar to the word for "reddish."

48. See *CAD* U/W, 130.

49. See Scurlock and Andersen 2005, 9.61.

50. See Scurlock and Andersen 2005, 9.40.

51. This will have been delivered in three batches; see BAM 578 iv 16.

52. See Scurlock and Andersen 2005, 6.39, 6.118, 9.39.

53. See Scurlock and Andersen 2005, 6.139.

54. See Scurlock and Andersen 2005, 6.151, 6.183.
55. See Scurlock and Andersen 2005, 6.108.
56. See chapter 3, n. 109.
57. See Scurlock and Andersen 2005, 6.113.
58. See Scurlock and Andersen 2005, 13.18.
59. The parallel has LAL.
60. This section is summarized by the commentary Civil 1974, 336:6.
61. The commentary Civil 1974, 336:8–9 has DIŠ *ga-bi-du al-pi tu-ub-bal ta-sa-ku ma-kut*.
62. Restored from the commentary, Civil 1974, 336:9.
63. See Scurlock and Andersen 2005, 6.104.
64. As the commentary, Civil 1974, 336:6–7 explains, the spleen is under the aegis of the planet Jupiter.
65. See Civil 1974, 336:8–9: "you dry (and) grind an ox liver—the lobe."
66. According to the commentary Civil 1974, 336:9, rawhide looks like the face of a falcon. It is also to note that the root for chewing, *kss*, is a pun on a word for falcon.
67. See Scurlock and Andersen 2005, 6.105.
68. See Scurlock and Andersen 2005, 6.106.
69. The commentary Civil 1974, 336:10–11 would seem to indicate that in at least some versions of this treatment, the spleen came specifically from an adult male goat. The choice of animal was due to the fact that the goatfish was the symbol of Ea, god of healing. The less expensive dog spleen will, however, have worked as well or better, and our text consequently recommends dog.
70. The commentary Civil 1974, 336:12–13 explains the choice as related to Marduk's proud boast of being an *ušumgallu* dragon and a *labbu* monster.

10

GENITOURINARY TRACT

Hot dry climates are not kind to the human genitourinary tract. In addition, ancient Mesopotamians seem to have suffered the attentions of *Schistosomiasis hematobium*. Ancient physicians examined the urine for color, consistency, and smell and listened to complaints of blood in the urine, discharge, inability to urinate and incontinence. They also had to deal with impotence, priapism, orchitis, and Ishtar's revenge (venereal disease). For more details, see Scurlock and Andersen 2005, chapters 4–5.

A. URINARY TRACT

TEXT 1: BAM 396 i–iii

BAM 396 has a unique way of indicating that there is more than one treatment available for a given condition. Instead of the usual repeated KI.MINs to indicate dittography, this text has KI.2, KI.3, etc., etc. Wasserman 1996, 2 has a list of the recitations that will have accompanied each treatment. The parallel of the beginning of column i of BAM 396 with *AMT* 59/1 i 29–32 indicates that these treatments were the fifteenth to twenty-first for constriction of the urethra. The first column of BAM 396 once contained twenty-one potions (i 1′–9′) for constriction of the urethra, in addition to a potion (i 10′–13′) for dribbling of the urine, two potions (i 14′–22′) for priapism, and a potion (i 23′–31′) and a wash (i 23′–31′) for terminal hematuria. Some at least of these conditions were probably caused by *Schistosomiasis hematobium*. For details, see Scurlock and Andersen 2005, 109–10.

Columns ii and iii preserve potions (ii 0′–15′, 23′–31′, iii 6–32), washes (ii 5′–12′, 16′–18′), baths (ii 5′–12′, iii 21–32), salves (ii 16′–22′), an aliment (ii 25′–31′) and a steam bath (iii 1–3) for stones. Noticeable in many of the treatments for stones is the frequency of shells used in the preparations. The hoped for result was that the stone would be passed by the patient. Note that that modern nonsurgical treatments for stones vary with the type but some types of calcium stones, uric acid stones, and Cystine stones respond to supplemental alkali, calcium lactate, or phosphates. Such treatment is not recommended for

Struvite stones due to Proteus infections. Lines ii 19′–22′ are probably due to a Proteus infection, since the urine stinks and, sure enough, the treatment does not include any shells.

Of particular interest are lines i 19′–22′ (cf. iii 21–32) which have the patient take his potion every other day. Lines i 23′–31′ are interesting in that they use half the preparation as a urethral irrigation using a bronze tube and the other half as a potion; lines ii 5′–12′ use it three ways as a potion, wash, and bath, lines ii 16′–18′ as a salve and a wash, lines iii 21–32 as a potion and a bath. It is not unusual to combine treatments, but usually each part of the treatment uses its own plant medicines.

Lines ii 25′–31′ envisage management of the illness with a once a month potion. Lines iii 1–3 heat the plant medicine on a baked brick and have the patient sit over it. The remark in lines iii 7–9 that the sun was not to see the plant (i.e., it was to be picked before sunrise) is cited from a vademecum (see chapter 2, text 1). Lines iii 12–13 are concerned about the purity of the medicine. If an impure person saw it, the impurity would pass into the potion.

i

1′. KI.16 IM.SAḪAR.GI$_6$.KUR.RA *ina* A NAG-*ma i-ne-eš*

2′. KI.17 ZÍD ^{Ú}NAM.TAL NITA ZÍD ^{Ú}GÍR *uḫ-ḫa-aḫ*
3′. *ina* KAŠ *ba-lum pa-tan* NAG-*ma i-ne-eš*

4′. KI.18 ZÍD.DA ŠE ZÍD ^{Ú}GÍR *ina* KAŠ NAG-*ma i-ne-eš*

5′. KI.19 ^{Ú}*im-ḫur-lim* KI.MIN

6′. KI.20 ^{Ú}GEŠTIN.KA$_5$.A ḪÁD.DU *ta-sàk ana* A KAŠ *u* Ì.GIŠ ŠUB
7′. *ina* UL *tuš-bat* NAG-*ma i-ne-eš*

8′. KI.21 ^{Ú}*a-ar*-KÙ.BABBAR *ina* KAŠ *u* GA ḪE.ḪE
9′. *ba-lu pa-tan* NAG-*ma i-ne-eš*

10′. DIŠ NA *ta-at-ti-kám ša* KÀŠ GIG 1 *qa* DÈ *ṣú-pur* UDU.NÍTA
11′. 1 *qa* DÈ NAM.TAL NITA
12′. *ba-lum pa-tan* KI A NAG.NAG U$_4$.5.KÁM*
13′. *ka-la* U$_4$-*mi* NAG.NAG-*ma i-ne-eš*

14′. DIŠ NA *ša-a-ši-tu-nam un-nu-ut ù ma-gal* ZI.ZI-*bi*[1]
15′. NUMUN ^{GIŠ}ŠINIG NUMUN ^{Ú}EME.UR.GI$_7$

16′. ^{ŠEM}ŠEŠ *ta-sàk ana* KAŠ SAG ŠUB
17′. *ina* UL *tuš-bat ina* Á.GÚ.ZI.GA
18′. *ba-lum pa-tan* NAG-*ma i-ne-eš*

19′. KI.2 ^{Ú}SIKIL ^{Ú}ḪAB ^{ŠEM}IM.DI ^{Ú}EME.UR.GI$_{7}$
20′. ḪÁD.DU *t*[*a*]-*sàk šum-ma i-na* GEŠTIN *šum-ma i-na* GA
21′. *šum-ma ina* KAŠ NAG.NAG *la i-sà-dar*
22′. *ina* U$_{4}$.3.KÁM* U$_{4}$.1.KÁM NAG-*ma i-ne-eš*

23′. DIŠ NA ^{UZU}ÉLLAG-*su* GU$_{7}$-*šu* MURUB$_{4}$-*šú* TAG.TAG-*šú ù* KÀŠ-*šú* GIN$_{7}$ KÀŠ ANŠE BABBAR
24′. EGIR KÀŠ-*šu* MÚD *ú-kal-la-ma* NA BI *mu-ṣa-am* GIG
25′. 2 GÍN ^{ŠEM}ŠEŠ 2 GÍN ILLU *ba-lu-ḫi-im*
26′. 2 (variant: 1/3) *qa* A.GEŠTIN.NA TÉŠ.BI *ina* ^{DUG}ÚTUL *tu-šab-šal*
27′. ŠED$_{7}$ Ì.GIŠ BÁRA.GA *ma-al-ma-liš* ḪE.ḪE
28′. *mi-iš-lam ina* MUD ZABAR
29′. [Š]È[2] *muš-tin-ni-su*[3] *ta-ša-pak*
30′. [*mi-i*]*š-lam ina* KAŠ SAG ḪE.ḪE
31′. [*ina* UL *tu*]*š-bat ba-lum pa-tan* NAG-*ma i-ne-eš*[4]

---

ii
0′. [DIŠ NA *ina* (GÌŠ-*šú* NA$_{4}$ ŠUB-*a* NA BI) [NA$_{4}$ G(IG)]
1′. ⌈Ú NUMUN⌉ x x […]
2′. Ú NUMUN EME.UR.GI$_{7}$ ḪÁD.D[U *ta-sàk*]
3′. *ina* KAŠ SAG *tara-sà-an* KI NU TAG.G[E][5]
4′. *ba-lum pa-tan* NAG-*ma i-*[*ne-eš*]

5′. KI.2 ^{ŠEM}ŠEŠ $^{\text{NA}_4\text{.Ú}}$NÍG.BÙR.BÙR ^{Ú}*a-ar*-KÙ.BABBAR[6]
6′. NUMUN ^{Ú}EME.UR.GI$_{7}$ NUMUN ^{Ú}GÍR *uḫ-ḫa-*[*aḫ*][7]
7′. $^{\text{NA}_4}$PÈŠ.ANŠE ŠIKA NUNUZ GA.NU$_{11}$$^{\text{M[(UŠEN)]}}$
8′. Ú.ḪI.A *an-nu-ti* TÉŠ.BI *ta-sàk*
9′. *ina* KAŠ SAG *ba-lu pa-tan* NAG-*šu*[8]
10′. *ina* MUD ZABAR ŠÈ *mùš-tin-ni-su*[9] MÚ
11′. *ina* A.ŠEG$_{6}$ *ir-ta-na-ḫaṣ*
12′. *ù tur-ra-am tu-ba-ḫar-ma*[10] *i-n*[*e-eš*]

13′. KI.3 ^{Ú}EME.UR.GI$_{7}$ ḪÁD.DU *ta-sàk*
14′. *ina* KAŠ.SAG *tara-sà-an ina* UL *tuš-bat*
15′. *ba-lu pa-tan* NAG-*ma i-n*[*e-eš*]

16′. KI.4 Ì ^{GIŠ}ERIN A.GEŠTIN.NA ḪE.ḪE ⸢ŠÉ⸣[Š][11]
17′. *ina* MUD ZABAR ŠÈ *mùš-tin-ni-su* D[UB-*ak*]
18′. *ina* U$_4$.3.KÁM *ú-ga-am-ma-ra-am-ma i-*[*ne-eš*]

19′. KI.5-*ma ù* KÀŠ-*šú ú-ṣa-nu* ^{ŠEM}ŠEŠ *ta-s*[*àk*]
20′. KI *ku-ru-un* KAŠ.Ú.SA *ù* GA KÚM ḪE.Ḫ[E]
21′. *ša-ap-ti-šu* ŠÉŠ-*ma* KÉŠ.D[A]
22′. NA$_4$ *i-ša-aḫ-ḫu-uḫ*

23′. KI.6 ^{ŠEM}ŠEŠ *ta-sàk ana* KAŠ 3.KÁM *sa-bi-*⸢*i*⸣[12]
24′. *ina* UL *tuš-bat ina še-ri* NAG-*ma né-eš*

25′. DIŠ NA NA$_4$ GIG A ^{GIŠ}ERIN ^{GIŠ}ŠU.ÚR.MÌN ^{ŠEM}L[I][13]
26′. GI.DÙG.GA ŠEM.ḪI.A *ka-li-šu-nu* ḪI.[ḪI]
27′. *ina* ITI! 1-*at-tu* NAG!-*ma i-na-a-ḫ*[*i-i*][14]
28′. IGI *mùš-tin-ni-su* NU *tuš-bat*
29′. *ru-ub-ṣu i-de-ek-ke-e-m*[*a*]
30′. GIG *là-zu ú-ṭa-ab-šu*
31′. SUḪUŠ ^{Ú}EME.UR.GI$_7$ GU$_7$-*ma i-ne-*[*eš*]

---

iii

1. KI.2 $^{\text{Ú.GIŠ.Ú}}$GÍR *uḫ-ḫa-a*[*ḫ ina*]
2. SIG$_4$.A[L.UR$_5$.R]A *tu-*⸢*um*⸣-[*ma-am-ma*]
3. *ina* UGU TUŠ-*ma* [*i-ne-eš*]

---

4. KI.3 NUMUN ^{Ú}EME.UR.GI$_7$ ^{Ú}ÚKUŠ.T[I.GI.LA]
5. ḪÁD.DU *ta-sàk ina* Ì.GIŠ Š[UB …]

---

6. KI.4 ^{Ú}ÚKUŠ.GÍL[15] *ina* KAŠ NAG-*ma* [*i-ne-eš*]

---

7. KI.5 ^{Ú}EME.UR.GI$_7$ *ša ina* ZI-*ka* ^{d}UTU [(NU IGI.DU$_8$)]
8. ḪÁD.DU *ta-sàk ana* KAŠ ^{LÚ}KÚRUN.NA [ŠUB-*di*]
9. *ina* UL *tuš-bat ba-lum pa-tan*[16] [NAG-*ma i-ne-eš*]

---

10. KI.6 ^{Ú}GEŠTIN.KA$_5$.A *ana* KAŠ ^{LÚ}⸢KÚRUN.NA⸣ [(ŠUB-*di*)][17]
11. *ina* UL *tuš-bat* [NAG-*ma i-ne-eš*]

---

12. KI.7 *ḫa-lu-la-a* ḪÁD.DU *ta-sàk ina* U[(L *tuš-bat* LÚ)]

13. NU SIKIL NU IGI[18] NAG-[*ma i-ne-eš*]

---

14. KI.8 ŠIKA NUNUZ GA.NU$_{11}$^{MUŠEN} ^{Ú}[(NÍG.BÙR.BÙR)]
15. ^{Ú}*nu-ṣa-ba* $^{\text{GIŠ.Ú}}$GÍR *uḫ-ḫa-aḫ* ⸢^{Ú}⸣[...]
16. ^{Ú}*a-zal-lá* U$_4$.7.KÁM Ú$^{\text{ḪI.}}$[^{A} ŠEŠ^{MEŠ}]
17. *ina* A ZÚ.LUM *ù* KAŠ.SAG ḪE.ḪE
18. NAG-*ma i-ne-*[*eš*]

---

19. KI.9 NUMUN ^{Ú}GÍR *ḫa-aḫ* ^{Ú}NÍG.BÙR.BÙR TÉŠ.BI *ta-s*[*àk*]
20. *ana* GEŠTIN ŠUB *i-na* UL *tuš-bat* NAG-*ma né-eš*

---

21. KI.10 $^{\text{NA}_4}$*za-la-qu* $^{\text{NA}_4}$KA.GI.NA *mu-ṣa-am*
22. AN.ZAḪ $^{\text{NA}_4}$PEŠ$_4$.ANŠE ^{ŠEM}ŠEŠ
23. ŠIKA ^{GIŠ}NU.ÚR.MA ŠIKA NUNUZ GA.NU$_{11}$$^{\text{M[(UŠEN)]}}$
24. AN.ZAḪ GI$_6$ NITA *ù* MUNUS
25. ^{Ú}*a-ar*-KÙ.BABBAR NUMUN ^{GIŠ}ŠINIG KA.A.AB.[(BA)]
26. ^{Ú}NÍG.BÙR.BÙR ^{Ú}*tar-muš* ^{Ú}GÍR *uḫ-ḫa-a*[*ḫ*]
27. NUMUN ^{Ú}EME.UR.GI$_7$ ^{Ú}EME.UR.GI$_7$
28. NUMUN Ú DIDLI TÉŠ.BI[19] *ta-ša-*[(*qa*)]-*a*[(*l*)]
29. *ta-sàk ina* Ì.GIŠ *u* Ì.GIŠ BÁRA.GA[20] ḪE.ḪE
30. *ana* IGI ⸢MUL.ÙZ⸣[21] *tuš-bat ina še-ri* NAG.NA[G]
31. *la i-sa!-a-dar ù* A KÚM
32. *ir-ta-na-ḫaṣ-*⸢*ma i-ne-eš*⸣

TRANSLATION

(i 1′)[22] If sixteen, if you have him drink black alum (mixed) with water, he should recover.

(i 2′–3′) If seventeen, if you have him drink male *pillû* flour (and) *ḫaḫḫinu*-thorn flour (mixed) with beer on an empty stomach, he should recover.

(i 4′) If eighteen, if you have him drink barley flour (and) *ašāgu*-thorn flour (mixed) with beer, he should recover.

(i 5′) If nineteen, *imḫur-lim* ditto (if you have him drink it mixed with beer, he should recover).

(i 6′–7′) If twenty, you dry (and) grind "fox grape." You pour (it) into water, beer and oil (and) leave (it) out overnight under the stars. If you have him drink (it), he should recover.

(i 8′–9′) If twenty-one, you mix "silver blossom" (*nuṣābu*) in beer and milk. If you have him drink (it) on an empty stomach, he should recover.

(i 10′–13′) If a person is sick with dribbling of the urine, you have him repeatedly drink 1 *qû*-measure of ashes of wether hoof (and) 1 *qû*-measure of male *pillû* ashes (mixed) with water on an empty stomach. If you have him repeatedly drink (it) for five days, all day, he should recover.

(i 14′–18′) If a person is compressed with regard to the *šašitūna* and he continually has an erection, you grind *bīnu*-tamarisk seed, *lišān kalbi* seed (and) myrrh. You pour (it) into first-quality beer (and) leave (it) out overnight under the stars. In the morning, if you have him drink (it) on an empty stomach, he should recover.

(i 19′–22′) If two, you dry (and) grind *sikillu*, *šammi buʾšāni*, *suʾādu*, (and) *lišān kalbi*. You have him drink (it) repeatedly (mixed) either with wine or with milk or with beer. He is not to do this two days in a row but, if you have him drink (it) one day in every three, he should recover.

(i 23′–31′) If a person's kidney region hurts him, his pelvic region continually hurts him intensely and his urine is as white as the urine of a donkey (and) after his urine he shows blood, that person is sick with *mūṣu*.[23] You boil 2 shekels of myrrh, 2 shekels of *baluḫḫu*-aromatic (and) 2 (variant: 1/3) *qû*-measures of vinegar together in a *dīqaru*-bowl. You let (it) cool. You mix (it with) an equal quantity of pressed-out oil. You pour half of it into his urethra[24] via a bronze tube. You pour the other half into first-quality beer. [You] let (it) sit out overnight [under the stars]. If you have him drink (it) on an empty stomach, he should recover.[25]

(ii 0′–4′) [If a person] produces a stone [from] his penis, that person is sick with [stones]. You dry (and) [grind …] seed, […] (and) *lišān kalbi* seed. You steep (it) in first-quality beer which has not touched the ground.[26] If he drinks (it) on an empty stomach, he [should recover].

(ii 5′–12′) If two, you grind together these plants: myrrh, *pallišu*-plant stone,[27] silver blossom (*nuṣābu*), *lišān kalbi* seed, *ḫaḫḫinu*-thorn[28] seed, *biṣṣuru* shell, (and) a fragment of ostrich egg shell. You have him drink (it) in first-quality beer on an empty stomach. You blow (the mixture) into his urethra[29] via a bronze tube. He should bathe over and over again in (the mixture) boiled in water. Also, if you heat (it) up for him again,[30] ⸢he should recover⸣.

(ii 13′–15′) If three, you dry (and) grind *lišān kalbi*. You steep (it) in first-quality beer. You let (it) sit out overnight under the stars. If you have him drink (it) on an empty stomach, ⸢he should recover⸣.

(ii 16′–18′) If four, you mix *erēnu*-cedar oil (and) vinegar (and) rub (him) gently (with it). You ⸢pour⸣ (it) into his urethra via a bronze tube. (You do this for two days.) On the third day, if (the treatment) finishes (it) off completely, he [should recover].

(ii 19′–22′) If five (a person is sick with stones) and his urine stinks,[31] ⌜you grind⌝ myrrh. You mix (it) with *kurunnu* beer, beerwort and hot milk. If you rub (it) on the lips (of) his (penis), the concentrated stone should fall out.

(ii 23′–24′) If six, you grind myrrh. (You pour it) into third quality beer merchant's beer. You leave (it) out overnight under the stars. If you have him drink (it) in the morning, he should recover.

(ii 25′–31′) If a person is sick with stones, you mix *erēnu*-cedar infusion, *šurmēnu*-cypress, ⌜*burāšu*⌝-juniper, "sweet reed" (and) *labanātu*-incense. If you have him drink (it) once a month, he should find relief.[32] You should not leave (it) overnight in his urethra. It ⌜may⌝ call up "shit" but a chronic illness will make it better for him. (If) he eats *lišān kalbi* root, he ⌜should recover⌝.

(iii 1–3) If two, you ⌜heat up⌝ *ḫaḫḫinu*-thorn [on] a baked brick. If you have him sit over it, [he should recover].

(iii 4–5) If three, you dry (and) grind *lišān kalbi* seed (and) ⌜*tigilû*⌝. You ⌜pour⌝ (it) into oil [...].

(iii 6) If four, you char *irrû*.[33] If you have him drink (it mixed) with beer, [he should recover].

(iii 7–9) If five, you dry *lišān kalbi*, which, when you pulled it up, the sun did not see. You grind (it and) [pour (it)] into *kurunnu* beer. You leave (it) out overnight under the stars. [If you have him drink (it)] on an empty stomach,[34] [he should recover].

(iii 10–11) If six, you pour "fox grape" into *kurunnu* beer. You let (it) sit out overnight under the stars. [If you have him drink (it), he should recover.]

(iii 12–13) If seven, you dry (and) grind a *ḫalulaya*-insect. You let (it) sit out overnight under the stars (but) an impure person must not see it.[35] [If] you have him drink (it), [he should recover].

(iii 14–18) If eight, you mix a fragment of ostrich egg shell, *pallišu*-plant stone, *nuṣābu*, *ḫaḫḫinu*-thorn, [...] (and) *azallû* for seven days in date infusion and first-quality beer. If you have him drink (it), ⌜he should recover⌝.

(iii 19–20) If nine, you ⌜grind⌝ together *ḫaḫḫinu*-thorn seed (and) *pallišu*-plant stone. You pour (it) into wine. You let (it) sit out overnight under the stars. If you have him drink (it), he should recover.

(iii 21–32) If ten, you weigh out *zalaqqu* stone, magnetic hematite, *mūṣu* stone, *anzaḫḫu*-frit, *biṣṣuru* shell, myrrh, a fragment of pomegranate (peel), a fragment of ostrich egg shell, male and female black *anzaḫḫu*-frit, "silver blossom" (*nuṣābu*), *bīnu*-tamarisk seed, *imbû tamtim*, *pallišu*-plant stone, *tarmuš*, *ḫaḫḫinu*-thorn, *lišān kalbi* (and its) seed, seed of "lone plant" together.[36] You grind (them). You mix (it) with oil or pressed-out oil.[37] You let (it) sit out overnight under the goat star. You have him drink (it) repeatedly in the morning. He does not do this more than once in a row but, if he bathes repeatedly (in it mixed) with hot water, he should recover.

B. PENIS AND TESTICLES

1. GENERAL

TEXT 2: BAM 396 iv

Column iv deals with problems with the penis and testicles. The preserved section has a bandage (iv 1–2) for "wind blasting" (an STD), a potion (iv 3–5) for bleeding due to trauma, a wash and a potion of the same composition (iv 6–12) for discharge of "semen" (actually mostly pus) and potions (iv 13–21, 24–27) and salves (iv 15–21) for sore or burning testicles.

Of particular interest is the use in lines iv 13–19 of scorpions to treat pain. Since the sting produces numbness, putting them in a potion is a logical, if unexpected, treatment. The preparation method for the salve is even more interesting. Decoctions are normally made in alcohol or water. This is an oil made by burying a live scorpion for two weeks in a copper vessel. Presumably, the scorpion would try to sting its way out of its trap, thus producing a venom-laced oil. By comparison with this, the ground lizards and insects of lines iv 15–21, 24–27 seem perfectly unremarkable. Lines iv 22–23 have a charming transfer rite whereby a fish gets a mouthful of urine, and hopefully mysteriously burning testicles.

iv

1. [KI].2 PA ^{GIŠ}ŠINIG SIG$_7$ ^{Ú}IN.UŠ GÚ.NÍG.ÀR.RA
2. TÉŠ.BI GAZ LAL-*ma i-ne-eš*

---

3. [(DIŠ N)]A *ina* GÌŠ-*šú* MÚD *ú-tab-ba-kám* GIN$_7$ MUNUS-*ma* ^{GIŠ}TUKUL *ma-ḫ*[(*i-i*)]*ṣ*
4. GÚ.NÍG.ÀR.RA[38] ^{Ú}NU.LUḪ.ḪA NAGA.SI
5. *ina* KAŠ *si-bi*[39] NAG.NAG-*ma i-ne-eš*

---

6. DIŠ NA *i-na-aṭ-ma i-na* DU-*šu re-ḫu-us-su* DU-*ma* NU ZU
7. [(GIN$_7$ *šá ana*)] SAL.LA-*šu* DU-*ma ma-aṣ-ra-aḫ*
8. ⸢KÀŠ⸣-*šu* Ù.BU.BU.UL[40] *ma-li*
9. IM.SAḪAR.NA$_4$.KUR.RA NAGA.SI[41] *ina* Ì.GIŠ ḪE.ḪE
10. *ina* MUD ZABAR ŠÈ *mùš-tin-ni-šu* DUB
11. *ù ina* Ì.GIŠ *ù* KAŠ ḪE.ḪE[42]
12. NAG-*ma i-ne-eš*[43]

---

13. DIŠ NA ŠIR-*šú* GIG GÍR.TAB ḪÁD.DU *ta-sàk*

14. *ina* KAŠ NAG-*ma i-ne-eš*

---

15. DIŠ ⸢NA⸣ T[AB?] ⸢ŠIR⸣ DIDLI ‹GIG› GÍR.TAB TI.LA ^{DUG}KAL Ì.GIŠ DIRI
16. [*ina* Š]À ŠUB U_4.14.KÁM *ina* GAN URUDU *te-tem-me-er*
17. E_{11}-*ma* ‹‹⸢KAŠ⸣ NAG-*šu-m*[*a*]›› *in-du-ḫal-la-ta-am*
18. ḪÁD.DU *ta-sàk ana* ŠÀ ḪE.ḪE BIR(!)-*šu ù ša-pu-li-šu* ŠÉŠ
19. *ù* ÍB.TAK_4 NAG-*ma i-ne-eš*

---

20. KI.2 EME.ŠID *ša* EDIN *tur-ár ta-sàk ina* Ì.GIŠ ŠÉŠ
21. *i-na* KAŠ NAG-*ma i-ne-eš*

---

22. KI.3 MU.ÙR.RA.KU_6 TI.LA DIB-*bat* KÀŠ!-*šu*
23. *ana* ⸢KA⸣-*ša iš-tan ana* ÍD BAR-*ši-ma i-ne-eš*

---

24. KI.4 É.GI_4.A.^{d}UTU SA_5 *in-du-ḫal-la-ta ša* A.ŠÀ
25. *ina* GA *ù* ^{G}[^{IŠ}GEŠTI]N *tu-šab-šal* NAG-*ma né-eš*

---

26. KI.5 *ia-ra-ra qá-ta-an-tú ša* A.ŠÀ
27. [*ina*] Ì.GIŠ? ⸢*tu-šab-šal*⸣[44] NAG-*ma i-ne-eš*

TRANSLATION

(iv 1–2) If two (wind "blasts" a person's penis), you crush together fresh *bīnu*-tamarisk leaves, *maštakal* (and) *kiššēnu*. If you bandage him (with it), he should recover.

(iv 3–5) If a person pours blood from his penis like a (menstruating) woman, he was wounded with a weapon,[45] you grind together *kiššēnu*-bean (or *ḫallūru*-chick pea),[46] *nuḫurtu* (and) *uḫḫūlu qarnānu*. You leave (it) out overnight (mixed) with beer merchant's beer.[47] If you have him drink (it) on an empty stomach, he should recover.

(iv 6–12) If a person has a condition of discharge so that when he walks his semen flows and he does not know (it) like one who goes to a woman (and) the "duct of his urine" (urethra) is full of narrow (i.e., small)[48] *bubuʾtu* (vesicles),[49] you grind[50] alum (and) *uḫḫūlu qarnānu* (and) mix (it) with oil. You pour (it) via a bronze straw into his urethra. Then you mix (it) with oil and beer. If you have him drink (it) (on an empty stomach),[51] he should recover.[52]

(iv 13–14) If a person's testicle is sore,[53] you dry (and) grind a scorpion. If you have him drink (it mixed) with beer, he should recover.

(iv 15–19) If a person ⸢has a burning sensation⸣ in one testicle,[54] you put a live scorpion ⸢into⸣ a *kallu*-bowl which you have filled with oil. You bury (it) for fourteen days in a copper *kannu*-vessel. You take (it) out and then[55] you mix in an *anduḫalatu*-lizard which you have dried (and) ground. You rub his loins and inguinal region gently (with it) and, if you have him drink what is left over, he should recover.

(iv 20–21) If two, you char (and) grind a steppe-dwelling *ṣurāru*-lizard. You rub him gently (with it mixed) with oil and if you have him drink (it mixed) with beer, he should recover.

(iv 22–23) If three, you capture a live *girītu*-fish. He urinates into its mouth and if he releases it into the river, he should recover.

(iv 24–25) If four, you boil a red *kallāt* Shamash-insect (and) an *anduḫal-atu*-lizard from the field in milk and ⸢wine⸣. If you have him drink (it), he should recover.

(iv 26–27) If five, you boil a thin *iararu*-insect from the field in oil(?). If you have him drink (it), he should recover.

2. PRIAPISM

TEXT 3: BAM 159 i 1–20

BAM 159 i 1–20 consists of a hot wash (i 1–8) for an uncertain illness, the potion for trauma (i 9–11) which we have already seen and two potions (i 12–20) for priapism. The second reference is possibly a case of acute bacterial prostatitis. For the rest of this text, see chapters 5, 9, and 11.

i

1. [...] a ${}^{\text{GIŠ}}$*šu-nim*
2. [...]${}^{\text{ŠEM}}$ŠEŠ Ú.BABBAR
3. [...] NUMUN ${}^{⸢\text{Ú}⸣}$[... ${}^{\text{Ú}}$*eli*]-⸢*kul*⸣-*la* ${}^{\text{Ú}}$*tar-muš*$_8$
4. NUMUN ${}^{\text{Ú}}$*úr-né-e* NUMUN ${}^{\text{GIŠ}}$GEŠTIN.KA$_5$.A NA$_4$ *ga-bi-i*
5. NAGA.SI SUḪUŠ ${}^{\text{GIŠ}}$NAM.TAR NÍTA ${}^{\text{NA}_4}$PEŠ$_4$.ANŠE
6. [...]x 12 Ú.ḪI.A ŠEŠ [*m*]*al-ma-liš tú-šam-ṣa*
7. ÀR-*en* SIM *ina* Ì+GIŠ *ḫal-ṣi* ŠEG$_6$-*šal baḫ-ru-su*
8. *ina* MUD ⸢URUDU⸣ *ana* GÌŠ-*šú* DUB-*ak-ma* TI

---

9. DIŠ NA *ina* GÌŠ-*šu* MÚD *ú-tab-ba-ka* GIN$_7$ MUNUS ${}^{\text{GIŠ}}$TUKUL *ma-ḫi-iṣ*
10. *ana* [T]I-*šú* ⸢GÚ⸣.GAL[56] ${}^{\text{Ú}}$NU.LUḪ.ḪA NAGA.SI 1-*niš* SÚD

11. [(*ina* KAŠ ^{LÚ}KÚRUN.NA)] *ina* UL *tuš-bat ina še-rim* NU *pa-tan* NAG-*ma* TI

---

12. 5 GÍN ^{ŠEM}[(Š)]EŠ 5 GÍN NA$_4$ *ga-bi-i*
13. 5 GÍN NAGA.SI 5 GÍN KA.A.AB.BA 5 GÍN GÚ.TUR
14. 5 Ú *ma-gal* ZI.MEŠ *lu* [(*ina*)] GEŠTIN *lu ina* KAŠ NAG

---

15. DIŠ NA *ša-a-ši-tu-na un-nu-*⸢*ut*⸣ *u ma-gal* ZI.MEŠ
16. B[(Ú)]N-*šú ḫe-sa-at* NA BI UD.DA SÁ.SÁ
17. *ana* TI-*šú* NUMUN ^{Ú}EME.UR.GI$_7$ NUMUN ^{GIŠ}*bi-ni*
18. NUMUN ^{Ú}GÍR.LAGAB ŠEM.ḪI.A ^{ŠEM}ŠEŠ 1-*niš* SÚD
19. *lu ina* GEŠTIN *lu ina* GA *lu ina* KAŠ SAG
20. NU *ú-sa-dir ina* U$_4$.3.KÁM U$_4$.1.KÁM NAG

TRANSLATION

(i 1–8) You take these twelve plants in equal proportions: [...], *šunû*-chaste-tree, [...], myrrh, "white plant," [...], [...] seed, ⸢*elikulla*⸣, *tarmuš*, *urnû*-mint seed, "fox grape" seed, alum, *uḫḫūlu qarnānu*, male *pillû* root, *biṣṣur atāne*-shell (and) [...]. You mill grind (and) sift (it). You boil (it) in pressed-out oil. If you pour (it) while still hot into his penis via a copper tube, he should recover.

(i 9–11) If a person pours blood from his penis like a (menstruating) woman, he was wounded with a weapon, [57] (to cure him), you grind together *ḫallūru*-chick peas,[58] *nuḫurtu* (and) *uḫḫūlu qarnānu*. You decoct (it)[59] in beer (and) leave (it) out overnight under the stars. If you have him drink (it) on an empty stomach, he should recover.

(i 12–14) 5 shekels of myrrh, 5 shekels of alum, 5 shekels of *uḫḫūlu qarnānu*, 5 shekels of *imbû tamtim*, (and) 5 shekels of *kakku*-lentils (are) five plants for cases where a person continually has a great erection. You have him drink (it mixed) either with wine or with beer.

(i 15–20) If a person is compressed with regard to the *šašitūna* and he continually has an erection (and) his urethra is pressured (and) that person has been "gotten" by *ṣētu*, to cure him, you grind together *lišān kalbi* seed, *bīnu*-tamarisk seed, *dadānu* seed, *labanātu*-incense, (and) myrrh. You have him drink (it mixed) either with wine or with milk or with first-quality beer. He should not do this for two days in a row but one day in every three.

3. IMPOTENCE

Men's answer to the female curse of barenness, impotence has many potential causes, some of them purely psychiatric. The ancient physician had many rituals to deal with this last aspect of the problem. For an example, see below, chapter 16, text 8. For more on impotence, see Scurlock and Andersen 2005, 111–13.

TEXT 4: BAM 272

BAM 272 consists of aliments (0′–6′, 20′–23′), a ritual (0′–6′), potions (0′–23′) and a salve (12′–14′) for impotence. Of interest is the masculinity ritual of lines 0′–6′, which requires the manufacture of a miniature cupid's bow using a needle and rodent tendon and knocking it with a reed arrow. However silly these treatments may sound, the blood and ox slaver possibly and the horse urine definitely will have contained testosterone. Note that estrogen was first synthesized from mares' urine. So we are dealing essentially with hormone enhancement therapy.

0′–1′. [(DIŠ KI.MIN ^{Ú}*úr-na-a šá* KUR-*e* ^{Ú}*imḫur-lim* ^{Ú}*imḫur*)-*ešra* (^{Ú}*ṣa-ṣu-um-tú* PI.TI SU.DIN.MUŠEN GURUN $^{\text{GIŠ.Ú}}$G)ÍR.LAGAB (^{GIŠ}ḪAŠḪUR ^{GIŠ}GI 7 Ú.MEŠ ŠEŠ-*tim* 1-*niš* SÚD)]

2′. [(MÚD MUŠEN *ḫur-ri*)] NÍTA! *ana* Š[(À *tu-maš*!-*šar*)]

3′. [(ŠÀ BURU$_5$.ḪABRUD.DA^{MUŠEN})] *i-*ʾ*a-*[(*lut ina* KAŠ SAG)]

4′. [(NU *pa-tan* NAG)]-*šú* ^{GIŠ}BAN *šá* GISSU^{60} [(DÙ-*u*)]*š*

5′. [(SA PÉŠ.ÙR.R)]A *ma-ta-an-ša* G[I (DIRI-*ši*)]

6′. [(*ina* SAG NÍT)]A *u* ⸢MUNUS⸣ *šá ṣa-lu* GAR-[*a*]*n*-[*ma* SILIM-*im*]

7′. [U$_4$-*ma* ANŠ]E.KUR.RA NÍTA KÀŠ.MEŠ-*šú ina* KASKAL-*ni*

8′. [*iš-t*]*i-nu si-ḫi-ir mi-*⸢*du*⸣*-u*ʾ*-*⸢*ri*⸣

9′. [KÀŠ.M]EŠ-*šú* TI-*qí ina* KAŠ ḪE.‹ḪE› NU *pa-tan* [N]AG-*m*[*a* KI.MIN]

10′. [DIŠ KI.MIN] *šá-rat ra-pal-te šá* GUD.NÍTA GI$_6$ ta x x [...]

11′. [o o *t*]*u-bal* SÚD *lu ina* KAŠ *lu ina* GEŠTIN.SUR NU *pa-*⸢*tan*⸣ [NAG-*ma* KI.MIN]

12′. [DIŠ KI.MIN] MÚD UDU.MÁŠ *ina* ^{DUG}⸢BUR⸣.ZI NU AL.ŠEG$_6$.GÁ *ta-ma*[*ḫ-ḫar*]

13′. [*mi-iš-l*]*a ina* Ì.GIŠ ḪE.ḪE ⸢LI⸣.DUR-*ka* GÌŠ-*ka* ŠÉŠ!-*áš*!

14′. [*ù m*]*i-iš-la-ma ina* A.MEŠ ⸢GAZ⸣ NA[G-*ma* KI.MIN]

15′. [(*ana* ŠÀ.ZI.GA TUK)]U AL.TI.⸢RÍ.G⸣[A^{MUŠ}]^{EN} DIB-*bat t*[*a-ba-qa-an*]

16′. [(MÚD.MEŠ NU *t*)]⸢*u-še-ṣa*⸣*-a tu-bal* SÚD KI ZÍD.ŠE.SA.[A ḪE.ḪE NAG-*ma* KI.MIN]

17′. [(*ana* ŠÀ.⸢ZI.GA⸣ TUK)]U BURU$_5$.⸢ḪABRUD⸣^{MUŠEN} NÍTA *šá ana* U$_5$ [ZI-*ú* DIB-*bat* (⸢*kap*⸣-*pí*)]

18′. [(*ta-ba-q*)]*a*-[(*a*)]*n* MÚD.MEŠ [(NU *t*)*u-še-ṣa-a*]

19′. [(*tu*!-*bal* SÚD)] *ina* KAŠ.SAG NU *p*[(*a*)-*tan* NAG-*ma* KI.MIN]

20′. [(DIŠ NA *ni-iš* ŠÀ-*šú e-ṭir-ma ni-iš* ŠÀ-*bi* NU TUKU-*ši*[61] 7 P)]A.MEŠ $^{\text{GIŠ.Ú}}$[(GÍR *ina* A^{MEŠ} ŠUB-*di* MÚD BURU$_5$.ḪABRUD.RU.D)A (NITA)]

21′. [(*ana* ⸢ŠÀ A⸣.MEŠ ŠUB-*ma* ŠÀ BURU$_5$.ḪABRUD.RU.DA NÍTA *i-al-lu-ut ru-pu-uš-ti* GU$_4$ TI-*qí ana* A.ME *ta-nam-di*)]

22′. [(*ina* UL *tuš-bat iš-tu* ^{d}UTU *it-tap*)]-*ḫa ina* UG[(U PA.MEŠ $^{\text{GIŠ.Ú}}$GÍR GUB-*su-ma*)]

23′. [(*ana* IGI ^{d}UTU NAG-*ma* ŠÀ.ZI.GA)][62]

Translation

(0–6′) Alternatively, you grind together these seven plants: wild *urnû*-mint, *imḫur-lim*, *imḫur*-[*ešra*], *ṣaṣumtu*, a bat's PI.TI, the fruit of a *dadānu*-tree (and) "swamp apple." You let *ḫurri*-bird blood fall into it. He should swallow the heart of the *ḫurri*-bird. You have him drink (it) on an empty stomach, (mixed) with first-quality beer. You make a (miniature) bow from a spear point or needle.[63] You use a *arrabu*-rodent tendon as its bowstring. You nock it with a ⸢reed⸣ (arrow). [If] you place (it) at the head of the man and woman while they are sleeping, [things should go back to normal].

(7′–9′) [When] a male horse urinates in the road, you take all of the crystalized residue of his ⸢urine⸣,[64] mix it with beer and if you have him drink (it) on an empty stomach, [ditto (he should be able to get an erection)].

(10′–11′) [Alternatively], you [...], dry (and) grind hair from the loins of a black bull. [If you have him drink] (it mixed) either with beer or drawn wine on an empty stomach, [ditto (he should be able to get an erection)].

(12′–14′) [Alternatively], you ⸢collect⸣ the blood of an adult male goat in an unbaked *pursītu*-vessel. You mix ⸢half⸣ (of it) with oil (and) anoint your navel (and) your penis (with it) [and] (the other) ⸢half⸣ you crush in water [and if] you ⸢drink⸣ (it) [ditto (you should be able to get an erection)].

(15′–16′) In order to have the ability to get an erection, you capture a *diqdiqqu*-bird. [You pluck (it)] but do not bleed (it). You dry, grind, (and) [mix (it)] with roasted grain flour. [If you have him drink it, ditto (he should be able to get an erection)].

(17′–19′) In order to have the ability to get an erection, [you capture] a male *ḫurri*-bird which [has an erection] for copulation. You pluck (its) wings but do not ⌜bleed⌝ (it). You dry (and) grind (it and) [if you have him drink (it)] on an empty stomach (mixed) with first-quality beer, [he should be able to get an erection].

(20′–23′) If a person's ability to get an erection is taken away so that he does not have (it), you pour seven *ašāgu*-thorn leaves/branches into water. You pour the blood of a male *ḫurri*-bird into the water and he should swallow the heart of the male *ḫurri*-bird. You take ox slaver (and) pour (it) into the water. You let (it) sit out overnight under the stars. After the sun has risen, you have him stand on the *ašāgu*-thorn leaves/branches and, if you have him drink (it) before Shamash, he should be able to get an erection.

4. SEXUALLY TRANSMITTED DISEASES

STDs were as common in ancient Mesopotamia as anywhere else. The physician had to be prepared to treat urethritis, vaginitis, and skin lesions of venereal origin. Unlike his Hippocratic counterpart, the *āšipu* was prepared to believe that person-to-person transmission via venereal contact was the source of the "wind blasting" that he was treating. For more on this subject, see Scurlock and Andersen 2005, chapter 4.

TEXT 5: BAM 580 iii 15′–25′

BAM 580 is interesting in that it appears to differentiate between chancroid and syphilitic ulcers. For more, see Scurlock and Andersen 2005, 94–97. The general approach, used also for nonsuppurating ulcers, was to cut or scrape the surface of the ulcer with a sharp, freshly broken flint blade and then to daub on (iii 15′–25′) the medicine and bandage it over.

iii

15′. DIŠ GIG MIN (= *ina* SU NA È) *ul-la-nu-ma ḫa-ri-is* ŠÀ-*ba-šu* KAK.MEŠ DIRI KAK.MEŠ-*šú* IDIM/BAD K[ÚM]

16′. *u* DU-*ak lam-ṣa-at ḫi-la-a-ti* NÍTA MU.NI IM *iš-biṭ-su-ma si-ḫi-*[*ip-ti*]

17′. ^{d}PA.BIL.SAG DUG$_4$.GA GAR-*an ana* ZI-*šú* GIG *ša-tu ina na-ag-la-pi te-né-*[*eṣ-ṣi*]

18′. ^{NA_4}GUG ^{NA_4}ZA.GÌN MUNUS *saḫ-lé-e* GAZI^{SAR} *qa-lu-te* IM.GÚ NÍG.NÍGIN.NA ÚḪ-^{d}[ÍD]

19′. IM.BABBAR *ba-áš-lu* SAḪAR UDUN ^{Ú}*di-ša* 9 Ú$^{ḪI.A}$ ŠEŠ 1-*niš* GAZ *ana* IGI GIG MAR LÁL-*s*[*u*]

20′. DIŠ GIG MIN *ul* GU$_7$-*šú* IGI UZU.MEŠ-*šú-ma* GAR-*in* MÚD-*šú-ma* MÚD.[BABBAR]

21′. *šur-du-ma* DU-*ak lam-ṣa-at ḫi-la-a-te* MUNUS MU.NI IM *iš-*[*biṭ-su*]

22′. *si-ḫi-ip-ti* ^{d}MAŠ.TAB.BA *qí-ba* GAR-*an ana* ZI-*šú* GIG *ša-tu*

23′. *tu-na-kap-šu* IM.BABBAR *ba-aš-la* SAḪAR UDUN GAZ SIM ^{NA_4}PEŠ$_4$.Í[D.DA]

24′. *tur-ár* SÚD *ana* IGI GIG MAR LAL-*su šum$_4$-ma ina* ŠÀ GÌR.PAD.D[U …]

25′. BAD-*te ta-sar-ri-im tu-še-lam-ma ana* [IGI GIG MAR]

TRANSLATION

(iii 15′–17′) If a sore ditto (comes out on a person's body), it has been itching for a long time, the inside of it is full of *sikkatu* (peg-shaped lesions), it encloses its *sikkatu*, it is hot and it flows, it is called a male suppurating *lamṣātu*-lesion.[65] If "wind" has "blasted" him, ⸢overwhelming⸣ by Pabilsag; you may make a (favorable) prognosis. To cure him, you ⸢make an incision⸣ in the sore with a knife. You crush together these nine plants: carnelian, "female"/delicate lapis lazuli, *saḫlû*-cress,[66] roasted *kasû*, riverbank silt, ⸢*ru'tītu*⸣-sulphur, cooked *gaṣṣu*-gypsum, "dust" from an oven (and) *dīšu*. You daub (it) on the surface of the sore (and) bandage him.

(iii 20′–25′) If a sore (comes out on a person's body), it does not hurt him, it is placed only on the surface of his flesh (and) its blood (and) pus flows freely, it is called a female suppurating *lamṣātu*-ulcer.[67] If "wind" has ⸢"blasted" him⸣, overwhelming by the twin gods; you may make a (favorable) prognosis. To remove it, you prick that sore. You crush (and) sift cooked *gaṣṣu*-gypsum (and) "dust" from an oven. You char (and) grind ⸢*išqillatu*⸣-shell. You daub (it) on the surface of the sore (and) bandage him. If it [has entered] into the bone, you cut (the bone) open. You bring up (the pus) and then [you daub the surface of the sore].

NOTES

1. These symptoms appear also in BAM 111 ii 15′–16′//BAM 159 i 15.

2. The use of ŠÈ as a pseudo-ideogram for *ana* is idiosyncratic, to say the least but see also ii 10′.

3. Instead of ŠÈ *muštinnisu* *AMT* 66/7 iii 20 has *ana* GÌŠ-*šú*.

4. *AMT* 66/7 iii 20–22 replaces BAM 396 i 30–31 with: 1/2-*tú* KAŠ.SAG ŠUB-*di* 1 *šu-ši* *ina* Ì.GIŠ *ḫal-ṣi u* KAŠ NU *pa-tan* NAG [2 *šu-ši ina* GEŠTIN KALA]G.GA ḪE.ḪE *e-nu-ma* TAG-*šú* NU *pa-tan* [NAG-*ma* TI].

5. BAM 111 iii 17 has: NU KÙ.BI NU TAG.GA̱.

6. *AMT* 66/11+65/6+Sm 126+K 11230:18′ has ^{ŠEM}BULUḪ.

7. *AMT* 66/11+65/6+Sm 126+K 11230:19′ has ^{Ú}GÍR.LAGAB.

8. Collated by Geller.

9. BAM 111 iii 12′ and *AMT* 66/11+65/6+Sm 126+K 11230:21′ substitute *ana* GÌŠ-*šú*.

10. BAM 111 iii 13′–14′ and *AMT* 66/11+65/6+Sm 126+K 11230:22′ have: E$_{11}$-*šú* UŠ MUNU$_{6}$ DUL-*šú*.

11. Geller thought he saw NÍG.BÙR.BÙR on the tablet but Köcher's copy indicates traces of a ŠÉŠ which makes much better sense in the context.

12. Collation by Geller.

13. Collated by Geller.

14. Erle Leichty and Grant Frame kindly collated this line for me on the original tablet in Philadelphia and report that "NAG is better than BÚN, but the sign is not perfectly clear. We also both think *ina* ITU.1-*at-tu* is the best—we both think the first vertical (the one of the ITU) is actually two wedges, one on top of the other."

15. *AMT* 34/3:1–2 has [^{Ú}ÚKUŠ.T]I.GI.LA.

16. *AMT* 34/3:3–4 has [*l*]*a-am* GÌR-*šú ana* KI GAR-*nu*!

17. Collated by Geller.

18. *AMT* 34/3:6 has KI *la* [GAR-*nu*].

19. BAM 115:8′ has *mal-ma-liš*.

20. BAM 115:8′ has KAŠ SAG apparently instead of Ì.GIŠ *u* Ì.GIŠ BÁRA.GA.

21. Collation by Geller.

22. Geller adds a line before Köcher's line 1′ which consist of the fragments of the fifteenth potion.

23. See Scurlock and Andersen 2005, 5.20, 5.54.

24. *AMT* 66/7 has: "into his penis."

25. *AMT* 66/7 has a more complicated instruction for the potion: You pour the other half into first-quality beer. You have him drink one sixth with pressed-out oil and beer on an empty stomach. You mix [the other two sixths] with ⸢strong⸣ [wine] (and) when it hurts him intensely, [if you have him drink (it)] on an empty stomach, [he should recover].

26. BAM 111 iii 17 has: "which an impure person has not touched."

27. *AMT* 66/11+65/6+Sm 126+K 11230:19 has *baluḫḫu*-aromatic.

28. *AMT* 66/11+65/6+Sm 126+K 11230:20 has *dadānu*-thorn.

29. BAM 111 iii 12′ and *AMT* 66/11+65/6+Sm 126+K 11230:22 have "penis."

30. BAM 111 iii 13′–14′ and *AMT* 66/11+65/6+Sm 126+K 11230:23 have "You have him come out (and) cover him with malt UŠ (perhaps a hearing error for IŠ/SAḪAR)."

31. See Scurlock and Andersen 2005, 5.23, 5.50.

32. Alternatively, one could read the end of ii 27′ as *ma-li*(!) *a-ḫ*[*e-e*] and translate: "You have him drink (it) once a month. You should not leave as much as a half portion overnight in

his urethra." Suggestion courtesy M. Stol.

33. *AMT* 34/3:1–2 has ⌈*tigilû*⌉ and it is ground.
34. *AMT* 34/3:3–4 has: "before he puts his foot to the ground (in the morning)."
35. *AMT* 34/3:6 has: "[it is] not [to be put] on the ground
36. BAM 115: 8′ has: "in equal quantities."
37. BAM 115: 8′ has: "first-quality beer" instead of the oil.
38. BAM 159 i 9–11//BAM 182:6′ have GÚ.GAL.
39. BAM 182: 6′ has KAŠ ^{LÚ}KÚRUN.NA.
40. *AMT* 61/1:5′ adds SIG-*ta*. This is neither *sīkta* or *šiqta* since both "powder" and "scales" are, by definition bone dry, hardly possible in this context.
41. *AMT* 61/1:6′ adds SÚD.
42. *AMT* 61/1:7′ adds NU *pa-tan*.
43. *AMT* 61/1:8′ adds ⌈Ú⌉.ḪI.A RA-*su-ma* [TI].
44. After a suggestion of Geller, BAM VII p. 40.
45. See Scurlock and Andersen 2005, 5.17, 14.23.
46. So BAM 159 i 9–11//BAM 182:6′.
47. BAM 182:6′ has: "*kurunnu* beer."
48. So *AMT* 61/1:5′.
49. See Scurlock and Andersen 2005, 4.20.
50. So *AMT* 61/1:6′.
51. So *AMT* 61/1:7′.
52. *AMT* 61/1: 8′ also recommends using the plants as a medicinal bath.
53. See Scurlock and Andersen 2005, 5.77.
54. See Scurlock and Andersen 2005, 5.80.
55. The scribe had the patient drinking the scorpion (mixed with) beer and then realized that he had forgotten to put in part of the procedure and erased the phrase.
56. BAM 396 iv 4 substitutes GÚ.NÍG.ÀR.RA.
57. See Scurlock and Andersen 2005, 5.17, 14.23.
58. BAM 396 iv 4 substitutes *kiššēnu*-bean.
59. See chapter 3, n. 109.
60. *AMT* 73/2:7 has ^{GIŠ}IGI.DÙ.
61. So *KAR* 70 obv. 22-27 (Biggs 1967, 53; cf. Schwemer 2011, 121). BAM 272: 20′ probably had simply *ana* ŠÀ.ZI.GA TUKU as in *LKA* 99d ii 11.
62. See also KUB 4.48 iii 1–6 (Biggs 1967, 55).
63. *AMT* 73/2:7 has "spear point."
64. Testosterone was first synthesized from human urine.
65. See Scurlock and Andersen 2005, 4.32.
66. For the translation of *saḫlû* as "cress," see Stol 1983–84, 24–32.
67. See Scurlock and Andersen 2005, 4.25.

11

NEUROLOGY

Neurology occupies its own section of the Diagnostic Series (tablets 26–30), suggesting that it was a subspecialty of the *ašipu*'s craft. Ancient physicians describe grand mal seizures, petit mal seizures, simple partial seizures, and complex partial seizures, as well as the more unusual sensory seizures and gelastic seizures. In addition, they were aware of what we call status epilepticus and phases of seizures including the post-ictal state, narcolepsy, cataplexy, stroke, and coma. They also distinguished between various grades ("hurting," "afflicting," "touching") and qualities ("squeezing," "pounding," "burning," "gnawing," "jabbing," "stinging," "needling") of pain, described numbness and paralysis (distinguishing between flaccid and spastic) and abnormal movement (including what are probably resting and intention tremors and pendular and jerking nystagmus). Ancient physicians were careful observers and, since neurology is one of the few specialties in modern medicine that is still largely clinical, their observations are exceptionally accessible to us today. For more on this subject, see Scurlock and Andersen 2005, chapter 13.

A. HEADACHES

The ancient physician distinguished between mild headaches, attributed to the *mukīl rēš lemutti* and severe headaches, caused by ghosts. They have left us very nice descriptions of tension headaches and migraine. For details, see Scurlock and Andersen 2005, 311–14 and Scurlock 2008, 195–202.

TEXT 1: BAM 11 (= *KAR* 188)

BAM 11 consists of "eighteen treatments for headache," specifically shaved head bandages (1–15,19–24, 30–35) and amulets (16–18, 25–27). Noticeable is the frequent use in these bandages of flours, beerwort, and sesame residue and the fact that many of the bandages went on wet (in leather to prevent seepage) and/or hot. Amulets were bound on the temples, which would have applied external pressure. The red wool used in amulets symbolized the blood vessels.

In other texts, headaches are also treated with fumigants, salves, potions, and enemas.

1. DIŠ LÚ SAG.KI.DIB.BA TUKU.TUKU NUMUN ÚKUŠ.GÍL NUMUN ÚKUŠ.TI.GI.⸢IL⸣ NUMUN ^{Ú}EME.UR.GI$_7$ NUMUN ^{Ú}*e-di*
2. NUMUN ^{GIŠ}KIRI$_6$[1] NUMUN *kiš-ša-ni* TÉŠ.BI GAZ SIM *ma-al-ma-liš* ḪE.ḪE *i+na* A.GEŠTIN.NA *tara-bak*
3. ZÍD ŠE.SA.A ZÍD ZÍZ.AN.NA *a-na pa-ni ta-ša-ba-aḫ i+na* KUŠ *te-ṭer-ri* SAG.DU-*su tu-gal-lab* LAL-*ma* TI.LA

---

4. DIŠ KI.MIN ^{GIŠ}ERIN ^{GIŠ}ŠUR.MÌN ^{GIŠ}ŠEM.GÍR GI.DÙG.GA ^{ŠEM}LI ^{ŠEM}KU$_7$.KU$_7$ ^{ŠEM}*šu-pu-uḫ*-[(*ru*)]
5. ^{ŠEM}MUG ŠEM.SAL ^{ŠEM}IM.DU ^{ŠEM}ḪAB ILLU *ba-lu-ḫi* TÉŠ.BI GAZ [SIM]
6. *i+na* GEŠTIN.SUR.RA *ta-rab-bak* ZÍD ŠE.SA.A ZÍD ZÍZ.AN.NA *ana* IGI *ta-ša-ba-aḫ* [KI.MIN]

---

7. DIŠ KI.MIN NUMUN ^{GIŠ}ÍLDAG ^{Ú}*ak-tam* NUMUN ÁB.DUḪ ^{Ú}*am-ḫa-ra* GAZI^{SAR} NUMUN ^{GIŠ}[(ḪAB ^{Ú}LAG A.ŠÀ 1-*niš*) GAZ SIM]
8. *i+na* GEŠTIN.SUR.RA *ta-rab-ba-ak* [KI.MIN]

---

9. DIŠ KI.MIN ^{Ú}ḪAR.ḪAR ^{Ú}KUR.KUR ^{Ú}*ak-tam* NUMUN ÁB.DUḪ ZÍD GIG KAŠ.Ú.SA S[(IG$_5$ ^{ŠE})^{M}... (*ina* KAŠ *tara-bak* LAL-*ma* TI)]

---

10. DIŠ KI.MIN ^{ŠEM}KU$_7$.KU$_7$ ^{ŠEM}LI ŠEM.^{d}NIN.IB ZÍD GIG [(KAŠ.Ú.SA 1-*niš* GAZ SIM)]
11. *i+na* KAŠ SAG *ta-la-aš tu-ba-ʾa-a-rù* SAG.D[(U-*su* SAR-*ab* LÁL-*ma*) TI]

---

12. DIŠ KI.MIN ^{ŠEM}KU$_7$.KU$_7$ ^{ŠEM}LI ŠEM.^{d}NIN.IB N[(UMUN ^{Ú}ÁB.DUḪ KA.A.AB.BA)]
13. ^{ŠEM}MUG TÉŠ.BI GAZ SIM *i+na* KAŠ [(*tara-bak* SAG.DU-*su* SAR-*ab* LAL-*ma* TI)]

---

14. DIŠ KI.MIN PA ^{GIŠ}GIŠIMMAR *ša i+na-zu-zu* ŠU.TI ‹(*ina* UD.DA)› *t*[*u-bal* (GA)Z S(IM)]
15. *i+na* A GAZI^{SAR} *ta-la-aš* LA[(L)]

---

16. DIŠ LÚ ZI-*ib* SAG.KI TUKU PA! ^{GIŠ}⸢GIŠIMMAR⸣ [...]

17. *i+na* SÍG.ḪÉ.ME.DA *tara-kas* [...]

---

18. DIŠ KI.MIN SA MAŠ.DÀ SÍG.ḪÉ.ME.DA ^{SAL}*pa-ri*[(*š-tú* NU.NU) $^{NA(_4}$ZA.GÌN ^{NA_4}ZÚ GI_6 È *i+na* SAG.KI^{II}-*šú* KEŠDA)]

---

19. *ana* ZI-*ib* SA SAG.KI *nu-uḫ-ḫi* DUḪ ŠE.[(GIŠ.Ì SUMUN.MEŠ ^{ŠEM}GÚR.GÚR ^{ŠEM}ḪAB ^{ŠEM}BULUḪ GAZI^{SAR} *ta-pa-aṣ*)]
20. *i+na* ZÌ.KUM KAŠ.Ú.SA ‹(SIG_5)› *ù* KAŠ SA[G (ŠEG$_6$-*šal tara-bak* LAL)]

---

21. DIŠ LÚ GIDIM$_4$ DIB-*su-ma* SAG.KI.DIB.BA TUKU.TUKU x[...]
22. *tu-ba-aḫ-ḫa-ar ba-aḫ-ru-su* [...]

---

23. DIŠ LÚ GIDIM$_4$ DIB-*su-ma* SAG.KI.DIB.BA TUKU.TUKU ^{GIŠ}GEŠ[TIN.KA$_5$.A? ...]
24. *i+na* A GAZI^{SAR} *ta-la-aš* [LAL]

---

25. DIŠ KI.MIN Ì SUMUN *ša* ^{GIŠ}IG KÁ.GAL *i+na* È-*ka ana* ZAG-*k*[*a* GUB-*zu* TI-*qí*]
26. GI_6 U_4 BI DUR NU.NU *i+na* ^{SÍG}ÀKA NIGIN-*m*[*a i-na* SAG.KI-*šú* KEŠDA]

---

27. DIŠ KI.MIN SUḪUŠ ^{GIŠ}DÌḪ NIGIN-*ma ta-na-saḫ* SÍG.ḪÉ.ME.DA NU.NU [...]

---

28. DIŠ KI.MIN LAG A.ŠÀ.GA ^{GIŠ}ZA.BA.LAM ZÍD ŠE.SA.A DUḪ ŠE.GIŠ.Ì [...]
29. ^{ŠEM}LI TÉŠ.BI GAZ SIM 1/3 SÌLA.TA.ÀM *i+na* KAŠ.SAG x[...]

---

30. DIŠ LÚ ZI-*ib* SAG.KI TUKU *ù* SU!-*šú* GU$_7$-*šú* ^{GIŠ}PA MES.MÁ.GAN.NA ḪÁD.DU G[AZ SIM ZÍD GÚ.GAL]
31. ZÍD GÚ.TUR ZÍD ^{ŠE}IN.NU.ḪA *i+na šur-šum-mi* KAŠ.SAG LAL.LAL-*su-ma* T[I.LA]

---

32. DIŠ LÚ ZI-*ib* SAG.KI TUKU *ù ri-mu-tú* TUKU PA ^{GIŠ}ŠE.DÙ.A ḪÁD.DU GAZ SIM Z[(ÍD ŠE.MUŠ$_5$)]
33. *saḫ-lé-e ṭe*$_4$-*ne-e-ti* ZÍD ŠE.SA.A TÉŠ.BI ḪE.ḪE *i+na* A GAZI^{SAR} *tara-bak* LAL.L[(AL-*ma* TI)]

---

34. DIŠ LÚ ZI-*ib* SAG.KI TUKU *ù šim-ma-tú* TUKU [GIŠ]PA MA.NU ḪÁD.DU *ta-sàk* ZÍD GI([G)]

35. *saḫ-lé-e* [Ú]ḪAR.ḪAR *i+na* KAŠ [LÚ]KÚRUN.NA *ta-rab-bak* LAL.LAL-*su-ma* TI.LA

---

36. 18 *bu-ul-ṭú ša* SAG.KI.DIB.BA (label as part of the colohon)

TRANSLATION

(1–3) If a person continually has a headache,[2] you crush together (and) sift *irrû* seed, *tigilû* seed, *lišān kalbi* seed, "lone plant" seed, seed of garden plants/cultivated(?) flax,[3] (and) *kiššēnu* seed. You mix (them) in equal quantities. You decoct (it)[4] in vinegar. You scatter roasted grain flour (and) emmer flour on it. You massage (it) into leather. You shave his head. If you bandage (him with it), he should recover.

(4–6) Alternatively, you crush together (and) sift *erēnu*-cedar, *šurmēnu*-cypress, *asu*-myrtle, "sweet reed," *burāšu*-juniper, *kukru*, *šupuḫru*-cedar, *ballukku*-aromatic, *šimeššalû*-tree, *suādu*, *ṭūru*-aromatic, (and) *baluḫḫu*-aromatic resin. You decoct (it) in drawn wine. You scatter roasted grain flour (and) emmer flour on it. You massage (it) into leather. [Ditto (You shave his head. If you bandage (him with it), he should recover)].

(7–8) Alternatively, [you crush] together [and sift] *adaru*-poplar seed, *aktam*, *kamantu*-henna(?), *amḫāru*, *kasû*, *ḫurātu* seed, (and) *kirbān eqli*. You decoct (it) in drawn wine. [Ditto (You scatter roasted grain flour and emmer flour on it. You massage (it) into leather. You shave his head. If you bandage (him with it), he should recover)].

(9) Alternatively, you decoct *ḫašû*-thyme, *atā᾽išu*, *aktam*, *kamantu*-henna(?), wheat flour, winnowed beerwort, (and) [...]-aromatic in beer. If you bandage (him with it), he should recover.

(10–11) Alternatively, you crush together (and) sift *kukru*, *burāšu*-juniper, *nikiptu*, wheat flour, (and) beerwort. You make (it) into a dough with first-quality beer. You heat (it). You shave his head. If you bandage (him with it), [he should recover].

(12–13) Alternatively, you crush together (and) sift *kukru*, *burāšu*-juniper, *nikiptu*, *kamantu*-henna(?), *imbû tamtim*, (and) *ballukku*-aromatic. You decoct (it) in beer. You shave his head. If you bandage (him with it), he should recover.

(14–15) Alternatively, you take a palm frond which sways (without any wind). You ‹(sun)› dry, ⸢crush (and) sift (it)⸣. You make (it) into a dough with *kasû* juice. You bandage (him with it).

(16–17) If a person experiences pulsation of the temples,[5] [you take] a palm frond [...]. You bind (it) on him with red-dyed wool. [...]

(18) Alternatively, you thread red-dyed wool which a post-menopausal woman has spun with [...], lapis and black obsidian. You bind (it) on his temples.

(19–20) To calm pulsating temporal blood vessels,[6] you pulverize old sesame residue, *kukru*, *ṭūru*-aromatic, *baluḫḫu*-aromatic (and) *kasû*. You boil (and) decoct (it) in *isqūqu*-flour, ‹(winnowed)› beerwort and first-quality beer (and) bandage (him with it).

(21–22) If a ghost afflicts a person so that he continually has a headache,[7] you [...]. You heat (it) up. [You bandage (him with it)] while it is still hot.

(23–24) If a ghost afflicts a person so that he continually has a headache, you [... "fox] gra[pe"? ...]. You make (it) into a dough with *kasû* juice (and) [bandage (him with it)].

(25–26) Alternatively, [you take] used grease from the door of the main gate, [(the one which) stands] on your right when you are going out. [...] (that) night (and) that day, you twine (it) together into a cord. You wrap (the grease) in a tuft of wool and [you bind (it) on his temples].

(27) Alternatively, you wrap and then uproot the root of a *baltu*-thorn. You twine (it) together with red-dyed wool [...]

(28–29) Alternatively, you crush together (and) sift *kirbān eqli*, *supālu*-wood, roasted grain flour, sesame residue, [...] (and) *burāšu*-juniper. 1/3 of a *qû*-measure each in first-quality beer [...].

(30–31) If a person experiences pulsating of the temples and his body hurts him, you ⸢crush⸣ (and) [sift] dried *musukkannu*-tree leaves. (You mix it with) [*ḫallūru*-chickpea flour], *kakku*-lentil flour, (and) *inninu*-barley flour. If you continually bandage him with (it mixed) with beer dregs, [he should recover].

(32–33) If a person experiences pulsating of the temples and *rimūtu*-paralysis, you dry, crush (and) sift *šigūšu*-flour, mill ground *saḫlû*-cress,[8] (and) roasted grain flour. You mix (them) together. You decoct (it) in *kasû* juice. If you repeatedly bandage (him with it), he should recover.

(34–35) If a person experiences pulsating of the temples and numbness, you dry (and) grind *eʾru*-tree leaves, wheat flour, *saḫlû*-cress (and) *ḫašû*-thyme. You decoct (it) in *kurunnu* beer. If you repeatedly bandage (him with it), he should recover.

(36) Eighteen treatments for headache.

B. SEIZURES

For ancient Mesopotamian descriptions of seizures, see Scurlock and Andersen 2005, 314–22. The majority of ancient Mesopotamian texts dealing with seizures mention only amulets. Since, however, these contain plant medicines, some of which (e.g., water lilies) are known to be central nervous system depressants, we may be reasonably sure that, unless aroma therapy is more effective than we think, these amulets were meant to accompany treatments by other means. The stock phrase is "in beer, in oil, in a leather bag," which would suggest administration as a potion or salve and indeed, such treatments are occasionally attested.

TEXT 2: BAM 159 iii 25–34

BAM 159 iii 25–34 contains a rare potion (iii 25–27) for seizures. What is most interesting is its bedfellows, which are grouped together because they use the same plant medicines. To note is that a heart in spasm (iii 28–29) would indeed benefit from the same types of drugs used to deal with seizures. All are formatted as pharmacist's preparations.

25. NUMUN ^{GIŠ}*bi-ni* NUMUN ^{GIŠ}MA.NU NUMUN ^{Ú}[...] NUMUN ^{Ú}*a-zal-lá*
26. ^{Ú}*tar-muš*$_8$ ^{Ú}*imḫur-lim* ^{Ú}*imḫur*-20 7 Ú
27. AN.TA.ŠUB.BA *lu ina* KAŠ *lu ina* GEŠTIN NAG

---

28. ^{Ú}*a-ra-ri-a-nu* NUMUN ^{GIŠ}*bi-ni* NUMUN ^{Ú}*a-zal-l*[(*á*)]
29. 3 Ú *ḫu-ṣa* GAZ ŠÀ-*bi* TUKU.MEŠ-*ši ina* KAŠ N[(AG)]

---

30. ^{Ú}*tar-muš*$_8$ ^{Ú}*imḫur-lim* ^{Ú}*imḫur*-20 SUḪUŠ ^{GIŠ}[(ḪAB)]
31. 4 Ú ZI.KU$_5$.RU.DA *ina* KAŠ [(NAG)]
32. ÉN ⸢*id*⸣-*di*-^{d}*É-a* [(ŠID-*nu*)][9]

---

33. NUMUN ^{GIŠ}*bi-ni* NUMUN ^{GIŠ}MA.NU [^{Ú}(ḪAR.ḪAR)]
34. 3 Ú SAG.ḪUL.ḪA.ZA [(*ina* KAŠ ⸢NAG⸣)]

Translation

(iii 25–27) *Bīnu*-tamarisk seed, *eʾru*-tree seed, [...] seed, *azallû* seed, *tarmuš*, *imḫur-lim* (and) *imḫur-ešra* are seven plants for AN.TA.ŠUB.BA. You have him drink (it mixed) either with beer or with wine.

(iii 28–29) *Arariānu*, *bīnu*-tamarisk seed (and) *azallû* seed are three plants for (cases where) he continually has a crushing sensation in the chest.[10] You have him drink (it mixed) with beer.

(iii 30–32) *Tarmuš*, *imḫur-lim*, *imḫur-ešra*, (and) *ḫurātu*-madder root are four plants for "cutting of the breath" magic. You have him drink (it mixed) with beer. You recite the recitation Iddi-^{d}Ea.[11]

(iii 33–34) *Bīnu*-tamarisk seed, *e᾿ru* seed and *ḫašû*-thyme are three plants for the *mukil rēš lemutti*-demon. You have him drink (it mixed) with beer.

C. STROKES

The fact that strokes are described in ancient Mesopotamian therapeutic texts is one more indication that a significant number of people lived into their sixties. For more on strokes, see Scurlock and Andersen 2005, 327–30.

TEXT 3: BAM 398 = BE 31.56

BAM 398 shares with BAM 396 the peculiar way of designating more than one treatment for the same condition. It consists of bandages (1–18, 22–29) and a salve (19–21) for paralysis due to a stroke. This is followed by bandages (30–36, rev. 28′–37′) and salves (rev. 4′–41′) for numbness of the limbs and baths (rev. 42′–52′), bandages (rev. 46′–52′) and salves (rev. 46′–52′) for numbness of the flesh. The former is probably peripheral neuropathy (see below). The latter sounds strange, but may be a reference to a patient with tuberculoid leprosy (chapter 7, text 3) or hypothyroidism (chapter 14, texts 4–7).

obv.

1. [(DIŠ LÚ *ši-pir mi-šit-ti šup-šu-ḫi u*)] *ri-mu-tim* ŠÀ-*šu* [...]
2. [...] ^{GIŠ}MA.NU
3. [... ^{Ú}]ÚKUŠ.GÍL ^{Ú}ḪAR.ḪAR NUMUN ^{Ú}[...] ^{Ú}⌜*si*⌝-*ḫu*
4. [^{Ú}*a*]*r-ga-an-nu-um* ^{Ú}*ba-ri-ra-tum*
5. [... ŠÀ]-*bi* Ú.ḪI.A *an-nu-ut-ti tuš*!-*te-m*[*éd*]
6. *ina* ^{DUG}ÚTUL GIN$_7$ *rib-ki tara-bak*
7. *ina* GA *u* KAŠ.SAG *tu-šab-šal* LAL.LAL-*su-ma* [TI]

---

8. DIŠ 2 NUMUN *ú-ra-an-nu-um* NUMUN ^{GIŠ}ŠE.NU ^{ŠEM}GÚR.GÚR
9. ^{ŠEM}LI ^{ŠEM}ŠE.LI *šur-šum-mi* KAŠ *la-bi-ru-t*[*i*]
10. ḪÁD.DU GAZ SIM *ina* A GAZI^{SAR} *em-mu-ti ta-la-*[(*aš*)]
11. *ina* KUŠ *te-ṭer-ri ba-aḫ-ru-us-su* ŠU.BI.DIDLI.ÀM[12]

---

12. DIŠ 3 ZAG.ḪI.LI^{SAR} *bu-tu-un-tú* KAŠ.Ú.SA SIG$_5$

13. ZÍD ŠE.SA.A ^{Ú}*ḫa-ši-i* ^{Ú}*ba-ri-ra-*[(*tú*)]
14. *ina* KAŠ.SAG *ina* ^{URUDU}ŠEN.TUR[13] *tara-bak ina* KUŠ *te-ṭer-ri*
15. ŠU.BI.DIDLI.ÀM[14]

---

16. DIŠ 4 ZAG.ḪI.LI^{SAR} ZÍD ŠE.SA.A ^{Ú}NU.LUḪ.ḪA ^{Ú}ḪAR.ḪAR PA ^{GIŠ}ŠINIG
17. ḪÁD.DU GAZ SIM *ina* KAŠ.SAG *ina* ^{URUDU}ŠEN.TUR *tara-bak*
18. ZÍD.ZÍZ *ana* IGI *ta-šá-ba-aḫ ina* KUŠ *te-ṭer-ri* ŠU.BI.DIDLI.ÀM

---

19. DIŠ 5 ZAG.ḪI.LI^{SAR} GAZI^{SAR} PA ^{GIŠ}*šu-šum* Ú.^{d}UTU
20. TÉŠ.BI *ta-sàk ana* A ŠUB-*di ina* IM.ŠU.RIN.NA *te-sek-ker*
21. GÌR^{II}-*šú tu-maš-šá-ʾ-ma ù* Ì.GIŠ ŠÉŠ-*su-ma* TI.LA

---

22. DIŠ 6 *šur-šum-mi tu-bal ta-sàk* ŠEM.^{d}NIN.IB ^{Ú}ḪAR.ḪAR
23. ^{Ú}KUR.KUR *te-ṭe-en ina* KAŠ.SAG *ina* ^{URUDU}ŠEN.TUR *tara-bak*
24. ZÍD ZÍZ *ana* IGI *ta-šá-ba-aḫ ina* KUŠ *ba-aḫ-ru-us-su* ŠU.BI.DIDLI.ÀM

---

25. DIŠ 7 ^{GIŠ}PA *šu-šum ina* A GAZI^{SAR} *ta-la-a-aš*
26. *tara-bak-ma* LAL-*su-ma* TI.LA

---

27. DIŠ 8 ^{GIŠ}ŠINIG ^{Ú}IN.UŠ ^{GIŠ}ŠÀ.GIŠIMMAR ḪÁD.DU GAZ SIM
28. ^{ŠEM}GÚR.GÚR ^{ŠEM}LI *ta-sàk* TÉŠ.BI ḪE.ḪE
29. *ina* ZÍD GIG *ù šur-šum-mi tara-bak* LAL-*su-ma* TI.LA

---

30. DIŠ LÚ *šim-ma-*[*at* GAB]A-*ri* TUKU.TUKU-*a*
31. *ana šim-ma-*[*at maḫ-ḫ*]*i-ri* ZI-[*ḫi*] *ṭú-ba-am šur-ši-i*
32. ^{Ú}*ak-tam* ^{Ú}*ḫu-up-*⸢*ši-lu*⸣*-ru-gu ina* SU.BIR$_4$^{KI}
33. GURUN ^{GIŠ}*kal-ba-n*[*u*] ^{Ú}*ṣa-ṣu-u*[*n-tú*] PA ^{GIŠ}GEŠTIN.GÍR
34. Ú.ḪI.A *an-nu-ut-ti* ḪÁD.DU GAZ SIM
35. *ù* IM.GÚ.EN.NA [… *tara-b*]*ak*
36. […] *baḫ-*[*ru-us-su* LAL-*s*]*u-ma* TI.LA

37–rev. 3′. *fragmentary*

---

rev.

4′. [ÉN] É.NU.⸢RU⸣
5′. [*ši-i*]*m-ma-tum ši-im-ma-tum*
6′. [*ši-im*]*-ma-tum šim-mat* GÍR.TAB
7′. [*ta*]*-az-qú-ti zu-qá-qí-pa-ni-iš*

8′. [*ta-am-ḫ*]*a-ṣi ina qar-ni-ki tu-šar-di-i ina si-im-ba-ti-ki*
9′. [GURUŠ] *ina su-un* KI.SIKIL *tu-še-li-i*
10′. [KI.SIKIL] *ina su-un* GURUŠ *tu-še-li-i*
11′. [*ṣi-i-i*]*m šim-ma-tum ki-ma ši-iz-bi ina tu-le-e*
12′. *ki-ma zu-ʾ-ti ina ša-ḫa-ti*
13′. *ki-ma me-e ša-te-e ina na-kap-ti*
14′. *ki-ma ši-na-a-ti ina bi-ri-it pu-ri-di*
15′. *ṣi-i-im šim-ma-tum ki-ma ši-iz-bi ina tu-le-e ir-ti-ša*
16′. *ki-ma ú-pa-ṭi ina na-ḫi-ri ù ḫa-si-si*
17′. *am-mi-ni šim-ma-tum* GURUŠ *u* KI.SIKIL *ta-kas-sà-si*
18′. *ki-ma ina ši-in-ni pu-u la i-bit-tu*$_4$
19′. *šim-ma-tum ay i-bit ina* SU GURUŠ *u* KI.SIKIL
20′. *ši-ip-tum ul ya-at-tu-un*
21′. *ši-pat* ^{d}*É-a ù* ^{d}*Asal-lú-ḫi ši-pat* MAŠ.MAŠ DINGIR.MEŠ ^{d}AMAR.UTU
22′. *šu-nu id-du-ú-ma a-na-ku ú-ša-an-ni* TU$_6$ ÉN É.NU.RU[15]

23′. KA.INIM.MA *šim-ma-tum*.KÁM*

24′. KÌD.KÌD.BI ŠE.KAK ^{GIŠ}DÌḪ ŠE.KAK ^{GIŠ}Ú.GÍR ŠE.KAK ^{GI}ŠUL.ḪI
25′. ŠE.KAK ^{GIŠ}GÍR ŠE.KAK ^{GIŠ}MA.NU ^{GI}PA.ÚR GI *ú-ra-an-nu-um*
26′. *ta-sàk* TÉŠ.BI *ina* Ì.GIŠ ḪE.ḪE *ka-a-a-na a-di i-nu-uḫ-ḫu*
27′. ŠÉŠ.ŠÉŠ-*su-ma* TI.LA[16]

28′. DIŠ 2 *ú-ra-an-nu-um* NUMUN ^{GIŠ}ŠE.NU ^{Ú}*su-pa-lam* ^{GIŠ}ŠINIG
29′. ^{Ú}IN.UŠ ^{ŠEM}GÚR.GÚR ^{ŠEM}LI ^{ŠEM}ŠE.LI ^{Ú}NU.LUḪ.ḪA
30′. ŠEM.GAM.MA KA.GÍR A.AB.BA[17] ŠEM.^{d}NIN.IB
31′. ZAG.ḪI.LI^{SAR} *ṭe*$_4$*-ne-e-ti* ZÍD ŠE.SA.A KAŠ.Ú.SA SIG$_5$
32′. ŠE.KAK ^{GIŠ}ŠUR.‹MÌN?› PA ^{GIŠ}A.AB.BA[18] ^{Ú}ḪAR.ḪAR ^{Ú}KUR.KUR
33′. ^{Ú}*úr-ne-e* ^{Ú}*ba-ri-ra-tum* ZÍD ZÍZ.AN.NA TÉŠ.BI ḪE.ḪE
34′. *ina šur-šum-mi e-pu-ti ina* A GAZI^{SAR} *em-mu-ti ta-la-aš*
35′. GIN$_7$ *ra-bi-ki tara-bak ina* KUŠ *ši-ip-ki te-ṭer-ri*
36′. *ba-aḫ-ru-us-su* LAL.LAL-*su u* ÉN *an-ni-tú* ŠID.ŠID-*nu*
37′. *ka-a-a-na tu-maš-ša-ʾ-šu-ma* TI[19]

38′. DIŠ 3 ^{GI}PA.ÚR.GI ^{GI}ŠUL.ḪI ŠE.KAK ^{GI}ŠUL.ḪI
39′. ŠE.KAK ^{GIŠ}Ú.GÍR ^{GIŠ}ŠINIG NUMUN ^{GIŠ}MA.NU NUMUN *ú-ra-an-nu-um*
40′. ^{Ú}*kám*-ka-du ta-sàk ina* A ÍD NAG SAG.DU KUR.GI^{MUŠEN}
41′. *ina* Ì ^{GIŠ}ŠUR.MÌN NUMUN ^{Ú}*kám*-ka-du* ḪE.ḪE ŠÉŠ.ŠÉŠ-*su-ma* TI[20]

42′. DIŠ LÚ *šim-ma-at* UZU GIG A.GAR.GAR *ru-ub-ṣi ši-ib-ra-ti*
43′. *it-ti* ^{Ú}IN.UŠ ^{GIŠ}GAN.U$_5$ *ana* ŠÀ A.GAR.GAR ŠUB-*di*
44′. *ina* A PÚ *ka-la* U$_4$-*mi ina* ^{IM}ŠU.RIN.NA *te-še-kir ina* MUL *tuš-bat*
45′. *ina* Á.GÚ.ZI.GA *ana* ^{DUG}*nam-ḫar ta-tab-bak i-ra-aḫ-ḫa-aṣ*[21]

46′. DIŠ 2 A.GAR.GAR *ta-ḫaš-šal ina* A GAZI^{SAR} *ta-la-a-aš ta-aṣ-ṣa-na-mid-su*
47′. *ina* Á.GÚ.ZI.GA DU$_8$-*šu ina* A ^{GIŠ}ŠE.NU *i-ra-aḫ-ḫa-aṣ*
48′. E$_{11}$-*ma* ^{Ú}*ak-tam* ŠEM.^{d}NIN.IB *ta-sàk* Ì.GIŠ.ERIN.NA *ina* Ì.GIŠ ŠÉŠ[22]

49′. DIŠ LÚ *šim-ma-at* SA.MEŠ GIG *i-ra* [...] *ina* ^{IM}ŠU.RIN.N[A *te-še-ker*]
50′. [MAŠ].SÌLA LAL.LAL-*id-su-ma* ⌈*tu-šar*⌉-[*ḫa-as-su*] ⌈*ina* ŠÀ⌉ A ^{GIŠ}ŠE.NU
51′. [E$_{11}$]-*ma* KI.A.^{d}ÍD KA.A.AB.BA $^{\text{NA}_4}$*mu*-[(*ṣa*)]
52′. ŠEM.^{d}NIN.IB Ì.GIŠ.ERIN.NA *ina* Ì.GIŠ ŠÉŠ.ŠÉŠ-*su*-[(*ma* TI)][23]

Translation

(obv. 1–7) If you want to soothe the effects of a stroke and the limpness from it,[24] you combine these plants: *eʾru*-tree [seed], *irrû* [seed], *ḫašû*-thyme, [*urânu*] seed, *sīḫu*-wormwood, ⌈*argannu*⌉, *barirātu*, and [...]. You decoct (it) till decocted in a *diqāru*-bowl. You boil (it) in milk and first-quality beer. If you continually bandage him (with it), [he should recover].

(obv. 8–11) If two, you dry, crush, (and) sift *urânu* seed, *šunû*-chastetree seed, *kukru*, *burāšu*-juniper, *kikkirānu*-juniper berries, (and) old beer dregs. You make (it) into a dough with hot *kasû*-juice. You work (it) into leather. Ditto (If you bandage him (with it) while it is still hot, he should recover).

(obv. 12–15) If three, you decoct *saḫlû*-cress, *buṭuttu*-cereal, winnowed beerwort, roasted grain flour, *ḫašû*-thyme (and) *barirātu* in first-quality beer in a *tamgussu*-vessel.[25] You work (it) into leather. Ditto (If you continually bandage him (with it), he should recover).

(obv. 16–18) If four, you dry, crush (and) sift *saḫlû*-cress, roasted grain flour, *nuḫurtu*, *ḫašû*-thyme (and) *bīnu*-tamarisk leaves. You decoct (it)[26] in first-quality beer in a *tamgussu*-vessel. You sprinkle emmer flour on it. You work (it) into leather. Ditto (If you continually bandage him (with it), he should recover).

(obv. 19–21) If five, you grind together *saḫlû*-cress, *kasû*, *šūšu*-licorice leaves, (and) "sunflower." You pour (it) into water. You bake (it) in an oven.

You massage his feet (with it) and then, if you rub him gently (with) oil, he should recover.

(obv. 22–24) If six, you dry (and) grind (beer) dregs. You mill-grind *nikiptu*, *ḫašû*-thyme, (and) *atāʾišu*. You decoct (it) in first-quality beer in a *tamgussu*-vessel. You sprinkle emmer flour on it. Ditto (If you bandage him (with it) in leather while it is still hot, he should recover).

(obv. 25–26) If seven, you make a dough of *šūšu*-licorice leaves with *kasû* juice. You decoct (it) and then, if you bandage him (with it), he should recover.

(obv. 27–29) If eight, you dry, crush (and) sift *bīnu*-tamarisk, *maštakal*, (and) palm heart. You grind *kukru* (and) *burāšu*-juniper. You mix (them) together. You decoct (it) in wheat flour and (beer) dregs. If you bandage him (with it), he should recover.

(obv. 30–36) If a person continually has ⸢numbness⸣ of the ⸢front part of the body⸣, to remove the ⸢numbness⸣ of the ⸢front part of the body⸣ and to cause him to experience improvement, you dry, crush (and) sift *aktam*, which is *ḫupšilurgu* in Hurrian,[27] *kalbānu* fruit, ⸢*ṣaṣuntu*⸣ (and) *amurdinnu* leaves. ⸢You also decoct⸣ (it) with river bank clay (and) [...] If [you bandage] ⸢him⸣ (with it) ⸢while it is still hot⸣, he should recover.

(obv. 37–rev. 3′) *(fragmentary)*

(rev. 4′–27′) É.NU.RU [recitation]: ⸢Numbness⸣, numbness, ⸢numbness⸣, numbness from a scorpion (sting), [you] stung like a scorpion. [You] ⸢struck⸣ with your horns; you let flow with your tail. You made [the young man] go out from the lap of the young woman; you made [the young woman] so out from the lap of the young man. ⸢Come out⸣, numbness, like milk from the breast, like sweat from the armpit, like irrigation water from the temples, like urine from between the thighs! Come out, numbness like the milk from her breast, like dirt from the nostrils and openings of the ears! Why, numbness, do you gnaw at young man and young woman? Just as chaff does not remain overnight in the teeth, so may the numbness not remain overnight in the flesh of young man and young woman. The spell is not mine; it is the spell of Ea and Asalluhi, the spell of the exorcist of the gods, Marduk. They know it and I (merely) repeat it. Spell and É.NU.RU recitation.

Recitation for numbness.

Its ritual is as follows: you grind these plants: *baltu*-thorn shoots, *ašāgu*-thorn shoots, *qān šalāli* shoots, *asu*-myrtle shoots, *eʾru*-tree shoots, reed blades, (and) *urânu* root. You mix (it) together with oil. If you continually and constantly rub him gently (with it) until it calms down, he should recover.

(rev. 28′–37′) If two, you mix together *urânu*, *šunû*-chastetree seed, *supālu*, *bīnu*-tamarisk, *maštakal*, *kukru*, *burāšu*-juniper, *kikkirānu*-juniper berries, *nuḫurtu*, *ṣumlalû*, *asu*-myrtle(!), *imbû tamtim*, *nikiptu*, ground *saḫlû*-cress, roasted grain flour, winnowed beerwort, *šurmēnu*-cypress (?), *kušabku*-tree leaves,[28] *ḫašû*-thyme, *atā'išu*, *urnû*-mint, *barirātu*, (and) emmer flour. You make a dough with baked beer dregs (and) boiled *kasû* juice. You decoct (it) till decocted. You work (it) into *šipku*-leather. You repeatedly bandage him (with it) while it is still hot and you repeatedly recite this recitation. If you continually massage him (with it), he should recover.

(rev. 38′–41′) If three, you grind reed blades, *qān šalāli* with the shoots, *ašāgu*-thorn shoots, *bīnu*-tamarisk, *e'ru*-tree seed, *urânu* seed, (and) *kamkādu* (and) have him drink (it mixed) with river water. (You grind) the head of a goose in *šurmēnu*-cypress oil. You mix (it with) *kamkādu* seed. If you repeatedly rub him gently (with it), he should recover.

(rev. 42′–45′) If a person is sick with numbness of the flesh, (you take) broken-up gazelle pellets (made) with *maštakal* (and) *kiškānu*-tree outer bark.[29] You pour (it) into the gazelle dung. You bake (it) for an entire day in well water in an oven. You leave (it) out overnight under the stars. In the morning, you pour (it) into a *namḫaru*-vat. He should bathe (in it).

(rev. 46′–48′) If two, you crush gazelle dung. You make a dough with *kasû* juice. You repeatedly bandage him (with it). In the morning, you take (it) off him. He should bathe in *šunû*-chastetree infusion. (After) he comes out, you grind *aktam* (and) *nikiptu*. You rub him gently (with it mixed with) *erēnu*-cedar oil (and) with oil.

(rev. 49′–52′) If a person is sick with numbness of the muscles, [you bake ...] in an oven. You repeatedly bandage his ⸢shoulders⸣ (with it) and then ⸢you bathe⸣ [him] with *šunû*-chastetree infusion. After [he comes out], if you repeatedly rub him gently (with) *kibrītu*-sulphur, *imbû tamtim*, *mūṣu*-stone, *nikiptu* (and) *erēnu*-cedar oil (mixed) with oil, he should recover.

D. PERIPHERAL NEUROPATHY

Peripheral neuropathy refers to pain, numbness, itching and paralysis due to damage to the long nerves running through the arms and legs. For more, see Scurlock and Andersen 2005, 338–39.

TEXT 4: BAM 122

BAM 122 is part of a series dealing with problems in the legs and feet that impede mobility. It contains baths (1–15), bandages (1–7, 16–rev. 10′), a salve (rev. 11′–17′), a potion (rev. 18′–19′) and a fumigant (rev. 20′–23′) for peripheral neuropathy. The physician might also arrange for a sauna.

1. DIŠ NA *kin-ṣa-šú* DU$_8$.DU$_8$ 2 GÍN GAZI^{SAR}
2. A ^{GIŠ}ŠE.NU A SAR MUNU$_6$
3. ^{Ú}*ak-tam* ŠEG$_6$-*šal*
4. GÌR^{II}-*šú*[30] *ir-ta-na-ḫaṣ*
5. ^{ŠEM}LI ^{ŠEM}GÚR.GÚR ^{ŠEM}BAL
6. DUḪ.LÀL *ina* Ì.UDU ḪE.ḪE
7. *ina* KUŠ *te-ṭer-ri* LAL-*id*

---

8. DIŠ NA GÌR^{II}-*šú šim-ma-tú* TUKU
9. GU$_7$.MEŠ-*šú* SA GÌR^{II}-*šú sa-ag-gu-ma*
10. GÌR^{II}-*šú* BAL.BAL-*šu* PA ^{GIŠ}*bi-ni*
11. ^{Ú}[…] ^{ŠEM}GÚR.GÚR ^{ŠEM}LI
12. 1-*niš ta-ḫaš-šal ina* A MUNU$_6$ *ina* NINDU
13. BAD-*ir ul-tu ib-taš-lu*
14. KI.MIN *a-di* 7-*šú* TU$_5$-*šú*
15. *ta-sa-dar-šum-ma* TI-*uṭ*

---

16. DIŠ LÚ GÌR^{II}-*šú šim-ma-tú ú-kal-la*
17. KÚM-*ma* TUKU-*a ù a-na a-tál-lu-ku* DUGUD-*šú*
18. ^{Ú}*kam-ka-da* ^{GIŠ}*úr-nu-u*
19. ^{GI}ŠUL.ḪI ^{Ú}EN.DI
20. *ta-ḫaš-šal* MUN *a-ma-an*
21. BA.BA.ZA.^{d}ÍD ÚḪ.^{d}ÍD
22. ^{Ú}*imḫur-lim* SUḪUŠ ^{GIŠ}NAM.TAR.NÍTA
23. [*ina*] ⸢KAŠ⸣.BIR$_8$.MEŠ Ú.ḪI.‹A› *an-*[*nu-ti* …]
24. […]-*bi-tu* […]
25. […] x […]

rev.

1′. [… *ú*]-*kal-ma* TI-*u*[*ṭ*]

2′. DIŠ NA ⸢SA⸣ GÌR^{II}-*šú ša-gu-ma*
3′. *a-tál-lu-ka la i-le-*ʾ*i*
4′. *ana* SA.MEŠ GÌR^{II}-*šú pu-uš-šu-ḫi*
5′. ZAG.ḪI.LI PA ^{GIŠ}*šu-ši*
6′. *ta-ḫaš-šal ta-nap-pi*
7′. *ina* KAŠ *pu-ut-ti ina* ^{DUG}ÚTUL
8′. GIN$_7$ *ra-bi-ki tu-ra-ba-ak* ⸢*te*!-*ṭe*$_4$!⸣-*er-ri*
9′. NÍG.LAL-⸢*ma*⸣ SA GÌR$^{\text{II.MEŠ}}$-*šú*
10′. *i-pa-šú-ḫa* GÌR^{II}-*šú i-qa-li-la*[31]

11′. [DIŠ NA] GÌR^{II}-*šú* DUGUD.MEŠ [GU$_7$]-*šú*
12′. [*a-tál-lu-ka*] *la i-le-ʾi*
13′. NA BI GÌ[R!^{II} GIG … GÌR^{II}]-*šú*
14′. ŠÉŠ-*ma muš-šú-a-te*
15′. ḪÁD.A GAZ KI Ì+GIŠ ^{ŠEM}GÚR.GÚR
16′. *ina* ^{NA_4}LA.ḪA.AN G[Ì]R$^{⸢II⸣}$-*šú*
17′. ŠÉŠ.MEŠ-*ma* TI-*uṭ*

18′. ^{Ú}TE.GÍL!.LA ^{Ú}*pu-qut-tú*
19′. ^{Ú}⸢*ka-zal-lá*⸣ *ina* KAŠ NAG[32]

20′. A.ÉSIR.ḪÁD.A x[…] KA.A.AB.BA
21′. ^{Ú}*kur-ka-*[*n*]*am* ^{Ú}*tar-muš*$_8$
22′. ^{Ú}*imḫur-lim* ^{Ú}*imḫur*-20
23′. BULUḪ Ì *ina* DÈ

Translation

(obv. 1–7) To loosen up a person's shins, you boil 2 shekels of *kasû*, *šunû*-chastetree infusion, watered malt[33] (and) *aktam*. He should repeatedly bathe his feet (variant: shins) (with it). You mix *burāšu*-juniper, *kukru*, *balukku*-aromatic, (and) wax with sheep fat. You work (it) into leather (and) bandage (him with it).

(obv. 8–15) If a person's feet are numb (and) hurt him, the muscles of his feet are stiff so that his feet shift constantly under him,[34] you crush together *bīnu*-tamarisk leaves, […], *kukru* (and) *burāšu*-juniper. You bake (it) in an oven in malt water until it boils. You do it again. If you have him bathe (with it) on seven consecutive days, he should recover.

(obv. 16–rev. 1′) If numbness grips a person's feet, they are feverish and it is difficult for him to walk,[35] you crush *kamkādu*, *urnû*-mint, *qān šalāli*, (and) *suʾādu*. You [decoct] ⸢these⸣ plants: *amānu*-salt, *papasītu*-sulphur, *ruʾtītu*-sulphur, *imḫur-lim*, (and) male *pillû* root [in] *ḫīqu*-beer. […] If [he] keeps it there, he should recover.

(rev. 2′–10′) If the muscles of a person's feet are so stiff that he cannot walk, to relax the muscles of his feet,[36] you crush (and) sift *saḫlû*-cress (and) *šūšu*-licorice leaves. You decoct (it) till decocted in freshly opened beer in a *diqāru*-bowl. You work (it into cloth). If you bandage (him with it), the muscles of his feet should relax (and) his feet should (seem) lighter.

(rev. 11′–17′) [If a person's] feet continually feel heavy, hurt(?) him (and) he cannot [walk], that person [has sore] ⌜feet⌝!. You gently rub his [feet with ...]. Then, you dry (and) crush rubbing plants (and mix it) with *kukru* oil in a stone *laḫannu*-vessel. If you repeatedly gently rub his feet (with it), he should recover.

(rev. 18′–19′) You have him drink *tigilû*, *puquttu*, (and) *kazallu* (mixed) with beer.

(rev. 20′–23′) Bitumen, [...], *imbû tamtim*, *kurkānu*-turmeric, *tarmuš*, *imḫur-lim*, *imḫur-ešra*, *baluḫḫu*-aromatic (and) oil over coals.

Notes

1. Collation for NUMUN ^{GIŠ}KIRI$_6$ by M. Geller for M. Stol produced NUMUN GADA. SAR.SAR; BAM 482 i 2 has instead NUMUN ^{Ú}ḪUR.SAG NUMUN ḪAB.
2. See Scurlock and Andersen 2005, 13.145.
3. BAM 482 i 2 substitutes seed of *azupīru* (and) seed of *ḫurātu*-madder(?).
4. See chapter 3, n. 109.
5. See Scurlock and Andersen 2005, 8.47.
6. See Scurlock and Andersen 2005, 13.149.
7. See Scurlock and Andersen 2005, 13.153
8. For the translation of *saḫlû* as "cress," see Stol 1983–84, 24–32.
9. For the recitation, see Böck 2007, 46–47, 167.
10. See Scurlock and Andersen 2005, 8.14.
11. For the text of this recitation, see Böck 2007, 46, 167.
12. Lines 1, 8–11 restored from BAM 138 ii 1–8//*AMT* 82/2 iii! 7–8.
13. For *ina* ^{URUDU}ŠEN.TUR *AMT* 82/2 iii! 12 has [*ina*] ^{DUG}ÚTUL GIN$_7$ *rib-ki*
14. Restored from *AMT* 82/2 iii! 11–12
15. Böck 2007, 261–313 treats this recitation as VIIIq. See *STT* 136 = Böck 2007, text VIIIe.
16. Duplicated by *AMT* 92/6:5–7; cf. BAM 159 vi 51–54.
17. The signs are a bit out of order; the parallel *AMT* 98/3:9 has ^{ŠEM}GÍR KA-*tam-tim*
18. Instead of ^{GIŠ}ŠUR.‹MÌN?› PA ^{GIŠ}A.AB.BA, the parallel has ^{GIŠ}DIḪ $^{\text{GIŠ.Ú}}$GÍR KA.A.AB.BA.
19. Restored from *AMT* 98/3:8–12.
20. Duplicated by *AMT* 92/6:2–4.
21. Duplicated by *AMT* 92/4+*AMT* 92/9+BM 20179 iii 12′–iv 2.
22. Duplicated by *AMT* 92/4+*AMT* 92/9+BM 20179 iv 3–4.
23. Restored from *AMT* 92/4+*AMT* 92/9+BM 20179 iv 5–6
24. See Scurlock and Andersen 2005, 13.53.
25. Instead of the *tamgussu*-vessel" *AMT* 82/2 iii! 12 has a *diqāru*-bowl.
26. See chapter 3, n. 109.
27. See *KADP* 4:9. This entry appears as Uruanna I 104 in Böck's unpublished edition.
28. Instead of *šurmēnu*-cypress(?) and *kušabku*-tree leaves, the parallel has *baltu*-thorn, *ašāgu*-thorn and *imbû tamtim*.
29. According to Uruanna II 321, *bukānu* (GIŠ.GAN) is equivalent to *siḫpu*, which is the inner bark of the *kiškānu*-tree (see *CAD* S, 238–39). U$_5$ is *rikbu*, which means "upper part" or "top level," hence the outer bark of the tree. This has nothing to do with the inflorescence of date palms. Stol forthcoming considers this a variety of truffle.

30. BAM 405:12′ substitutes *kin-ṣi-šú*.

31. Duplicated by *AMT* 68/1 rev. 8–11.

32. See BAM 81:8′–9′ reading ÚTI.GI.LA.A and BAM 257:11–16 reading ÚTI.GI.LA and adding Ú*kur-ka-nu-u* (treatments for *maškādu* and *sagallu*),

33. For this medicament and malt products in general, see Stol 1989, 328.

34. See Scurlock and Andersen 2005, 13.48, 13.267.

35. See Scurlock and Andersen 2005, 19.351.

36. See Scurlock and Andersen 2005, 11.7.

12

OBSTETRICS AND GYNECOLOGY

A. GYNECOLOGY

As is still the case today, women were generally treated in the same way and with the same medicines as men but with exceptions. As we know from rare references to dosages, these were adjusted for female patients. It was also unethical to give a woman something which might accidentally cause an abortion if she happened to be pregnant. There were, of course, special problems relating to menstruation and childbirth that only women have, and these occupied a separate section of the diagnostic series, suggesting the possibility of specialization. Certainly specialists were the midwives who attended the typical, unproblematic childbirth. The female doctors who practiced in the harems of Assyrian kings will also have specialized in treating women and children. Ancient physicians seem to have performed pelvic examinations to check up on pregnant women. They also played the game of predicting the sex of the child for anxious parents. For more details, see Scurlock and Andersen 2005, chapter 12.

1. IRREGULAR BLEEDING; VENEREAL DISEASE

Menstruation is not called by us "the curse" for nothing. Ancient physicians had to deal with inadequate and excessive flow. For more details, see Scurlock and Andersen 2005, 260. The sexually transmitted diseases treated by ancient physicians in their female patients include crabs and vaginitis. For more details, see Scurlock and Andersen 2005, 20, 93 and text 9 below (BAM 240).

TEXT 1: BAM 237 (= *KAR* 194), i, iv

BAM 237 is a four-column text dealing with gynecology. The preserved parts of column i begin with a salve (i 1′–3′) and an amulet (i 4′–8′) for irregular bleeding which, along with a missing potion, was to be accompanied by a ritual (i 9′–20′). The recitation also doubled for use with another amulet (i 18′–24′). BAM 237 continues with vaginal suppositories (i 25′, 33′–36′, 39′,

40′–46′), a fumigant (i 26′–27′), potions (i 28′–30′, 32′, 37′–38′, 40′–42′) and amulets (i 31′, 40′–42′, 47′–48′) for irregular bleeding. Columns ii-iii are mostly taken up with garbled Sumerian É.NU.RU recitations[1] accompanying potions (ii 16′–17′, 23′–24′, 34′–35′) and amulets (ii 36′, 41′–47′, iii 1–5) for irregular bleeding. Column iv has potions (iv 1, 3–5, 8), vaginal suppositories (iv 2, 6–7), again for irregular bleeding. This is followed by a vaginal suppository (iv 9–10), douches (iv 1–12), and potions (iv 13–14) for puerperal fever. This is followed by vaginal suppositories (iv 15–28) and potions (iv 15–28) for genital crabs and a vaginal suppository (iv 29–33), a potion (iv 34–38), and an amulet (iv 39–43) for vaginitis.

Lines i 4′–8′ are of an interesting type of amulet that puts burls of medicinal plants between the magical stones bound onto the affected area. The ritual of lines i 9′–20′ is an extremely interesting example of the interplay between medical treatment, exorcism, and prayer in the healing of illness. At one level we have an exorcistic ritual in which symbols of obstruction—a potsherd that stands up in the road, a door, the hands behind the back—signal to listening spirits the desired stoppage of the woman's bleeding. These instructions are connected with the patient by sprinkling her with water in which the potsherd has been washed and by putting some of the medicine by the door before which the woman is praying. There is also a religious ritual which begins with a censer to summon the goddess Ishtar to act as guarantor for the proceedings. The patient is required to kneel and say her prayers. A simple offering of sweets and a libation (of beer) followed by prostration completes the religious ritual. Mediating the two rituals is the physician, who is no mere administrator of medicines, although he does this, but also an exorcist, making all the requisite arrangements and seconding the woman's prayers with an efficacious recitation. The latter consists essentially of epithets, but calls Ishtar a knotter, of obvious relevance to the problem at hand.

The amulet in lines i 22′–24′ is quite specific about the area on which the amulet is to be bound, suggesting that the intent was to put pressure on the areas under it. To note is that the date stones of line i 25′ are a significant source of plant estrogen, which means that this is essentially hormone therapy of a sort still used today, and for this problem. Lines i 26′–27′ are interesting for an unusual procedure, in which the woman is asked to sit over a brazier in which a medicinal plant is burning. The alum of lines i 33′, 36′, 43′–44′ will certainly have stopped the patients' bleeding. In the bad old days of straight razors, men used to keep alum handy to repair the damage caused by inept strokes. Lines iv 9–10 and iv 29–33 have an usual type of suppository in which knots made in cloth and sprinkled with plant medicines are inserted one by one into the vagina.

i

1′. [... IM].KAL IM.KAL.GUG ⸢IM.SAḪAR⸣.[NA$_4$.KUR.RA]

2′. $^{\mathrm{NA_4}}$KA.GI.NA.⸢DIB.BA⸣ [NA$_4$ KÙ.BABBAR NA$_4$] KÙ.SIG$_{17}$ $^{\mathrm{NA_4}}$AN.ZAḪ GI$_6$ EME PÉŠ.A.ŠÀ.GA 20 Ú.[$^{\mathrm{HI.A}}$] ⸢*an*⸣-*nu-ti*

3′. TÉŠ.BI SÚD *ina* LÀL Ì.NUN *u* Ì AMAR ḪE.ḪE ÉN 3-*šú ana* ŠÀ ŠID-*nu-ma* LI.DUR-*sa* KÁ GAL$_4$.LA-*šá* ŠÉŠ-*aš*

4′. $^{\mathrm{NA_4}}$*ḫal-ta* $^{\mathrm{NA_4}}$ŠUBA Á.ZI.DA $^{\mathrm{NA_4}}$ŠUBA Á.GÙB.BA $^{\mathrm{NA_4}}$*šu-u* NITA *u* MUNUS

5′. $^{\mathrm{NA_4}}$GUG MÚD.MEŠ $^{\mathrm{NA_4}}$*ka-pa-ṣa* $^{\mathrm{NA_4}}$*iá-ni-ba* $^{\mathrm{NA_4}}$*zib-tum* 9 NA$_4$.MEŠ *an-nu-ti*

6′. *ina* SÍG ḪÉ.ME.DA SÍG ZA.GÌN.NA SÍG GA.RÍG.AK.A SA ÁB RI.RI.GA SA MAŠ.DÀ *šá* NITA *u* MUNUS

7′. ^{Ú}*aš-lam* NITA ^{SAL}MUD[2] TÉŠ.BI NU.NU È-*ak* 7 *u* 7 KA.KEŠDA KEŠDA Ú DILI NUMUN ^{Ú}*tu-lal*

8′. *ina* SÍG ḪÉ.ME.DA *ina bi-rit* KA.KEŠDA *u* NA$_4$.MEŠ *tála-pap* ÉN 3-*šú ana* UGU ŠID-*ma ina* MURUB$_4$-*šá* KEŠDA

9′. ŠIKA E.SÍR.KA.LÍM GUB.BA TI-*qí* A TU$_5$ Ì ŠÉŠ SÍG ḪÉ.ME.DA NIGIN-*mi*

10′. *ina* É *ina* EGIR ^{GIŠ}IG *ina* KI *par-si* GAR-*an-ši* KI.TA *ša* É A *ta-sa-laḫ-ši* NÍG.NA ^{ŠEM}LI

11′. ^{Ú}KUR.KUR GAR-*an-ši* MUNUS BI *i-kám-mis-ma* Á-*šá ana* EGIR-*šá ú-tar* ÉN 3-*šú* ŠID-*nu*

12′. 3-*šú še-gu-ú i-šá-si* NU *uš-kìn* GIN$_7$ *an-na-a tuš-tál-li-mu* NINDA.Ì.⸢DÉ.A⸣ LÀL Ì.NUN.NA

13′. GAR-*an* BAL-*tú* BAL-*qí uš-kìn* 3 U$_4$ GUR.GUR-*ár* GIN$_7$ *an-nam* DÙ.DÙ-*šu* [*maš-q*]*i*!-*tu* NAG-*ši*

14′. *nap-šel-tu* ŠÉŠ-*si* NA$_4$.MEŠ KEŠDA-*si ina* 4 U$_4$-*me* ^{GIŠ}*si-ḫa* ^{GIŠ}*ár-ga-n*[*u* $^{\mathrm{GI}]\mathrm{Š}}$*ba-ri-ra-*[*ta*]

15′. *ana* IGI ^{GIŠ}IG *ta-sa-raq* MUNUS BI *ana* IGI ^{GIŠ}IG *še-gu-u i-ša-si ana* IGI ⸢^{d}*Iš*⸣-[*tar*]

16′. *še-gu-u i-ša-si* ÉN 3-*šú* ŠID-*nu-ma i-*[*šá-lim*]

17′. KA.INIM.MA MUNUS *ša na-aḫ-šá-te* GIG *bul-ṭu* [*lat-ku*][3]

18′. ÉN ^{d}INNIN AN.KI.BI.DA.KE$_4$ ^{d}INNIN *la-gal-la-*[*i-tum*]

19′. *ka-ad-ra-a-a-i-tum šu-gal-li-tum* : *ka-ad-ra-a-a-i-tum te-li-tum* [...]

20′. ^{d}*iš-ta-ri-tum ù an-ki-bi-i-tum ke-ṣi-ru ša* AN-*e* TU$_6$ [ÉN]

21′. KA.INIM.MA MUNUS *ša na-aḫ-šá-te* GIG

22′. DÙ.DÙ.BI ^{Ú}NINNI NITA SÍG ḪÉ.ME.DA SA ÁB RI.RI.GA ^{SAL}TAR-*tum* NU.NU 14 KA.KEŠDA K[EŠDA]

23′. $^{\text{NA}_4}$*at-bar ina* EGIR KA.KEŠDA *ina* SÍG ḪÉ.ME.DA NIGIN-*mi* KA.KEŠDA *ina* KI.TA ḪÁŠ-*šá* GAR-*a*[*n*]

24′. *ina* MURUB$_4$-*šá* KEŠDA-*ma na-aḫ-šá-tu* TAR-*sa*

25′. NA$_4$ ZÚ.LUM *tur-ár* SÚD ^{SÍG}ÀKA NIGIN *ana* ŠÀ.TÙR-*šá* GAR-*an*

26′. GÌR.PAD.DU NAM.LÚ.U$_{19}$.LU *ina* DÈ *ta-sár-raq* MUNUS BI *ina* UGU TUŠ-*ši* A.MEŠ-*šá ana* UGU DU-*ku*

27′. *šum-ma* NU TAR-*su* GUR-*ma* TUŠ-*ši* MIN

28′. ^{Ú}*el-lu-ra* SAḪAR *ḫi-ri-iṣ ma-gar-ri* ⸢^{GIŠ}GIGIR⸣ TI *ana* KAŠ SAG ŠUB *ina* UL *tuš-bat*

29′. *ina še-rim la pa-tan* NAG-[*ši-ma*] ⸢*na*⸣-*aḫ-šá-tu* TAR-*sa*

30′. ^{Ú}*el-*⸢*lu-ra*⸣ SÚD *ina* KAŠ NAG MIN

31′. SÍG ḪÉ.ME.DA SA ÁB RI.RI.GA NU.NU AN.BAR $^{\text{NA}_4}$*at-bar tála-pap ina* MURUB$_4$-⸢*šá*⸣ [KEŠDA] ⸢MIN⸣

32′. ^{Ú}NU.LUḪ.ḪA SÚD *ina* KAŠ NAG MIN

33′. IM.SAḪAR.BABBAR.KUR.RA SÚD ^{SÍG}ÀKA NIGIN *ana* ŠÀ.TÙR-*šá* GAR-*an* MIN

34′. NUNUZ TU^{MUŠEN} SÚD ^{SÍG}ÀKA NIGIN *ana* ŠÀ.TÙR-*šá* GAR MIN

35′. NUNUZ TU.KUR$_4$^{MUŠEN} SÚD ^{SÍG}ÀKA NIGIN *ana* ŠÀ.TÙR-*šá* GAR MIN

36′. IM.SAḪAR.GI$_6$.KUR IM.SAḪAR.BABBAR.KUR SÚD ^{SÍG}ÀKA NIGIN *ana* ŠÀ.TÙR-*šá* GAR MIN

37′. ^{Ú}*im-ḫur-20* : ^{Ú}*imḫur-lim* SÚD *ina* KAŠ NAG MIN

38′. SI ÙZ *ša* NIGIN BIL ^{Ú}NÚMUN *tur-ár ina* KAŠ NAG MIN

39′. ^{Ú}IN.NU.UŠ A.GAR.GAR.^{d}ÍD SÍG ḪÉ.ME.DA SÍG BABBAR *ta-lá-pap si-ik-ti* $^{\text{NA}_4}$*at-bar* SUD *ana* ŠÀ.TÙR-*šá* GAR MIN

40′–41′.[4] $^{\text{NA}_4}$GUG.ZÚ : $^{\text{NA}_4}$GUG $^{\text{NA}_4}$*ka-pa-ṣa ta-sàk ina* KAŠ SAG NAG MIN $^{\text{NA}_4}$*at-bar* NUMUN ^{Ú}IN.NU.UŠ SÚD SÍG ḪÉ.ME.DA
42′. SA ÁB RI.RI.GA NIGIN *ina* MURUB$_4$-*šá* KEŠDA : *ana* ŠÀ.TÙR-*šá* GAR-*an* MIN

43′. KI.A.^{d}ÍD IM.SAḪAR.BABBAR.KUR.RA IM.SAḪAR.GI$_6$.KUR.RA IM.SAḪAR.NA$_4$.KUR.RA AN.ZAḪ GI$_6$: AN.ZAḪ SÚD
44′. ^{SÍG}ÀKA NIGIN *ana* ŠÀ.TÙR-*šá* GAR MIN

45′. $^{\text{NA}_4}$KA.GI.NA.DIB.BA AN.BAR KUG.GAN $^{\text{NA}_4}$*u$_5$-ri-za* $^{\text{NA}_4}$*ka-pa-ṣu* $^{\text{NA}_4}$*šu-a*
46′. $^{\text{NA}_4}$*iá-ár-tú* SÚD ^{SÍG}ÀKA NIGIN *ana* ŠÀ.TÙR-*šá* GAR MIN

47′. $^{\text{NA}_4}$*iá-ár-tú šá* 7 GÙN-*šá* $^{\text{NA}_4}$AN.BAR $^{\text{NA}_4}$*zik-tum* $^{\text{NA}_4}$SAG.LI.MUD NUMUN ^{Ú}IN.NU.UŠ
48′. *ina* SA ÁB RI.RI.GA SA U$_8$ RI.RI È-*ak* 14 KA.KEŠDA KEŠDA *ina* MURUB$_4$-*šá tara-kas* MIN

iv

1. NUMUN ^{Ú}*a-zal-le-e* Ú.KUR.RA ^{Ú}ḪUR.SAG SÚD *ina* KAŠ [NAG]

2. SUḪUŠ ^{GIŠ}GIŠIMMAR SUḪUŠ ^{GIŠ}ŠINIG SUḪUŠ $^{\text{GIŠ.Ú}}$GÍR *tur-ár* SÚD *ina* SÍG ZA.GÌN.NA NIGIN *ana* ŠÀ.TÙR-*šá* GAR-*an*

3. IM.SIG$_7$.SIG$_7$ IM.KÙ.SIG$_{17}$ IM.KAL.LA IM.SAḪAR.NA$_4$.KUR.RA *ina* KAŠ NAG

4. NUMUN ^{GIŠ}*šu-šum* NU.LUḪ.ḪA ^{ŠEM}LI SÚD *ina* KAŠ NAG

5. NUMUN $^{\text{GIŠ.Ú}}$GÍR NUMUN ^{GIŠ}DÌḪ SUḪUŠ ^{GIŠ}NAM.TAL NÍTA *ta-sàk ina* KAŠ NAG

6. *ka-mun* ^{GIŠ}ŠINIG NIM.UR$_4$.UR$_4$ MUŠ.DÍM.PÚ.RU.NU ŠÈ EME.DIR
7. *tur-ár* SÚD *ina* SÍG ḪÉ.ME.DA NIGIN-*mi ana* ŠÀ.TÙR-*šá* GAR-*an*

8. NUMUN ^{GIŠ}MA.NU NUMUN ^{Ú}*pu-qut-te* NUMUN ^{Ú}ŠAKIRA SÚD *ina* KAŠ NA[G]

---

9. DIŠ MUNUS Ì.KÚM GIG 1 *qa* DÈ ^{GIŠ}ÁSAL 1 *qa* DÈ ^{Ú}*am-ḫa-ra* ḪE.⌜ḪE⌝
10. 14 KEŠDA.MEŠ NÍG.MU$_4$ KEŠDA 1.TA.ÀM *ana* ŠÀ.TÙR-*šá* GAR-*an*

---

11. NUMUN ^{Ú}EME UR.GI$_7$ ^{Ú}NÍNDA $^{\text{NA}_4}$PEŠ$_4$.ANŠE *ta-sàk ana muš-tin-ni-ša* DUB-*ak*

---

12. Ú BABBAR *ta-sàk ina* Ì+GIŠ ḪE.ḪE *ina* MUD ZABAR *ana muš-tin-ni-ša* DUB-*ak*

---

13. ^{Ú}IN.NU.UŠ ḪÁD.DU SÚD *ina* KAŠ NAG NU.LUḪ.ḪA ḪÁD.DU SÚD *ina* KAŠ NAG

---

14. NUMUN *pú-qut-te* ḪÁD.DU SÚD *ina* KAŠ NAG SI DÀRA.MAŠ ḪÁD. DU SÚD *ina* KAŠ NAG

---

15. [DIŠ MUNUS *a*]*l-lu-tú* GIG KA.A.AB.BA *ta-sàk* ^{SÍG}ÀKA NIGIN *ana* ŠÀ.TÙR-*šá* GAR-*an*
16. [… *t*]*a-sàk* ^{SÍG}ÀKA NIGIN *ana* ŠÀ.TÙR-*šá* GAR-*an*
17. […]x RA SÚD ^{SÍG}ÀKA NIGIN IM.SAḪAR.NA$_4$.KUR.RA SÚD $^{\text{SÍ[G]}}$ÀKA NIGIN
18. [P]A ^{GIŠ}NU.ÚR.MA SÚD ^{SÍG}ÀKA NIGIN BAR ^{GIŠ}*al-la-an* SÚD $^{\text{SÍ[G]}}$ÀKA NIGIN
19. KA.MÚRGU! LÚ.U$_{19}$.LU SÚD ^{SÍG}ÀKA NIGIN TÚG GI$_6$ *tur-ár* SÚD ^{SÍG}ÀKA NIGIN ‹PA›.PA-*a-n*[*u tu*]*r-ár* SÚD
20. ^{SÍG}ÀKA NIGIN ^{GIŠ}ŠINIG *tur-ár* SÚD ^{SÍG}ÀKA NIGIN NUMUN ^{Ú}KI.^{d}I[M] *tur-ár* SÚD
21. ^{SÍG}ÀKA NIGIN NUMUN ^{GIŠ}ŠE.NU *tur-ár* SÚD ^{SÍG}ÀKA NIGIN DÈ[5] ^{GIŠ}Á[SA]L *ta-sàk*
22. ^{SÍG}ÀKA NIGIN DÈ ^{GIŠ}ERIN SÚD ^{SÍG}ÀKA NIGIN DÈ ^{Ú}NÚMUN [SÚD] ^{SÍG}ÀKA NI[GIN]
23. DÈ ^{Ú}*a-la-me-e ta-sàk* ^{SÍG}ÀKA NIGIN ŠIKA SÁḪAR SÚD ^{SÍG}ÀKA NIGIN NUN[UZ G]A.NU$_{11}$$^{\text{[MUŠEN]}}$
24. SÚD ^{SÍG}ÀKA NIGIN NUMUN ^{GIŠ}ESI *ta-qàl-lu* SÚD ^{SÍG}ÀKA NIGIN *ga-bi* [… SÚD]
25. ^{SÍG}ÀKA NIGIN BI.RI GUD IZI *qal-liš tu-kal-lam* ^{Ú}ḪAR.ḪAR ⌜Ú⌝[…]
26. 1-*niš* SÚD *ina* KAŠ NAG ILLU *a-bu-ka-tum* SÚD *ina* KAŠ NAG ^{Ú}*im-ḫur-lim* ^{Ú}[*im-ḫur*-20]

27. SÚD *ina* KAŠ NAG NUMUN GI.ZÚ.LUM SÚD ^{SÍG}ÀKA NIGIN Ì.UDU [...]
28. ^{SÍG}ÀKA NIGIN *ana* ŠÀ.TÙR-*šá ina* [...] x

---

29. DIŠ MUNUS Ú.ḪI.A *ze-ru-te šu-ku-ul* A.MEŠ *ina* ŠÀ GAL$_4$.LA-*šá ma-gal* DU-*ku* [...] TUKU-*ú*
30. *ana* ⸢*ša*⸣ GIG-*ša* NU GÍD.DA BÍL.LÁ ^{Ú}*ur-ba-te* GÌR.PAD.DU *tur-ár* NA[$_4$ ...]x *ta-qa-lu*
31. GURUN ^{GIŠ}*ṣa-da-ni* LAG A.ŠÀ.GA SUḪUŠ ^{Ú}*qúl-qúl-li-a-ni* 6 Ú[.ḪI.A *an-n*]*u-ti*
32. TÉŠ.BI *tuš-te-med ana* 15-*šú ni-ba ina* TÚG.ḪI.A *ḫal-li tu*-[*šar*]-*kas*
33. 1.TA.ÀM *ana* ŠÀ GAL$_4$.LA-*šá* GAR-*an-ma* A[.MEŠ TAR]-*su*

---

34. DIŠ KI.MIN *ma-áš-qi-sa* UGU *ku-pi-ti* UGU UGA$^{\text{⸢MUŠEN⸣}}$ [...] BAR ^{GIŠ}KÍN
35. NUNUZ KIŠI$_9$ SA$_5$ Ì.UDU BAR.GÙN.NA[6] KUR-*i ša* ZAG.LU ŠIKA SILA.LÍM ⸢Ì⸣.[UDU... GÌR.PAD.D]U BA.AL.GI
36. ^{ŠEM}LI ^{Ú}*imḫur-lim* KA.A.AB.BA ^{Ú}AN.KI.NU.DI SUḪUŠ ^{GIŠ}[...] ⸢SUḪUŠ⸣ ^{Ú}ḪAR.ḪAR
37. SUḪUŠ ^{GIŠ}GI.ZÚ.LUM.MA *pa-pa-si*-^{d}ÍD SUḪUŠ ^{Ú}KU$_6$ *ku-li-l*[*i*[7] ...] ⸢Ì⸣. UDU ^{ŠEM}GIG
38. 25 Ú.ḪI.A *an-nu-ti* TÉŠ.BI SÚD *ina* KAŠ NU *pa-tan* NAG-*ši-m*[*a* A.] MEŠ-*šá* TAR-⸢*su*⸣

---

39. DIŠ KI.MIN *tu-ka-ṣar-ši* $^{\text{NA}_4}$*ḫal-ta* $^{\text{NA}_4}$ŠUBA Á.ZI.DA $^{\text{NA}_4}$ŠU[BA] ⸢Á⸣. [GÙB.BA...]
40. ⸢$^{\text{NA}_4}$⸣GUG *ša* MÚD *la-tik-ta* 7 *ḫi-ir-ṣi šá* ^{GIŠ}MA.NU *tu-pa-la-áš* [...]
41. [KEŠD]A.KEŠDA-*ma ina* SÍG ḪÉ.ME.DA SÍG BABBAR *tu-šá-kak* 7 KEŠDA.MEŠ *ta-ka-ṣa-ar* [...]
42. [ÉN *k*]*i-a-am* ŠID-*nu* ÉN *šal-lu-ur-za* KEŠDA DAM.GAL.LA KUR *šal-l*[*u-ur-za* ...]
43. [... *ḫar-ra-g*]*i-ri ḫar-ra-gi-ri ḫar-ra-gi-ri šá-ḫi-ma-za-a-te* x [...]

---

44. [KA.INIM.MA DIŠ MUNUS A].⸢MEŠ⸣ *ina* ŠÀ GAL$_4$.LA-*šá* DU-[*ku*]

TRANSLATION

(i 1′–3′) (For irregular bleeding), you grind together these twenty plants: [...] *kalû*-mineral, *kalgukku*-mineral, ⸢alum⸣, magnetic hematite, [silver], gold, black *anzaḫḫu*-frit (and) tongue of a fieldmouse. You mix (it) with honey, ghee and calf fat. You recite the recitation three times over it and then you rub (it) gently on her umbilical area (and) the mouth of her vulva.

(i 4′–8′) You thread these nine stones: *ḫaltu*-stone, right handed *šubû*-stone, left-handed *šubû*-stone, male and female *šû*-stone, blood red carnelian, *kapāṣu*-shell, *ianibu*-stone (and) *zibtu*-stone on red-dyed wool, lapis wool, carded wool, tendons from a dead cow, tendons from a male and female gazelle, male *ašlu*-rush (and) *daʾmātu*-clay which you have twined together. You tie seven and seven knots. You wind "lone plant" and *tullal* seed into burls with red-dyed wool between the knots and the stones. You recite the recitation over it three times and bind (it) on her hips.

(i 9′–16′) You take an upstanding potsherd from a crossroads. You wash (it) with water, rub (it) with oil (and) wrap (it) in red-dyed wool. You put it in the house, behind the door in an isolated place. Below the house, you sprinkle her with (some of the wash) water. You set out a censer (burning) juniper and *atāʾišu* for her. That woman[8] kneels so as to put her hands behind her. You recite the recitation three times. She utters a *šegû* prayer three times (but) does not prostrate herself. When you have completed this, you put out *mersu*-confection (made with) honey and ghee. You pour out a libation. (Then), she prostrates herself. You keep doing this for three days. You have her drink the ⸢potion⸣. You gently rub the salve on her. You bind the stones on her. On the fourth day, you scatter *sīḫu*-wormwood, *argannu* (and) *barirātu* before the door. That woman utters a *šegû* prayer before the door. She utters a *šegû* prayer before Ishtar. If you recite the recitation three times, she [should get well].

(i 17′) Recitation for a woman who is sick with *naḫšātu* (irregular bleeding).[9] This is a [tested] treatment.

(i 18′–20′) Recitation: Goddess of heaven and earth at the same time. Ishtar is a *lagallu* priestess, an impetuous one, a *šugallitu*,[10] an impetuous one, a pure one, [...], a goddess and of heaven and earth at the same time, knotter of heaven. Spell and Recitation.

(i 21′) Recitation for a woman who is sick with *naḫšātu* (irregular bleeding).

(i 22′–24′) Its ritual: You have a woman past childbearing age twine together male *ašlu*-rush, red-dyed wool (and) tendons from a dead cow. You ⸢tie⸣ fourteen knots. You wrap *atbar*-stone in red-dyed wool behind the knots. You position the knots below her lower abdominal (hypogastric) region. If you bind (it) on her hips, the irregular bleeding should stop.

(i 25′) You char (and) grind date stone, wrap (it) in a tuft of wool and insert (it) into her vagina.

(i 26′–27′) You scatter "human bone" over coals. You have that woman sit over it (so that) her waters flow onto it. It they do not stop, you have her sit (over it) again. Ditto (The irregular bleeding should stop.)

(i 28′–29′) You pour *illūru* (and) dust which you have taken from the track of a chariot wheel into first-quality beer. You let (it) sit out overnight under the stars. In the morning, [if] you have [her] drink (it) on an empty stomach, the *naḫšātu* (irregular bleeding) should stop.

(i 30′) You grind *illūru*. (If) you have her drink (it mixed) with beer, ditto[11] (the irregular bleeding should stop)

(i 31′) You twine together red-dyed wool (and) tendons from a dead cow. You wind iron (and) *atbar*-stone into burls. (If) [you bind it] on her hips, ⸢ditto⸣ (the irregular bleeding should stop).

(i 32′) You grind *nuḫurtu*. (If) you have her drink (it mixed) with beer, ditto (the irregular bleeding should stop).

(i 33′) You grind "white" alum (and) wrap (it) in a tuft of wool. (If) you insert (it) into her vagina, ditto (the irregular bleeding should stop)

(i 34′) You grind *summatu*-dove egg (and) wrap (it) in a tuft of wool. (If) you insert it into her vagina, ditto (the irregular bleeding should stop).

(i 35′) You grind *sukanninu*-turtledove egg (and) wrap (it) in a tuft of wool. (If) you insert (it) into her vagina, ditto (the irregular bleeding should stop).

(i 36′) You grind "black" and "white" alum (and) wrap (it) in a tuft of wool. (If) you insert (it) into her vagina, ditto (the irregular bleeding should stop).

(i 37′) You grind *imḫur-ešra* (var: *imḫur-lim*). (If) you have her drink (it mixed) with beer, ditto (the irregular bleeding should stop).

(i 38′) You roast a goat horn that curls (and) char *elpetu*-rush. (If) you have her drink (it mixed) with beer, ditto (the irregular bleeding should stop).

(i 39′) You wind *maštakal* (and) *agargarītu*-sulphur in red-dyed wool (and) white wool. You sprinkle (it with) powdered *atbar*-basalt. (If) you insert (it) into her vagina, ditto (the irregular bleeding should stop).

(i 40′–42′) You grind obsidian (flecked) carnelian (variant: carnelian) (and) *kapaṣu*-shell. (If) you have her drink (it mixed) with first-quality beer, ditto (the irregular bleeding should stop). You grind *atbar*-stone (and) *maštakal* seed. You wrap (it) in red-dyed wool (and) tendons from a dead cow (and) tie (it) on her hips or you (wrap it in a tuft of wool and) insert (it) into her vagina. Ditto (The irregular bleeding should stop).

(i 43′–44′) You grind *kibrītu*-sulphur, "white" alum, "black" alum, alum (and) black *anzaḫḫu*-frit (variant: *anzaḫḫu*-frit) (and) wrap (it) in a tuft of wool. (If) you insert (it) into her vagina, ditto (the irregular bleeding should stop).

(i 45′–46′) You grind magnetic hematite, iron, *lulû*-antimony, *urizu*-stone, *kapaṣu*-shell, *šû*-stone (and) *ayartu*-coral (and) wrap (it) in a tuft of wool. (If) you insert (it) into her vagina, ditto (the irregular bleeding should stop).

(i 47′–48′) You thread seven colored *ayartu*-coral, iron, *ziktum*-stone, SAG. GIL.MUD-stone (and) *maštakal* seed onto tendons from a dead cow (and) tendons from a dead sheep. You tie fourteen knots. (If) you bind (it) on her hips, ditto (the irregular bleeding should stop).

(columns ii and iii are badly preserved)

(iv 1) (For irregular bleeding), you grind *azallû* seed, *nīnû*-mint (and) *azupīru* (and) [have her drink] (it mixed) with beer.

(iv 2) You char (and) grind datepalm root, *bīnu*-tamarisk root (and) *ašāgu*-thorn root. You wrap (it) in lapis colored wool (and) insert (it) into her vagina.

(iv 3) You have her drink *da*ʾ*mātu*-clay, "gold clay," *kalû*-clay, (and) alum (mixed) with beer.

(iv 4) You grind *šūšu*-licorice seed, *nuḫurtu* (and) *burāšu*-juniper (and) have her drink (it mixed) with beer.

(iv 5) You grind *ašāgu*-thorn root, *baltu*-thorn root, (and) male *pillû* root (and) have her drink (it mixed) with beer.

(iv 6–7) You char (and) grind *kamun bīni*-fungus, a *ḫamītu*-wasp, a *pizzal-urtu*-gecko (and) lizard droppings. You wrap (it) in red-dyed wool (and) insert (it) into her vagina.

(iv 8) You grind *e*ʾ*ru*-tree seed, *puquttu*-thorn seed (and) *šakirû* seed (and) ⌈have her drink⌉ (it mixed) with beer.

(iv 9–10) If a woman is sick with puerperal fever, you mix 1 *qû* of ashes of *ṣarbātu*-poplar (and) 1 *qû* of ashes of *amḫaru*. You tie fourteen knots in worn rags (and sprinkle them with the mixture). You insert them one by one into her vagina.

(iv 11) You grind *lišān kalbi* seed, *illūru*, (and) *biṣṣur atāne*-shell (and) pour it into her urethra.

(iv 12) You grind "white plant," mix (it) with oil (and) pour (it) into her urethra by means of a bronze tube.

(iv 13) You dry (and) grind *maštakal* (and) have her drink (it mixed) with beer. You dry (and) grind *nuḫurtu* (and) have her drink (it mixed) with beer.

(iv 14) You dry (and) grind *puquttu*-thorn seed (and) have her drink (it mixed) with beer. You dry (and) grind stag horn (and) have her drink (it mixed) with beer.

(iv 15–28) [If a woman] is sick with ⌈crabs⌉,[12] you grind *imbû tamtim*, wrap (it) in a tuft of wool (and) insert (it) into her vagina. ⌈You grind⌉ […], wrap (it) in a tuft of wool (and) insert (it) into her vagina. You grind ⌈*nīnû*-mint?⌉ (and) wrap (it) in a tuft of wool. You grind alum (and) wrap (it) in a tuft of wool. You grind *nurmû*-pomegranate ⌈leaves⌉ (and) wrap (it) in a tuft of wool. You grind *allānu*-oak bark (and) wrap (it) in a tuft of wool. You grind a human vertebra (and) wrap (it) in a tuft of wool. You char (and) grind a black cloth (and) wrap (it) in a tuft of wool. You ⸢char⸣ (and) grind *arariānu*(?) (and) wrap (it) in a tuft of wool. You char (and) grind *bīnu*-tamarisk (and) wrap (it) in a tuft of wool. You char (and) grind *qutru* seed (and) wrap (it) in a tuft of wool. You char (and) grind *šunû*-chastetree seed (and) wrap (it) in a tuft of wool. You grind *ṣarbātu*-poplar ashes (and) wrap (it) in a tuft of wool. You grind *erēnu*-cedar ashes (and) wrap (it) in a tuft of wool. You [grind] *elpetu*-rush ashes (and) ⸢wrap⸣ (it) in a tuft of wool. You grind *alamû* ashes (and) wrap (it) in a tuft of wool. You grind a fragment of a porous water jar (and) wrap (it) in a tuft of wool. You grind an ⸢ostrich egg⸣ (and) wrap (it) in a tuft of wool. You roast (and) grind *ušû*-tree seed (and) wrap (it) in a tuft of wool. You grind [...] (and) wrap (it) in a tuft of wool.

You grind together ox spleen that you have lightly exposed to fire, *ḫašû*-thyme, (and) [...] (and) have her drink (it mixed) with beer. You grind *abukkatu* resin (and) have her drink (it mixed) with beer. You grind *imḫur-lim* (and) [*imḫur-ešra*] (and) have her drink (it mixed) with beer.

You grind *buṣinnu* seed (and) wrap (it) in a tuft of wool. [You grind ...] fat, wrap (it) in a tuft of wool (and) insert (it) into her vagina. [...]

(iv 29–33) If a woman has been given plants of hatred to eat (and) much fluid runs from her vagina (and) she has [...] in order that her illness not be prolonged,[13] you meld together ⸢these⸣ six plants: *emṣu*-sourdough,[14] *urbātu*-rush, bone which you have charred, [...]-stone which you have roasted, *ṣadānu* fruit, *kirbān eqli*, (and) *qulquliānu* root. You tie fifteen-count[15] (knots) in a loincloth (and sprinkle them with the mixture). If you insert (them) one by one into her vagina, the fluid should ⸢stop⸣.

(iv 34–38) Alternatively, her potion (is the following). You grind together these twenty-five plants: *kupītu*-bird skull, *āribu*-crow skull, [...], *kiškānu*-tree bark, red ant eggs, "fat" of a wild multi-colored snake(?!) from the right side, potsherd from a crossroads, [...] fat, ⸢bone⸣ of a *raqqu*-tortoise, *burāšu*-juniper, *imḫur-lim*, *imbû tamtim*, *ankinūtu*, [...] root, *ḫašû*-thyme root, *buṣinnu* root, *pappasītu*-sulphur, *šimru* root, *kulīlu*-dragonfly, [...] (and) "fat" of *kanaktu*-aromatic. If you have her drink (it) on an empty stomach (mixed) with beer, her [fluid] should stop.

(iv 39–43) Alternatively, you tie knots for her. You thread *ḫaltu*-stone, right (and) [left] swirling *šubû*-stone, tested carnelian the color of blood, seven blocks of *eʾru*-tree which you have bored through (and) knotted [...] on red-dyed wool (and) white wool. You tie seven knots. [While you are tying them], you recite [a recitation] ⸢as follows⸣: Šallurza Bind! Queen ⸢Šallurza⸣ [...] ⸢*ḫarragiri*⸣ *harragiri harragiri šaḫimazate* [...].

(iv 44) [Recitation for cases where fluid] flows from a [woman's] vagina.[16]

2. PREGNANCY TESTS

TEXT 2: UET 7.123

UET 7.123 consists exclusively of pregnancy texts. The most usual variety involves examining a tampon (1–12) which has been left in the vagina overnight to look for color changes. It was also possible to test for queasy stomach with a potion (1–7). For more details, see Scurlock and Andersen 2005, 262.

obv.

1. […] 1/2 GÍN Ú.BABBAR 4-*tú* NA$_4$ *gab-u*
2. [… *ana* ŠÀ.T]ÙR-*šá* GAR-*an mu-šú gab-bi*
3. […]x-*nu-tú* LUḪ-*si ki-*⸢*i* SÍG⸣.ÀKA SA$_5$-*at lu* MÚD *ul-lu-ḫa-tú*
4. [MUNUS BI PEŠ$_4$ *k*]*i-i* SÍG.ÀKA *ši-i* SIG$_7$-*at* MUNUS BI NU PEŠ$_4$ *ki-i* ŠÀ-*bi* ŠÀ.TÙR-*šú*
5. […]-*šú ki pi-it* GÌR[17] *u-ṣi* GUR-*ma*[18] *dul-la-šá e-pu-uš me-ru-šú*
6. […] *maš-qit* NAG-*šú* ki x x x *su-ši maš-šit in-na-áš-šú* GÚR.GÚR
7. LI ḪAR.ḪAR NU.LUḪ.ḪA *u* ILLU ⸢LI.TAR⸣ 2-*šú* 3-*šú* NAG *ù* ḪAL-*šú* PEŠ$_4$

---

8. DIŠ KI.MIN SULLIM^{SAR} *ina* SÍG.ÀKA NIGIN-*mi ana* [ŠÀ].TÙR-*šá* GA 3 U$_4$ ÍL-*ši-ma*
9. *šúm-ma* SULLIM^{SAR} GIN$_7$ ŠEŠ *ib-tar-rù* MUNUS BI PEŠ$_4$

---

10. DIŠ KI.MIN Ú.BABBAR NAGA.SI *ina* SÍG.ÀKA NIGIN-*mi ana* ŠÀ.TÙR-*šá* GAR 3 U$_4$ ÍL-*ma*
11. *ina šal-šú* U$_4$-*me* SÍG.ÀKA *ina* A LUḪ-*si šúm-ma* SÍG.ÀKA […]
12. *šúm-ma* SÍG.ÀKA SIG$_7$ SA$_5$? ZÁLAG MUNUS BI […]

---

13. DIŠ KI.MIN NA$_4$ *gab-u Mi-ṣir-a-a* x […]
14. *lu* ILLU.ME IGI.IGI MUNUS BI […]
15. ⸢LI⸣ NAGA ZÁLAG-*ma* […]

rev.

1′. […]-*šú* SA$_5$ SU-*šú* x […]

2′. […] un gi is sa nu […]

3′. [o o o] x NU SUM-*su* 1 *šá* GÚR.GÚR SIG$_7$ *k*[*ab-ba-ra*? o]x *šá* É ni […]

4′. 2.⸢TA⸣.ÀM DÈ *ina* A SILA$_{11}$ *tu-kap-par*$_5$ DUḪ.LÀL Ì *ḫal-ṣa ta-sal-làḫ-ma* ‹‹*ma*›› ⸢GIN$_7$?⸣ SUD

5′. 1-*šú* 2-*šú* 3-*šú ana* ŠÀ.TÙR-*šá* GAR-*an* NITA-*šú* NU TE-*šú a-di*

U$_4$.2.KÁM* EGIR *šá iz-zi-zu*

6′. *mím-ma gáb-bi* NU SUM-*su šá qer-bit-si* ZI-*ḫu u* SAL.ŠÀ.ZU LÁ-*šú mál-tak-ta-šú*

7′. *ki-i* PEŠ$_4$ *u ki-i* NU PEŠ$_4$ Ú *ú-sa-bu ina* IZI ⸢BÍL⸣ *a-na di-ik-me-en-na* GUR-*ru*

8′. *ina* Ì *ḫal-ṣa* KÚM SÚD *tu-lam lu ina* A *tu-kap-par*$_5$ 1 *maš-šit* DÙ-*uš ma-la* BURU$_{14}$-*tú*[19]

9′. *ta-máṣ-ṣi ki-i* ŠURUN-*su saḫ-pu-ma ta-at-tar-ṣu-uš u maš-šit šá* GÚR.GÚR SIG$_7$

10′. *kab-ba-ra šá iṭ-pu-pu ta-ad-da-áš-šum-ma iz-zi-zu maš-šit* AN.TA

11′. SUM-*šum-ma* ÍL-*ši ki-i* ŠURUN-*su maš-šit i-man-za-qu u ina* IGI A.MEŠ *ta-at-tam-ḫa-ḫu*

12′. [MUNUS.B]I PEŠ$_4$ *ki-i maš-šit bal-ṭa-tú u ru-bu-us-su la-man-za-qu ul* PEŠ$_4$

13′. [o o ŠURU]N-*su na-ṭi-pè-e ki-i la saḫ-pa maš-šit šá* GÚR.GÚR SIG$_7$ *kab-ba-ra*

14′. [*šá iṭ-pu-pu š*]*u-a-tú* SUM-*su u* [*mal-ta*]*k-tú ta-lat-tak* GABA.RI 1-*en* GIŠ.DA

15′. [...-T]U.TU ZI-*ḫi*

Translation

(obv. 1–7) You [wrap] one half shekel "white plant," a quarter shekel alum (and) [one shekel *tarmuš* in a tuft of wool]. You insert (it) [into] her ⸢vagina⸣. [She keeps it in place] all night. [The next morning], (you take it out and) you wash (it). If the tuft of wool is red or streaked with blood red, [that woman is pregnant]. If that tuft of wool is green, that woman is not pregnant.[20]

If the inside of her vagina is [...] and her [...] protrudes when she is walking, do her workup over again. Her pregnancy is [...]. You have her drink the potion. If [...] her, a tampon should be worn. You have her drink *kukru*, *burāšu*-juniper, *ḫašû*-thyme, *nuḫurtu*, (and) ⸢*abukkatu*⸣ resin ‹once›, twice, (or) three times. If she vomits, she is pregnant.[21]

(obv. 8–9) Alternatively, you wrap *šambaliltu*-fenugreek in a tuft of wool and insert (it) into her ⸢vagina⸣. She wears it for three days and then, if the *šambaliltu*-fenugreek is speckled like myrrh/*šegušša*-cereal,[22] that woman is pregnant.

(obv. 10–12) Alternatively, you wrap "white plant" (and) *uḫḫūlu qarnānu* in a tuft of wool and insert (it) into her vagina. She wears (it) for three days and then, on the third day, you wash the tuft of wool with water. If the tuft of wool is [..., she is ...]. If the tuft of wool is green, red? and shiny, that woman [is ...].

(obv. 13–15) Alternatively, [you wrap] Egyptian alum and [… If …] or exudation is repeatedly seen, that woman […]. If the *burāšu*-juniper and *uḫḫūlu* look brighter (in color) […].

(rev. 1′–15′) [If …] her […] is red and her body is […] is not to be given to her. [You make] one (tampon) of fresh thick *kukru* from […]. In two batches, you make ashes into a dough with water. (With one batch), you wipe (her) off. (The other batch), you sprinkle with honey (and) pressed-out oil and, when you have sprinkled (it), you insert (it) once, twice, three times into her vagina. Her man should not approach her. For two days afterward,[23] nothing whatsoever should be given to her; they should remove whatever is inside her and the midwife should keep watch over her. (This is) her test to see whether she is pregnant or not pregnant.

You roast *usābu*-plant over a fire. You reduce (it) to ashes. You grind (it and) soften (it) in hot pressed-out oil or (you make it into a dough) with water. You wipe (her) off (with it). You make a tampon; you may use as much as you wish.

If her womb looks abnormal (lit. has "turned over/fallen flat on its face") so that she (lies) stretched out, then you give her the tampon of fresh *kukru* as thick as necessary to fill her up and afterwards you give her the above tampon (of ashes) and she wears it.

If her womb sucks the tampon and it is softened by the waters, [that woman] is pregnant. If the tampon stays in its original condition and her womb does not suck (it), she is not pregnant; [the fruit of] her ⸢womb⸣ has been plucked out.

If (her womb) looks normal (lit. has not "turned over/fallen flat on its face"), you give her the aforementioned tampon of fresh *kukru* as thick [as necessary to fill her up] and you perform the ⸢test⸣.

Copy of a writing board. Excerpted by […]-Marduk.

What is interesting about the reverse of this text is that the writer keeps going back over material already covered, as if he were writing this in haste as the situation developed. Rearranged so that it actually makes sense, rev. 1′–15′ reads as follows:

[If …] her […] is red and her body is […] is not to be given to her.

[You make] one (tampon) of fresh thick *kukru* from […]. (This is) her test to see whether she is (still) pregnant or no (longer) pregnant. If her womb sucks the tampon and it is softened by the waters, [that woman] is (still) pregnant. If the tampon stays in its original condition and her womb does not suck (it), she is no (longer) pregnant; [the fruit of] her ⸢womb⸣ has been plucked out.

If (her womb) looks normal (lit. has not "turned over/fallen flat on its face"), you give her the aforementioned tampon of fresh *kukru* as thick [as necessary to fill her up] and you perform the ⌜test⌝.

If her womb looks abnormal (lit. has "turned over/fallen flat on its face") so that she (lies) stretched out, then you give her the tampon of fresh *kukru* as thick as necessary to fill her up and (after)wards you give her the following tampon and she wears it. You roast *usābu*-plant over a fire. You reduce (it) to ashes. In two batches, you grind (it) and soften the ashes in hot pressed-out oil or you make the ashes into a dough with water. (With one batch), you wipe (her) off. (The other batch), you make a tampon; you may use as much as you wish. You sprinkle (it) with honey (and) pressed-out oil and, when you have sprinkled (it), you insert (it) once, twice, three times into her vagina. Her man should not approach her. For two days afterwards, nothing whatsoever should be given to her; they should remove what is inside her and the midwife should keep watch over her.

The situation described is of a woman whose pregnancy has gone wrong. The doctors do not know whether she has had a miscarriage, which is why a pregnancy test is being administered. If her womb has not "turned over/fallen flat on its face" (i.e., everything seems normal), then she has either lost the child or is still pregnant. However, there may be clear indications of something more seriously wrong in the womb. In this case, the woman and her womb need to be disinfected with ashes. In addition, if she is still pregnant, the pregnancy will need to be terminated. As with ancient Roman practice (followed by Islamic law), the priority of the doctor was the mother's life, not that of the foetus.

B. OBSTETRICS

1. MISCARRIAGES

For details on problems experienced during pregnancy including miscarriages, see Scurlock and Andersen 2005, 268–69.

TEXT 3: BAM 235

BAM 235 consists of vaginal suppositories (1–3, 7–9), a potion (4–6) and an amulet (10–18) to stop a woman from bleeding. Lines 1–3 and 7–9 contemplate what appears to be spotting—small amounts of bright blood. The woman of lines 4–6 was "hit with a weapon," probably literally and in the stomach while pregnant. The desire, then, is to prevent miscarriage. Lines 10–18 have a very charming recitation about this problem. Marduk is invoked in his capacity as patron of childbirth. The carnelian, lapis and plants mentioned in the recitation will have been used in the broken treatments that end the passage.

1. [x] šu GU-*šá pe-lu-*[*ti* DU-*ku* …]
2. $^{[N]A_4}$KUR-*nu* DIB SÚD *ina* ^{SÍG}ÀKA NIGIN-*mi ana* ŠÀ.T[ÙR-*šá* GAR-*an-ma*]
3. [MÚ]D.MEŠ-*šá* T[AR-*su*]

---

4. [DIŠ M]UNUS ^{GIŠ}TUKUL *maḫ-ṣa-at* MÚD BURU$_5$.[ḪABRUD.DA]
5. ⸢Ú⸣NU.LUḪ.ḪA 1-*niš* SÚD *ina* KAŠ NAG-*ši* […]
6. [NÍG].NA GAR-*an še-gu-ú i-šá-si-m*[*a* …]

---

7. [x] šá GU-*šá pe-lu-ti* DU-*ku* ni iḫ […]
8. [^{NA_4}AN].ZAḪ ^{Ú}NÚMUN 14 *rik-si* […]
9. [1.T]A.ÀM *ana* ŠÀ GAL$_4$.LA-*šá* GAR-*an* […]

---

10. [TU]$_6$! ÉN ^{NA_4}GUG MÚD-*šá a-tap* ^{NA_4}G[UG]
11. [*ina ta*]-*mir-ti*[24] ^{NA_4}GUG A.MEŠ [(*ub-ba-lu*)]
12. [(*man*)]-*nu liq-bi ana re-mi-ni-i* ^{d}AM[(AR.UTU)]
13. [*ina t*]*a-mir-ti* ^{NA_4}GUG [(*li-is-ki-ru*)]

13a. ‹(ÍLDAG ^{NA_4}ZA.GÌN [*i-sek-ki-ru*] *aš-la ub-bal*)›

---

14. [K]A.INIM.MA MÚD MUNUS [(TAR-*si*)]

---

15. [DÙ.(D)]Ù.BI SÍG BABBAR SÍG SA$_5$ ⸢1-*niš*⸣ NU.NU 7 KEŠ[(DA KEŠDA)]
16. [(^{GIŠ}ḪA)]B^{SAR} ŠUB ‹(*e-ma* KA.KEŠDA)› ÉN 7-*šú* ŠID-*n*[(*u*)] *ina* MURUB$_4$-[(*šá* KEŠDA-*ma ina-aš*)]
17. […] *ina* ^{SÍG}ÀKA […]
18. […] ^{NA_4}KA.G[I.NA.DIB.BA …]

---

19. […] ur ma MÚD […]
20. […] x x x […]

TRANSLATION

(1–3) [If ..] her vein(s) [let flow] bright red (blood) [...] you grind magnetic hematite (and) wrap (it) in a tuft of wool. [If you insert (it)] into [her] ⸢vagina⸣, her ⸢blood⸣ should ⸢stop⸣.

(4–6) [If] a ⸢woman⸣ was struck with a weapon, you grind together *ḫurri*-bird blood (and) *nuḫurtu* and have her drink (it mixed) with beer. You set up a ⸢censer⸣ [burning ...]. If she utters a *šêgu*-prayer, [...].

(7–9) [If ...] her vein(s) let flow bright red (blood) [...], [you make] fourteen strings of [...], ⸢*anzaḫḫu*⸣-frit (and) *ašlu*-rush. [...] You insert (them] into her vagina [one] ⸢by one⸣.

(10–13) ⸢Spell⸣ (and) Recitation: Carnelian (color) (is) her blood. Will they dry up the waters [in] the carnelian ⸢*tamirtu*-irrigation district⸣ (with) a ⸢carnelian⸣ branch canal? ⸢Who⸣ can tell (it) to merciful Marduk? Let them dam up the carnelian ⸢*tamirtu*-irrigation district⸣! ‹(*Adāru*-wood, (and) lapis lazuli, [will dam up the canal]; *ašlu*-rush will dry up the waters)›.[25]

(14) ⸢Recitation⸣ for stopping a woman's bleeding.

(15–18) Its ⸢ritual⸣: You twine together white wool (and) red wool. You tie seven ⸢knots⸣. You dribble *ḫurātu* (on the knots). ‹Whenever (you tie one of the) knots›, you recite the recitation seven times. If you tie (it) on her hip region, she should recover. [You wrap ...] in a tuft of wool [...] ⸢magnetic hematite⸣ [...].

(19–20) (*fragmentary*)

TEXT 4: SpTU 3.84:56–78

SpTU 3 no. 84 is concerned with sorcery. Among the problems potentially caused by a witch was miscarriage. This text contains a salve (56–57), ritual (58), and amulet (59–61) for this problem.

The potsherd of line 58 is standing on edge at a crossroads to signal obstruction, meaning that the baby will not be able to leave the womb prematurely. Burying it at the inner threshold will prevent evil influences from crossing into the house. The amulet of lines 59–61 is accompanied by a charming recitation addressed to the baby. Lines 62–77 raise an issue which is often dealt with separately, namely the miscarriage-causing demoness Lamashtu. In this case, the witch seems to have put the patient in Lamashtu's way.

56. *ana* ^{MUNUS}PEŠ$_4$ UŠ$_{11}$.ZU NU TE-*ma ša* ŠÀ-*šá* NU *na*!-*de*-⸢*e*⸣ [(^{NA_4}KUR-*nu* DIB KUG.GAN SAḪAR ^{NA_4}ŠUBA *ù* ^{GIŠ}GEŠTIN.KA$_5$.A ḪÁD.DU SÚD)]

57. *ina* MÚD BURU$_5$.ḪABRUD.DA NÍTA *ina* Ì ^{GIŠ}ŠUR.MÌN ḪE.ḪE-*ma* U[(GU ŠÀ-*ša em-ši-ša ù* SAG.DU-*sa* ŠÉŠ-*ma kiš-pu* NU T)E-*ši*]

---

58. DIŠ KI.MIN ŠIKA SILA.LÍMMU.BA *za-qip-ti* TI-*qí-ma* ‹*ina*› KUN$_4$ *b*[*ít*-(*a-ni-tú te-te-mer-ma* GABA *kiš-pi tur-rat*)]

---

59. DIŠ KI.MIN $^{\text{NA}_4}$*šu-u* NÍTA *u* MUNUS *ina* ŠU^{II} 15-*šú* KEŠDA ÉN *a-šib ek-let* [(3-*šú ana* UGU ŠID)-*n*(*u-ma kiš-pu* NU TE.MEŠ-*šú*)]

---

60. ÉN *a-šib ek-let la a-mi-ru* ZÁLAG ^{d}UTU-*ši* È-*am-ma* I[GI(-*m*)*a*(*r* ZÁ)LA(G ^{d}UTU)-*ši*]
61. *lu-u né-ḫe-e-ti* GIN$_7$ A.ME *a-gam-me lu-u ṣal-la-ta* GIN$_7$ *ár-m*⸢*é-e*⸣ [(*šá* MAŠ.DÀ EN *i-nap-pa-ḫu* ^{d}UTU *pa-šìr*)-*k*(*a*) TU$_6$ É(N)]

---

62. ÉN *ez-ze-et šam-rat ì̀l-at na-mur-rat u ši-i bar-ba-rat* DU[(MU.MUNUS ^{d}*A-nu*)]
63. GÌR-*šá an*-[(*zu*)]-*ú* ŠU^{II}-*šá lu-ʾ-tú pa-an* UR.MAḪ *da-pi-nu pa-n*[(*u-šá šak*)-*nu*]
64. *iš-tu a*-⸢*pi*⸣ *i-lam-ma uš-šu-rat pi-rit-su bu-ut-tu-qa* [(*di-da-a-šu*)]
65. *kib-si* GUD *il-lak kib-si* UDU.NÍTA UŠ-*di ina* UZU *u* MÚD ŠU^{II}-[(*šá šak-na*)]
66. *a-pa-niš* KU$_4$-*ub ṣi-ra-niš i-ḫal-lu-up* É KU$_4$ É È *bi*-[(*la-ni*)]
67. DUMU.MEŠ-*ki-na lu-še-niq u* DUMU.MEŠ-*ki-na lut*-[(*tar-ra*)]
68. *ana* KA DUMU.MUNUS.MEŠ-*ki-nu lu-uš-tak-ka-nu tu-la-a iš-mé-ši-ma* É-[(*a* AD-*šá*)]
69. *am-ma-ki* DUMU.MUNUS ^{d}*A-nu mu-ut-tar-ra-at* LÚ-*ut-tum tal-ma-di*-[(*ma*)]
70. *am-ma-ki ina* UZU *u* MÚD ŠU^{II}-*ki šak-na am-ma-ki* É KU$_4$-*bi* É È
71. *mu-uḫ-ri šá* ^{LÚ}DAM.GÀR *qá-an-na-šú u ṣi-di-is*-[(*su*)]
72. *mu-uḫ-ri šá* ^{LÚ}SIMUG *si-mir si-mat* ŠU^{II}-*ki u* GÌR-*k*[(*i*)]
73. *mu-uḫ-ri šá* ^{LÚ}KÙ.DIM *in-ṣab-ti si-mat* GEŠTU^{II}-*ki*
74. *mu-uḫ-ri šá* ^{LÚ}BUR.GUL $^{\text{NA}_4}$GUG *si-mat* GÚ-*ki*
75. [(*mu-u*)]*ḫ-ri šá* ^{LÚ}NAGAR ^{GIŠ}GA.ZUM ^{GIŠ}BAL *du-di-it-ti šid-di*
76. [(*ù ki-ri-is*)]-*su si-mat qé-e-ki* : *ú-tam-mi-ki* ^{d}*A-nu* AD-*ki*
77. [(*An-tum* AMA)]-*ki ú-tam-mi-ki* ^{d}*É-a* DÙ-*ki* TU$_6$ ÉN

---

78. [(ÉN *an-ni*)]-*ti ana* UGU *nap-šal-ti* ŠID-*nu*

TRANSLATION

(56–57) If (you want) sorcery not to approach a pregnant woman, (and) for her not to have a miscarriage, you grind magnetite, *guḫlu*-antimony, dust, *šubû*-stone (and) dried "fox grape." You mix (it) with the blood of a male shelduck (and) cypress oil and, if you rub (it) on her heart, her hypogastric region and her (vulva's) "head," sorcery will not ⸢approach⸣ [her].

(58) Alternatively, you take a potsherd (found) standing on edge at a crossroads and, if you bury (it) in the inner threshold, sorcery will be kept at bay.

(59) Alternatively, you bind masculine and feminine *šû*-stone on her right hand. If you recite the recitation: "He who lives in the darkness" three times over it, the sorcery will not approach her.

(60–61) "He who lives in the darkness, never seeing the light of the Sun, you have come out and seen the sunlight. May you be as calm as swamp water; may you sleep like the kids of a gazelle, until the rising of the Sun who releases you (from sleep)." [Spell (and)] ⸢recitation⸣.

(62–77) Recitation: "She is furious, she is raging, she is a goddess, she is brilliant and she is a wolf, the daughter of Anu. Her foot is that of Anzu; her hands are dirty; her face has the appearance of the face of a ferocious lion. She comes up from the swamp and, as a result, her hair is loose, her *dīdu*-cloths are cut off. She walks in the tracks of oxen; she follows the tracks of sheep. Her hands are placed in flesh and blood. She comes in through the window; she slips in through the door pivot. She enters the house; she leaves the house, (saying): 'Bring me your sons so that I may suckle them and your children so that I may rear them; let me put the breast into the mouth of your daughters.' Ea, her 'father', heard her and (said): 'Instead, Daughter of Anu, directress of mankind, of your taking ‹(the bread of tears and wailing)›[26] as (your) provision and instead of having your hands laid in flesh and blood, instead of entering houses (and) leaving houses, receive from the merchant his *qannu* and his travel provisions; receive from the iron smith the bracelets appropriate to your hands and feet; receive from the silver smith the earrings appropriate to your ears; receive from the seal-cutter the carnelian appropriate to your neck; receive from the carpenter the comb, spindle, *tudittu*-pin,[27] distaff, and the *kirissu* appropriate to your thread. I have made you swear by Anu, your father, Antu, your mother, (and) Ea who created you." Spell and Recitation.

(78) You recite this recitation over the salve.

TEXT 5: FARBER 2014, PL. 9 (4R^{2} 56) ii 28–33 COMPLETED BY *LKU* 33

Surprisingly common in ancient Mesopotamia is a tendency to sympathize with demonic attackers. As may be gathered from this recitation, Lamashtu was an Elamite lady of very exalted parentage who got banished to the swamp for bad behavior. As we learn from lines 23–31, she caused miscarriages in the form of a fever. The descriptions of the symptoms of this fever ennumerated in diagnostic texts are consistent with typhoid, which is indeed responsible for a high miscarriage rate among pregnant women with the disease. For details, see Scurlock and Andersen 2005, 483–85.

Farber 2014, pl. 9 (4R^{2} 56) ii 28–33

ii

28. ÉN ^{d}DIM$_{10}$.ME DUMU.AN.NA MU.PÀD.DA DINGIR.RE.E.NE.KE$_{4}$
29. [(^{d}I)]N.NIN NIR.GÁL NIN SAG.GI$_{6}$.GA
30. [(ZI.AN.N)]A ḪÉ.PÀ ZI.KI.A ḪÉ.PÀ
31. [(*E-la-ma-t*)]*i ra-bu-ú up-ru-u-šá*
32. [(*iš-tu* GIŠ.GI *i-l*)]*am-ma šá-niš uṣ-ṣa-am-ma*
33. [(*ez-ze-et šam-rat*!) *g*]*a-aš-rat gaṣ-ṣa-at g*[(*áp*)]-*š*[(*á-at*)]
34. [(*i-la-at*)] *n*[(*a-mur-rat*)]

LKU 33

2′. [GÍR^{II}]-*šá An-zu-ú*(?) [ŠU-*s*(*u lu-*ʾ*u-ti*)]
3′. [...] ru ki *su-q*[*u*? ...(x *pu-uz-zu-ra-a*)*t*?]
4′. [GISSU B]ÀD *ma-an-za-zu-šú a*[(*s-kup-pa-tu*)*m* (*mu-šá-b*)*u-š*(*á*)]
5′. [*ar-ra-k*]*a*?-*a*? *ṣu-up-ra-šú u*[*l gu-ul-l*(*u-ba šá-ḫa-ta-šá*)]
6′. [*la*] ⸢*i*⸣-*šá-rat u qal-lat* DUMU.MUNUS ^{d}A[-*ni*(*m* x) o o (x *ri-tum* ši b)u?]
7′. [^{d}]⸢*A*⸣-*num* AD-*ša* ⸢^{d}⸣[(*An-tum* AMA-*š*)*á*-(*m*)*a*]
8′. [*i*]-*na ep-še-ti-šá la ba-na-a-t*[*i* (*u*)*l-tu* AN-(*e*)]
9′. ⸢*ú*⸣-*še-ri-du-niš-šim-ma ul i*[(*d-du-ú pa-rak-k*)*a*-(*šá ina* K)I?-*tim*]
10′. [*ka*]*p-pi šak-na-at-ma ki-ma li-l*[*i-ti*]
11′. ⸢*a*⸣-*na mu-ši mu-šá a-na ka-ṣa-a-ti ka-ṣa-a-t*[*i*]
12′. *i-tur a-na sin-niš-ti šá né-re-bu-šú pit-r*[*u-su*]
13′. ⸢DUMU⸣.MUNUS ^{d}*A-nim* U$_{4}$-*me-šam-ma e-ra-a-ti i-man-*[(*nu*)]
14′. [*ar-k*]*i a-li-da-a-ti it-ta-na-al-l*(*ak*)]
15′. [I(TU)]-*ši-na i-man-ni* U$_{4}$-*me-ši-na ina i-ga-ra uṣ-ṣ*[(*ar*)]
16′. *a-*[(*na*)] ⸢*a-li-da*⸣-*a-ti na-da-a-ti šip-tú*

17′. *b*[*i-l*]*a-a-ni* DUMU.MEŠ-*ki-na lu-še-niq*
18′. ⸢*a-na*⸣ KA DUMU.MUNUS.MEŠ-*ki-na tu-la-a lu-uš-tak-kan*
19′. ⸢*na-šat*⸣ *ina qa-ti-šá um-ma ku-uṣ-*‹(*ṣa*)› *ḫur-ba-šá* ‹(*ma-ma-a*)› *ma-la ta-pil-tim* ‹(*ka-tim-ta*)›
20′. *nab-li mu-ḫa-am-me-ṭu-ti ma-li zu-mur-ša*
21′. *az-zu-za-a i-zar-ri im-ta*
22′. *a-na šur-su-ru i-zar-ri im-ta*
23′. ⸢*i*⸣*-mat* MUŠ *i-mat-su i-mat* GÍR.⸢TAB⸣ *i-mat-su*
24′. [(GUR)]UŠ.MEŠ *šug-gu-šú ú-šag-ga-áš*
25′. KI.SIKIL.⸢MEŠ *ḫu*⸣*-ub-bu-lu ú-ḫa-bal*
26′. DUMU.MEŠ *nu-up-pu-ṣu ú-nap-*⸢*pa-aṣ*⸣
27′. ⸢*ba-tu-la-ti*⸣ *i-šaq-q*[(*a-a*! A.MEŠ *pu-uš-qí*)]
28′. [(*ana* É *pe-ti-i ir-ru-ub*)]
29′. [*ana*] ⸢É⸣ *ed-li i-*[(*ḫal-lu*)*-u*(*p ṣer-ra-niš*)]
30′. [*i-ḫal-lu-u*]*p*] *ṣe-ra-niš* G[A *im-ti ú-še-*(*naq ṣu-ḫa-ra*)]
31′. [MÚD] ⸢ŠÀ⸣*-bi-šú ip-ta-šá-áš pa-*[(*ni-šu/šá*)]
32′. [*šer-ru*] *i*!*-bak-ki ma-ka-le-e* [*i-*(*mat mu-ú-ti*)]
33′. [*La-maš*]*-tum ù La-ba-ṣi pa-ni-šú ip-š*[(*u-uš*)]
34′. [*ku-u*]*s-su ki-ḫu-le-e ina qa-ti-šú i*[(*ṣ-bat*)]
35′. [*e*]*-pi-ir ki-ḫu-le-e ina qa-ti-šú iš-bu-u*[(š)]
36′. [*šin-n*]*a* UR.GI$_7$ *šin-na-a-šá ṣu-up-ra a-re-e ṣu-up-ra-a-*[(*šá*)]
37′. [*šeb-ret*] ⸢*du-di*⸣*-it-ta-šá pe-ti tu-lu-šá*
38′. [*al-lu-ḫap-pu* ŠU].MEŠ-*šá ru-um-mu ki-rim-mu-šá*
39′. [*ina* GA (*mu-t*)]*i ru-um-mu-ka ir-ta-a-šá*
40′. [...] TUKU *ṣir-ti ina tu-le-e-šá*
41′. [...].MEŠ-*šú a-na* UGU *e-ra-a-tú bur-ra-tú* KA[(Š$_4$-*um*)]
42′. [... ED]IN *i-rap-pu-uš*
43′. [...] *ki-ma ṣu-ḫa-ru*
44′–45′. (very fragmentary; for the continuation see Farber 2014, 87–94)

Translation

Farber 2014, pl. 9 (4R^2 56) ii 28–34

(ii 28–34) Recitation: Lamaštu, daughter of Anu, by whom the gods swear, Inanna, trustworthy lady, lady of the black-headed people—may you be made to swear by heaven; may you be made to swear by earth. She is an Elamite; she has a large topknot.[28] She comes up from the swamp and then again goes out again. She is overpoweringly strong; she is teeth-gnashingly angry. She is huge; she is a goddess; she is brilliant. She is furious; she is raging.

LKU 33

(2′–5′) Her [feet] are (those of) Anzû; ⌜her⌝ [hand] is dirty. ... She is secretive. The [shadow] of the wall is her emplacement. The threshold is her dwelling place. Her nails [are long.] Her armpits are not ⌜shaved⌝.

(6′–10′) She is [un]just and of low standing, the daughter of ⌜Anu⌝. ... Anu her father (and) Antu her mother, at her deeds which were not pleasing, made her come down ⌜from⌝ [heaven]. They did not set up her dais on ⌜earth⌝. She is endowed with ⌜wings⌝ and [flies] like a ⌜*lilītu*⌝.[29]

(11′–18′) Night turns to night and morning to morning for the woman whose entrance ⌜blocks itself off⌝. The daughter of Anu daily counts the pregnant women; she goes around after those (about to) give birth. She counts up their [months]; she marks the days (of their confinement) onto the wall. For the lying-in women giving birth (this) is (her) recitation: "Bring me your sons so that I can give them suck; let me put the breast into the mouth of your daughters."[30]

(19′–26′) She holds in her hands fever, cold, chills (and) frost. They (the hands) are full of ambiguous[31] (and) hidden things. Her body is covered with burning flames. Now and then, she spits venom; suddenly, she spits venom. Her venom is snake venom; her venom is scorpion venom. She murders the young men, ruins the young women (and) smites the children.

(27′–30′) She makes adolescent girls ⌜drink⌝ the water of distress. She enters the open house; she slips in the locked house past the door pivot. She ⌜slips in⌝ like a snake. She suckles the infant on [her poisonous] ⌜milk⌝.

(31′–35′) She has smeared his/her face with his heart's [blood]. [The infant] wails for food (but it is) deadly poison. ⌜Lamaštu⌝ and Labaṣu have smeared his face with poisonous venom.[32] She has seized the ⌜chair⌝ from a place of mourning; she has gathered the ⌜dust⌝ from a place of mourning.

(36′–39′) Her teeth are the [teeth] of a dog; her talons are the talons of an eagle. Her *tudittu*-pin [is broken], her breast exposed. Her [hand]s [are an *aluḫappu*-net]; her hold is limp.[33] Her breasts are bathed [in] ⌜deadly⌝ [milk].

(40′–45′) *(fragmentary)*

2. DIFFICULT CHILDBIRTH

The Akkadian term used for this has literally to do with narrowness. Indeed, the disjunction between human babies and the birth canal is the cause of many deaths in childbirth. For more details, see Scurlock and Andersen 2005, 270–71.

TEXT 6: YOS XI 86:1–28

What is interesting about this Old Babylonian childbirth recitation is that it recognizes that a baby is formed in the "fluids of intercourse." The word used is "creation" and indeed the creation of the universe was imagined as having taken place in the same way. Marduk was the patron of childbirth, but not due to any connection with original creation—it is Ea and not Marduk who was responsible for the first humans. Instead, the mercy for which Marduk was proverbial betokened the release of the prisoner: "(It lies with you, Marduk) to keep the pregnant woman well together with her foetus, to cause (her) to give birth, to make (people) obtain an heir ... to treat the infant tenderly ... to lead a laden boat in the river."[34] It is perhaps not irrelevant in this particular context that the Akkadian word for "womb" and "mercy" are the same (*rēmu*). The remainder of this text is a Sumerian recitation against the baby-snatching demoness Lamashtu.

1. *i-na me-e* ⸢*na*⸣*-a-ki-im*
2. ⸢*ib-ba*⸣*-ni* ⸢*e-ṣé*⸣*-em-tum*
3. *i-na ši-i-ir* [*ši*]*-ir-ḫa-nim*
4. *ib-ba-*⸢*ni*⸣ [*l*]*i-il-li-du-*⸢*um*⸣
5. *i-na me-e* A.AB.BA *ša-am-ru-tim*
6. *pa-al-ḫu-ú-tim*
7. *i-na me-e ti-a-am-tim ru-qú-ú-tim*
8. *a-*⸢*šar ṣe-eḫ*⸣*-ru-um ku-us-sà-a i-da-a-šu*
9. ⸢*qé*⸣*-er-bi-is-sú la-a uš-na-wa-ru*
10. *i-in ša-am-ši-im*
11. *i-mu-ur-šu-ú-ma* ^{d}*Asal-lú-ḫi ma-ri* ^{d}EN.KI
12. *ip-*⸢*ṭù*⸣*-ur ma-ak-sí-i-šu*
13. *ku-uṣ-ṣú-ru-ú-tim*
14. *ṭù-ú-da-am iš-ku-un-šum*
15. *pa-a-da-na-am ip-te-e-šum*
16. [*pu-ut*]*-*⸢*tu*⸣*-ku-um* ⸢*ṭù*⸣*-ú-*⸢*du*⸣
17. *pa-a-da-nu u*[*s-sú-k*]*a-ku-um*
18. *wa-aš-ba-at-ku-*⸢*um*⸣ [^{d}Š]À*-a-*⸢*zu*⸣*-tum*
19. *ba-a-ni-a-*⸢*at*⸣ [o]-x-*mi-i-*⸢*im*⸣
20. *ba-ni-a-at ka-li-i-ni*
21. *a-na ši-ga-ri-im*
22. *ta-aq-ta-bi wu-uš-šu-r*[*a*]*-*⸢*at*⸣
23. [*pa-a*]*ṭ*!*-ru sí-ik-ku-ru-*[*ka*]
24. [*ru-u*]*m-ma-a da-la-t*[*u-ka*]

25. [*li-i*]*m-ḫa-aṣ* [*da-al-tam*]
26. ⸢*ki*⸣*-ma da-di-*[*im*]
27. *šu-ṣí ra-ma-an-*⸢*ka*⸣
28. KA.INIM.MA MUNUS.Ù.TU.DA.K[AM]

TRANSLATION

(1–28) From the fluids of intercourse was created a skeleton; from the tissue of the muscles was created an offspring. In the turbulent and fearful sea waters, in the distant waters of the ocean where the little one's arms are bound, whose midst the eye of the sun does not illumine, Asalluhi, the son of Ea, saw him. He loosened his many-knotted bonds. He made a path for him; he opened a way for him, (saying): "Paths are ⸢opened⸣ for you; ways are ⸢alotted⸣ to you." [The divine] ⸢midwife⸣ sits (waiting) for you, she who created [...], she who created all of us. She has told the lock bar: "You are released. [Your] door bolts are ⸢loosened⸣; [your] doors are ⸢left unlocked⸣." [Let him] knock at [the door]. "Let yourself out like a favorite child." Recitation for a woman who is about to give birth.

TEXT 7: BAM 248

BAM 248 is, for the most part a collection of recitations, which accompanied what are essentially oil- or stick-assisted massages (i 52–53, 68–69, iii 7–9, iii 46–53, iv 4–5, 8–9) for a woman having difficulty giving birth. At the end, a number of potions (iv 12–16, 21–30), salves (iv 17–20), and eating meats high in fat (iv 24–30) are also suggested, presumably to be used as a last resort if nothing else has worked. At the very end an amulet (iv 31–38) is provided for the woman and a short section designed to keep "hand" of god from the newborn child is appended (see chapter 13).

Lines i 37–50 are interesting in noting the observation that "clouds" are formed in the womb and the breasts swell with milk when a woman becomes pregnant. They also include one of many references in this text (i 62–66, ii 14–iii 5, iii 54–iv 1) to the baby as a boat loaded with a male or female child moored at the quay of death (the Netherworld) to pick up a human soul and then floating across the amniotic fluid to be unloaded at the quay of life (the Upperworld). For more details, see Scurlock 1991, 146–47 and Kilmer 2007, 159–65. Lines ii 14–iii 5 contain an interesting explanation (cf. iii 46–53) for the use of specific substances put into the oil. These all invoke what we would call the principle of gravity to ensure that the baby falls to the floor.

Lines iii 10–35 give an example of the curious myth of Sîn and the cow (cf. i 37–50, iii 36–45, iii 54–iv 1; cf. also text 8), a humorous, not to say disrespectful, account of how a male god came to be patron of something only women do, namely childbirth. The "real" reason is that normal childbirth takes place after exactly ten lunar months. In any case, this tale is a good example of a historiola or story, which both explains the origin and ensures the efficacy of the ritual to which it is attached.

The salve-filled reed of iii 46–53 would have been used not only to massage the woman but also to cut the umbilical cord. Particularly interesting in iv 31–38 is the making of an amulet from a plant which has been harvested using a ritual which was probably fairly typical of medicinal plants meant to be used singly. Note that the plant needs to be told why it is being picked and to be compensated for this. The prohibition on looking back or speaking to anyone is to ensure that the plant does not take back, or someone else acquire, its healing properties. For the ancient Mesopotamian commentary to this text, which has been extensively used to reconstruct broken portions of this text, see chapter 4, text 4.

i

1–35. (fragmentary)

---

36. [KA.INIM.MA MUNUS] *šup-šu-*[(*qat a-la-da*)]

---

37. [ÉN ÁB.GAL ^{d}ŠEŠ.KI A.RI.A *l*]*e*?*-qí-ma ib-ri* DÙ-*uš* ⸢*ma*⸣-[(*la-at* GIN$_7$ *na-a-di*)][35]
38. [(*ina qar-ni-šú qaq*)]-*qa-ru* [(*ṭe-ra-at*)]
39. [*ina* KUN-*šú ú-šeš-še-ra tur-bu-ʾi*][36] ^{d}ŠEŠ.KI [*iṣ-bat* (*ḫar-ra-na*) *ana* IGI] ^{d}EN.LÍL
40. [*i-bak-ki il-la-ka di-ma-šú am-mi-ni-mi* ^{d}ŠEŠ].KI
41. [(*i-bak-ki el-la-me-e*) *il-la-ka* (*di-ma*)]-*šu*!
42. [...] KAL
43. [(*aš-šum* ÁB-*ia la a-lit-ti*) *aš-šum u-ni-qí la pe-ti*]-*ti*
44. [*ina* KAR] *pu-uš-qí* [*k*]*a-lat* ^{GIŠ}MÁ
45. [*ina* KAR] *dan-na-te ka-*⸢*lat*⸣ ^{GIŠ}MÁ.GUR$_8$
46. [*man-nam lu-uš*]-*pur a-*⸢*na*⸣ *ri-*[*mi*]-*ni* ^{d}AMAR.UTU
47. [*ina* KAR] *pu-uš-qí lip-ru-ru* ^{GIŠ}MÁ
48. [*ina* KAR] *dan-na-te li-maš-ši-ra* ^{GIŠ}MÁ.GUR$_8$
49. [*ṣa-a* G]IN$_7$ MUŠ *ni-šil-pa-a ki-ma ni-ra-ḫi*
50. [MUNUS LA.R]A.AḪ ⸢SILIM⸣-*ma* ⸢*šer*⸣-*ru lim-*⸢*qu*⸣-*tam-ma* ZÁLAG IGI

---

51. [(KA.INIM.MA)] MUNUS LA.RA.AḪ.A.KÁM

---

52. [*ina* GI.SA]G.KUD[37] GI DÙG.GA Ì.GIŠ *ta-tab-bak*
53. [...] ⸢me/ši⸣ nu *ina* UGU ŠÀ-*šá* ḪÁŠ!-[*šá* EŠ] *šer-ru uš-*[*te-še*]*-ra*

---

54. ÉN ši x [(o)] e LA.RA.AḪ
55. x x x x LA.RA.AḪ
56. [*šuḫ*]*-ri-ri* [(o o o o)] da? ab ba *nap-ri-šá*
57. [*š*]*uḫ-ri-ri* [(o o o)] ta? rik *li-ṣa-a*
58. x x x x [(*Na-ḫu*)]*-un-de-e Na-ru-un-di*
59. [(*na*)]*-am-*[(*l*)]*i-*[*su*] *ki-ma ṣa-bi-ti*
60. ⸢*ni-ši-il*⸣-[*pa-a*] *ki-ma ni-ra-ḫi*
61. *ana-ku* ^{d}[*Asal-lú-ḫi* ...] ma a *li-mur-šu* ÉN

---

62. ÉN *ina* KAR *mu-ti k*[*a-lat*] ^{GIŠ}MÁ
63. *ina* KAR *dan-na-ti* [*k*]*a-l*[*at*] ^{GIŠ}MÁ.GUR$_8$
64. *ul-tu* AN-[*e*] [*ur-da-an*]*-ni*
65. *ana* ^{d}*Be-let-ì-lí re-e-me qí-bi-ma*
66. *ur-ḫu li-ši-ir ana* ŠÀ [*dan-na*]*-ti*[38] *li-ṣa-a* [*li-mur*] ^{d}UTU-*ši*

---

67. KA.INIM.MA MUNUS LA.RA.AḪ.A.KÁM

---

68. DÙ.DÙ.BI Ì [(BUR) ...] *ana* ŠÀ x [...]x
69. *ta-maḫ-ḫa-aṣ* [TA *e-la-an ana*] *šap-la-an* [*tu-maš-šá-ʾ-ma*] SI.SÁ

---

ii
1–13. (broken away)
14–29. (very fragmentary)
30. ⸢*uš*⸣*-šu-rat* ⸢*ḫur*⸣*-da-as-sa* [...]
31–43. (very fragmentary)
44. *i-*[(*na kit-tab-ri-šú*) GUB]*-za*! ^{d}AMAR.UTU
45. *qí-*[(*ip nap-šá-a-tum*)] *ši-pat* TI.LA
46. *an-nu-ú me-ḫu-ú* ⸢*la-ma*⸣*-ku kul-dan-ni*
47. *i-na* ib/lu [...] *liš-li-ma* ^{GIŠ}MÁ
48. *i-na* ib/lu [...] *liš-te-še-ra* ^{GIŠ}MÁ.GUR$_8$
49. *dan-nu lip-pa-ṭir mar-kas-sa*
50. *ù ed-lu lip-pi-ti* KÁ-*šá*
51. DUR *ša* ^{GIŠ}MÁ *a-na* KAR *šul-me*
52. DUR *ša* ^{GIŠ}MÁ.GUR$_8$ *a-na* KAR TI.LA
53. *meš-re-e-tu lip-te-ṭi-ra li-ir-mu-ú* SA.MEŠ

54. *ka-an-ga-tum lup-taš-ši-ra li-ṣa-a nab-ni-tu*
55. GÌR.PAD.DU *a-ḫi-tum bi-nu-ut a-me-*⸢*lu*⸣*-ti*
56. *ár-ḫiš li-ta-ṣa-am-ma li-ta-mar* ZÁLAG ^{d}UTU-*ši*
57. *ki-ma ti-ik* AN-*e a-a i-tur a-na* EGIR-*šú*
58. *ki-ma ma-qit* BÀD *a-a i-ne-ʾ* GABA-*su*
59. *ki-ma pi-sa-an-ni šur-di-i a-a i-si-tu mu-*⸢*ú*⸣*-šá*
60. *an-ni-ta* ^{d}*Asal-lú-ḫi ina še-mé-e-šu*
61. *ik-kud it-ta-id ba-laṭ-sa*
62. *ina zik-ri ša* ^{d}*É-a ú-šar-bi šum-šu*
63. *id-di* ÉN *ša* TI.LA *tu-ú ša šul-*[(*me*)]
64. *ú-*⸢*ram*⸣*-mi* ⸢DUR⸣ *ip-ta-ṭar ki-ṣ*[*ir-šá*]
65. *ed-le-e-ti ba-ba-a-ti up-*[*te-et-ta*]
66. *up-te-eṭ-ṭi-ra meš-r*[*e-e-tu ir-mu-ú* SA.MEŠ]
67. *kan-ga-tum up-taš-ši-ra ú-*[*ṣa-a nab-ni-tu*]
68. GÌR.PAD.DU *a-ḫi-*[*t*]*u bi-nu-ut* [*a-me-lu-ti*]
69. *ár-ḫiš* [*l*]*i-ta-ṣa-am-ma i-ta-mar* [ZÁLAG ^{d}UTU-*ši*]
70. *ki-ma ti-ik* AN-*e ul i-tur* [*a-na* EGIR-*šú*]

iii

1. *ki-ma ma-qit* BÀD *ul i-né-ʾ* [GABA-*su*]
2. *ki-ma* ^{GIŠ}PÍSAN *šur-di-i ul i-si-tu* [*mu-ú-šá*]
3. ÉN *šá* ^{d}*Asal-lú-ḫi ni-ṣir-tu šá* [(*Eri*$_4$)-*du*$_{10}$]
4. *an-nu ke-nu šá* ^{d}*É-a i-di-tum* ÉN *ša* ^{d}*Ma-mi* [(*i-ri-šú*)]
5. ^{d}40 LUGAL *id-di-nu ana šu-te-šur* [(ŠÀ.TÙR)]

---

6. KA.INIM.MA MUNUS LA.RA.AḪ.A.K[(ÁM)]

---

7. DÙ.DÙ.BI ^{NA_4}*ti-ik-*AN-*e* SAḪAR *sa-mit* BÀD ŠUB-*t*[(*i*)]
8. SAḪAR ^{GIŠ}PÍSAN *šur-di-i ina* Ì BUR ḪE.ḪE TA *e-la-niš*
9. *ana šap-la-niš tu-maš-šá-ʾ-ma* MUNUS BI SI.SÁ

---

10. ÉN 1-*et* ÁB *šá* ^{d}30 GÉME-^{d}EN.ZU.NA *šum-šá*
11. *ti-iq-na-a-te tuq-qù-na-at*
12. *bi-nu-tam kaz-bat i-mur-ši-ma* ^{d}30 *i-ra-am-ši*
13. *nam-ru šá* ^{d}30 *šu-ba-ḫi iš-ta-kan-ši*
14. *uš-te-eṣ-bi-is-si-ma pa-an su-kul-lim*
15. *re-é-ú-tu il-la-ka* EGIR-*šá*
16. *ina nu-ru-ub šam-me i-re-ʾu šam-me*
17. *ina šub-bé-e maš-qé-e i-šaq-qu-ši me-e*
18. *ina pu-zur ka-bar-ri la a-mar re-ʾ-i*

19. *ana* UGU ÁB *iš-ta-ḫi-iṭ mi-ru ek-du* (*ḫe-pí*) ‹*zib*›*-ba-tuš-šá* ÍL-*ši*
20. U$_4$.MEŠ-*šá ina qu-ut-ti-i ár-ḫi-šá ina ga-ma-ri*
21. ÁB *ig-ta-lit ú-ga-al-lit*
22. *re-é-a-šá ap-pa-šu qá-di-is-su ka-par-ru ana ka-li-šú-nu sap-*⸢*du*⸣*-šú*
23. *ana ik-kil-li-šá ana ri-gim ḫa-li-šá ne-pal-síḫ* ^{d}ŠEŠ.KI-*ru*
24. ^{d}30 *ina* AN-*e iš-tam-me ri-gim-šá iš-ši qa-as-su šá-ma-me*
25. 2 ^{d}LAMMA.MEŠ AN-*e ú-ri-da-nim-ma* 1-*et* Ì ^{GIŠ}BUR *na-šá-at*
26. *šá-ni-tum ú-šap-pa-la me-e ḫa-li il-pu-tam* Ì ^{GIŠ}BUR *pu-us-sa*
27. *me-e ḫa-li ú-sap-pi-ḫa ka-la zu-um-ri-šá*
28. *šá-na-a il-pu-tam* Ì ^{GIŠ}BUR *pu-us-sa*
29. *me-e ḫa-li ú-sap-pi-ḫa ka-la* SU-*šá*
30. *šal-la-ti-iš-šu ina la-pa-ti*
31. *bu-ru* GIN$_7$ *ú-za-li im-ta-qut qaq-qar-šú*
32. AMAR.GA *iš-ta-kan šu-um bu-ú-ri*
33. *ki-ma* GÉME-^{d}EN.ZU.NA *i-šá-riš i-li-da*
34. *li-li-id ár-da-tum mu-šap-šiq-tum*
35. *šab-su-tum a-a ik-ka-li e-ri-tu li-ši-ir*

---

36. ÉN *Na-ru-un-di Na-ḫu-un-di u Na-nam-gi-ši-ir*
37. 1-*et* ÁB *šá* ^{d}30 GÉME-^{d}30 *šum-šá*
38. *ana ik-kil-li-šá ana ri-gim ḫa-li-šá*
39. ^{d}ŠEŠ.KI-*ru* ^{d}30 *iš-te-mi ri-gim-šá*
40. *man-nu-um-ma Na-ru-un-di man-nu-um-ma Na-ḫu-un-di*
41. ÁB-*mi* EN *šup-šu-qat a-la-da*
42. EN *me-e* BA.AN.DU$_8$.DU$_8$-*ka ana* UGU-*ḫi-šá i-di-ma*
43. *šá* ÁB E.GI-^{d}EN.ZU.NA *lip-pe-tu-ú pa-nu-šá*
44. *li-ṣa-a* GIN$_7$ MUŠ *ki-ma* MUŠ.TUR *liš-šá-li-la*
45. *ki-ma ma-qit* BÀD *li-is-su a-na ku-tal-li-šú a-a id-di* TU$_6$ ÉN

---

46. DÙ.DÙ.BI SAḪAR.SILA.LÍM.MA SAḪAR KUN$_4$ *maḫ-ri-tú*
47. SAḪAR *pi-sa-an-ni e-li-i ù šap*(!)*-li-i*
48. SAḪAR *pi-sa-an-ni* ^{GIŠ}IG GI.NÍG.GAL.GAL.LA
49. *ap-pa ù il-da ta-šar-ri-im*
50. SAḪAR.ḪI.A *šu-nu-ti a-na* ŠÀ Ì.GIŠ ŠUB-*di*
51. ÉN *an-ni-tú* 7-*šú ana* ŠÀ ŠID-*nu*
52. GI.NÍG.GAL.GAL.LA DIRI-*ma ina* UGU ŠÀ-*šá zaq*(!)*-pi*
53. TA *e-le-nu ana šap-la-nu tu-maš-šá-*ʾ

---

54. ÉN ÁB GAL ^{d}30 *šá* ^{d}30 *ana-ku*

55. *e-ru-ú e-ra-ku-ma nu-uk-ku-pu ú-nak-kap*
56. *ina* SI.MU *qaq-qa-ru ṭe-ra-ku*
57. *ina* KUN.MU *uš-te-eš-še-ra tur-bu-ʾ-i*
58. *ina* KAR *mu-ti ka-lat* ^{GIŠ}MÁ
59. *ina* ⸢KAR⸣ *dan-na-ti ka-lat* ^{GIŠ}MÁ.GUR$_{8}$
60. [...] ^{d}40 EN ÉN
61. [*ina* KAR *mu-t*]*i lip-ṭu-ru* ^{GIŠ}MÁ
62. [*ina* KAR *dan-na-ti li*]*-ram-ma-a* ^{GIŠ}MÁ.GUR$_{8}$
63. [*ki-ma* GÉME-^{d}EN.ZU.NA *šá i-šá-riš i-l*]*i*!*-du-u l*[*i*!*-li-id*]
64. [*ár-da-tum mu-šap-šiq-tum* PEŠ$_{4}$*-tum*] ⸢*li*⸣*-ši-*[*ir šab-šu-tum a-a ik-ka-li*]

iv

1. *ár-ḫiš lit-ta-ṣa-am-ma li-mu-ra* ZÁLAG ^{d}UTU-*ši* TU$_{6}$ ÉN

---

2. ÉN *lu-us-ma ki-ma* MAŠ.DÀ *ni-ir-ru-ba* GIN$_{7}$ MUŠ.TUR
3. *ana-ku* ^{d}*Asal-lú-ḫi šab-sa-ku a-maḫ-ḫar-ka* TU$_{6}$ ÉN

---

4. DÙ.DÙ.BI ^{GIŠ}PA ^{GIŠ}MA.NU *šá* ŠU *re-ʾ-i ta-maḫ-ḫar*
5. ÉN 7-*šú ana* UGU ŠID *ina* UGU ŠÀ-*šá ta-par-rik-ma ár-ḫiš* Ù.TU

---

6. ÉN *šup-šuq-ta re-mi* ⸢*ka*⸣-[*an-g*]*a-tú*
7. ^{d}ŠÀ(!).ZU(!)[39] *šab-su-ta-šá-ma at-ta šum-li-is-si* TU$_{6}$ ÉN

---

8. DÙ.DÙ.BI ^{GIŠ}PA ^{GIŠ}MA.NU *šá* ŠU *re-ʾ-i*
9. ÉN 7-*šú* ŠID-*nu-ma* TA SAG ŠÀ-*šá ana šap-la-an* ŠÀ-*šá tuš-ga-ra-ár*

---

10. ÉN *za-la-aḫ iz-za-la-aḫ za-la-aḫ* AL.TI.LA TU$_{6}$ ÉN

---

11. KA.INIM.MA MUNUS LA.RA.AḪ.A.KÁM

---

12. ^{Ú}I[(N.NU.U)]Š ZÍD ŠE.SA.A *ina* Ì.GIŠ *u* KAŠ NAG-*ši-ma uš-te-šer*

---

13. DIŠ MUNUS Ù.TU-*ma uš-tap-šiq* ^{GIŠ}GEŠTIN.KA$_{5}$.A ^{Ú}EME.UR.GI$_{7}$
14. ^{Ú}*tuḫ-lam* SÚD ^{DUG}LA.ḪA.AN KAŠ ^{LÚ}KÚRUN.NA DIRI-*ma*
15. Ú.ḪI.A *an-nu-ti ana* ŠÀ SÌG-*aṣ la pa-tan* NAG-*ma ár-ḫiš* Ù.TU

---

16. DIŠ KI.MIN ŠÈ EME.DIR *šá* IZ.ZI SÚD *ina* KAŠ *la pa-tan* NAG-*ma* KI.MIN

---

17. DIŠ KI.MIN SAḪAR *ni-pil-ti* UR.GI$_{7}$ SÚD *ana* ŠÀ Ì.GIŠ SÌG-*aṣ* ŠÀ-*šá*

ŠÉŠ KI.MIN

---

18. DIŠ KI.MIN *qin-ni* SIM.MAḪ^{MUŠEN} SÚD *ina* Ì.GIŠ ḪE.ḪE ŠÉŠ KI.MIN

---

19. DIŠ KI.MIN SUḪUŠ ^{GIŠ}NAM.TAR NÍTA *šá* IM.SI.SÁ SÚD *ina* Ì.GIŠ ḪE.ḪE
20. *7-šú ana m*[(*u*)]*q-q*[(*à*)]*l-pi-ti pa-pa-an* ŠÀ-*šá* ŠÉŠ-*ma* KI.MIN

---

21. DIŠ KI.MIN ^{GIŠ}GEŠTIN.KA$_5$.A SÚD *ina* KAŠ *la pa-tan* NAG-*ma* : ^{Ú}EME.UR.GI$_7$ KI.MIN

---

22. DIŠ KI.MIN ^{Ú}EME.UR.GI$_7$ ^{Ú}KUR.RA^{SAR} SÚD *ina* KAŠ NU *pa-tan* NAG-*ma* KI.MIN

---

23. DIŠ KI.MIN U$_5$ ARGAB^{MUŠEN} SÚD KI.MIN

---

24. DIŠ KI.MIN ^{Ú}EME.UR.GI$_7$ ^{Ú}IN.NU.UŠ SÚD KI.MIN
25. DIŠ KI.MIN UZU NÍG.BÚN.NA$^{\text{KU}_6}$ GU$_7$-*ma* KI.MIN
26. DIŠ KI.MIN UZU ŠAḪ BABBAR GU$_7$-*ma* KI.MIN
27. DIŠ KI.MIN UZU ^{MUNUS}KA$_5$.A GU$_7$-*ma* KI.MIN
28. DIŠ KI.MIN ^{Ú}KUR.KUR SÚD *ina* KAŠ NAG-*ma* KI.MIN
29. DIŠ KI.MIN IM KAL.GUG SÚD *ina* KAŠ NAG-*ma* KI.MIN
30. DIŠ KI.MIN *al-la-an-ka-niš ina* ZÚ-*šá i-mar-raq-ma* KI.MIN
31. DIŠ KI.MIN ŠE.GAG *ta-šab-bu-uš ina* KI.TA Ú.GÍR
32. *šá* UGU *pi-ti-iq-ti a-ṣu-ú ta-tab-bak*
33. *ki-a-am* DUG$_4$.GA-*ma um-ma at-ta-ma*
34. NÍG.BA-*ka maḫ-ra-ta* Ú *šá* TI *id-nam-ma*
35. *šá* MUNUS NENNI DUMU.MUNUS NENNI *šá* ŠÀ-*šá liš-te-šer*
36. *an-nam* DUG$_4$.GA-*ma* SUḪUŠ-*su u* SUḪUR-*su* ⸢ZI⸣-*ma*
37. *ana* EGIR-*ka* NU IGI.BAR KI LÚ.NA.ME NU DU$_{11}$.DU$_{11}$-*ub*
38. DUR NU.NU-*ú tara-kas ina* ^{UZU}ÚR 150–*šá* KEŠDA-*ma* TI

39–45. (see chapter 13, text 3)

Translation

(i 1–35) *(fragmentary)*

(i 36) [Recitation for a woman] who is having difficulty giving birth.[40]

(i 37–50) [Recitation: The cow of Sîn] took in [the semen] and so made clouds;[41] she was full as a waterskin (i.e., her udders filled with milk). The earth was rooted up with her horn. [With her tail, she made the sandstorm pass along.] Sîn [took] the road; [before] Enlil, [he cries (and) his tears come. Why] does ⸢Sîn⸣ cry, the pure-in-rite's tears [come]? [...] Because of my cow which has not yet given birth, [because of my she-goat which has not yet] ⸢been opened⸣.

The boat is ⸢detained⸣ [at the quay] of difficulty ("narrows"); the *magurru*-boat is held back [at the quay] of hardship. [Whom should I] ⸢send to merciful⸣ Marduk? May the boat be loosed [from the quay] of difficulty; may the *magurru*-boat be freed [from the quay] of hardship. [Come out to me] ⸢like⸣ a snake; slither out to me like a little snake. May the ⸢woman having difficulty having birth⸣ bring (her pregnancy) to term[42] so that the infant may fall to the earth and see the sunlight.

(i 51) Recitation for a woman who is having difficulty giving birth.

(i 52–53) [Its ritual. ...] You pour oil and "sweet reed" [into] a ⸢hollow reed⸣. [...] You rub (it) gently] over her abodmen (and) hypogastric region. The infant should ⸢come out straight away⸣.

(i 54–61) Recitation: [...] having difficulty [....] having difficulty. ⸢Abate!⸣ [...] Fly! ⸢Abate!⸣ [...] Let it come out. [...] "(Who is it), Naḫundi; (who is it), Narundi?" Run like a gazelle; slither like a snake. I am [Asalluhi]. May [...] see him. Recitation

(i 62–66) Recitation: The boat is ⸢detained⸣ at the quay of death; the *magurru*-boat is ⸢held back⸣ at the quay of hardship. [Come down] to me from heaven. Command Belet-ili to have mercy so that it may go straight down the road. May it come out from (the quay of) ⸢hardship⸣; [may it see] the sun.

(i 67) Recitation for a woman who is having difficulty giving birth.

(i 68–69) Its ritual: You whisk *pūru*-oil into [...]. [If you massage (her) in a] ⸢downwards direction⸣, she should give birth straight away.

(ii 14–iii 5) [...] Her loincloths are loosened [...] Stand beside her, Marduk. Entrust life, the spell of life. (With) this storm I am surrounded; reach me.[43]

May the boat be safe in [...]. May the *magurru*-boat go aright in [...]. May her massive mooring rope be loosened, and may her locked gate be opened. (May) the mooring rope of the boat (be moored) to the quay of health, the mooring rope of the *magurru*-boat to the quay of life. May the limbs be relaxed; may the sinews be slackened. May the sealed woman be loosened; may the offspring come out, a separate body, a human creature. May he come out promptly and see the light of the sun.

Like a rain shower (which can never go back to the heavens), may the (foetus) not be able to return to what is behind him. Like one who has fallen from a wall, may he not be able to turn his breast. Like a leaky drainpipe (which cannot hold water), may none of the (mother's) waters remain.

When Asalluhi heard this, he became exceedingly concerned for her life. At the command of Ea, he exalted his name. He cast the recitation of life (and) the spell of health. He loosed (her) mooring rope; he undid [her] ⸢knotting⸣. The locked gates [were] ⸢opened⸣. The ⸢limbs⸣ were relaxed; [the sinews slackened]. The sealed woman was loosened; [the offspring came out], a ⸢separate⸣ body, a [human] creature. He came out promptly and saw [the light of the sun].

Like a rain shower, he did not return [backwards]. Like one who had fallen from a wall, he did not turn [his breast]. Like a leaky drainpipe, none [of her waters] remained. The recitation of Asalluhi, the secret of ⸢Eridu⸣, the true yes of Ea, the renowned spell which Mami requested (and which) ⸢king⸣ [Ea] gave to help make the foetus come out straight away.

(iii 6) Recitation for a woman having difficulty giving birth.

(iii 7–9) Its ritual: you mix hailstone, dust from the parapet of an abandoned wall (and) dust from a leaky drainpipe with *pūru*-oil. If you massage (her) in a downward direction, that woman should give birth straight away.

(iii 10–35) One cow of Sîn, "Maid of Sîn" (was) her name, she was richly adorned; she was luxuriant in shape. Sîn saw her and loved her. He put the shining *šubaḫu* of Sîn on her. He had her take the lead of the herd, going as herdsman after her. They pastured her on grass among the juiciest grasses; they gave her water to drink in the most satisfying of watering places. Concealed from the herd boy, without the herdsman seeing, a vigorous fat (bull) mounted the cow; he reared up (over) her tail(?).[44]

At the coming to an end of her days (and) the completion of her months, the cow became frightened; it frightened her herdsman. His face was downcast; all the herd boys mourned with him. At her bellowing; at her cries in labor, he threw himself to the ground.[45]

In heaven, the moon-crescent Sîn, heard her cry. He raised his hand towards heaven. Two protective divinities came down from heaven and one of them was carrying oil in a *pūru*-vessel. The other one brought down the water of giving birth.[46]

They smeared the oil from a *pūru*-vessel onto her forehead. They sprinkled the water of giving birth over her whole body. A second time, they smeared the oil from a *pūru*-vessel onto her forehead (and) sprinkled the water of giving birth over her whole body. While (they were) smearing it on a third time, the calf fell on the ground like a young gazelle. He made the calf's name "Suckling Calf." Just as "Maid of Sîn" gave birth straightaway, so may the adolescent who is having difficulty give birth. May the midwife not be kept waiting; may the pregnant woman give birth straightaway.[47]

(iii 36–45) Narundi, Naḫundi and Nanam-gišir. (There was once) a cow of Sîn, "Maid of Sîn" (was) her name. At her bellowing, at her cries in labor, the moon crescent, Sîn, heard her cry. "Who is it, Narundi; who is it, Naḫundi?" "(It is) a cow, oh lord, who is having difficulty giving birth. Lord, pour down water from your bucket over her so that the sight of the cow "Bride of Sîn" may be opened." May he come out like a snake; may he slither out like a little snake.[48] Like one who has fallen off a wall, may he not be able to throw his cheek towards his back.[49] Spell and Recitation.

(iii 46–53) It's ritual: you pour dust from a crossroads, dust from a former threshold, dust from the upper and lower drainpipe (and) dust from a door drain into oil. You trim a thick reed at the top and base. You recite this recitation seven times over it. You fill the thick reed (with the oil) and you massage it in a downwards direction over her protruding belly.

(iii 54–iv 1) I am the great cow of Sîn, belonging to Sîn; I am pregnant and ready to gore. With my horn, I root up the earth; with my tail, I make the sandstorm pass along. The boat is detained at the quay of death; the *magurru*-boat is held back at the quay of hardship. [At the command of] Ea, lord of spells, may the boat be loosed [from the quay] of ⌜death⌝; [may] the *magurru*-boat be freed [from the quay of hardship. Just like "Maid of Sîn" who] ⌜gave birth⌝ [straight away], ⌜so may⌝ [the adolescent who is having difficulty give birth]. May [the pregnant woman] ⌜be all right⌝. [May the midwife not be kept waiting;] may (the baby) come out promptly and see the light of the sun. Spell (and) Recitation.

(iv 2–3) Recitation: Run to me like a gazelle; flee to me like a little snake. I, Asalluhi, am the midwife; I will receive you. Spell (and) Recitation.

(iv 4–5) Its ritual: you take a stick of *eʾru*-wood from a shepherd. You recite the recitation seven times over it. If you lay (it) across her abdomen, she should give birth quickly.

(iv 6–7) Recitation: (As for) the sealed woman who is made (too) narrow of womb,[50] you Marduk (= DINGIR.ŠÀ.ZU) are her midwife (ŠÀ.ZU); make her give birth. Spell and Recitation.

(iv 8–9) Its ritual: you recite the recitation seven times over a stick of *eʾru*-wood (purchased from) a shepherd and you roll (it) over her epigastrium in a downwards direction.

(iv 10) Recitation: *zalaḫ izzalaḫ zalaḫ*,[51] may she live.

(iv 11) Recitation for a woman having difficulty giving birth.

(iv 12) If you have her drink *maštakal* (and) roasted barley flour (mixed) with oil and beer, she should give birth straight away.

(iv 13–15) If a woman has difficulty in giving birth,[52] you grind together "fox grape," *lišān kalbi* (and) *tuḫlu*. You fill a *laḫannu*-vessel with *kurunnu*-beer and whisk these plants into it. If you have her drink (it) on an empty stomach, she should give birth promptly.

(iv 16) Alternatively, you grind droppings of a lizard from the wall. If you have her drink (it mixed) with beer on an empty stomach, ditto (she should give birth promptly).

(iv 17) Alternatively, you grind dust pawed up by a dog. You whisk (it) into oil. You rub her abdomen gently ditto (with it. She should give birth promptly).

(iv 18) Alternatively, you grind swallow's nest. You mix (it) with oil. You rub (it) gently ditto (on her. She should give birth promptly).

(iv 19–20) Alternatively, you grind male *pillû* root from the north side. You mix (it) with oil. If you rub her abdomen gently (with it) seven times downwards, ditto (she should give birth quickly).

(iv 21) Alternatively, you grind "fox grape." If you have (her) drink (it mixed) with beer on an empty stomach, ditto (she should give birth promptly). Alternatively, (you do this with) *lišān kalbi*.

(iv 22) Alternatively, you grind *lišān kalbi* (and) *nīnû*-mint. If you have (her) drink (it mixed) with beer on an empty stomach, ditto (she should give birth quickly).

(iv 23) Alternatively, you grind *rikibti arkabi*. Ditto (If you have her drink it mixed with beer on an empty stomach, she should give birth promptly).

(iv 24–38) Alternatively, you grind *lišān kalbi* (and) *maštakal*. Ditto (If you have her drink it mixed with beer on an empty stomach, she should give birth promptly). Alternatively, if you have her eat tortoise meat, ditto (she should give birth promptly). Alternatively, if you have her eat white pig meat, ditto (she should give birth promptly). Alternatively, if you have her eat vixen meat, ditto (she should give birth promptly). Alternatively, you grind *atāʾišu*. If you have her drink (it mixed) with beer, ditto (she should give birth promptly). Alternatively, you grind *kalgukku*-clay. If you have her drink (it mixed) with beer, ditto (she should give birth promptly). Alternatively, if she crushes *allān kaniš*-oak with her teeth, ditto (she should give birth promptly).

Alternatively, you gather a shoot. You pour (it) out below an *ašāgu*-thorn which has sprouted on brickwork (and) you say as follows: "You have received your gift. Give me the plant of life so that the foetus of so and so daughter of so and so may come out straight away." You say this, and then you pull out its root and its crown without looking behind you or speaking to anyone whatsoever. You spin (it) into a band (and) tie it. If you bind (it) on her left thigh, she should recover.

(iv 39–45) *(see chapter 13, text 3)*

3. POSTPARTUM COMPLICATIONS

A woman's problems do not cease with the birth of her child. She may suffer from bloating, diarrhea and urinary tract infection or, more seriously, uterine atony and child-bed (puerperal) fever. For more details, see Scurlock and Andersen 2005, 281–82.

TEXT 8: LAMBERT 1969, PL. 5

This text, copied by an incompetent Middle Assyrian scribe, is an excerpt text that contains a fumigant (1–13) and a vaginal suppository (1–13) to be administered on the first day, a bath and a fumigant (14–18) for the second day plus a supplemental if there is no improvement, a bath (19–26) or a bandage (27–31), all for uterine antony. For more on this condition and treatment, see Scurlock and Andersen 2005, 282 and Scurlock 2005, 311. The rest of the text is taken up with more childbirth recitations: another version of the Cow of Sîn and one which compares the woman giving birth to a warrior on the field of battle. To this day in Morocco, women who die in childbirth are considered martyrs. By contrast, in Christian Europe, despite the best efforts of the church, it was the custom to deny Christian burial to women who died before being "churched."

1. MUNUS Ù!.TU-*ma em-rat šit-t*[*u*…]
2. ŠÀ.MEŠ-*ša es-lu* A.MEŠ-*ša u* MÚD.M[EŠ-*šá* …]
3. GUR.MEŠ-*ru ana šup-šu-ri-ša* ^{ŠEM}GÚR.GÚR ⸢^{ŠEM}LI⸣
4. ^{Ú}KUR.KUR ^{ŠEM}GAM.ME GI.DÙG.GA ^{ŠEM}BAL!
5. ^{ŠEM}ŠEŠ ^{ŠEM}ḪAB ILLU *a-bu-ka-ta*
6. ILLU ^{ŠEM}BULUḪ SUḪUŠ ^{Ú}KUR.KUR 11 Ú.ḪI.A
7. *an-nu-ti* TÉŠ!.BI *tu-sa-maḫ* DÈ $^{\text{GIŠ.Ú}}$GÍR
8. *ana* ^{DUG}KÍR!(text LID×SA) *te-si-ip* Ú.‹ḪI.A› *šá-šu-nu ana* ŠÀ ŠUB-*di*
9. MUNUS *šá-ši ina* UGU *tu-še-ša-ab ina* TÚG.ḪI.A *tu-šer-ši*
10. ^{GIŠ}*si-ḫa* ^{GIŠ}*ar-ga-na* ^{Ú}*ba-ri-ra-ta*
11. ZAG.ḪI.LI.A^{SAR} KAŠ.Ú.SA *ina* Ì AMAR KÙ.GA
12. ḪE.ḪE *ina* ^{SÍG}ÀKA!(text ÍL) NIGIN-*ma ana* ŠÀ GAL$_{4}$.LA-*šá* GAR.GAR-*ma*
13. *ur-ra u* GI$_{6}$ *an-na-a* DÙ.MEŠ-*uš-ma* DÙG-*ba* IGI-*mar*

---

14. *ina* 2 U$_{4}$.ME x x x *tu-šab-šal* E$_{11}$-*la-ma*
15. MUNUS *ina* ⸢UGU⸣ [*t*]*u-še-*⸢*ša*⸣*-ab ina* TÚG.ḪI.A *tu-šer-ši*
16. KAŠ *ana* UGU ⸢*qí*⸣*-ri tu-sa-laḫ* ⸢*qut*!⸣*-ru*[53]
17. *ana* KA.MEŠ-*šá u na-ḫi-ri-ša e-ru-ub*
18. Ì.DÙG.GA ŠÉŠ.MEŠ *še-ḫa* NU IGI-*mar-ma* TI

---

19. *šum*$_{4}$*-ma* DÙG-*ba* NU IGI-*mur* ^{URUDU}ŠEN.TUR A.MEŠ *u* KAŠ DIRI
20. ^{ŠEM}ERIN.NA ^{ŠEM}ŠUR.MÌN.NA ^{ŠEM}*dáp-ra-na*
21. ^{ŠEM}GÚR.GÚR ^{ŠEM}LI ^{ŠEM}GAM.ME ^{Ú}KUR.KUR
22. ^{Ú}*si-ḫa* ^{Ú}*ar-ga-na* ^{Ú}*ba-*⸢*ri*⸣*-ra-ta*

23. GAZI^{SAR} NUMUN *šu-ši* 11 Ú.ḪI.A! *an-nu-ti*
24. TÉŠ.BI *ana* ŠÀ ŠUB-*di tu-šab-šal ta-šá-ḫal*
25. *ina* ŠÀ RA-*si* E$_{11}$-*ma* Ì.GIŠ ŠÉŠ *ana* É
26. *pag-ri tu-še-rab-ši še-ḫa* NU IGI DU$_{8}$-*ma*

---

27. ⸢ŠEŠ⸣.MEŠ ŠIM.MEŠ DÙ.A.BI-*šu-nu* ^{GIŠ}*ba*!(SU)-*ri-ra-*[*t*]*a*
28. KI KAŠ.Ú.SA GIBIL ḪE.ḪE *ana* ^{DUG}MAŠ? *te-se-ep*
29. *ina* IM.‹ŠU›.RIN.NA *te*!-*se-kér* E$_{11}$-*ma ina* TÚG.ḪI.A
30. *te-ṭe*$_{4}$-*ri* ^{UZU}*em-ši-e-ša* ^{UZU}*šu-ḫe-e-ša u*
31. ^{UZU}*ra-pal-te-ša* LÁL-*id-ma* TI

---

32. *ṭup-pu ši-it ša-bu-ša-ta la ga-am-rat*

---

33. MUNUS ^{MUNUS}LA.‹RA.›AḪ-*tu šap-šu-qa-at* Ù.TU.MEŠ-*da*
34. Ù.TU.MEŠ *šap-šu-qa-at še-er-ra ku-na-at*
35. *še-er-ra ku-na-at ana qa-tu-ú* ZI-*te* ŠU.RA ^{GIŠ}SAG.KUL
36. *sa-ni-iq*! KÁ *ana ti-nu-qí la-lu-ú ši-it* SILA$_{4}$-*mu*
37. *ba-ni-tu ú-bu-ḫa-at* BA.MEŠ[54] *mu-ú-te*
38. *ki-i* ^{GIŠ}GIGIR *ú-bu-ḫa-at* BA.MEŠ *ta-ḫa-zi*
39. *ki-i* ^{GIŠ}APIN *ú-bu-ḫa-at* BA.MEŠ ^{GIŠ}TIR.MEŠ
40. *ki-i* UR.SAG *mu-ut-taḫ-iṣ ina* MÚD.MEŠ-*šá ṣa-la-at*
41. *šam-ṭa-a* IGI.MEŠ-*šá ul ta-da-gal ka-at-ma šap-ta-šá*
42. *ul ta-pa-te ši-mat mu-te u ši-ma-ta ša-pa-a* IGI.MEŠ-*šá*
43. *ú-ya* GÙ-*ša*[55] *ig-ta-na-lu-uṭ ul* ŠE.GA-*a*
44. GEŠTU.MEŠ-*šá ul sa-qa-at* GABA-*sa sà-pu-ḫu ku-lu-lu-šá*
45. *pu-ṣu-ni ul pa-ṣu-na-at bu-ul-ta ul ti-šu*
46. GUB-*za ma-am-ma* DUG$_{4}$.GA.MEŠ-*ši re-ma-nu-ú* ^{d}AMAR.UTU
47. *an-nu-ú te-šu-ú la-a-ma-ku-ma ku-ul-da-a-ni*
48. *še-li kak-ka ša-ti bu-nu-*⸢*ut*⸣ DINGIR.MEŠ
49. *bu-nu-ut* LÚ×U$_{19}$.LU *lu-ú-ṣa-ma li-mur* AN.BAR$_{7}$[56]
50. ÉN É.NU.RU *ši-ip-tu ša mu-ul-tap-ši-iq-te*

---

51. *Gi-Se-en*$^{\text{d}30}$ GÉME *ša* ^{d}30 *a-la-da šap-šu-qa-at še-er-ra*
52. *ku-na-at še-er-ra ku-na-at ana qa-tu-ú* ZI-*te* ŠU.⸢RA⸣ *si-ku-rum*
53. *sa-ni-iq* KÁ-*bu ana* NU TI-*qí la-lu-ú* IGI.DU$_{8}$-*ši-ma* ^{d}30
54. *i-*⸢*ra-*ʾ⸣*-ši ana nu-ru-ub* Ú.MEŠ *ir-ta-na-*ʾ*u ina sa-ḫi* x (x)
55. NAG.MEŠ-[*ši* A].MEŠ *ana* UGU ^{GUD}ÁB *il-ti-ki-iṭ bu-ru*
56. *ek-du* U$_{4}$.MEŠ-*ša ana mu-le-e* ITU.MEŠ-*ša ana* [*ga-ma-ri*]
57. *ta-aḫ-ti-me-iš ta-ḫa-al bu-ur-tu ina i*[*k-ki-li-ša*]

58. *ina* GÙ.MEŠ *ḫi-li-ša* ^{d}30 *na-na-ar* AN-*e* [...]
59. 2-*ši-na* DUMU.MUNUS ^{d}*A-ni*[*m* T]A AN-*e ú-ri-da-a-ni* 1-*te na-ša-at* A.MEŠ [*ḫ*]*i-i-li ša-ni-tu*
60. *na-ša-at* Ì *pu-ú-ri* A.MEŠ *ḫi-li* ‹‹li›› *il-pu-ut* SAG.KI.MEŠ-*sa* Ì *pu-ú-ri* x ú pi
61. DÙ!.A.BI SU.MEŠ-*ša* GIN_7-*ma Gi-i*-^{d}30 GÉME *ša* ^{d}30 *e-eš-ri-ši* Ù.TU-*du lu* Ù!.TU-*id*
62. *ar-da-a-tu* MUNUS LA.RA.AḪ.MEŠ ÉN! É.NU.RU

TRANSLATION

(1–13) (If) a woman gives birth and subsequently she is distended, [her] excrement [. . .], her insides are constipated, (and) her waters and [her] blood have gone back [inside her].[57]

To make her release (it), you gather together these eleven plants: *kukru*-aromatic, *burāšu*-juniper, *atā'išu*, *ṣumlalû*, "sweet reed," *ballukku*-aromatic, myrrh, *ṭūru*-aromatic, *abukkatu* resin, *baluḫḫu*-aromatic resin, (and) *atā'išu* root. You gather *ašāgu*-thorn coals into (an overturned) pottery drum (and) you pour those plants onto them. You have that woman sit over it. You wrap her in a cloth.

You mix *sīḫu*-wormwood, *argānu*, *barirātu*, *saḫlû*-cress,[58] (and) beerwort in fat from a pure cow. You wrap (it) in a tuft of wool and insert (it) repeatedly into her vagina and, if you continually do this day and night, she should experience improvement.

(14–18) On the second day, you boil [...] (and bathe her with it). After she comes out (of the bath), you have the woman sit over (the fumigants). You wrap her in a cloth. You sprinkle beer onto hot bitumen. The smoke should enter her mouth and nostrils. You repeatedly rub her gently with sweet oil. If she does not experience delirium, she should recover.

(19–26) If she does not experience improvement, you fill a *tamgussu*-vessel with water and beer. You pour these eleven plants together into it: *erēnu*-cedar, *šurmēnu*-cypress, *daprānu*-juniper, *kukru*-aromatic, *burāšu*-juniper, *ṣumlalû*, *atā'išu*, *sīḫu*-wormwood, *argānu*, *barirātu*, *kasû*, (and) *šūšu*-licorice seed. You boil (it and) filter (it and) bathe her with it. When she comes up (out of the bath), you rub her gently with oil. You have her enter a slaughterhouse. If she does not experience delirium, she should recover.

(27–31) You mix the aforementioned plants, all of them (*erēnu*-cedar, *šurmēnu*-cypress, *daprānu*-juniper, *kukru*-aromatic, *burāšu*-juniper, *ṣumlalû*, *atā'išu*, *sīḫu*-wormwood, *argānu*, *barirātu*, *kasû*, and *šūšu*-licorice seed) with roasted beerwort. You collect it into a [...]-vessel. You bake (it) in an oven. You take (it) out and massage (it) into cloth. If you bandage her hypogastric region, her buttocks and her coccyx (with it), she should recover.

(32) That tablet is collected (but) not finished.

(33–50) The woman in travail is having difficulty giving birth; she is having difficulty giving birth. The infant is stuck fast; the infant is stuck so fast as to end (her) life.[59] The door bolt is secure; the door is fastened against the suckling kid—that one (f) and the lamb to be plucked. The creatress is enveloped in the dust(!) of death. Like a chariot she is enveloped in the dust(!) of battle; like a plow she is enveloped in the dust(!) of the (olive-)grove. Like a warrior in the fray, she is cast down in her blood. Her eyes are weakened; she cannot see. Her lips are closed; she cannot open (them). Her eyes are clouded (with) a deathly fate or fates.[60] Her wail of "uya" continually trills; her ears do not hear. Her breast is not tight(ly corsetted); her headcloths are scattered. She is not covered with a cloak, (yet) she is not ashamed. Merciful Marduk,[61] stand by and say something to her. (With) this confusion am I surrounded, so reach me.[62] Bring forth that sealed up one, a creation of the gods, a creation of man. Let it come out and see the light. É.NU.RU spell; a spell for a woman in travail.

(51–62) Gi-Sîn, the maid of Sîn was having difficulty giving birth. The infant was stuck fast; the infant was stuck fast. The bolt was secure so as to bring life to an end; the door was closed so as not to accept the baby.

Sîn saw her and loved her. They pastured her among the juiciest grasses; they gave [her water] to drink in the [...] meadows. A vigorous bull mounted the cow. At the filling of her days (and) the [completion] of her months, the cow knelt down and went into labor. At [her bellowing]; at her cries in labor, Sîn, the moon-crescent of heaven [...]. Two daughters of Anu came down from heaven. One of them was carrying the water of giving birth. The other one was carrying oil in a *pūru*-vessel and water of giving birth. They smeared oil from a *pūru*-vessel onto her forehead. [They sprinkled] the water of giving birth over her whole body.

Just as Gi-Sîn, the maid of Sîn, gave birth straightaway, so may the adolescent who is having difficulty give birth. May the midwife not be kept waiting; may the pregnant woman be all right.

TEXT 9: BAM 240 (KAR 195)

This text contains treatments for a woman who is pregnant or who has just given birth. Included are a wash (6′–9′) and a tampon (6′–9′) for spotting, a bandage (17′–19′), a wash (17′–19′) and a potion (17′–19′) for urinary tract infection, a tampon (20′–22′) and a wash (23′–24′) for herpes, a bandage (25′), aspirants (26′, 28′) and a potion (27′) for bloating, a salve and a potion (29′)

for condylomata, a powder (30′), a bandaged-over daub (31′–32′), bandages (39′–42′, 50′–51′, 61′–63′), tampons (43′–49′, 52′–54′, 56′–57′, 64′–65′), washes (43′–46′, 52′–53′, 61′–63′), a potion (55′), baths (58′–63′), and rubs (56′–57′, 64′) for puerperal fever, aliments (33′–35′) and a potion (36′–38′) for diarrhea and a tampon (67′–68′) for reactive arthritis. The text ends with remarks on the ominous significance of births (69′–70′) and ends with a tampon (71′–74′) to prevent a miscarriage.

What is interesting about lines 11′–16′ is that they avowedly supplement medical treatment with something to take the patient's mind off of her problem. Unlike the ancient Greeks physicians, ancient Mesopotamians had no embarrassment about speaking of a woman's "mind." The magic circle of lines 61′–63′ was designed to ensure that the medicines went to work right away.

1′. [..] ^{Ú}x[...]

2′. [DIŠ] KI.MIN *si-si*[*k-ti* ...]
3′. 1-*niš ta-sàk* [...]

4′. DIŠ ^{MUNUS}PEŠ$_4$-*ma* ⸢ŠÀ.MEŠ⸣ [...]
5′. ZAG.ḪI.LI *ta-ma-ši-*[*id* ...]

6′. GEŠTIN SUR.RA KAŠ KALAG.GA NAG [...]
7′. *it-ti qí-líp* ZÚ.LUM.MA *ina* Ì.UDU x x [...]
8′. *za-mar* x x *ši-i* SA$_5$ *i-tab-ba-ka* A GAZI^{SAR} ⸢KÁ ŠÀ.TÙR-*šá*⸣ [ŠÉŠ-*aš*]
9′. *saḫ-lé-e ina* Ì.UDU ḪE.ḪE *ana* ŠÀ.TÙR-*šá* GAR-*ma kal* U$_4$-*me ú-k*[*al*]

10′. *a-nu-ú šá pi-i ṭup-*⸢*pi*⸣

11′. *ta-ḫap-šá la-bi-ra it-ti gu-un-ni li-taḫ-ḫi-ḫu-ma pur-qa liš-ši*
12′. *mu-un-da šá* GÚ.TUR ^{ŠEM}ḪAB *ina* GA *li-taḫ-ḫi-ḫu-ma pur-qa liš-ši*
13′. *mu-ṣip-ti la-bir-ta ina* GA *li-taḫ-ḫi-ḫu-ma pur-qa liš-ši*
14′. *gul-gul* NAM.LÚ.U$_{19}$.LU *ina* IZI *li-ir-ri-‹ru›*[63]*-ma ina* ^{SÍG}*pu-šik-ki liš-ši*
15′. EN *ina ṭè-mi-šá* ⸢*iṭ*⸣*-ṭi-*⸢*ra di-ú*⸣ [*di-lip-t*]*u*$_4$ *ana muḫ-ḫi la i-qar-ru-ub*

16′. *a-gan-nu-ú šá šum-ʾ-ut-tu*

17′. DIŠ MUNUS Ù.TU-*ma e-la-an ú-ri-šá ú-sa-ḫal-ši em-ša-ša* TAG.MEŠ-*ši*
18′. MUNUS BI Ì.RA DIB-*si e-ra-a šá* KAŠ.ÚS.SA *baḫ-ru-su* LAL-*si* EME UR.GI$_7$

19′. GEŠTIN.KA$_5$.A SÚD *ina* KAŠ ŠEG$_6$-*šal ta-šá-ḫal ana* GAL$_4$.LA-*šá ta-ak-ra* ^{Ú}*imḫur-lim ina* GEŠTIN NAG-*ši*

20′. DIŠ MUNUS IM *iš-biṭ-ma ma-lit ù* SU-*šá* KÚR.KÚR *ana* TI-*šá* ^{GIŠ}GÚR.GÚR GAZI^{SAR} Ú.KUR.RA

21′. ^{ŠEM}LI ^{Ú}ḪAR.ḪAR ^{Ú}NU.LUḪ.ḪA *saḫ-lé-e* NUMUN GADA Ú *a-ši-e* ^{ŠEM}ḪAB

22′. Ú BABBAR 11 Ú.ḪI.A ŠEŠ *ina* KAŠ SAG *u* Ì ŠEG$_6$-*šal* ÍL-*ma ina-eš*

23′. DIŠ KI.MIN ^{GIŠ}*ḫa-šu-u* ^{Ú}NU.LUḪ.ḪA ^{GIŠ}ŠE.NÁ.A ZÚ.LUM.MA ^{Ú}*a-ṣú-ṣi-im-tú*

24′. 5 Ú *an-nu-ti ina* KAŠ SAG ŠEG$_6$-*šal ana* ŠÀ.TÙR-*šá* DUB

25′. DIŠ MUNUS Ù.TU-*ma* IM *ud-du-pat* ^{GIŠ}GÚR.GÚR ^{GIŠ}LI SÚD *ina* KAŠ.ÚS.SA SIG ḪE.ḪE *e-ma* GAL$_4$.LA-*šá* LAL-*ma ina-eš*

26′. DIŠ MUNUS Ù.TU-*ma ṣi-im-rat u* IM *ud-du-pat* SAḪAR ^{URUDU}NÍG.KALAG.GA *tu-še-ṣe-en-ši-ma ina-eš*

27′. DIŠ KI.MIN ^{ŠEM}LI SÚD *ina* KAŠ SAG NAG-*ši-ma ina-eš*

28′. DIŠ MUNUS *e*ʾ*(em)-re-et-ma u* IM *ud-du-pat* DIM$_{10}$.ME DIB SAḪAR ^{URUDU}NÍG.KALAG.GA-*e tu-še-ṣe-en-ši*

29′. DIŠ MUNUS Ù.TU-*ma* SU-*šá bir-di* DIRI DÚR-*šá ma-qit* PA ^{GIŠ}ḪA.LU.ÚB *ina* Ì EŠ *ina* KAŠ NAG

30′. DIŠ MUNUS MIN-*ma* LI.DUR-*sa* DU$_8$-*at* IR *a-la-ka la i-kal-la* $^{\text{NA}_4}$PEŠ$_4$ *tur-ár* SÚD *ana* IGI ŠUB

31′. DIŠ KI.MIN ^{Ú}GÍR.LAGAB ^{Ú}ŠAKIRA ^{Ú}EME.UR.GI$_7$ ^{Ú}ḪAB ^{Ú}SIKIL ḪÁD.A *mál-ma-liš* SÚD

32′. $^{\text{NA}_4}$PEŠ$_4$ ḪE.ḪE-*ma* Ì ^{GIŠ}ERIN *ana* IGI LI.DUR-*šá ta-sár-raq* LAL-*id*

33′. DIŠ MUNUS MIN-*ma ir-ru-šá* SI.SÁ ^{GIŠ}GÚR.GÚR SÚD NINDA.Ì.DÉ.A ZÌ.KUM Ì.NUN GU$_7$ *ir-ru-šá ik-*[…]-*ru*

34′. DIŠ MUNUS MIN-*ma re-du-ut ir-ri* TUKU ZÌ.KUM ZÍD ZÍZ.ÀM Ì.UDU ÉLLAG UDU Ì.UDU GUD KI.A.⌈^{d}⌉[ÍD]

35′. ŠE.LÚ^{SAR} SÚD KI Ì.UDU *tu-sa-maḫ ina* DUḪ.LÀL ŠUB-*ma* ŠEG$_6$-*šal* GU$_7$-*ši-ma* [...]

36′. DIŠ ⌈^{MUNUS}⌉*ḫa-riš-tú* ŠÀ.SI.SÁ DIB-*si* NÍG.ÀR.RA ZÍZ.ÀM ZÚ.LUM.MA x [...]

37′. [*ina*] ^{DUG}NÍG.DÚR.BÙR *tàra-sà-an ina ši-mi-tan tu-*[...]

38′. NAG-*ši-ma* [...]

39′. DIŠ MUNUS Ù.TU-*ma* KÚM *ir-ri* TUKU.[TUKU]-*ši i-ár-ru* ŠÀ *ši-*[...]

40′. MÚD *ḫa-riš-ti-šá ina* ŠÀ-*šá it-t*[*e-es*]-*ki-ru* MUNUS BI *ina* Ù.TU-*š*[*á* ...]

41′. ZÍD ^{ŠE}GIG ZÍD GAZI^{SAR} B[ÍL].MEŠ ZÍD ^{GIŠ}ŠE.NU ^{ŠEM}GÚR.GÚR ^{GIŠ}L[I ...]

42′. DUḪ.ŠE.GIŠ.Ì ŠÈ TU$^{\text{MUŠEN.MEŠ}}$ [*ina*] $^{\text{NA}_4}$NA.ZAG.ḪI.LI SÚD *ina* KAŠ.ÚS.SA [...]

43′. DIŠ MIN KAŠ.Ú.SA SIG ^{GIŠ}GÚR.GÚR ^{GIŠ}LI ^{ŠEM}BULUḪ GAZI^{SAR} BÍL.MEŠ ^{Ú}NU.LAḪ.Ḫ[A ...]

44′. *saḫ-lé-e* BÍL.MEŠ *bu-ṭu-tú ina* ŠÀ DUB-*aq ina* Ì ḪE.ḪE *ina* TÚG *šú-nu-ti tála-pap ana* Š[À.TÙR-*šá* GAR-*an*]

45′. ÍL-*ma ú-kal* GIN$_7$ *ši-i i-te-mu pa-gar-šá it-tan-pa-ḫu ú-na-kar-ma* LÀ[L ...]

46′. 1-*niš tuš-tab-bal ina* MUD A.BÁR *ana pag-ri-šá i-nap-paḫ-ma ina-*[*eš*]

47′. DIŠ MIN ^{GIŠ}GÚR.GÚR ^{GIŠ}LI GAZI^{SAR} ^{GIŠ}ERIN.SUMUN ^{ŠEM}MUG ^{Ú}NU.LAḪ.ḪA ^{GIŠ}MAN.DU ^{GIŠ}*ti-iá-tú*

48′. ^{ŠEM}ḪAB ILLU ^{ŠEM}BULUḪ ^{Ú}*an-daḫ-šum* ^{Ú}*šu-un-ḫu* ^{Ú}MAŠ.TAB.BA KAŠ.ÚS.SA SIG

49′. 1-*niš te-ṭe*$_4$-*en ina* Ì ^{ŠEM}GÍR *u* KAŠ ŠEG$_6$-*šal lap-pa tála-pap* Ì SUD *ana* ŠÀ.TÙR-*šá* GAR-*an*

50′. DIŠ MIN ZÍD ^{ŠE}GIG ZÍD GAZI^{SAR} BÍL.MEŠ ZÍD ^{GIŠ}ŠE.NÁ.A ^{GIŠ}LI ^{ŠEM}BULUḪ ZÍD ŠE.MUŠ$_5$ ⌈ZÍD⌉ GÚ.GAL

51′. ZÍD ^{ŠE}GÚ.TUR DUḪ.ŠE.GIŠ.Ì ŠÈ TU^{MUŠEN} NUMUN GADA ZÍD ^{GIŠ}*ḫa-ru-bi* KAŠ.ÚS.SA SIG *mál-ma-liš* ⌈SÚD⌉ ḪE.ḪE LAL

52′. DIŠ MIN ^{Ú}ḪAR.ḪAR ^{Ú}NU.LUḪ.ḪA Ú *a-ši-e* ^{GIŠ}GÚR.GÚR ^{GIŠ}LI GAZI^{SAR} Ú BABBAR NUMUN GADA

53′. 1-*niš* BÍL-*lu*$_4$ SÚD KI KAŠ.ÚS.SA ILLU LI.DUR *ina* Ì ŠEG$_6$-*šal ana* ŠÀ.TÙR-*šá* DUB *ina* ^{SÍG}ÀKA NIGIN *ina* ŠÀ.TÙR GAR-*an*

54′. DIŠ MIN ^{Ú}*a-zu-ki-ra-ni* SÚD *ina* Ì *u* KAŠ *ina* ŠÀ.TÙR!-*šá* GAR-*an* ^{GIŠ}MAN.DU ^{ŠEM}BULUḪ ^{GIŠ}LI KI KAŠ.ÚS.SA ḪE.ḪE MIN

55′. DIŠ MIN ^{GIŠ}GÚR.GÚR Ú *a-ši-e saḫ-lé-e* MUN ^{ŠEM}ḪAB ŠEM.ḪI.A DÙ.A.BI *ina* KAŠ ḪE.ḪE ⸢NAG⸣-*ma ina-eš*

56′. DIŠ MIN ^{GIŠ}GÚR.GÚR ^{GIŠ}LI GAZI^{SAR} Ú *a-ši-e* ^{ŠEM}ḪAB ^{GIŠ}MAN.DU *sik-ka-tú* KAŠ.Ú.SA SIG 1-*niš* ḪE.ḪE

57′. MUNUS ⸢ÍL⸣ KAŠ AL.ŠEG$_6$.GÁ *sú-un-šá ú-maš-šá-ʾ* ÍL-*ma ina-eš*

58′. ^{GIŠ}*šu-šum* ^{GIŠ}ŠE.NÁ.A ^{Ú}*ak-tam* GAZI^{SAR} GI DÙG ^{GIŠ}LUM.ḪA ^{GIŠ}*ár-gan-nu ina* A ŠUB ŠEG$_6$ *ina* ŠÀ RA.MEŠ-*si*

59′. DIŠ MUNUS MIN-*ma* KÚM *li-ʾ-ba u tir-ku ina* UZU.MEŠ-*šá u* SA.MEŠ-*šá* KAB^{ME} *qer-bi-nu*

60′. MÚD.BABBAR *ú-kal ana šup-šú-ḫi ina*! A GAZI^{SAR} *ina* A ^{GIŠ}*bu-uṭ-na-nu* RA.MEŠ

61′. A.GAR.GAR *ša* IGI MU.AN.NA *ina* NINDU BAD-*ir* RA-*si* Ì *u* KAŠ *ana* ŠÀ.TÙR-*šá* DUB-*ak*

62′. 1 *qa* ZÍD ^{GIŠ}*šu-še* 1 *qa* ZÍD DUḪ.ŠE.GIŠ.Ì 1 *qa* ZÍD MUNU$_6$ 1 *qa* ZÍD ^{GIŠ}GÚR.GÚR 1 *qa* ^{ŠEM}LI

63′. *ina* A GAZI^{SAR} SILA$_{11}$-*aš ina zì-sur-ri tu-kàṣ-ṣa ina ruq-qí* LAL-*id*

64′. DIŠ KI.MIN GA GA.RAŠ^{SAR} *tu-kàṣ-ṣa-ma* EŠ-*aš ana* ŠÀ.TÙR-*šá* GAR-*an*

65′. DIŠ MUNUS MIN-*ma* ⸢ŠÀ-*bi-šá*⸣ SÌG.SÌG-*si qer-bi-nu* MÚD.BABBAR TUKU GAZI^{SAR} ^{GIŠ}GÚR.GÚR BÍL ZAG.ḪI.LA SÚD ḪE.ḪE ALLA DÙ *ana* ŠÀ.TÙR-*šá* GAR-*an*

66′. ^{Ú}ḪAR.ḪAR ^{Ú}[…] Ì.UDU ÚKUŠ.GÍL ḪÁD.DU SÚD *ina* Ì *u* KAŠ NAG-*ši*

67′. DIŠ MUNUS MIN-*ma qer-bi-s*[*a* … *mi-na*]-*tu-šá ik-te-ner-ra-a* MUNUS BI a tur ri ti šá

68′. ^{Ú}GUR$_5$.UŠ SIG$_7$[-*su*] ⸢SÚD⸣ *ina* ⸢^{SÍG}ÀKA⸣ N[IGIN-*mi*] *ana* ŠÀ.TÙR-*šá* GAR-*an*

69′. DIŠ MUNUS *qer-bi-sa re-ḫu-tam im-ḫur-ma* DUMU.NÍTA [Ù.TU] *gi-mil-li* [DINGIR]

70′. DIŠ MUNUS *qer-bi-sa re-ḫu-tam im-ḫur-ma* NU Ù.TU *šib-sat* DINGIR NU DÙG-*ub* [ŠÀ]

71′. DIŠ MUNUS *ina* ŠÀ TUKU-*at ka-la-a la i-le-ʾ-e ana* MUNUS *nu-uḫ-ḫi* GÌR.PAD.DA G[ÍD.DA]

72′. SAL.ÁŠ.GÀR GÌŠ.NU.ZU *ki-lal-la-*⸢*an*⸣ x [...] ⸢NÍG⸣.ÀR.RA *ina* A *ta-maḫ-ḫa-a*[*ṣ*]

73′. GÌR.PAD.DU GÍD.DA *šú-nu-ti ina* ŠÀ x[...] x x [...]

74′. *ina* GAL$_4$.LA-*šá* GAR-*an tu-u*[*l* ...]

75′. ^{Ú}*ku-li-*[*la-nu*?]

76′. ^{Ú}[...]

TRANSLATION

(1′–3′) *(fragmentary)*

(4′–5′) If a woman is pregnant and her insides [...], you ⸢comb out⸣ *saḫlû*-cress [...]

(6′–9′) (Alternatively), you have her drink drawn wine (and) strong beer. [...] with date rind in sheep fat [...]. (If) suddenly that [...] pours out red (liquid),[64] you [gently rub/wash?] the entrance to her vagina with *kasû* juice. You mix *saḫlû*-cress with sheep fat (and) insert (it) into her vagina and she keeps (it) there all day.

(10′) These are (copied) in accordance with a tablet.

(11′–15′) Let them moisten an old blanket with average quality (oil) and let her wear (it as) a *burqa*.[65] Let them moisten groats made from *kakku*-lentils (and) *ṭūru*-aromatic with milk and let her wear (it as) a *burqa*. Let them moisten an old *muṣiptu*-garment with milk and let her wear (it as) a *burqa*. Let them(!) char a human skull with fire and let her wear (it wrapped) in a piece of combed wool. (She should do this) until it escapes from her mind; *diʾu* and ⸢sleeplessness⸣ must not approach (her).

(16′) This is supplemental.

(17′–19′) If a woman gives birth and subsequently her pubic region stings her (and) her lower abdomen (hypogastric region) continually hurts her intensely, "striking" afflicts that woman.[66] You bandage her with hot dregs of beerwort. You grind *lišān kalbi* (and) "fox grape." You boil (it) in beer, filter (it) and pour(?) (it) into her vulva. You have her drink *imḫur-lim* (mixed) with wine.

(20′–22′) If "wind" blasts a woman and she is about to give birth[67] and her body looks worse and worse,[68] to cure her, you boil these eleven plants: *kukru*, *kasû*, *nīnû*-mint, *burāšu*-juniper, *ḫašû*-thyme, *nuḫurtu*, *saḫlû*-cress, flax seed, *šammi ašî*, *ṭūru*-aromatic, (and) "white plant" in first-quality beer and oil. If she wears (it), she should recover.

(23′–24′) Alternatively, you boil these five plants: *ḫašû*-thyme, *nuḫurtu*, *šunû*-chastetree, dates (and) *aṣuṣimtu* in first-quality beer. You pour (it) into her vagina.

(25′) If a woman gives birth and subsequently is inflated with "wind," you grind *kukru* (and) *burāšu*-juniper. You mix (it) with winnowed beerwort. If you completely bandage her vulva (with it), she should recover.

(26′) If a woman gives birth and subsequently becomes distended and is inflated with "wind,"[69] if you have her smell dust from a copper kettledrum, she should recover.

(27′) Alternatively, you grind *burāšu*-juniper. If you have her drink (it mixed) with first-quality beer, she should recover.

(28′) If a woman is colicky and puffed up with "wind," if you have her smell dust from a copper kettledrum, she should recover.

(29′) If a woman gives birth and subsequently her body is full of *birdu*-nodules (and) her anus has prolapsed,[70] you rub her gently with *ḫaluppu*-tree leaves (mixed) with oil (and) have her drink (it mixed) with beer.

(30′) If a woman (gives birth) and subsequently her umbilical area (feels) supple (but) she cannot stop sweat from coming,[71] you char (and)grind *išqil-latu*-shell[72] (and) pour (it) on it.

(31′–32′) Alternatively, you dry (and) grind *dadānu*-thorn, *šakirû*, *lišān kalbi*, *šammi bu᾽šāni*, (and) *sikillu* in equal proportions. You mix (it) with *išq-illatu*-shell (and) *erēnu*-cedar resin. You scatter (it) on her umbilical area (and) bandage (it) over.

(33′) If a woman (gives birth) and subsequently she has loose bowels,[73] you grind *kukru* (and) have her eat (it) with *mersu*-confection made with *isqūqu*-flour (and) ghee. Her bowels should […]

(34′–35′) If a woman (gives birth) and subsequently she has flowing of the bowels,[74] you grind *isqūqu*-flour, emmer flour, sheep kidney fat, ox fat, *kibrītu*-sulphur (and) *kisibirrītu*-coriander. You mix (it) together with sheep fat, pour (it) into wax (and) boil (it). If you have her eat (it), [she should recover].

(36′–38′) If loose bowels afflict a woman in confinement,[75] you soak emmer groats, dates (and) [… in …] in a *namzītu*-vessel. In the evening, you […]. If you have her drink it […].

(39′–42′) If a woman gives birth and subsequently she [continually] has internal fever, she vomits and [...], the blood of her confinement has been ⸢locked⸣ up inside her; that woman, while giving birth [...].[76] You grind wheat flour, powdered ⸢roasted⸣ *kasû*, powdered *šunû*-chastetree, *kukru*, *burāšu*-juniper, [...], sesame residue, (and) "dove dung" with a stone pestle. [You mix (it)] with beerwort (and) [bandage her with it].

(43′–46′) Alternatively, [you ...] winnowed beerwort, *kukru*-aromatic, *burāšu*-juniper, *baluḫḫu*-aromatic, roasted *kasû*, *nuḫurtu* (and) [...]. You pour roasted *saḫlû*-cress (and) *buṭuttu*-cereal into it. You mix (them) with oil (and) wind them into burls with a cloth. [You insert it] into [her] ⸢vagina⸣. She takes (it) up and keeps (it) there. As soon as it has changed (color)[77] and her body has become swollen, she takes it out. Then you have her mix together honey (and) [...]. If she blows (it) into her body with a lead tube, she should recover.

(47′–49′) Alternatively, you mill-grind together *kukru*, *burāšu*-juniper, *kasû*, *šupuḫru*-cedar, *ballukku*-aromatic, *nuḫurtu*, *suʾādu*, *tiyātu*, *ṭūru*-aromatic, *baluḫḫu*-aromatic resin, *antaḫšum*-vegetable, *šunḫu*, *šammi ašî* (and) winnowed beerwort. You boil (it) in *asu*-myrtle oil and beer (and) wind (it) into a burl. You sprinkle (it) with oil (and) insert (it) into her vagina.

(50′–51′) Alternatively, you grind (and) mix wheat flour, roasted *kasû* flour, *šunû*-chastetree flour, *burāšu*-juniper, *baluḫḫu*-aromatic, *šigūšu* flour, *ḫalluru*-chick pea flour, *kakku*-lentil flour, sesame residue, "dove dung," flax seed, *ḫarubu*-carob flour, (and) winnowed beerwort in equal proportions. You bandage (her with it).

(52′–53′) Alternatively, you roast together (and) grind *ḫašû*-thyme, *nuḫurtu*, *šammi ašî*, *kukru*-aromatic, *burāšu*-juniper, *kasû*, "white plant," (and) flax seed. You boil (it) with beerwort (and) *abukkatu* resin (mixed) with oil (and) pour (it) into her vagina. You wrap (it) in a tuft of wool (and) insert (it) into her vagina.

(54′) Alternatively, you grind *azukirānu* (and) insert (it) into her vagina (mixed) with oil and beer. You mix *suʾādu*, *baluḫḫu*-aromatic resin, (and) *burāšu*-juniper with beerwort ditto (and insert it into her vagina).

(55′) Alternatively, you mix *kukru*, *šammi ašî*, *saḫlû*-cress, salt, *ṭūru*-aromatic, (and) assorted incense. If you have her drink (it), she should recover.

(56′–57′) Alternatively, you mix together *kukru*-aromatic, *burāšu*-juniper, *kasû*, *šammi ašî*, *ṭūru*-aromatic, *suʾādu*, *sikkatu*-yeast, (and) winnowed beerwort. The woman wears (it). She should massage her lap with boiled beer. If she wears (it), she should recover.

(58′) You pour *šūšu*-licorice, *šunû*-chastetree, *aktam*, *kasû*, "sweet reed," *barirātu*, (and) *argannu* into water. You boil (it and) repeatedly bathe her with it.

(59′–60′) If a woman (gives birth) and subsequently she (has) fever (and) *li'bu* and dark spots accumulate(?) on her flesh and her veins (and) inside she contains pus,[78] to soothe it, you repeatedly bathe her with *kasû* juice (and) with *buṭnānu* infusion.

(61′–63′) You bake (gazelle) dung from the early part of the year in an oven (and) bathe her (with it). You pour oil and beer into her vagina. You make 1 *qû* of powdered *šūšu*-licorice, 1 *qû* of powdered sesame residue, 1 *qû* of malt flour, 1 *qû* of *kukru*-aromatic flour, (and) 1 *qû* of *burāšu*-juniper flour into a dough with *kasû* juice. You let (it) cool in a magic circle (and) bandage (her) over the canal (with it).

(64′) Alternatively, you cool *karāšu*-leek with milk and rub her gently (with it). You insert (it) into her vagina.

(65′) If a woman ditto (gives birth) and subsequently her insides give her a sharp pain (and) she has pus within, you grind (and) mix *kasû*, roasted *kukru* (and) *saḫlû*-cress. You form an acorn-shaped suppository (and) insert (it) into her vagina.

(66′) You dry and grind *ḫašû*-thyme, [...] (and) *irrû* "fat." You have her drink (it mixed) with oil and beer.

(67′–68′) If a woman (gives birth) and subsequently inside [...] (and) her ⌈limbs⌉ become shrunken,[79] that woman [...]. You grind fresh *šarmadu*, wrap (it) in a tuft of wool (and) insert (it) into her vagina.

(69′) If a woman's womb receives the semen and [she gives birth to] a son, (it means) [divine] favor.

(70′) If a woman's womb receives the semen and she does not give birth, (it means) divine anger (and) ⌈unhappiness⌉.

(71′–74′) If a woman has something in her womb but cannot retain (it),[80] to calm the woman, you stir both long bones of a virgin she-goat (and) [...], mill-ground, into water. [You wrap] those long bones [in a tuft of wool] (and) insert (it) into her vuvla. ⌈She should be able to give birth.⌉

(75′–76′) *(fragmentary)*

Notes

1. See Finkel, 1980, 37–52.

2. This is a pseudo ideogram for *da'mātu*-clay. MUD is *da'mu*: "blood colored" and the determinative indicates a feminine.

3. See Finkel 1980, 50.

4. Line i 41′ is a glossenkeil line (an explanatory gloss). Glosses appear either on a separate line or actually in the line to which they belong and are marked by a glossenkeil, rendered in transliteration by a colon (:).

5. See *CAD* Ṭ, 110–11.

6. This would be a popular name for a plant. Alternatively, the signs have been read

backwards by the scribe and are actually DÀRA.MAŠ: "stag." Suggestion courtesy M. Stol.

7. Alternatively, one could read ÚḪA.‹LÚ›.UB *li-li-*[...]. Suggestion courtesy M. Stol.

8. The verbs are consistently masculine singular.

9. See Finkel 1980, 37–52.

10. The epithet points to the Ishtar of OB Zabalam. See Krebernik 2012, 256–57.

11. The text has a MIN sign (two wedges) under the section to be repeated, an almost exact analogue to our "ditto" sign.

12. See Scurlock and Andersen 2005, 2.25.

13. See Scurlock and Andersen 2005, 4.21.

14. *CAD* U/W, 212b takes this as an instruction to dry the rush.

15. Akkadian *nību* seems to function similarly to Turkish *tane*, indicating that something is being counted.

16. See Scurlock and Andersen 2005, 4.22.

17. For the reading *purīdu* for GÌR, see *CAD* P.

18. The expression, fairly common in medical texts, indicates that an action or procedure is to be repeated.

19. $BURU_{14}$ has a reading *erištu*, here for *erištu*: "wish."

20. See Scurlock and Andersen 2005, 12.17. The translation is restored from the similar BM 42313+43174 rev. 29–32.

21. Literally "and her vomiting"—the construction is an Aramaicism.

22. The text consistently omits determinatives, which make it unclear whether this is ŠEM. ŠEŠ or ŠE.$MUŠ_5$.

23. Literally: "after that stands."

24. For the restoration, see Collins 1999, 181–82.

25. Compare: "A cloud, a cloud, a red cloud has risen and covered (another) red cloud. Red rain has risen and fecundated the red earth. A red flood has risen and filled a red canal. Let the red farmer bring a red plow and a red hod and let him dam up the red water" (CT 23.37 iii 65–67 [*CAD* S, 131b s.v. *sāmu* mng e]).

26. For the expression, see chapter 16, text 4 ii 16′.

27. See Klein 1983, 255–84 ("toggle pin").

28. She is an Elamite because she comes up (*e-lam-ma*) from the swamp. The large topnot is a distinctive mark of Elamite dress which may be seen on Assyrian reliefs showing Elamite prisoners.

29. Farber 2014, 83, 155 differently.

30. See Scurlock and Andersen 2005, 19.232, as here corrected.

31. Reading *ta-pil-tim* (from *apālu*: to answer; cf. *tapalu*: pair). Differently Farber 2014, 84, 155.

32. Farber 2014, 84, 157 differently.

33. In other words, she drops the child.

34. *Šurpu* (Reiner 1958), tablet IV: 24–25, 28–29, 31.

35. Collation M. Geller, courtesy M. Stol.

36. The restoration is based on KUB 4.13:17.

37. Suggestion courtesy M. Stol.

38. Alternatively, this could be a reference to the mother: [*e-ri*]*-ti*: "pregnant woman." Suggestion courtesy M. Stol. Usually however, by this point, the mother is referred to as "the woman having difficulty having birth." The restoration supposes a completion of the quay motif of the preceding lines.

39. See *CAD* A/1, 293a.

40. See Scurlock and Andersen 2005, 12.60.

41. Alternatively, one could take this as *ep-ri*: "dust" and connect it with the following phrases. Suggestion courtesy M. Stol. In this case what was understood to be forming in the womb was "human clay."

42. Literally: "deliver safely," "bring to completion." Suggestion courtesy M. Stol.

43. The unborn child is here speaking from the womb. See Finkel 1980, 45.

44. Compare Lambert 1965, 287 obv. 20–25; Lambert 1969, pl. 5: 53–56.

45. Compare Lambert 1965, 287 obv. 25–29; Lambert 1969, pl. 5: 56–57.

46. Compare Lambert 1965, 287 obv. 29–31; Lambert 1969, pl. 5:57–60 (with two daughters of Anu instead of the protective divinities).

47. Compare Lambert 1965, 287 obv. 32–36; Lambert 1969, pl. 5:60–62; KUB 4.13:6–12. For this recitation, see also Röllig 1985, 260–73.

48. For more on the foetus as a snake in the womb, see Civil 1974, 294 ad ll. 3–5.

49. If the baby actually did this, it would result in a breech birth.

50. *CAD* R, 263b s.v. *rēmu* takes this as an irregular imperative meaning "have mercy."

51. This is probably meant to evoke MUNUS LA.RA.AḪ, the woman having difficulty giving birth.

52. See Scurlock and Andersen 2005, 12.59.

53. The reading follows *CAD* Q, 326b s.v. *qutru* mng 1c.

54. BA.MEŠ (= *qištū* "gifts" or *zittū* "portions") in lines 37–39 is interpreted by Lambert as a scribal mistake for the expected SAḪAR.MEŠ (*epru* "dusts").

55. For the reading, see *CAD* R, 334a.

56. The text has AN.BAR$_7$ (= *muṣlālu* "noon"), which Lambert emends to the expected IZI.GAR (= *nūru* "light").

57. See Scurlock and Andersen 2005, 12.122.

58. For the translation of *saḫlû* as "cress," see Stol 1983–84, 24–32.

59. *CAD* Q, 178b misconstrues *kânu* to refer to a mother's alleged emotional attachment to the foetus, making it her fault that she is about to die. As Lambert already realized, the infant (*šerru*), which has a feminine plural and is therefore grammatically feminine, is the subject of the sentence.

60. This means that either she or the baby or both may die. Pace *CAD* Š/1, 489b and Š/3 11a, this has nothing to do with *šimtu*: "paint, varnish, brandmark."

61. This deity, the head of the Babylonian pantheon and an important god in Assyria as well was, like the Moon God, a patron of childbirth.

62. The unborn child is here speaking from the womb. See Finkel 1980, 45.

63. The emendation is the suggestion of Stol 2007a, 2.

64. See Scurlock and Andersen 2005, 12.46.

65. *purqa* is presumably from *parāqu*, a West Semitic loanword meaning: "to isolate." The *CAD* P, 521b translates this passage: "she should wear it in a *p.* manner." The obvious suggestion is that the reference is to what is still called a *burqa*.

66. See Scurlock and Andersen 2005, 12.120.

67. What the text literally says is that she is in a state of fullness (from *malû*: "to be full"). What this means is that she is as full as she can be, meaning that the baby is fully grown and ready to be born. Compare the French *plein*, said of a pregnant woman.

68. See Scurlock and Andersen 2005, 4.15.

69. See Scurlock and Andersen 2005, 12.116

70. See Scurlock and Andersen 2005, 4.27, 10.73.

71. See Scurlock and Andersen 2005, 12.123.

72. Pace *CAD* I/J, *išqillatu* means "shell" and not "pebble."

73. See Scurlock and Andersen 2005, 12.117.

74. See Scurlock and Andersen 2005, 12.118.

75. See Scurlock and Andersen 2005, 12.58.

76. See Scurlock and Andersen 2005, 6.78, 12.124.

77. See chapter 12, text 2 rev. 1′–15′.

78. See Scurlock and Andersen 2005, 10.61, 12.125.

79. If the restoration is apt, the reference will be to arthritis and, given the context, perhaps "sausage digits." See Scurlock and Andersen 2005, 11.20. Alternatively, it would be possible to restore [*nap-šá*]-*tu-šá* in which case she would be continually short of breath. Suggestion courtesy M. Stol.

80. See Scurlock and Andersen 2005, 12.51.

13

PEDIATRICS

A. INFANTILE SEIZURES

The ancient physician was a careful observer, who has left to us a very wide description of birth defects. A tablet of the diagnostic series (no. 40) was devoted exclusively to the medical problems of infants. For more details, see Scurlock and Andersen, 2005, chapter 17. Treatments specifically and exclusively designed for infants or toddlers are relatively rare and usually scattered among prescriptions for adults with similar problems. So, for example, BM 78963: 45–46 (see chapter 8, text 3) deals with an infant with *su'ālu* cough.

Seizures are not uncommon among infants, although not everything that looks like a seizure actually is one. For details, see chapters 13 and 19 in Scurlock and Andersen 2005, 316–17 and 442–44.

TEXT 1: K 3628 + 4009 + SM. 1315

K 3628+ is interesting in that it represents an extract text (rev. 20–23) which apparently was designed to find salves (obv. 3–4, 11–15, 17–19, 23, rev. 13–16), fumigants (obv. 20–23) and an amulet (obv. 25–rev. 12) for (mostly) neurological conditions affecting infants, namely, AN.TA.ŠUB.BA Lugalurra, "hand" of god, "hand" of Ishtar, *lilû*-demon, and evil *alû*-demon. Unfortunately, the first two sections and all but the end of the third are lost. These sections were extracted from tablets that contained other treatments (obv. 5, 16, 24, rev. 17) for the same conditions. Periodically, the symptoms that allowed the physician to recognize the condition in question are given (obv. 6–9, rev. 18–19), quoted from the Diagnostic and Prognostic Handbook (SA.GIG), as our text tells us explicitly (obv. 10). Since we have the tablet from which these were quoted, these sections can be restored in their entirety. As luck would have it, another text allows us to guess what was in the missing section on "hand" of god (see below, text 3).

Mūṣu stone (obv. 12, 19) is probably bezoar (ox bile stone), something that is used in modern Chinese medicine[1] as an anticonvulsant. The amulet (obv. 25–rev. 12) is particularly interesting in that it provides a rare example where a text is actually written onto the object used as an amulet, in this case a clay cylinder seal of which actual examples have been discovered (see below, text 2).

obv.

1. (traces)
2. (traces)
3. [Ú.ḪI].⌜A *an*⌝-[*nu-ti a-na* ŠU.DINGIR.RA] LÚ.TUR Š[ÉŠ.MEŠ-*su-ma* TI]

---

4. [# *n*]*ap-šal*-⌜*a*⌝-*t*[*i an-na-ti ša*] LÚ.TUR ŠU.DINGIR.⌜RA⌝ [DIB-*su*]

---

5. ⌜*ni-pi-ši*⌝ *qu-ta*-⌜*ri*⌝ [*ù maš-qa-a-ti š*]*a* DIŠ LÚ.TUR ŠU.DINGIR.RA NU TE-*e ul am-r*[*u*]

---

6. DIŠ LÚ.TUR *ib-ta-n*[(*ak-ki u* GÙ)].GÙ-*si ek-ke-em-tum* ŠU ^{d}15 DUMU. MUNUS ^{d}*A-nim*
7. DIŠ LÚ.TUR *tu-la*-[(*a i-niq-ma*) Š]UB-*tu* ŠUB-*su* ŠU ^{d}15 : ^{d}30[2]
8. DIŠ LÚ.TUR *ina* ⌜KI⌝.[(NÁ-*šú*)] *ina* ⌜NU⌝ ZU-*ú is-si* ŠU ^{d}*Iš-tar*[3]
9. [(DIŠ)] LÚ.TUR *ina* ⌜KI⌝.[(NÁ-*šú is-si-ma*)] ⌜*mim-ma*⌝ *šá i-mu-ru i-qab-bu* ŠU ^{d}15 *ik-ri-bu* DIB.MEŠ-*šú*[4]

---

10. [SA].GIG *ša* LÚ.[TUR ŠU] ⌜^{d}INNIN⌝ DIB-*su ul-tu* ŠÀ-*bi* DIŠ LÚ.TUR *la-ʾ-ḫu* ZI.MEŠ-*ḫa*

---

11. [G]ÌR.PAD.DU LÚ.U$_{18}$.⌜LU⌝ *ina* Ì.GIŠ *ka-a-a-na* ŠÉŠ.MEŠ-*su*

---

12. $^{[NA]}{}_{4}$*mu-ṣu* ^{Ú}*ṣa-ṣu-un-tu* GÌR.PAD.DU ŠAḪ SÚD *ina* Ì ŠÉŠ.MEŠ-*su*

---

13. [BAR] MUŠ UM.ME.DA GÍR.TAB *saḫ-lé-e* TÚG.NÍG.DÁRA.ŠU.LÁL SÍG ŠAB NAGA.SI *ina* Ì ŠÉŠ.MEŠ-*su*

---

14. [Ú.ḪI.A] *an-nu-ti a-na* ŠU ^{d}INNIN LÚ.TUR ŠÉŠ.MEŠ-*su-ma* TI

---

15. [3 *nap*]-*šal-a-ti ša* LÚ.TUR ŠU ^{d}INNIN DIB-*su*

---

16. *ni-pi*-[*š*]*i* A.UGU *qut*-PA *ù maš-qa-a-ti ul am-ra*

---

17. DIŠ *a-na* [(L)]Ú.TUR LÍL.LÁ.EN.NA NU TE-*e*
18. GÌR.PAD.DU L[(Ú)].U$_{18}$.LU *ina* Ì *ka-a-a-na* ŠÉŠ.MEŠ-*su*

19. DIŠ KI.MIN ^{NA_4}⸢*mu*⸣-*ṣa* ⸢^{Ú}*ṣa*⸣-*ṣu-un-tú* GÌR.PAD.DU ŠAḪ SÚD *ina* Ì ŠÉŠ.MEŠ-*su*

20. DIŠ KI.MIN SÍG ⸢UR⸣.GU.LA ⸢SÍG UR⸣.GI$_7$ SÍG ⸢ÙZ *ina* DÈ⸣ SAR-*šú*

21. DIŠ KI.MIN BAR [MUŠ] UM.M[E.D]A GÍR.TAB *saḫ-lé-e* TÚG.NÍG. DÁRA.ŠU.⸢LÁL⸣
22. ⸢SÍG⸣.[ŠAB] NAGA.SI *ina* DÈ SAR-*šú*

23. *n*[*ap-šal-a-t*]*i u qut*-PA ⸢*ša*⸣ *a-na* LÚ.TUR LÍL.LÁ.EN.NA NU TE-*e*

24. [*ni-pi-ši* A.UGU] *u maš-qa-a-ti* NU *am-ra*

25. [ÉN É BA.AN.GE].E BA.AN.ŠÚ
26. [BI.ZA.AḪ A]N.NÉ BI.ZA.⸢AḪ⸣
27. [DINGIR.RE.E.NE.KE$_4$ A.ŠÀ].⸢GA⸣ BA.AN.Ú[S]
rev.
1. ⸢^{d}⸣*A*-⸢*nu*⸣ *ina* AN-*e i*[*g-ru-uš*]
2. *u er-ṣe-tum ina ra-ma-ni-šá-ma ig-ru-uš* [TU$_6$ ÉN][5]

3. ÉN MUL.KAK.SI.SÁ MU.NE *mu-šá-lil* [(MURUB$_4$)]
4. *muš-te-ʾ-u ur-ḫe*-⸢*e-ti*⸣ *mu-šak-lil m*[(*im*+*ma* MU-*šú*)]
5. ^{GIŠ}TUKUL.DINGIR *šá ina pa-an* ^{GIŠ}⸢TUKUL⸣ *na-an-du-ru t*[(*e-bu-ú*)]
6. *a-na* NENNI A NENNI NU ⸢TE⸣-*ḫi* NU [(DIM$_4$-*qa*)]
7. LÚ.ZI.ZI LÚ.ZI.ZI NAM.BA.TE.GÁ.E.D[(È TU$_6$ ÉN)][6]

8. 2 KA.INIM.MA LÚ.TUR A.LÁ.ḪUL ŠÚ.[ŠÚ-*šú*]

9. DÙ.DÙ.BI ^{NA_4}KIŠIB ⸢IM⸣ *kul-la-ti* [DÙ-*uš-ma*]
10. ÉN *an-ni-tú ina* UG[U] SA[R-*ár-ma*]
11. *ina* IZI IN.BUBBU *ta-ṣa*[*r-ra*]*p* ⸢*šum*$_4$⸣-*ma ina* GÚ-*šú* G[AR-*an*]
12. *šum*$_4$-*ma ina* SAG ^{GIŠ}NÁ-*šú tal-lal-ma mim-ma lem-nu* NU TE-*š*[*ú*][7]

13. DIŠ *mim-ma lem-nu ana* LÚ.TUR NU TE-*e* NUMUN ^{GIŠ}MA.NU NUMUN ^{Ú}ŠAKIRA
14. NUMUN ^{Ú}KU$_6$ TÚG.NÍG.DÁRA.ŠU.LÁL *ina* Ì.GIŠ ḪE.ḪE
15. [*l*]*a*-[*a*]*m* UBUR *ana* KA-*šú* GAR-*nu* ŠÉŠ-*su-ma* TI-*uṭ*[8]

---

16. [KA.INIM.MA] *ù nap-šal-tu ša* LÚ.TUR A.LÁ.ḪUL ŠÚ.ŠÚ-*šú*
17. [SA.G]IG *ne-pe-ši qut*-PA *u maš-qa-a-ti ul am-ru*

---

18. [DIŠ *ṣi*]-*biṭ be-en-nim šá ina* MU.7.KÁM* Ù.TU IGI *i-a-az-za*
19. *i-ta-na-šá-áš ina* ŠUB-*šú* ŠU^{II}-*šú ana* EGIR-*šú* NIGIN-*mi*
20. [*ni-i*]*s-ḫu bul-ṭi ša* LÚ.TUR AN.TA.ŠUB.BA ^{d}LUGAL.ÙR.RA
21. [ŠU DINGIR ŠU] ^{d}INNIN LÍL.LÁ.EN.NA *ù* A.LÁ.ḪUL DIB-*su* AL.TIL
22. [… SA].GIG KI *ši-lu-ši-tú* AN.⸢TA.ŠUB⸣.BA
23. […] GIŠ.ZU.MEŠ ⸢IGI⸣-*r*[*u*…]

TRANSLATION

(obv. 1–3) (*two unreadable lines*) ⸢These plants⸣ [are for "hand" of god. If you repeatedly] ⸢gently rub⸣ the infant (with it), [he should recover.]

(obv. 4) [These X] ⸢salves⸣ [are for (cases where)] "hand" of god [afflicts] an infant.

(obv. 5) The rituals, fumigants [and leather-bag amulets] ⸢for⸣ (cases where) you do not want "hand" of god to approach an infant were not looked at.

(obv. 6–9) If an infant continually wails and screams, the thieving one,[9] "hand" of Ishtar, daughter of Anu.[10] If an infant sucks the breast and then a *miqtu*-seizure falls on him, "hand" of Ishtar (var. Sîn).[11] (infantile seizures) If a young child screams in his bed without knowing (it), "hand" of Ishtar. If a young child screams in his bed and says whatever he sees, "hand" of Ishtar; (unfulfilled) vows afflict him.[12] (nightmares)

(obv. 10) (Quoted from) [SA].GIG (Diagnostic and Prognostic Series) on (the subject of) ["hand"] of Ishtar afflicting an ⸢infant⸣ excerpted from "If an infant" (tablet 40).

(obv. 11) You continually and repeatedly rub him gently with "human bone" (= "lone plant") (mixed) with oil.

(obv. 12) You grind *mūṣu*-⸢stone⸣, *ṣaṣuntu* (and) pig bone. You repeatedly gently rub him (with it mixed) with oil.

(obv. 13) You repeatedly rub him gently (with) snake [skin], scorpion stinger, *saḫlû*-cress,[13] "soiled rag" (= *sikillu*), bristles, (and) *uḫḫulu qarnānu* (mixed) with oil.

(obv. 14) These [plants] are for "hand" of Ishtar. If you repeatedly gently rub the infant (with them), he should recover.

(obv. 15) [Three] ⸢salves⸣ for (cases where) "hand" of Ishtar afflicts an infant.

(obv. 16) The ⸢rituals⸣, amulets, fumigants and leather-bag amulets (for "hand" of Ishtar) were not looked at.

(obv. 17–18) If you do not want the *lilû* demon to approach an infant, you continually and repeatedly rub him with "human bone" (= "lone plant") (mixed) with oil.

(obv. 19) Alternatively, you repeatedly rub him with *mūṣu*-stone, *ṣaṣuntu* (and) pig bone (mixed) with oil.

(obv. 20) Alternatively, you fumigate him with lion hair, dog hair, (and) goat hair over coals.

(obv. 21–22) Alternatively, you fumigate him with [snake] skin, scorpion ⸢stinger⸣, *saḫlû*-cress, "soiled rag" (= *sikillu*), ⸢bristles⸣, (and) *uḫḫūlu qarnānu* over coals.

(obv. 23) ⸢Salves⸣ and fumigants for if you want "hand" of *lilû* not to approach an infant.

(obv. 24) [The rituals, amulets], and leather-bag amulets (for "hand" of *lilû*) were not looked at.

(obv. 25–rev. 2) Recitation: The house that was in good condition got "gotten." Heaven was lost, was lost. The gods were driven overland. Anu came near from heaven and the earth came near all by itself.

(rev. 3–7) Sirius is his name, one who utters the battle cry, seeker-out of paths, one who brings everything to fruition, the *mīṭu*-mace which is more furious than all other weapons. May an attacker not approach (or) come near so-and-so, son of so-and-so. May no attackers approach. Spell (and) recitation.

(rev. 8) Two recitations for an evil *alû*-demon "getting" an infant.

(rev. 9–12) Its ritual. [You make] a cylinder seal of potter's clay and then ⸢you write⸣ this recitation on it and then you ⸢bake⸣ (it) in a straw fire. If you either ⸢put⸣ (it) on his neck or you hang (it) on the head of his bed, "anything evil" should not approach ⸢him⸣.

(rev. 13–15) If you do not want "anything evil" to approach an infant, you mix *eʾru*-tree seed, *šakirû* seed, *šimru* seed, (and) "soiled rag" (= *sikillu*) with oil. If you gently rub him (with it) ⸢before⸣ putting the breast to his mouth, he should recover.

(rev. 16–17) [Recitation] and salve for (cases where) an evil *alû*-demon "gets" an infant. ⸢SA.GIG⸣ (the Diagnostic and Prognostic series), rituals, fumigants (and) leather-bag amulets were not looked at.

(rev. 18–19) ⸢Affliction⸣ of *bennu* that is observed in the seventh year (after) birth: he makes senseless noises, (his stomach) is continually upset (and) during his falling spell he winds his hands behind him.[14]

(rev. 20–23) ⸢Excerpt⸣ of treatments for an infant whom AN.TA.ŠUB.BA Lugalurra, ["hand" of god, "hand"] of Ishtar, *lilû*-demon or evil *alû*-demon afflicts. Finished. [… (and)] ⸢SA.GIG⸣ with the excerpts on AN.TA.ŠUB.BA [on tablets (and)] writing boards were looked at. […]

TEXT 2: CAMPBELL THOMPSON[15] 1940, 110 NO. 38

K 3628+ lines rev. 3–12 (see above, text 1) describes the manufacture of a clay cylinder inscribed with the following recitation:

Sirius is his name, one who utters the battle cry, seeker-out of paths, one who brings everything to fruition, the *mīṭu*-mace which is more furious than all other weapons. May an attacker not approach (or) come near so-and-so, son of so-and-so. May no attackers approach. Spell (and) recitation.

A number of actual examples of such cylinders have been found at Nineveh and Kalḫu, one of them inscribed with the requisite name. They are hollow so that they could be strung on a thread and are quite tiny. Campbell-Thompson, 1940, 110 no. 38 is only 1 1/4 inches long with a diameter of 7/16 inches.

1. ÉN MUL.KAK.SI.SÁ MU.NE
2. *mu-šá-lil qab-li*
3. *muš-te-ʾ-u ur-ḫi-tú*
4. *mu-šak-lil mim+ma šum-šú*
5. ^{GIŠ}*me-ṭu šá ina* IGI ^{GIŠ}TUKUL
6. *na-an-dúr* ZI-*u*
7. *a-na* ^{m}(blank) A DINGIR-*šú*
8. NU TE-*ḫi* NU DIM$_4$
9. LÚ.ZI.ZI KI.MIN NAM.BA.TE.GÁ.DÈ
10. TU$_6$ ÉN

TEXT 3: BAM 248 iv 39–43

BAM 248 is largely devoted to difficult childbirth (see chapter 12). At the very end, there is an amulet (iv 39–40) for "hand" of god, and a fumigant (iv 41) and salves (iv 42–43) for the *lilû* demon affecting infants.

39. DIŠ *a-na* LÚ.TUR ŠU.DINGIR.RA NU TE-*e* ŠÈ ŠAḪ ŠÈ UR.GI$_7$ GI$_6$
40. *il-la-at* ANŠE ḪE.ḪE *ina* ^{SÍG}ÀKA ⸢NIGIN⸣-*mi ina* GÚ-*šú* GAR-*ma* TI-*uṭ*
41. DIŠ *a-na* LÚ.TUR LÚ.LÍL.LÁ NU TE-*e* SÍG UR.GU.LA SÍG ÙZ *ina* DÈ SAR-*šú*
42. DIŠ KI.MIN GÌR.PAD.DU LÚ.U$_{18}$.LU *ina* Ì.GIŠ *ka-a-a-na* ŠÉŠ.ME-*su*

43. DIŠ KI.MIN ^{NA_4}*mu-ṣu* ^{Ú}*ṣa-ṣu-tú* GÌR.PAD.DU ŠAḪ *ina* Ì ŠÉŠ.ME-*su*

---

44. ÉN A IDIM.TA BA.GIN.NA.TA MU.UN.DA.ÚS.SA
45. LIBIR.RA.BI GIN$_7$ AB.SAR-*ma* BA.AN.È

TRANSLATION

(iv 39–40) If you do not want "hand" of god to approach an infant, you mix pig dung, "excrement of a black dog" (= *nikiptu*)[16] (and) donkey slaver. You wrap (it) in a tuft of wool (and) put (it) on his neck.

(iv 41) If you do not want the *lilû* demon to approach an infant, you fumigate him with lion hair (and) goat hair over coals.

(iv 42) Alternatively, you continually and repeatedly rub him gently with "human bone" (= "lone plant") (mixed) with oil.

(iv 43) Alternatively, you repeatedly rub him gently with *mūṣu*-stone, *ṣaṣuntu* (and) pig bone (mixed) with oil.

(iv 44–45) The recitation: A IDIM.TA BA.TA.GIN.NA.TA[17] follows thereafter. Written in accordance with its original and then collated.

B. CHOKING

This does not sound like a serious problem, but for an infant, it can be fatal. There are also infectious diseases that obstruct the airway. For details, see Scurlock and Andersen 2005, 414.

TEXT 4: BM 62376

BM 62376[18] describes a cold water wash and an aspirant for choking in an infant. To judge from the LÍL sign carefully drawn in monumental script on the left edge, the problem was supposed to be the result of a *lilû*-demon actually trying to strangle the child. *Lilû*-demons were the spirits of young men who died without having had the opportunity to marry and to have children. In this case, one such demon was taking matters, literally, into his own hands. Interesting is the involvement of the concerned adults in a bit of magic designed to encourage the plants to do their work (14–16)

1. DIŠ LÚ.TUR GÚ.⌜MUR⌝-*su ḫa-niq*
2. *šá-niš* GUB-*ma ina šu-ba-as-su im-qut*

3. LÚ.TUR BI *ina* A.MEŠ *ka-ṣu-tu*
4. RA.MEŠ A.MEŠ *ka-ṣu-tu*
5. *it-ti muḫ-ḫi-šú* SAG.DU-*šú*
6. MAŠ.SÌLA^{II}-*šú ù nap-šá-ti-šú*
7. *tu-sal-la-aḫ* EGIR-*šú*
8. ^{Ú}*ši*!-*bur-a-tú* ^{Ú}*na-na-ḫa*
9. ^{Ú}*ka-mu-nu mun-zi-qa*
10. *ina* KAŠ DÙG.GA *ú-na-ṣab*
11. *re-*⸢*eḫ*⸣*-ti* Ú.ḪI.A *an-nu-*⸢*ti*⸣
12. *šá ina* KAŠ DÙG.GA *bal-lu ina pi-šú*
13. *ù muḫ-ḫi-šú* GAR.GAR-*an-ma*
14. *k*[*am* DUG$_4$].DUG$_4$ *šal-ḫa šu-ṣi-*⸢*i*⸣
15. *at-tu-nu um-ma e-pu-šú*
16. *iš-ta-lim*

l.e. LÍL

Translation

(1–16) If an infant's pharynx is constricted or he stands up and then falls down on his seat,[19] you repeatedly wash that infant with cold water. You sprinkle cold water on his the top of his head, his head, his shoulders and his throat. Afterwards, he should suck up *šibburratu*, *nanaḫa*-mint, *kamūnu*-cumin (and) raisins (mixed) with sweet beer. You repeatedly put the rest of these plants which were mixed with sweet beer to his mouth and the top of his head and say ⸢as follows⸣: "Sprinklings, make (it) go out!" You-all say: "They do (it); he has gotten well."

Notes

1. See Kee Chang Huang 1993, 139.
2. See Scurlock and Andersen 2005, 13.177.
3. See Scurlock and Andersen 2005, 17.165.
4. See Scurlock and Andersen 2005, 17.166.
5. Restorations are based on I. Finkel's unpublished edition of ḪUL.BA.ZI.ZI as quoted in Farber 1989b, 128.
6. See Ebeling 1953, 403–4; cf. Farber 1989b, 128.
7. See Farber 1989b, 128.
8. See Farber 1989b, 67.
9. For more on this menace, see Stol 1993, 10, 37 and Geller and Wiggerman 2008, 150, 153–56.
10. This is cited from DPS 40:28.
11. See Scurlock and Andersen 2005, 13.177. This is cited from DPS 40:60.
12. See Scurlock and Andersen 2005, 17.165–166, 19.10. These two lines are cited from

DPS 40:112–113.

13. For the translation of *saḫlû* as "cress," see Stol 1983–84, 24–32.

14. See Scurlock and Andersen 2005, 3.272 (cysticercosis) and 13.200 (complex partial seizures).

15. This British Assyriologist's name is correctly given as R. Campbell Thompson, not R.C. Thompson as often in the literature.

16. The equation is given in *KADP* 2 iv 6′.

17. See van Dijk, Goetze and Hussey 1985, 32.

18. This is a hastily written, hollow, school text in IM.GÍD.A format.

19. See Scurlock and Andersen 2005, 3.55, 17.159.

14

POISONING, IMAGINARY AND OTHERWISE; ENDOCRINE DISORDERS

A. POISONING

1. *KIŠPŪ*

In addition to trying to counteract the real or imagined attempts to hex enemies (using figurines or animal surrogates, examples of which were occasionally found by the distraught victims), ancient Mesopotamians viewed poisoning by sorcerers as the source of a variety of illnesses with prominent salivation or production of phlegm, mucus, or semen. Included are probably cases of actual and deliberate or accidental poisonings with muscarinic mushrooms. For more details, see chapters 15 and 19 in Scurlock and Andersen 2005, 356–58, 500–501, 503 and the "Unsolved Puzzles" appendix, pp. 563–566.

TEXT 1: BM 42272:1–31

BM 42272 begins with potions (1–9, 19–22) and a recitation (10–18) for *kišpu* and curse. It follows with potions (23–31) for excess salivation. For the rest of this text see chapter 6, text 2. Extremely interesting is the little recitation to the Pleiades, which is attested in a few other versions. The direct impersonation of divinities suggests Egyptian influence, although the worry that an unjustified curse will come back to haunt the speaker is purely Mesopotamian.

1. ⸢Ú⸣.KUR.RA ^{Ú}KUR.KUR ^{Ú}⸢LAG.A.ŠÀ.GA ^{Ú}⸣x[...]
2. 5 Ú.MEŠ UŠ$_{11}$.BÚR.RU *ina* [...]

---

3. ^{Ú}*tar-muš* ^{Ú}*imḫur-lim* ^{Ú}*imḫur*-20 Ú ‹DILI› Ú.KUR.R[(A ^{Ú}KUR.KUR)]
4. ^{Ú}*úr-nu-ú* ^{Ú}*ti-iá-a-ti* Ú.⸢ḪAR⸣.‹ḪAR› *saḫ*-[(*lu-u* ^{Ú}SAG.ŠUR)]
5. GAZI^{SAR} ^{Ú}⸢*ak*⸣-*tam* ^{GIŠ}GEŠTIN.KA$_5$.A ^{Ú}‹(LUḪ)›.MAR.TU [(^{Ú}EME.UR.GI$_7$)]
6. NUMUN ^{Ú}MIN MUN ‹(*eme*)›-*sal-lim* ^{Ú}SIKIL ^{GIŠ}ŠINIG NUMUN

^{GIŠ}[(*bi-nu* ^{ŠEM}LI)]
7. NUMUN ^{ŠEM}LI ^{Ú}*a-zal-lá* NUMUN ^{Ú}MIN ^{Ú}IN.[(NU.UŠ)]

---

8. 25 Ú.ḪI.A ŠÀ.DÙG.GA ÚŠ.BÚR.RU.DA *u* NAM.ÉRI[(M BÚ)]R.R[U.DA]
9. GABA.RI ^{m}*Ì-lí-rím*!*-ni*[1]

---

10. ÉN *ana-ku* [(*nu*)]-⸢*bat-tum*⸣ *a-ḫat* ^{d}AMAR.UTU ^{d}*Za-ap-pi i-ra-an-*⸢*ni*⸣
11. ^{d}*Bal-*⸢*lum ú*⸣*-li-dan-ni* ^{d}LÚ.ḪUŠ.‹(A)› ⸢*ana*⸣ *li-qu-ti-*[(*šú il-qa*)]*-an-ni*
12. ⸢*áš*⸣*-ši* ŠU.SI^{MEŠ}.MU *ina bi-rit* ^{d}*Za-ap-pi u* ^{d}[(*Ba*)]*l-lum ú-šeš-šib*[2]
13. ⸢*ú*⸣*-še-*⸢*eš*⸣*-šib ina* IGI.MU ^{d}15 GAŠAN GAL-*tum a-pi-lat* ⸢*ku*!*-mu-ú-a*⸣ *aḫ-*[*ḫat*] ⸢^{d}AMAR.UTU⸣
14. *um-m*[*i*] U$_4$.15.KÁM* AD-*a* U$_4$-*mu*[3] KI-*ya-a-ma lip-šu-ru ka-la* [(*ta-ma*)]-*a-ti*
15. *ma-mi*[*t*] *šá at-tem-mu-ú la ú-qàr-ra-ab re-mé-nu-ú* ^{d}A[(MAR.UTU) TU]$_6$.ÉN[4]

---

16. DÙ.DÙ.⸢BI⸣ *ina nu-bat-ti* ÉN *an-ni-ti ana* UGU Ú UŠ$_{11}$.BÚR.RU.DA
17. *u* N[AM.É]RIM.BÚR.RU.DA ŠID-*ma* U$_4$.3.KÁM* U$_4$.7.KÁM* U$_4$.16.KÁM* ⸢DÙ⸣-*ma*[5]
18. *mim-ma* [*lem-nu*] *ù* NAM.ÉRIM *pa-áš-ru*

---

19. ^{Ú}[...] ^{Ú}ḪAR.ḪAR ^{Ú}[o o o G]AZI^{SAR} *saḫ-lu-ú*
20. ^{Ú}[... NUMU]N ^{Ú}*úr-nu-ú* [...] ⸢*šá*⸣ NAM.ÉRIM
21. ^{Ú}[(*imḫur-lim*)] ^{Ú}*imḫur*-20 ^{Ú}*tar-muš* [(SUḪUŠ $^{\text{GI)}}$]^{Š}ḪAB 4 Ú [(ZI.KU$_5$.RU.DA)]
22. NAM.[ÉRIM.BÚR.R]U.DA *ina* KAŠ NAG-*šú* ÉN *Id-di-*^{d}*É-*[(*a*) Š]ID-*nu*[6]

---

23. DIŠ NA *il-la-tu-šú il-la-ku* NU TAR.MEŠ *ana* TI-*šú* ^{Ú}[*imḫu*]*r-lim*
24. ^{Ú}*t*[*ar*]*-muš* ^{Ú}*eli-kul-la* NUMUN ^{Ú}IN.NU.UŠ *ba-lu pa-tan a-ḫi-a-nu* NAG

---

25. DIŠ NA *il-la-tu-šú ina* KI.NÁ *lu ina kal* U$_4$-*mi lu ina kal* GI$_6$ DU.MEŠ-*ma*
26. NU TAR.M[EŠ] *ana* TI-*šú* ^{Ú}ḪAR.ḪAR ^{Ú}KUR.KUR 1/2 GÍN *an-nu-ḫa-ra* ^{GIŠ}ŠINIG
27. ILLU $^{\text{[Š]EM}}$BULUḪ ^{ŠEM}GÚR.GÚR ⸢^{ŠEM}LI⸣ *ina* KAŠ NAG-*šú*

---

28. DIŠ NA [*il*]*-la-tu-šú* DU.MEŠ-*ma* A.ZU *u* MAŠ.MAŠ TAR-*ú la i-le-ʾ-i*
29. *ana* T[I-*šú*] ^{Ú}*imḫur-lim* ^{Ú}*imḫur*-20 ^{Ú}*tar-muš* ^{Ú}NU.LUḪ.ḪA ^{Ú}ḪAR.ḪAR
30. [^{Ú}KUR.KU]R ^{Ú}EME.UR.GI$_7$ ^{Ú}IN.NU.UŠ NAGA.SI ⸢*an*⸣*-nu-ḫa-ra*

31. [10 Ú].ḪI.[A *a*]*n-nu-tim* 1-*niš* SÚD *ina* Ì.GIŠ BÁRA.GA LÀL *u* GEŠTIN N[U *p*]*a-tan* NAG-*ma* DIN

BM 42272

(1–2) *Nīnû*-mint, *atāʾišu*, *kirbān eqli*, [...] (and) [...] are five plants to dispel *kišpu*. [You have him drink] (it mixed) with [...].

(3–9) *Tarmuš*, *imḫur-lim*, *imḫur-ešra*, "lone plant," *nīnû*-mint, *atāʾišu*, *urnû*-mint, *tiyātu*, ⸢*ḫašû*-thyme⸣, *saḫlû*-cress,[7] *karāšu*-leek,[8] *kasû*, *aktam*, "fox grape," *šiburratu*, *lišān kalbi*, *lišān kalbi* seed, *emesallim*-salt, *sikillu*, *bīnu*-tamarisk, *bīnu*-tamarisk seed, *burāšu*-juniper, *burāšu*-juniper seed, *azallû*, *azallû* seed, (and) *maštakal* are twenty-five plants to make the heart happy, to dispel *kišpu* and curses; copy of Ili-rimanni. (They are to be mixed with beer and used in a potion).

(10–15) I am the *Nubattum* (seventh of the month), sister of Marduk. The Zappu (Pleides) conceived me; Balu gave me birth; Luḫušû (Nergal's panther) adopted me. I raised my fingers; I stationed (them) between the Zappu and Balu. I stationed before me Ishtar (the Bowstar), great lady, the one who answers for me. (I am) the ⸢sister⸣ of Marduk. The fifteenth of the month (is) my mother; my father (is) the (first) day (variant: month). May they reconcile all persons I have cursed/enemies[9] with me. May the curse which I have uttered not approach (me), merciful ⸢Marduk⸣. ⸢Spell and recitation⸣.[10]

(16–18) Its ritual: You recite this spell in the evening over the plants to dispel *kišpu* and curse and if you do this (again) on the third, the seventh and the sixteenth day. "Anything [evil]" and curse will be loosened. [11]

(19–22) [...], *ḫašû*-thyme, [...], *kasû*, *saḫlû*-cress, [...], *urnû*-mint ⸢seed⸣ (and) [...] are [plants] for a curse. [*Imḫur-lim*], *imḫur-ešra*, *tarmuš* (and) *ḫurātu*-madder [root] are 4 ⸢plants⸣ for [*zikurudû*] (and) ⸢to dispel a curse⸣. You have him drink (it mixed) with beer (and) recite the recitation: "Ea cast (it)."

(23–24) If his saliva flows (and) will not stop, to cure him, you have him drink ⸢*imḫur-lim*⸣, ⸢*tarmuš*⸣, *elikulla* and *maštakal* seed separately on an empty stomach.

(25–27) If a person's saliva continually flows when he sleeps either all day or all night and will not stop, to cure him, you have him drink *ḫašû*-thyme, *atāʾišu*, 1/2 shekel of *annuḫāru*-alum, *bīnu*-tamarisk, *baluḫḫu* resin, *kukru*, (and) *burāšu*-juniper (mixed) with beer.

(28–31) If a person's saliva continually flows and the *asû* and *āšipu* cannot stop (it), to ⸢cure⸣ [him], you grind these [ten] ⸢plants⸣ together: *imḫur-lim*, *imḫur-ešra*, *tarmuš*, *nuḫurtu*, *ḫašû*-thyme, ⸢*atāʾišu*⸣, *lišān kalbi*, *maštakal*, *uḫḫūlu qarnānu*, (and) *annuḫāru*-alum. If you have him drink (it mixed) with pressed-out oil, honey and wine ⸢on an empty stomach⸣, he should recover.

2. ALCOHOL

Drinking wine (or more usually beer) to excess was as much a plague of ancient Mesopotamian society as it is of our own. Alcoholism, properly speaking, was attributed by ancient Mesopotamians to the baleful influence of ghosts. For more details, see Scurlock and Andersen 2005, 360–363 and 500–503.

TEXT 2: BAM 59 AND BAM 438

BAM 59 consists of two potions (1–20) for *kišpu* followed by a potion for alcoholism which is duplicated by BAM 575 iii 51–54 (text 3). Lines 1–12 duplicate BAM 438 obv.16–27 whose preceding lines (5–14) list symptoms which may be indicative of congestive heart failure.[12] Generally such references in witchcraft texts are associated with ghosts and may, therefore, refer specifically to congestive heart failure in an alcoholic patient. Lines 13–20 of BAM 59 would seem to be treating what we would call depression or, in this case, a vague sense of having been cursed. Again, it is possible that an alcoholic patient is involved.

BAM 438

obv.

5. [DIŠ NA *a-ka-li*]-*šú muṭ-ṭu ana da-ba-bi* ŠÀ-*šú l*[*a* ÍL-*šú*]
6. [*ḫu-u*]*ṣ* GAZ ŠÀ TUKU.MEŠ-*ši mi-na-ti-šú it*-[*ta-na-áš-pa-ka* EME-*šú*]
7. *it-te-nen-bi-iṭ* NUNDUN.MEŠ-*šú ú-na-áš-šak* GEŠTU^{II}-*šú* G[Ú.GÚ-*a*]
8. ŠU^{II}-*šú i-šam-ma-ma-šú bir-ka-šú kin-ṣa-šú i-kàs-s*[*a-sa-šú*]
9. SAG ŠÀ-*šú it-ta-na-áz-qar ana* MUNUS DU-*ka mu*[*ṭ-ṭu*]
10. *ana* MUNUS ŠÀ-*šú* NU ÍL-*šú ḫur-ba-šu* ŠUB.ŠUB-[*su*]
11. *i-kab-bir i-ba-aḫ-ḫu* ÚḪ *ana* KA-*šú it-ta-na*-[-*di*]
12. *ik-ka-šú* LÚGUD.DA.MEŠ KI.NÁ NU ÍL-*š*[*i*]
13. *pi-qa la pi-qa ú-ta-ṣal* NA BI *ka*-[*šip*]
14. NU.MEŠ-*šú* DÙ-*ma ina* ÚR LÚ.ÚŠ *šu-nu*-[*lu*]

TRANSLATION

(5–14) [If a person]'s [appetite] is diminished, he ⸢does not⸣ [have] the heart to speak, he continually has a crushing sensation in his heart, his limbs are continually [tense, his tongue] is continually cramped, he bites his lips, his ears [continually] ⸢ring⸣, his hands go numb, his knees (and) his shins give him a gnawing pain, his upper abdomen (epigastrium) continually protrudes, his desire to go to a woman ⸢is diminished⸣, (and) he cannot get an erection for a woman, chills keep falling on [him], he is now fat (and now) thin, he continually lets his spittle ⸢fall⸣ from! his mouth, his breath is continually short, he cannot stand the bed, (and) he is incessantly sluggish, that person is ⸢hexed⸣; figurines of him were manufactured and made to ⸢lie⸣ in the lap of a corpse.

BAM 59

1. ^{Ú}*tar-muš*$_8$ ^{Ú}*imḫur-lim* [(^{Ú}*imḫur*-2)0 (^{Ú}SIKIL ^{Ú}*el-kul-la*)]
2. ^{ŠEM}BULUḪ ^{Ú}*ak-tam* ^{Ú}KUR.KUR ^{GIŠ}[(ḪAŠḪUR ^{GIŠ}GI ^{Ú}*la-pat ar-ma-ni*)]
3. $^{\text{NA}_4}$*gab-bé-e* KA.A.AB.BA ^{Ú}NU.L[(UḪ.ḪA ^{Ú}DÚR.NU.LUḪ.ḪA)]
4. ^{Ú}ḪAR.ḪAR ^{Ú}*úr-nu-u* ‹(^{Ú}KUR.ZI)› ^{Ú}*šib*-[(*bur-ra-tú* ^{Ú}ḪUR.SAG)]
5. Ú.KUR.RA ^{Ú}*šu-mut-tú* ŠE.KAK ^{GIŠ}[(DÌḪ ŠE.KAK $^{\text{GIŠ.Ú}}$GÍR)]
6. [(ŠE)].KAK GI.ŠUL.ḪI ^{GIŠ}*bi-nu* NUMUN ^{GIŠ}*bi-n*[(*u* ^{Ú}IN$_6$.ÚŠ)]
7. NU[(M)]UN ^{Ú}IN.NU.UŠ ^{ŠEM}LI NUMUN [(^{ŠEM}LI)]
8. MUN KÙ.PAD MUN *A-ma-ni* ZÚ.LUM.MA N[(UMUN ^{GIŠ}ḪA.LU.ÚB)]
9. $^{\text{ŠE[(M)]}}$MAN.DU ^{Ú}*kul-ka-nam* GAZI^{SAR} 3[(7 Ú UŠ$_{11}$.BÚR.RU).DA]
10. *š*[*a i*]*na* ŠU^{II} *šu-ṣu-u lu-u ina* KAŠ SAG [(*lu*) *ina* ^{GIŠ}GEŠTIN]
11. *lu-u ina* A.MEŠ *lu ina* Ì+GIŠ *lu ina ḫi-qa-a*-[(*ti* NAG.MEŠ)]
12. *lu ta-bi-lam ana* KA-*šú* [(ŠUB-*di*)]

---

13. [(^{Ú}*tar-muš* ^{Ú}*imḫur*)]-⸢*lim*⸣ ^{Ú}*imḫur*-20 ⸢Ú⸣ [(DILI)]
14. [(^{Ú}KUR.KUR Ú.KUR)].RA ^{Ú}*úr-n*[(*u-ú*)]
15. [(^{Ú}*ti-iá-tú saḫ*)]-*lu-u* GAZI^{SAR} ⸢Ú!⸣[(⸢*ak-tam*⸣)]
16. [(^{GIŠ}GEŠTIN.KA$_5$.A)] ⸢^{Ú}⸣LUḪ.MAR.TÚ ^{Ú}[(EME.UR.GI$_7$)]
17. [(NUMUN) ^{Ú}EME.U(R.G)]I$_7$ MUN *eme-sal-lim* [(^{Ú}SIKIL)]
18. [(^{GIŠ}ŠINIG)] NUMUN [(^{GIŠ})]*bi-nu* ^{ŠEM}LI
19. [(NUMUN ^{ŠEM}LI ^{Ú}*a*)]-*zal-lá* NUMUN [(^{Ú})]*a-zal-lá* ^{Ú}[(IN$_6$.ÚŠ)]

---

20. [(25)] Ú DÙG ŠÀ-*bi* [(ŠÀ.DÙG)].⸢GA⸣ NAM.RÍN [(BÚR)]

---

21. DIŠ NA KAŠ.SAG NAG-*ma* SAG.[(DU-*su* DIB.DIB-*su*)]
22. INIM.MEŠ-*šú im-ta-na-aš*-⸢*ši ina* D⸣[(UG$_4$.DUG$_4$-*šú ú-pa-áš-šaṭ*)]
23. *ṭè-en-šú la ṣa-bit* ⸢NA⸣ BI I[(GI^{II}-*šú* GUB-*za*)]
24. [(*ana* TI-*šú*)] ^{Ú}*imḫur-lim* ^{Ú}*imḫur*-2[(0 ^{Ú}*tar-muš* ^{Ú}ḪAR.ḪAR)]
25. [(Ú)] SIKIL [(Ú DILI KA.A.AB.BA ^{Ú}NU.LUḪ.ḪA NUMUN)]
26. [(^{Ú}NÍG.GÁN.GÁN ^{Ú}*kam-ka-du* ^{Ú}*eli-kul-la* 11 Ú.ḪI.A ŠEŠ)]
27. [(1-*niš* SÚD *ina* Ì.GIŠ *u* KAŠ *ana* IGI ^{d}*Gu-la tuš-bat ina še-rim*)]

28. [(*la-am* ^{d}UTU MÚ-*ḫi la-am ma-am-ma iš-ši-qu-šú* NAG-*ma ina-eš*)]

TRANSLATION

(1–12) *Tarmuš*, *imḫur-lim*, ⌜*imḫur-ešra*⌝, *sikillu*, *elkulla*, *baluḫḫu*-aromatic, *aktam*, *atāʾišu*, "swamp apple," *lapat armanni*, alum, *imbû tamtim*, *nuḫurtu*, *tiyātu*, *ḫašû*-thyme, *urnû*-mint, ‹(*samīdu*)› *šibburatu*, *azupīru*, *nīnû*-mint, *šumuttu*-vegetable, *baltu*-thorn shoots, *ašāgu*-thorn shoots, *qān šalāli*-reed shoots, *bīnu*-tamarisk, *bīnu*-tamarisk seed, *maštakal*, *maštakal* seed, *burāšu*-juniper, *burāšu*-juniper seed, KÙ.PAD-salt, *Amanum* salt, dates, *ḫaluppu*-tree seed, *suʾādu*, *kurkānû*-turmeric, (and) *kasû* are thirty-seven plants to loosen *kišpu* ⌜which are⌝ readily available. You have him drink (it) repeatedly (mixed) either with first quality beer or [with wine] or with water or with oil or with *ḫīqu*-beer or you pour (it) dry into his mouth.

(3–20) *Tarmuš*, *imḫur-lim*, *imḫur-ešra*, "lone plant," *atāʾišu*, *nīnû*-mint, *urnû*-mint, *tiyātu*, *saḫlû*-cress, *kasû*, *aktam*, "fox grape," *šiburratu*, *lišān kalbi*, *lišān kalbi* seed, *emesallim*-salt, *sikillu*, *bīnu*-tamarisk, *bīnu*-tamarisk seed, *burāšu*-juniper, *burāšu*-juniper seed, *azallû*, *azallû* seed, (and) *maštakal* are twenty-five plants to make the heart happy (and) to dispel curses. (They are to be mixed with beer and used in a potion).

(21–28) If a person drinks beer and as a result his head continually afflicts him, he continually forgets his words (and) slurs them when speaking, he is not in full possession of his faculties, (and) that person's eyes stand still,[13] to cure him, you grind together these eleven plants: *imḫur-lim*, *imḫur-ešra*, *tarmuš*, *ḫašû*-thyme, *sikillu*, "lone plant," *imbû tamtim*, *nuḫurtu*, *egemgirû* seed, *kamkādu* (and) *elikulla*. You leave (it) out overnight in oil and beer under Gula's star. If you have him drink (it) in the morning before the sun rises (and) before anybody kisses him, he should recover.

TEXT 3: BAM 575 iii 49–54

BAM 575 is part of the subseries of UGU dealing with the gastrointestinal tract. Among many other treatments, it has two potions for alcohol poisoning. The occular paralysis of lines iii 51–54 is characteristic of Wernicke disease, a thiamine defficiency often seen in alcoholics. It would appear that people normally rose at sunrise and that it was usual to greet the morning with kisses.

iii

49. DIŠ NA KAŠ.SAG NAG-*ma* SUḪUŠ.MEŠ-*šú pa-al-qa di-ig-la ma-a-ṭi*

ana TI-*šú* NUMUN ^{Ú}SIKIL NUMUN Ú.DILI NUMUN ^{GIŠ}*b*[*i-ni*]

50. NUMUN ^{Ú}*am-ḫa-ra* NUMUN ^{Ú}IN$_6$.ÚŠ 5 Ú.ḪI.A ŠEŠ 1-*niš* SÚD *ina* GEŠTIN SÌG-*aṣ* NU *pa-tan* NAG-*ma ina-e*[*š*]

---

51. DIŠ NA KAŠ.SAG NAG-*ma* SAG.DU-*su* DIB.DIB-*su* INIM.MEŠ-*šú im-ta-na-aš-ši ina* DUG$_4$.DUG$_4$-*šú ú-pa-áš-šaṭ*

52. *ṭè-en-šú la ṣa-bit* LÚ BI IGI^{II}-*šú* GUB-*za ana* TI-*šú* ^{Ú}*imḫur-lim* ^{Ú}*imḫur*-20 ^{Ú}*tar-muš* ^{Ú}ḪAR.ḪAR

53. Ú SIKIL Ú DILI KA.A.AB.BA ^{Ú}NU.LUḪ.ḪA NUMUN ^{Ú}NÍG.GÁN.GÁN ^{Ú}*kam-ka-du* ^{Ú}*eli-kul-la* 11 Ú.ḪI.A ŠEŠ

54. 1-*niš* SÚD *ina* Ì+GIŠ *u* KAŠ *ana* IGI ^{d}*Gu-la tuš-bat ina še-rim la-am* ^{d}UTU MÚ-*ḫi la-am ma-am-ma iš-ši-qu-šú* NAG-*ma ina-eš*

TRANSLATION

(iii 49–50) If a person drinks fine beer and as a result he is unsteady on his foundations (and) his eyesight is diminished,[14] to cure him, you grind together these five plants: *sikillu* seed, "lone plant" seed, ⸢*bīnu*⸣-tamarisk seed, *amḫara* seed, (and) *maštakal* seed. You whisk (it) into wine. If you have him drink (it) on an empty stomach, he should recover.

(iii 51–54) If a person drinks beer and as a result his head continually afflicts him, he continually forgets his words (and) slurs them when speaking, he is not in full possession of his faculties, (and) that person's eyes stand still,[15] to cure him, you grind together these eleven plants: *imḫur-lim*, *imḫur-ešra*, *tarmuš*, *ḫašû*-thyme, *sikillu*, "lone plant," *imbû tamtim*, *nuḫurtu*, *egemgirû* seed, *kamkādu*, (and) *elikulla*. You leave (it) out overnight in oil and beer under Gula's star. If you have him drink (it) in the morning before the sun rises (and) before anybody kisses him, he should recover.

B. ENDOCRINE DISORDERS: GRAVES' DISEASE AND HYPOTHYROIDISM

A number of diseases are caused by an excess or insufficiency of essential hormones. In ancient Mesopotamian texts, it is possible to recognize references to Primary Adrenocortical Deficiency, Testosterone Deficiency, and Graves' Disease. For more details, see Scurlock and Andersen 2005, 160–62.

Graves' Disease is primarily caused by excess production of thyroid hormone. It may be recognized by nervousness, peu d'orange lesions on the legs or feet, warm and moist skin, weight loss despite well-maintained appetite, a characteristic stare with infrequent blinking and lid lag, excessive sweating, diffuse itching, emotional lability, and sinus tachycardia (rapid heart rate). K 2351+ lines 6–11 (text 4) are certainly a reference to Graves' disease For more details, see Scurlock and Andersen 2005, 161–62.

A common problem associated with the treatment of Graves' Disease is that having too little thyroid hormone is just as much of a problem as having too much. It is thus possible for treatment for Graves' Disease to actually induce hypothyroidism. Moreover, some patients present with the symptoms of hypothyroidism and hyperthyroidism at the same time. The ancient physician was well aware of this problem, which is described in the sequenced references of *STT* 89:8–61.[16] These references begin with the potentially treatable stages of hypothyroidism for which K 2351+:1–5, BAM 453: 7′–10′ (texts 4–5) and BAM 449 iii 13′–23′ (text 6) provided treatments, progress via less and less favorable prognoses (BAM 449 iii 24′–27′) to terminal stages for which the best chance for survival was that the stone charms of BAM 361:35–48 (text 7) could prevent their appearance.

In one of the references in text 6, (BAM 449 iii 13′–27′), the diagnosis suspects the involvement of something poisonous in soured milk. Since soured milk is used as a carrier in one of the treatments for Graves' Disease in text 5 (K 2351+:22–27), this diagnosis is more than accurate.

TEXT 4: K 2351 + 10639 (= *AMT* 13/4) + 8184 + 5859 (+) K 3293 (= BAM 460) (COPY: AMD 8/1 PL. 122)

K 2351 + consists of potions (6–21), amulets (6–21), salves (6–21), and an aliment (22–27) for Graves' Disease. Graves' Disease has spontaneous remission, particularly if anti-thyroid drugs are applied. To note is that one of the plant medicines, *šūšu* (= Glycyrrhiza, sp.) is used in Chinese medicine[17] for hyperthyroidism. Framing these references are a potion (1–5) and a lost treatment (BAM 543:7′–10′) for hypothyroidism. Symptoms for these treatable cases may be reconstructed from *STT* 89:8–17 and include "sluggish" feet, meaning a prolongation of the relaxation phase of the deep tendon reflexes (the so-called hung-up reflex), "numb" arms (or what we call carpal tunnel), "binding," and "afflicting" flesh (muscle stiffness and cramping), pins and needles (paresthesias), and being easily frightened (paranoia). Also of note is a reference to Pemberton's sign (K 2351+: 6) in which the patient with Graves' disease is able to raise his arms above his head whereas the patients with hypothyroidism who try this (K 2351+:1; BAM 453:7′) become dizzy. Common to both sets of treatments are transfer rites in which the patient is asked to stand on dried bitumen (1–5, 22–27) and/or to look on carnelian and gold (1–5) while taking his medicine.

1. DIŠ NA IGI^{II}-*šú* NIGIN-*du* ⸢Á⸣[^{II}-*šú i-šam-ma-ma-šú* …]
2. ⸢Ú⸣*ur-né-e* ^{Ú}KU$_{6}^{18}$ ⸢Ú?⸣[…]
3. ⸢3⸣ ŠE.TA.ÀM *ina* Ì+GIŠ BÁRA.[GA ḪE.ḪE *ina* UL] ⸢*tuš*⸣-*bat ina* Á.GÚ.Z[I.GA L(Ú BI)]
4. IGI ^{d}UTU *ina* UGU ESIR ⸢ḪÁD GUB⸣-[*ma* NAG-*ma* ^{NA_4}]GUG KÙ.SIG$_{17}$ IGI.DU$_{8}$-*m*[*a*]
5. ZI.KU$_{5}$.RU.DA *šá* [(NENNI DUMU NENNI)] *pa-še-er*

---

6. DIŠ NA Á^{II}-*šú ina* UGU SAG.DU-*š*[*ú* GAR.GAR-*an* (Á.MEŠ-*šú*)] *i-šam-ma-ma-šu*
7. GÌR^{II}-*šú mu-ne-e* ŠUB.ŠUB [(UZU.MEŠ-*šú*) *i-n*]*a* ^{d}UTU.È *i-mi-mu-šú*
8. ⸢*ana*⸣ MUNUS *a-la-ka mu-uṭ-ṭù* [(NINDA GU$_{7}$-*m*)*a* U]GU-*šú* NU DU-*ak*
9. IGI^{II}-*šú it-ta-na-za-za* IGI x[…]x *na-da-ta-šú-um-ma*
10. *i-te-ki-ik* DUG$_{4}$-*šú* LÙ.⸢MEŠ⸣ [KA-*šú it-ta-na-a*]*ṣ-bat a-wa-tam i-qab-bu-šum-ma*
11. *i-ma-aš-ši* ŠÀ-*šú it-ta-na-a*[*d-la-aḫ* NA BI ALA]M^{II}-*šú ep-šu-ma ana* LÚ.ÚŠ *paq-du*
12. ALAM^{II}-*šú šá* Ì.UDU *ep-šu-m*[*a*] ⸢UR.GI$_{7}$⸣ *šu-k*[*u-lu* ALA]M^{II}-*šú šá* E⸢SIR.ḪÁD.DU *ep-šu-ma*⸣
13. *ana* ^{d}*Bil-gi paq-du-u na-áš-*[*pa-r*]*a-at* ZI.KU$_{5}$.RU.D[A …]
14. NA BI EN UR.GI$_{7}$ *šá* N[U].M[EŠ-*š*]*ú* ⸢*i*⸣-*ku-lu* TI.LA UR.[GI$_{7}$ …]
15. *la-ma* TE-*šu-ma* BA.[ÚŠ] ^{Ú}*imḫur-lim* ^{Ú}*tar-mu*[*š* …]
16. NUMUN ^{GIŠ}*šu-ši* NUMUN ^{GIŠ}ÁŠ.D[UG$_{4}$?.GA?] ^{GIŠ}*šim-ri* ^{GIŠ}ḪAŠḪUR ^{GIŠ}GI TÉŠ.BI […]
17. TÉŠ.BI AL.GAZ 1 G[ÍN LÀ]L.KUR.RA 1 ⸢GÍN⸣ Ì.NUN 2 GÍN Ì+GIŠ BÁ[RA.GA […]
18. *ana* 1/3 ‹*qa*› KAŠ SAG ŠUB-*m*[*a*] ⸢*ta*⸣-*sàk ina* UL *tuš-*[*b*]*at ina* Á.GÚ.ZI.G[A …]
19. ÉN *i-ri-pa-*[*a*]*ḫ* NAM.TAR *i-ri-pa-aḫ* NAM.GAL *bir-bi*[*r* …]
20. 3-*šú* ŠUB-*di-*[*ma*] NAG-*šu-ma ana* IGI ^{d}UTU KI.ZA.ZA-*ma* […]
21. ^{NA_4}NÍR *ina* G[Ú-*šú*] GAR-*an-ma* Ì+GIŠ ^{GIŠ}ŠUR.MÌN ŠÉŠ-*ma* EGI[R-*šú* …]

---

22. DIŠ KI.MIN NUMUN [^{GIŠ}Š]INIG NUMUN ^{Ú}*ka-zal-la* NU[M(UN ^{Ú}*a-mu-š*)*i* …]
23. ⸢Ú⸣[GEŠTI]N.KA$_{5}$.A ^{Ú}IN.NU.UŠ ^{Ú} ⸢*tar*⸣-[(*muš*) ^{Ú}(*imḫur-lim*) …]
24. [^{Ú}*u*]*r-ne-e* NUMUN ^{GIŠ}*pu-qut-te* 5 [(ŠE.TA.ÀM *ina*) …]
25. [# GÍN] LÀL.KUR.RA 2 GÍN Ì.N[(UN TÉŠ.BI ḪE.ḪE *ana* ŠÀ GA.⸢ḪAB⸣) …]

26. [*ina* (Á)].GÚ.ZI.GA *ina* UG[(U ESIR.ḪÁD.DU G)UB-*ma* …]
27. […] 7-*šú ana* ŠÀ ŠUB-*m*[(*a* LÚ BI *tu-šá-kal-ma*) *pa-še-er*]

TEXT 5: BAM 453:7′–10′

7′. [DIŠ NA (GÌR^{II}-*šú i-ra-ʾu-ba*)][19] UZU DIB.DIB-*su* IGI^{II}-*šú iṣ*-[(*ṣa-nun-du* ⸢GÌR⸣^{II}-*šú* ⸢*it-te*⸣-*n*[*e*]*n-ṣi-la*)]
8′. [GIN$_7$ ^{GIŠ}TUKUL (SÌG-*iṣ*) *m*]*i-na-tu-šú ú-za-qá*!-[*tu-šú* GU$_7$ (*u* NAG-⸢*ma*⸣)]
9′. [(UGU-*šú* GUB-*za* UZU.MEŠ-*šú i*)*k*]-*ta-na-su-šú i-sa-a-šú i-ša*[(*m-ma-ma-šú*) …]
10′. [… *ú*]-*pal-la-aḫ-šú* NA BI *ana* x[…][20]

TRANSLATION

K 2351 + 10639 (= *AMT* 13/4) + 8184 + 5859 (+) K 3293 (= BAM 460)

(1–5) If a persons eyes seem to spin, [his] arms [are continually numb …]. You [mix] three grains each of *urnû*-mint, *šimru*, (and) […] with pressed-out oil. You leave (it) out overnight [under the stars]. In the ⸢morning⸣, that person should ⸢stand⸣ on dried bitumen before Shamash [and then you have him drink (it) and], if he looks at carnelian (and) gold, so-and-so son of so-and-so's "cutting of the breath" should be dispelled.

(6–21) If a person [can continue to put] his arms over ⸢his⸣ head (without getting dizzy), his arms (feel) numb, his feet (look like they) are spotted with *munû*-lesions, his flesh (feels) hot ⸢in⸣ the morning, his going to a woman is diminished, he eats bread ⸢and then⸣ it does not agree with him, his eyes continually stand still, [sweat?] pours off him so that he scratches, his words are troubled, [his mouth is continually] seized, when they say something to him, he forgets it (and) his heart is continually troubled, [that person]'s ⸢figurines⸣ have been manufactured and then entrusted to a dead person. Figurines of him made of fat have been manufactured ⸢and then⸣ given to a dog ⸢to eat; figurines⸣ of him made of dried bitumen have been manufactured and then entrusted to Bilgi (the fire). ⸢Messages⸣ of "cutting of the breath"[21] […]. (If) that person is the owner of the dog that ate [his] ⸢figurines⸣, he will live; (if) [that] dog […]. Before it approaches him so that he ⸢dies⸣, you […] together (and) crush together *imḫur-lim*, *tarmuš*, […], *šūšu*-licorice seed, ⸢*araru*⸣(?),[22] *šimru*, (and) "swamp apple." You pour (it and) 1 ⸢shekel⸣ of wild ⸢honey⸣, 1 shekel of ghee, 2 shekels of pressed-out oil, (and) [...] into 1/3 ‹*qû*› of first quality beer ⸢and then⸣ you grind (it). You leave (it) out overnight under the stars. In the morning, you cast the spell: ⸢*i-ri-pa-aḫ*⸣, fate demon, *i-ri-pa-aḫ* , greatness, *bir-bi*[*r* ... three times (and)] three times and then you have him drink (it) and then he prostrates himself before Shamash and then you put [...] (and) *ḫulālu*-chalcedony on [his] ⸢neck⸣ and then you rub him gently with *šurmēnu*-cypress oil and then ⸢afterwards⸣ [...]

(22–27) Alternatively, you mix together five grains each of ⸢*bīnu*-tamarisk⸣ seed, *kazallu* seed, *amuššu*-onion seed, [...], "fox grape," *maštakal*, *tarmuš*, *imḫur-lim*, [...], ⸢*urnû*-mint⸣, (and) *puquttu* seed with [...], [#] ⸢shekels⸣ of wild honey (and) 2 shekels of ghee. [You pour?] (it) into ⸢sour⸣ milk [and you leave (it) out overnight under the stars]. [In] the morning, he should ⸢stand⸣ on dried bitumen [and] you cast [the spell: ...] seven times over it and, if you have that person eat (it), [it should be dispelled].

BAM 453

(7′–10′) [If a person]'s feet tremble, his flesh continually afflicts him, his eyes seem [continually] to ⸢spin⸣, his feet are continually sluggish, [as if] he had been struck [with a weapon], his limbs ⸢give him a stinging pain⸣, [he eats] and drinks and it stays down, his flesh continually "binds" him, his arms(!)[23] are numb (and) [...] frightens him, in order to [...] that person [...]

TEXT 6: BAM 449 iii 13′–27′

The patients of this text are riding the bubble between treatable and terminal cases of hypothyroidism. The symptoms listed in lines iii 13′–16′ are paralleled by *STT* 89:18–22, and involve patients with a dreaded complication, namely, intestinal obstruction due to adynamic ileus. The "loud growling noise," known to us as high pitched borborgymi, will have been osculated by the physician. Particularly dangerous was the vomiting of blood (*STT* 89:43–47) and/or "*miḫḫu*-beer" (*STT* 89:34–37), which modern physicians describe as feculant vomitus (orange-brown in color and foul-smelling due to bacterial overgrowth). Either of these meant death in ten days or less unless the vomiting could be stopped. Merely vomiting (without blood or feculant vomitus) was much less cause for alarm as *STT* 89:38–42 explains by contrast. As BAM 449 iii 24′–27′ (= *STT* 89:23–27) warn, however, even with white (that is, uncolored sputum), the patient could be in a hopeless state, stiff and racked with pain, out of his mind and unable to remember anything. This stuporous state (myxedema coma) is frequently fatal. A month of this, and it would be all over.

iii

13′. [(DIŠ NA KI.MI)]N *it-ta-n*[(*a-a*)]*d-la-aḫ it-te-nen-biṭ* IGI^{II}-*šú ir-ru-ru*

14′. [(*u* U)Z]U.MEŠ-*šú i-šam-ma-mu-šú ši-in-na-šu ka-li-ši-na* GU$_7$.MEŠ-*šú*

15′. [(NINDA)] GU$_7$ KAŠ NAG-*ma i-le-ḫi-ib ana* LÚ BI ZI.KU$_5$.RU.DA *ša* GA.ḪAB DÙ-*su*

16′. *šum-ma* KIN-*šú il-ta-bir* ÚŠ *la-ma* TE-*šu-ma* BA.ÚŠ ^{Ú}*úr-né-e*

17′. ^{Ú}*imḫur-lim* NUMUN ^{Ú}GADA NUMUN Ú DILI TÉŠ.BI AL.GAZ *ina* Ì+GIŠ BÁRA.GA ḪE.ḪE *ina* UL *tuš-bat*

18′. *ina* Á.GÚ.ZI.GA *ana* IGI ^{d}UTU *ina* UGU ESIR.ḪÁD.DU GUB-*ma*

19′. NAG-*ma* KÙ.SIG$_{17}$ KÙ.BABBAR IGI.DU$_8$-*ma pa-še-er*

20′. DIŠ NA KI.MIN ^{Ú}*a-ta-i-ši* NUMUN ^{Ú}*a-zal-le-e* ^{Ú}*úr-ne-e* NUMUN ^{Ú}*ka-zal*

21′. NUMUN ^{Ú}GEŠTIN.KA$_5$.A NUMUN ^{Ú}IN$_6$.ÚŠ TÉŠ.BI 3 ŠE.TA.ÀM LÀL.KUR.RA Ì+GIŠ *u* KAŠ.SAG ḪE.ḪE

22′. *ina* UL *tuš-bat ina* Á.GÚ.ZI.GA IGI 20 NAG *ina* UGU ESIR.ḪÁD.DU GUB-*ma*

23′. ^{NA_4}ZA.GÌN ^{NA_4}GUG KÙ.SIG$_{17}$ KÙ.BABBAR IGI.DU$_8$-*ma pa-šer*

24′. DIŠ NA SA ÚR ZAG-*šú* TAG.TAG-*su ši-ḫat* UZU TUKU.TUKU *mi-na-tu-šú ma-an-ga*

25′. UŠ$_4$-*šú* KÚR.KÚR *ma-la* DÙ-*šú i-ma-aš-ši* ÚḪ-*su pe-ṣa-a-at*

26′. *ana* NA BI *ana* IGI ^{d}*Gu-la ep-šú ep-šú-šú*

27′. *ina* U$_4$.27.KÁM U$_4$.28.KÁM DUG$_4$.BI AL.TIL ŠU ZI.KU$_5$.RU.DA BA.ÚŠ

TRANSLATION

(iii 13′–19′) If a person is continually troubled and cramped, his flesh goes numb, all of his teeth continually hurt him, and if he eats bread and drinks beer, he makes a loud growling noise, "cutting of the breath" with soured milk has been practiced against that person. If it is prolonged, he will die.[24] Before it approaches him so that he dies, you crush together *urnû*-mint, *imḫur-lim*, flax seed, (and) "lone plant" seed. You mix (it) with pressed out oil. You let (it) sit out overnight under the stars. In the morning, he should stand on dried bitumen before Shamash and then you have him drink (it) and, if he looks at gold (and) silver, it (the "cutting of the breath") should be dispelled.

(iii 20′–23′) Alternatively, you mix three grains each of *atāʾišu*, *azallû* seed, *urnû*-mint, *kazallu* seed, "fox grape" seed, (and) *maštakal* seed with wild honey, oil, and first quality beer. You leave (it) out overnight under the stars. In the morning, you have (him) drink (it) before Shamash. He should stand on dried bitumen and, if he looks at lapis, carnelian, gold, (and) silver, it should be dispelled.

(iii 24′–27′) If the muscles of a person's "right" thigh continually hurt him intensely, he continually has wasting of the flesh, his limbs are stiff, his mentation is altered (and) he forgets whatever he does (but) his phlegm is white, rituals have been performed against him before Gula. On the twenty-seventh or twenty-eighth day, his affair is over; "hand" of "cutting of the breath"; he will die.[25]

TEXT 7: BAM 361:35–48

BAM 361 duplicates a series of stone charms whose avowed purpose was to ward off ghosts, bad omens, bad dreams, failure of sexual performance, and what we still call grave signs, a sort of magical preventative medicine. Lines 35–38 (= *STT* 89:57–61) were concerned with pneumonia, a normally unexciting and treatable illness but, in the context of hypothyroidism, potentially fatal. Lines 39–43 (= *STT* 89:48–51) describe a patient with a fever, suffused eyes and blood flowing out of the mouth, probably a description of sepsis. Finally, lines 44–48 (= *STT* 89:52–56) concern a patient with advanced hypothyroidism. The enlarged and cramped tongue is characteristic, as is cold intolerance, lethargy, and disturbed sleep. This condition was treatable by ancient physicians, but nobody really wanted his patient to reach this stage.

35. $^{[\text{NA}]_4}$KUR $^{\langle\text{NA}_4\rangle}$NÍR[26] $^{\text{NA}_4}$ŠUBA
36. [($^{\text{NA}_4}$)]ZA.GÌN $^{\text{NA}_4}$[*a*]-*ár-tum*

---

37. [5] NA$_4$.MEŠ *bi-rit* MAŠ.SÌLA.[(MEŠ-*šú* GU$_7$)]-*šú*
38. [(*ù* Z)]Ú.MEŠ-*šú* MÚD *i-ḫi-i*[(*l-la* GÚ)].BA GAR

---

39. [($^{\text{NA}_4}$PEŠ$_4$)].A.AB.BA $^{\text{NA}_4}$AN.ZAḪ

---

40. [(2 N)]A$_4$.MEŠ *ta-*⌈*lam*⌉*-me* 15-*šú* KÚM
41. *ta-lam-me* 150-*šu* ⌈ŠED$_7$⌉
42. [(IGI)]^{II}-*šú i-bar-ru-r*[(*a*)]
43. MÚD *ina* KA-*šú* DU-*ku ina* GÚ-*šú* GAR-*an*

---

44. $^{\text{NA}_4}$URUDU $^{\text{NA}_4}$*su-u* (variant A: $^{\text{NA}_4}$*šu-u*, var. B: $^{\text{NA}_4}$ŠUBA) $^{\text{NA}_4}$*ka-pa-ṣu*

⸢SA$_5$⸣

---

45. [(3)] NA$_4$.MEŠ DIŠ LÚ ŠÀ.MEŠ-*šu*
46. [*i*]*t-te-ne-en-me-ru* (variants: *it-te-nen-bi-ṭu*) EME-*šú*
47. [(DI)]B.DIB-*bat ina ka-ṣa-a-ti* NÁ-*al*
48. [(*ina* GI)]$_6$ *i-gal-lu-uṭ* (variant: MUD-*ud*) *ina* DUR GÚ BA.GAR

Translation

(35–38) *Šadānu*-hematite, *ḫulālu*-chalcedony, *šubû*-stone, lapis, (and) *ayartu*-coral are [five] stones (to prevent the situation that) the area between the lungs hurts him and his teeth ooze blood. It is to be worn on the neck.

(39–43) Sea *biṣṣūru*-shells (and) *anzaḫḫu*-frit are two stones (to prevent the situation that) his "right" buttock is hot (and) his "left" buttock is cold, his eyes become dimmed, (and) blood flows from his nose/mouth.[27] You put (it) on his neck.

(44–48) Copper bead, *sû*-stone (variants: *šû*-stone or *šubû*-stone) and red *kapaṣu*-shell are three stones (to prevent the situation that) his insides are continually colicky (variant: cramped), his tongue is continually seized, he lies down (to sleep) in the cold of the morning (and) at night he jerks (variant: shudders). It is to be put on the neck on a band.

Notes

1. See Abusch and Schwemer 2011, 216–17.

2. Duplicate substitutes *a-šá-kan*.

3. CT 51 202 iv 7 has: AMA *šá-pat-tú* AD *a-ra-aḫ* and similarly Craig, *ABRT* 2.11 iii 25.

4. For BA 10/1 81 no. 7, see Koch 2003, 89–99 with discussion of a previous treatment by Stol (1992, 245–77).

5. 81-7-27,205: 13-15 gives the procedure as follows: KA.INIM.MA NAM.ÉRIM.BÚR.RU.DA.KÁM KÌD.KÌD.BI *lu ana* UGU A.MEŠ *lu ana* UGU KAŠ.SAG ÉN 3-*šú* ŠID-*nu-ma* NAG-*šu*.

6. For the recitation, see Böck 2007, 46–47, 167.

7. For the translation of *saḫlû* as "cress," see Stol 1983–84, 24–32.

8. As Schwemer 2007, 114 points out, citing Campbell Thompson 1949, 90, lexical texts indicate that SAG.ŠUR is to be interpreted as *karāšu*.

9. To note is the interesting word games involved. "Persons you have cursed" (*tamâti*) are also your enemies (*ayyābū*). But A.AB.BA is the Sumerogram for Akkadian *tantu*, "sea," which in the plural is *tamāti*.

10. For the astronomy, see Koch 2003, 89–99.

11. 81-7-27, 205:13–15 gives the procedure as follows: Recitation to dispel a curse. Its ritual: you recite the recitation three times either over water or over first quality beer and then you give (it) to him to drink.

12. See Scurlock and Andersen 2005, 8.28.

13. See Scurlock and Andersen 2005, 13.91, 16.81.

14. See Scurlock and Andersen 2005, 15.13, 16.80.

15. See Scurlock and Andersen 2005, 13.91, 16.81.

16. This is edited in Abusch and Schwemer 2011 as no. 12.1. To note is that the *-ma* clauses are incorrectly translated obscuring the fact that 13–17 and 18–22 describe treatable conditions.

17. See Duke and Ayensu 1985, 327.

18. Abusch and Schwemer 2011 prefer to read ^{Ú}*ḫa-š*[*e-e*...], although the trace is not good for the *š*[*e*].

19. The same symptom appears in BAM 452:10′.

20. Restored from similar symptoms in *STT* 89:8–11 and 13–16 (see Abusch and Schwemer 2011, no. 12.1).

21. Abusch and Schwemer 2011, 417 suggest (with many question marks) that *upšašû* was also mentioned.

22. As suggested by Abusch and Schwemer 2011, 417.

23. This should be "arms" as in the other passages.

24. This entry and its friends originally languished in the Unsolved Puzzles Appendix of Scurlock and Andersen 2005. This was Ap. 70.

25. See Scurlock and Andersen 2005, Ap. 69.

26. The first two stones are omitted from the duplicate, and the summary has 3 NA_4.MEŠ.

27. See Scurlock and Andersen 2005, Ap. 72.

PART 3

HOLISTIC HEALING

15

PRAYERS AND STONE CHARMS

1. SPECIFIC MEDICAL PROBLEMS

TEXT 1: BM 50346

BM 50346 is a typical extract text which records a stone charm to be used in cases of ghost-induced pain. Like many of the stone lists, its focus is on which stones are to be used for what purpose. Other texts allow us to fill in details about the type of cord used and whether or not burls with plants in them were included. For pain, numbness and varicose veins, the practice was to bind the charm onto the affected part suggesting that pressure was intended to be applied, which, in the case of varicose veins at least, is likely to have been effective.

1. [^{NA_4}G]UG ^{NA_4}ZA.GÌN ^{NA_4}NÍR
2. $^{N[A_4]}$MUŠ.GÍR ^{NA_4}BABBAR.DIL ^{NA_4}BABBAR.MIN$_5$
3. ^{NA_4}DÚR.MI.NA ^{NA_4}KUR-*nu* DIB
4. ^{NA_4}AN.ZAḪ ^{NA_4}AN.ZAḪ.BABBAR
5. ^{NA_4}AN.ZAḪ GI$_6$ ^{NA_4}*mu-ṣa*
6. ^{NA_4}KÙ.BABBAR ^{NA_4}KÙ.SIG$_{17}$ ^{NA_4}⸢URUDU⸣
7. ^{NA_4}*an-na-ku* ^{NA_4}DÚR.MI.NA.BÀN.DA
8. ^{NA_4}MUŠ ^{NA_4}ŠIM.BI.ZI.DA
9. ^{NA_4}ZÁLAG ^{NA_4}*ka-pa-ṣa*

---

10. 21 NA$_4$ ŠU.GIDIM.MA *a-šar*
11. GU$_7$-*šú* KEŠDA-*su*

TRANSLATION

(1–11) ⸢Carnelian⸣, lapis, *ḫulālu*-stone, *muššaru*-stone, *pappardilû*-stone, *papparmīnu*-stone, *turminû*-stone, magnetic hematite, *anzaḫḫu*-frit, white *anzaḫḫu*-frit, black *anzaḫḫu*-frit, *mūṣu*-stone, a silver bead, a gold bead, a ⸢copper⸣ bead, a tin bead, *turminabandû*-stone, "snake"-stone, kohl, *zalāqu*-stone, (and) *kapāṣu*-shell: Twenty-one stones for "hand" of ghost. Wherever it hurts him, you bind (it) on him.

B. DIVINE FAVOR

TEXT 2: *STT* 95+295

STT 95 is a fascinating glimpse into the relationship between religion and science in ancient Mesopotamia. In addition to the medical treatments for various conditions caused by divinities of the pantheon, there were things for the patient to do to regain divine favor, a particular problem where the patient was depressed, anxious, or stressed with or without any other symptoms. If we were to engage divine assistance in being healed or comforted, we would use prayer, perhaps reinforced by a church visit to light a candle. Ancient Mesopotamian practices are similar, but with interesting variations.

In the first place, the religious approach and the medical approach are inextricably linked in ancient Mesopotamia. So the patient's symptoms are enumerated and treatment in the form of a salve or potion and/or amulet containing plant medicines (for use in a salve or potion) is usually prescribed. In addition, and interwoven with this, are recitations (35–40, 49–52, 70–74, 84–97), personal prayers (1–6), modified mourning rites (63–65), censors (1–6, 49–52, 84–86), libations (35–40, 49–52, 84–97), food offerings (42–43, 59–61, 68–69, 70–74), gifts (63–65), and stone charms (32–34, 48, 68–69, 124–125).

Lines 1–12 are for Marduk stress. The personal prayer to Marduk might, then, be classed actually as therapy. The *šigû* prayer was always recited aloud, literally "cried out," allowing the patient to vent bottled up feelings. For an actual example of such a prayer, see below, text 3. Patients with Marduk-connected fevers and venereal disease (13–23) received medical treatment; the Marduk-stressed got leather-bag amulets (24–31) and a stone charm (32–34).

The moon god Sîn (35–41) was honored with a libation of water and a recitation said by the exorcist who plays here the role of intercessor. The more usual libation for Sîn was milk; the water was to signal a cooling of the divine wrath. Shamash (42–46) was assumed to be angry because of an unfulfilled vow of food offerings that were then to be given in addition to the treatment. Just to make sure that the god got the message, used grease from the Shamash temple found its way into one of the amulets (46).

Interestingly, Adad (47–48) gets a stone charm with only one stone (48) in contrast to Marduk's seven, perhaps reflecting the relative importance of the divinities in question. Belet-ili (49–54) is given a set prayer but, as with the approach to Marduk, said by the patient himself, reflecting the closeness that worshippers felt to these divinities. In stark contrast, Nergal (59–62), god of the underworld, is approached with a full-fledged offering ceremony not accompanied by prayer. His name cannot even be mentioned without the addition of an aprotropaic formula (57–58). Nergal's apples feature also in the annual mourning rites for Tammuz. Like the sweet halvah and the action of extinguishing the brazier, the idea was to cool anger and sweeten tempers. To note is also that Nergal, like Hades, was married by a love match, and that apples were, in ancient Mesopotamia as in Greece, a love charm.

Gula (63–69) was the goddess of healing and, as such, received the most expensive offering, a gold dog figurine. Self-laceration with an obsidian blade invoked the doctor's scalpel, but also was a modified mourning rite used to put pressure on divinities to cease being angry. A less expensive alternative to the gift of the gold dog figurine was to keep the figurine as a charm and instead to feed an offering of halvah to Gula to one of her dogs. The temple of Gula at Isin doubled as a sort of animal shelter where dogs were fed and encouraged to lick patients as part of therapy.

Ishtar's stress (70–83) was dealt with by appeasing the goddess with abasement and praise. The patient did the kneeling but the seven-fold recitation was performed by the exorcist, again acting as intercessor. Personal-god anxiety (84–97) allowed for a more direct approach and the application of some behavioral psychology in which the patient takes charge of the ritual and "becomes brave and becomes strong." The libation of water was, again, to cool wrath. In the same category probably belong some of the ingredients of the amulets, salves, and potions for personal god anxiety (98–155), which shade off into a type of quasi-legitimate magic known as Egalkura of which 114–117, 126–129, and 130–144 are particularly clear examples. Egalkura rituals were designed to help people win legal cases and engage successfully with authorities, both high-stress situations. So, for example, the animal wombs of lines 118–119 are rubbed on the face because the word in Akkadian for "womb" is the same as the word for "mercy" and the magnetic hematite of lines 121–122 are, literally, for attraction. The seven stones for a divine intercessor (124–125) differ from Marduk's seven stones in that carnelian, *muššaru*-stone, silver, and gold replace *zalāqu*-stone, *ašpû*-jasper, *abašmu*-stone, and green obsidian. The leftovers from flour offerings to Nusku (145–148) signal intercession.

i

1. [DIŠ N]A *i-sà-m*[*u-ma* NU DUG$_4$.DUG$_4$-*m*(*a ù* UMUŠ-*šú la*)] ⸢*ṣa*⸣-*bit* NA BI ⸢*ki-mil*⸣-[*ti* (LUGAL DINGIR.M)]EŠ
2. ⸢UGU⸣-*šu* [(GÁL)]-*š*[(*i*)]
3. *ana* IGI ^{d}MES NÍG.NA ^{ŠEM}[(L)]I ŠE[(M.GIG *u* ZÍ)]D.DA GAR-*un*! *ši*-⸢*gu*⸣-*ú* GÙ[(-⸢*si-ma*⸣)]
4. *ma-la* ŠÀ-*šú* DIB-*tu*
5. *lid-bu-ub-ma lu-uš-ke-en* ^{Ú}[(ḪAR.ḪUM.BA.⸢NU$_{11}$⸣ *u* IM BABBAR *ina* Ì)] ŠÉŠ-*su-ma ki-mil*!-*ti*!

6. ^{d}AMAR.UTU DU$_{8}$-*at*

---

7. DIŠ NA *ina ma-ka-*⸢*li*⸣-*šu* ŠÀ-⸢*šú* GAZ⸣.M[(E)]-*šú ina* É *ṣal-te* ⸢*ina* SILA *pu*⸣-[(*úḫ-pu*)-*u*]*ḫ-ḫu-ú* GAR-⸢*šu*⸣
8. *šá* NA BI *ki*!-*mil-ti* ^{d}MES U[(G)]U-*šú* GÁ[(L)-*š*]*i ana* BÚR-*ri* ^{G}[(^{IŠ}ŠUR.MÌN ^{ŠEM}ŠE.L)]I.BABBAR
9. ⸢$^{NA_{4}}$⸣KUR-*nu*.DI[(B)].⸢BA⸣
10. ^{Ú}*u*$_{5}$-⸢*ra*⸣-*nu* ^{Ú}IN.NU.U[(Š *k*)]*i-ṣir* ^{GIŠ}MA.NU NUMUN ^{GIŠ}ŠINIG
11. 7 Ú.[ME]Š[1] *an-nu-te*
12. *ina* KUŠ *ina* Ì *ina* KAŠ *me-e-lu lat-*⸢*ku ni-ṣir*⸣-*ti* ⸢^{LÚ}⸣MAŠ.MAŠ *mu-du-ú mu-*⸢*da-a li*⸣-*kal-lim*

---

13. DIŠ NA SA.SAL.LA-*šú* KÚM.KÚM ŠU^{II}-*šú* GÌR^{II}-*šú* IR ŠUB.MEŠ-*a* ⸢GÌR^{II}⸣-*šú ú-zaq-qa-ta-šu*
14. ŠU ^{d}ALAD *šá*!-*ni* ^{d}AMAR.UTU *ina* ŠU ^{d}ALAD KAR!-*šú* ⸢^{Ú}⸣[*a*]-*ra-ri-ia-nu*
15. ^{Ú}*a-zal-lá* NUMUN ^{GIŠ}*bi-ni ina* KUŠ *ina* Ì *ina* KAŠ

---

16. DIŠ NA *ina* KI.NÁ-*šú* LUḪ.LUḪ-*ut* ŠÀ-*šú e-šu-u ina* KI.NÁ-*šú* A.RI.A-*su* DU-*ak*
17. NA BI DIB-*tì* ^{d}AMAR.UTU
18. *u* ⸢^{d}⸣EŠ$_{4}$.DAR UGU-*šú* GÁL-*ši ana* TI.LA-*šú* ^{Ú}*tar-muš* ‹(Ú DILI)›[2] ^{Ú}ḪAR.ḪUM.BA.ŠIR ‹(*ki-ṣir*)›
19. ^{GIŠ}MA.NU[3] ILLU ^{GIŠ}DÌḪ[4]
20. $^{NA_{4}}$AT.BAR *ḫi-ṣib*! $^{NA_{4}}$GUG ^{Ú}SIKIL ‹(PA)› ^{GIŠ}ŠE.NÁ.⸢A⸣ (erasure)
21. ^{Ú}IN.NU.UŠ ^{Ú}NÍG.BÙR.BÙR ^{Ú}*a-za-la* ^{Ú}EME.UR.GI$_{7}$ ^{GIŠ}DÌḪ *šá* IZ.ZI[5]
22. 1-*niš* ^{SÍG}⸢ÀKA⸣ NIGIN-*mi* MÚD ^{GIŠ}ERIN SUD *ina* KUŠ[6]

---

23. [DIŠ K]I.MIN(!) ^{ŠEM}LI ^{MUN}*a-ma-nim ina* Ì+GIŠ ^{GIŠ}ŠUR.MÌN ŠÉŠ-*su*

---

24. [DIŠ] ⸢UGU⸣ LÚ.GIG *na-áš-pa-ru-ú e-ki-is-su*[7] *ki-mil-te*
25. [^{d}AMAR.UTU] UGU-*šú* GÁL-*u ana ki-mil-ti* ^{d}AMAR.UTU BÚR-*ri* ⸢^{Ú}⸣*imḫur-lim*
26. [*e-p*]*é-ri né-med* KÁ ^{d}KU SAḪAR ‹É›.SAG.ÍL
27. x x x la še nu um ma[8] ^{Ú}MUD *ina* KUŠ

---

28. DIŠ KI.MIN(!) ^{NA}[$_{4}$…] NA$_{4}$ *ú-ri*(!)-*ṣa* ^{Ú}⸢*ḫa*⸣-*šá-nu* ⸢Ì.KU$_{6}$⸣
29. *ina* KUŠ

---

30. *ana ki-mil-ti* [(^{d}AMAR.UTU BÚR)]-*ri* ^{Ú}*nu-ṣa-ba* ^{NA_4}PEŠ$_4$.ANŠE NA$_4$ *ga-bi-i*
31. *ina* ⸢KUŠ⸣

---

32. DIŠ KI.MIN ^{NA_4}ZA.GÌN ^{NA_4}AN.BAR ^{NA}[($_4$ZÁ)]LAG ^{NA_4}*aš-pu-ú* ^{NA_4}*àb-aš-*⸢*mu*⸣ ⸢^{NA_4}⸣[(KUR-*nu*)] DIB
33. ^{NA_4}ZÚ SIG$_7$[9] 7 NA$_4$.MEŠ *an-nu-*⸢*ti*⸣ *ina* ⸢DUR⸣ È-*ak* ^{Ú}SIKIL
34. *ina bi-ri-šu-nu tál!-pap ina* ⸢GÚ-*šú*⸣ GAR-⸢*an*⸣

---

35. DIŠ NA *ina* KI.NÁ LUḪ-*ut* UZU.MEŠ-*šú* ⸢*ú*⸣-[... *ki-mil-te*]
36. [^{d}]30 UGU-*šú* GÁL-*ši a-na* BÚR-*ri* ^{Ú}NU.LUḪ ^{Ú}⸢*an-ki-nu-te*⸣
37. ESIR ḪÁD.A(!) ^{GIŠ}MÁ.GUR$_8$ IM KI.A.ÍD SUḪUŠ ^{GIŠ}⸢*šú-ši*⸣ *šá* UGU *ba-ri-ti*[10]
38. *ina* KUŠ GAG.GAG *ina* GÚ-*šú* GAR A-⸢UGU⸣ *lat-ku ana* ^{d}30 A BAL-*qí*
39. UR$_5$.GIN$_7$ DUG$_4$.GA ÉN *ú-*⸢*šá!*⸣-[*an-nu*] ⸢*na!*⸣-*mir-tú ag-gu* ŠÀ-*ka* ⸢*li*⸣-*nu-ḫa*
40. *ka-bat-ta-ka lip-pa-áš-ra* DUG$_4$.GA-*ma ina* GÚ-*šú* GAR-*ma* ŠE.GA

---

41. *ana ki-mil-ti* ^{d}30 BÚR-*ri* Ú DILI ⸢^{NA_4}⸣ZÁLAG ^{Ú}LAL SUḪUŠ ^{GIŠ}*šú-ši ina* KUŠ

---

42. DIŠ NA GÌŠ-‹*šu*› SÌG.SÌG-*šú i-te-e*[*b*]-*bi* KI A-*šú* MURUB$_4$.MEŠ-*šú* GU$_7$.MEŠ-*šú šá* NA BI [...]
43. *ki-mil-ti* ^{d}UTU UGU-*šú* GÁL-*ši* LÚ BI *qí-bit* ⸢*el*⸣ *ma-ka-le-e u ma-ka-la-a* ^{d}UTU SUM-*ma ki-mil-ti* ^{d}UTU DU$_8$-*su*

---

45. *ana ki-mil-ti* ^{d}UTU BÚR-*ri* ŠIKA E.SÍR LÍM.MA ⸢^{Ú}⸣*ḫa-mi-ma* ^{Ú}NÍG.BÙR.BÙR *ina* ⸢KUŠ⸣

---

46. DIŠ KI.MIN! ^{Ú}*am-ḫa-ra* KUG.GAN ^{NA_4}BAL ⸢Ì⸣.SUMUN ⸢BÁRA ^{d}⸣UTU *ina* KUŠ

---

47. [*ana*] *ki-mil-ti* ^{d}IM BÚR-⸢*ri*⸣ ^{Ú}KUR.KUR ⸢^{NA_4}ALGAMES⸣ [^{Ú}SIKIL *ina* KUŠ]

---

48. [DIŠ K]I.MIN NA$_4$ ⸢ALGAMEŠ⸣ *ina* GU ⸢GADA⸣ È *ina* ⸢GÚ⸣-[*šú* GAR]

---

ii

49. DIŠ NA ⸢UGU⸣-*šú* Š[ED$_7$-*ma*] ⸢*liq*⸣ KA-*šú šá-bu-ul* [DIB-*ti* ^{d}MAḪ

UGU-*šú* GAL-*tú-ši*]

50. NA BI ⸢NÍG.NA⸣ $^{\text{[Š]EM}}$LI IGI ^{d}MAḪ GAR-*an* KAŠ BAL-[*qí uš-ken*]
51. ⸢UR$_5$.GIN$_7$⸣ DUG$_4$.GA ^{d}MAḪ *ana ṣi-it* ŠÀ *šá at-ti-ma* x x [...]
52. x x TE-⸢*ma*⸣ *ki-mil-ti* ^{d}MAḪ ⸢DU$_8$⸣-*su*

---

53. *ana ki-mil-ti* ^{d}MAḪ [(B)]ÚR-*r*[*i*] UZU.DIR.KUR.RA ⸢SA!⸣ MAŠ.DÀ *ina* K[(UŠ)]

---

54. DIŠ KI.MIN ^{Ú}‹(*nu*)›-*ṣa-bu* [(^{GIŠ}ḪAŠ)]ḪUR ^{GIŠ}⸢GI⸣ SA! MAŠ.DÀ *ina* KUŠ

---

55. *ana ki-mil-ti* ^{d}⸢NIN⸣.IB BÚR-*ri* ^{Ú}⸢*túl*⸣-*lal* ^{Ú}NAM.TI.LA ^{ŠEM}ŠE[.LI]
56. NA$_4$ ZÚ.LUM.MA *ina* KUŠ

---

57. DIŠ NA (⸢*ḫé*⸣-*pí eš-šú*) *eṭ-re-et ki-mil-ti* ^{d}U.⸢GUR⸣ UGU-*šú* ⸢GÁL⸣-*ši*
58. ⸢^{d}U⸣.GUR ⸢*liš-šir*⸣ INIM.GAR *ù* ŠÀ ^{d}U.GUR *li-nu-uḫ-ma ṭé-ma-at ni-ši li-ṭ*[*é*]*m*

---

59. *ana* [*ki-mil*]-*ti* ^{d}U.GUR BÚR-*ri* [(*ana*)] IGI GUNNI GI.DU$_8$ GAR-*an* ⸢*eq-qí-i*⸣ *ú-ṭaḫ-ḫa*
60. NINDA.Ì.D[É].⸢A⸣ LÀL Ì.NUN.NA GAR-*an* UGU ⸢GUN⸣NI *šu-a-tu* ^{GIŠ}ḪAŠḪUR *ta-sár-raq ina* [(Ì)] BÁRA.GA
61. *ú-na-aḫ* BÚR-*ir*

---

62. DIŠ [K]I.MIN $^{\text{NA}_4}$[*m*(*u-ṣ*)]*u* ^{Ú}KUR.KUR *ina* KUŠ : DIŠ KI.MIN $^{\text{NA}_4}$ZA.GÌN.KUR.RA *ina* K[(UŠ)]

---

63. DIŠ NA DUL.DUL-⸢*tam*⸣ [(*ḫur*)]-*ba*-⸢*šu*⸣ ŠUB.ŠUB-*su ki-mil-ti* ^{d}*Gu-la* UGU-*šú* GÁL-*ši*
64. NA BI UR.GI$_7$ KÙ.⸢SIG$_{17}$ DÙ⸣-*ma ana* ^{d}*Gu-la lid-din* ŠU-*su ina* $^{\text{NA}_4}$ZÚ
65. *iṣ-ṣi-ma* ⸢DIB!⸣-*tim* ^{d}*Gu-la paṭ-rat*

---

66. *ana ki-mil-ti* ^{d}*Gu-la* BÚR-*ri* ^{Ú}*a-ra-ri-*<*ya*>*-na*[11] A!.[(ZAL.LÁ)]
67. A.ÉSIR ḪÁD.DU.A ^{Ú}DILI *ina* KUŠ

---

68. DIŠ KI.MIN[12] UR.GI$_7$ ZI ‹(KÙ.SIG$_{17}$)› *ina* GÚ-*šú* [(GAR)-*a*]*n-ma ù* ‹(*ana*)› UR.GI$_7$ *šá* KÁ ‹(É)› ^{d}*Gu-la*
69. NINDA.Ì.DÉ.A LÀL [(Ì.NUN.N)]A *ú-ṭaḫ-ḫa-ma* BÚ[(R)]

---

70. DIŠ NA ŠÀ-*bi* ŠÀ-*bi* DUG$_4$.GA ŠÀ-[(*šú* NU)] GU$_7$-*šú* ⸢NINDA⸣ NU ⸢GU$_7$!⸣ [(A/KAŠ NU NAG)]
71. *i-da-mu-um* NA BI DIB [(DINGIR-*šú*)] ^{d}15-[(*šú*)]
72. UGU-*šú* GÁL-*ši ana* IGI ^{d}15 KE[(ŠDA KEŠDA NA *ina* GÌR-*šú* DU$_{10}$)] GAM-*ma*
73. ÉN ⸢SIKIL-*tum*⸣ [(^{d}15 7-*šú*)] ⸢ŠID⸣-[(*nu*)]

---

74. ÉN *an*-[*ni-tú* (*ina* GÌR^{II}-*šú tu-šaq-ma-su-ma* 7-*šú* ŠID)][13]

75–78. very fragmentary

---

79. [DIŠ KI.MI]N ^{NA_4}AN.ZAḪ ^{NA_4}PEŠ$_4$! NA$_4$ *ga-bi-i* NUMUN Ú[KUŠ *ina* KUŠ]

---

80. ⸢DIŠ KI.MIN⸣ MUN! *eme*!-*sal*!-*lim* ⸢ŠURUN⸣ ^{d}*Še-riš* KA.A.AB.⸢BA⸣ [(GI.DÙG.GA)][14]
81. ^{NA_4}AN.ZAḪ ⸢*ina* KUŠ⸣

---

82. DIŠ KI.MIN SUḪUŠ! $^{Ú!}$⸢*u*$_5$⸣-*ra-an-ni* MU-‹*šú*› EŠ-*aš*
83. DIŠ KI.MIN DÚR‹MI.NA› DIB AN.BAR BABBAR.DIL *ina* K[UŠ]

---

84. DIŠ NA *nu-ul-la-ti*! KI ŠÀ-*šú i-ta-mu at-mu-šú i-šá-an*-[(*ni*)]
85. ‹(*za-mar ṣa-lil*)› *za-mar e-er*
86. *u* UMUŠ-*šú* NU DIB-*al* DIB-*ti* DINGIR-*šú* UGU.BI GÁL NA BI *ina* [(U$_4$ ŠE.GA)]
87. *li-te*!-*lil lim-te-es*-[(*si*)]
88. TÚG-*su li-bi-ib níg*-⸢*na-ki*!⸣ 1 ⸢$^{ŠEM!}$⸣ LI *ana* IGI DINGIR-*šú* 1 *e*-[*re-ni*]
89. *ana* IGI DINGIR URU-*šú* G[AR-(*un*)][15]
90. [(A.MEŠ)] BAL-*qí* [(*lik*)]-*mis*! *lit*!-*nen u* UR$_5$.GIN$_7$ DUG$_4$.GA[16]

91–97 [ÉN] *ú*-[*šá-an-nu na-mir-tú* (*ag-gu* ŠÀ-*ka li-nu-ḫa* A.MEŠ *ta-ni-iḫ-ti lim-ḫu-ru-ka* 3-*šú* DUG$_4$.GA-*ma* KI.ZA.ZA) o-*šú* (GUR.GUR-*ma* DIB-*ti* DINGIR-*šú* DU$_8$-*su*)][17]

---

iii

98. DIŠ KI.MIN [...]

---

99. DIŠ KI.MIN ^{Ú}[...]
100. [...]
101. ^{Ú}*nam-ru*[*q-qu*]

---

102. DIŠ KI.MIN ^{Ú}*šu*-[…]
103. DIŠ KI.MIN ^{Ú}*a-ra-r*[*u-ú* …]

---

104. DIŠ KI.MIN ^{Ú}DILI NA$_4$! ZÁLAG ^{Ú}*nu-ṣa-bu* ⸢x x-x⸣ *ina* [KUŠ]

---

105. *ana ki-mil-ti* DINGIR-*šu* BÚR-*ri* Ì.SUMUN BÁRA ^{d}UTU $^{\text{NA}_4}$[(KUR-*nu* DIB)]
106. $^{\text{NA}_4}$*mu-ṣa* URUDU KUG.GAN[18] MÚD ^{GIŠ}ERIN Ú ‹DILI› *ina* K[(UŠ)]

---

107. *ana ki-mil-ti* DINGIR URU-*šú* BÚR-⸢*ri*⸣ ŠIKA! SILA LÍM.MA MUN *A-ma-ni*[(*m*)]
108. ^{ŠEM}LI ‹(PA)› ^{GIŠ}ŠINIG *ina* KU[Š][19]

---

109. *ana* DINGIR URU-*šú* KI-*šú* SILIM-*mi* ÉR! IGI GUD *šá* GÙB PA ^{GI}[^{Š}*p*]*i*[*š-ri*(?)]
110. ZÍD! ^{GIŠ}*šú-ši* IM GÚ.EN.NA *ina* KUŠ

---

111. DIŠ KI.MIN ^{Ú}EME.UR.GI$_7$ ^{Ú}KUR.KUR ^{Ú}ḪAB *ina* KUŠ
112. DIŠ KI.MIN G[ÌR] NAGA.GA$^{\text{MUŠEN!}}$ ^{Ú}IN.NU.UŠ *ina* ⸢KUŠ⸣

---

113. *ana ki-mil-ti* DINGIR.MEŠ DÙ.A.BI BÚR-*ri* ^{Ú}ÁB!.DUḪ! KA ⸢*tam*⸣-*tim* [*ina* KUŠ]

---

114. *ana* DINGIR ŠÀ.DIB!.BA SILIM-*me*! GUNNI *šá* GI.DÙG.GA SAḪAR NU ‹ŠUB› ŠÀ.TUR *ana* ŠÀ [NU ŠUB]
115. *li-pu-uḫ*! ^{d}GIŠ.BAR DINGIR ŠÀ.DIB.BA *ú-sal-lam* LÚ BE *šá* U[Š$_{11}$ZU]
116. *šu-ku-lu ina* Ì GI.[DÙG.GA]
117. SU-*ka* ⸢ŠÉŠ-*ma* DINGIR LUGAL⸣ [ID]IM NUN EN DUG$_4$.DUG$_4$[-*ka* SILIM-*mu*]

---

118. *ana* DINGIR *ana* ⸢LÚ⸣ A[(RḪU)]Š [(T)]UK[(U-*e*)] ARḪUŠ ÁB ‹(*u* UDU)› ARḪUŠ ⸢U$_8$⸣ ‹(*u* ÙZ)› Ú.⸢ZÚG⸣ *ina* GA SÚD IGI-⸢*ka*⸣[20]
119. ⸢ŠÉŠ⸣-*ma* DINGIR ARḪUŠ TUKU-*ku*

---

120. DIŠ KI.MIN ⸢$^{\text{NA}_4}$⸣[(AN)].⸢ZAḪ!⸣ $^{\text{NA}_4}$ÀB.AŠ.MU SUḪUŠ ^{GIŠ}DÌḪ.BABBAR *ina* KUŠ

---

121. *ana* DINGIR ^{d}ALAD ^{d}LAMMA![21] TUKU-*e tas-lit*-[*su še-me*]-*e*[22]

122. ^{NA_4}KA.⸢GI⸣.NA DIB.BA *ni-kip*-[(*tú* NITÁ *u* MUNUS AN)].BAR ^{GIŠ}ŠÀ.GI *ina* KUŠ

---

123. DIŠ KI.MIN ^{NA_4}GUG ^{NA_4}ZA.GÌN ^{NA_4}⸢NÍR ^{NA_4}MUŠ⸣.GÍR ^{NA_4}AN.BAR ^{NA_4}KÙ.BABBAR ^{NA_4}KÙ.SIG$_{17}$
125. 7 NA$_4$.ME *an-nu-tim ina* SÍG ^{MUNUS}ÁŠ.GÀR GÌŠ.NU.ZU BABBAR *u* GI$_6$ ‹(NU.NU)› È *ina* GÚ-*šú* GAR-*an*[23]

---

126. *ana* ⸢*ṭa*⸣-*pul-ti* LÚ *la qá-bi-i* ŠU.SI ḪUL-*tim*! EGIR-*šú* ⸢BA⸣.RA *ta-ra-ṣi*
127. ^{Ú}*imḫur-lim* ^{Ú}*ḫa-šu-tú* ^{Ú}KUR.KUR ‹$^{(NA_4)}$›ŠURUN ^{d}*Še-riš ina* KUŠ

---

128. DIŠ KI.MIN ^{Ú}*imḫur-lim* $^{GIŠ!}$ḪAŠḪUR.$^{GIŠ!}$PÈŠ *ina* Ì BUR SÚD IGI.MEŠ-*šú* ŠÉŠ.MEŠ *ina* KAŠ NAG.MEŠ
129. *e-ma* DU-*ku ma-gir ṭa-pul-ta-šú ul iq-qa-bi*

---

130. DIŠ NA *gi-na-a šu-dur ur-ra u* GI$_6$ *ina-ziq* ZI.GA *sad-ra*[(*t-su*[24] *iš-d*)]*i-iḫ-šú* KUD-⸢*is*⸣
131. EME.SIG.MEŠ-*šú* GU$_7$.MEŠ ⸢*da*!-*bi-ib*!⸣ *it-ti-šú* ⸢*kit*⸣-[(*tú* NU)] ⸢DUG$_4$.MEŠ⸣
132. ŠU.SI ḪUL-*tim* EGIR-*šú* LAL-*ma*
133. *ina* É.GAL-*šú*[25] *la maḫ-ra-šú* MÁŠ.GI$_6$.MEŠ-*šú* [(*pár-da ina* MÁŠ)]. GI$_6$-*šú* ÚŠ.MEŠ IGI!-*ma*[*r*]
134. GAZ ŠÀ GAR-*šú* D[I]B[26] DINGIR *u* ^{d}‹(EŠ$_4$)›.DAR UGU-*šú* GÁ[(L-*a*)] DINGIR-*šú u* ^{d}‹(EŠ$_4$)›.DAR-⸢*šú*⸣
135. KI-*šú ze-nu-u*[27]
136. KI LÚ.DINGIR *u* ENSI[28] DI-*šú* ‹(EN 7-*šú*)› NU S[(I.SÁ DUG$_4$.GA)]
137. *la* ŠE.GA[29] GAR-*šú ana* EŠ.BAR-*šú* TAR-*si-im-ma* D[(I.KU$_5$-*šú ana šu-t*)]*e-šu-ri*[30]

iv

139. [KÌD.K]ÌD.BI[31] ^{Ú}*tar-muš* ^{Ú}*imḫur-lim* ^{Ú}*imḫur*-20 ^{Ú}⸢*eli-kul*⸣-*la*! ^{Ú}LÚ.U$_{19}$.LU[32] KA! *tam-t*[*im*][33]
140. [(^{GIŠ}Š)]INIG GIŠ BÚR ^{Ú}*er-kul-la*[34] 7 Ú.ḪI.A *an-nu-te* ^{SÍG}ÀKA ⸢NIGIN⸣ *ina* KUŠ *ina* Ì ⸢BÁRA⸣[35]
141. [(IN)]IM.GAR-*šú* SI.SÁ MÁŠ.GI$_6$.MEŠ-*šú* SIG$_5$.MEŠ *qá-bu-ú u š*[*e-mu-u*][36] GAR!-*šú*
142. DINGIR *u* EŠ$_4$.DAR KI-*šú* SILIM-*mu*[37]
143. [(ÉN)] *a-la-aḫ-sa šu-la-aḫ ba-ši-in-ti*
144. ÉN A.RA.ZU! ŠU.TE.MA.AB ŠID-*nu*[38]

---

138. DIŠ KI.MIN Ì.SUMUN *ša* É ^{d}KU *mu-ṣa* EREN [S]UD[39] *ina* ^{SÍG}ÀKA NIGIN *ina* KUŠ[40]

---

145. DIŠ NA! GAZ ŠÀ TUKU U$_4$ GI$_6$ *pu-luḫ-tú* TUKU DINGIR-*šú* KI-*šú* *ze-ni*[41] *ši-qit-tú*
146. KA.A.AB.BA
147. $^{\text{NA}_4}$BABBAR.DIL $^{\text{NA}_4}$*èš-me-qu ḫa-ḫe-e* UDUN ^{ZÍD}MA.AD.GÁ *šá* IGI
148. ^{d}NUSKU *ina* KUŠ

---

149. ^{Ú}*imḫur-lim* Ú.KUR.RA NUMUN NINNI$_5$ ^{Ú}*a-zal-lá ina* KUŠ

---

150. DIŠ (*ḫe-pi*) x si ŠÀ DINGIR-*šú* KI-*šú ze-ni né-um* ŠÀ *ana* TUKU-*e* ^{Ú}*er-kul-la* ^{Ú}ḪAR?!.ḪAR
151. ^{ŠEM}ŠEŠ ^{ŠEM}GÚR.GÚR ^{Ú}*ár-zal-la* ^{Ú}UKUŠ.GÍL NUMUN ^{GIŠ}MA.NU *ina* KUŠ

---

152. DIŠ NA *ana* DUG$_4$ KA-*šú* NU ÍL-*šú u i-ṣa-mu* DINGIR-*šú* KI-*šú ze-ni* ‹‹NUMUN››
153. NUMUN ^{GIŠ}GURUN ^{GIŠ}NAM.TAR
154. ^{Ú}EME.UR.GI$_7$ ^{GIŠ}*si-ḫa* $^{\text{NA}_4}$ZÚ GI$_6$ $^{\text{NA}_4}$ZÁLAG *ina* KUŠ

---

155. ^{Ú}ḪAŠḪUR ^{GIŠ}GI ^{Ú}SIKIL ^{GIŠ}*bi-nu* GI.⸢DÙG.GA⸣ *ina* KUŠ

TRANSLATION

(1–6) [If] a ⸢person⸣ ⸢turns so red (in the face)⸣ (with anger) [that he cannot speak] and he is not in full possession of his faculties, the wrath of the king of the gods is upon him. He should set up before Marduk an incense burner (burning) *burāšu*-aromatic, *kanaktu*-aromatic, and flour. He should continually utter a *šigû*-prayer. He should say as much as his heart prompts and then he should prostrate himself.[42] If you rub him gently with *ḫarmunu* and *gaṣṣu*-gypsum, (mixed) with oil, the wrath of Marduk should be dissipated.

(7–12) If when a person eats, his heart continually crushes him (and) in the house quarrel and in the street disturbance are inflicted upon him, the anger of Marduk is upon that person,[43] to loosen (the anger of Marduk), (you use) these seven plants: *šurmēnu*-cypress, *kikkirānu*, magnetic hematite, *uriānu*, *maštakal*, a block of *eʾru*-wood, (and) *bīnu*-tamarisk seed as an amulet, (mixed) with oil (as a salve) or (mixed) with beer (as a potion). Tested prophylactic, a secret of *ašipūtu*. An expert may ‹not› show it to a nonexpert.

(13–15) If a person's upper back is continually hot, his hands and his feet continually produce sweat, (and) his feet sting him, "hand" of a *šēdû*, deputy of Marduk.[44] To save him from the "hand" of a *šēdû*, (you use) *arariānu*, *azallû* (and) *bīnu*-tamarisk seed as an amulet, (mixed) with oil (as a salve) or (mixed) with beer (as a potion).

(16–22) If a person continually jerks in his bed, his heart(beat) is confused (and) his semen flows in his bed, the anger of Marduk and Ishtar is upon that person.[45] To cure him, you wrap together[46] *tarmuš*, ‹("lone plant")›[47] *ḫarmunu*, ‹(a block of)› *eʾru*-tree,[48] *baltu*-thorn resin,[49] *atbaru*-basalt, a broken piece of carnelian, *sikillu*, *šūnû*-chastetree leaves,[50] *maštakal*, *pallišu*-stone, *azallû*, *lišān kalbi*, (and) *baltu*-thorn from a wall[51] in a tuft of wool. You sprinkle (it) with *erēnu*-cedar resin (and put it) in a leather bag.

(23) ⸢Alterntively⸣, you rub him gently (with) *burāšu*-juniper (and) *Amanim*-salt (mixed) with *šurmēnu*-cypress oil.

(24–27) If the patient's guardian angel is taken away from him,[52] the anger of [Marduk] is upon him. To dispel the wrath of Marduk, (you put) *imḫur-lim*, ⸢dust⸣ from the foundations[53] of the Marduk gate, dust of the Esagil [...] (and) "dark-red plant" in a leather bag

(28–29) Alternatively, (you put) [...], *urizu*-stone, *ḫašānu*, (and) fish oil in a leather bag.

(30–31) To ⸢dispel⸣ the wrath of Marduk, (you put) *nuṣābu*, *biṣṣur-atāne*-shell, (and) alum in a leather bag.

(32–34) Alternatively, you thread these seven stones: lapis, iron, ⸢*zalāqu*⸣-stone, *ašpû*-jasper, *abašmu*-stone, magnetic hematite, (and) green obsidian on a band. You wind *sikillu* into burls between them. You put (it) on his neck.

(35–40) If a person jerks in his bed (and) his flesh [itches], the [wrath] of Sîn is upon him.[54] To dispel it, you sew up *nuḫurtu*, *ankinūtu*, dried bitumen from a *magurru*-boat,[55] clay, *kibrītu*-sulphur, (and) *šūšu*-licorice root from a balk in a leather bag (and) put (it) on his neck. (This is) a tested prophylactic. You pour a libation of water to Sîn (and) say as follows: "I have ⸢altered⸣ the brightness;[56] may your angry heart calm down; may your anger be appeased." You say this and, if you put it on his neck, he should find favor.

(41) To dispel the wrath of Sîn, (you put) "lone plant," *zalāqu*-stone, *ašqulālu*, (and) *šūšu*-licorice root in a leather bag.

(42–43) If a person's penis continually gives him a stabbing pain, he gets up (in the night to urinate and) with his water, his hip region continually hurts him, that person's [...]; the wrath of Shamash is upon him.[57] That person (has made an unfulfilled) promise for a food offering. So, if he gives a food offering to Shamash, the wrath of Shamash should be dispelled for him.

(45) To dispel the wrath of Shamash, (you put) a potsherd from a crossroads, *ḫamimu*, (and) *pallišu*-plant in a leather bag.

(46) Alternatively, (you put) *amḫaru*, *lulû*-antimony, spindle-stone, (and) used grease from the dais of Shamash in a leather bag.

(47) [To] dispel the wrath of Adad, (you put) *atāʾišu*, *algamešu*-stone, (and) [*sikillu* in a leather bag].

(48) ⸢Alternatively⸣, you thread *algamešu*-stone on linen thread (and) [put] (it) on [his] neck.

(49–52) If the top of a person's head is ⸢cold⸣ and his ⸢palate⸣ is dried up, [the wrath of Belit-ili is upon him]. That person sets up an incense burner (burning) *burāšu*-juniper before Belit-ili. He pours a libation of beer. [He prostrates himself.] He says as follows. [...] to the child whom you yourself [...]. The wrath of Belit-ili should be dispelled from him.

(53) To ⸢dispel⸣ the wrath of Belit-ili, (you put) *kamun šadê*-fungus (and) gazelle tendon in a ⸢leather bag⸣.

(54) Alternatively, (you put) *nuṣābu*, "swamp apple," (and) gazelle tendon in a leather bag.

(55–56) To dispel the wrath of Ninurta, (you put) *tullal*, "life plant," ⸢*kikkirānu*⸣-juniper berries, [...] (and) date stone in a leather bag.

(57–58) If a person's [...] was taken away, the wrath of Nergal is upon him. O Nergal, may an omen from a chance utterance come straightaway and may the heart of Nergal calm down so that he may ⸢issue⸣ orders for mankind.

(59–61) To dispel the ⸢wrath⸣ of Nergal, before a brazier you set up a reed altar. He offers an *eqû*. You put out *mersu*-confection (made with) honey and ghee (on the reed altar). You scatter apples on that brazier. He extinguishes (it) with pressed-out (oil). (The wrath) should be dispelled.

(62) ⸢Alternatively⸣, (you put) ⸢*mūṣu*⸣-stone (and) *atāʾišu* in a leather bag. Alternatively, (you put) mountain lapis in a ⸢leather bag⸣.

(63–65) If a person continually covers himself (and) ⸢chills⸣ continually fall upon him, the wrath of Gula is upon him. That person should make a gold dog (figurine) and should give it to Gula. If he cuts himself with an obsidian blade, the wrath of Gula should be dispelled.

(66–67) To dispel the wrath of Gula, (you put) *arariyānu*, *azallû*, dried bitumen, (and) "lone plant" in a leather bag.

(68–69) Alternatively, you put a standing dog ‹(of gold)› on his neck and then, if he also offers *mersu*-confection (made from) honey (and) ⸢ghee⸣ ‹(to)› a dog at the gate of the Gula ‹(temple)›, (the wrath) ⸢should be dispelled⸣.

(70–74) If a person says: "My insides, my insides!" (but) his stomach does not hurt him, he cannot eat bread (and) he cannot drink water/beer (and) he moans, the anger of Ištar[58] is upon him.[59] You set up an offering arrangement before Ishtar. You have the person sit on his feet and you recite the recitation: "Purest Ishtar" seven times. You have the person sit on his feet and you recite this recitation seven times.

(75–78) *Very fragmentary*

(79) ⸢Alternatively⸣, (you put) *anzaḫḫu*-frit, *biṣṣūru*-cowrie, alum (and) ⸢*irru*⸣ seed [in a leather bag].

(80–81) Alternatively, (you put) *emesallim*-salt, ox dung, *imbû tamtim*, "sweet reed" and *anzaḫḫu*-frit in a leather bag.[60]

(82–83) Alternatively, root of *urânu* is (its's) name. You rub ⸢him⸣ gently (with it). Alternatively, (you put) magnetic *turminnû*-breccia, iron (and) *papardillû*-stone in a ⸢leather bag⸣.

(84–97) If a person ponders untruths with his heart, he repeats his words, ‹(he is now sleeping)›, now awake, and he cannot make up his mind (to do anything), the anger of his god is upon him.[61] On a favorable day, that person should purify and wash himself. He should put on a new garment. He should set up one incense burner (burning) *burāšu*-juniper before his god (and) one (burning) ⸢*erēnu*-cedar⸣ before the god of his city. [62] He should pour out a libation of water. He should kneel.[63] He should pray, and you have him say as follows: "I have ⸢altered⸣ the brightness;[64] may your angry heart calm down. May the water that brings relaxation beseech you." He says (this) three times and prostrates himself. If he repeats this [seven?] times, the wrath of his god should be dispelled from him.

(98–103) *Very Fragmentary*

(104) Alternatively, (you put) "lone plant," *zalaqqu*-stone, *nuṣābu* and ... [into a leather bag].

(105–106) To dispel the wrath of his god, (you put these) plant(s): used grease from the dias of Shamash, magnetic hematite, *mūṣu*-stone, copper, *lulû*-antimony, (and) *erēnu*-cedar resin in a leather bag.

(107–108) To dispel the wrath of the god of his city, (you put) a potsherd from a crossroads, *Amanim*-salt, *burāšu*-juniper (and) *bīnu*-tamarisk ‹(leaves)›[65] in a leather bag.

(109–110) To reconcile the god of his city with him, (you put) a tear from the left eye of an ox, ⸢*pišru*-wood(?)⸣ leaves, powdered *šūšu*-licorice (and) clay from a river bank in a leather bag.

(111–112) Alternatively, (you put) *lišān kalbi*, *atāʾišu*, (and) *šammi buʾšāni* in a leather bag. Alternatively, (you put) a "crows-foot" (and) *maštakal* in a leather bag.

(113) To dispel the wrath of all the gods, (you put) *kamantu*-henna(?) (and) *imbû tamtim* [in a leather bag].

(114–117) To calm an angry god, he should light a brazier on which neither sweet reed nor dust nor (even so much as) a *šassuru*-insect[66] [has been allowed to fall].[67] The fire god will pacify the angry god. That person who has been fed ⸢witchcraft⸣: if you gently rub your body with [sweet] reed oil, god, king, ⸢notable⸣, prince (and) [your] adversary in court [will come to be at peace (with you)]

(118–119) For a god to have mercy on a person, you grind the "womb" (afterbirth) of a cow ‹(or sheep)›, the "womb" (afterbirth) of a ewe ‹(or she-goat)› that has just given birth[68] in milk. If you gently rub your face (with it),[69] the god will have mercy on you.

(120) Alternatively, (you put) *anzaḫḫu*-frit, *abašmû*-stone, (and) white *baltu*-thorn root in a leather bag.

(121–122) In order for a person to have a personal god, *šēdû*, (and) *lamassu* (and) to have [his] prayers ⌜heard⌝,[70] (you put) magnetic hematite, [male and] ⌜female⌝ *nikiptu*, iron (and) reed pith in a leather bag.

(124–125) Alternatively, you thread these seven stones: carnelian, lapis, *ḫulālu*-chalcedony, *muššaru*-stone, iron, silver, (and) gold onto (a band spun from) white and black wool from a virgin she goat. You put (it) on his neck.

(126–127) For disparaging things not to be said about a person (and) for bad things never ever to be said[71] about him behind his back, (you put) *imḫur-lim*, *ḫašūtu*, *atā ʾišu*, (and) a coprolite in a leather bag.

(128–129) Alternatively, you grind *imḫur-lim* (and) *tinānu* ("fig-like") apple in *pūru*-oil. You have him repeatedly gently rub his face (with it). You have him drink (it mixed) with beer. Wherever he goes, he should find favor (and) disparaging remarks should not be made about him.

(130–144) If a person is continually made sad, he is upset day and night, he is having serious financial losses one after the other and making no profit, people slander him, the person who talks with him does not tell him the truth, people say bad things about him behind his back so that they will not see him in his palace,[72] his dreams are troubled, in his dream he continually sees dead persons, a crushing sensation in his chest is established for him, the anger[73] of god and goddess is upon him, his god and his goddess are angry with him,[74] he cannot get an answer to his problems out of ecstatic or dream interpreter (variant: diviner or seer)[75] ‹(even after seven attempts)›[76] and nobody listens to what he says, in order to obtain a fetwa for his case and to have it judged fairly,[77] this is its ritual.[78] You wrap these seven plants: *tarmuš*, *imḫur-lim*, *imḫur-ešra*, *elikulla*, *amilānu*, *imbû tamtim*, *bīnu*-tamarisk, *pišru* wood, (and) *erkulla* in a tuft of wool (and sew it up)[79] into a leather bag (or you use it mixed) with *pūru*-oil. The things he hears said around him should be favorable, his dreams should be good, people should listen to him; ‹(that person)›'s[80] god and goddess should be at peace with him.[81] You recite the recitations *alaḫ sašulaḫ bašinti* (and) A.RA. ZU ŠU.TE.MA.AB (seven times over it).

(138) Alternatively, you ⌜sprinkle⌝ used grease from the Marduk temple (and) *mūṣu*-stone with *erēnu*-cedar.[82] You wrap (it) in a (white) tuft of wool (and put it) in a leather bag.

(145–148) If a person (continually) has crushing of the heart (and) day and night he has fearfulness, his god is angry with him.[83] ‹(In order to make his god at peace with him)›,[84] (you put) *šiqittu*, *imbû tamtim*, *pappardillu*-stone,[85] *ešmeku*-stone, oven slag (and) *maṣḫatu* flour which has been offered to Nusku in a leather bag.

(149) (Alternatively, you put) *imḫur-lim*, *nīnû*-mint, *ašlu*-rush seed, (and) *azallû* in a leather bag.

(150–151) If [...], the heart of his god is angry with him. To make him have a change[86] of heart. (you put) *erkulla*, *ḫašû*-thyme, myrrh, *kukru*-aromatic, *arzallû*, *irrû*, (and) *eʾru*-tree seed in a leather bag.

(152–154) If his mouth does not rise to the words and he is thirsty, his god is angry with him. To dispel (it), (you put) fruit seeds, *pillû*, *lišān kalbi*, *sīḫu*-wormwood, green obsidian, (and) *zalāqu*-stone in a leather bag.

(155) (Alternatively, you put) "swamp apple," *sikillu*, *bīnu*-tamarisk, (and) "sweet reed" in a leather bag.

TEXT 3: K 2581

K 2581 is a precious example of instructions for private prayer. The rest of the text contains treatments for fever, for which see chapter 16, text 3. The prayer in question is what might be termed a penitential prayer or confession of guilt, performed in a kneeling position with the arms behind the back as if bound. Quite naturally, it shades off into a nonscripted prayer from the heart.

rev.

5′. DIŠ NA *ana* DINGIR-*šú ši-gu-ú* GÙ-*si ina* ITI.DU$_6$ U$_4$.1[6.KÁM]

6′. *ši-gu-ú il-si* NA BI DINGIR-*šú* KI-*šú i-šal-*[*lim*]

7′. DIŠ NA *ana* DINGIR-*šú ši-gu-ú* GÙ-*si ina* U$_4$ ŠE.GA *in*[*a še-rim*]

8′. *ina li-la-ti-šú sir*$_4$*-qa še-eb-ḫu i-sar-*[*raq*]

9′. *sir*$_4$*-qa šu-ú šu-luḫ-ḫa ul i-*[*sal-laḫ*]

10′. [N]A BI *ina* EGIR *rik-si i-kám*-*⸢*mis*⸣*-ma* Á-*šú ana* EGIR-*š*[*ú* GUR-*ma*]

11′. *kám** DUG$_4$.GA *an-nu-ú* ⸢*gil*⸣*-lat u ḫi-ṭi-ti* [*e-tep-pu-šú*]

12′. *e-gu ana* DINGIR.MU *aḫ-ṭu ana* ^{d}15.MU *ú-qal-lil ana-*[*ku*]

13′. *i-ta-ka lu* ⸢*e*⸣*-ti-iq a-sak-ka-ka lu* [*a-kul*]

14′. *an-zil-la-ka lu ú-kab-bi-i*[*s*]

15′. *mim-mu-ú* ‹*e*›*-te-ep-pu-šú ana-ku lu-ú i-du-*⸢*ú*⸣

16′. DINGIR.MU *pu-ṭur* ^{d}15.MU *us-si-*[*ḫi*]

17′. *šuk-na-ni ḫi-ṭa-ti-ya*$_5$ *a-na* SIG$_5$.[MEŠ-*ti*]

18′. *an-nam* 7-*šú* DUG$_4$.GA-*ma i-k*[*ám*-mis-ma*]

19′. [*ḫi*]*-ṭi-šú* DU$_8$*-ma ma-la* ŠÀ-*b*[*i-šú* DIB KUR-*ád*][87]

20′. [NA]M.BÚR.[BI]

TRANSLATION

(rev. 7′–20′) If a person wishes to cry a *šigû*-prayer to his god, on a propitious day ⸢in⸣ the [morning] (and) in the evening, ⸢he scatters⸣ a sprinkled scatter-offering. This is a scatter-offering. He does not [perform] a ritual hand washing (with it). That ⸢person⸣ kneels behind the offering arrangement and then [he puts] his arm(s) behind ⸢his⸣ (back) [and then] he says as follows: "This is the misdeed and sin [which I have committed]. I was negligent; I sinned against my god; I belittled my goddess. I have crossed your boundary, [eaten] what is sacred/offensive to you, trod on what is abomination to you. Whatever I have done, I know very well (that I have done something wrong). My god, release (it); my goddess, ⸢remove⸣ (it). Make my sins into good deeds." [If] he says this seven times and then ⸢kneels⸣, his ⸢sin⸣ should be dispelled and [he should be able to achieve] whatever ⸢he wants⸣. ⸢NAM.BÚR.BI⸣

NOTES

1. The duplicates have Ú.ḪI.A.
2. Added from BAM 205:22′//BAM 320:27′. *STT* 280 ii 3 substitutes ^{Ú}ḪAR.ḪAR.
3. Added from BAM 205:22′//BAM 320:28′. *STT* 280 ii 4 substitutes [(*ki*)]-*ṣir* ^{GIŠ}*bi-ni*.
4. For ILLU ^{GIŠ}DÌḪ BAM 205:22′//STT 280 ii 4 substitute ^{GIŠ}DÌḪ SIG$_7$-*su*. BAM 320:28′ omits ^{GIŠ}DÌḪ.
5. BAM 205:26′//STT 280 ii 6–7//BAM 320:32′ have $^{\text{GIŠ.Ú}}$GÍR *ša* (UGU) É.[SIG$_4$] and add 14 Ú.ḪI.A ŠEŠ.
6. BAM 205:27′//STT 280 ii 7 have *ina* MÚD ^{GIŠ}ERIN ḪE.ḪE *ina* KUŠ. BAM 320:33′ has *ina* MÚD ^{GIŠ}ERIN ḪE.ḪE *ina* KAŠ.
7. For the expression, see also SpTU 2.22 i 24.
8. The last part of this could be ŠE.NU DUB-*ma*, in which case you are to pour out the dust [by??] a chaste-tree and then put the "dark red plant" into the leather bag. Suggestion courtesy M. Stol.
9. BM 56148+ ii 42–43 (Schuster-Brandis 2008, 290) omits $^{\text{NA}_4}$ZÚ SIG$_7$.
10. Stadhouders, personal communication, suggests *ba-t*[*i*]*q*?-*ti*.
11. *CAD* A/2, 234a.
12. BAM 315 iii 42 has: *ana* DIB ^{d}ME.ME BÚR.
13. *KAR* 92 rev. 9–33 continues with the accompanying recitation.
14. BM 56148+ vi 26 (Schuster-Brandis 2008, 299), omits KA.A.AB.BA and $^{\text{NA}_4}$AN.ZAḪ.
15. BAM 316 vi 8′–9′ has: NÍG.NA ^{ŠEM}LI *ana* IGI ^{d}UTU *liš-ku-un* / NÍG.NA ^{ŠEM}ŠEŠ! *ana* IGI DINGIR URU-*šú liš-ku-un*.
16. BAM 316 vi 10′ has: *liq-bi*.
17. BAM 317 rev. 3 has: NU *tuš-ken*.
18. For URUDU KUG.GAN, BAM 315 substitutes *lu-lu-tú*.
19. BAM 315 ii 30–32 adds: DIB DINGIR URU-*šú* DINGIR URU-*šú* ARḪUŠ [TUKU]

ŠU.SI ḪUL-*tim ár-rat* KA UN.MEŠ NU TE-*šú*.

20. BAM 315 iv 20//BAM 316 i 13′ have: IGI.MEŠ-*šú*.

21. Reading follows Schuster-Brandis 2008, 177.

22. BAM 316 iii 2′ adds: *u* DU$_8$-*ár ár-ni-šú*.

23. At the end, BAM 316 iii 7′ has: GAR-*an-ma* DINGIR *zi-nu-ú* SILIM-*im*.

24. BAM 316 ii 5′ has: *sa-dir-šú*.

25. BAM 316 ii 7′//BAM 315 iii 4 have: *ina* É.GAL GUB-*zu*.

26. BAM 316 ii 9′ has: *amat* and BM 64174: 5 (Geller 1988, 21–22) has: *šib-sat*.

27. BAM 316 ii 10′–11′ adds: *kiš-pi ep-šú-šú* KI DINGIR *u* ^{d}*Eš*$_4$*-dar šu-zu-ur* / [U]R$_5$.MEŠ-*šú dal-ḫa* DINGIR MAN IDIM NUN *šu-zu-qú-šú*. BAM 316 iii 8–9 has the first additional sentence.

28. BAM 316 ii 12′ has: ^{LÚ}ḪAL *u* LÚ.DINGIR.RA and BM 64174: 6 (Geller 1988, 21–22) has: ^{LÚ}ḪAL *u da-gi-li*.

29. BM 64174: 6 (Geller 1988, 21–22) has: NU *še-mu-ú*.

30. BAM 316 ii 15′–16′ adds: MÁŠ.GI$_6$.MEŠ-*šú ana* SIG$_5$-*tim* A.RÁ-*šú ana ṣú-di* / ŠU.SI SIG$_5$-*tim* EGIR-*šú ana* LAL-*ṣi*

31. BAM 316 ii 17′ has ḎÙ.DÙ.BI.

32. BAM 316 ii 18′ has ^{Ú}LÚ-*a-nu*.

33. BAM 316 ii 19′ has KA.A.AB.BA.

34. BAM 316 ii 19′ has this in a different order.

35. BAM 316 ii 19′ has GAG.GAG and omits the oil; ii 22′ adds: NA BI DINGIR-*šú u* ^{d}*Eš*$_4$*-dar-šú* KI-*šú* SILIM-*mu*. Abusch 1999, 96 suggests reading DÙ!.⌜DÙ!-*pí*!⌝ to harmonize the texts.

36. BAM 316 ii 23′ has: ŠE.GA GAR-*an-šú*.

37. BAM 316 ii 24′–25′ add: DINGIR MAN IDIM *u* NUN KI-*šú* GUB-*zu e-em ana di-nim* DU-*ku di-in-šú* SI.SÁ.

38. BAM 316 ii 21′ has: 7-*šú ana* UGU ŠID-*nu* GÚ BA.GAR. The full recitation appears in BM 56148+ i 49–51 (Schuster-Brandis 2008, 288).

39. Reading courtesy H. Stadhouders.

40. This line actually appears vertically on the side of the tablet in approximately this location. It cannot actually fall between 137 and 139, so I have inserted it at the first possible place after 137, which is here.

41. BAM 316 iii 14′//BAM 317 rev. 17 add: DINGIR-*šú* (KI-*šú*) *ana* SILIM-*me*.

42. Maul and Strauß 2011, 35 iv 1–4 restores [*l*]*a uš-ken* in the duplicate. This is clearly incorrect. Failure to prostrate oneself before the king of the gods was hardly a tactic designed to assuage his anger. See below.

43. See Scurlock and Andersen 2005, 8.15, 16.17, 19.111.

44. See Scurlock and Andersen 2005, Ap. 92.

45. See Scurlock and Andersen 2005, 4.7, 8.1, 13.71, 19.112.

46. BAM 205:26′//STT 280 ii 6–7//BAM 320:32′ add: "these fourteen plants."

47. Added from BAM 205:22′//BAM 320:27′. *STT* 280 ii 3 substitutes *ḫašû*-thyme.

48. Added from BAM 205:22′//BAM 320:28′. *STT* 280 ii 4 substitutes "⌜a block⌝ of *bīnu*-tamarisk.

49. For the *baltu*-thorn resin, BAM 205:22′//STT 280 ii 4//BAM 320:28′ substitute "fresh *baltu*-thorn." BAM 320:28′ omits the *baltu*-thorn.

50. Added from BAM 205:22′//STT 280 ii 4.

51. BAM 205:26′//STT 280 ii 6–7//BAM 320:32′ have: "*ašāgu*-thorn from a ⌜wall⌝" and add: "these fourteen plants."

52. For the expression, see also SpTU 2.22 i 24.

53. Alternatively, one could read this as Ì.SUMUN in which case you are to use both dust and "used grease" from the gate of the Marduk temple. Suggestion courtesy M. Stol.

54. See Scurlock and Andersen 2005, 3.267.

55. Recycling bitumen from old boats has a long history. For a discussion of this and other uses of bitumen, see Stol 2012, 48–60.

56. He has made the moon god so angry that it has dimmed his light.

57. See Scurlock and Andersen 2005, 5.48, 19.107.

58. BAM 316 iv 4 and *KAR* 92 rev. 6 have: "his god and his goddess."

59. See Scurlock and Andersen 2005, 16.25, 19.36.

60. BM 46148+ vi 26 (Schuster-Brandis 2008, 299), omits *imbû tamtim* and *anzaḫḫu*-frit.

61. See Scurlock and Andersen 2005, 16.93, 19.37.

62. BAM 316 vi 8′–9′ has: "He should set up an incense burner (burning) *burāšu*-juniper before Shamash (and) one (burning) myrrh before the god of his city."

63. BAM 317 rev. 3 instructs the exorcist not to prostrate himself during the proceedings. Presumably, if he did so, the benefits of the ritual would go to him rather than to the suppliant.

64. He has made the moon god so angry that it has dimmed his light.

65. Added from BAM 315 ii 31–32, which predicts: "The wrath of the god of his city should be dispelled from him. The god of his city [should have] mercy (on him). Bad rumors and curses in the mouth of the people should not approach him.

66. See *CAD* Š/1, 146–47. Suggestion courtesy M. Stol.

67. In other words, a brand-new brazier. Similarly, a number of medical texts require a new millstone "on which vegetables have never (before) fallen (and which) salt (and) vinegar have not touched" (BAM 480 i 10–11//BAM 3 i 15–17//BAM 4 i 7′–9′).

68. The term *mussuku* is almost always used for humans, but not here unless an ARḪUŠ has been omitted.

69. BAM 315 iv 20//BAM 316 i 13′ have: "If he gently rubs his face (with it)."

70. BAM 316 iii 2′ adds: "and to dispel his sins."

71. Literally: "a finger of evil not to be pointed after him." BAM 316 iv 7 has the expected formulation. This scribe has attempted more Sumerian than he knows. The Sumerian prefixes BA.RA have been attached to the Akkadian infinitive to render the absolute impossibility of any finger pointing ever taking place while the amulet is worn.

72. BAM 316 ii 7′ has: "in the palace where he stands."

73. BAM 316 ii 9′ substitutes "word" (as in unfavorable judgement).

74. BAM 316 ii 10′–11′ adds: "sorcery has been performed against him, he has been cursed before god and goddess, his ⌈liver omens⌉ are confused, god, king, patron and prince cause him grief. The parallel BAM 316 iii 8–9 has the first additional sentence.

75. BAM 316 ii 12′ has: "diviner or estatic" and BM 64174: 6 (Geller 1988, 21–22) has: "diviner or seer."

76. Added from BAM 316 ii 12′.

77. BAM 316 ii 15′–16′ adds: "to make his dreams good, to turn his behavior around and to have people say good things behind his back."

78. See Scurlock and Andersen 2005, 16.95.

79. So BAM 316 ii 19′.

80. So BAM 316 ii 22′.

81. BAM 316 ii 24′–25′ add: "god, king, patron and prince should side with him and whenever he goes for judgment, his case should be judged fairly."

82. The copy has "(and) a red tuft of wool," which does not sound right.

83. See Scurlock and Andersen 2005, 8.17, 16.18.

84. Added from BAM 316 ii 14′//BAM 317 rev. 17.

85. BAM 311:6′ has *zalāqu*-stone.
86. Literally: "turning round"
87. For the reading, see von Soden 1987, 71.

16

HEALING RITUALS

A. TEETH

TEXT 1: BAM 542 iii 1–19

If there were any doubt that the tooth worm (see Scurlock and Andersen 2005, 420–21) had to do with rotten teeth, this charming series of rituals ought to put it to rest. Lines iii 1–3 describe a transfer rite in which the illness of the tooth is given to a skull by spitting out a mouthful of malt lumps onto it. In lines iii 4–7, the worm's "wish" was: "Put me among the teeth and set me in the jaw so that I may suck the blood of the tooth and chew up the chewed up (food particles collected) in the jaw!" For more, see chapter 5, text 9. In lines iii 8–12 and iii 17–19, a model jaw receives the patient's evil, which is spat onto it. The evil is then transferred to the Netherworld (the hole to the West) and sealed in so that it cannot come back.

iii

1. [*a-n*]*a ma-ḫar* ^{d}UTU A KÙ.GA ŠUB.ŠUB ÉN *an-ni-ta* 3-*šú* [*ana* UGU ŠID-*nu*]
2. *e-ma* ŠID-*ú* LAGAB MUNU$_6$ KA-*šú* DIRI-*ma ana* UGU *gul-gul-*[*li* ŠUB]
3. *gul-gul-lu* GIG ZÚ.MU *tab-li* 7-*šú* DUG$_4$.G[A-*ma* TI]

---

4. ÉN *ši it-ta-ag-ru-ma* ^{GIŠ}IG UZU ^{GIŠ}SAG.KUL GÌR.PAD.DU *iš-tu a-a-nu* [*tul-tum iš-tu*]
5. GÌR.PAD.DU UGU ZÚ *it-ta-bak* KÚM : UGU SAG.DU *it-ta-bak i*[*m-tú*]
6. *man-na lu-uš-pur ana* DUMU.NITA *šá* KUR.RA ^{d}AMAR.UTU *li-lap-pi-tu$_4$ tul-*[*tum*]
7. [*t*]*ul-tum ki-ma šik-ke-e lit-ta-ṣi ṣer-ra-niš* TU$_6$ É[N][1]

---

8. DÙ.DÙ.BI *la-áš-ḫa šá* IM.KI.GAR DÙ *ana* ŠID.MEŠ
9. ZÚ.MEŠ-*šú áš-na-an tu-rat-ta* KI ZÚ-*šú*
10. [G]IG-*ti* ZÍZ.AN.NA GI$_6$ *ti-ret-ti* Ì+GIŠ KA-*šú* DIRI *ana* ŠÀ *la-áš-ḫi* MÚ-*aḫ* ÉN 3-*šú*

11. [ŠID]-*nu*! *ana* ḪABRUD *šá* ^{d}UTU.ŠÚ.A GAR-*an ina* IM IN.BUBBU BAD-*ḫi*
12. [*ina* ^{NA}]^{4}KIŠIB ^{NA_4}ŠUBA *u* ^{NA_4}KA.GI.NA KÁ-*šú ta-bar-ram*

---

13. [(ÉN DUMU.NI)]TA É.MAḪ DUMU.NITA É.MAḪ DUMU.NITA GAL-*u šá* ^{d}50 *at-ta-ma*
14. [(*iš-tu*$_4$ É.KUR) *tu*]-*ri-dam-ma ina* MURUB$_4$ AN-*e* KI MUL.MAR.GÍD.DA GUB-*az*
15. [(DUG$_4$.GA-*ma ka-li*) o o]-KAL-*an-ni li-is-ku-ta at-ta-ma*
16. [(*ina*) …]x UZU.UR$_5$.ÚŠ : UZU.UR$_5$: NU GU$_7$! TU$_6$ ÉN

---

17. [(DÙ.DÙ.BI) *la-áš-ḫa šá* IM.KI.GAR DÙ]-*uš ana* ŠID.MEŠ ZÚ.MEŠ-*šú* ZÍZ.AN.NA *tu-rat-ta*
18. [KI ZÚ-*šú* GIG-*ti* ZÍZ.AN.NA G]I$_6$ *te-ret-ti* LÀL *u* Ì BÁRA.GA KA-*šú* DIRI
19. [*ana* ŠÀ *la-áš-ḫi* MÚ-*aḫ* ÉN 3-*šú* ŠID *ana* ḪABRUD *š*]*á* ^{d}UTU.ŠÚ.A GAR-*a*[*n*]

TRANSLATION

(iii 1–3) […] You repeatedly pour out pure water before Shamash. [You recite] this recitation three times [over it]. When you recite, he fills his mouth with malt lumps and [he pours (it) out] onto the skull. [If] he says: “Skull, take away the illness of my tooth,” [he should recover].

(iii 4–7) “They granted it (the worm)’s wish[2] with the (following) result. The door is the flesh. The bolt is the bone. From where [is the worm? From] the bone. Over the tooth, it poured out fever. Over the head, it poured out ⸢poison⸣. Whom can I send to the son of the Ekur, Marduk. Let them strike the ⸢worm⸣. May the worm leave through the door pivot like a mongoose!”

(iii 8–12) For the recitation: “They granted it’s wish,” its ritual (is as follows). You make a jaw out of potter’s clay. You fix in (it) emmer corns in proportion to the number of his teeth. Where he has a ⸢sore⸣ tooth, you fix in a black emmer corn. You have him fill his mouth with oil and blow (it) onto the jaw. ⸢You recite⸣ the recitation three times and place (it) in a hole to the West. You close the hole with clay (and) straw (and) seal its mouth [with] a seal of *šubû*-stone or magnetic hematite.

(iii 13–16) “You are the son of the Emah, son of the Emah, eldest son of Enlil. [You] came down from the Ekur; in the midst of the heavens, you stand as the Wagon Star. If you speak, all who […] me should remain silent. In […] may the omen/orders not be “eaten.”

(iii 17–19) For the recitation: "Son of the Emah," [its ritual (is as follows)]. ⸢You make⸣ [a jaw out of potter's clay]. You fix in (it) emmer corns in proportion to the number of his teeth. [Where he has a sore tooth], you fix in a ⸢black⸣ [emmer corn]. You have him fill his mouth with honey and pressed-out oil [and blow it onto the jaw. You recite the recitation three times] and place (it) [in a hole] ⸢to⸣ the West.

TEXT 2: BAM 30 (= *LKA* 136)

BAM 30 consists of toothpaste (12′–13′), amulets (2′–11′, 22′–28′, 31′–32′, 36′–43′), a stone charm (44′–46′), and rituals (14′–21′, 29′–30′, 33′–35′, 47′–53′) for bruxism. Grinding one's teeth at night is usually stress related. For details, see Scurlock and Andersen 2005, 368 and 422–23.

All of the rituals involve transferring the problem to a human skull. Since skulls have teeth but cannot gnash, this seemed a good plan. The most elaborate ritual is in lines 14′–21′ where a skull is taken from and then returned to a grave and honored with offerings in addition to the more usual kissing (29′–30′, 33′–35′, 47′–53′) of the skull by the patient. The offerings are *kispu*, that is, the sorts of things one gives to the dead. For more details on *kispu*, see Tsukimoto 1985. In order to receive its offerings, the skull is placed on a chair spread with a blue garment, the color of the Netherworld. For more on the use of chairs and other soul emplacements for ghosts, see Scurlock 2002a, 1–6. The seven and seven times yields fourteen, the Netherworld's number.

Lines 33′–35′ are an interesting variant. In all transfers, there is a two-way street in which good influences come to the patient in return for the evils he is giving away. It is unusual for this to be expressed directly, except in the legomena. Here, however, the lack of teeth grinding of the dead person is transferred to the patient by washing the skull and having the patient drink the wash water. Similarly, in lines 47′–53′, the skull spends seven days at the patient's bedside and gets a licking.

1′. […] SILIM-*im*

2′. […] x ^{d}15-*šú* MAŠKIM-*šu*
3′. […] ku IGI-*mar ana* TI-*šú*
4′. […] x ^{Ú}LÚ.U$_{19}$.LU *ina* KUŠ

5′. ÉN É.NU.RU DA.RA.SIG$_5$.GA IGI DA.RA.SIG$_5$.GA
6′. A.RA.ZU ḪÉ.EN.SIG$_5$.GA IGI ^{d}EN.KI ^{d}ASAL.LÚ.ḪI
7′. U$_4$.ŠÚ.UŠ ŠUB ḪÉ.EN.DAR.DAR.RA.GIM TU$_6$ ÉN

8′. KA.INIM.MA DIŠ NA ZÚ.MEŠ-*šú i-gaṣ-ṣa-aṣ*

9′. KÌD.KÌD.BI SAḪAR ⸢KÁ⸣ KI.MAḪ
10′. ⸢*la*⸣-*bi-ru*-⸢*ti*⸣ TI-*qí*
11′. *ina* ⸢*šu-pi-i*⸣ GAG(!).GAG-*p*[*i ina*] GÚ-*šú* GAR-*an*[3]

12′. DIŠ KI.MIN MUN *A-ma-nim* ^{ŠEM}LI
13′. TI-*qí-ma* 1–*niš* SÚD UGU ZÚ.MEŠ-*šú ta-kap-par*

14′. DIŠ KI.MIN *gul-gul* LÚ.U$_{18}$.LU TI-*qí-ma*
15′. *ina* UGU ^{GIŠ}GU.ZA *ina* TÚG *ḫaš-ma-ni tu-wa-aṣ-ṣa*
16′. *gul-gul-la šu-a-tú ina* UGU GAR-*an*
17′. *ina še-rim u ši-me-tan* 3 U$_4$-*me ki-is-pa ta-kas-sip*
18′. ÉN 7-*šú ana* ŠÀ *gul-gul-li* ŠID-*nu*
19′. *gul-gul-la šu-a-tú ina* IGI KI.NÁ-*šú*
20′. 7-*šú u* 7-*šú tu-šá-aš*-⸢*šaq*⸣-*šu-ma ina-eš*
21′. *gul-gul-la* : *šú-a-tú* : *a-šar* [*ta*]*š-šá-a tu-tar-š*[*i*]

22′. DIŠ KI.MIN ^{Ú}ḪAR.ḪUM.BA.ŠIR KA *tam-tim*
23′. KI.A.^{d}ÍD ŠÈ ^{d}NISABA ^{Ú}*ka-man*-[*tu*]
24′. *ni-kip-tú* NÍTA *u* MUNUS LÚ.U$_{19}$.LU ÚḪ-^{d}ÍD *ina* [(KUŠ)]

25′. DIŠ KI.MIN KA.A.AB.BA ŠÈ ^{d}NIS[ABA]
26′. ^{Ú}ḪAR.ḪUM.BA.ŠIR *ni-kip-tú ina* [KUŠ]

27′. DIŠ KI.MIN $^{\text{NA}_4}$KUR-*nu* DIB KA.‹(A)›.A[(B.BA)]
28′. *ni-kip-tú* GÌR.PAD.LÚ.U$_{19}$.LU *ina* [(KUŠ)][4]

29′. [DIŠ K]I.MIN 3 U$_4$-*me ina* IGI KI.NÁ-*šú gul-gul* [LÚ.U$_{18}$.LU]
30′. [7-*šú u*] 7-*šú ina-šiq-ma* [*ina-eš*]

31′. [DIŠ KI.MIN] ^{Ú}*er-kul*-[*la* …]

32′. DIŠ KI.MIN SAG.DU ^{GIŠ}BAL ^{GIŠ}ME[S …]

33′. DIŠ KI.MIN *gul-gul* NAM.LÚ.U$_{19}$.LU *ki-ma* SAG D[Ú NAM.LÚ.U$_{18}$.LU]
34′. A LUḪ-*si* 3-*šú* A.MEŠ-*šá i-al-lut*

35′. *ina* KI.NÁ-*šú tu-šá-aš-šaq-šú*

36′. DIŠ KI.MIN ^{NA_4}KUR-*nu* DIB KA.A.AB.BA
37′. NUMUN ^{GIŠ}ḪA.LU.ÚB GÌR.PAD.DU LÚ.U$_{19}$.LU *ina* KUŠ[5]

38′. DIŠ KI.MIN SAḪAR KASKAL TÚG.NÍG.DÁRA.ŠU.LÁL
39′. GÌR.PAD.DU LÚ.U$_{19}$.LU
40′. *tim-bu-ut-ti* A.ŠÀ *ina* KUŠ[6]

41′. DIŠ KI.MIN SAḪAR *up-pat* TÚG.NÍG.DÁRA.ŠU.LÁL
42′. *gul-gul* LÚ.U$_{19}$.LU *tim-bu-ut-ti* A.ŠÀ *ina* KUŠ

43′. DIŠ KI.MIN BAR GU$_4$.UD^{KU_6} *ina* KUŠ

44′. DIŠ KI.MIN SAG.DU ^{GIŠ}BAL ^{GIŠ}MES
45′. ^{NA_4}ÁŠ.GÌ.GÌ ^{NA_4}PA *šá* 7 GÙN.MEŠ-*šá*
46′. ^{NA_4}ZÁLAG *ina* DUR *ina* GÚ-*šú* GAR-*an*

47′. DIŠ NA *ina i-tu-li-šú* ZÚ.MEŠ-*šú*
48′. *i-gaṣ-ṣa-aṣ gul-gul* LÚ.U$_{19}$.LU
49′. TI-*qí ina* A LUḪ-*si* Ì+GIŠ ŠÉŠ
50′. 7 U$_4$.MEŠ *ina* SAG ^{GIŠ}NÁ-*šu* GAR
51′. *ina* IGI *i-tu-li-šú*
52′. 7-*šú ina-ši-iq*
53′. 7-*šú i-le-ek-ma* TI-*uṭ*[7]

54′. DIŠ NA *ina* KI.NÁ-*šú* GÙ.GÙ-*si iṣ-ṣi-ni-iḫ* (catchline)

Translation

(1′) [If …] he should get well.

(2′–4′) [If …] his goddess, his *rābiṣu*-demon […] he experiences […]. To cure him, (you put) […] (and) *amīlānu* in a leather bag.

(5′–7′) *Pseudo Sumerian recitation asking Enki and Asalluhi to be receptive to the patient's prayers.*

(8′) Recitation for cases where a person gnashes his teeth.[8]

(9′–11′) Its ritual: you take earth from the mouth of an old grave. You sew (it) up in a wrapper and put (it) [on] his neck.

(12′–13′) Alternatively, you take *Amanim* salt (and) *burāšu*-juniper (and) grind (them) together. You wipe (it) onto his teeth.

(14′–21′) Alternatively, you take a human skull and you spread a garment of blue-green wool on a chair. You put that skull on it. In the morning and evening for three days you make *kispu* offerings. You recite the recitation seven times into the skull. If you have him kiss that skull before he goes to bed seven and seven times, he should recover. You return that skull to the place from which ⌈you got it⌉.

(22′–24′) Alternatively, (you put) *ḫarmunu*, *imbû tamtim*, *kibrītu*-sulphur, *zê* Nisaba (straw), ⌈*kamantu*-henna(?)⌉, male and female *nikiptu*, *amilānu*, (and) *ru*ʾ*tītu*-sulphur in a leather bag.[9]

(25′–26′) Alternatively, (you put) *imbû tamtim*, *zê* Nisaba, *ḫarmunu*, (and) *nikiptu* in [a leather bag].

(27′–28′) Alternatively, (you put) magnetic hematite, *imbû tamtim*, *nikiptu*, (and) "lone plant" (= "human bone")[10] in a leather bag.

(29′–30′) ⌈Alternatively⌉, if he kisses a [human] skull [seven and] seven times for three days before he goes to bed, [he should recover].

(31′) [Alternatively], (you put) *erkulla* (and) [… in a leather bag].

(32′) Alternatively, (you put) the head of a spindle of *mēsu* wood (and) [… in a leather bag].

(33′–35′) Alternatively, you wash a human skull with water as if it were the head of a [(living) person]. He swallows the wash water three times. You have him kiss it (the skull) before he goes to bed.

(36′–37′) Alternatively, (you put) magnetic hematite, *imbû tamtim*, *ḫaluppu*-tree seed (and) "lone plant" (= "human bone")[11] in a leather bag.

(38′–40′) Alternatively, (you put) dust from a road, *sikillu* (= "soiled rag"), "lone plant" (= "human bone"),[12] (and) *timbut eqli*-insect in a leather bag.

(41′–42′) Alternatively, (you put) dust stirred up by an *uppatu*-insect, *sikillu* (= "soiled rag"), human skull, and *timbut eqli*-insect[13] in a leather bag.

(43′) Alternatively, (you put) the skin of an *arsuppu*-fish in a leather bag.

(44′–46′) Alternatively, you put the head of a spindle of *mēsu*-wood, *ašgigû*-stone, seven-colored *ayyartu*-shell (and) *zalaqqu*-stone on a band on his neck.

(47′–53′) If a person gnashes his teeth when he lies down to sleep,[14] you take a human skull. You wash (it) with water (and) anoint (it) with oil. You put (it) at the head of his bed for seven days.[15] Before he goes to sleep, he kisses (it) seven times. If he (also) licks (it) seven times, he should recover.

(54′) If a person repeatedly cries out (and) laughs in his sleep[16] … (*catch-line*)

B. FEVERS

TEXT 3: K 2581 AND *AMT* 53/7+K 6732

K 2581 contains lizard salves (obv. 1–19) and a ritual (obv. 20–28) for fever. The parallel to obv. 20–28, *AMT* 53/7+K 6732, is not only much better preserved, but also more fulsome, and so we have substituted that version. This is followed in K 2581 by a potion (rev. 3′–4′) for urinary tract problems and instructions (rev. 5′–20′) for the ritual performance of a *šigû* prayer to calm the heart of an angry god. The connection between these is that angry gods can cause fever, and among the angry gods who did so was Marduk, for whom a *šigû* prayer was in order. See chapter 15, text 3.

The fever ritual is specifically for *liʾbu ṣibit šadî*, for which see Scurlock and Andersen 2005, 482–83. A frog was chosen for the simple reason that it lives in the swamps whence fevers of the type included under this rubric typically came. The trick, then, was to get the disease into the frog by spitting into its mouth. It was then to be taken to the waterless steppe and tied up in the expecation that it would try to go home, leaving the illness behind it in the steppe where it would die.

K 2581

obv.

1. [(DIŠ NA KÚM DIB-*su* ^{Ú}GAMUN)]^{SAR} ^{Ú}[(*ka-man-tú*)]
2. [(^{Ú}*kám**-*ka-du*) *ni-k*(*ip*)]-⌈*tu*$_4$⌉ [(N)]ITA *u* MUNUS ^{ŠE}[(^{M}GÚR.GÚR ^{ŠEM}LI ^{Ú}ḪUR.SAG^{S})^{AR}]
3. [(^{GIŠ}GEŠTIN.KA$_5$.A)] ^{Ú}UZU.DIR.KUR.RA ⌈1⌉-[(*niš* SÚD *ina* Ì.GIŠ ḪE.ḪE)]
4. [(*ana* URUDU.ŠEN.TUR D)]UB-*ak* EME.ŠID DIN-*su* DIB [(*ana* ŠÀ ŠUB-*di*)]
5. [(*ina* IZI ŠEG$_6$)-*š*]*al* E$_{11}$-*ma ta-na-suk tu-kaṣ*-[(*ṣa* ŠÉŠ-*su-ma* DIN)]

---

6. [...]-*ma* ŠÉŠ-*su*^{MEŠ} [...]

---

7. [DIŠ U$_4$.1].KÁM* DIB-*su* U$_4$.1.KÁM* *ú-maš-šar-šú ina* AN.BAR$_7$ *qaq*-[*qar*]
8. [(GISS)]U UD.DA TI-*qí si-i-ri šá sip-pi ana sip*-[(*pí*)]
9. [(SAḪ)]AR KUN$_4$ *maḫ-ri-ti* SAḪAR *šá-pal* ⌈*pi*!⌉-*sa-an-ni* SAḪAR K[(I.MAḪ)]

10. [(^{Ú}KUR.ZI)] SÚD *ina* Ì.BUR ‹(ḪE.ḪE)› *ina* BUR ^{NA_4}ALGAMES *ina* IZI ŠEG$_6$-*šal*
11. [(EME.ŠID)] DIN-*su ana* ŠÀ ŠUB-*di a-di i-ár-ru-u tu-kal-la*
12. [(E$_{11}$-*ma*)] *ta-na-suk* TU$_6$ *ana* ŠÀ-*bi* UR$_5$.GIN$_7$ ŠID-*nu*

---

13. [(ÉN *ki*)] TAB UD.DA *e-me-em u* GIN$_7$ GISSU *ur-ra* GIN$_7$ *sip-pi*
14. [(*sip*)]-⌜*pa*⌝ NU KU.NU *mur-ṣu* NENNI A NENNI *a-‹a› iq-rib-šú*
15. [(GIN$_7$ KU)]N$_4$ *li-kab-bi-su-ši!-ma man-ma-an a-a ir-šú*
16. [(GIN$_7$ *pi-s*)]*a-an-ni ana ur-ri u te-bé-e-šú la iz-zi-bu*
17. [(GIG)] *a-a in-ne-zib* GIN$_7$ ÚŠ NU BAL-*u* ÉLLAG-*su mar-ṣu*
18. [(ÉLLAG-*su*)] *a-a i-ni* ‹(TU$_6$ ÉN)› 7-*šú* ‹(*ana* ŠÀ)› ŠID-*ma* ŠÉŠ-*su*
19. [(EME)].ŠID TI-*su ina* GI.SAG.KUD ŠUB *ina* TÚG GI$_6$ KÁ-*šú* KEŠDA *ina* GÚ-*šú* GAR-[(*ma* TI)]

AMT 53/7+K 6732

1. DIŠ NA TA GÌR^{II}-*šú* EN MAŠ.SÌLA-*šú i-ta-rak* ‹(NA BI)› *li-ib* KUR [(DIB-*su*)]
2. DÙ.DÙ.BI BIL.ZA.ZA SIG$_7$ *ina* A DIB-*bat ina* U$_4$-*um iṣ-ṣab-tu-šú*[17] *i*[(*na še-rim*)]
3. *la-am* GÌR^{II}-*šú ana* KI GAR-*nu* TA SAG.[(DU)]-*šú* EN ‹‹*ina*›› GÌR^{II}-*šú tu-maš-*[*šá-a-šú*]
4. *ù ki-a-am ta-qab-bi* BIL.ZA.ZA *ṣib-*<*tu*>*-um šá ṣa-ab-tan-an-ni at-ta* ZU!-[*ú ana-ku* NU ZU-(*ú*)]
5. BIL.ZA.ZA *li-*ʾ*-bu šá ṣab-tan-ni* [*at-ta* ZU *ana-ku* NU ZU]
6. *un-du at-ta tap-pi-du-ma a-na* A.MEŠ-*ka* GUR[-*ra*]
7. *na-mi-šú tu-tar-ra* 3-*šú tu-šaq-ba-*[*šú-ma*] 3-*šú* ÚḪ-*su ana* KA-*šú* ŠUB
8. *ana* EDIN TI-*qí-šu-ma ina* D[UR SÍG.ḪÉ.M]E.DA SÍG.BABBAR GÌR-*šú tara-kas-*[*ma*]
9. KI ^{GIŠ}DÌḪ *tara-kas* [*lu* KI $^{GIŠ.Ú}$GÍR *tara*]-*kas* TI-[*uṭ*]

K 2581

rev.

1′. Ú (blank) SAR ⌜SIG$_7$-*su*⌝ [...]
2′. ^{Ú}NAM.TI.LA x[...]

3′. DIŠ NA *ina* GÌŠ-*šú* MÚD *ú-tab*[*-ba-ka*]

4′. 1/2 GÍN ^{GIŠ}*bu-ú-lu ina* KAŠ *lu ina* [GEŠTIN NAG]

5′–20′. See chapter 15, text 3.

21′. [GIŠ].ŠINIG Ú.IN$_6$.ÚŠ GIŠ x [...]

22′. [o o] IM.BABBAR x [...]

23′. [o o] x *li-šú* [...]

24′. [o o o] na [...]

Translation

K 2581

(obv. 1–5) If fever afflicts a person, you grind together *kamunu*-cumin, *kamantu*-henna(?), *kamkādu*, male and female ⌜*nikiptu*⌝, *kukru*, *burāšu*-juniper, *azupīru*, "fox grape" (and) *kamūn šadê*-fungus. You mix (it) with oil (and) pour (it) into a *tamgussu*-vessel. You drop a live *ṣurāru*-lizard into it (and) boil (it) over a fire. You take (it) out and throw (it) away. You let (it) cool. If you rub him gently (with it), he should recover.

(obv. 6) [...] repeatedly rub him gently [...]

(obv. 7–12) [If one day] it afflicts him (and) one day it releases him, at noon, you take dust from shade (and) sunlight. You grind (it and) plaster from both doorposts, dust from the front threshold, dust from below a reed basket, dust from a tomb (and) *samīdu* (and mix it) with *pūru* oil. You boil (it) over a fire in a *pūru*-vessel (made) from *algamešu*-stone. You drop a live *ṣurāru*-lizard into it (and) keep it there until it vomits. You have him recite over it as follows.

(obv. 13–19) "The shade brings (shade) in proportion to the heat of the sunlight (The hotter the sun, the cooler the shade). Just as one door-post does not approach the other, so may the sickness never approach the patient, so-and so, son of so-and-so. Just as should anyone step on the threshold, (he will never obtain anybody as a wife), so may (the illness) not obtain anybody (as a wife).[18] Just as a drainpipe can never abandon[19] its runnel and its riser so may the sick person not be given up on. Just as a dead person does not change his kidney (i.e., toss and turn), so may the sick person not change his kidney: ‹(spell and recitation)›." You recite (this) ‹(over it)› seven times and then rub him gently (with it). You drop a live *ṣurāru*-lizard into a reed straw. You tie its mouth with a black cloth. If you put (it) on his neck, he should recover.

AMT 53/7+K 6732

(1–9) If from his feet to his shoulders it throbs, the *li'bu* of the mountain afflicts ‹(that person)›.[20] Its ritual: he catches a green frog in the water. On the day that it afflicts him,[21] in the morning before he puts his foot on the ground, you ⸢massage⸣ [him] from head ‹(to)› foot, (saying): "O frog, the affliction that seized me you know (but) [I do not know]; O frog, the *li'bu* that seized me [you know but I do not know]. When you hop off and return to your waters, you will return (the evil) to its steppe." You have [him] say this three times [and] three times he spits his spittle into its mouth. You take it to the steppe and you tie its foot with a ⸢band⸣ of ⸢red-dyed⸣ (and) white wool [so that] you fasten (it) to a *baltu*-thorn [or to an *āšagu*-thorn]. He should recover.

K 2581

rev.

1′–2′. [...], fresh [...], [....], "life" plant [...]

3′-4′. If blood [pours] from a person's penis, [you have him drink] 1/2 shekel of *būlu* (mixed) with beer or with [wine].

5′–20′. *See chapter 15, text 3.*

21′–24′. *Bīnu*-tamarisk, *maštakal*, [...], [...], *gaṣṣu*-gypsum [...]

TEXT 4: FARBER 2014, PL. 55–56 (*KAR* 239) ii–iii

We have already met Lamashtu in chapter 6, text 2 and chapter 12, texts 4–5. This particular ritual is a classic case of the use of a figurine to get the message to a represented demon. In addition to the figurine itself, a surrogate body, Lamashtu gets a donkey loaded with provisions, but only on condition that she go off into the desert. Just to make sure that she understands that this is a binding contract, she is tied up and surrounded with a magic circle, so forcing her to swear to fulfil her side of the bargain. The poor piglet evokes a similar rite with another daughter of Anu, the goddess Ishtar—it represents a lover, which is why the heart is put in Lamashtu's mouth.

ii

1′. *k*[(*i-ma bu-*)...(*7-šú iḫ-bu-us-su*)]

2′. *ina su-*⸢*li-i*⸣ [...*i-t*(*a?-ar i-na*)]

3′. *šá-ḫa-ta-ti* [...*it-ta-n*(*a-áš-šab*)]

4′. *dan-na-at šak-ṣa-*[*at* ...(.MEŠ]

5′. ⸢*šu*⸣-*ḫar-rat* U$_4$-*me* [… *mu-ša-*(*di-rat* U$_4$-*me*)]
6′. [*mu*]-*ḫum-maṭ ṣe-e-ti ṣú-ḫar* [*ib-b*(*a-la-kat*])
7′. *im-ḫur* UR.MAḪ *me-lam-me-šu uš-*[(*te-di-ša*)]
8′. *im-ḫur* UR.BAR.RA *la-ḫa-ba* [(*i-nu*)]
9′. *e-bir* ÍD *ana me du-lu-uḫ-ḫa-a iš-*[(*ta*)-*kan*] ‹(*il-lik ḫar-ra-nu a-lak-ta-šá ip-ru*)-*us*›
10′. *i-mid* IZ.ZI *lu-ḫum-ma-a ip-ta-*[(*šá*)-*aš*]
11′. *i-mid* ^{GIŠ}ŠINIG *it-ta-bak ú-ri-*[(*šá*)]
12′. *i-mid* ^{GIŠ}GIŠIMMAR *ul-tam-me-ṭa u$_4$-ḫi-in-*[(*ni-šá*)]
13′. *i-mid* ^{GIŠ}*al-la-nu u* ^{GIŠ}*bu-uṭ-nu ša* KUR-*e ḫa-ma-di-ru-*[(*tu ul-ta-lik*)]
14′. *il-ta-na-*⸢*at*⸣-*ti* MÚD.MEŠ *niš-pu-tim ša a-me-*[(*lu-ti*)]
15′. UZU *ša la a-*⸢*ka*⸣-*li* GÌR.PAD.DU *ša la ga-*[(*ra-a-ṣi*)]
16′. *tal-tam-de-e* DUMU.MUNUS ^{d}*A-nim ša*(sic) (var. *a-kal*) *dim-ma-ti u* ⸢*bi*⸣-[(*ki-ti*)]
17′. *tal-ta-na-ti-i* MÚD.MEŠ *niš-pu-tim š*[(*a a-me-lu-ti*)] ‹(UZU *šá la a-ka-li* GÌR.PAD.DU *šá la ka-ra-a-ṣi*)›
18′. *li-ṣad-di-ki* ^{d}*A-num* AD-*ki* : *li-ṣad-*⸢*di*⸣-[(*ki*)] *An-tum* [(AMA-*ki*)]
19′. *us-ḫi* ^{GIŠ}GAG·.MEŠ-*ki qu-ub-bi-ri qé-e-k*[(*i*)]
20′. GIN$_7$ *sér-rim* EDIN KUR-*ki ru-up-d*[*i*] (var. *ru-uk-bi*)
21′. *lid-din-ki maš-maš a-ši-pu* ^{d}*Asal-lú-*[(*ḫi*)]
22′. ^{GIŠ}GA.ZUM ‹$^{\text{(GIŠ)}}$›*tu-di-it-ta* ^{GIŠ}BAL *šid-du u ki-*[(*ri-is-su*)]
23′. *ana* ‹(*pa-an*)› *na-maš-še-e* EDIN IGI-*ki šuk-ni*
24′. *lu pa-áš-šá-ti* Ì+GIŠ *mi-iḫ-ri*
25′. *lu-ú šak-na-a-ti še-e-ni šá du-ur-da-*[(*a-ri*)]
26′. *lu-ú na-šá-a-ti na-a-di ana ṣu-me-k*[(*i*)]
27′. *lid-din-ki* ^{LÚ}LUNGA NÍG.ÀR.RA MUNU$_6$ BAP[(PIR)]
28′. *pa-ti-ḫa-ta li-mel-*⸢*li*⸣-[(*ki*)]
29′. *nar-ṭa-ba ana la-ḫ*[(*a-mi*)] *lid-*[(*din-ki*)]
30′. *ú-tam-me-ki* DUMU.MUNUS ^{d}[*A-nim* (*A-num* AD-*ki An-tum* AMA-*ki*)]
31′. KI.MIN ^{d}EN.LÍL *u* ^{d}[(NIN.LÍL ^{d}É-*a ù* ^{d}DAM.GAL.NUN.NA)]
32′. KI.MIN ^{d}ŠÀ.ZU ⸢NUN⸣.[(M)E *ù* (^{d}*Ṣar-pa-ni-tum*)]

(the remainder of the column is missing)[22]

iii

1′. *n*[*a-as-ḫa-a-ti* (*šu-ṣa-a-ti*)]
2′. *ṭa*[(*r-da-a-ti u kuš-šu-da-a-ti*)]
3′. [(*d*)*u-p*(*u-ra-ti lu-u ta-at-tal-ki*)]
4′. […(x.NA MU.UN.ZI.ZI)]
5′. (incomprehensible)

6′. KA.INIM.MA ^{d}⸢DIM$_8$⸣.[(ME.KE$_4$)]

7′. ⸢KÌD.KÌD.BI⸣ [(NU)] DUMU.[(MUNUS ^{d})]*A-nim šá* IM PA[($_5$ DÙ-*uš*)]
8′. ⸢ANŠE *šá* IM PA$_5$ DÙ-[(*uš*)]
9′. *ṣu-de-e* DIRI 14 NINDA ZÍD ŠE.MUŠ$_5$ TUR[.TUR]
10′. *ina* ŠU.SAR *ta-šá-kak ina* GÚ-*šá* GAR-[(*an*)]
11′. *bu-uḫ-ra ta-tab-bak* A *u* KAŠ.MEŠ [(BAL-*qí-ši*)]
12′. ŠAḪ.TUR KUD-*is* ŠÀ [(*ana*) K]A DUMU.MUNUS ^{d}⸢*A*⸣-[(*nim* GAR-*an*)]
13′. ‹(3 U$_4$-*me*)› 3-*šú* ÉN *kal* U$_4$-*m*[(*e a-na pa-ni-šá* ŠID-*nu*)]
14′. *ina* U$_4$.3.[K]ÁM *ina qid-da-at* [U]$_4$-*me a-na* [(EDIN È-*ši-ma*)]
15′. IGI-*šá ana* ^{d}UTU.ŠÚ.⸢A⸣ [(GAR-*an*)]
16′. *ina* [EGIR.MEŠ-*šá* ZÌ.SU(R).R]A-*a šá* [Z]ÍD Š[E.M]UŠ$_5$ *i-na* I[GI.MEŠ-*šá* ḪUR-*i*(*r*)]
17′. *i*[*t-ti* (^{GIŠ}DÌḪ)] ⸢$^{GIŠ!}$⸣Ú.GÍR *tar-*[*kas-si*)]
18′. [(*niš* AN-*e* KI-*tim u* ^{d}*A-nun-na-ki tu-tam-ma-ši*)][23]

Translation

(ii 1′–8′) Like a [...], she robbed him seven times. [Seven times?] she returns to the street. She continually sits in the corners. She is mighty; she is intractable. [...] She [shatters?] the stillness of the day. She ⸢darkens⸣ the daylight; she [causes] burning with *ṣētu*-fever; she ⸢springs like a trap on⸣ the infant. She took from the lion her divine radiance; he assigned (it to) her. She took from the wolf the (evil) eye for infecting (people) with *liʾbu*-fever.[24]

(ii 9′–13′) She crosses a river, she ⸢causes⸣ confusion in the water. ‹(She goes on a road, she ⸢blocks off⸣ its traffic)›. She leans on a wall, she ⸢smears (it)⸣ with mud. She leans on a *bīnu*-tamarisk, it loses its foliage. She leans on a datepalm, she strips off its dates. She leans on an *allānu*-oak or a wild *buṭnu*-terebinth, she makes it shrivel up.

(ii 14′–17′) She continually drinks the dried(?)[25] blood of men, flesh that is not to be eaten, bones that are not to be cracked. You, daughter of Anu, have continually taken the bread of tears and wailing as (your) provision; you continually drink the dried(?) blood of men, ‹(flesh that is not to be eaten, bones that are not to be cracked)›.

(ii 18′–20′) Let Anu, your father, provision you. Let Antu, your mother, provision you. Pull up your (tent) poles; roll up your (tent) ropes. Wander/Ride off to your mountain like the wild ass of the steppe!

(ii 21′–23′) Let the *mašmašu*, *āšipu* of Asalluhi, give you comb, *tudittu*-pin, distaff and *kirissu*-clasp.[26] Head for the wild beasts of the steppe!

(ii 24′–29′) May you be smeared with the oil of *miḫru*-offerings; may you have put on shoes (that last) for ever and ever; may you carry the waterskin for your thirst. May the Brewer God give you groats, malt and beer bread; may he fill a leather pouch for you; may he give you beerwort for making beer.

(ii 30′–iii 5′) I have made you swear, Daughter of [Anu], by Anu, your father (and) Antum, your mother. Ditto (I have made you swear) by Enlil and Ninlil, Ea, and Damgalnunna. Ditto (I have made you swear) by Marduk the sage and Sarpanitum. ... [...] You are extracted. You are made to go out. You are expelled and driven away. You are banished. You must leave. [...].

(iii 6′) Recitation for Lamashtu.

(iv 7′–18′) Its ritual: You make a Lamashtu of clay from the river bank. You make a donkey of clay from the river bank. You load[27] (it) with provisions. You thread fourteen breads made from *šig*ūšu flour on palm fibre. You put (it) on her neck. You pour out hot broth (for her). You pour out water and beer for her. You cut the throat of a piglet. You put the heart in the mouth of the Daughter of Anu. You recite the recitation three times every day for three days before her. On the third day, in the late afternoon you take her out into the steppe and you make her face the setting sun. ⸢You draw a magic circle⸣ made of ⸢*šigušu*-flour behind⸣ [her] (and) in ⸢front of⸣ [her]. You tie her to a *baltu*-thorn (or) an *ašāgu*-thorn. You make her swear an oath by heaven, earth and the Anunnaki.

TEXT 5: FARBER 2014, PL. 8 (4R^2 56) i 11–29

This text is a fine example of the marriage between ritual dromena and legomena. Again, Lamashtu is provided with a husband and provisions on the condition that she go away and leave the patient alone. We do not need to guess this from the ritual actions since the legomena say so directly. The only thing left unexplained is the "marriage" to a black dog. What is meant is that the figurine of Lamashtu and a figurine of a black dog are tied to one another. To note is that, despite the close fit, it was possible to use this same recitation in a completely different context, as in text 6, below.

i

11. É[(N ^{d}DI)]M$_{10}$.ME DUMU.AN.NA MU.PÀD.DA DINGIR.RE.E.NE.KE$_4$
12. [(^{d}IN.NIN NIR)].GÁL NIN SAG.GI$_6$.GA
13. [(ZI.AN.NA ḪÉ.P)]À ZI.KI.A ḪÉ.PÀ
14. [(*ú-šá-ḫi-iz-k*)]*i* UR.GI$_7$ GI$_6$ *qal-la-ki*

15. [(*aq-qí-ki*)] A.MEŠ PÚ *pu-uṭ-ri at-la-ki*
16. [(*i-si-i ù re-e-q*)]*í ina* SU ^{LÚ}TUR DUMU DINGIR-*šú an-ni-i*
17. [(*ú-tam-mi-ki* ^{d}*A-num*)] ⸢*ù*⸣ *An-tum* KI.MIN ^{d}EN.LÍL *u* ^{d}NIN.LÍL
18. [(KI.MIN ^{d}AMAR.UTU)] *ù* ^{d}*A-nu-ni-tum* (var. *Ṣar-pa-ni-tum*)
19. [(KI.MIN DINGIR.MEŠ)] GAL.MEŠ *šá* AN-*e u* KI-*tim*
20. [(*šum-ma ana*)] É *an-ni-i ta-tur-rim-ma* TU$_6$ ÉN

---

21. KA.INIM.MA KÚM *la-az-za ù* ^{d}DIM$_{10}$.ME ZI-*ḫi*

---

22. DÙ.DÙ.BI *La-maš-tú ki-ma šá* É *ṣi-bit-ti* DÙ-*uš*
23. *ter-ṣa ta-tar-ra-aṣ* 12 NINDA ZÍD NU SIM *ana* IGI-*šá* GAR-*an*
24. A.MEŠ PÚ BAL-*qí-ši* UR.GI$_7$ GI$_6$ *tu-šaḫ-ḫas-si*
25. 3 U$_4$.ME *ina* SAG ^{LÚ}GIG *tu-še-šeb-ši*
26. ⸢ŠÀ ŠAḪ⸣.TUR *ana* KA-⸢*šá*⸣ GAR-*an ba-aḫ-ru ta-tab-bak-ši*
27. [(^{GIŠ}GAN)] Ì+GIŠ SUM-[*ši* ...] *tu-ṣa-ad-di-ši*
28. [(NINDA ḪÁD.DA GAR-*ši še-ru* AN.ZAḪ *ši-me*)]-*tan*
29. [(ŠID-*tú* ŠID-*ši ina šal-ši* U$_4$-*me ina* U$_4$.GURUM.MA È-*ši-ma*)]
30. [(*ina* UB BÀD *te-qeb-be*)*r-ši*]

(i 11–20) Recitation: Lamashtu, daughter of Anu, by whom the gods swear, ⸢Inanna⸣, trustworthy lady, lady of the black-headed people—may you be made to swear by heaven; may you be made to swear by earth. I have married you to a black dog, your slave; I have poured out for you well water (as a libation). Let up! Go away! Withdraw and distance yourself from the body of the infant, son of his god! I have made you swear by Anu and Antu. Ditto (I have made you swear) by Enlil and Ninlil. Ditto (I have made you swear) by Marduk and Anunītum (variant: Ṣarpanitum). Ditto (I have made you swear) by the great gods of heaven and earth. If you ever return [to] this house (may you be punished)![28] Spell and Recitation.

(i 21) Recitation to remove a persistent fever and Lamashtu.

(i 22–30) It's ritual: You make a Lamashtu represented as imprisoned. You arrange offerings; you put twelve breads made from unsifted flour before her. You pour out well water for her (as a libation). You marry her to a black dog. For three days you have her sit at the head of the patient. You put the heart of a piglet in [her] mouth. You pour out hot broth for her. You give [her] a wooden šikkatu-vessel full of oil. You provide her with [provisions]. You put out dried bread for her. You recite the spell (every day) in the morning, noon, and evening. On the third day in the late afternoon you take her out and bury [her] in the corner of a wall.

TEXT 6: *STT* 281 iv 1–15

In this text, we meet again the recitation of text 5 along with three others to accompany a salve. Most of this consists of "plant" medicines but the sources of some of them are intended to match the contents of the recitations. So the bitumen comes from a boat, signaling travel away by boat back to Elam, and the fat is specifically from a pig as in the piglet whose heart Lamashtu eats in the rituals.

1. ⸢ESIR.ḪÁD.A⸣ [(GIŠ.M)]Á MIN ⸢*sik!?-kán!?*⸣[29]
2. MIN ⸢^{GIŠ}GISAL!⸣ MIN *ú-nu-ut* ^{GIŠ}MÁ
3. DÙ!.A.BI SAḪAR KAR SAḪAR *né-ber*
4. Ì.ŠAḪ Ì.KU$_{6}$ *nap-ṭu* Ì.NUN.NA
5. *an-ki-nu-tú ak-tam* $^{\text{Ú}!}$*áp-ru-šú* ‹(^{Ú}*a-zal-lá*)›
6. KUŠ AN[(ŠE)] *kur-‹ru›*[30] *ša* ^{LÚ}AŠGAB ‹(TÚG)›.NÍG.DÁRA!.ŠU.LAL
7. [Ì.(NUN.BAR.ḪUŠ)].KU$_{6}$ Ì.ŠA[(Ḫ)] BABBAR!
8. Ì *šu-e* Ì [...] MÚD *ere-nu*
9. 22? *nap* ^{d}DIM$_{8}$.ME
10. ÉN ⸢*a-nam!-di!*⸣ *šip-tú la-zu ‹(mi›)-lik-ki* (= Farber 2014, Lam. II 1–26)
11. ÉN ^{d}DIM$_{8}$ ⸢DUMU⸣ AN.NA (= Farber 2014, Lam. I 11–21)
12. ÉN *ez-ze-*⸢*et! šam-rat*⸣ (= Farber 2014, Lam. II 84–111 or 119–127)
13. ÉN ⸢*ez-ze-et!*⸣ *ul* ⸢*i*⸣*-lat* (= Farber 2014, Lam. I 37–45)
14. 4 ÉN.MEŠ *ana* ŠÀ *nap* ŠID
15. LÚ.TUR! EŠ TI

TRANSLATION

(iv 1–15) Dried bitumen from a boat, a rudder(?!), an oar and from boat implements, dust from quay (and) river crossing, pig fat, fish oil, hot bitumen, ghee, *ankinūtu*, *aktam*, *aprušu*, *azallû*, donkey hide, tanner's depilatory paste, "soiled rag" (*sikillu*), NUN.BAR.ḪUŠ-fish oil, white pig fat, sheep fat, [...] fat, (and) *erēnu*-cedar resin are a salve for Lamashtu. You recite four recitations: "I will cast a spell (against) your persistently (bad) advice";[31] "Lamashtu, daughter of Anu," "She is furious, she is angry" (and) "She is furious; she is not a goddess" over the salve. (If) you gently rub the infant (with it), he should recover.

C. MISCELLANEOUS

TEXT 7: SpTU 5 NO. 248

This interesting text consists of a collection of three rituals for a woman who is able to get pregnant, but who is plagued by frequent miscarriages. All of them involve transfer rites in which the woman's problem is given away. The first ritual promises the birth of a son; the "masculine" lone-stone and the choice of the right hand (which is used to release masculine birds in apotropaic rituals)[32] indicates that the woman's problem in this case was specifically the failure to bring male children to term. The second ritual seems to have been designed for a child of either sex, whereas the choice of a female animal swaddled like a baby would seem to indicate that the third ritual was meant to deal with the specific problem of girls not coming to term.

obv.

1. x x x x x *sin-niš-tu*$_4$ *la mu-še-šèr-tu*$_4$ *it-ti ri-bi šá* ^{d}UTU-*ši*
2. *ta-pa-ra-as ina* KUŠ *gal-la-bu-us te-ep-pu-ši-ma ina* ^{KUŠ}*na-áš-tu-qa*
3. *eš-še-tu*$_4$ *ina* GÚ-*šú ta-šak-kan* ^{NA_4}URUDU ^{NA_4}ZA.GÌN ^{NA_4}AŠ *zi-ka-ri* ^{NA_4}*šá-da-nu* DIB.BA
4. *u* ^{NA_4}*iṣ-bi-tú ina sa-mu-tú ta-šak-kak* 3 *li-ip-pi* ^{SÍG}ḪÉ.ME.DA *ta-lap-pa-ap*
5. *ina* ŠU^{II} 15-*šú ta-šak-kan u* NINDA *ku-ri-tú* UDU NÍTA *a-di* UZU-*šú* 2 *qa* ŠE.NUMUN
6. *it-ti-i ta-nam-di-is-su ina re-ši-šú i-ba-a-tú ina še-e-ri la-ma* ^{d}UTU
7. *na-pa-a-ḫu ul-tu* UGU *i-ga-ri tu-šá-qal-la-al-šú il-lak-ma ina a-šar pa-ar-su*
8. *ina* UGU KASKAL^{II} *pa-rik-tu*$_4$ NINDA.ḪI.A UZU *u* ŠE.NUMUN *ta-šak-kan-ma na-bu-ú it-tan-nu-nu*
9. *la na-bu-ú in-da-ḫar-ú-*ʾ*-in-ni* 5-*šú i-qab-bi e-ma* ʾ*-iq-ta-bu-ú*
10. TÚG-*su i-šaḫ-ḫaṭ-ma* A.MEŠ *tu-ra-am-ma-ak-šú i-te-eb-‹be›-e-ma*
11. TÚG-*su* 2-*ú il-lab-ba-áš u le-es-su a-na ku-tal-li-šú ul i-na-an-di*
12. *a-na* ÍD *il-lak-ma a-na* ÍD *ur-rad* A.MEŠ *a-na mu-qal-pi-tu*$_4$ 3-*šú ib-bak*
13. *u* ÉN *ana* UGU-*ḫi-šú ta-man-nu* ÉN *eš-re-tu*$_4$ *šu-šu-ru mu-ka muḫ-ra-an-ni-ma*
14. *ár-nu šèr-tú gíl-lat ḫi-ṭi-tu*$_4$ *lum-nu mi-neš-tu*$_4$ *šá zu-um-ri-ia it-ti* A.MEŠ-*ka*
15. *a-na qid-da-tu*$_4$ *ta-bal* ÍD.MEŠ *lim-la-*ʾ *a-gam-mu li-ṭe-e-pi-a ṭa-ab-a-ta*
16. [*l*]*i-še-ṣa-*ʾ *ri-kis lum-ni-ia* ÍD *eš-re-ta*$_5$ *šu-šu-ru mu-ka šu-ši-ra-an-ni-ma*

17. *dà-lí-lí-ka lud-lul* TU$_6$ *ul ya-a-tu-un* ÉN ^{d}IDIM *u* ^{d}*Asal-lú-ḫi*
18. ÉN ^{d}*Da-mu u* ^{d}*Gu-la* ÉN ^{d}NIN.GÌRIM *be-let* ÉN TE ÉN

---

19. 3-*šú ta-qab-bi* ⸢NAGA⸣ *ta-nam-di-is-su ù* ÉN *a-na* UGU-*ḫi-šú* ŠID-*nu*

---

20. ÉN NAGA NAGA ^{d}30 *i-*⸢*ri*⸣*-ka* ^{d}UTU *ú-rab-bi-ka*
21. ^{d}*Ad-da-a ina ur-p*[*e*]*-e-ti* A.MEŠ ⸢*iš-ta-qí-ka* i x x *ka-am-ma* x x ŠU^{II}-*a-a* x⸣
22. *šá ka-šap* DÙ-*šu uš-taḫ-ḫi-iṭ šá kaš-šap-tu*$_4$ DÙ-*šu uš-taḫ-ḫi-iṭ*
23. *šá e-piš* DÙ-⸢*šu*⸣ *uš-taḫ-ḫi-iṭ šá e-piš-tu*$_4$ DÙ-*šu uš-taḫ-ḫi-iṭ*
24. *šá muš-te-pi-šú* DÙ-*šu uš-taḫ-ḫi-iṭ ka-šap u kaš-šap-tu*$_4$ *e-piš u e-piš-tu*$_4$
25. ⸢*la i-di?*⸣*-nu lu-ú it-tu-um-ma lu-ú en-de-tu-nu i-gàr* TE ÉN

---

26. TA ÍD *il-lam-ma ana* UGU-*ḫi a-tu-nu* BÁḪAR *il-lak-ma a-tu-nu i-ḫaṣ-ṣí-in-ma*
27. *ki-a-am i-qab-bi* ⸢*a*⸣*-tu-nu el-let* DUMU.MUNUS ^{d}*A-nim ra-bi-tu*$_4$ *šá ina* ŠÀ-*bi-šú na-an-ḫu-za-at*
28. ⸢IZI⸣ ḪÁŠ *šá*! *ina* ŠÀ-*bi-šú* ^{d}⸢GIŠ⸣.BAR *qar-du ir-mu-ú šu-bat-su šal-ma-ti-ma*
29. *ú-de-e-ka šal-mu šat* ⸢*ana*⸣ *šat ta-ma-al-li-ma u ta-re-qa u a-na-ku ir-re-e-ma*
30. *šá ina* ŠÀ-*bi-ia ul ú-*[*š*]*al-lam šal-ma-nu-ut-ka bi-in-nim-ma la šal-ma-nu-ta-ma*
31. *le-qé-e ú-du-ú* g/zi? x mu TA ŠÀ-*ka la il-la-ʾ u ana-ku šá ina* ŠÀ-*bi-ia*
32. *lis-lim-ma* TUKU.TUKU?-*šú lu-*⸢*mu*⸣*-ur ina* É *áš-bak pa-ni lu-ú maḫ-rat* TE ÉN

---

33. *a-na* ^{GIŠ}KIRI$_6$ *ur-rad-ma* ^{GIŠ}GIŠIMMAR *i-ḫaṣ-ṣi-in-ma* ^{GIŠ}GIŠIMMAR *ma-ḫi-rat kal šá-a-ri mu-uḫ-ra-an-ni-ma*
34. *ár-nu šèr-tú gíl-lat ḫi-ṭi-ti u a-na-ku ina* É *áš-ba-ak u*$_8$*-ú-a-a-a la ṣa-la-la*
35. *di-ʾu di-lip-tu*$_4$ *ṣi-it še-er-ra* ÌR *u* GÉME *ma-la ba-šu-ú ina* EDIN-*ya a a-mu-ut*
36. *la i-te-nu-ú i-ta-ri u ši-i qer-bé-et-ma qid-da-at maḫ-rat*
37. *a-šar* ⸢*ḫar-pu*⸣ *up-ul tu-šab-šú a-šar up-ul tu-šab-šú ḫar-pu*
38. *iṣ-ṣi* [*nap-ṣ*]*a zum-bi tu-šar-šú iṣ-ṣi la na-šu-ú tu-šar-šú in-bi*
39. *la ṭu-ub* ŠÀ *la ṭu-ub* UZU *u ḫa-mu* DINGIR-*yá u* ^{d}15-*ya šá ina la e-de-e*
40. *a-tam-ma-ru ú-kab-bi-*⸢*su*⸣ *ul i-di mu-ḫur mu-ḫur-an-ni-ma da-li-li-ka lud-lul* TE ÉN

---

41. ÉN ^{d}UTU *at-ta-ma šá ka-liš kib-rat* ZALAG *šá e-liš u šap-liš* EN-*šú-nu at-ta-ma*
42. *šá e-piš u e-piš-tú di-nim-šú-*⸢*nu*⸣ *ta-pa-ar-ra-as šá kaš-šap u kaš-šap-tú* EŠ.BAR-*šú-nu ta-*⸢*aq-bi*⸣
43. *šá ḫi-bé-el u ḫi-bil-ti ár-nu-šú-*[*nu*] *tu-qát-ta*$_5$ *ub-be-ak-ka la mu-šal-in-*[*du*]
44. *šá en-de-et ár-nu šá e-piš u* ⸢*e*⸣*-piš-tú ú-kal-lu-šú u šu-lum šá kaš-šap u* [*kaš-šap-ti*]
45. *ú-šá-az-ba-lu-uš bil-tu*$_4$ *šá še-er-ri ul-la-du-ma* x[…]
46. *la ú-rab-bu-ú še-er-šu-ma la ú-rap-pa-šú kim-is-su* x[…]
47. *la ip-pal-la-su kim-is-su* [*š*]*á tab-lat-ma* AN.TA […]
48. *at-ta-ma* ^{d}UTU *šá ka-liš kib*!*-ra*[*t* ZAL]AG *šá* ^{MUNUS}*sin-*[*niš-tú la mu-šal-lim-tu*$_4$]
49. [*e*]*-pu-uš di-in-šú šá kaš-šap* [*u kaš-šap-tú* EŠ.BAR-*šú-nu qí-bi*]

rev.

1′. […] šu x[…]
2′. […] ⸢*še*⸣*-er-ri ul-la-*⸢*du*⸣ […]

3′. [ÉN] ^{d}⸢É⸣-[*a a*]*t-ta-ma ba-nu-ú ka-la-mu* x[…]
4′. ⸢x x⸣ nu *at-ta-ma ub-be-ak-ka* ^{MUNUS}*sin-niš-t*[*u*$_4$ *la mu-šal-lim-tu*$_4$]
5′. *šá en-de-et ár-nu a-na ap-si-i a-na ma-ḫar-ka* […]
6′. ^{MUNUS}*sin-niš-tú e-pu-uš di-nim-šu-ma pu-uṭ-ru* ⸢*ár*⸣*-nu-šú* ⸢*gíl-lat-su*⸣
7′. *u bil-lat-su* ÍD.MEŠ *liš-šá-ʾ a-gam-ma li-ṭe-pi-a ṭa-ab-a-*[*ta*]
8′. *li-še-ṣa-ʾ ri-kis lu-um-*⸢*ni*⸣*-šú ár-nu e-piš e-piš-*⸢*tú*⸣
9′. *kaš-šap kaš-šap-tú i-mid-da a-na* ^{MUNUS}*sin-niš-tú šu-zu-bu*
10′. *pu-uṭ-ru ina ṣú-ḫar-ri-šú lu-rab-bi še-er-ri*
11′. *lu*$_4$*-rap-pí-iš kim-mit-su da-li-li-ka lid-lul* TE ÉN

12′. *ana* MUNUS NU SI.SÁ SI.SÁ DÙ.⸢DÙ⸣.BI *ana* IGI ^{d}*Gu-la* NÍG.NA ^{ŠEM}LI GAR-*an*
13′. *mi-iḫ-ḫa* BAL-*qí-ma kám** DUG$_4$.GA

14′. ^{d}NIN.KAR.RA.AK.A GAŠAN [*šu*]*r-bu-tu* AMA *rem-ni-*⸢*ka*⸣
15′. *im-mer-tú šá* ^{d}GÌR *u* [^{d}D]UMU.ZI *mi-ra-a-a lim-ḫu-ra-an-ni-ma*
16′. *mi-ra-šú lid-di-na l*[*a*] *mu-še-ši-ru-ti lim-ḫu-ra-an-ni-ma*
17′. *mu-še-ši-ru-sa lid-di-na*

18′. 3-*šú* DUG$_4$.GA-*ma ina š*[*e-r*]*im ana* IGI ^{d}UTU *ina* UGU SIG$_4$.ḪI.A *ab-ra* SAR-*aḫ*

19′. $^{\text{GIŠ.ŠEM}}$LI DUB-*aq* ⸢U$_8$⸣ PEŠ$_4$ *mu-šal-lim-ti*
20′. *ana* IGI *nis-ḫi lis-si-ma* 2 G[URU]Š.MEŠ *i-na-áš-šu ù* MUNUS.PEŠ$_4$ *ana* ŠÀ GEŠTU^{II} U$_8$ PEŠ$_4$ *kám** DUG$_4$.GA

21′. *im-mer-tú šá* ^{d}GÌR [*u*] ⸢^{d}⸣DUMU.ZI *mi-ra-a-a tab-li-ma mi-ḫir-ki bi-la*
22′. *la mu-še-ši-ru-t*[*i t*]*ab-li-ma mu-še-ši-ru-ut-ka bi-la*

23′. *ana* ŠÀ GEŠTU$^{\text{II.MEŠ}}$ *ki-lal-*⸢*le*⸣*-e* 3.TA.ÀM ŠID-*nu ki-ma* ŠID-*ú ina šap-la-an* U$_8$ *uṣ-ṣi*
24′. *u*! *ina 7-i-tú* DU-*šá ana* [EDI]N IGI.MEŠ-*šú* NIGIN-*ma* ÚḪ-*su ana* KA U$_8$ ŠUB-*ma ana* EDIN È-*ma* TAG$_4$-*šú*

25′. *ana* [MUNUS NU SI.SÁ SI.SÁ DÙ.DÙ.BI …]x.MEŠ tu šu x x x
26′. […]x x x ⸢2.TA.ÀM NINDA.MEŠ⸣ *ina* SILA.LIMMU.BA GAR-*an ù ina bi-rit* SILA.LIMMU.BA
27′. TÚG ⸢*i-ša-ḫáṭ*⸣ *u* GAR.GAR-*ma na-aq-bi-ta an-ni-ta* DUG$_4$.GA

28′. *na-šu-ma am-ta-ḫar na-šá-ku-ma lim-ḫu-ru-in-ni* 3-*šú* ÉN *an-ni-tú* DUG$_4$.GA
29′. *u* 3-*šú* NINDA.MEŠ GAR-*an let-su a-na ku-tal-li-šú ul i-nam-di*

30′. *ḫa-am-ṣi-ir-ta* GAZ-*ma a-qar-tú* TA ^{GIŠ}ERIN *ina* ŠU^{II}-*šú* DIB-*si* ^{ŠEM}MUG SAG.DU-*su* KEŠDA-*ma*
31′. *ina* ^{SÍG}GA.ZUM.AK.A *ta-kar-rik ina* SILA.LIMMU.BA GAR-*an na-aq-bi-ta an-ni-tú* DUG$_4$.GA
32′. *na-šu-ma am-ta-ḫar na-šá-ku-ma lim-ḫu-ru-in-ni* DUG$_4$.GA-*ma* SILA DIB NU DIB

33′. *an-nam u an-nam ina la-pat* AN-*e* DÙ.DÙ-*uš-ma ina* SILA.LIMMU.BA GAR-*an-ma na-aq-bi-tú an-ni-tú* DUG$_4$.GA
34′. *na-šu-ma am-ta-ḫar na-šá-ku-ma lim-ḫu-ru-in-ni* DUG$_4$.GA-*ma* SILA DIB NU DIB

35′. MUNUS.ANŠE PEŠ$_4$ *tuš-za-az-ma* ŠE.BAR MUNUS *ina up-ni-šú* ÍL-*ma šu-pal* MUNUS.ANŠE PEŠ$_4$ *i-ḫal-lu-um-ma*
36′. MUNUS.ANŠE 3-*šú ú-šá-kal-ma na-aq-bi-ta an-ni-ta a-na* MUNUS.ANŠE ⸢DUG$_4$⸣.GA *ša* ŠÀ-*ki li-mut-ma*
37′. *šá*! ŠÀ-*iá lib-luṭ* 3-*šú ina šu-pal* MUNUS.ANŠE *i-ḫal-lu-pí ù* 3-*šú* ŠE.BAR MUNUS.ANŠE *ú-šá-áš-šá*

38′. ZALAG.BAR ŠE.MUŠ$_5$ *ina* SILA.LIMMU.BA GAR-*an-ma ina ap-ti tal-lal-ma* MUNUS.PEŠ$_4$ x *ù tu-lu ú-lap-pat-ma*

39′. *ina* U$_4$-*um ḫi-li-šá* MUNUS.TUR *i-ṭe*$_4$*-en-ma ina* A *ḫi-li-šá i-la-aš-šu-uš-ma* NU NITA DÙ-*uš*

40′. ⸢*ù*⸣ NU MUNUS DÙ-*uš* EN *mi-šil* GI$_6$ *ina* ‹É› *te-ru-ba ina mi-šil* GI$_6$ *ana* SILA ŠUB-*di lu ana* KASKAL ŠUB-*uš-šú*

41′. DIŠ ⸢TÚG-*šu*⸣ i-x x [...]-*ma ana* É-*šú* KU$_4$-*ub* 3 *ne-pi-šá* GABA.RI ^{URU}KAR.EN.KUR.KUR

42′–44′. Colophon

Translation

The First Ritual

(1–5) (Ritual for) ⸢making bring to term(?)⸣ a woman who does not bring (her children) to term. At the setting of the sun, you isolate (her). You do her shaving onto a piece of leather and then you put (it) around her neck in a new leather bag. You thread copper beads, lapis, masculine lone-stone, magnetic hematite, and *iṣbitu*-stone on red (wool). You wind three burls of red-dyed wool. You put (it) on her right hand.

(5–11) And you give her bread, the short (bone) of a male sheep with its meat (still on it), (and) 2 *qû*-measures of seed grain besides. It spends the night at her head. In the morning, before the sun comes up, you suspend it from a wall. She goes and then you place the bread, meat, and seed grain in a secluded place, at a crossroads, and then she says five times: "The ones with names have given (them) to me; the ones without names have received (them) from me." When she has said (this), she takes off her garments and then you bathe her with water. She gets up (out of the water) and then dresses in another garment. And she does not look down behind her.[33]

(12–18) She goes to the river and she goes down to the river. She draws water three times in a downstream direction and you recite (this) recitation over it. Recitation. "You flow in a straight line (and) your waters make (things) flow in a straight line. Receive (evil) from me and so carry away the sin, crime, offense, wrongdoing, evil, (and) weakness from my body downstream with your water. May the rivers fill up (with it). May the marshes add good things. May they make the bond of my evil depart. River, you flow in a straight line (and) your waters make (things) flow in a straight line (*ʾšr*); cause me to give birth easily (*ʾšr*) so that I may sing your praises. The spell is not mine; it is the recitation of Ea and Asalluhi. It is the recitation of Damu and Gula, the recitation of Ningirim, the mistress of recitations." Spell (and) recitation.

(19) You say (this) three times. You give her ⌜soap-plant⌝ and you recite (this) recitation over it.

(20–25) Recitation. "Soap-plant, soap-plant, Sîn conceived you; Shamash made you grow; Addâ gave you water to drink from the clouds. [...]. What the sorcerer did, I have washed off. What the sorceress did, I have washed off. What the caster (of spells) did, I have washed off. What the castress (of spells) did, I have washed off. What the person who has (sorcery) done, I have washed off. The sorcerer and sorceress, caster and castress ⌜did not give(?) (it to me). May it (stay) with (you); may it be imposed on you." Spell (and) recitation.

(26–32) She comes up from the river and then she goes to a potter's oven and then takes shelter in the oven and then she says as follows. "Pure oven, eldest daughter of Anu, from whose womb fire is withdrawn; hypogastric region inside which the heroic fire god makes his home. You are in good condition and your implements are in good condition. Year after year, you become full and then you become empty. But I am pregnant and then I do not bring to term what is in my womb. Please give me your things which are well formed and so take away the things which are not well formed. [...] implements do not come out of your womb. And may what is in my womb be in good health and so may I experience continually obtaining (progeny)(?). Where I live may it be pleasing." Spell (and) recitation.[34]

(33–40) She goes down to a garden ⌜and⌝ takes shelter (under) a date palm and (says): "Date palm, who receives every wind, receive from me sin, crime, offense (and) wrongdoing and, where I live, (receive from me having to say) wah!, not sleeping, *diʾu*, restlessness, (and) loss of infants, slaves and slave girls as many as there may be so that I may not die in my steppe. They inalterably keep coming back; it (the misfortune) is close by, downstream (and) in front. Where there is an ⌜early harvest⌝, you cause there to be a late harvest. Where there is a late harvest, you cause there to be an early harvest. You cause the ⌜broken⌝ tree to have flies (to pollinate it). You cause the tree that does not bear (fruit) to have fruit. Unhappiness (and) ill health and whatever insignificant little thing of my god and goddess I saw and stepped upon without realizing it; I don't know (what)—receive, receive it from me so that I may sing your praises." Spell (and) recitation.

(41– rev. 2′) Recitation: "Shamash, you are the one who entirely lights the four quarters. You are the lord of (those) above and below. You decide the case of caster and castress (of spells); you pronounce the decision of sorcerer and sorceress; you bring to an end the punishment of the wronged man and woman. She seeks you out, the woman who does not bring (her children) to term, on whom punishment was imposed, whom caster and castess (of spells) detain, and whom the greeting of sorcerer [and sorceress] make bear a load, who gives birth to infants and then [...], who does not raise her infant and does not widen her relations, [...], who does not look upon her relations, who is taken away and [...]. Shamash, you are the one who entirely ⸢lights⸣ the four quarter[s]; make the judgement of the ⸢woman⸣ [who does not bring (her children) to term (and) pronounce the decision] of the sorcerer [and sorceress]! [...] who gives birth to infants [...][35]

(rev. 3′–11′) "[Ea], you are the one who created everything. You are the one who [...]. She seeks you out, the woman [who does not bring (her children) to term] on whom punishment was imposed. Before you [...] to the *apsû* (Ea's home and the repository of sweet water), make the woman's judgement and cancel her sin, ⸢her offense⸣ and her load. May the rivers carry (them) off. May the marshes add good things. May they make the bond of her evil depart. Make the woman escape the punishments that the caster and castress, the sorcerer and sorceress imposed; cancel (them). May she raise the infants among her male children. May she widen her relations. May she sing your praises." Spell (and) recitation.[36]

The Second Ritual

(rev. 12′–13′) Ritual for making bring to term a woman who does not bring (her children) to term. You set out a censer (burning) juniper before Gula (goddess of healing). You pour out a libation of *miḫḫu*-beer and she (the patient) says as follows.

(rev. 14′–17′) "Ninkarrak, ⸢exhalted⸣ mistress, your merciful mother, may the pregnant ewe of ⸢Šakkan⸣ and Dumuzi (gods of domestic animals) receive my pregnancy from me and give me her pregnancy. May she receive from me (my) inability to give birth right away and give me her ability to give birth right away."

(rev. 18′–20′) She says (this) three times and then in the ⸢morning⸣ before Shamash you ignite a brush pile on top of bricks. You scatter juniper. One should secure(?) a pregnant ewe which brings (its young) to term to an uprooted (pole) and then two ⸢young men⸣ carry it and the pregnant woman says as follows into the ears of the pregnant ewe.[37]

"Pregnant ewe of Šakkan and Dumuzi, take my pregnancy away and so bring me your equivalent. Take away (my) inability to give birth right away and so give me your ability to give birth right away."

(rev. 23′–24′) She recites (this) three times each into both ears (and), when she recites (it) she comes out from below the ewe. And when she comes out the seventh time, facing the [steppe], she spits into the ewe's mouth and then she goes out to the steppe and then leaves it (there).

THE THIRD RITUAL

(rev. 25′–27′) [Ritual] for [making bring to term a woman who does not bring her children to term]. [...] She places two breads (of) each (kind) at a crossroads and she takes off her garment in the midst of the crossroads and puts it back on again and then she says this spoken prayer.

(rev. 28′–29′) "They brought (the evil) and I received (it); I brought (it back) so let them receive (it back) from me." She says this recitation three times and three times she puts out bread. She does not look down behind her.

(rev. 30′–32′) You kill a female mouse and then you have it grasp jewelry(?) (made) from cedar in its hands. You fasten *ballukku*-aromatic to its head and then you swaddle (it) with carded wool. You put (it) at a crossroads and then she says this spoken prayer. "They brought (the evil) and I received (it); I brought it (back) so let them receive (it back) from me." She says (this) and does not take (to get home) the road she took (to get there).

(rev. 33′–34′) You repeatedly do this and this at dawn and then you put (the bread and mouse) at a crossroads and she says this spoken prayer. "They brought (the evil) and I received (it); I brought (it back) so let them receive (it back) from me." She says (this) and does not take (to get home) the road she took (to get there).

You station a pregnant she-ass and then the woman holds barley in the cup of her hand and then crawls under the pregnant she-ass and then she feeds the she-ass three times and then ⸢says⸣ this spoken prayer to the she-ass. "May what is within you die so what is within me may live." She crawls three times under the she-ass and three times she raises up barley to the she-ass.

(rev. 38′–42′) At noon(?), you put *šigūšu*-grain at the crossroads and then you hang (it) from a window and then the pregnant woman rubs womb(?) and breast (with it). Then, on the day of her labor pains, a girl grinds (it) and then they make it into a dough with the water of her labor pains and then you make a figurine of a man ⸢or⸣ you make a figurine of a woman. You go indoors until midnight. At midnight, you throw (it) into the street or they throw it into a road. She [...] and then enters her house. 3 rituals copied from (tablets from) Kar-bel-matate.

TEXT 8: *KAR* 70:1–10

This is a curious ritual diagnostic for impotence which relies for its efficacy on the fact that pigs are very smart.

1–4. Garbled Sumerian recitation.

---

5. KA.INIM.MA *maš-taq-ti* [Š]À.ZI.GA

---

6. DÙ.DÙ.BI NÍG.LAG.GA ZÍZ.AN.NA *u* IM KI.GAR 1-*niš* ḪE.ḪE NU NITA *u* MUNUS DÙ-[*u*]*š*
7. *ana* UGU *a-ḫa-meš* ŠUB-*di-šu-nu-ti ina* SAG.DU LÚ GAR-*an-ma* [ÉN]
8. 7-*šú* ŠID-*nu tu-nak-ka-ram-ma ana* ŠAḪ *tu-q*[*ar-rab*]
9. *šum*$_4$-*ma* ŠAḪ *iq-te-ru-ub* ŠU ^{d}EŠ$_4$.DAR *ana pa-a*[*n* NU.MEŠ]
10. ŠAḪ *la iq-ru-ub* NA BI *kiš-pu* DIB-[*su*]

TRANSLATION

(1–4) *Garbled Sumerian recitation.*

(5) A recitation to test potency.

(6–10) Its ritual: You mix together dough (made with) emmer flour and clay from the clay pit. You make a figurine of a man and a woman. You put them down next to one another. You put (them) at the head of the person('s bed) and you recite [the recitation] seven times. You remove (them) and ⸢present⸣ (them) to a pig. If the pig approaches, it is "hand" of Ishtar (but if) the pig does not approach the [figurines], sorcery afflicts that person.

TEXT 9: BAM 323

This text consists of rituals (1–38, 39–64, 79–88, 89–107), salves (65–69, 75–78), and amulets (65–69, 75–78) for "hand" of ghost. Of the rituals, three (1–38, 39–64, 79–88) involve the manufacture of figurines, which are given presents and pressured in various ways to return to the Netherworld where they belong. To this end, the great gods of the pantheon and in particular the god of the sun and justice, Shamash, are enlisted as guarantors of the efficacy of the ritual. The treatment of the situation as a sort of legal case makes a great deal of sense in this context, since families were obligated to care for diseased love ones, and Shamash was the enforcer both of the proper provision of funerary offerings and of the quid pro quo expected of the ghostly recipients. For a discussion of the wide variety of rituals deployed against ghosts, see Scurlock 2006. For the range of diseases potentially caused by ghosts, see Scurlock and Andersen 2005, 204–6, 311–14, 328, 355–56, 361–63, 437–39, 464–65, 471–72, 488–89, 495–98, 501–3, 526, 839.

Since, moreover, ghosts visited the living periodically, it was possible to persuade them to take away evils with them to the Netherworld. Only one's closest relatives could be asked such a favor, as in lines 79–88.

Lines 89–107 describe what is perhaps the most interesting ritual, since it involves modified mourning rites—dressing in sackcloth and self laceration, practices that in ancient Mesopotamia, as in ancient Israel, were designed to show extreme contrition in the face of heavenly powers and to excite their pity.

1. DIŠ NA GIDIM DIB-*su-ma* ÚS.MEŠ-*šú lu a-l*[*u-u lu gal-lu-u*]
2. *lu* SAG.‹ḪUL›.ḪA.ZA DIB-*su lu mim+ma lem-nu* DIB.DI[B]-⸢*su*⸣ *lu* […]
3. ⸢SAḪAR⸣ URU ⸢ŠUB⸣-*i* SAḪAR É ŠUB-*i* SAḪAR É DINGIR ⸢ŠUB⸣-*i* [SAḪ]AR ⸢KI⸣.MAḪ SAḪAR *uš-š*[*i*]
4. SAḪAR ÍD ŠUB-*ti* SAḪAR ⸢KASKAL 1-*niš* TI-*qí*⸣ KI MÚD GUD [Ḫ]E.ḪE NU *mim+ma lem-nu* DÙ-*uš*
5. KUŠ UR.MAḪ MU$_4$.MU$_4$-*su* ^{NA_4}GUG È *ina* GÚ-*šú* GAR KUŠ.A.GÁ.LÁ DIB-[*su*]
6. ⸢*u*⸣ *ṣú-de-e* SUM-*šú* U$_4$.3.KÁM 9 ŠUK-*su* ÚTUL *ṣir-pe-ti ana* IGI-*šú* GAR-*an*
7. *ina* ÙR É LÚ.GIG GUB-*sú-ma* ZÍD ŠE.SA.A *ina* A *u* KAŠ ⸢SÌG⸣-*aṣ-ma* BAL-*qí-šú*
8. 3 *sil-ti* GIŠ.ERIN.NA *i-ta-ti-šú* ⸢*tu-zaq-qap*⸣
9. ZÌ.SUR.RA NIGIN-*šú* DUG.NÍG.DÚR.BÙR NU AL.ŠEG$_6$.GÁ
10. UGU-*šú tu-kat-tam ina*! U$_4$ (coll. Schwemer) DUG.NÍG.DÚR.BÙR! ^{d}UTU *li-mur-šú ina* GI$_6$ MUL.MEŠ *li-mu-ru-šú*
11. U$_4$.3.KÁM MAŠ.MAŠ U$_4$-*mi* 22 NÍG.⸢NA⸣(coll.).NÍG.NA ^{ŠEM}LI *ana* IGI ^{d}UTU GAR-*an*
12. *ina* GI$_6$ ZÍD ZÍZ.ÀM *ana* IGI MUL.MEŠ GI$_6$-*tim* DUB-*aq*
13. *ana* IGI ^{d}UTU *u* MUL.MEŠ U$_4$.3.KÁM *ana muḫ-ḫi* (eras.) *im-ta-‹na›-an-nu*

---

14. ⸢ÉN GIDIM⸣ *mim+ma lem-nu iš-tu* U$_4$-*mi an-ni-i ina* SU! NENNI A NENNI ZI-*ta*$_5$ *šu-ṣa-a-ta*
15. *ṭar-da-*⸢*ta u kuš-šu-da*⸣*-ta* (eras.) DINGIR *šá-kin-ka*
16. ^{d}15 *šá-kin-ta-ka* ⸢*ina* SU⸣ NENNI A NENNI GIG *is-su-ḫu-ka*

---

17. *ina* U$_4$.3.KÁM *ina* U$_4$.GURUM.MA KEŠDA *ana* IGI ^{d}UTU ⸢KEŠDA⸣
18. LÚ.GIG NU ÍL-*ma ana* IGI ^{d}UTU *ki-a-am tu-šad-bab-*⸢*šú*⸣

---

19. ⸢ÉN⸣ ^{d}UTU *mu-tál* ^{d}*A-nun-na-*⸢*ki*⸣ *e-tel* ^{d}*Í-gì-gì mas-su-ú ṣi-ru mut-tar-ru-*⸢*u te-ni-še*$_{20}$*-e*⸣*-ti*
20. *da-a-a-‹an›* AN-*e u* KI-*tim la e-nu-u qí-bi-tuš-šú*
21. ⸢^{d}UTU⸣ *muš-te-šir ek-le-ti šá-kin nu-ri a-na ni-ši*
22. ⸢^{d}UTU⸣ *ina e-re-bi-ka* ZÁLAG *ni-ši ú-ta-aṭ-ṭi* ^{d}UTU *ina a-ṣi-ka i-nam-mi-*

ra kib-ra-a-ti

23. *e-ku-tum al-mat-tum ki*(coll.)-*gul-la-tum* ⸢*ù ru*⸣-*ut-tum*
24. *ṣi-iṭ*(coll)-[(*k*)]*a uš-taḫ-ḫa-na ka-la ab-ra-a-tum*
25. *b*[(*u-lum šik-na-a*)]*t* ZI-*tim a-šu*!(text:*ṣu*)-*ú ṣe-e-ri*
26. [(*it-ta-nab-ba-l*)]*a-ka nap-šat-si-na meš-re-ta*
27. [(*di-in-ḫab-lim ù ḫa-bi*)]*l-ti ta-da-an* EŠ.BAR-*ši-na tuš-te-šer ana-ku* NENNI A NENNI ⸢*šu-nu-ḫu kám-sa-ku*⸣
28. [(*šá i-na šib-sat* DINGIR *u* ^{d})]15 *iʾ-il-tum i-ʾ-i-la-an-ni*
29. [(UDUG MAŠKIM GIDIM LÍL)].LÁ *ḫi-mi-tum ṭi-mi-tum šim-mat* UZU *ṣi-da-nu*
30. [(*šá-áš-šá-ṭu mi-qit*) *ṭ*]e_4-*mi iš-qu-lu-nim-ma* U_4-*mi-šam-ma ud-dam-ma-mu-nin-ni*
31. [(^{d}UTU DI.KU_5 *at-ta*)]-⸢*ma*⸣ ZI-*tim ub-lak-ka di-nu* LÚ.GIG *šá* DIB-*an-ni ana di-ni kám-sa-ku*
32. [(*di-nu di-in* EŠ)].BAR-*a-a* TAR-[(*us a-di d*)]*i-in* EŠ.BAR-*a-a tu-šar-šu-ú*
33. [(*ana* ⸢*di-ni šá*⸣)-*nim-ma a*]-*a* ⸢SUM⸣-*in* [EŠ.BAR-*š*]*u iš-tu di-ni* EŠ.BAR *tuš-ter-šu-ú*
34. [(*iʾ-il-ti ú-ta*)]*š-ši-ra-an*-⸢*ni*⸣ [*ina*] ⸢SU⸣.MU (coll) *it-tap-ra-šú e-ma tak-la-ku* DINGIR.MEŠ *lim-tag-ru pu-ka*
35. [AN-*u liḫ*]-⸢*du*⸣(coll.)-*ka* KI-*tim li-riš-ka* TU_6 ÉN

---

36. [*ki-a-am tu*]-*šad-bab-šu ana* DUG GAR-*an-šu-ma tu-tam-ma-šu*
37. [*niš* KI-*tim lu-u ta-ma-ta*$_5$] *niš* AN-⸢*e*⸣ *lu-u ta-ma-ta*$_5$ *niš* ^{d}UTU *lu-u ta-ma-ta*$_5$ DUG_4.GA-*ma* KÁ-*šú* BAD-*ḫi*
38. [o o o o] x x x x *ina ḫar-bi na-du-ti te-qé*-⸢*ber-šú*⸣

---

39. [DIŠ NA GI]DIM DIB-⸢*su-ma*⸣ ÚS.M[EŠ-*šú lu* (LÍ)]L.LÁ.EN.NA *lu* KI.SIKIL.LÍL.LÁ.EN.NA
40. [(*lu* AN.TA)].ŠUB.BA *lu mim+ma lem-nu* [(DIB-*su*)]-*ma ina* SU-[(*šú*) NU DU_8-*ar* (K)]ÀŠ ANŠE.KUR.RA *tu-šam-ḫar*
41. [(*ina* Z)ÍD I]N.NU.ḪA ḪE.ḪE NU GIDIM *u mim+ma lem-nu šá* DIB-*š*[*ú*] DÙ-*uš*
42. MU-*šú* SAR-*ár* ZAG-*šú* KA-*šú* GÙB-*šú* GU.DU-⸢*su*⸣ DIB-*su*
43. [U(RUDU.MÚRU.ŠÈR)].ŠÈR ŠUB-*šú* GAG ^{GIŠ}MA.NU *ina* KA-*šú te-ret-ti*
44. [SÍG Ù]Z *ta-kar-šu-ma ana* ⸢IGI⸣ ^{d}UTU *ta*-⸢*dan*⸣-*šú*

---

45. ÉN ^{d}UTU LUGAL ⸢*mi-šá-ri*⸣ [(*ṭè-en-k*)]*a lis*-⸢*kip*⸣
46. ABGAL DINGIR.MEŠ ⸢^{d}AMAR.UTU⸣ [(*di-ni-k*)]*a* DA.KÚR![38]

47. ^{d}*Nin-geštin-*<(*an*>*-na*! *ú-suk-ka-tum* [(*na-gi-ir* ^{GI}NÍNDA.NA-*k*)]*i*
48. *i-na a-ru-ti* KI-*tim* A.⸢MEŠ⸣-*k*[(*a*! *lip-ru-us-ka*)]
49. ⸢^{d}⸣*Nin-*⸢*giš-zi-da* GU.ZA.LÁ⸣ KI-*tim* ⸢DAGAL-*tú*⸣ [(GABA-*ka li-né-i*)]
50. ⸢^{d}⸣[(AR)]A[39] ⸢SUKKAL⸣ *Eri-du*$_{10}$ ⸢*lit-ru*⸣-[(*ka*)]
51. [^{d}30 EN] AGA *màḫ-rit da-*[o o o o]
52. [^{d}NIN.URT]A[40] ⸢EN⸣ GIŠ.⸢TUKUL⸣ GÚ-*ka* [*lik-kis* x x]
53. [o o o o o (o)] o o (x) da? ru x [o o o o]
54. [(long gap)] KI.A.[^{d}ÍD o o o]
55. [(long gap)] ⸢ŠÀ⸣-*bi* ŠÉŠ.⸢ŠÉŠ-*su*⸣ [o o o o o o]
56. (traces)
57. [o o (o) NU BI *ana* ŠÀ ^{URUDU}]ŠEN.TUR *šá* 7 GÍN URUDU ⸢ŠUB⸣-*šú* IGI-*šú* ‹*ana*› GÙB!-[*šú* GAR]
58. [o o o o o o]x *ina* SAG LÚ.GIG DÙ-*uš ana* ŠÀ KU$_4$-*šú* U$_4$.3.K[AM]
59. [o o o o o o o (o)] *ki-*⸢*ma*⸣ x (x) x U$_4$ *ù*! (text: ši) GI$_6$-*tam* ŠID-*tú šá ana* IGI DINGIR ⸢*tam-ta*⸣-[*nu-u*]
60. [o] x x x [o o o o o o] x ZÍD ŠE.MUŠ$_5$ *ana* UGU-*šú* BIR-*aḫ*
61. *ina* U$_4$.3.KÁM U$_4$-*mi* G[IN$_7$] ^{d}UTU.[ŠÚ].A [*in*]*a*! EDIN PÚ BAD-*ma qé-te-ber-šú*
62. IGI-*šú a-na*! ^{d}UTU.ŠÚ.A GAR-*a*[*n-ma l*]*a*? GUR-*ár* ZÌ.SUR.RA-*a šá* ZÍD ŠE.MUŠ$_5$ ⸢NIGIN⸣-[*šú*]
63. TU^{MUŠEN} ⸢KUD⸣-*is* MÚD-⸢*šú*⸣ [*a-n*]*a* UGU-*šú* BAL-*qí*
64. *zi-pà-de-*⸢*e*⸣ [*tu-ta*]*m-*[*m*]*a-šú ana* EGIR-*ka* NU IGI.BAR

---

65. DIŠ NA GIDIM DI[(B-*su-ma*)] ⸢x x x x x x⸣[41] *ma-a-ad*(coll.)
66. *ḫa-a-a-at-t*[(*a-šú*)] *qer-bi-š*[*ú*] U$_4$ *u* ⸢GI$_6$⸣ NU ḪUN.ḪUN
67. GÙ-*š*[(*ú* GIN$_7$ G)]Ù ANŠE GIDIM *a-ḫu-ú ina ḫar-ba-te iṣ-bat-su* ‹(*ana* TI-*šú*)›
68. [(SU)]-*šú ina* KAŠ.Ú.SA *tu-kar tu-kaṣ-ṣa* ⸢^{Ú}⸣GEŠTIN.KA$_5$.A ‹(ḪÁD.A)› SÚD *ina* Ì[42] ‹(ḪE.ḪE)› ŠÉŠ-*su*
69. $^{N[A_4...]}$.KÙ ^{NA_4}*ár-zal-lu ia*$_4$*-artu* ‹(*šá* 7 GÙN.MEŠ-*šá*)› ^{NA_4}GUG SA$_5$ ^{NA_4}ZÚ GI$_6$ ^{NA_4}*aš-pu-u* ‹(^{NA_4}AN.Z)ÁḪ … (^{Ú}*tar-muš*)› [(*ina* KUŠ)]

---

70. ÉN UDUG ḪUN.GÁ A.LÁ ḪUN.GÁ GIDIM ḪUN.GÁ GAL$_5$.LÁ ḪUN.GÁ DINGIR ḪUN.GÁ MAŠKIM ḪUN.GÁ
71. ^{d}DIM$_9$.ME ḪUN.GÁ ^{d}DIM$_9$.ME.A MIN ^{d}DIM$_9$.ME.LAGAB MIN TU$_6$.DUG$_4$.GA ^{d}EN.KI.GA.KE$_4$
72. UR.SAG ^{d}ASAL.LÚ. DUMU ERIDU^{KI}.GA.KE$_4$ DUG$_4$.GA ^{d}NIN.GÌRIM NIN.TU$_6$.TU$_6$.KE$_4$
73. ZI.AN.NA ḪÉ.PÀ ZI.KI.A ḪÉ.PÀ

---

74. ÉN *an-ni-tú ana me-eli nap-šal-ti u maš-qa-ti* ŠID-*nu*

---

75. DIŠ NA ŠU.GIDIM$_4$.MA DIB-*su* ^{LÚ}MAŠ.MAŠ ZI-*šú la i-le-ʾi* ^{Ú}LÁL ^{Ú}*an-ki-nu-te* ‹(Ú DILI)›
76. ^{Ú}AŠ.TÁL.TÁL ^{Ú}ḪUR.SAG SIG$_7$ GURUN ^{GIŠ}MAŠ.ḪUŠ GURUN ^{GIŠ}DÌḪ ‹(NUNUZ $^{\text{GIŠ.Ú}}$GÍR)›[43] ^{Ú}*ár-zal-la*
77. ^{Ú}*tar-muš* ^{Ú}*eli-kul*!-*la* NUMUN ^{GIŠ}ŠINIG GÌR.PAD.DU LÚ.U$_{19}$.LU 1-*niš* *ina* Ì (variant: Ì ^{GIŠ}ERIN)
78. ŠÉŠ-*su-ma ina* KUŠ DÙ.DÙ *ina* GÚ-*šú* GAR-*an* TI-*uṭ*

---

79. DIŠ NA! GIDIM AD-*šú u* AMA-*šú* DIB.DIB-*su ina* ITI.NE U$_4$.27!.KAM
80. IM KI.GAR TI-*qí* NU NITA *u* MUNUS DÙ-*uš* ⌜NU⌝ NITA *šu-ra šá* KÙ.SIG$_{17}$ GAR-*šu* [(NU MUNUS) ^{GIŠ}]PA? (variant: GESTU^{II}) KÙ.SIG$_{17}$ GAR-*ši*
81. $^{\text{NA}_4}$GUG (variant: $^{\text{NA}_4}$ZA.GÌN) *ina* SÍG.ḪÉ.ME.DA È *ina* GÚ-*šá* GAR *tu-ṭaḫ-ḫad-su-nu-ti*
82. *tu-kab-bat-su-nu-ti tu-kán-na-šu-nu-ti* NU.MEŠ *šú-nu-ti* 3 U$_4$-*mi*
83. *ina* SAG LÚ.GIG *tu-še-eš-šeb-šu-nu-ti* TU$_7$ KÚM.MA *ta-tab-bak-šu-nu-ti*
84. *ina* U$_4$.3.KÁM U$_4$.29.KÁM *e-nu-ma* GIDIM *uš-taš-še-ru* ^{GIŠ}MÁ.ŠÀ.ḪA DÙ-*uš*
85. *ṣú-de-šú-nu te-es-siḫ ana* IGI ^{d}UTU *ta-dan-šu-nu-ti*
86. *ana qid*!-*da-ti* IGI-*šú-nu* GAR-*an u kam* DUG$_4$.GA

---

87. *ina* ZU NENNI A NENNI ŠÁR KASKAL.GÍD *i-si-a re-e-qá re-e-qá i-si-a i-si*(coll.)-*a*!
88. ZI DINGIR.MEŠ GAL.MEŠ ⌜*tùm*⌝-*ma-tu-nu*[44]

---

89. DIŠ NA SAG.‹(KI)›.DIB.BA TUKU.TUKU-*ši* GEŠTU^{II}-*šú* ⌜*i-ša-gu-ma* IGI^{II}-*šú*⌝ *i-bar-ru-ra*
90. SA.GÚ-*šú* GU$_7$.MEŠ-*šu* Á-*šú šim-ma-ti* TUKU.TUKU-*ši* ÉLLAG-*su ú-maḫ-ḫa-s*[(*u*)]
91. ŠÀ-*šú da-li-iḫ* GÌR^{II}-*šú ri-mu-tú* TUKU.TUKU-*ši*
92. NA BI GIDIM *ri-da-ti* ÚS.MEŠ-*šú ana* TI.LA-*šu*

---

93. *ina* U$_4$.15.KÁM U$_4$-*um* ^{d}30 *u* ^{d}UTU 1-*niš* GUB-*zu*
94. NA BI TÚG.ŠÀ.ḪA MU$_4$.MU$_4$ *ina* NA$_4$.ZÚ SAG.KI-*šú te-eṣ-ṣi-ma*
95. MÚD-*šu ta-tab-bak ina* ŠÀ GI.⌜ÙRI⌝.GAL TUŠ-*eb-šu*
96. IGI-*šu ana* IM.SI.SÁ GAR-*an ana* ^{d}30 *ana* ^{d}UTU.ŠÚ.A

97. NÍG.NA ^{ŠEM}LI GAR-*an* GA ÁB BAL-*qí ana* ^{d}UTU (coll.) ^{d}UTU.È NÍG.NA ^{GIŠ}ŠUR.MÌN GAR-*an*
98. KAŠ SAG BAL-*qí* NA BI UR$_5$.GIN$_7$ DUG$_4$.GA

---

99. *ana* GÙB-*ya* ^{d}30 U$_4$.SAKAR AN-*e* GAL.MEŠ *ana* ZAG-*ya a-bi ṣal-mat* SAG.DU ^{d}UTU DI.KU$_5$
100. DINGIR.MEŠ *ki-lal-la-an a-bi* DINGIR.MEŠ GAL.MEŠ TAR-*su* EŠ.BAR *ana* UN.MEŠ DAGAL.MEŠ
101. IM ḪUL-*tim i-di-pan-ni-ma* GIDIM *ri-da-a-ti* ÚS.MEŠ-*an-ni*
102. *lu ‹na›-as-sa-ku e-šá-ku u dal-ḫa-ku ana di-ni-ku-nu šu-zi-ba-ni-ma la aḫ-ḫa-bil*
103. 7-*šú* DUG$_4$.GA-*ma iš-tu* GI.ÙRI.GAL È-*ma* TÚG.BI *ú-na-kar* TÚG DADAG MU$_4$.MU$_4$ *ana* ^{d}30 UR$_5$.GIN$_7$ DUG$_4$.GA

---

104. ÉN ^{d}NANNA GIŠ.NU$_{11}$.GAL.AN.KI.KE$_4$ TU.RA NU.DÙG.GA ZU.MU.TA BA.Z[I]
105. 3-*šú* ⸢DUG$_4$⸣.GA-*ma ana* ^{d}UTU UR$_5$.GIN$_7$ DUG$_4$.G[A]

---

106. ^{d}UTU ⸢DI.KU$_5$ GAL A!⸣.A SAG.GI$_6$.GA IM.ḪUL.GAR.RA.BA I.BÍ.GIN$_7$ AN.ŠÈ ḪÉ.È
107. KA.TAR.ZU! GA.AN.SI.IL : 3-*šú* DUG$_4$.GA-*ma* NU x [(x x)][45]

---

108. ⸢^{Ú}*al*⸣-*la-an-ka-niš* ^{Ú}*nu-ṣa-bu* ⸢^{Ú}⸣[... ^{Ú}]⸢*eli-kul*⸣-[*la* ...]
109. ⸢SUḪUŠ ^{GIŠ}⸣[DÌ]Ḫ *šá* UGU KI.MAḪ NUMUN ^{GIŠ}ŠINIG [...]

TRANSLITERATION

1–13. If a ghost afflicts a person (and) continually pursues him or an *alû*-⸢demon⸣, [or a *gallû*-demon], or a *mukīl rēš lemutti*-demon afflicts him or anything evil ⸢continually⸣ afflicts him or [pursues him(?)], you take together dirt from an abandoned town, dirt from an abandoned house, dirt from an abandoned temple, ⸢dirt⸣ from a sepulcher, dirt from ⸢foundations(?)⸣, dirt from an abandoned canal (and) dirt from a road. You mix (them) with ox blood. You make a figurine of whatever evil thing (it is).

You clothe it with the skin of a lion. You thread carnelian (and) put (it) on its neck. You provide [it] with a waterskin and give it travel provisions. For three days, you put out nine dishes of barley gruel before it as its food ration. You stand it up on the roof of the patient's house and then you stir flour made from roasted grain into water and beer and then you pour out a libation for it. You plant three *erēnu*-cedar shavings around it. You surround it with a magic circle. You put an unbaked fermenting vessel over it as a cover. Let Shamash see the fermenting vessel by day; let the stars see it by night. For three days, by day, the *āšipu* sets up twenty-two censers (burning) *burāšu*-juniper before Shamash; by night, he scatters emmer flour before the stars of the night. Before Shamash and the stars, for three days, he repeatedly recites over it.

(14–16) Recitation: "Ghost (or) whatever is evil—from this day forward, you are extracted from the body of NN son of NN; you are expelled; you are driven away and banished. The god who set you (on), the goddess who set you (on)—they have removed you from the body of NN, son of NN, the patient."

(17–18) On the third day, in the late afternoon, you set up an offering table before Shamash. The patient raises the figurine and then you have him say as follows before Shamash.

(19–35) Recitation: "Shamash, noblest of the Anunnaki, lordliest of the Igigi; august leader, ruler of the people, judge of heaven and earth, whose command is unalterable; Shamash, who keeps the darkness in order (and) who establishes light for the people; Shamash, at your setting, the light of mankind is darkened; Shamash, at your rising, the regions brighten. The homeless girl, the widow, the waif, and the female companion—all mankind warms itself (at) your emergence; the wild animals, living creatures, beasts of the steppe, continually bring you their lives and limbs. You decide the case of the wronged man and woman; you make their decisions go aright. I am NN, son of NN; I kneel in exhaustion; I, who as a result of the anger of god and goddess, an obligation has bound. An *utukku*-demon, a *rābiṣu*-demon, a ghost (and) a *lilû*-demon have weighed out for me paralysis, twisting, numbness of the flesh, dizziness, *šaššaṭu* (and) insanity and daily they cause me to twist. Shamash, you are the judge and I have brought you my life. I kneel for judgment of the case concerning the sickness that afflicts me. Judge my case; make a decision about me. Until you cause my case to be decided, [may] you not give [a decision] for [any other] case. After you have caused my case to be decided, (and after) my obligation has let me go (and) fled [from] my ⸢body⸣, wherever I put my trust, let (those) gods come to agree with what you say. [May the heavens be pleased with] you; may the earth rejoice in you."

(36–38) [You] have him speak [thus]. You put it (the figurine) in a jar and then you make it swear. You say: "[By earth may you swear]; by ⸢heaven⸣ may you swear; by Shamash may you swear," and then you close its (the pot's) mouth. [...] You bury it (the pot) in an abandoned waste.

(39–44) [If] a ⸢ghost⸣ afflicts [a person] and continually pursues [him, or] a *lilû*-demon or an *ardat lilî*-demon, or AN.TA.ŠUB.BA or anything evil afflicts him and [can not be dispelled(?)] from his body, you have (him—the patient) collect(?) horse urine. You mix (it) with flour (made from) ⸢*inninnu*⸣-cereal.

You make a figurine of the ghost or anything evil which afflicts ⌜him⌝. You write its name (on it). You have it hold its mouth with its right hand and its rear end with its left. You put a ⌜copper⌝ chain on it. You nail a peg of *e*ʾ*ru*-tree wood into its mouth. You rub it with ⌜goat⌝ [hair] and bring suit against it[46] before Shamash.

(45–53) Recitation: "May Shamash, the king of justice, overthrow your plans. (May) the wisest of the gods, Marduk, and your lawsuit become mutual enemies.[47] May Ningeštianna, the woman who has just given birth, the herald of the reed measuring rod, cut off water from your (clay) pipe (laid in) the earth. [May] Ningizzida, chair bearer of the broad Netherworld turn back your breast. May Usmû, *sukkallu*-official of Eridu, lead (you) away. [May Sîn, lord] of the corona, [… May Ninurta], lord of the weapon, [cut] your throat. […]"

(54–64) […] ⌜sulphur⌝ […] You continually rub him [with] it. […] You put [that figurine into a] *tamgussu*-vessel of seven shekels' copper (weight). [You turn] its face [to its] left. At the head of the patient you make a […]. You make it (the figurine in the *tamgussu*-vessel) enter it (i.e., what you have made). For three days, […] as soon as […], the recitation which you have ⌜recited⌝ day and night before the god, […] You scatter *šigūšu*-flour over it. On the third day, ⌜when⌝ the sun is ⌜setting⌝, you dig a pit in the steppe and bury it. You make it ⌜face⌝ the setting sun [so that it will] ⌜not⌝ return(?).[48] You surround [it] with a magic circle of *šigūšu*-flour. You cut the throat of a dove. You pour its blood ⌜over⌝ it. [You] ⌜make⌝ it ⌜swear⌝ a ritual oath; you must not look behind you.

(65–69) If a ghost afflicts a person and …,[49] his confusional states[50] are numerous and (a confusional state) is (always) nearby, he gets no rest day or night, (and) his cry is like the cry of a donkey, a strange ghost has seized him in the waste land. ‹(To cure him)›, you rub his body with beerwort. You let (it) cool. You ‹(dry)› (and) grind "fox grape." ‹(You mix)› (it) with oil[51] (and) gently rub him (with it). (You put), […], *arzallu*-stone, ‹(seven-colored)› *ayyartu*-shell, red carnelian, black obsidian, jasper, ‹(⌜*anzaḫḫu*⌝-frit, […] (and) *tarmuš*)› in a leather (bag).

(70–73) Recitation: "*utukku*-demon, relent; *alû*-demon, relent; ghost, relent; *gallû*-demon, relent; evil god, relent; *rābiṣu*-demon, relent; *lamaštu*-demon, relent; *labāṣu*-demon, relent; *aḫḫāzu*-demon, relent. By the spell pronounced by Enki (and) the hero, Asalluhi, son of Eridu, (and) at the command of Ningirim, mistress of spells. By heaven are you made to swear; by earth are you made to swear."

(74) You recite this recitation over amulets, salves, and potions.

(75–78) If "hand" of ghost afflicts a person (and) the *āšipu* is not able to remove it, you rub him gently with *ašqulālu*, *ankinūtu*, *ardadillu*, fresh *azupīru*, fruit of the *kalbānu*, fruit of the *baltu*-thorn, ‹(fruit of the *ašāgu*-thorn)›, *arzallu*, *tarmuš*, *elikulla*, *bīnu*-tamarisk seeds, (and) "human bone" (mixed) together with oil (variant: *erēnu*-cedar oil) and then you lace (it) in a leather (bag and) put (it) on his neck. He should recover.

(79–86) If the ghost of a person's father or mother continually afflicts him, on the twenty-seventh(!) of Abu, you take clay from a potter's pit. You make a figurine of a man and a woman. You put a reed (made) of gold on the male figurine. You put a ⸢staff⸣ (variant: ear) (made) of gold on the female figurine. You thread carnelian (variant: lapis) on red wool. You put (it) on her (the female figurine's) neck. You abundantly fit them (the figurines) out. You honor them, you treat them with care. For three days, you seat those figurines at the head of the patient. You pour out hot broth for them. On the third day, the twenty-ninth, when the ghosts are (customarily) provided with food offerings, you make a sailboat. You assign their travel provisions. You bring suit against them before Shamash. You make them face downstream and you say as follows:

(87–88) "From the body of NN, son of NN, be 3,600 double hours distant, be far away, be distant, be distant. By the great gods are you made to swear."

(89–92) If a person continually has headaches, his ears roar, his eyes become dimmed, his neck muscles continually hurt him, his arm(s) are continually numb, his lower back gives him a jabbing pain, his heart is troubled, (and) his feet continually have *rimūtu*-paralysis, a pursuing ghost continually pursues that person. To cure him,

(93–98) On the fifteenth, the day when Sîn and Shamash stand together, you dress that person in sackcloth. You make an incision in his temple with a flint knife and draw his blood. You have him sit in a reed enclosure.[52] You have him face north. To Sîn, towards the setting sun, you set up a censer (burning) *burāšu*-juniper. You make a libation of cow's milk. To Shamash, (towards) the rising sun, you set up a censer (burning) *šurmēnu*-cypress. You pour out a libation of beer. That person says as follows:

(99–103) "To my left is Sîn, moon crescent of the great heavens. To my right is the father of the black headed ones, Shamash, the judge, both gods, fathers of the great gods, makers of decisions for the widespread people, an evil wind has blown upon me and a pursuing ghost continually pursues me. I am truly grieved, confused and troubled. ‹I kneel?› for your judgment; save me so that I may not be wronged." He says (this) seven times and then he emerges from the reed enclosure and removes his garment. He puts on a clean garment. To Sîn, he says as follows:

(104–105) Recitation: "Nanna, light of heaven and earth, ⸢remove⸣ the unpleasant sickness from my body." He says (this) three times and then, to Shamash, he ⸢says⸣ as follows:

(106–107) "Utu, great judge, father of the black-headed ones, let the evil wind that put it there(?) go up like smoke to heaven and let me praise you." : If he says this three times, it (the ghost) will not [...]."[53]

(108–109) *Allān kaniš*, *nuṣābu* [...], ⌈*elikulla*⌉, [...] root of a ⌈*baltu*⌉-thorn which (was growing) on a grave, *bīnu*-tamarisk seeds [...]

NOTES

1. See Farber 1990, 319; Collins 1999, 268–69.
2. From *magāru*. The reference is to the tooth worm recitation (chapter 5, text 9) where the worm asks to be allowed to suck the blood out of teeth.
3. For the reading, see *CAD* Š/3, 328a.
4. BAM 311:90′ replaces GÌR.PAD.DU LÚ.U_{19}.LU with Ú DILI.
5. BAM 311:91′ replaces GÌR.PAD.DU LÚ.U_{19}.LU with Ú DILI.
6. BAM 311:93′ replaces GÌR.PAD.DU LÚ.U_{19}.LU with Ú DILI and TÚG.NÍG.DÁRA. ŠU.LÁL with ^Ú^SIKIL.
7. BAM 157 obv. 6′–9′ replaces 7 U_4.MEŠ with *ina* 3 U_4.ME *ú-mi-šam-ma*.
8. See Scurlock and Andersen 2005, 16.3, 18.24.
9. BAM 311: 87–89 indicates that this is specifically for teeth gnashing during sleep.
10. BAM 311 consistently gives the "real" name of the plant in lieu of the fanciful *Deckname*.
11. BAM 311 consistently gives the "real" name of the plant in lieu of the fanciful *Deckname*.
12. BAM 311 consistently gives the "real" name of the plant in lieu of the fanciful *Deckname*.
13. Uruanna gives a number of different plants as equivalents. For references, see *CAD* T, 417–18.
14. See Scurlock and Andersen 2005, 16.4, 18.26
15. BAM 157 obv. 6′–9′ replaces "seven days" with "daily for three days."
16. See Scurlock and Andersen 2005, 16.16.
17. K 2581 obv. 22 has: *ina* KI.NÁ-*šú*.
18. A similar superstition attends marriages in our own culture, and is why we carry the bride over the threshold.
19. The *CAD* T, 390a emends(?) *iz-zi-bu* to *iz-zi-qa* and translates: "just as a basket does not groan at its lowering and raising." However, the word being translated "lowering" (*urḫu*) means "road/path." Böck 2011, 84 takes the "basket" (*pisannu*) to be a doorpost. However, *pisannu* is rarely used for parts of a door, and when it is, it is the socket which is being referred to. A third option, and the one taken here, is to take *pisannu* as meaning "drainpipe," which makes perfect sense in the context.
20. See Scurlock and Andersen 2005, 13.17, 19.217.
21. K 2581 obv. 22 has: "In his bed."
22. The duplicates give different lists of gods:
    RS 25.456A++ (Nougayrol 1969, 397 and Farber 2014, 92) gives:
    ii 23′. ^d^MÁ *ù* ^d^AMA.ZA.ḪA.NU.DÁ)]
    ii 24′. [*be*]-*let* DINGIR.MEŠ *be-let šu-ur-bu-ti*
    ii 25′. [^d^15 *kab-t*]*a-at* DINGIR.MEŠ *qa-rit-ti*
23. Restored after K 132 ($4R^2$ 55 rev. 31–33, Farber 2014, 141 lines 126–129). Note the similar procedures in KAL 4.36–37, both of them almost certainly also Lamashtu texts.
24. Differently Farber 2014, 89 lines 178–180.
25. For the translation, see Civil 1982, 2 n. 4.
26. For a discussion of the gifts given to Lamashtu, see Farber 1987b, 85–105. It is there

argued that *šiddu* is some sort of rolled carpet. However, it seems odd that a carpenter should provide a textile rather than something made of wood.

27. Literally "fill."

28. PBS 1/2 113 i 3–11 adds: Be blocked off from this street!

29. The duplicate has ^{GIŠ}ZI.GAN.

30. Suggestion courtesy M. Stol.

31. For the bad advice in question, see chapter 12, text 5: "For the lying-in woman giving birth (this) is (her) recitation: 'Bring me your sons so that I can give them suck; let me put the breast into the mouth of your daughters.'" (*LKU* 33:16′–18′).

32. Maul 1994, § VIII.1.2: 63–66, 81–82.

33. The family ghosts (who have names) are to give their names (i.e., live boys) to the patient and the forgotten ghosts (who have no names) are to take the patient's no-names (the stillborn male children symbolized by the offerings) in return.

34. The choice of a potter's oven is dictated by the patient's problem; it is in some sense also a womb from which foetuses (pots) regularly emerge, sometimes "whole" (also "well" in Akkadian) and sometimes cracked or broken. We may presume that the potter was paid for his oven to compensate him for the hoped-for loss of crockery.

35. This recitation was apparently meant to be recited to the setting sun to accompany the amulets.

36. This recitation was apparently meant to be recited to the river to accompany the river section.

37. As the third ritual makes clearer, she is supposed to crawl under the suspended ewe.

38. *STT* 214–217 rev. iv 51 and K 2506+ rev. v 4 (Schwemer 2009, 176 n. 6) have *li-kìr*. Schwemer's reads *li-rim* in the parallels and li_x(DA)-rim_x(AŠ) in the main text, and translates "cover your lawsuit (in darkness)."

39. For more on this divinity, see Schwemer 2011, 126 n. 279.

40. For the restoration of the gods' names, see Schwemer 2011, 126.

41. BAM 385 i 23′//BAM 471 ii 26′ have *i-mi-im i-ka-aṣ-ṣa* at this point.

42. Dupl. substitutes MÚD ^{GIŠ}ERIN : Ì BÚR.

43. So from BAM 221 iii 16 while BAM 385 iv 8 substitutes this for the ^{GIŠ}DÌḪ.

44. For the edition of this section, together with its parallel K 4508+6648:1–13, see Farber 1977, 210–17.

45. Schwemer 2009, 172 interprets the end of the line as a prohibition on proskinesis. However, the supplicant would hardly fail to show proper respect to the god of justice! Prohibitions of this sort do exist but they are, to my knowledge, in a context of a continuing ritual in which the proskinesis is postponed until the proper moment. So certainly in BAM 237 i 11′–13′ where the woman is supposed kneel and utter her prayer but to delay proskinesis until the *mersu*-confection and the libation have been offered.

46. The translation follows Schwemer's interpretation of this form as being from *dânu* rather than *nadānu*; see Schwemer 2007a, 206–7.

47. The duplicate has Marduk becoming hostile to his lawsuit.

48. Schwemer 2011, 126 interprets this odd phrase as the more typical: "You put its arms behind its back." However, since the figurine has not only been put in a container, but also buried, this would be difficult.

49. BAM 385 i 23′//BAM 471 ii 26′ have "He gets hot, he gets cold" at this point.

50. See Scurlock and Andersen 2005 315, 318.

51. Dupl. substitutes: *erēnu*-cedar resin (variant: *pūru*-oil).

52. See Schwemer 2009, 172–73 for a discussion of the *urigallu*.

53. A translation and discussion of lines 93–107 appears in Reiner 1995, 136–38. Schwemer

2011, 128 n. 288 restores the instruction that the patient is not to prostrate himself. As noted above, there are situations where this instruction appears, but it is specifically in the context of prostrating oneself at the appropriate moment, not refusing to show proper respect to the god of justice!

SOURCE LIST

DPS

A previous edition and French translation of DPS was published by R. Labat, *TDP*. A scored edition and German translation of DPS 15–33 with many new texts was published by Heeßel (2000). On pp. 140–46, Heeßel very generously also published a list of texts forming DPS 3–14 that were previously known and those that he had newly discovered. Several new duplicates were added by Scurlock.

DPS 3 is a combined edition made up of:

A: BM 33424 (coll.) = lines 1–32a, 93–123

B: BM 46139 (coll.) = lines 1–8

C: MLC 2639 (Goetze, JCS 2 [1948] 305–308 (coll.) = lines 10–123

D: VAT 14554 (*LKU* 90) (coll.) = lines 35–50

E_1: VAT 14553 (*LKU* 91) (coll.) = lines 69–85 (+) E_2: W17360k (*TDP* II:LXVII) = lines 73–89

F: W 17360ac (AUWE 23:323) = lines 86–98

G: VAT 14552 (*LKU* 89) (coll.) = lines 111–123

H: BM 40744 = lines 34–49, 85–98

DPS 4 is a combined edition made up of:

A = K 2723+K 3872 obv.+K 4051 (*TDP* IV–V) (coll.)+

A_2 = K 3872 rev. (*AMT* 107/1)

A_3 = K 10602+

A_4 = K 13842+

A_5 = K 10592(+)

A_6 = K 19432 (coll.) = lines 1–72, 84–142

B = AO 6682 (*TDP* VI–VIII) (coll.) = lines 1–45, 105–143

C = ND 4405/35 (CTN 4.77) (coll.) = lines 1–13

D = VAT 14550 (*LKU* 79) (coll.) = lines 2–16

E = W 22761 (SpTU 3.88) line nos. follow translit. = lines 21–39, 54–92, 123–138
F = *LKU* 77 = lines 41–70
G = VAT 14567 (*LKU* 94) = lines 48–64, 88–104
H = W 17360c (*TDP* LXVI) (coll.) = lines 83–94
3A = BM 33424 (coll.) = DPS 3:143 = line 1

DPS 5 is a combined edition made up of:
A = K 6629 (*AMT* 75/2) (coll.) = lines 1–17
B = K 6737 (CT 37/50) (coll.) = lines 18–26a, 50–60
C = K 13985 (*TDP* IX) (coll.) = lines 27–34, 61–67
D = K 10570 (*TDP* IX) (coll.) = lines 35–49, 67–80
E = W 17360g (*TDP* LXVI) = lines 61–68
F = K 3957+K 6347+K 9350 (*AMT* 105/2) (coll.) = lines 81–99
G = K 7099 (CT 37/50) (coll.) = lines 100–126
4A = K 2723+K 3872 obv.+K 4051 (*TDP* IV–V) (coll.) = DPS 4:143 = line 1
4B = AO 6682 (*TDP* VI–VIII) (coll.) = DPS 4:143 = line 1

DPS 6 is a combined edition made up of:
A = K 2243+Rm 248+Rm 481 (*TDP* X–XI) (coll.) = lines 1–33, 94′–110′ (comes in at $B_2$2)
B_1 = K 10343(*TDP* XI)+ (coll.) = lines 97–109
B_2 = K 12539+K 12897(both *KMI* 35)(+) (coll.) = lines 15–31, 94′–110′ (follows $B_5$10)
B_3 = K 12899(+) (coll.) = 43′–51′(follows B_5 obv.); 68″–83″ (follows B_4 rev.)
B_4 = K 13959 (CT 28:18&TBP 31)+ (coll.) = 55′–62′ (follows B_3 9), 65′–67′ (comes in at C11)
B_5 = K 18289 (coll.) = lines 32–42, 83″–93″ (comes in at $E_2$6+$E_1$2)
C = BM 34071 obv. = lines 18–36, 56′–66′ (comes in at $B_4$2)
D = VAT 14557(*LKU* 95) (coll.) = lines 18–32
E = K 4977 (*TDP* X)+K 11858 (*TDP* XI) = 78″–92″ (comes in at B_3 rev. 11 and goes to $B_5$10)
F = W 17360p (*TDP* LXVII) = 82′–87″ (comes in at $E_2$5+$E_1$1 and goes to $E_2$10+$E_1$6)

DPS 7 is made up of:
A = K 2949+K 12856 (CT 37:37&*KMI* 41) (coll.) (first and last sections)
B = K 2952+K 3678 (CT 37:40) (coll.) (follows A and is followed by A)

C = BM 34071 rev. (coll.) (placement uncertain; probably in the central section)
6A = K 2243+Rm 248+Rm 481 (*TDP* X–XI) (coll.) = DPS 6:110″ = line 1
6B = B_2 = K 12539+K 12897(both *KMI* 35) = line 1 = DPS 6:110″ = line 1

DPS 8 is:
K 4080+Sm 552+K 9254+K 11774 (*TDP* XII)+K 14851 (*AMT* 69/6) (coll.)

DPS 9 is a combined edition made up of:
A = AO 6681 (*TDP* XIII–XIV) (coll.) = lines 1–79
B = K 261 (*TDP* XV–XVII) (coll.) = lines 1–79
C = VAT 14561 (*LKU* 99) (coll.) = line 30–49

DPS 10 is a combined edition made up of:
A = AO 6679 (= *TDP* XIX–XX) (coll.) = lines 1–54b
B = K 3687+K 6389+Sm 951 (= *TDP* XXI–XXIII = *AMT* 106/2, 107/2) (coll.) = lines obv. 1–31, rev. 1–18
C = *LKU* 86 = lines 23–41
D = VAT 14544 (*LKU* 75) (coll.) = lines 42–54b
9A = AO 6681 (*TDP* XIII–XIV) (coll.) = line 1
9B = K 261 (*TDP* XV–XVII) (coll.) = line 1

DPS 11 is a combined edition made up of:
A = BM 65698 (*TDP* XXIV–XXVIII) (coll.) = lines obv. 1–56, rev. 1–60
B = W 22307/1 (SpTU 1.34) = lines 1–36
C = Sm 1210 (TBP = AfO Beih3.29) (coll.) = lines rev. 42–48
10A = AO 6679 (= *TDP* XIX–XX) (coll.) = line 1
10B = K 3687+K 6389+Sm 951 (= *TDP* XXI–XXIII = *AMT* 106/2, 107/2) (coll.) = line 1

DPS 12 is a combined edition made up of:
A = Sm 232 (*TDP* XXIX) (coll.) = lines 1–27
B = K 6704 (coll.) = lines 18–35
C = W 22307/56 (SpTU 1:35) = lines 36′–48′
D = A 3442 (*TDP* XXXI) (Oriental Institute tablet; i–ii not copied by Labat) (coll.) = lines 49″–55″, 57″–107″, 109″–134″
E = BE 35828 (*TDP* XXX) = lines 64″–104″, 106″–134″
F = K 7286+Sm 856 = lines 56″–82″, 113″–122″
G_1 = VAT 14537 (*LKU* 85)+G_2 = VAT 14598 (*LKU* 83) (coll.) = lines 61″–87″, 111″–134″

11A = BM 65698 (*TDP* XXIV–XXVIII) (coll.) = line 1

DPS 13 is a combined edition made up of:

A = K 18019 (coll.) = lines 1–7
B = A 3506 (*TDP* XXXII–XXXIV) (coll.) = lines 4–117
C = K 5670 (coll.) = lines 22–32
D = K3743 (CT 37:41) (coll.) = lines 31–48, 161–181
E = K 19906 (coll.) = lines 36–42
F = K 9250 (coll.) = lines 42–62
G_1 = K 1756 (+) G_2 = K 3693+K 6290+Rm 102 (CT 37:38–39) (coll.) = lines 54–110, 119–141
H = W17360n (*TDP* LXVII) = lines 85–90
I = VAT 14551 (*LKU* 88) (coll.) = lines 111–119
J = VAT 14564 (*LKU* 102) (coll.) = lines 142–160
K = BM 40857 (coll.) = lines 31–40, 73–86, 92–116, 130–154
12E = BE 35828 (*TDP* XXX) = line 1
12G_1 = VAT 14537 (*LKU* 85) = line 1

DPS 14 is a combined edition made up of:

A = K 2006+K 3795+K 4014+K 4083+K 4094a+K 11294+K 14000(+)K 3826 (TDPXXXV–XXXVI) (coll.) = lines 1–41, 78–122, 168′–193′, 237′–266′
A_2 = (+)K 3826 (CT 37.44+*TDP* XXXVI) (coll.) = lines 53–73, 123–150, 207′–224′
B = VAT 14542 (*LKU* 73) (coll.) = lines 2–13
C = VAT 303+VAT 404+VAT 579+VAT 589 (BAM VII pls. 31–34) (coll.) = lines 35–84, 89–146, 173′–220′, 228′–247′, 257′–266′
D = VAT 14543 (*LKU* 74) (coll.) = lines 52–63
E = VAT 14545 (*LKU* 76) (coll.) = lines 85–93
F = BM 38655 (BAM VII pl. 35) (coll.) = lines 106–115, 191′–206′
G = VAT 14540 (*LKU* 70) (coll.) = lines 143–167, 217′–232′
H = VAT 14541 (*LKU* 71) (coll.) = lines 149–163
I = VAT 14547 (*LKU* 82) (coll.) = lines 172′–186′
J = VAT 14548 (*LKU* 84) (coll.) = lines 190′–197′
K = W 17360o (*TDP* LXVII) = lines 242′–252′
L = *LKU* 65 = lines 255′–266′

DPS 15 is a combined edition based on Heeßel 2000, 150–70.

A = A 3440 (*TDP* LXIV–LXV) (coll.) = lines 1′–73′
B = K 12371 (Heeßel 2000, 449) = lines 1′–12′
C = VAT 14566 (*LKU* 81) (coll. Heeßel 2000, 471) = lines 43′–62′

D = VAT 14565 (*LKU* 80) (coll. Heeßel 2000, 471) = lines 48′–64′
E = K 8161 (+) Sm 1059 (Heeßel 2000, 449) (coll.) = lines 74′–92′
14A = K 2006+K 3795+K 4014+K 4083+K 4094a+K 11294+K 14000(+)K 3826 (TDPXXXV–XXXVI) (coll.) = line 1
14C = C = VAT 303+VAT 404+VAT 579+VAT 589 (BAM VII pls. 31–34) (coll.) = line 1

DPS 16 is a combined edition based on Heeßel 2000, 171–93
A = W 22307/5 (SpTU 1.37) = lines 1–17, 19–35
B = W 22651 (SpTU 2.44) = lines 1–30, 73′–101′
C = W 17360d (*TDP* LXVI) = lines 1–17
D = *LKU* 68a = lines 17–26
E = W 17360t (*TDP* LXVIII) = lines 17–34, 101′
F = EHE 110 (Scheil, *RA* 14:123, 125) = lines 36′–94′
G = *LKU* 68b = lines 41′–48′
H = *LKU* 68c = lines 49′–66′, 69′–80′
15E = K 8161 (+) Sm 1059 (Heeßel 2000, 449) = line 1

DPS 17 is a combined edition based on Heeßel 2000, 194–217
A = A 3437 (*TDP* XXXVII–XXXIX) (coll.) = lines 1–56, 62–105
B = K 3962 (*TDP* XL–XLIII) (coll. Heeßel 2000, 471) (coll.) = lines 1–40, 44–105
C = K 12624 (*TDP* VIII) (coll. Heeßel 2000, 471) = lines 1–8
D = *LKU* 66 = lines 20–35
E = K 3706+K 6202 (*AMT* 50/4)+K 8035+K 9113 (Heeßel 2000, 450–51) = lines 25–105
F = *LKU* 67 = lines 50–64
G = W17360y (*TDP* LXVIII) = lines 52–58
H = VAT 14562 (*LKU* 100) = lines 88–101
16B = W 22651 (SpTU 2.44) = line 1
16D = D = *LKU* 68a = line 1
16E = W 17360t (*TDP* LXVIII) = line 1

DPS 18 is based on Heeßel 2000, 218–25
K 2536+K 1101+K 12145 (Heeßel 2000, 452–53)

DPS 19/20 is a combined edition based on Heeßel 2000, 226–45
A = VAT 14555 (*LKU* 92)+W 17360l (*TDP* LXVII)+W 17360z (AUWE 23, no. 320) = lines 1′–17′
B = K 6422 (*TDP* XXIX) (coll. Heeßel 2000, 471) = lines 11′–35′

C = K 5860 (Heeßel 2000, 454)+ K 6717 (*TDP* XII) (coll. Heeßel 2000, 471) = lines 36′–49′

D = K 7009+BM 30011 (Heeßel 2000, 455–56) = lines 37′–83′, 91′–100′

E = K 2274+K 6284+K 7940+K 9134+K 11780 (Heeßel 2000, 457) = lines 84′–124′

F = W 17360v (*TDP* LXVII) = lines 84′–91′

G = VAT 14556 (*LKU* 93) = lines 104′–119′

DPS 21 is based on Heeßel 2000, 246–49

A = *LKU* 78 = lines 1–23

19/20E K 2274+K 6284+K 7940+K 9134+K 11780 (Heeßel 2000, 457) = line 1

DPS 22 is a combined edition based on Heeßel 2000, 250–71

A = AO 6678 (*TDP* XLV–XLVII) (coll.) = lines 1–78

B = K 2603 (*TDP* XLIV) (coll.) = lines 1–23

C = K 2203+K 3257 (Heeßel 2000, 458) (coll.) = lines 1–18

D = BM 68023+BM 68040 (Heeßel 2000, 459) (coll.) = lines 1–16, 69–78

E = K 3700+K 8673+K 11604 (*AMT* 2/4)+ K 11896+K 12227 (Heeßel 2000, 460–61) (coll.) = lines 23–78

DPS 23 is based on Heeßel 2000, 272–75

A = VAT 14539 (*LKU* 64) = 1–13, 14′–18′

22 D = BM 68023+BM 68040 (Heeßel 2000, 459) (coll.) = line 1

DPS 26 is a combined edition based on Heeßel 2000, 278–96. It was previously edited and translated into English by Stol 1993, 56–74 and translated by Kinnier Wilson and Reynolds 1990, 189–97.

A = *STT* 91+ *STT* 287 = lines 1′–53′, 57′–90′

B = BM 47753 (Stol 1993, 156–57) (coll. Heeßel 2000, 471) = lines 2′–56′, 62′–90′

DPS 27 is a combined edition based on Heeßel 2000, 297–306. It was previously translated into English by Stol 1993, 74–81.

A = AO 6680 (*TDP* XLVIII–XLIX) (coll.) = lines 1–36

B = A 3441 (*TDP* L–LI) (coll.) = lines 22–36

C = W 22743/1 (SpTU 3.89) = lines 16–36

26A = *STT* 91+ *STT* 287 = line 1

26B = BM 47753 (Stol 1993, 156–57) (coll. Heeßel 2000, 471) = line 1

DPS 28 is a combined edition based on Heeßel 2000, 307–17. It was previously translated into English by Stol 1993, 81–90.

A = AO 6680 (*TDP* XLVIII–XLIX) (coll.) = lines 1–13, 17–43
B = A 3441 (*TDP* L–LI) (coll.) = lines 1–43
C = W 22743/1 (SpTU 3.89) = lines 1–26
D = ND 4405/58 (CTN 4.70) = lines 30–43

DPS 29 is a combined edition based on Heeßel 2000, 318–38

A = BM 42310+BM 42401+BM 42623+BM 43121+BM 43231+BM 43318+BM 43351+BM 43416+BM 43647+unnumbered fragments (Heeßel 2000, 462–63) = lines 1–37, 55′–86′
B = BM 46563 (Heeßel 2000, 464) = lines 4–32
C = VAT 14596 (BAM 402 = *LKU* 58) (coll. Heeßel 2000, 471) = lines 38′–54′
28A = AO 6680 (*TDP* XLVIII–XLIX) (coll.) = line 1
28B = A 3441 (*TDP* L–LI) (coll.) = line 1
28D = ND 4405/58 (CTN 4.70) = line 1

DPS 30 is based on Heeßel 2000, 339–40

A = VAT 14538 (*LKU* 72)
29A = BM 42310+BM 42401+BM 42623+BM 43121+BM 43231+BM 43318+BM 43351+BM 43416+BM 43647+unnumbered fragments (Heeßel 2000, 462–63) = line 1

DPS 31 is a combined edition based on Heeßel 2000, 242–352

A = BM 38530 (Heeßel 2000, 466–467) (coll.) = lines 1–15, 41″–56″
B = IM 44568 (BAM 416) = lines 16′–40′
30A = VAT 14538 (*LKU* 72) = line 1

DPS 32 is represented only by the catchline of DPS 31.

31B = IM 44568 (BAM 4.416) = line 1

DPS 33 is a combined edition based on Heeßel 2000, 353–74. It was previously edited and translated into German by von Weiher in SpTU 4, 81–88.

A = W 23292 (SpTU 4.152) = lines 1–123
B = BM 121082 (CT 51.148) (coll.) = lines 21–32

DPS 34 is represented only by the catchline of DPS 33.

33A = W 23292 (SpTU 4.152) = line 1

DPS 36 is a combined edition made up of:

A = BM 92694 (*TDP* LII–LVI) (coll.) = lines 1–115
B = BM 65450+BM 76497 (coll.) = lines 14–66, 85–109
C = W17360f (*TDP* LXVI) = lines 76–88
D = K 7071 = lines 104–115

DPS 37 is a combined edition made up of:
A = A 3438 (*TDP* LVII) = lines 1–30
B = W 17360q (*TDP* LXVIII) = lines 24–27
36A = BM 92694 (*TDP* LII–LVI) (coll.) = line 1

DPS 40 is a combined edition made up of:
A = BM 92690 (*TDP* LVIII–LXII) (coll.) = lines 1–67, 73–122
B = BM 46228 (*TDP* LXIII, variants only) (coll.) = lines 1–123
C = VAT 14563 (*LKU* 101) (coll.) = lines 1–10
D = VAT 14549 (*LKU* 87) (coll.) = lines 5–22

TEXT BIBLIOGRAPHIES

In the interest of saving space, only editions of all or important sections of text, more or less full translations and the most important duplicates (those from which the text has been restored or with significant variants) are, in principle, given here. An = sign indicates a duplicate. A ~ sign indicates a parallel.

PART I: FOUNDATIONS

CHAPTER 2: PHARMACOLOGY

TEXT 1: BAM 1 (= *KAR* 203), COL. i 17–67

The most recent edition is Attia and Buisson 2012, 22–51. For the remainder of the text, see chapter 5, text 7.

Sections of this text appear verbatim in a number of other vademecum texts. Like many vademeca, its entries are also cited in medical commentaries and therapeutic texts.

Line 18 = BAM 380:26//BAM 381 iii 19.
Lines 19–20 = BAM 380:25//BAM 381 iii 17–18.
Lines 21–29 = CT 14.35 (K 4180+):22–30.
Lines 22–29 = CT 14.27 (K 4430):1′–8′.
Line 22 is cited in a therapeutic text, *AMT* 31/1+59/1 (= BAM VII pls. 1–2) i 19.
Line 23 is cited in *AMT* 31/1+59/1 (= BAM VII pls. 1–2) i 22 and i 32b.
Line 24 is cited in *AMT* 31/3+59/1 (= BAM VII pls. 1–2) i 25a.
Line 25 is cited in *AMT* 31/1+59/1 (= BAM VII pls. 1–2) i 30b.
Lines 30–35 = Scheil 1916, 37:18–23.
Line 35 = BAM 423 i 8′.
Line 36 = BAM 423 i 12′.
Line 40 = BAM 423 i 31′.

Line 53 ~ BAM 379 iii 24.
Line 59 is cited in two nonvademecum texts, BAM 318 iii 29 (therapeutic text) and BRM 4.32:19 (medical commmentary).
Line 62 = BAM 426 ii 14′; it is also cited in therapeutic texts BAM 494 ii 42//*AMT* 16/4:3′.
Lines 63–65 = BAM 426 ii 28′–30′.
Line 66 = BAM 423 i 25′; BAM 426 ii 31′.
Line 67 = BAM 426 ii 41′.

TEXT 2: SpTU 3.106 (OBVERSE)

For a transliteration and translation of the *Šammu šikinšu* series as a whole, see Stadhouders 2011, 17–21; 2012, 1–21.

The text is duplicated by BAM 379 i 18′–46′ and CTN 4.196+195 ii 21′–34′. More information about individual plants appears in other *Šammu šikinšu* texts (*KADP* 33; *STT* 93) as well as medical commentary BRM 4.32, various vademeca (BAM 1; BAM 380//BAM 381//STT 92) and Uruanna.

TEXT 3: BAM 378 ii–iii AND *STT* 108: 1–3, 13–35, 47–48

For an edition of the *Abnu šikinšu* series as a whole, as well as numerous stone lists, see Schuster-Brandis 2008, 17–47.

STT 108:1–3 = *STT* 109:1–3.
BAM 378 col. ii 0′–15′ = *STT* 108:4–12//STT 109:4–13.
STT 108:13–35 = *STT* 109:14–39.
BAM 378 iii 1′–19′ = *STT* 108:36–46//STT 109:40′–49′.
STT 108:47–48 = *STT* 109:50′.

TEXTS 4–5: CT 14.21–22 vii–viii 17–30, 42–51

Exact duplicates of URU.AN.NA texts are few and far between, but individual entries from this text appear also in *KADP* 1 i 19–21, *KADP* 2 i 38–40 and CT 37.32 iv 25′–33′, which have been used to restore broken passages.

CHAPTER 3: THE THERAPEUTIC SERIES

TEXT 1: BECKMAN AND FOSTER 1988, NO. 9

Restorations are based on the lines from the series that it cites. I have collated the catalogue fragments from photographs made for me in the Yale Babylonian Collection by Gojko Barjamovic.

TEXT 2: BAM 480

For an edition of this text, see Worthington 2005 (including a list of the many duplicates) and 2007. For a partial German translation (iii 8–25, iii 57–iv 4), see Heeßel 2011c, no. 2.3.2.

AMT 1/3:16′–17′ = iv 32–33.
BAM 3 i 1–10 = i 1–5; i 11–19 = i 7–12; i 20–22 = ii 19–20; i 23–25 = ii 23–25; ii 38–39 = ii 65; ii 40–41 = ii 67–68; ii 27–29 = iii 8–9; ii 14–17 = iii 22–25; ii 18–23 = iii 26–31; ii 7–8 = iv 5; ii 43–46 = iv 23–24; iii 42–46 = iv 26–29.
BAM 4 i 1′–12′ = i 1–15; iv 1′–2′ = iv 49′–50′.
BAM 9:23–34 = iii 8–15; 12–13 = iv 19–20.
BAM 10:20–29 = iii 10–13.
BAM 12:11′–12′ = i 30–31; 14′–15′ = i 32; 24′–25′ = i 54′; 38′–39′ = i 55′; 41′–42′ = i 57′; 44′–45′ = i 58′.
BAM 156:41–47 = iv 16–20.
BAM 481:6′–9′ = iii 17–19.
CTN 4.123:5′ = i 43′; 6′–7′ = i 45′; 8′–9′ = i 47′–48′.
Jastrow 1913 (Scurlock 2003, 16–17) obv. 1–6 = i 1–5; obv. 9–17 = ii 4–9; obv. 18–26 = iii 8–13; obv. 27–30 = iii 29–31; obv. 31–34 = iv 26–28; obv. 35–42 = iv 32–36; obv. 43–rev. 3′ = iv 38–41.
OECT 11.71:7′–8′ = iii 26–28; 9′–10′ = iii 32–33; 11′–13′ = iii 36–37; 14′–16′ = iii 42–44.

TEXT 3: BAM 156

A German translation of lines 1–24 appears in Maul 2011, text 2.5.13.

BAM 9:12–13 = 45–47.
BAM 52:39–44 = 21–24.

BAM 67:1′–9′ = 21–24.
BAM 480 iv 16–20 = 41–47.
BAM 494 iii 24′–28′ = 25–31; iii 31′–35′ = 32–39.
BAM 579 i 40–44 = 21–24.
Herrero 1975, 41–53 ii 1–6 = 1–10; ii 8–14 = 11–18.

CHAPTER 4: MEDICAL TEXT COMMENTARIES

TEXT 1: SpTU 1.47

The text is edited in the original text publication volume. A German translation of lines 1–11, 13–15 appears as Frahm 2011, text 6.1.

TEXT 2: BRM 4.32 AND TCL 6.34 i

For a German translation of lines i 1′–8′ of TCL 6.34, see Böck 2011, text 2.10.4. Restorations in the text are from *AMT* 35/3 i 1′–6′ and BAM 178:1′–7′. For a German translation of lines 1–4, 7–8, 10, 15–16 of BRM 4.32, see Frahm 2011, text 6.2. For the whole text and TCL 6.34, see Geller 2010, 168–76.

TEXT 3 (GHOSTS): SpTU 1.49

The text is edited in the original text publication volume.

TEXT 4 (DIFFICULT CHILDBIRTH): CIVIL 1974, NO. 2

This text is edited in Civil 1974, 329–36. For lines 1–3, 6–15, 17, 21, 30–36, 38–40, 43–44, 46, 48, 51, see Veldhuis 1989, 239–48, text c. A German translation of lines 8–9, 11–12, 40–43 is to be found in Frahm 2011, text 6.3. For an extensive discussion, see Cavigneaux 1987, 252–55.

PART 2: THERAPEUTICS

CHAPTER 5: EYES, EARS, NOSE, AND MOUTH

TEXT 1: SpTU 2.50

The text is edited in the original text publication volume.

BM 54641+BM 54826 (Fincke 2009, 84–93) obv. 19′–20′ = 15–17; rev. 4 = 18–19; rev. 1 = 20–21; rev. 5 = 22–23; rev. 9 ~ 24.
BM 132097 (Geller 1988, 22–23) obv. 11′–14′ = 5–9; obv. 16′ = 27–28.
BAM 159 iv 28′–29′ = 18–19; iv 26′–27′ = 20–21.
Heeßel and Al–Rawi 2003, 223 ii 4–5 = 22–23.

TEXT 2: BAM 159 iv 0′–v 9

For more of this text, see chapter 5, text 8; chapter 9, texts 3–6, 8; chapter 10, text 3 and chapter 11, text 2.

AMT 18/4:1′–5′ = iv 16′–22′.
BAM 18:3–4 ~ iv 23′–25′.
BAM 20:9′–10′ = iv 0′–1′; 11′–17′ = iv 2′–7′.
BAM 22:23′–24′ = v 5–6.
BAM 510 i 18′–20′ = iv 2′–7′.
BAM 513 i 8′–10′ = iv 2′–7′.
BAM 515 i 10, i 57′ = iv 0′–1′; ii 45–47 = iv 2′–7′.
BAM 518:8′ = iv 0′–1′; 6′–7′ = iv 8′–10′; 9′–12′ = iv 11′–15′.
BAM 521:10′–12′ = iv 16′–22′
BM 54641+BM 54826 (Fincke 2009, 84–93) rev. 1 = iv 26′–27′; rev. 4 = iv 28′–29′; rev. 8 = v 3–4.
Heeßel and Al-Rawi 2003, 223 ii 20–21 = iv 0′–1′.
SpTU 2.50:20–21 = iv 26′–27′; 18–19 = iv 28′–29′.

TEXT 3: BAM 503

The “hand” of ghost sections are treated in Scurlock 2006 as nos. 339, 316, 159, 136a, 145, 149a, 150, 146–147, 137a, 138, 139a, 140–142, 151, 148, 152–154, 132–135, 161–162, 160 for which see also the review in Schwemer

2009, 168–77. For a discussion and a German translation of i 28′–40′ and ii 58′–72′, see Heeßel 2011c, text 2.4.1.

BAM 3 iv 33–34 = i 31′–32′; iii 50–52 = ii 61′–62′; iv 12–13 = ii 63′–65′; iv 14–16 = ii 67′–71′; iv 28–30 = iv 29–31.
BAM 506:22′–23′ ~ i 22′–23′; 14′–17′ = i 41′–ii 2; 18′ = ii 6; 19′–21′ ~ ii 9–12; 26′–27′ = ii 16–17; 32′–37′ = ii 31′–36′.
BAM 507:2′–5′ = ii 16–17; 6′–14′ = ii 31′–36′.
BAM 508 iv 1–2 = i 28′–29′; iv 18–34 = ii 22′–36′.
BAM 512:4′–5′ = iv 18–19.
BM 41289 ii 4′–13′ = iv 11–19.
BM 41373 i 1–4 = iii 48′–51′; i 6–10 = iii 52′–56′.
BM 76023+83009 i 1′–5′ = i 20′–23′.
CT 51.199:1–4 = i 28′–29′; 5–13 ~ i 31′–32′; 14–20 = ii 31′–36′.
CTN 4.113 ii 4–8 = iv 11–14.
Heeßel and Al-Rawi 2003, 223 i 43–45 = i 31′–32′; i 30–36 = ii 63′–66′.
Labat 1959, 1–18 rev. 29–30 = i 31′–32′; rev. 18–21 = ii 63′–66′.
Labat 1957, 109–22 v 13′–16′ = i 17′–18′; ii 11′–20′ = ii 53′–57′; ii 1′–7′ = iii 12–15; iv 10′–14′ = iv 11–14; iii 17–18 ~ iv 19; iii 4–9 = iv 29–31.

TEXT 4: *AMT* 105/1 iv 7–20

AMT 35/5:1′–8′ = iv 8–16.
AMT 38/5:2′–6′ = iv 7–11.
Labat 1957, 109–22 v 18–19 = iv 7–8.

TEXT 5: SpTU 1.45 REVERSE

The text is edited in the original text publication volume.

BAM 543 i 68′ ~ rev. 16′–17′.
BM 42634+42635+43163:7–12//BM 43496+43652 (Finkel 2000, no. 13) obv. 7′–12′ = rev. 22′.
SpTU 1.44:34 ~ rev. 16′–17′.

TEXT 6: SpTU 1.44:16–83

Apart from the edition in SpTU 1, a discussion and a German translation of lines 1–12, 26–39, 69–83 appears as Heeßel 2011c, text 2.4.3.

AMT 54/3 i 1′–6′ = 55–61; ii 1′–11′ = 69–76.
BAM 28 rev. 3′–13′ = 69–76.
BAM 29:1′–36′ = 62–76.
BAM 533:36–47 = 55–61; 50–56 = 65–67.
BAM 536:1′–9′ = 52b-61.
BAM 537 rev. 1′–8′ = 55–61.
BAM 543 ii 24–28 = 16–19; ii 11–23 = 20–28; ii 6–10 = 31–33; i 68′ = 34; i 63′–67′ ~ 35–39; iv 11–13 = 40–41; iv 22′–23′ = 44–45; ii 46′–49′ = 51–54; iii 43′–iv 5 = 55–76.
BM 66560 obv. 2′–9′ = 24–31; rev. 1′–11′ = 46–54.
BM 67158:4′–8′ = 48–50.
BM 76515 obv. 13–15 = 48–50.
CTN 4.114 obv. 1′–4′ = 29–30.
Heeßel and al-Rawi 2003, 223 ii 35–47 = 35–39.

TEXT 7: BAM 1 i 1–16

For the rest of this text, see chapter 2, text 1.

Sections of this text appear verbatim in a number of other vademecum texts. Like many vademeca, its entries are also cited in medical commentaries and therapeutic texts.

Lines 1–15 = CT 14.23 (K 259):1–15.
Line 2 is cited in BAM 538 ii 48′ (therapeutic text).
Line 3 = CTN 4.194:8.
Line 4 = CTN 4.194:7.
Line 11 = CTN 4.194:9.
Line 12 is cited in BAM 159 v 15–16 (therapeutic text)
Line 15 = CTN 4.194:10.
Line 16 is cited in BAM 159 v 23–25 (therapeutic text).

TEXT 8: BAM 159 v 10–16

For more of this text, see chapter 5, text 2; chapter 9, texts 3–6, 8; chapter 10, text 3; chapter 11, text 2.

BAM 543 i 1–2 = v 10–14

TEXT 9: CT 17.50

For bibliography and a French translation, see Bottéro 1978–79, 88–89. For a more recent German transliteration and translation which also puts the text into its greater context, see Dietrich and Loretz 2000, 491–504. See also Dietrich 2000, 209–20.

AMT 23/6:1′–7′ = 10–26
BAM 538 iv 31′–39′ = 5–26.

CHAPTER 6: FEVER

TEXT 1: BAM 147

A discussion and German translation of obv. 1–24, rev. 5′–25′ appears in Böck 2011 as text 2.8.4.

AMT 19/2 ii 2′–5′+*AMT* 63/2:9′–11′ = rev. 1′–4′
BAM 148 obv. 1–33 = obv. 1–33, rev. 3′–27′ = rev. 1′–25′.
BM 35512 rev. 11–14 = obv. 25–33.
BM 42272:72 = rev. 3′–4′; 54–62 = rev. 5′–16′.
K 2581 obv. 7′–19′ = rev. 5′–16′.

TEXT 2: BM 42272:32–85

AMT 19/2 ii 4′–5′+*AMT* 63/2:11′ = 72.
BAM 147 rev. 5′–16′ = 54–62; rev. 3′–4′ = 72.
BAM 148 rev. 7′–18′ = 54–62, rev. 5′–6′ = 72.
BAM 149:10′–13′ = 49–51.
BAM 315 i 38–41 = 32–36; i 33 = 74; i 34–35 = 76–77; i 36 = 80.

BM 35512 obv. 1–23 = 32–72; 24–26 = 74–77.
K 2581 obv. 1′–5′ = 32–36; obv. 7′–19′ = 54–62.
K 3628+4009+Sm. 1315 (chapter 13, text 1) obv. 11′ ~ 70–71.

TEXT 3: TSUKIMOTO 1999, 199–200:1–36

This text, probably from Middle Babylonian Emar, was first published and edited in the work by which it is cited here. Corrections to the recitations appear in Finkel 1999 and Böck 2007, 62, 295–96. The text is discussed and translated into German as Schwemer 2011, text 2.2.2. For lines 37–97, see chapter 7, text 3.

TEXT 4: BAM 106 OBV. 1–10

AMT 39/4 rev. 3′–9′ = obv. 1–7.
BAM 52:101 (catchline) = obv. 1.
BAM 107:1–8 = obv. 4–8
BAM 108 rev. 2′–22′ = obv. 1–10.
BAM 109:1–16 = obv. 4–8
BM 42298 (Finkel 2000, no. 181):23–25 = obv. 1–4.

TEXT 4: BAM 107

AMT 39/4 rev. 6′–9′ = 1–8.
BAM 106 obv. 4–8 = 1–8.
BAM 108 rev. 7′–17′ = 1–8.
BAM 109:1–16 = 1–8.

TEXT 5: BAM 145 (= *KAR* 199)

BAM 146:29′–42′ = 1–23.

TEXT 6: BAM 480 iii 8–21

See chapter 3, text 2 and chapter 7, text 7.

BAM 3 ii 27–29 = iii 8–9.
BAM 9:23–30 = iii 8–13.
BAM 10:20–29 = iii 10–13.
BAM 481:6′–9′ = iii 17–19.
Jastrow 1913 (Scurlock 2003, 16–17) obv. 18–26 = iii 8–13.

CHAPTER 7: SKIN AND BONES

TEXT 1: BAM 33

For a German translation of lines 1–8, see Böck 2011, text 2.9.5.

AMT 6/1:9–11 = 1–7.
BM 41294(+)41284 (Fincke 2011b, 187–88) ii 8′–11′ = 1–7; i 4′–9′ = 9–18.
Labat 1959, 1–18 obv. 30–33 = 1–7.

TEXT 2: BAM 156:25–40

See chapter 3, text 3. A discussion of lines 25–31 appears in Böck 2003, 170.

BAM 494 iii 24′–28′ = 25–31; iii 29′–35′ ~ 32–39.

TEXT 3: TSUKIMOTO 1999, 199–200:37–97

This text, probably from Middle Babylonian Emar, was first published and edited in the work by which it is cited here. Corrections to the recitations appear in Finkel 1999. For a discussion, see Böck 2007, 64–65. The text is translated in Schwemer 2011, text 2.2.2. For lines 1–36, see part 2, chapter 6, text 3.

TEXT 4: BAM 32

For a German translation of lines 5′–12′ see Böck 2011, text 2.9.3.

BAM 417 obv. 1–13 = 1′–15′.
CTN 4.116:16–17 = 16′–17′

TEXT 5: *AMT* 16/5 ii 1–10

The text is unedited and has no known duplicates.

TEXT 6: BAM 480 iii 57–IV 8

See chapter 3, text 2 and chapter 6, text 6.

BAM 3 ii 7–8 = iv 5.

TEXT 7: BAM 124 i 1–ii 50

A German translation of lines i 1–18, ii 34–35 appears as Böck 2011, text 2.11.2.

AMT 73/1 i 11–14+*AMT* 15/3 i 21–24 = i 1–7.
AMT 73/1 i 15–27 = i 8–23.
AMT 73/1 i 28–34+*AMT* 18/5 obv. 1′–8′ = i 24–32.
AMT 73/1 ii 1′–*AMT* 74/1 ii 23′ = ii 25–50.

TEXT 8: BAM 124 ii 51–iv 35

A discussion and German translation of iii 44–59 appears as Böck 2011, 2.11.3. For iv 22–26 and 28–33, see Böck 2007, 58, 312.

AMT 32/5 rev.(!) 10′–11′ = iii 1–2; rev.(!) 7′–9′ = iii 41–43.
AMT 32/5 rev.(!) 14′–15′ +*AMT* 43/3:3′–4′ = iii 3–5.
AMT 32/5 rev.(!) 12′–13′+*AMT* 43/3:1′–2′ = iii 6–8.
AMT 42/6 obv. 3–6 = iii 60–iv 1.
AMT 75/1 iii 31–32 = iii 18–21.
AMT 93/2 rev. 3–5 = iii 1–2.
BAM 125:1–34 = iii 44–60.
BAM 127:1–14 = iii 60–iv 27.
BAM 128 iv 1′–33′ = iv 10–34.
BAM 131 rev. 4′–6′ = iii 3–5; rev. 1′–3′ = iii 6–8.
BAM 181:1–16 = ii 51–iii 6; l.e. 1–2 = iii 12–13.
BM 30918:18–35 = iii 44–59.

CT 23.1–2:15–20 = iii 60–iv 9.

CHAPTER 8: HEART AND LUNGS

TEXT 1: BAM 388

BAM 445:10–25 ~ i 12–19f.
TCL 6.34 iii 3–16 = i 3–19f.

TEXT 2: BAM 548

For references, and a German translation of i 1–18, see Heeßel 2011c, text 2.4.6.

AMT 49/1 iv 11′ (catchline) = i 1.
AMT 80/1 i 1–28 = i 1–28.
AMT 81/1 iv 1′–5′ = iv 12′–15′.
BAM 552 iv 4′–17′ = iv 2′–15′.

TEXT 3: BM 78963

BAM 42:24–35 ~ 25–31.
BAM 43:4′–5′ ~ 22–24.
BAM 44:5′–6′ = 20–21; 11′–12′ ~ 22–24; 22′–32′ and 33′–39′ ~ 25–31.
BAM 52:39–44 ~ 1–3; 88 ~16.
BAM 67:1′–9′ ~ 1–3.
BAM 159 iii 28–29 = 84.
BAM 161 vii 13–16 ~ 22–24.
BAM 259 obv. 1–rev. 6 ~ 25–31.
BAM 316 iv 2 = 84.
BAM 579 i 40–44 ~ 1–3.
BM 32277+ ii 1′–4′ ~ 25–31
BM 76515 rev. 7′–8′ = 4–6.
Heeßel and Al-Rawi 2003, 229 iv 7–10 ~ 22–24; iv 24–44 ~ 25–31.

TEXT 4: BAM 558

BAM 44:14′–15′ = i 14′–15′.
BAM 174 obv. 11′–20′ = iv 7–14.
BAM 389:10′–13′ = i 18′–22′.
BM 47672:11′–15′ = i 18′–22′.
Heeßel and Al-Rawi 2003, 229 iv 14–19 = i 14′–15′.

TEXT 5: BAM 55

BAM 56 rev. 8′–11′ = 1–17.
BAM 57:1′–14′ = 1–17.
BAM 575 iii 30–36 = 1–17.

TEXT 6: BAM 39

AMT 49/4 rev. 1–9 = 1′–9′.
BAM 520 ii 8′–10′ ~ 1′–2′.

CHAPTER 9: GASTROINTESTINAL TRACT

TEXT 1: *AMT* 76/1

Individual treatments appear in Scurlock 2006 as nos. 312, 200, 197–98, 304b, 308b, 309–11 for which see also the review in Schwemer 2009, 168–76.

TEXT 2: *STT* 96

The text has not been edited and has no known duplicates.

TEXT 3: BAM 159 ii 20–48

For more of this text, see chapter 5, texts 2 and 8; chapter 9, texts 4–6, 8; chapter 10, text 3; and chapter 11, text 2.

BAM 73 ii 1–7 = ii 20–27.

BAM 482 iv 7–8 ~ ii 46–48

TEXT 4: BAM 159 v 33–47

For more of this text, see chapter 5, texts 2 and 8; chapter 9, texts 3, 5–6 8; chapter 10, text 3 and chapter 11, text 2.

BAM 579 iv 1–11 ~ v 37–47

TEXT 5: BAM 159 v 48–vi 33

For more of this text, see chapter 5, texts 2 and 8; chapter 9, texts 3, 4, 6, and 8; chapter 10, text 3; and chapter 11, text 2.

BAM 70:2′–6′ = vi 1–4.
BAM 85:2′–8′ = vi 25–33.
BAM 86:3′–8′ = vi 26–33.
BAM 108 obv. 1–7 = vi 1–4.
BAM 110:3′–11′ = vi 1–4.
BAM 168:66–69 = vi 1–4.
BM 29254:1–7 = vi 24–28.

TEXT 6: BAM 159 ii 49–iii 24, 47–56

For more of this text, see chapter 5, texts 2 and 8; chapter 9, texts 3–5, 8; chapter 10, text 3; and chapter 11, text 2.

TEXT 7: BAM 578

The recitation of lines ii 29–38 is edited in Michalowski 1981, 1–18. Medical aspects of the text are discussed in Haussperger 2001,108–22. A German translation of i 1–14, 16, 18, 20–26, ii 20–22, 29–49, 67–70, iii 4–12, 16, 19–22, iv 5, 16, 26–29, 31–34, 45–46 is to be found in Böck 2011 as text 2.7.3.

AMT 14/7:1–2 (catchline) = iv 47.
BAM 52:97–100 = i 70–ii 1.

BAM 60:1′–3′ = i 14–16; 3′–6′ = i 18–19; 7′–12′ = i 38–40.
BAM 62:1–4 = i 70–ii 1.
BAM 64 i(!) 9′–16′ = i 14–19; ii(!) 2′–13′ = iii 16–24.
BAM 159 i 29–37 = i 38–41; i 38–42 = i 50–52.
BAM 174 rev. 1–3 ~ i 65–66.
BAM 575 iv 54 (catchline) = i 1.
BAM 579 i 34–37 ~ i 65–66.
BM 38583:12′–24′ ~ iii 21–24.
BM 76510 rev. 1′–5′ = i 39–41.
Labat and Tournay 1945–46, 113–22:1–3 = ii 13.

TEXT 8: BAM 159 i 21–ii 19

For more of this text, see chapter 5, texts 2 and 8; chapter 9, texts 3–6; chapter 10, text 3; and chapter 11, text 2.

BAM 60:7′–12′ = i 29–35.
BAM 160:2′–8′ = ii 11–16.
BAM 578 i 38–41 = i 29–37; i 50–52 = i 38–42.
BM 76510 rev. 1′–5′ = i 31–37.

TEXT 9: BAM 77

BAM 78:1–6 = 20′–24′.

CHAPTER 10: GENITOURINARY TRACT

TEXT 1: BAM 396 i–iii

The text is edited in BAM VII as no. 1; for specific suggestions for improvements to this text, see the reviews of BAM VII in Böck 2008, 324, Buisson 2006, 185–88 and Scurlock 2009, 38–40. There is also a German translation of i 10′–18′ and 23′–31′ in Geller 2011 as text 2.6.1.

AMT 34/3:1–12 = iii 6–27.
AMT 59/1 i 29–30 = i 1′–3′; i 31–32 = i 6′–9′.
AMT 66/7 iii 18–22 = i 23′–31′.

AMT 66/11+65/6+Sm 126+K 11230 (BAM VII no. 16):17–23 = ii 0′–12′.
BAM 111 iii 15′–18′ = ii 0′–4′; iii 8′–14′ = ii 5′–12′.
BAM 115:2′–4′ = ii 25′–31′; 5′–9′ = iii 21–32.

TEXT 2: BAM 396 iv

AMT 61/1 (BAM VII no. 2A): 5′–8′ = iv 6–12.
BAM 159 i 9–11 = iv 3–5.
BAM 182 obv. 6′ = iv 3–5.

TEXT 3: BAM 159 i 1–20

For more of this text, see chapter 5, texts 2 and 8; chapter 9, texts 3–6, 8; and chapter 11, text 2.

BAM 111 ii 15′–20′ = i 15–20.
BAM 161 v 21–25 = i 12–14.
BAM 182 obv. 6′ = i 9–11.
BAM 396 iv 3–5 = i 9–11.

TEXT 4: BAM 272

The text and its duplicates are edited in Biggs 1967, 52, 53, 53–54, 55, 63–64.

AMT 73/2:3–8 = 0′–6′.
KAR 70:22–27 = 20′–23′
LKA 99d ii 1–5 = 0′–6′; ii 6–17 = 15′–23′.

TEXT 5: BAM 580 iii 15′–25′

This section of the text has no known duplicate.

CHAPTER 11: NEUROLOGY

TEXT 1: BAM 11 (= *KAR* 188)

The text is edited in Heeßel 2009, 13–28. Lines 21–35 are treated in Scurlock 2006 as nos. 55–56, 62–64, 99–100, and 105. A German translation appears in Heeßel 2011c, text 2.3.1.

AMT 20/1 i! 1–2 = 9; i! 5–9 = 10–15; i! 36′–37′ = 32–33; i! 42′–43′ = 34–35.
BAM 9:35–39 = 4–6; 61–63 = 19–20.
BAM 480 iv 50′//BAM 4 iv 2′ [catchline] = 1.
BAM 482 i 1–4 = 1–3; i 7–14 = 4–9; i 17–22 = 10–15; ii 17–18 = 18; ii 2–3 = 19–20; i 49′–50′ = 32–33; i 54′–55′ = 34–35.
Jastrow 1913 (Scurlock 2003, 16–17) rev. 4′–7′ = 4–6, rev. 13′–15′ = 19–20.

TEXT 2: BAM 159 iii 25–34

For more of this text, see chapter 5, text 8; chapter 9, text 3–6, 8; and chapter 10, text 3. A German translation of lines iii 25–27 appears in Böck 2011 as text 2.10.5.

BAM 316 iv 2 = iii 28–29
BM 42272:21–22 = iii 30–32.
BAM 185 v 50–52 = iii 33–34.
BM 78963:84 = iii 28–29.
SpTU 1.60 rev. 14′–16′ = iii 30–34.

TEXT 3: BAM 398 (= BE 31.56)

For lines obv. 1–35 and rev. 24′–41′, see Limet 1986, 83–87. A German translation appears in Böck 2011, text 2.10.11.

AMT 82/2 iii! 7–8 = obv. 1, 8–11; iii! 11–12 = obv. 12–15.
AMT 92/6:5–7 = rev. 24′–27′; 2–4 = rev. 38′–41′.
AMT 98/3:8–12 = rev. 28′–37′.
BAM 138 ii 1–8 = obv. 1 (the symptoms) and obv. 8–11 (the treatment).
BAM 159 vi 51–54 = rev. 24′–27′.
AMT 92/4+*AMT* 92/9+BM 20179 iii 12′–iv 6 = rev. 42′–52′.

TEXT 4: BAM 122

A German translation of lines 1–24 appears in Böck 2011 as text 2.11.6–7.

AMT 68/1 rev. 8–11 = rev. 2′–10′.
AMT 70/7 ii 7′–10′ = obv. 8–15; ii 3′–6′ ~ obv. 16–rev. 1.
BAM 405:12′–13′ = obv. 1–7.
BAM 406 rev. 8′–10′ ~ obv. 8–11.

CHAPTER 12: OBSTETRICS AND GYNECOLOGY

TEXT 1: BAM 237 (= *KAR* 194) i AND iv

A German translation of i 9′– 29′, iv 9–10, 12–13 appears in Böck 2011 as text, 2.12.7.

BAM 241 ii 5′–8′ = iv 9–10.

TEXT 2: UET 7.123

The text is edited in Reiner 1982, 124–38. A German translation of obv. 1–12 appears in Böck 2011 as text 2.12.3.

BM 42313+43174 rev. 29–32 ~ obv. 1–7

TEXT 3: BAM 235

BAM 236 rev. 1′–9′ = 10–16.

TEXT 4: SpTU 3.84:56–78

This text is edited in von Weiher, SpTU 3 as no. 84. For a discussion, see Farber 1989a, 229–30.

BM 42327+BM 51246:1–13 (Farber 1989b, 112–15 §§ 39a–40) = 56–61.
Farber 1989b, pls. 14–15:14–39 = 62–78.

LKA 9 rev. 7′–13′, 15′ (Farber 1989b, 110–11 § 39) = 56–57.
Thureau-Dangin 1921, 163 rev. 13–29 = 62–77.

TEXT 5: FARBER 2014, PL. 9 (4R² 56) ii 28–34 COMPLETED BY *LKU* 33

The text is edited in Farber 2014 in scored transliteration, transcription and translation as Lamaštu Series I, lines 100-150, Texts C1 and n. These lines appear on pp. 82-87 (transliteration) and 154-157 (transcription and translation). 4R2 56 ii 28-33 was recopied as Farber 2014, pl. 9. *LKU* 33 was collated.

Farber 2014, pl. 24 ii 37–43 = ii 28–34
Farber 2014, pl. 43 iv 33 = ii 28
Farber 2014, pl. 53 i 1-7 = ii 28–34
Farber 2014, pl. 60 ii 8-13 = ii 28–34
Farber 2014, pls. 24–25 ii 42-45, ii 1′–iii 21 = i 1′–45′
Farber 2014, pls. 53–54 i 6-57 = i 2′–45′
Farber 2014, pl. 59 i 3′-10′ = i 7′–14′
Farber 2014, pl. 70 i 1′–5′ ~ i 13′–39′
Farber 2014, pls. 9–10 ii 1′–iii 9 = i 32′–45′

TEXT 6: YOS XI 86:1–28

Bibliography: The text is edited in van Dijk 1973, 502–7.

TEXT 7: BAM 248

For a general discussion of this text and some fragmentary duplicates to i 1–35, see Veldhuis 1989, 239–60. For the recitations involving the moon god's Cow in general, see Veldhuis 1991. A German translation of lines iv 13–17 appears in Böck 2011 as text no. 2.12.9. Particularly helpful in reconstructing the text is the ancient commentary, Civil 1974, 332 (chapter 4, text 4).

AMT 67/1 iii 1–29 = iii 10–39; iv 1–31 = iv 8–38.
BAM 249 i 8′–12′ = iv 13–16.
K 3485+K 18482 (Veldhuis 1989, 256–57):1–10 = iii 1–10.
K 8210 (Veldhuis 1989, 255) i 9′–14′ = i 36–41.
K 10443 (Veldhuis 1989, 256): 1–15 = ii 54–68.

VS 17.34 (van Dijk 1972, 343–44):1–10 ~ i 37–43.

TEXT 8: LAMBERT 1969, PL. 5

This is edited in Lambert 1969, 28–39. For further discussion, see Stol 2000, 130. An English translation appears in Foster 1996, 875.

TEXT 9: BAM 240 (= *KAR* 195)

A German translation of rev. 70′–74′ appears in Böck 2011 as text 2.12.2, of obv. 17′–22′ as text 2.12.8 and of obv. 26′–27′, 29′ and rev. 39′–42′, 50′–53′, 58′ as text 2.12.10.

CHAPTER 13: PEDIATRICS

TEXT 1: K 3628+4009+SM. 1315

BAM 183:12–13 = obv. 19; 10–11 = obv. 20.
BAM 248 iv 41 = obv. 20; iv 42–43 = obv. 17–19.
DPS 40:28 = obv. 6; 60 = obv. 7; 112 = obv. 8; 113 = obv. 9.
KAR 76:14–19 = rev. 3–7.
KAR 88 fragment 3 obv! i 10–14 = rev. 3–7.
STT 215 i 65–69 = rev. 3–7.

TEXT 2: CAMPBELL THOMPSON 1940, 110 NO. 38

The text is duplicated by Wiseman 1950, 197 no. 280:1–9 and Scheil 1898, 201:1–12. For bibliography, see Scheil 1898, 200–201.

TEXT 3: BAM 248 iv 39–43

For the rest of this text, see chapter 12, text 7.

BAM 183:8–11 = iv 39–41; 12–13 = iv 43.
K 3628+4009+Sm. 1315 obv. 20 = iv 41; obv. 17–19 = iv 42–43

TEXT 4: BM 62376

This text is unique and has no known duplicate.

CHAPTER 14: POISONING, IMAGINARY AND OTHERWISE; ENDOCRINE DISORDERS

TEXT 1: BM 42272:1–31

For the rest of this text see chapter 6, text 2.

BAM 59:13–20 = obv. 3–9.
BAM 159 iii 30–32 = obv. 21–22.
BAM 161 iii 1′–7′ = obv. 3–9.
BAM 190:1–8 = obv. 3–9.
BAM 430 vi 8–18 = obv. 3–8.
BAM 431 v 50′–vi 5′ = obv. 3, 6–8.
BAM 434 iii 52′–54′ = obv. 7–9.
ABRT 2.11 rev. iii 20–27 = obv. 10–15.
CT 51.202 iv 2–9 = obv. 10–15.
K 8447 (BA 10/1 81 no. 7)+89–4–26,133:1–8 (for anger) = obv. 10–15.
K 15239:3′–8′ = obv. 10–15.
81–7–27,205:1–15 (for curse) = obv. 10–17.
KAL 2 no. 49:1–8 = obv. 3–7.
SpTU 1.60 rev. 14′–15′ = obv. 21–22.

TEXT 2: BAM 438

This text is edited in Abusch and Schwemer 2011 as text no. 7.2 A.

TEXT 2: BAM 59

BAM 161 iii 2′–7′ = 14–20.
BAM 190 (KAL 2 no. 49):9–21 = 1–12; 1–8 = 13–20.
BAM 430 iv 7′–24′ = 1–9; vi 8–18 = 13–20.
BAM 431 iv 2–19 = 1–9; v 50′–vi 5′ = 13, 17–20.
BAM 434 iii 53′–54′ = 20.
BAM 437 obv. 1′–6′ = 3–8.

BAM 438 obv. 16–27 = 1–12.
BAM 575 iii 51–54 = 21–28.
BM 42272:3–9 = 13–20.

TEXT 3: BAM 575 iii 49–54

For an edition of this text and further context, see Heeßel 2002, 99–106.

TEXT 4: K 2351+10639 (= *AMT* 13/4)+8184+5859 (+) K 3293 (= BAM 460) (COPY: AMD 8/1 PL. 122)

Both K 2351+ and BAM 453 are edited in Abusch and Schwemer 2011, 2–11 as texts 10.4 A and C, respectively, except that the duplicate BAM 467 has been missed. Not clearly indicated is the fact that BAM 453 duplicates the last two sections of K 2351+ and provides its continuation.

BAM 467 right col. 1′–11′ = 1–9.
BAM 453:1′–7′ = 22–28.

TEXT 5: BAM 453:7′–10′

See text 4, above.

TEXT 6: BAM 449 iii 13′–27′

BAM 449 is edited in Abusch and Schwemer 2011 as text no. 10.3 A_1.

BAM 455 iii 4′–11′ = iii 13′–16′.
BAM 467 left col. 1′–11′ = iii 14′–19′.

TEXT 7: BAM 361: 35–48

BAM 361:35–48 are edited in Maul 1994, 109–11 and Schuster-Brandis 2008, 358, 364–65. A German translation of the entire text appears in Heeßel 2011c, no. 3.3.

K 3010 (+)(Schuster-Brandis 2008, pl. 33) v 13′–16′ = 39–43.
BAM 386 iv 11′–14′ = 44–48.
K 8785:11′–13′ = 44–48.

PART 3: HOLISTIC HEALING

CHAPTER 15: PRAYERS AND STONE CHARMS

TEXT 1: BM 50346

The text is edited as Scurlock 2006, no. 176, and in Schuster-Brandis 2008, 141.

TEXT 2: *STT* 95+295

I have benefited from the forthcoming edition by Henry Stadhouders in *Journal des Médicines Cunéiformes*, which is based on photographs of the original.

AMT 40/2+K 9085:1′–9′ = 1–12.
BAM 205:19′–27′ = 16–22.
BAM 314 obv. 8′–12′ = 59–61; obv. 4′–7′ = 63–65; obv. 1′–3′ = 68–69.
BAM 315 ii 17–20 ~ 30–31; ii 6–7 ~ 41; ii 8–12 ~ 46–47; iii 37–38 = 53–54; iii 35–36 = 62; iii 39–41 = 63–65; iii 42–43 = 68–69; ii 26–32 ~ 105–108; iv 19–21 = 118–120.
BAM 316 iv 3–6 = 70–73; vi 4′–13′ = 84–91ff; i 12′–14′ = 118–120; iii 1′–7′ = 121–125; iv 7–10 = 126–129; ii 5′–25′ ~ 130–144; iii 13′–16′ = 145–148.
BAM 317 rev. 27–30 = 7–12; rev. 1–3 ~ 91ff; rev. 16–18 = 145–148.
BAM 320:27′–33′ = 18–22.
BAM 376 iv 30–31 ~ 123, 125.
BAM 447:4′–6′ = 145–148.
BM 56148+ (Schuster-Brandis 2008, 281–318, pls. 9–27) vi 25 ~ 30–31; ii 42–43 ~ 32–34; i 39–40 ~ 35–40; vi 28 ~ 41; vi 30 ~ 47; vi 31–33 ~ 66–67; vi 26 ~ 80–81.
BM 64174:1–8 (Geller 1988, 21–22) = 130–140.
K 8907 obv. 8′–11′ = 1–6, 14′–17′ = 16–22.
KAL 4.35 iv 1–4 = 1–6; iv 5–17 = 84–91
KAR 92 rev. 4–8 = 70–74.

Labat 1950, 17–18 ii 28′–29′ = 121–122.
STT 280 ii 1–7 = 16–22.

TEXT 3: K 2581

For a discussion of rev. 5′–20′ of this text, see van der Toorn 1985,135–36 and the copy on pls. 1–2. Von Soden 1987, 71 argues for exchanging obverse and reverse. However, the order of treatments on the text seems more appropriate to the current assignments and indeed what is now the reverse is slightly curved, as would be expected. For the rest of the text, see chapter 16, text 3.

CHAPTER 16: HEALING RITUALS

TEXT 1: BAM 542 iii 1–19

CTN 4.196 ii 4′–9′ = iii 13–16.

TEXT 2: BAM 30 (= *LKA* 136)

A German translation of 8′–46′ appears in Heeßel 2011c, 57–59.

BAM 157 obv. 6′–9′ = 47′–53′.
BAM 311:87′–89′ = 22′–24′; 90′ = 27′–28′; 91′ = 36′–37′; 93′ = 38′–40′; 92′ = 43′.
BAM 372 iii 4′–5′ ~ 44′–46′.
BAM 376 ii 16′–17′ = 44′–46′.

TEXT 3: K 2581

For a copy of K 2581 and an edition of rev. 5′–20′ of this text, see van der Toorn 1985, 135–36 and pls. 1–2.

BAM 147 rev. 5′–16′ = obv. 7–19.
BAM 148 rev. 7′–18′ = obv. 7–19.
BAM 315 i 38–41 = obv. 1–5.
BM 35512 obv. 1–3 = obv. 1–5; obv. 14–19 = obv. 7–19.

BM 42272:32–36 = obv. 1–5; 54–62 = obv. 7–19.

TEXT 3: *AMT* 53/7+K 6732

K 2581 obv. 20–28 = 1–9.

TEXT 4: FARBER 2014, PL. 55–56 (*KAR* 239) ii–iii

The text is edited in Farber 2014 in scored transliteration, transcription and translation as Lamaštu Series I, lines 173–232, text m. These lines appear on pages 88–94 (transliteration) and 158–63 (transcription and translation). *KAR* 239 col. ii–iii was recopied as Farber 2014, pls. 55–56.

Farber 2014, pls. 26–27 iii 45–iv 34 = ii 1′–32′, iii 1′–16′
Farber 2014, pl. 57 i 25′–28′ = ii 1′–4′
Farber 2014, pl. 70 ii 1′–29′ ~ ii 4′–32′, iii 1′–5′
Farber 2014, pls. 2–3 ii 1′–28′ = ii 5′–32′
Farber 2014, pl. 10 iii 1′–iii 25′ = ii 10′–31′
Farber 2014, pl. 61 i 13′–16′ = iii 1′–5′

TEXT 5: FARBER 2014, PL. 8 ($4R^2$ 56) i 11–30

The text is edited in Farber 2014 in scored transliteration, transcription and translation as Lamaštu Series I, lines 11–31, Text C1. These lines appear on pp. 70–73 (transliteration) and 146–47 (transcription and translation). $4R^2$ 56 col. i 11–29 was recopied as Farber 2014, pl. 8. For a German translation, see Farber 1987a, 259.

Farber 2014, pl. 1 i 11–18 = i 11–18
Farber 2014, pl. 23 i 12–24 = i 11–22
Farber 2014, pl. 38 i 11–25 = i 11–30
Farber 2014, pl. 45 i 4′–12′ = i 11–20
Farber 2014, pl. 79 i 29–34 = i 11–20
Farber 2014, pl. 81: 9–18 = i 11–20
Farber 2014, pl. 50 i 1′–13′ = i 19–30

TEXT 6: *STT* 281 iv 1–15

The text appears in Farber 2014 as a parallel to Lamaštu Series III, lines 64–73, Text Ra. These lines appear on pages 135–36 (transliteration) and cf. 190–91.

Farber 2014, pl. 19 obv. 28′–35′ = iv 1–15
Farber 2014, pl. 31 obv. 13′– rev. 5 = iv 1–15
Farber 2014, pl. 35 obv. 14′–18′ = iv 1–15
Farber 2014, pl. 4 v 1″–5″ = iv 11–14

TEXT 7: SpTU 5 NO. 248

The text is edited in von Weiher, SpTU 5. For fuller discussion, see Scurlock 2002b, 209–23. For a German translation, see Hecker 2008, no. 2.2.12.

TEXT 8: *KAR* 70:1–10

This is edited in Biggs 1967, as no. 27. For a German translation, see Schwemer 2011, text no. 2.13.2.

TEXT 9: BAM 323

This text is edited in Scurlock 2006 as nos. 226, 218, 225, 223, 236, 289, 228, 91 and 333. Lines 45–52 are reedited by Schwemer 2009, 176 on the basis of *STT* 214–17 iv 50–55//SpTU 3.82 iv 17–19, a recitation which, as pointed out by Mayer (1991, 111), parallels this section of the text. There is also an unpublished parallel, K 2506+ rev. v 3ff.; see Schwemer 2011:126 w. n. 277. A German translation of the entire text appears in Schwemer 2011 as text no. 2.14.1.

BAM 221 iii 14′–18′ = 75–78.
BAM 228:23–32 = 89–97.
BAM 229:17′–26′ = 89–98.
BAM 385 i 23′–26′ = 65–67; iv 4–13 = 75–78.
BAM 471 ii 26′–29′ = 65–68; ii 29′–34′ = 69–71; iii 17′–20′ = 75–78.
BiOr 39.598–99:4–8 = 75–78.
Gray 1901, pl. 12:2′–15′ = 17–38

Gray 1901, pl. 20 obv. 1–12 = 39–46, rev. 1–5 = 62–64.
KAR 74:16–20 = 19–38.
K 4508+6648 (Farber 1977, 210–17): 1–13 = 79–83.

BIBLIOGRAPHY

Abusch, Tzvi. 1999. Witchcraft and the Anger of the Personal God. Pages 81–121 in *Mesopotamian Magic: Textual, Historical and Interpretative Perspectives*. Edited by Tzvi Abusch, and Karel van der Toorn. AMD 1. Leiden: Brill.

Abusch, Tzvi and Daniel Schwemer. 2011. *Corpus of Mesopotamian Anti-Witchcraft Rituals*. AMD 8/1. Leiden: Brill.

Adamson, P. B. 1981. Anatomical and Pathological Terms in Akkadian: Part III. *JRAS* 1981:125–32.

———. 1984. Anatomical and Pathological Terms in Akkadian: Part IV. *JRAS* 1984:3–18.

Arnaud, Daniel 1987. *Recherches sur le pays d'Aštata Emar* VI/4: *Textes de la bibliothèque: transcriptions et traductions*. Paris: Éditions Recherche sur les Civilizations.

Attia, Annie and Giles Buisson, editors. 2009. *Advances in Mesopotamian Medicine from Hammurabi to Hippocrates: Proceedings of the International Conference "Oeil Malade et Mauvais Oeil," Collège de France, Paris, 23rd June 2006*. CM 37. Leiden: Brill.

———. 2012. BAM 1 et consorts en transcription. *JMC* 19:22–51.

Beckman, Gary and Benjamin R. Foster. 1988. Assyrian Scholarly Texts in the Yale Babylonian Collection. Pages 1–26 in *A Scientific Humanist: Studies in Memory of Araham Sachs*. Edited by Erle Leichty, et al. Occasional Publications of the Samuel Noah Kramer Fund 9. Philadelphia: University Museum.

Beeson, Paul B. and Walsh McDermott. 1975. *Textbook of Medicine*. 14th ed. Philadelphia: Lippincot.

Biggs, Robert D. 1967. *ŠÀ.ZI.GA: Ancient Mesopotamian Potency Incantations*. TCS 2. Locust Valley, NY: Augustin.

Böck, Barbara. 2003. Hauterscheinungen in altmesopotamischer Divination und Medizin Teil 1. *AuOr* 21:161–84.

———. 2008. Babylonisch-assyrische Medizin in Texten und Untersuchungen: Erkrankungen des uro-genitalen Traktes, des Endarmes und des Anus. *WZKM* 98:295–346.

———. 2007. *Das Handbuch Muššuʾu "Einreibung" : Eine Serie Sumerischer und Akkadischer Beschwörungen aus dem 1 Jt. vor Chr.* BPOA 3. Madrid: Consejo Superior de Investigaciones Cientificás.

———. 2009. On Medical Technology in Ancient Mesopotamia. Pages 105–28 in *Advances in Mesopotamian Medicine from Hammurabi to Hippocrates: Proceedings of the International Conference "Oeil Malade et Mauvais Oeil," Collège de France,*

Paris, 23rd June 2006. Edited by Annie Attia and Giles Buisson. CM 37. Leiden: Brill.

———. 2011. Akkadische Texte des 2. und 1. Jt. v. Chr. 2: Therapeutische Texte 2.7.1–3, 2.8.1–4, 2.9.1–7, 2.10.1–13, 2.11.1–10, 2.12.1–11. Pages 69–114 in *Texte zur Heilkunde*. Edited by Bernd Janowski and Daniel Schwemer. TUAT 5. Gütersloh: Gütersloher Verlagshaus.

Borger, Rykle. 1957. Assyriologische und altarabische Miszellen 3. ŠU.DU$_8$.A = ikmî. *Or* 26:4–5.

———. 2010. *Mesopotamisches Zeichenlexicon*. Zweite, revidierte und aktualisierte Auflage. AOAT 305. Münster: Ugarit-Verlag.

Bottéro, Jean. 1978–79. Antiquités Assyro-Babyloniennes. *Annuaire* 1978–79:85–135.

Buisson, Giles. 2006. Review of *Renal and Rectal Disease Texts* by Markham J. Geller. *RA* 100:185–88.

Cadelli, Danielle. 1997. "Lorsque l'enfant paraît malade," in Enfance et éducation dans le Proche-orient Ancien. *Ktèma* 22:11–33.

Campbell Thompson, Reginald. 1940. A Selection from the Cuneiform Historical Texts from Nineveh (1927–32). *Iraq* 7:85–131.

———. 1949. *A Dictionary of Assyrian Botany*. London. British Academy.

Cavigneaux, Antoine. 1982. Remarques sur les commentaires à Labat *TDP* 1. *JCS* 34:231–39.

———. 1987. Aux sources du Midrash: l'hermanéneutique babylonienne. *AuOr* 5: 243–55.

———. 1988. Un texte médical bilingue. *NABU* 1988/24.

Civil, Miguel. 1974. Medical Commentaries from Nippur. *JNES* 33: 329–38.

———. 1982. Studies on Early Dynastic Lexicography I. *OrAnt* 21:1–26.

———. 2006. be$_5$/pe-en-zé-er = *biṣṣūru*. Pages 55–61 in *If a Man Builds a Joyful House: Assyriological Studies in Honor of Erle Verdun Leichty*. Edited by Anne Guinan et al. Leiden: Brill.

Cohen, Mark E. 1976. Texts from the Andrews University Archaeological Museum. *RA* 70:129–43.

Collins, Timothy Joseph. 1999. Natural Illness in Babylonian Medical Incantations. Ph.D. diss., University of Chicago.

Deller, Karlheinz. 1985. *kurru* "Mehlbrei." *Or* 54:327–30.

———. 1990. *šukkulu*, "abwischen," (*ZA* 70, 198–227). *NABU* 1990/3.

Dietrich, Manfried. 2000. Die unheilbringende Wurm. Beschwörung gegen den "Zahnwurm" (CT 17,50). Pages 209–20 in *Studi sul vicino oriente antico dedicata alla memoria di Luigi Cagni*. Edited by Simonetta Graziani. Naples: Instituto universitario orientale.

Dietrich, Manfried and Oswald Loretz. 2000. KTU 1.114 und seine mesopotamischen Parallelen Mythos und medizinisch-therapeutische Anweisung. Pages 491–504 in *Studien zu den ugaritischen Texten I: Mythos und Ritual in KTU 1.12, 1.24, 1.96, 1.100 und 1.114*. Edited by Manfried Dietrich and Oswald Loretz. AOAT 269/1. Münster: Ugarit-Verlag.

Dijk, Jan van. 1972. Une variante du thème de "l'Esclave de la Lune." *Or* 41:339–48.

———. 1973. Une incantation accompagnant la naissance de l'homme. *Or* 42:502–7.

———. 1975. Incantations accompagnant la naissance de l'homme. *Or* 44:52–79.

Dijk, Jan van, Albecht Goetze, and Mary I. Hussey. 1985. *Early Mesopotamian Incantations and Rituals*. YOS 11. Yale University: New Haven.

Duke, James A., and Edward S. Ayensu. 1985. *Medicinal Plants of China*. Algonac: Reference Publications.

Ebeling, Erich. 1953. Sammlungen von Beschwörungsformeln. *ArOr* 21:357–423.

Ebeling, Erich and Franz Köcher. 1953. *Literarische Keilschrifttexte aus Assur*. Berlin: Akademie-Verlag.

Farber, Walter. 1977. *Beschwörungsrituale an Ištar und Dumuzi*. Wiesbaden: Steiner.

———. 1979. Review of *Spätbabylonische Texte aus Uruk, Teil 1* by H. Hunger. *ZA* 69: 300–304.

———. 1982. Review of *Die Babylonisch-Assyrische Medizin in Texten und Untersuchungen* 6 by Franz Köcher. *BiOr* 39:591–99.

———. 1987a. Rituale und Beschwörungen in akkadischer Sprache B. Magische Rituale" Pages 255–81 in *Religiöse Texte*. Edited by Walter Farber et al. TUAT 2. Gütersloh: Gütersloher Verlagshaus.

———. 1987b. Tamarisken-Fibeln-Skolopender. Pages 85–105 in *Language, Literature and History: Philological and Historical Studies Presented to Erica Reiner*. Edited by Francesca Rochberg-Halton. AOS 67. New Haven: American Oriental Society.

———. 1989a. Lamaštu, Enlil, Anu-ikṣur: Streiflichter aus Uruks Gelehrtenstuben. *ZA* 79:224–41.

———. 1989b. *Schlaf, Kindchen, Schlaf!: Mesopotamische Baby-Beschwörungen und -Rituale*. Winona Lake, IN: Eisenbrauns.

———. 1990. Mannam lušpur ana Enkidu: Some New Thoughts on an Old Motif. *JNES* 49:299–321.

———. 2014. *Lamaštu: An Edition of the Canonical Series of Lamaštu Incantations and Rituals and Related Texts from the Second and First Millennium B.C.* Winona Lake, IN: Eisenbrauns.

Fincke, Jeanette C. 2000. *Augenleiden nach keilschriftlichen Quellen*. WMF 70. Würzburg: Königshausen & Neumann, 2000.

———. 2009. Cuneiform Tablets on Eye Diseases: Babylonian Sources in Relation to the Series DIŠ NA IGI^{II}-*šú* GIG. Pages 79–104 in *Advances in Mesopotamian Medicine from Hammurabi to Hippocrates: Proceedings of the International Conference "Oeil Malade et Mauvais Oeil," Collège de France, Paris, 23rd June 2006*. CM 37. Leiden: Brill.

———. 2011a. Neue Erkenntnnisse zur 21. Tafel der diagnostischen Omenserie SA.GIG und zur Überlieferung diagnostischer Omentexte in Hattuša. *BiOr* 68:472–76.

———. 2011b. Spezialisierung und Differenzierung im Bereich der altorientalischen Medizin. Pages 159–208 in *The Empirical Dimension of Ancient Near Eastern Studies*. Edited by Gebhard J. Selz. Wiener offene Orientalistik 6. Vienna: Lit.

Finkel, Irving. 1980. "The Crescent Fertile." *AfO* 27:37–52.

———. 1998. A Study in Scarlet: Incantations against Samana." Pages 71–106 in *Festschrift für Rykle Borger zu seinem 65. Geburtstag am 24. Mai 1994*. Edited by Stefan M. Maul. Groningen: Styx, 1998.

———. 1999. Magic and Medicine at Meskene. *NABU* 1999/30.

———. 2000. On Late Babylonian Medical Training. Pages 137–223 in *Wisdom, Gods and Literature: Studies in Assyriology in Honour of W. G. Lambert*. Edited by

Andrew R. George and Irving L. Finkel. Winona Lake, IN: Eisenbrauns.

Fossey, Charles. 1926. *Manuel d'Assyriologie*. Tome Deuxième: Évolution des cunéiformes. Paris: Conard.

Foster, Benjamin R. 1996. *Before the Muses*. 2nd ed. Bethesda: CDL.

Frahm, Eckart. 2011. Akkadische Texte des 2. und 1. Jt. v. Chr. 2: Therapeutische Texte 6.1–3. Pages 171–76 in *Texte zur Heilkunde*. Edited by Bernd Janowski and Daniel Schwemer. TUAT 5. Gütersloh: Gütersloher Verlagshaus.

Geller, Markham J. 1985. *Forerunners to UDUG-ḪUL*. FAS 12 Stuttgart: Steiner.

———. 1988. New Duplicates to SBTU II. *AfO* 35:1–23.

———. 2007. Textes médicaux du Louvre nouvelle édition. *JMC* 10:4–12.

———. 2010. *Ancient Babylonian Medicine: Theory and Practice*. Chichester: Wiley-Blackwell.

———. 2011. Akkadische Texte des 2. und 1. Jt. v. Chr. 2: Therapeutische Texte 2.5, 2.6.1–2.6.4. Pages 61–68 in *Texte zur Heilkunde*. Edited by Bernd Janowski and Daniel Schwemer. TUAT 5. Gütersloh: Gütersloher Verlagshaus.

Geller, Markham J. and F. A. M. Wiggerman. 2008. Duplicating Akkadian Magic. Pages 149–60 in *Studies in Ancient Near Eastern World View and Society Presented to Marten Stol on the Occasion of his 65th Birthday*. Edited by R. J. van der Spek. Bethesda: CDL.

George, Andrew. 1991. Babylonian Texts from the Folios of Syndey Smith. Part Two: Prognostic and Diagnostic Omens Tablet 1. *RA* 85:137–67.

Goetze, Albrecht. 1948. Texts and Fragments 6. *JCS* 2:305–8.

Gray, C. D. 1901. The Šamaš Religious Texts. Ph.D. diss., University of Chicago. Published in *AJSL* 17 (1900/1901):129–45, 222–43.

Haussperger, M. 2001. Krankheiten von Galle und Leber in der altmesopotamischen Medizin anhand des Textes BAM 578. *Würzburger medizin-historische Mitteilungen* 20:108–22.

Hecker, Karl. 2008. Akkadische Texte des 2. und 1. Jt. v. Chr. 2. Rituale und Beschwörungen. Pages 61–127 in *Omina, Orakel, Rituale und Beschwörungen*. Edited by Karl Hecker et al. TUAT 4. Gütersloh: Gütersloher Verlagshaus.

Heeßel, Nils. P. 2000. *Babylonisch-assyrische Dignostik*. AOAT 43. Münster: Ugarit-Verlag.

———. 2002. Ein neubabylonisches Rezept zur Berauschung und Ausnüchterung. Pages 99–106 in *Mining the Archives: Festschrift for Christopher Walker on the Occasion of His 60th Birthday, 4 October 2002*. Edited by Cornelia Wunsch. Dresden: ISLET.

———. 2009. The Babylonian Physician Rabâ-ša-Marduk: Another Look at Physicians and Exorcists in the Ancient Near East. Pages 13–28 in *Advances in Mesopotamian Medicine from Hammurabi to Hippocrates: Proceedings of the International Conference "Oeil Malade et Mauvais Oeil," Collège de France, Paris, 23rd June 2006*. Edited by Annie Attia and Giles Buisson. CM 37. Leiden: Brill.

———. 2010. Neues von Esagil-kīn-apli. Pages 139–87 in *Assur-Forschungen*. Edited by Stefan M. Maul and Nils P. Heeßel. Wiesbaden: Harrasowitz, 2010.

———. 2011a. Akkadische Texte des 2. und 1. Jt. v. Chr. 1: Diagnostische Texte." Pages 8–31 in *Texte zur Heilkunde*. Edited by Bernd Janowski and Daniel Schwemer. TUAT 5. Gütersloh: Gütersloher Verlagshaus.

———. 2011b. Akkadische Texte des 2. und 1. Jt. v. Chr. 2: Medizinisch-astrologische

Texte. Pages 169–70 in *Texte zur Heilkunde*. Edited by Bernd Janowski and Daniel Schwemer. TUAT 5. Gütersloh: Gütersloher Verlagshaus.

———. 2011c. "Akkadische Texte des 2. und 1. Jt. v. Chr. 2: Therapeutische Texte 2.0, 2.3.1–3, 2.4.1–6, 2.17.1–3." Pages 31–35, 45–61, 153–56 in *Texte zur Heilkunde*. Edited by Bernd Janowski and Daniel Schwemer. TUAT 5. Gütersloh: Gütersloher Verlagshaus.

Heeßel, Nils and Farouk Al-Rawi. 2003. Tablets from the Sippar Library XII: A Medical Therapeutic Text. *Iraq* 65:221–39.

Herrero, Pablo. 1975. Une tablette médicale assyrienne inédite. *RA* 69:41–53.

———. 1984. *La thérapeutique Mésopotamienne*. Paris: Editions Recherche sur les Civilizations, 1984.

Hunger, Hermann. 1976. *Spätbabylonische Texte aus Uruk 1*. Ausgrabungen der Deutschen Forschungsgemeinschaft in Uruk-Warka 9. Berlin: Gebr. Mann.

Jastrow, Morris. 1913. An Assyrian Medical Tablet in the Possession of the College of Physicians. *Transactions of the College of Physicians of Philadelphia* 1913:365–400.

Kämmerer, Thomas R. 1999–2000. Zur Kenntnis der Erkrankungen von Leber und Galle im alten vorderen Orient. Pages 165–69 in *Landscapes: Territories, Frontiers and Horizons in the Ancient Near East: Papers Presented to the XLIV Rencontre assyriologique Internationale, Venezia, 7–11 July 1997*. Edited by L. Milano et al. Padova: Sargon.

Kee Chang Huang. 1993. *The Pharmacology of Chinese Herbs*. Boca Raton: CRC.

Kilmer, Anne Draffkorn. 2007. Of Babies, Boats, and Arks. Pages 159–65 in *Studies Presented to Robert D. Biggs*. Edited by Martha T. Roth et al. AS 27. Chicago: The Oriental Institute of the University of Chicago.

Kinnier Wilson, J. V. 1956. Two Medical Texts from Nimrud. *Iraq* 18:130–46.

Kinnier Wilson, J. V. and E. H. Reynolds. 1990. Translation and Analysis of a Cuneiform Text Forming Part of a Babylonian Treatise on Eplepsy. *Medical History* 34:189–97.

Klein, Harald. 1983. Tudittum. *ZA* 73: 255–84.

Koch, Johannes. 2003. Neues vom Beschwörungstext BA 10/1, 81 No. 7 rev. 1–8. *WO* 33:89–99.

Köcher, Franz. 1966. Die Ritualtafel der magisch-medizinischen Tafelserie "Einreibung." *AfO* 21:13–20.

———. 1978. Spätbabylonische medizinische Texts aus Uruk. Pages 17–34 in *Medizinische Diagnostik in Geschichte und Gegenwart*. Edited by C. Habrich, et al. München: Werver Fritsch.

———. 1995. Ein Text medizinischen Inhalts aus dem neubabylonischen Grab 405. Pages 203–16 in *Uruk: Die Gräber*. Edited by R. M. Boehmer et al. AUWE 10. Mainz: von Zabern.

Kraus, F. R. 1939. *Texte zur babylonischen Physiognomatik*. AfOB 3. Berlin: Ernst Weidner.

———. 1987. Verstreute Omentexte aus Nippur im Istanbuler Museum. *ZA* 77:194–206.

Krebernik, Manfred. 2012. S/Šugallītu. *RlA* 13/3–4:256–57.

Labat, Renée. 1950. La pharmacopée au service de la piété (tablette assyrienne inédite). *Semitica* 3:5–18.

———. 1951. *Traité akkadien de diagnostics et pronostics médicaux*. Paris: Académie

Internationale d'Histoire des Sciences.
———. 1954. À propos de la chirurgerie babylonienne. *Journal Asiatique* 242:207–48.
———. 1956. Une nouvelle tablette de pronostics médicaux. *Syria* 33:119–30.
———. 1957. Remèdes Assyriens contre les affections de l'oreille, d'après un inédit du Louvre (AO. 6774). *RSO* 32:109–22.
———. 1959. Le premier chapitre d'un précis médical Assyrien. *RA* 53:1–18.
———. 1974. *Textes Littéraires de Suse*. MDP 57. Paris: Geuthner.
Labat, Renée and Jacques Tournay. 1945–46. Un texte médical inédit. *RA* 40:113–22.
Lambert, Wilfred G. 1965. "A Middle Assyrian Tablet of Incantations." Pages 283–88 in *Studies in Honor of Benno Landsberger on His Seventy-fifth Birthday*. AS 16. Chicago: The Oriental Institute of the University of Chicago.
———. 1969. A Middle Assyrian Medical Text. *Iraq* 31:28–39.
———. 1983. Kūšu. *RlA* 6/5–6:382.
Landsberger, Benno. 1967. Über Farben im sumerisch-akkadischen. *JCS* 21:139–73.
Leichty, Erle. 1973. Two Late Commentaries. *AfO* 24:78–86.
———. 1988. Guaranteed to Cure." Pages 261–64 in *A Scientific Humanist: Studies in Memory of Abraham Sachs*. Edited by Erle Leichty, et al. Occasional Publications of the Samuel Noah Kramer Fund 9. Philadelphia: University Museum.
Limet, Henri. 1986. Croyances, superstitions et débuts de la science en Mésopotamie. *Oikumene* 5:67–90.
Livingstone, Alasdair. 1986. *Mystical and Mythological Explanatory Works of Assyrian and Babylonian Scholars*. Oxford: Clarendon.
Maul, Stefan M. 1994. *Zukunftsbewältigung: Eine Untersuchung altorientalischen Denkens anhand der babylonisch-assyrischen Löserituale (Namburbi)*. Baghdader Forschungen 18. Mainz: von Zabern
———. 1997. Küchensumerisch oder hohe Kunst der Exegese? Überlegunen zur Bewertung akkadischer Interlinearübersetzungen von Emesal-Texten. Pages 253–67 in *Ana šadî Labnāni lū allik: Beiträge zu altorientalischen und mittelmeerischen Kulturen. Festschrift für Wolfgang Röllig*. Edited by Beate Pongratz-Leisten et al. AOAT 247. Neukirchen-Vluyn: Neukirchener Verlag.
———. 2011. Akkadische Texte des 2. und 1. Jt. v. Chr. 2: Therapeutische Texte 2.15.1–3. Pages 135–46 in *Texte zur Heilkunde*. Edited by Bernd Janowski and Daniel Schwemer. TUAT 5. Gütersloh: Gütersloher Verlagshaus.
Maul, Stefan and Rita Strauß. 2011. Ritualbeschreibungen und Gebete I. WVDOG 133 (= KAL 4). Wiesbaden: Harrassowitz.
Mayer, Werner R. 1991. "Akkadische Lexikographie: *CAD* S," *Or* 60:109–20.
Michalowski, Piotr. 1981. Carminative Magic: Towards an Understanding of Sumerian Poetics. *ZA* 71:1–18.
Myhrman, David W. 1902. Die "Labartu"–Texte, babylonische Beschwörungsformeln gegen die Dämonin "Labartu." *ZA* 16:141–200.
Nougayrol, Jean. 1969. La Lamaštu à Ugarit. *Ugaritica* 6:393–408.
Prechel, Doris and Thomas Richter. 2001. Abrakadabra oder Althurritisch. Betrachtungen zu einigen altbabylonischen Beschwörungstexten. Pages 333–72 in *Kulturgeschichten: Altorientalistische Studien für Volkert Haas zum 65. Geburtstag*. Edited by Thomas Richter, Doris Prechel, and Jörg Klinger. Saarbrücken: Saarbrücker Druckerei.

Reiner, Erica. 1958. *Šurpu: A Collection of Sumerian and Akkadian Incantations.* AfOB 11. Graz: Weidner.
———. 1982. Babylonian Birth Prognoses. *ZA* 72: 124–38.
———. 1995. *Astral Magic in Babylonia.* TAPS 85/4. Philadelphia: American Philosophical Society.
Riddle, John. 1985. *Dioscorides on Pharmacy and Medicine.* Austin: University of Texas, 1985.
Röllig, Wolfgang. 1985. Der Mondgott und die Kuh: Ein Lehrstück zur Problematik der Textüberlieferung im Alten Orient. *Or* 54:260–73.
Rutz, Matthew T. 2011. Threads for Esagil-kīn-apli: The Medical Diagnostic-Prognostic Series in Middle Babylonian Nippur. *ZA* 101:294–308.
Scheil, Vincent. 1898. Notes d'épigraphie et d'archéologie assyriennes: no. 39: La plus petite inscription cunéiforme connue. *Recueil de travaux relatifs à la philologie et à l'archéologie égyptiennes et assyriennes* 20:200–201.
———. 1916. Un document médical Assyrien. *RA* 13:35–42.
———. 1917. Tablette de pronostics médicaux. *RA* 14:121–31.
Schuster-Brandis, Anais. 2008. *Steine als Schutz- und Heilmittel: Untersuchung zu ihrer Verwendung in der Beschwörungskunst Mesopotamiens im 1. Jt. v. Chr.* Münster: Ugarit-Verlag.
Schwemer, Daniel. 2007a. *Abwehrzauber und Behexung: Studien zum Schadenzauberglauben im alten Mesopotamien.* Wiesbaden: Harrassowitz.
———. 2007b. *Rituale und Beschwörungen gegen Schadenzauber.* KAL 2. WVDOG 117. Wiesbaden: Harrassowitz.
———. 2009. Review of *Magico-Medical Means of Treating Ghost-induced Illnesses in Ancient Mesopotamia*, by JoAnn Scurlock. *BiOr* 66:168–77.
———. 2011. Akkadische Texte des 2. und 1. Jt. v. Chr. 2: Therapeutische Texte 2.1.1–2, 2.2.1–2, 2.13–14." Pages 35–45, 115–35 in *Texte zur Heilkunde.* Edited by Bernd Janowski and Daniel Schwemer. TUAT 5. Gütersloh: Gütersloher Verlagshaus.
Scurlock, JoAnn. 1991. Baby-Snatching Demons, Restless Souls and the Dangers of Childbirth: Medico-Magical Means of Dealing with Some of the Perils of Motherhood in Ancient Mesopotamia. *Incognita* 2:137–85.
———. 1995. *Upinzir* or *pizzer* : Creepy Medicine. *NABU* 1995/110.
———. 1999. Physician, Conjurer, Magician: A Tale of Two Healing Professionals. Pages 69–79 in *Mesopotamian Magic: Textual, Historical and Interpretive Perspectives.* Edited by Tzvi Abusch and Karel van der Toorn. AMD 1. Groningen: Styx.
———. 2002a. Soul Emplacements in Ancient Mesopotamian Funerary Rituals. Pages 1–6 in *Magic and Divination in the Ancient World.* Edited by L. Ciraolo and J. Seidel. AMD 2. Leiden: Brill.
———. 2002b. Translating Transfers in Ancient Mesopotamia. Pages 209–23 in *Magic and Ritual in the Ancient World.* Edited by Paul Mirecki and Marvin Meyer. Leiden: Brill.
———. 2003. Collation of the "Jastrow" Tablet. *JMC* 2:16–17
———. 2005. Ancient Mesopotamian Medicine. Pages 302–15 in *A Companion to the Ancient Near East.* Edited by Daniel C. Snell. Oxford: Blackwell.
———. 2006. *Magico-Medical Means of Treating Ghost-Induced Illnesses in Ancient Mesopotamia.* AMD 3. Leiden: Brill.

———. 2007. A Proposal for Identification of a Missing Plant: *Kamantu*/ÚÁB.DUḪ = *Lawsonia inermis* L./"henna." *WZKM* 97:491–520.
———. 2008. Some Mesopotamian Medicine for a Greek Headache. Pages 195–202 in *Studies in Ancient Near Eastern World View and Society Presented to Marten Stol*. Edited by R. J. van der Spek. Bethesda: CDL.
———. 2009. Corrections and Suggestions to Geller BAM VII Part 1: Urinary Tract Texts. *JMC* 13:38–48.
———. 2010. Advantages of Listening to Patients: The First Description of Parkinson's. *JMC* 15:57–60.
Scurlock, JoAnn and Burton R. Andersen. 2005. *Diagnoses in Assyrian and Babylonian Medicine*. Urbana: University of Illinois Press.
Scurlock, JoAnn and Farouk al-Rawi. 2006. A Weakness for Hellenism. Pages 357–82 in *If a Man Builds a Joyful House: Assyriological Studies in Honor of Erle Verdun Leichty*. Edited by Anne Guinan et al. Leiden: Brill.
Scurlock, JoAnn and Dafydd Stevens. 2007. A Ringing Endorsement for Assyro-Babylonian Medicine: The Diagnosis and Treatment of Tinnitus in 1st Millennium BCE Mesopotamia. *Audiological Medicine* 2007:1–12.
Soden, Wolfram von. 1987. Review of *Sin and Sanction in Israel and Mesopotamia*, by K. van der Toorn. *AfO* 34:69–72.
Stadhouders, Henry. 2011. The Pharmacopoeial Handbook *Šammu šikinšu*. *JMC* 18:3–51.
———. 2012. The Pharmacopoeial Handbook *Šammu šikinšu*. *JMC* 19:1–21.
Stol, Marten. 1979. *On Trees, Mountains and Millstones in the Ancient Near East*. MVEOL 21. Leiden: Ex Oriente Lux.
———. 1983–84. Cress and Its Mustard. *JEOL* 28:24–32.
———. 1989. Malz. *RlA* 7/5–6:322–29.
———. 1992. The Moon as Seen by Babylonians. Pages 245–74 in *Natural Phenomena*. Edited by Diederik J. W. Meijer. Amsterdam: Royal Netherlands Academy of Arts and Sciences.
———. 1993. *Epilepsy in Babylonia*. CM 2. Groningen: Styx.
———. 1998. Einige kurze Wortstudien" Pages 343–52 in *Festschrift für Rykle Borger zu seinem 65. Geburtstag am 24. Mai 1994*. Edited by Stefan M. Maul. Groningen: Styx.
———. 2000. *Birth in Babylonia and the Bible: Its Mediterranean Setting*. CM 14. Groningen: Styx.
———. 2007a. An Unusual Prescription: Oral Tradition? *JMC* 10:1–3.
———. 2007b. "Remarks on Some Sumerograms and Akkadian Words." Pages 233–42 in *Studies Presented to Robert D. Biggs*. Edited by Martha T. Roth et al. AS 27. Chicago: The Oriental Institute of the University of Chicago.
———. 2009a. Insanity in Babylonian Sources. *JMC* 13:1–12.
———. 2009b. "To be ill" in Akkadian: The Verb *Salā'u* and the Substantive *Sili'tu*." Pages 29–46 in *Advances in Mesopotamian Medicine from Hammurabi to Hippocrates: Proceedings of the International Conference "Oeil Malade et Mauvais Oeil," Collège de France, Paris, 23rd June 2006*. Edited by Annie Attia and Giles Buisson. CM 37. Leiden: Brill.
———. 2011. Pferde, Pferdekrankheiten und Pferdemedizin in altbabylonischer Zeit. Pages 363-402 in *Hippologia Ugaritica*. Edited by Oswald Loretz. AOAT 386.

Münster: Ugarit-Verlag.
———. 2012. Bitumen in Ancient Mesopotamia: The Textual Evidence. *BiOr* 69:48–60.
———. forthcoming. Trüffel. *RlA* 13.
Streck, Michael P. 2004. Dattelpalme und Tamarske in Mesopotamien nach dem akkadischen Streitgespräch. *ZA* 94:250–90.
Toorn, Karel van der. 1985. *Sin and Sanction in Israel and Mesopotamia: A Comparative Study*. Maastricht: van Gorcum.
Thureau-Dangin, François. 1921. Rituel et amulettes contre Labartu. *RA* 18:161–97.
Tsukimoto, Akio. 1985. *Untersuchungen zur Totenpflege* (kispum) *im alten Mesopotamien*. AOAT 216. Kevelaer: Butzon & Bercker.
———. 1999. By the Hand of Madi-Dagan, the Scribe and Apkallu-priest—A Medical Text from the Middle Euphrates Region. Pages 187–200 in *Priests and Officials in the Ancient Near East: Papers of the Second Colloquium on the Ancient Near East, The City and Its Life, Held at the Middle Eastern Culture Center in Japan (Mitaka, Tokyo), March 22–24*. Edited by Kazuko Watanabe. Heidelberg: Winter.
Veldhuis, Niek. 1989. The New Assyrian Compendium for a Woman in Childbirth. *ASJ* 11:239–60.
———. 1991. *A Cow of Sîn*. Library of Oriental Texts 2. Groningen: Styx.
Volk, Konrad. 1999. Kinderkrankheiten nach der Darstellung babylonisch-assyrischer Keilschrifttexte. *Or* 68:1–30.
Wasserman, Nathan. 1996. An Old-Babylonian Medical Text Against the Kurārum Disease. *RA* 90:1–5.
Weiher, Egbert von. 1983. *Spätbabylonische Texte aus Uruk* 2. Ausgrabungen der deutschen Forschungsgemeinschaft in Uruk-Warka 10. Berlin: Gebr. Mann.
———. 1988. *Spätbabylonische Texte aus Uruk* 3. Ausgrabungen der deutschen Forscungsgemeinschaft in Uruk-Warka 12. Berlin: Gebr. Mann.
———. 1993. *Uruk: Spätbabylonische Texte aus dem Planquadrat U 18*. SpTU 4. AUWE 12. Mainz: von Zabern.
———. 1998. *Uruk: Spätbabylonische Texte aus dem Planquadrant U 18*. SpTU 5. AUWE 13. Mainz: von Zabern.
Westenholz, Joan Goodnick and Marcel Sigrist. 2006. The Brain, the Marrow, and the Seat of Cognition in Mesopotamian Tradition. *JMC* 7:1–10.
Wilhelm, Gernot. 1994. *Medizinische Omina aus Ḫattuša in akkadischer Sprache*. StBoT 36. Wiesbaden: Harrassowitz.
Wiseman, Donald J. 1950. The Nimrud Tablets. *Iraq* 12:197 no. 280.
Wiseman, D. J. and J. Black. 1996. *Literary Texts from the Temple of Nabû*. Cuneiform Texts from Nimrud 4. The British School of Archaeology in Iraq.
Worthington, Martin. 2005. Edition of UGU 1 (= BAM 480 etc.). *JMC* 5:6–43.
———. 2006. Edition of BAM 3. *JMC* 7:18–48.
———. 2007. Addenda and Corrigenda to "Edition of UGU 1 (= BAM 480 etc.)" and "Edition of BAM 3." *JMC* 9:43–46.

INDEX OF TEXTS

Bold face indicates a text transliterated and translated. Nonbold face indicates a text cited as a duplicate or comparand, the reference to which will most likely be found in the source lists and footnotes. The line numbers given indicate the complete set of lines duplicated by any given text. For the exact tally of which lines in the duplicate match which lines in the main text and in what order, the source lists should be consulted. The locators are formatted as part.chapter.text no.

www.ingramcontent.com/pod-product-compliance
Lightning Source LLC
Chambersburg PA
CBHW021931220326
41598CB00061BA/879